a LANGE medical book

Concise Pathology

a LANGE medical book

Concise Pathology

First Edition

Parakrama Chandrasoma, MD, MRCP (UK)
Associate Professor of Pathology
University of Southern California
Director of Anatomic Pathology
Los Angeles County—University of Southern California Medical Center

Clive R. Taylor, MD, DPhil, MRCPath
Professor and Chairman of Pathology
University of Southern California
Director of Laboratories and Pathology
Los Angeles County—University of Southern California Medical Center

MYA THAUNG, MBBS

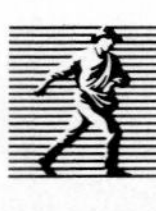

APPLETON & LANGE
Norwalk, Connecticut/San Mateo, California

0-8385-1320-4

Notice: Our knowledge in clinical sciences is constantly changing. As new information becomes available, changes in treatment and in the use of drugs become necessary. The authors and the publisher of this volume have taken care to make certain that the doses of drugs and schedules of treatment are correct and compatible with the standards generally accepted at the time of publication. The reader is advised to consult carefully the instruction and information material included in the package insert of each drug or therapeutic agent before administration. This advice is especially important when using new or infrequently used drugs.

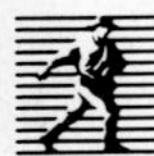

91 92 93 94 95 / 10 9 8 7 6 5 4 3 2 1

Prentice Hall International (UK) Limited, *London*
Prentice Hall of Australia Pty. Limited, *Sydney*
Prentice Hall Canada Inc., *Toronto*
Prentice Hall Hispanoamericana, S.A., *Mexico*
Prentice Hall of India Private Limited, *New Delhi*
Prentice Hall of Japan, Inc., *Tokyo*
Simon & Schuster Asia Pte. Ltd., *Singapore*
Editora Prentice Hall do Brasil Ltda., *Rio de Janeiro*
Prentice Hall, *Englewood Cliffs, New Jersey*

ISBN: 0-8385-1320-4
ISSN: 1048-0730

Production Editor: Charles F. Evans

PRINTED IN THE UNITED STATES OF AMERICA

To

Cherine
Shahin, Janak, Pradip
Chandrasoma

Sue
Matthew, Benedict, Jeremy, Emma
Taylor

...for many years of patience and support

and

to our colleagues and students at the University of Southern California who have provided a model environment in which to learn and to teach Pathology.

Table of Contents

Preface

THIS BOOK'S GOALS

The principal goal of the second-year pathology course in medical schools is to foster understanding of the mechanisms of disease (pathogenesis) as a foundation for dealing with a vast amount of clinical information the student will encounter in later clinical years. Important lesser goals are to teach students how to use the laboratory and to help them pass the examinations necessary to earn a medical degree, including the various Boards.

This book addresses these goals. In developing it, we have endeavored to present information at the level of the second-year medical student, guiding the reader logically and as concisely as possible through the mechanisms by which the normal in our bodies is converted to the abnormal. Since our objective is to use pathology to facilitate medical education, we stress mechanisms leading to disease rather than morphologic alterations used by pathologists to make pathologic diagnoses. Understanding these mechanisms is more a function of logic than of memory. We hope this book will leave students with a lasting knowledge of pathology and a desire to use pathology for the rest of their career as the scientific basis of the "art" of medicine.

ORGANIZATION & APPROACH

The study of pathology is traditionally divided into general and systemic pathology, and we preserve this distinction.

In the *general pathology* chapters (Part A), the pathologic changes occurring in a hypothetic tissue are considered. This idealized tissue is composed of parenchymal cells and interstitial connective tissue and is the prototype of every tissue in the body. General pathology explores and explains the development of basic pathologic mechanisms without detailing the additional specific changes occurring in different organs.

In the *systemic pathology* chapters (Part B), the pathologic mechanisms discussed in the general pathology section are related to the various organ systems. In each system, normal structure, function, and the symptoms and signs that arise from pathologic changes are discussed first. The diseases in each organ system are then considered, with emphasis given to those that are more common, so that the student can become familiar with most of the important diseases encountered in clinical practice.

We have divided this book into sections that cover a broad topic, eg, the endocrine system. Each section is divided into chapters, eg, pituitary gland, thyroid gland. Division into chapters is for the purpose of serving up smaller blocks of text than are usual in pathology books.

SPECIAL FEATURES

We have aimed to make this book as easy to study from as we believe is possible for a textbook of pathology. We have paid special attention to the following features that facilitate achievement of these objectives:

- The chapters are—with few exceptions—short enough to be assimilated in a reasonable length of time, enabling the student to set easily achievable goals.
- The text is concise. We have tried our best to use the minimum number of words to impart the necessary information.
- The text is comprehensive. The second-year student's needs are completely satisfied, both from the point of view of understanding the subject and passing examinations.
- The text is logical. We have presented the material in a logical sequence wherever possible. When doubt or controversy exists, we have indicated this clearly.
- The illustrations and tables are extensive and designed to visually reinforce the text in the more important areas.
- A glossary of about 500 pathologic terms is provided (Appendix I) to enable the student to develop a new vocabulary effectively. Terms are defined in the text when they are first introduced, but not thereafter. The glossary provides a mechanism for the student to obtain a concise definition of an undefined term that is encountered.
- It is our experience that most second-year students are faced with such a massive quantity of material that they rarely have time for additional reading beyond the course material and one standard textbook. We have therefore not given references in the text. We have, however, provided a list of references as Appendix II. These are arranged according to section to guide the interested student.

Acknowledgments

Original illustrations in this book are the work of Biomed Arts Associates, Inc., San Francisco, and in particular the following individuals: Laurel V. Schaubert, Susan Taft, Walter Denn, Gay Giannini, Ward Ruth, Hisako Moriyama, Michael Yeung, Terrence Schoop, Kenneth Rice, and Wendy Hiller.

—Parakrama Chandrasoma
—Clive R. Taylor
Los Angeles
January, 1991

Introduction: The Discipline of Pathology

WHAT IS PATHOLOGY?

Pathology is the study of disease. In its broadest sense, it is the study of how the organs and tissues of a healthy body—the basis of normal anatomy and physiology—change to those of a sick person. The study of pathology therefore provides an understanding of the disease processes encountered, their causes, and their clinical effects. In this way, pathology constitutes a logical and scientific basis of medicine. Pathology in this broad sense is what we aim to teach medical students.

In hospital practice, the term *pathology* is used in a narrower sense to denote that specialty of medicine concerned with the performance and interpretation of laboratory procedures. There are 2 main divisions of pathology in the hospital environment.

Clinical pathology is concerned with biochemical and microbiologic procedures performed on blood, tissue fluids, or other substances secreted or excreted by the body, such as sputum, urine, and cerebrospinal fluid. The hospital clinical pathology laboratory is divided into many sections—chemistry, microbiology, immunology, etc—to perform the many specific kinds of procedures. The results of these laboratory procedures, when used in conjunction with the clinical evaluation of the patient, facilitate diagnosis of specific diseases.

Anatomic pathology considers structural abnormalities of cells and tissues that can be detected by gross and microscopic examination of tissues removed from the patient. The anatomic pathology laboratory in a hospital includes subdivisions such as surgical pathology, cytology, hematopathology, and autopsy pathology.

In addition, specialized types of pathology have developed to serve specific needs. **Forensic pathology** is the application of medical knowledge to legal problems, such as determining whether death is due to natural or unnatural causes. **Blood banking** ensures the safety of collection, storage, and transfusion of blood components. **Experimental pathology** deals with basic scientific research into cellular processes.

WHO IS A PATHOLOGIST?

A pathologist may be a physician (MD) or a person with a doctorate (PhD) in pathology who has been trained in the proper performance and interpretation of laboratory procedures. Training as a physician pathologist takes many years. In the USA, a 5-year pathology residency follows the MD degree and covers all aspects of clinical and anatomic pathology. In England, pathology training also lasts for 5 years, being general in the first 2 years and more specialized in the last 3. Pathologists in small hospitals maintain a basic knowledge of all areas of pathology. In large academic medical centers, an individual pathologist may specialize in surgical pathology, hematopathology, chemical pathology, microbiology, immunology, and so forth. The PhD program in pathology provides training in the scientific methods of pathology. PhD pathologists play a vital role in basic scientific research and function in many hospital laboratories in their spheres of expertise.

Training in clinical pathology includes learning the methodology of chemical, microbiologic, and immunologic procedures and learning how to operate the various instruments so as to produce accurate results. Training in anatomic pathology deals with microscopic diagnosis of disease by recognizing deviations from normal of cells and tissues by light and electron microscopic study.

The end product of a pathologic procedure is a **pathology report** that contains the result of the procedure. This may be a number (in chemical tests), the name of a microorganism (in microbiology), or a diagnosis based on the microscopic features of a tissue section (in surgical pathology). Interaction with the laboratory in terms of ordering the most appropriate laboratory procedures and being able to interpret the pathology report correctly is a vital part of the training of all physicians.

Concise
Pathology

Causes of Disease.

Exogenous

Physical, Chemical, Biological.

Endogenous.

Neoplasm, Cell changes itself ← congenital / acquired. (mutation). mutation.

~~Immunity~~ secondary effect.

especially immunity.

physical → pressure effect

Blood supply

chemical → o

Chemical attack.

Oxygen supply

Nutrient supply

Maintain cell environment. (chemical changes).

Defence. system

~~Biogo~~ Biological → immune.

From Introduction to Human Diseases; Thomas H. Kent & Michael Noel Hart

Causes of Disease.

Exogenous Causes.

* Physical injury
  - Trauma
  - Heat-cold
  - Electricity
  - Pressure
  - Ionizing radiations.
* Chemical injury
  - Poisoning
  - Drug reactions
* Microbiologic injury
  - Bacteria
  - Fungi
  - Rickettsia
  - Viruses
  - Protozoa
  - Helminths

— " —

Endogenous Causes.

* Vascular Cause
  - Mechanical Obstruction
  - ~~Bleeding~~
  - Deranged flow
* Immunologic Cause (Biological)
  - Immune deficiency
  - Allergy
* Metabolic cause (Chemical)
  - Abnormal metabolism or deficiency of:-
    - Lipid
    - Carbohydrate
    - Protein
    - Mineral
    - Vitamins
    - Fluids.

— " —

Major Disease Categories

- Genetic and developmental diseases
- Acquired injuries and inflammatory diseases
- Hyperplasias and neoplasms.
- Miscellaneous or consequence.
- Functional Disturbance.
- Disorders due to organ.
- Idiopathic

Section I.
Effects of Injury on Tissues

All tissues in the body are composed of **parenchymal cells,** which are specialized to perform the functions of that particular tissue, and **interstitial connective tissue elements,** which act as the supporting framework of the tissue (Fig I–1). Human disease results from the action of various injurious agents on tissues. Injurious agents may act on parenchymal cells or interstitial connective tissue, causing biochemical or structural damage. Biochemical damage may result in abnormal function and disease without producing any structural alteration in tissue. Structural damage may sometimes be recognized only by microscopic examination of the tissue. In parenchymal cells, it results either in reversible changes short of cell death **(cell**

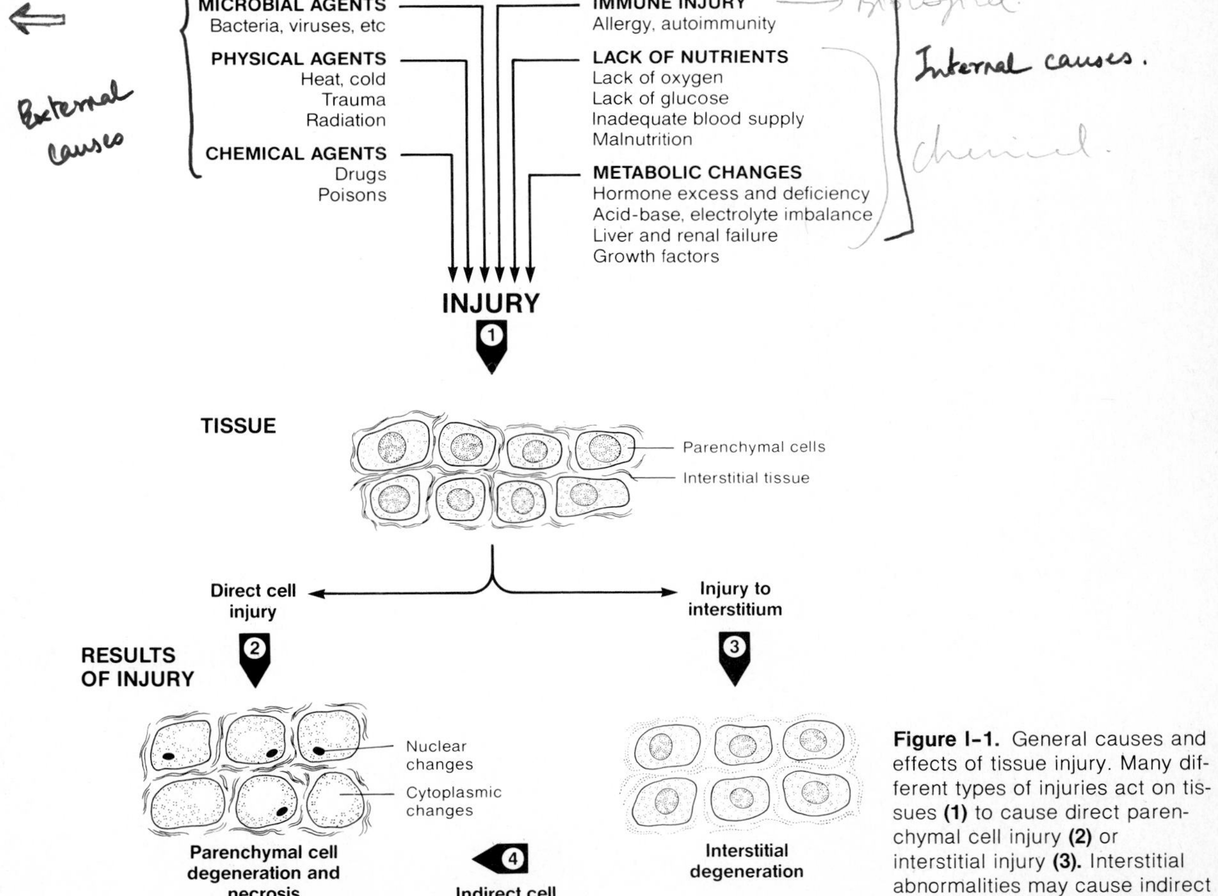

Figure I–1. General causes and effects of tissue injury. Many different types of injuries act on tissues **(1)** to cause direct parenchymal cell injury **(2)** or interstitial injury **(3).** Interstitial abnormalities may cause indirect parenchymal cell injury **(4).**

degenerations) or in irreversible cell death **(necrosis)**. These are discussed in Chapter 1. Interstitial tissue damage results in interstitial abnormalities (Chapter 2). Parenchymal cell damage may result from interstitial abnormalities and vice versa.

A variety of injurious agents act on human tissues (Fig I–1) to produce tissue damage either directly or indirectly.

Direct Injury

A noxious agent may act directly on the tissue and interfere with its structure or biochemical function. An example is a burn, in which the heat causes immediate direct destruction of cell membranes and other tissue components and coagulation of intracellular proteins.

Indirect Injury

An injurious agent may act at some site other than the tissue in question to produce an abnormality in the immediate environment of the cell or cause accumulation of some toxic substance, which in turn causes cell damage. Representative causes of indirect injury include accumulation of toxic products in kidney and liver failure or a change in extracellular pH, electrolyte concentrations, or core body temperature. These indirect injuries may result in cell damage in many different tissues throughout the body, eg, structural and functional abnormalities in the brain in liver failure (hepatic encephalopathy).

Cell Degeneration & Necrosis 1

THE NORMAL CELL (Fig 1–1)

The normal cell is a highly complex unit in which the various organelles and enzyme systems continuously carry out the metabolic activities that maintain cell viability and support its normal functions. Normal functioning of the cell is dependent on (1) the immediate environment of the cell; (2) a continuous supply of nutrients such as oxygen, glucose, and amino acids; and (3) constant removal of the products of metabolism, including CO_2.

CELLULAR INJURY

Injury to a cell may be nonlethal or lethal (Fig 1–2).

LETHAL INJURY

Lethal injuries to the tissues of a living individual cause cell death **(necrosis)**. Necrosis is accompanied by biochemical and structural changes (see below) and is irreversible. The necrotic cells cease to function; if necrosis is sufficiently extensive, clinical disease results.

Cell necrosis should be distinguished from the **death of the individual,** which is difficult to define. From a legal standpoint in many countries, an individual is considered dead when there is complete and irreversible cessation of brain function. Many individual cells and tissues in a legally

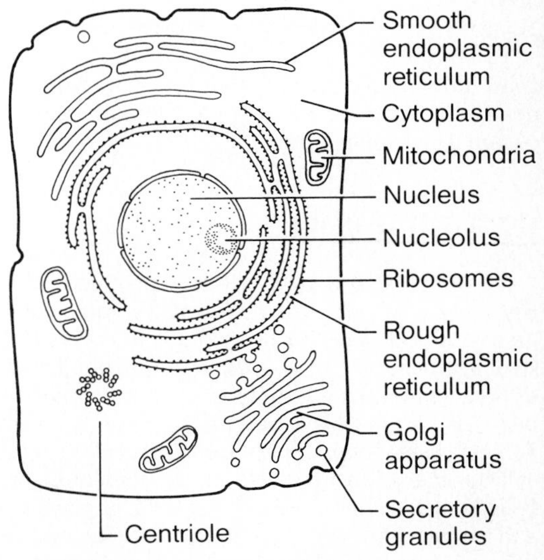

Figure 1–1. The normal cell.

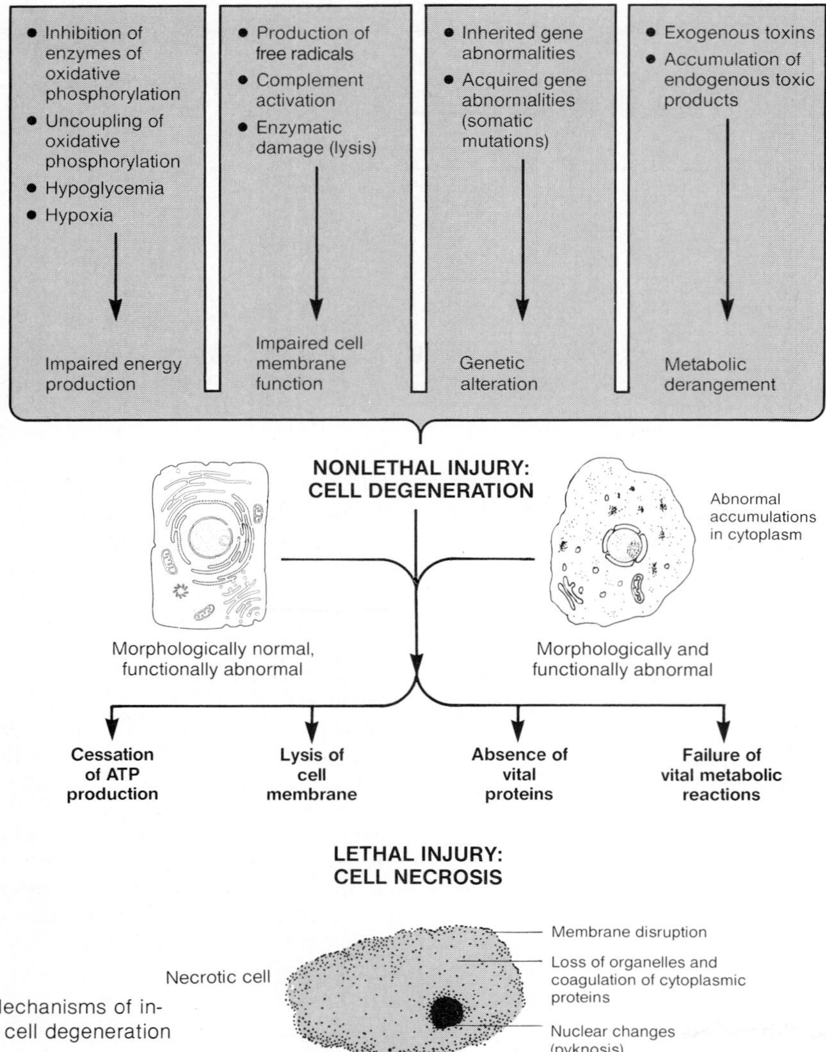

Figure 1-2. Mechanisms of injury leading to cell degeneration and necrosis.

dead individual remain viable for some time after death, however, and constitute a major source of organs for transplantation.

NONLETHAL INJURY

Nonlethal injury to a cell may produce **cell degeneration,** which is manifested as some abnormality of biochemical function, a recognizable structural change, or a combined biochemical and structural abnormality. Degeneration is reversible but may progress to necrosis if injury persists. When it is associated with abnormal cell function, cell degeneration may also cause clinical disease. It is worth remembering that cell degeneration and necrosis are ongoing phenomena in multicellular organisms and that in the healthy state, they are balanced by cell renewal, with dead cells being removed by the body's scavenging systems.

In its broadest sense, cell degeneration touches all of medicine, since all diseases can ultimately be traced to some cellular abnormality. In this chapter, the discussion of cell degeneration is limited mainly to those types of degeneration that cause a visible structural alteration in the cell.

MECHANISMS OF CELLULAR DEGENERATION & NECROSIS

IMPAIRED ENERGY PRODUCTION

Normal Energy Production

High-energy phosphate bonds of adenosine triphosphate (ATP) represent the most efficient energy source for the cell. ATP is produced by phosphorylation of ADP in the mitochondrial membrane, a reaction that is linked to the oxidation of reduced substances in the respiratory chain of enzymes. Oxygen is required (oxidative phosphorylation) (Fig 1–3).

Causes of Defective Energy (ATP) Production (Fig 1–3)

A. Hypoglycemia: Glucose is the main substrate for energy production in most tissues and is the sole energy source in brain cells. Lack of glucose in cells due to low glucose levels in blood (hypoglycemia) therefore results in deficient ATP production that is most profound in the brain.

B. Hypoxia: Oxygen reaches the cells via arterial blood but is ultimately derived from the atmosphere. Most of the oxygen carried in blood is bound to hemoglobin. Lack of oxygen in the cells (hypoxia) may result from (1) respiratory obstruction or disease, preventing oxygenation of blood in the lungs; (2) failure of blood flow in and out of the tissue, due either to generalized circulatory failure or to local vessel obstruction; (3) anemia (ie, decreased hemoglobin in the blood), resulting in decreased oxygen carriage by the blood; or (4) alteration of hemoglobin (as occurs in carbon monoxide poisoning), making it unavailable for oxygen transport and leading to the same result as anemia.

C. Enzyme Inhibition: Cyanide poisoning is a good example of interference with enzymes associated with oxidative phosphorylation. Cyanide inhibits cytochrome oxidase, the final enzyme in the respiratory chain, causing acute ATP deficiency in all cells of the body and rapid death.

D. Uncoupling of Oxidative Phosphorylation: Uncoupling of oxidation and phosphorylation occurs either through chemical reactions or through physical detachment of enzymes from the mitochondrial membrane. Mitochondrial swelling, which is a common change associated with many types of injury, causes uncoupling of oxidative phosphorylation.

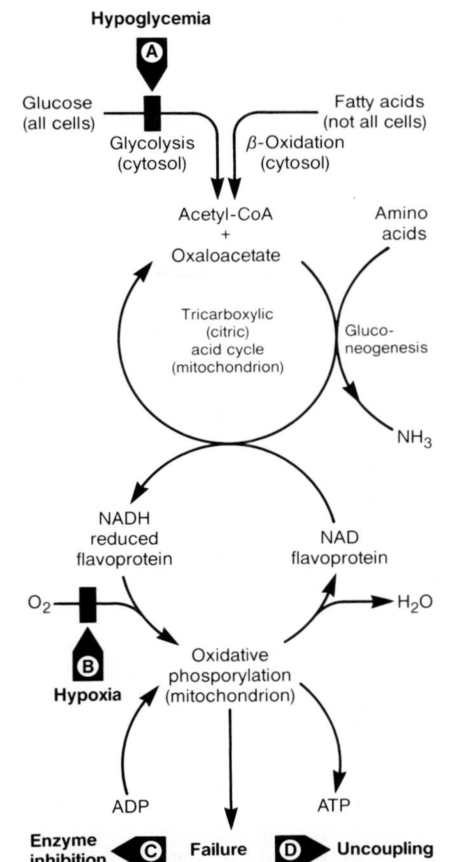

Figure 1–3. Main biochemical pathways involved in cellular ATP (energy) production. Abnormalities that result in failure of energy production are noted by letters that correspond to the text description.

Effects of Defective Energy Production

Generalized failure of energy production will first affect those cells with the highest demand for oxygen because of their high basal metabolic rate. Brain cells are maximally affected. The earliest clinical signs of hypoxia and hypoglycemia are due to neurologic dysfunction, leading to a disturbance of the normal level of consciousness.

A. Intracellular Accumulation of Water and Electrolytes: The earliest detectable biochemical evidence of diminished availability of ATP is dysfunction of the energy-dependent sodium pump in the plasma membrane. The resulting influx of sodium and water into the cell leads to **cloudy swelling**. (The cloudy appearance is due to the cytoplasmic organelles dispersed in the swollen cell.) Cloudy swelling is the earliest microscopic change of defective ATP production. **Hydropic change** is a more severe form of this phenomenon. Both are reversible. Changes also occur in the intracellular concentrations of other electrolytes (particularly K^+, Ca^{2+}, and Mg^{2+}), the concentrations of which are also maintained by energy-dependent activity of the plasma membrane. These electrolyte abnormalities may lead to disordered electrical activity and enzyme inhibition.

B. Changes in Organelles: Swelling of cytoplasmic organelles follows influx of sodium and water. Distention of the endoplasmic reticulum detaches the ribosomes and interferes with protein synthesis. Mitochondrial swelling causes physical dissociation (uncoupling) of oxidative phosphorylation, which further impairs ATP synthesis.

C. Switch to Anaerobic Metabolism: In hypoxic conditions, cellular metabolism changes from aerobic to anaerobic glycolysis. The conversion leads to the production of lactic acid and causes a decrease in intracellular pH. Chromatin clumping in the nucleus and further disruption of organelle membranes then occur. Disruption of lysosomal membranes leads to release of lysosomal enzymes into the cytoplasm, which damages vital intracellular molecules.

The exact point at which cell injury becomes irreversible and the degenerating cell becomes necrotic is unknown.

IMPAIRED CELL MEMBRANE FUNCTION

The Normal Plasma Membrane (Fig 1-4)

The plasma membrane of the cell is composed of a lipid bilayer in which several types of proteins are embedded. The membrane is supported by a framework of cytoplasmic filaments.

Causes of Plasma Membrane Damage

A. Production of Free Radicals: Free radicals are highly unstable particles with an odd number of electrons (an unpaired electron) in their outer shell. The excess energy attributable to the unstable configuration is released through chemical reactions with adjacent molecules. One of the best known interactions is that between oxygen-based free radicals and cell membrane lipids (lipid peroxidation), which leads to membrane damage.

Free radicals are produced in cells exposed to (1) powerful external energy sources, such as radiation, which cause ionization of cytoplasmic water and form hydroxyl ($OH^{\cdot}$) radicals; or (2) chemical poisons, such as carbon tetrachloride, which cause abnormal electron transfers ($CCl_3^{\cdot}$ free radical).

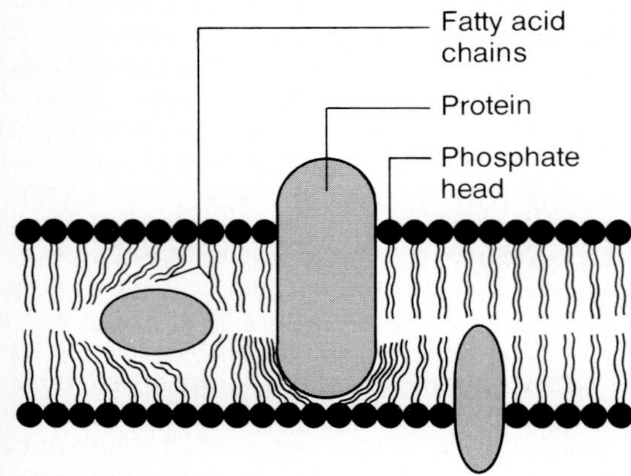

Figure 1-4. The cell (plasma) membrane, which is composed of a lipid bilayer made up of a phosphate head (circle) to which are attached 2 fatty acid chains (wavy lines). Membrane proteins may lie within the membrane or project on either side of it.

B. Activation of the Complement System: The final compounds of the activated complement pathway (Chapter 4), probably a complex of C5b, C6, C7, C8, and C9, exert a phospholipaselike effect that can enzymatically damage the plasma membrane. This phenomenon (complement fixation and activation) is an important component of the immune response that causes the death of cells recognized as "foreign."

C. Lysis by Enzymes: Enzymes with lipaselike activity damage cell membranes. For example, pancreatic lipases—when they are liberated outside the pancreatic duct in acute pancreatic inflammation—damage nearby cells and cause extensive necrosis. Some microorganisms—eg, *Clostridium perfringens,* one of the causes of gas gangrene—produce enzymes that damage plasma membranes and cause extensive necrosis.

Effects of Plasma Membrane Damage

A. Loss of Structural Integrity: Severe injury to the plasma membrane results in loss of structural integrity of the cell, leading to rupture and necrosis. In some cases, dissolution of part of the plasma membrane causes a localized defect in the cell wall that later closes over, as occurs in erythrocytes, in which loss of surface membrane followed by repair results in an intact erythrocyte that is smaller and rounder than normal (microspherocyte; see Chapter 25).

B. Loss of Function: The plasma membrane maintains the internal chemical composition of the cell by means of selective permeability and active transport. Damage to the plasma membrane may result in abnormal entry of water, causing cloudy swelling and hydropic change identical to that resulting from injury due to defective energy production; electrolyte imbalance in the cell, most commonly increased intracellular sodium and decreased potassium; and swelling and disruption of cytoplasmic organelles. These changes in the internal cell composition may result in a decline in cellular function.

C. Deposition of Lipofuscin (Brown Atrophy): Lipofuscin is a fine, granular, golden-brown pigment composed of phospholipids and proteins. It accumulates in the cytoplasm as a result of damage to the membranes of cytoplasmic organelles and is most commonly seen in myocardial cells (Fig 1-5), liver cells, and neurons. Lipofuscin causes no cellular functional abnormalities.

Lipofuscin deposition occurs in elderly individuals, those suffering from severe malnutrition, and those with chronic diseases. It is due to a lack of cellular antioxidants that normally prevent lipid peroxidation of organelle membranes. Lipo-

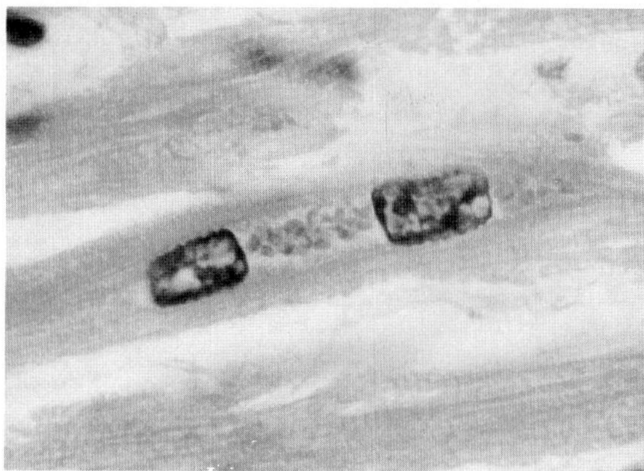

Figure 1-5. Myocardial fiber with lipofuscin pigment in the perinuclear region. On sections stained with hematoxylin and eosin, lipofuscin has a golden brown color.

fuscin is also called "wear and tear" pigment because of its association with aging and chronic diseases.

GENETIC ALTERATION

Normal Genetic Apparatus

Deoxyribonucleic acid (DNA) in the chromosomes represents the genetic basis of control of cellular function. DNA controls the synthesis of structural proteins (Fig 1-6), growth-regulating proteins, and enzymes.

Causes of DNA Abnormalities

Inherited genetic abnormalities are passed from generation to generation, frequently in predictable fashion according to mendelian laws (Chapter 15). **Acquired genetic abnormalities** are somatic mutations resulting from damage to genetic material by any of several agents, including ionizing radiation, viruses, and mutagenic drugs and chemicals.

Effects of DNA Abnormalities

The clinical and pathologic effects of genetic abnormalities depend on (1) the severity of damage, (2) the precise gene or genes damaged, and (3) when the damage was sustained. When genetic damage is inherited or occurs during gametogenesis or early fetal development, clinical effects may be present at birth (congenital genetic disease). Acquired genetic disease results when genetic damage occurs postnatally.

DNA abnormalities are manifested at a cellular level in several ways.

A. Failure of Synthesis of Structural Proteins: Severe damage to DNA in the nucleus—as occurs after high doses of radiation and some

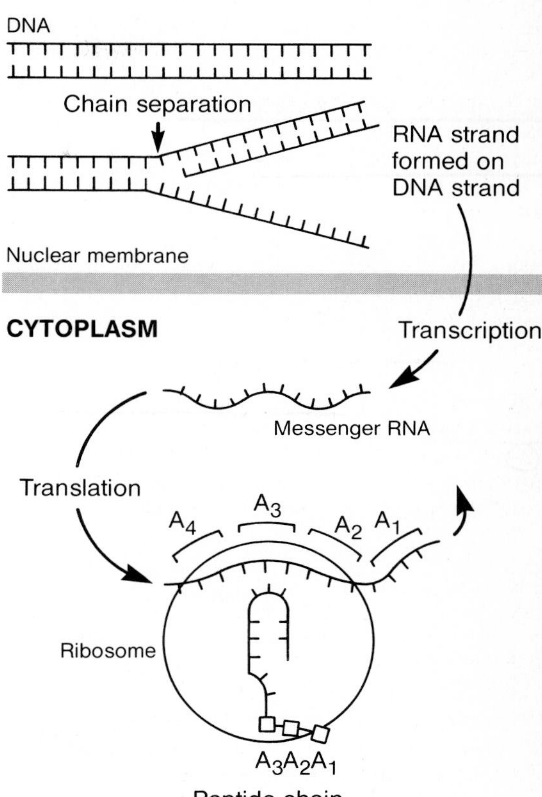

Figure 1-6. Protein synthesis. Nucleic acids are represented as lines with multiple short projections representing the bases. Changes in the nucleotide sequence will lead to synthesis of an abnormal protein or failure of synthesis of the protein.

viral infections—causes necrosis due to inhibition of synthesis of vital intracellular structural proteins. Less severe damage may result in a variety of effects, depending on the extent of inhibition and the type of protein synthesis that is inhibited.

B. Failure of Mitosis: Interference with mitosis in actively dividing cells (eg, bone marrow cells) may result in depletion of erythrocytes (anemia) and neutrophils (neutropenia). Similar depletion of cells may occur in intestinal mucosa, resulting in abnormal structure and function. Failure of mitosis in the testis may result in decreased spermatogenesis, leading to infertility.

C. Failure of Growth-Regulating Proteins: Changes in growth regulation that result from DNA damage may result in cancer. This is discussed in Chapter 18.

D. Failure of Enzyme Synthesis: Enzyme deficiency in the embryo may result in congenital diseases (inborn errors of metabolism) (Chapter 15). Acquired enzyme defects result in necrosis if a vital biochemical system is affected. Enzyme defects involving less vital biochemical reactions result in a variety of sublethal degenerative changes.

METABOLIC DERANGEMENTS

Exogenous Toxic Agents

Many exogenous injurious agents, including alcohol, drugs, heavy metals, and infectious agents, cause cellular degeneration and necrosis by interfering directly with various specific biochemical reactions. Individual injurious agents and their effects on cellular metabolism are discussed in Section III (Chapters 8–14).

Accumulation of Endogenous Substances (Table 1-1)

A. Fatty Change (Fatty Degeneration): Fatty change is the **accumulation of triglyceride** in the cytoplasm of parenchymal cells due to an acquired defect in the metabolism of triglycerides. Clinically significant fatty change, which is common in the liver and rare in the kidney and myocardium, occurs as a nonspecific response to many types of injury.

1. Normal triglyceride metabolism in the liver–The liver plays a central role in triglyceride metabolism (Fig 1-7). Free fatty acids are carried in the blood to the liver, where they are converted to triglycerides, phospholipids, and cholesteryl esters. After these lipids form complexes with specific lipid acceptor proteins (apoproteins), which are also synthesized in the liver cell, they are secreted into the plasma as lipoproteins. When triglycerides are metabolized normally, there is so little triglyceride in the liver cell that it cannot be seen in routine microscopic sections.

2. Causes of fatty liver–Accumulation of triglycerides in the cytoplasm of liver cells to an extent that they are visible on microscopic examina-

Table 1-1. Endogenous substances accumulating in tissues as a result of deranged metabolism.

Accumulated Substance	Effects in Parenchymal Cells	Effects in Interstitial Issues
Water	Cloudy swelling Hydropic change	Edema
Lipid Triglyceride	Fatty change	
Cholesterol		Atherosclerosis (Chapter 20) Xanthoma
Complex lipids (phospholipid)	Lipid storage diseases (Chapter 15)	
Protein		Amyloidosis
Glycogen	Glycogen storage diseases (Chapter 15)	
Mucopolysaccharide	Mucopolysaccharidoses (Chapter 15)	Myxoid degeneration
Minerals Iron	Hemochromatosis	Localized hemosiderosis
Calcium		Calcification
Copper	Wilson's disease	Wilson's disease
Pigments Bilirubin	Kernicterus	Jaundice
Lipofuscin	Brown atrophy	
Urate		Gout (Chapter 68)
Homogentisic acid		Alkaptonuria (Chapter 68)

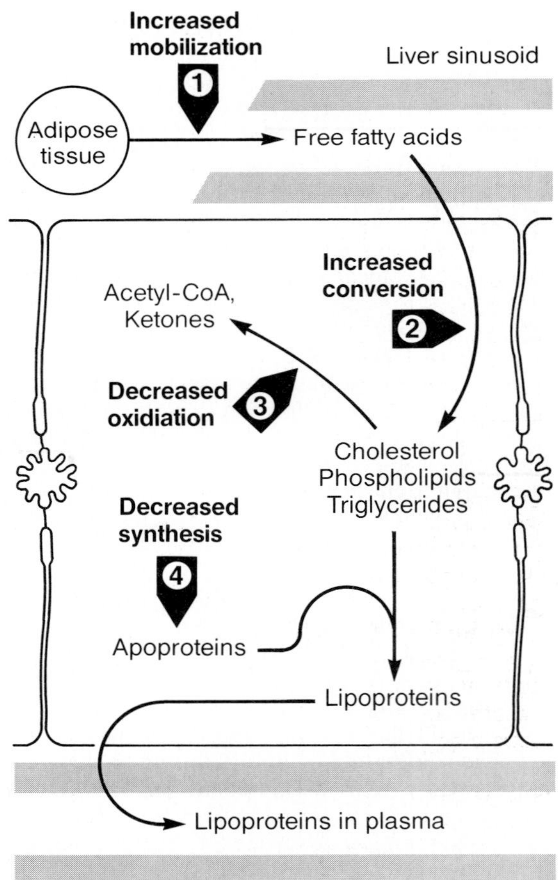

Figure 1-7. Fat metabolism in the liver cell. Numbers shown correspond with causes of fatty liver as described in the text.

tion (fatty liver) represents an abnormality of the metabolic pathway shown in Fig 1–7 and occurs in the following conditions: (1) When there is increased mobilization of adipose tissue, resulting in an increase in the amount of fatty acids reaching the liver, eg, in starvation and diabetes mellitus. (2) When the rate of conversion of fatty acids to triglycerides in the liver cell is increased because of overactivity of the involved enzyme systems. This is the main mechanism by which alcohol, a powerful enzyme inducer, causes fatty liver. (3) When oxidation of triglycerides to acetyl-CoA and ketone bodies is decreased, eg, in anemia and hypoxia. (4) When synthesis of lipid acceptor proteins is deficient. Protein malnutrition and several hepatotoxins, eg, carbon tetrachloride and phosphorus, cause fatty liver in this way.

3. Types of fatty liver–

a. Acute fatty liver–Acute fatty liver is a rare but serious condition associated with acute liver failure (Chapter 42). In acute fatty liver, triglyceride accumulates as small, membrane-bound droplets in the cytoplasm (microvacuolar fatty change, Fig 1–8).

b. Chronic fatty liver–Chronic fatty liver is much more common than acute fatty liver. It is associated with chronic alcoholism, malnutrition, and several hepatotoxins. Fat droplets in the cytoplasm fuse to form progressively larger fat globules (macrovacuolar fatty change, Fig 1–9). The distribution of fatty change in the liver lobule varies with different causes (Fig 1–10). Grossly, the fatty liver is enlarged and yellow, with a greasy appearance when cut. Even when severe, chronic fatty liver is rarely associated with clinically detectable liver dysfunction.

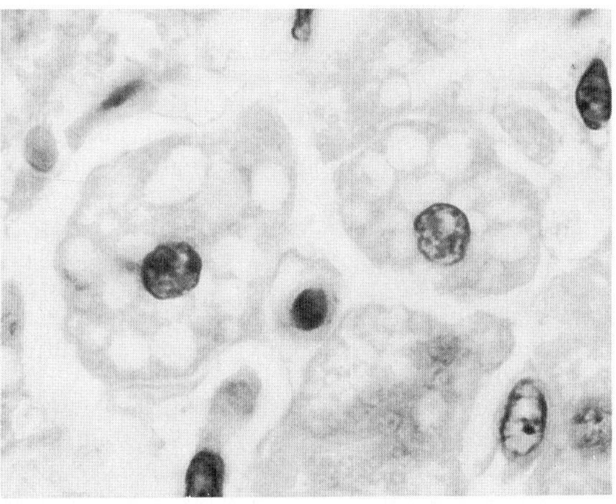

Figure 1-8. Acute microvacuolar fatty change of the liver in Reye's syndrome. The cytoplasm of the liver cells is filled with numerous small vacuoles representing the lipid that has been dissolved out of the tissue during processing. The nuclei are centrally located.

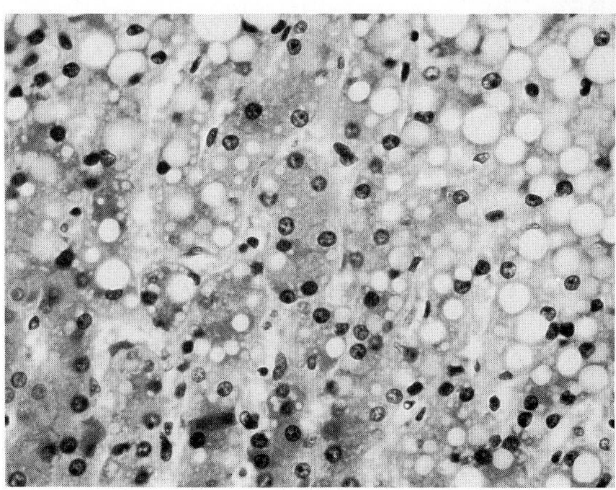

Figure 1-9. Macrovacuolar fatty change of the liver in alcoholism. The large fat globules in the cytoplasm appear as empty spaces that have displaced the nucleus to the side. The degree of fatty change varies from slight in the bottom left to marked at the top right of this photograph.

4. Fatty change of the myocardium–Triglyceride deposition in myocardial fibers occurs in chronic hypoxic states, notably **severe anemia**. In chronic fatty change, bands of yellow streaks alternate with red-brown muscle ("thrush breast" or "tiger skin" appearance); this usually causes no clinical symptoms. Toxic diseases such as diphtheritic myocarditis and Reye's syndrome produce acute fatty change. The heart is flabby and shows diffuse yellow discoloration; myocardial failure commonly follows.

5. Microscopic features of fatty change– Any fat present in tissues dissolves when various fat solvents are used to process tissue samples for microscopic sections. In routine tissue sections, therefore, cells in the earliest stages of fatty change have pale and foamy cytoplasm. As fat accumulation increases, cytoplasmic vacuoles appear. These represent the dissolved fat, and they grow progressively larger. Positive demonstration of fat requires the use of frozen sections made from fresh tissue. Fat remains in the cytoplasm in frozen sections, where it can be demonstrated by fat stains such as oil red O and Sudan black B.

B. Deposition of Iron (Hemochromatosis and Hemosiderosis):

1. Normal iron metabolism–(Fig 1–11) Iron metabolism is normally regulated so that the total amount of iron in the body is maintained within a narrow range. The body has no effective mechanism for eliminating excess iron, although women lose 10–15 mg of iron each month in menstrual blood. Iron overload is therefore rare in women, whereas iron deficiency is common.

2. Hemochromatosis and hemosiderosis– An increase in the total amount of iron in the

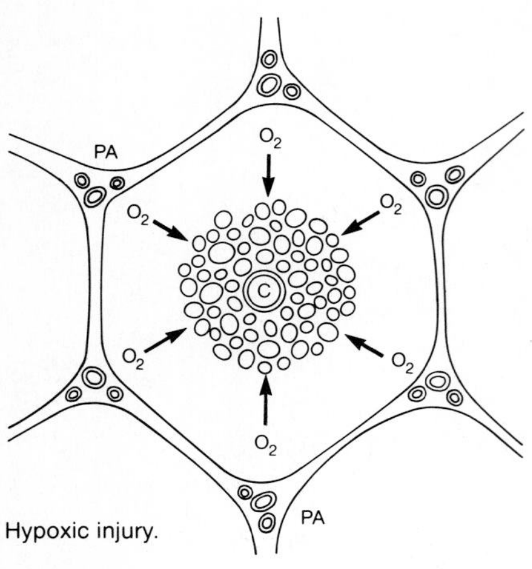

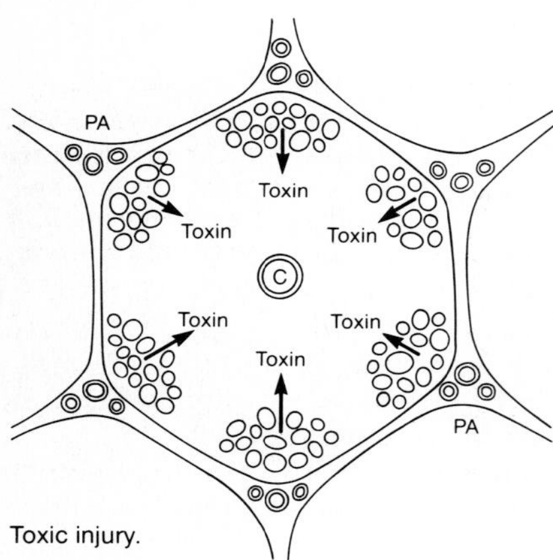

Figure 1-10. Distribution of fatty change (open circles) in the liver in hypoxic and toxic liver injuries. In hypoxic injury, fatty change is centrizonal; in toxic injury, fatty change occurs around the portal areas. The rules relating to this distribution, which are dependent on the mode of entry of oxygen and toxins into the liver lobule, are not without exception. Carbon tetrachloride, for example, causes centrizonal fatty change.

body is termed **hemochromatosis.** The excess iron accumulates in macrophages and parenchymal cells as ferritin and hemosiderin and causes parenchymal cell necrosis (Fig 1-12).

Deposition of hemosiderin primarily in tissue macrophages (histiocytes), with or without an increase in total body iron content and without parenchymal cell necrosis, is termed **hemosiderosis.**

3. Causes and effects of deposition of iron- **Localized hemosiderosis** is common in any tissue that is the site of hemorrhage. Hemoglobin is broken down and its iron is deposited locally, either in macrophages or in the connective tissue, as hemosiderin. Localized hemosiderosis has no clinical significance; its presence signifies only that hemorrhage has occurred at that site.

Generalized hemosiderosis is less common, occurring with relatively minor iron excess following multiple transfusions, excessive dietary iron, or excess absorption of iron in some hemolytic anemias. The excess iron is deposited as hemosiderin in macrophages throughout the body, notably in bone marrow, liver, and spleen. Generalized hemosiderosis can be diagnosed in bone marrow and liver biopsies and, apart from indicating the presence of iron overload of minor degree, has no clinical significance.

Hemochromatosis is uncommon, occurring both as an idiopathic (inherited) disease and as a secondary phenomenon following major iron overload. The distinction between generalized hemosiderosis and hemochromatosis is somewhat arbitrary, the major differences being the degree of iron overload and the presence of parenchymal cell damage or necrosis in hemochromatosis.

It is postulated that once intracellular storage mechanisms are exhausted, free ferric iron accumulates and undergoes reduction to produce toxic oxygen-based free radicals. The liver, heart, and pancreas are the most severely affected tissues in hemochromatosis (Chapter 43).

C. Deposition of Copper (Wilson's Disease): Copper is a trace mineral that is normally transported in the plasma as ceruloplasmin, composed of copper complexed with an $\alpha 2$-globulin, and "free" copper, which is loosely bound to albumin. Normally, copper absorption is balanced by excretion, mainly in bile.

In Wilson's disease, which is an inherited disorder, excretion of copper into bile is defective and leads to an increase in total body copper, with accumulation of copper in cells. The liver and basal ganglia of the brain (lenticular nucleus) are the most severely affected tissues; chronic liver failure and degeneration of the lenticular nucleus result—hence the alternative name **hepatolenticular degeneration.**

D. Accumulation of Bilirubin (Jaundice or Icterus):

1. Metabolism of bilirubin-(Fig 1-13.) Bilirubin is a bile pigment that is the catabolic end

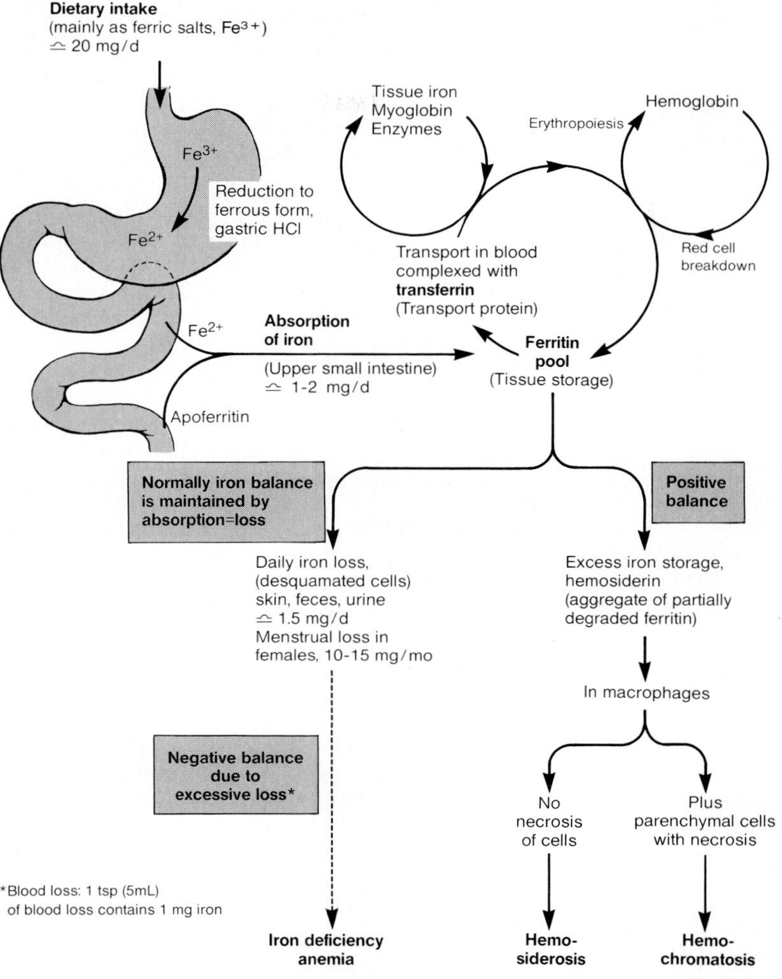

Figure 1-11. Iron metablism. Normally, iron loss is balanced by intestinal absorption. Negative balance due to a loss that cannot be compensated for by increased absorption leads to depletion of iron stores and anemia. Positive iron balance due to increased absorption or administration of excessive iron (usually in blood transfusions) leads to excessive iron storage.

product of the porphyrin ring of the hemoglobin molecule; it contains neither iron nor protein. Normally, it is formed in the reticuloendothelial system, where senescent erythrocytes are destroyed. Bilirubin is then transported in the plasma to the liver in an unconjugated form, bound to albumin. Unconjugated bilirubin, which is lipid-soluble, is also called **hemobilirubin** or **indirect bilirubin**. In the liver, bilirubin is conjugated enzymatically with glucuronide to form water-soluble diglucuronide **(conjugated** or **direct bilirubin, cholebilirubin),** which is excreted by liver cells into the bile and thence to the intestine. In the intestine, bacterial activity converts bilirubin to **urobilinogen,** which is disposed of in one of 3 ways: (1) directly excreted in feces (as stercobilin); (2) absorbed in the portal vein and reexcreted into bile by the liver in the enterohepatic circulation; or (3) excreted in urine, normally in small amounts (Fig 1–13).

2. **Causes of jaundice-**(See also Chapter 42.) An increase in serum bilirubin is called **jaundice,** or **icterus.** Jaundice is common and may result from 3 distinct mechanisms (Table 1–2): increased production, decreased excretion by the liver, or bile duct obstruction.

a. **Hemolytic jaundice (increased production)-**Increased destruction of erythrocytes, if sufficiently severe, overwhelms the capacity of the liver to conjugate bilirubin and results in accumulation of unconjugated bilirubin in serum. Because unconjugated bilirubin is lipid-soluble and bound to albumin in the blood, it is not excreted in the urine **(acholuric jaundice)**. Since hepatic conjugation is proceeding at its maximal rate, the conjugated bilirubin content of bile is increased, and levels of fecal stercobilin and urinary urobilinogen increase as a result (Fig 1–13).

b. **Hepatocellular jaundice (decreased uptake, conjugation, or excretion)-**Failure of the liver to take up, conjugate, or excrete bilirubin results in an increase in serum bilirubin. Usually, both conjugated and unconjugated bilirubin levels are elevated, the proportions depending on which

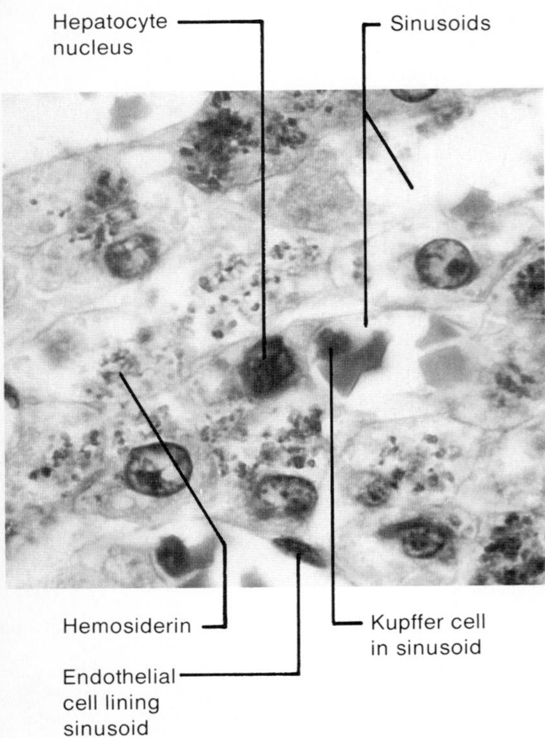

Figure 1-12. Hemochromatosis of the liver, showing hemosiderin pigment deposited in hepatocytes and Kupffer cells. Hemosiderin stains golden brown with hematoxylin and eosin and deep blue with Prussian blue stain.

metabolic failure predominates. Conjugated, water-soluble bilirubin is commonly present in urine. Urinary urobilinogen levels are usually elevated because liver dysfunction prevents normal uptake and reexcretion of urobilinogen absorbed from the intestine.

c. Obstructive jaundice (decreased excretion)-Biliary tract obstruction results in an accumulation of conjugated bilirubin proximal to the obstruction in the biliary tract and liver **(cholestasis)**. In a manner not clearly understood, reflux of conjugated bilirubin into the plasma occurs, causing jaundice; some conjugated bilirubin is then excreted in the urine. Failure of bilirubin to reach the intestine causes a decrease in fecal and urinary urobilinogen levels. In complete biliary obstruction, absence of bilirubin alters the normal color of the feces (clay-colored stools).

3. Effects of deposition of bilirubin-

a. Deposition in connective tissue-The increase in serum bilirubin leads to deposition of bilirubin in the connective tissue of the skin, scleras, and internal organs. The resulting yellow-green discoloration is characteristic of jaundice. No functional abnormality results from bilirubin accumulation in connective tissue.

b. Deposition in parenchymal cells-

(1) Basal ganglia-Kernicterus is an uncommon condition in which unconjugated bilirubin is deposited in the basal ganglia (nuclei) of the brain (Fig 1-14). It occurs only with an increase in unconjugated bilirubin, which is lipid-soluble and can cross the blood-brain barrier. It is especially common in premature babies, in whom bilirubin-conjugating enzymes are poorly developed and serum albumin levels low. Kernicterus occurs in the neonatal period, when the blood-brain barrier is relatively permeable to the entry of bilirubin (Fig 1-14). After the neonatal period, there is no risk of kernicterus even when there is marked unconjugated hyperbilirubinemia.

The most common cause of kernicterus is severe neonatal hemolysis, usually as a result of Rh blood group incompatibility between mother and baby (Chapter 25). In the newborn, the increased bilirubin load and failure of the liver to conjugate bilirubin result in accumulation of unconjugated bilirubin in the plasma. When plasma albumin is low, bilirubin-binding capability is rapidly exhausted, and free unconjugated bilirubin accumulates in the plasma and can enter the brain (Fig 1-14).

Intracellular accumulation of bilirubin in brain cells causes neuronal dysfunction and necrosis, which may cause death in the acute phase. Infants who survive the acute phase show the effects of neuronal loss.

(2) Liver-Accumulation of bilirubin in liver cells in obstructive jaundice results in toxic injury associated with cellular swelling. Bilirubin forms plugs of bile in bile ductules and canaliculi. Escape of bilirubin into the liver lobule produces bile "lakes" that may be associated with cell necrosis. Fibrosis ensues that may lead to **biliary cirrhosis** and **chronic liver failure** (Chapter 42).

E. Accumulation of Other Toxic Products: (Table 1-1.) Various other potentially toxic endogenous substances accumulate in cells and tissue fluids as a result of metabolic derangements. Many of these substances and their adverse effects are discussed in Chapter 2. Toxic substances that accumulate in hepatic and renal failure are discussed in the systemic pathology section.

NECROSIS OF CELLS

Necrosis may occur directly or may follow cell degeneration.

Morphologic Evidence of Necrosis

A. Early Changes: In early necrosis, the cell is morphologically normal. There is a delay of 1-

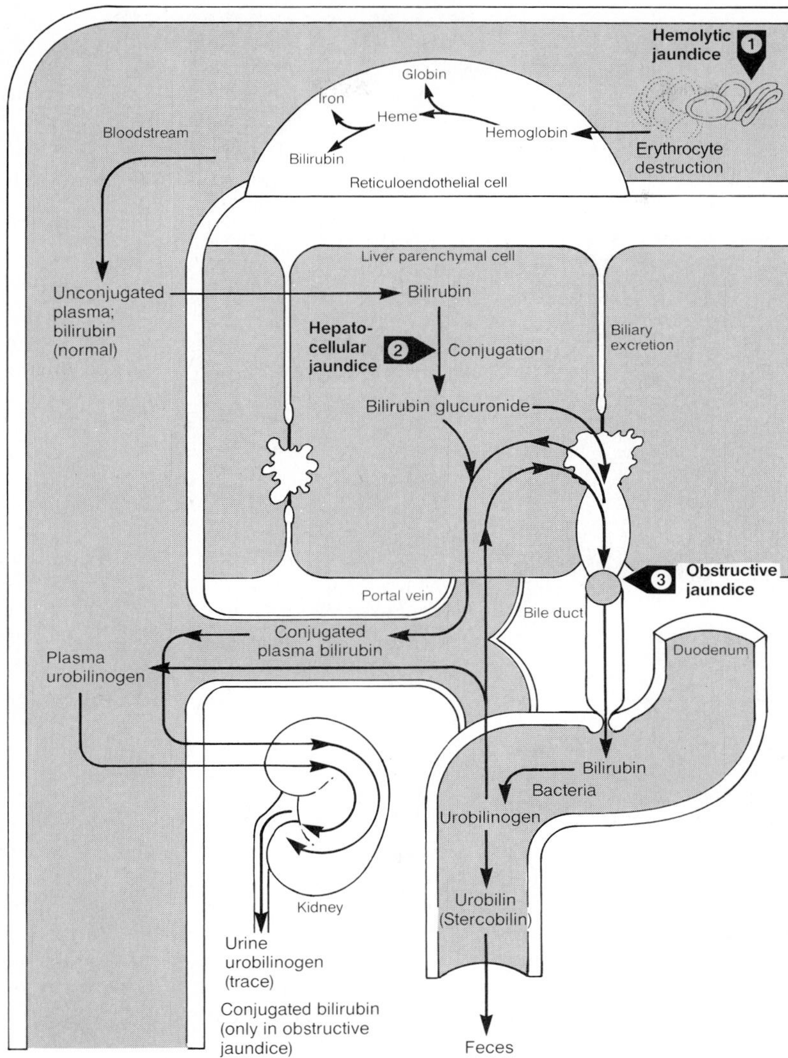

Figure 1–13. Bilirubin metabolism and causes of jaundice. In hemolytic jaundice **(1),** there is increased bilirubin formation due to increased hemoglobin breakdown. In hepatocellular jaundice **(2),** conjugation and excretion of bilirubin by the liver is defective. In obstructive jaundice **(3),** conjugated bilirubin refluxes into the blood. Note that conjugated bilirubin is present in plasma and urine only in patients with obstructive jaundice.

Table 1–2. Differential features of the different types of jaundice.

	Hemolytic Jaundice	Hepatocellular Jaundice	Obstructive Jaundice
Basic defect	Excessive production of bilirubin	Defective uptake, conjugation or excretion of bilirubin by liver cells	Obstruction of bile ducts
Elevation of serum bilirubin	Mild	Severe	Severe
Type of bilirubin in plasma	Unconjugated	Conjugated and unconjugated	Conjugated
Bile in urine	Absent	Present	Present
Urobilinogen in urine	Increased	Increased	Decreased (absent)
Stercobilin in feces	Increased	Variable	Decreased
Red cell survival	Decreased	Normal	Normal
Liver function tests	Normal	Abnormal	Variable
Bile ducts	May contain pigment stones	Normal	Obstructed, with proximal dilatation

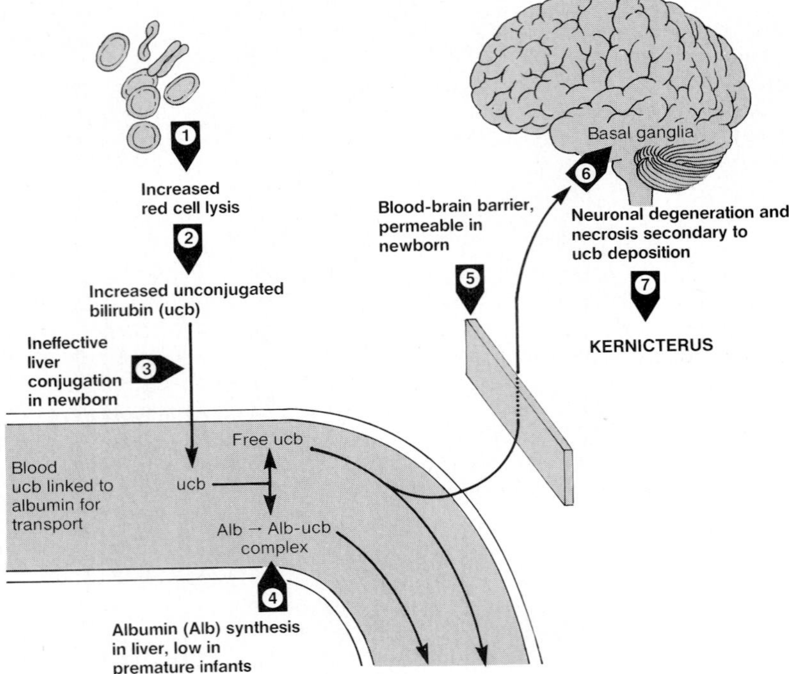

Figure 1-14. Factors involved in the pathogenesis of kernicterus. Increased hemolysis **(1)** leads to increased production of unconjugated bilirubin **(2),** which, in the neonate, is not cleared normally owing to immaturity of liver enzyme systems **(3).** Unconjugated bilirubin is normally complexed with plasma albumin, levels of which may also be low in neonates **(4).** Unconjugated bilirubin that is not complexed to albumin (Free ucb) can cross the blood-brain barrier in the neonatal period **(5),** causing toxic neuronal injury **(6)** and kernicterus **(7).**

3 hours before changes of necrosis are recognizable on electron microscopy and at least 6–8 hours before changes are apparent on light microscopy. For example, if a patient has a heart attack (myocardial necrosis caused by occlusion of a coronary artery) and dies within minutes, autopsy will reveal no structural evidence of necrosis; if, on the other hand, death occurs 2 days after the heart attack, changes due to necrosis are obvious.

B. Nuclear Changes: Nuclear changes are the best evidence of cell necrosis. The chromatin of the dead cell clumps into coarse strands, and the nucleus becomes a shrunken, dense, and deeply basophilic mass (ie, it stains blue with hematoxylin). This process is called **pyknosis** (Fig 1–15). The pyknotic nucleus may then break up into numerous small basophilic particles **(karyorrhexis)** or undergo lysis as a result of the action of lysosomal deoxyribonucleases **(karyolysis).** In rapidly occurring necrosis, the nucleus undergoes lysis without a pyknotic stage.

C. Cytoplasmic Changes: About 6 hours after the cell undergoes necrosis, its cytoplasm becomes homogeneous and deeply acidophilic—ie, it stains pink with an acidic stain such as eosin. This is the first change detectable by light microscopy, and it is due to denaturation of cytoplasmic proteins and loss of ribosomes. The RNA of the ribosomes is responsible for the basophilic tinge in normal cytoplasm. When specialized organelles are present in the cell, such as myofibrils in myocardial cells, these are lost early. Swelling of mito-

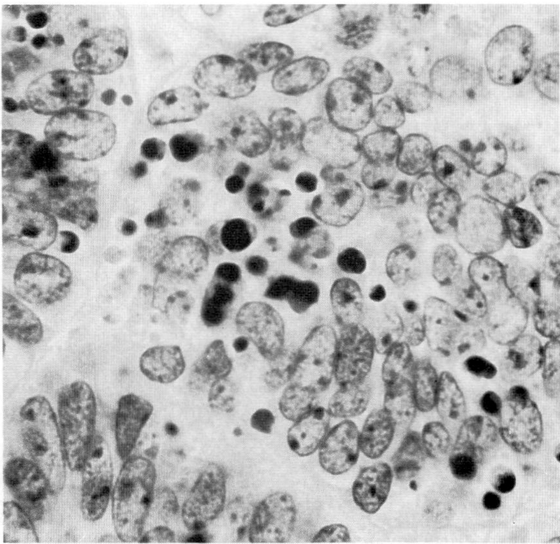

Figure 1-15. Cancer cells, showing nuclear pyknosis associated with cell necrosis. The pyknotic nuclei are dark and shrunken and contrast with the nuclei of adjacent living cells, which have a well-defined nuclear membrane and dispersed chromatin.

chondria and disruption of organelle membranes cause cytoplasmic vacuolation. Finally, enzymatic digestion of the cell by enzymes released by the cell's own lysosomes causes lysis **(autolysis)**.

D. Biochemical Changes: The influx of calcium ions into the cell is closely related to irreversible loss of viability of the injured cell and the appearance of morphologic changes of necrosis. In the normal cell, the intracellular calcium concentration is about 0.001 that of extracellular fluid. This gradient is maintained by the cell membrane, which actively transports calcium ions out of the cell. In experimental cell systems in which cell injury is induced by ischemia and a variety of different toxic agents, intracellular calcium accumulation occurs only when the cell is irreversibly damaged. Reversible cell degeneration is not associated with an increase in intracellular calcium concentration. Some authorities believe that the influx of calcium into the damaged cell is the biochemical event that results in cell necrosis.

Types of Necrosis

Different cells show different morphologic changes after they undergo necrosis; the differences reflect variations in cell composition, speed of necrosis, and type of injury (Fig 1-16).

A. Coagulative Necrosis: In this type of necrosis, the necrotic cell retains its cellular outline, often for several days. The cell, devoid of its nucleus, appears as a mass of coagulated, pink-staining, homogeneous cytoplasm (Fig 1-17).

The mechanism of coagulative necrosis is not well understood. Denaturation of cytoplasmic proteins renders them more resistant to the action of lysosomal enzymes, thereby delaying liquefaction.

Coagulative necrosis typically occurs in solid

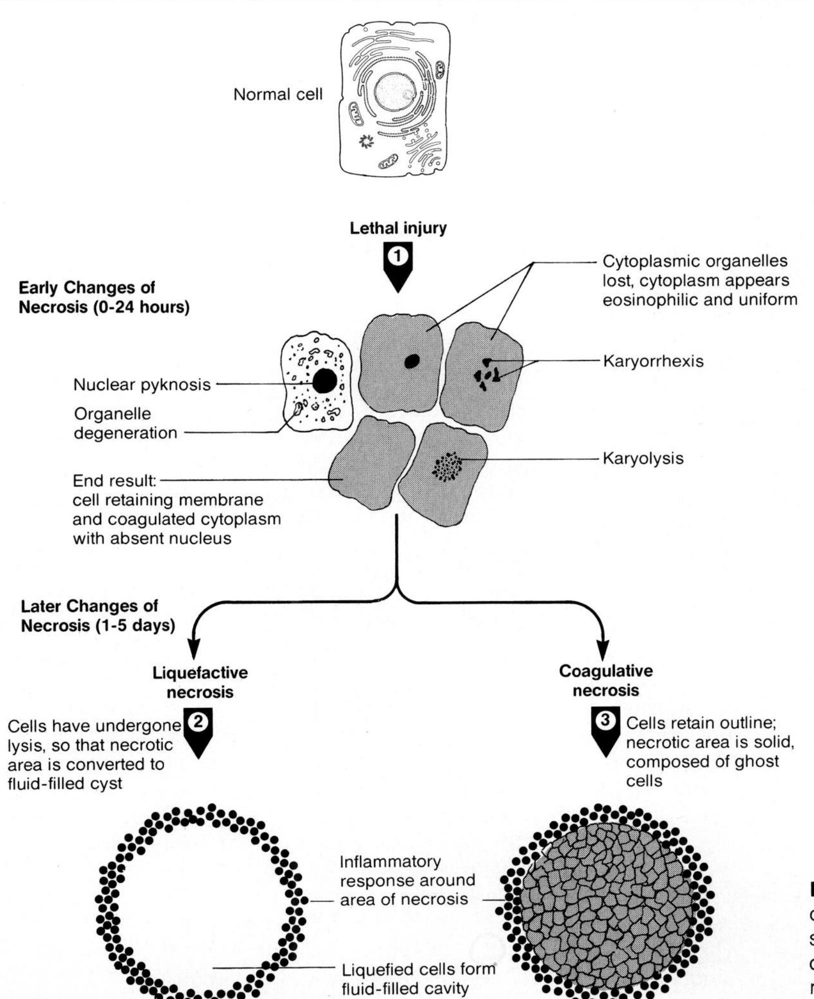

Figure 1-16. Necrosis of cells caused by letal injury **(1)**, showing early changes, and the difference between liquefactive necrosis **(2)** and coagulative necrosis **(3)**.

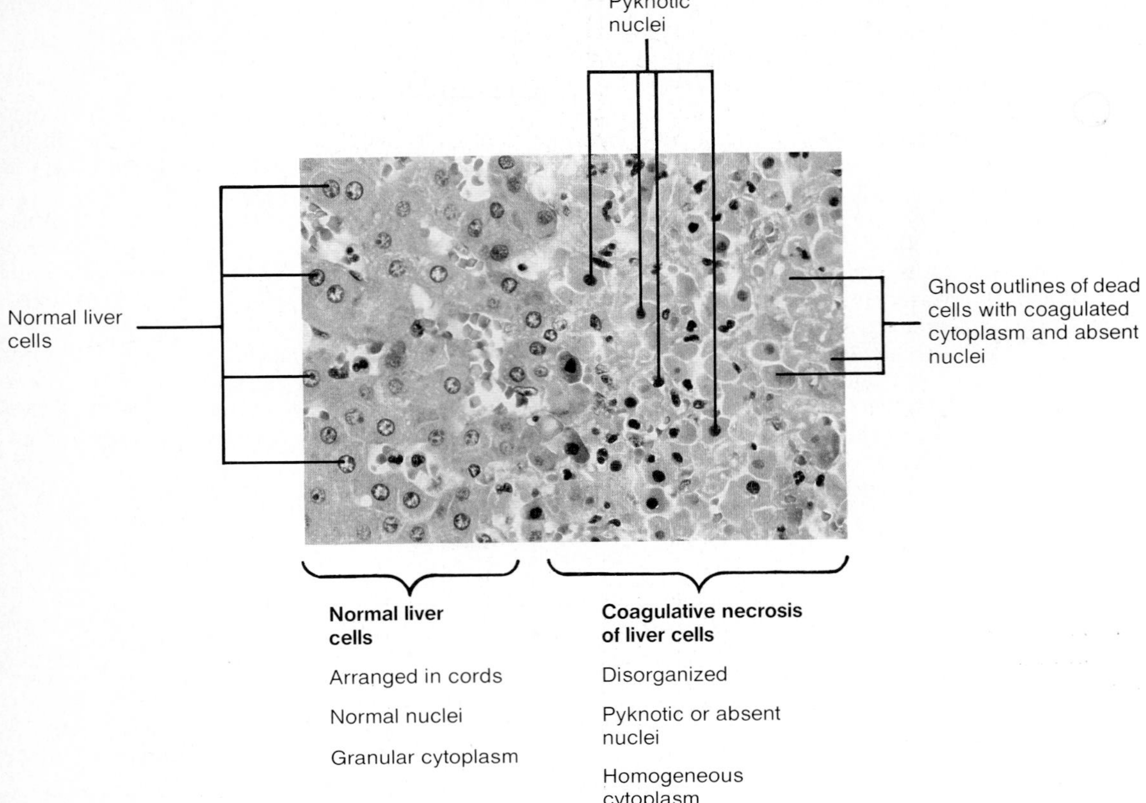

Figure 1–17. Coagulative necrosis of liver cells. The left half of the photograph shows normal liver cells and contrasts with the necrotic liver cells in the right half.

organs, such as the kidney, heart (myocardium), and adrenal gland, usually as a result of deficient blood supply and anoxia (Chapter 9). It is also seen with other types of injury, eg, coagulative necrosis of liver cells due to viruses or toxic chemicals, and coagulative necrosis of skin in burns.

B. Liquefactive Necrosis: Liquefaction of necrotic cells results when lysosomal enzymes released by the necrotic cells cause rapid liquefaction. Lysis of a cell as a result of the action of its own enzymes is **autolysis.** Liquefactive necrosis is typically seen in the brain following ischemia (Figs 1–18 and 1–19).

Liquefactive necrosis also occurs during pus formation **(suppurative inflammation)** as a result of the action of proteolytic enzymes released by neutrophils. Cellular lysis by enzymes derived from a source other than the cell itself is **heterolysis.**

C. Fat Necrosis:

1. Enzymatic fat necrosis–Enzymatic fat necrosis most characteristically occurs in acute pancreatitis and pancreatic injuries when pancreatic enzymes are liberated from the ducts into surrounding tissue. Pancreatic lipase acts on the triglycerides in fat cells, breaking these down into glycerol and fatty acids, which complex with plasma calcium ions to form calcium soaps. The gross appearance is one of opaque chalky white plaques and nodules in the adipose tissue surrounding the pancreas (Fig 1–20).

Rarely, pancreatic disease may be associated with entry of lipase into the bloodstream and subsequent widespread fat necrosis throughout the body; the subcutaneous fat and bone marrow are most affected.

2. Nonenzymatic fat necrosis–Nonenzymatic fat necrosis occurs in the breast, subcutaneous tissue, and abdomen. Many patients have a history of trauma. Nonenzymatic fat necrosis is also termed **traumatic fat necrosis** even though trauma is not established as the definitive cause. Nonenzymatic fat necrosis evokes an inflammatory response characterized by numerous foamy macrophages, neutrophils, and lymphocytes. Fibrosis follows, producing a mass that may be difficult to distinguish from a cancer.

D. Caseous and Gummatous Necrosis: Caseous (cheeselike) and gummatous (gum- or rubberlike) necrosis occur in infectious granulomas

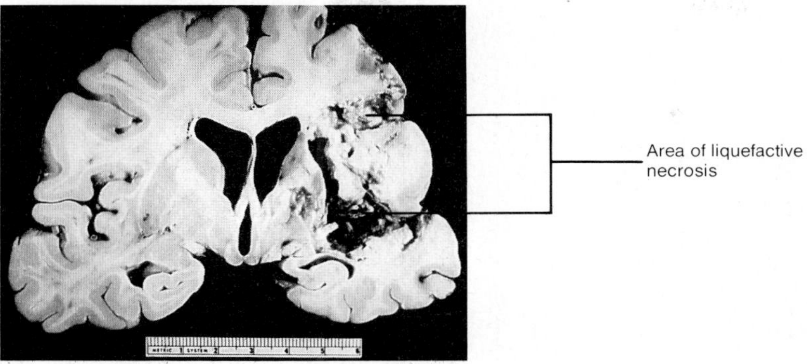

Figure 1-18. Cerebral infarct, showing liquefactive necrosis of the cerebral hemisphere. The involved area has been converted to a fluid-filled cyst that collapsed when the brain was cut and the fluid drained out.

(localized chronic inflammatory lesions; see Chapter 5).

E. Fibrinoid Necrosis: Fibrinoid necrosis is a type of connective tissue necrosis seen particularly in autoimmune diseases (eg, rheumatic fever, polyarteritis nodosa, and systemic lupus erythematosus). Collagen and smooth muscle in the media of blood vessels are especially involved. Fibrinoid necrosis of arterioles also occurs in accelerated (malignant) hypertension.

Fibrinoid necrosis is characterized by loss of normal structure and replacement by a homogeneous, bright pink-staining necrotic material that resembles fibrin microscopically (Fig 1–21). Note, however, that "fibrinoid" is not the same as "fibrinous," which denotes deposition of fibrin, as occurs in inflammation and blood coagulation. Areas of fibrinoid necrosis contain various amounts of immunoglobulins and complement, albumin breakdown products of collagen, and fibrin.

F. Gangrene: The term "gangrene" is widely used to denote a clinical condition in which extensive tissue necrosis is complicated to a variable degree by secondary bacterial infection.

1. Dry gangrene-(Fig 1–22.) Dry gangrene most commonly occurs in the extremities as a result of ischemic coagulative necrosis of tissues due to arterial obstruction. The necrotic area appears black, dry, and shriveled and is sharply demarcated from adjacent viable tissue. The secondary bacterial infection is usually insignificant. Treatments consists of surgical removal of dead tissue (debridement).

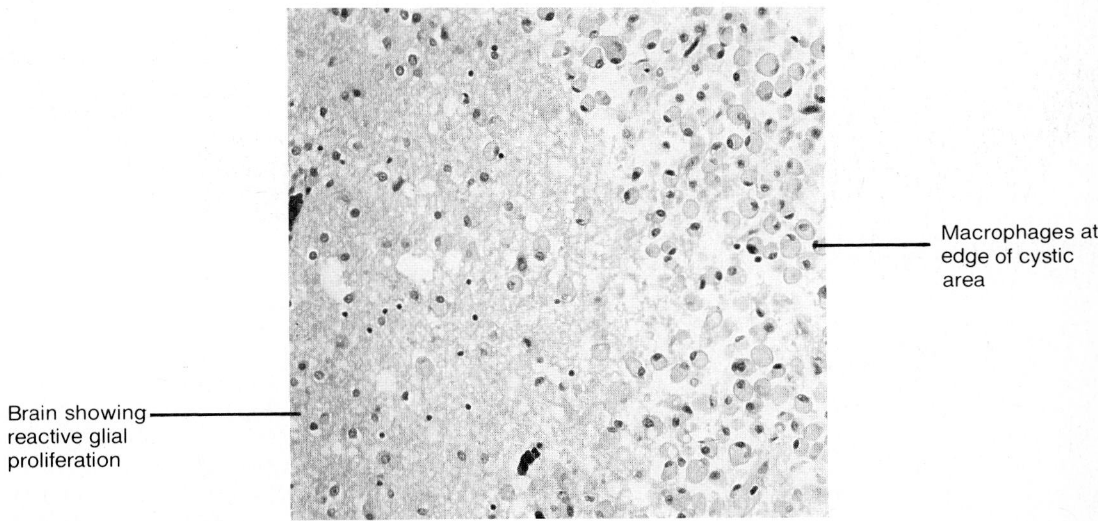

Figure 1-19. Edge of a cerebral infarct, showing the lining of the cystic cavity. Numerous macrophages with abundant foamy cytoplasm are present as a result of phagocytosis of the liquefied necrotic brain tissue.

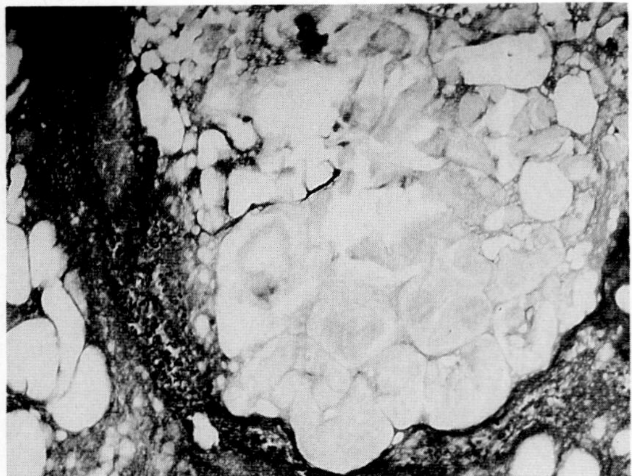

Figure 1-20. Fat necrosis in acute pancreatitis, showing a necrotic lobule of adipose tissue. Vague outlines of the fat cells remain, though the cells have lost their nuclei. The cytoplasm has a pale, amorphous appearance as a result of hydrolysis of triglyceride by lipase.

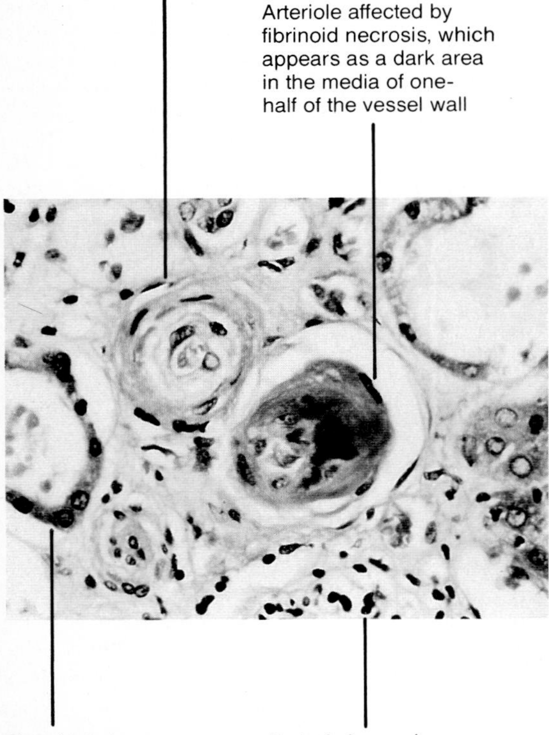

Figure 1-21. Fibrinoid necrosis of renal arteriole. In hematoxylin and eosin-stained sections, the necrotic area stains bright pink, resembling fibrin.

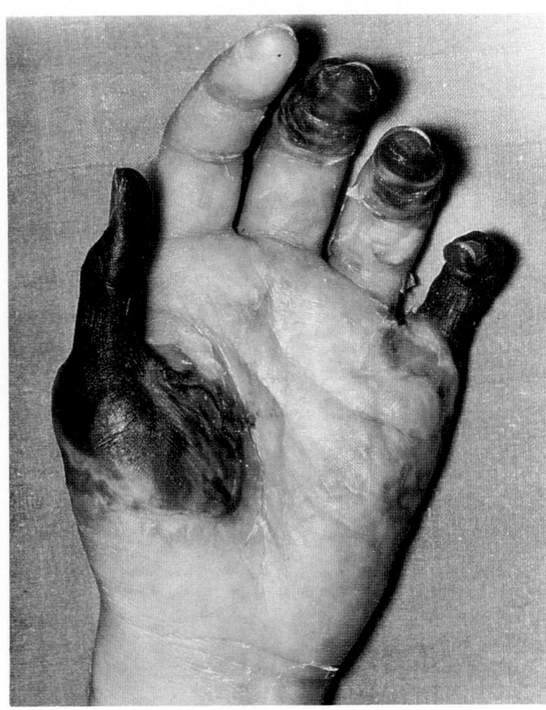

Figure 1-22. Dry gangrene of the hand, showing necrosis of the thumb and distal parts of 3 fingers. Note the black, dry, shriveled appearance. This resulted from inadvertent injection of a drug into the brachial artery by an intravenous drug user.

2. Wet gangrene-Wet gangrene results from severe bacterial infection superimposed on necrosis. It occurs in the extremities as well as in internal organs such as the intestine. Marked acute inflammation and growth of invading bacteria cause the necrotic area to become swollen and reddish-black, with extensive liquefaction of dead tissue (Fig 1–23). Wet gangrene is a spreading necrotizing inflammation that is not clearly demarcated from adjacent healthy tissue and is thus difficult to treat surgically. Bacterial fermentation produces a typical foul odor. The type of bacteria involved varies with the site and with other patient and environmental characteristics. Wet gangrene is associated with a high mortality rate.

3. Gas gangrene-Gas gangrene is a wound infection caused by *Clostridium perfringens* and other clostridial species. It is characterized by extensive necrosis of tissue and production of gas by the fermentative action of the bacteria. The gross appearance is similar to that of wet gangrene, with the additional presence of gas in the tissues. **Crepitus** (a crackling sensation on palpation over the site) can often be detected clinically, and gas may be seen on soft tissue radiographs. Gas gangrene is associated with a high mortality rate.

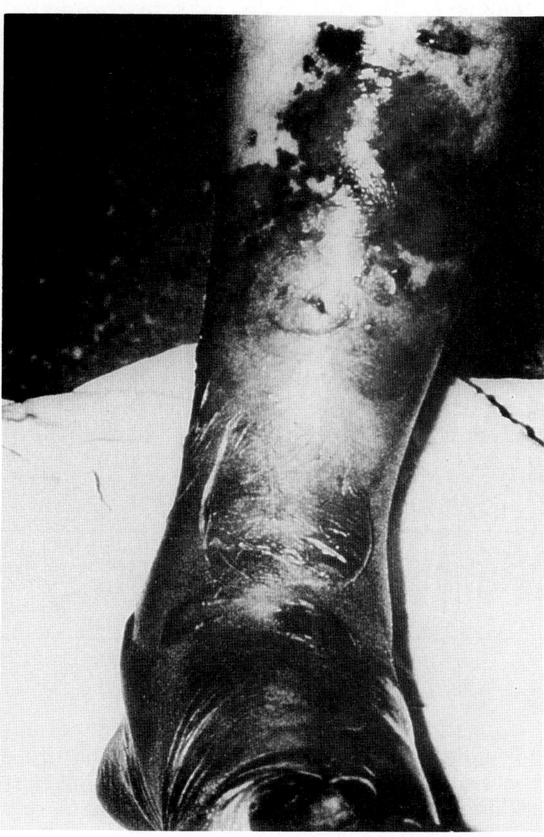

Figure 1-23. Wet gangrene of the leg. The entire leg below the knee is black and markedly swollen.

Table 1-3. Serum enzyme elevations in cell necrosis.

Enzyme	Tissue
Creatine kinase (MB isoenzyme)	Heart
Creatine kinase (BB isoenzyme)	Brain
Creatine kinase (MM isoenzyme)	Skeletal muscle, heart
Lactate dehydrogenase (isoenzyme 1)	Heart, erythrocytes, skeletal muscle
Lactate dehydrogenase (isoenzyme 5)	Liver, skeletal muscle
Aspartate aminotransferase (AST) (glutamic-oxaloacetic transaminase [GOT])	Heart, liver, skeletal muscle
Alanine aminotransferase (ALT) (glutamic-pyruvic transaminase [GPT])	Liver, skeletal muscle
Amylase	Pancreas, salivary gland

Clinical Effects of Necrosis

A. Abnormal Function: Necrosis of cells leads to functional loss that frequently causes clinical disease, as in heart failure resulting from extensive myocardial necrosis. The severity of clinical disease depends on the type of tissue involved and the extent of tissue destruction in relation to the amount and continued function of surviving tissue. Necrosis in the kidney, for example, does not cause renal failure even when an entire kidney is lost, because the other kidney can compensate. Necrosis of a small area of the motor cortex in the brain, however, results in muscle paralysis.

The clinical manifestations of necrosis vary. Abnormal electrical activity originating in areas of cerebral or myocardial necrosis may result in epileptic seizures or cardiac arrhythmias. Failure of peristalsis in an area of intestinal wall necrosis may cause functional intestinal obstruction. Bleeding into necrotic tissue often produces symptoms, eg, expectoration of blood **(hemoptysis)** with pulmonary necrosis.

B. Bacterial Infection: Bacterial infection in an area of necrosis or gangrene may disseminate throughout the body via the lymphatics or bloodstream. This potentially fatal development makes gangrene a serious condition that often requires surgical removal of the affected tissue.

C. Release of Contents of Necrotic Cells: Necrotic cells release their cytoplasmic contents (eg, enzymes) into the bloodstream, where their presence signifies that cell death has occurred. These enzymes may be detected by various tests (Table 1-3) whose specificity depends on distribution of the enzyme in different cells of the body; eg, elevation of the MB isoenzyme of creatine kinase (CK, or creatine phosphokinase [CPK]) is specific for myocardial necrosis, because this enzyme is found only in myocardial cells. Elevation of aspartate aminotransferase levels (AST, formerly called glutamic-oxaloacetic transaminase [SGOT]) is less specific, since this enzyme is present not only in myocardium but also in liver and other cells.

D. Systemic Effects: Cell necrosis is commonly associated with fever (due to release of pyrogens from the necrotic cells) and neutrophil leukocytosis (due to the associated acute inflammatory reaction).

E. Local Effects: Ulceration of epithelial surfaces and swelling of tissues due to edema may occur. Edema may lead to severe pressure effects in a confined space (eg, the cranial cavity).

2 Abnormalities of Interstitial Tissues

NORMAL INTERSTITIAL TISSUE

The normal function of parenchymal cells is largely dependent on the integrity of the interstitial tissues that make up the immediate microenvironment of the cells. Interstitial tissue occupies the space between the parenchymal cells, providing structural and nutritive support. It is composed of cells, water and electrolytes, ground substance, and fibrillary elements (Fig 2–1). The pH and the electrolyte composition of interstitial tissue are maintained within a narrow range and are in equilibrium both with those of plasma in capillaries and with those of the intracellular fluid compartment. The ground substances and supporting fibers of interstitial tissue are produced by specialized connective tissue cells derived from the mesoderm (mesenchymal cells), mainly fibroblasts.

MECHANISMS & RESULTS OF INJURY TO THE INTERSTITIUM

Interstitial injury may result from general abnormalities in plasma composition, which cause abnormal accumulation of substances in the interstitium, or from local changes in the tissue (eg, necrosis of parenchymal cells) that cause secondary changes in the composition of the interstitium.

Accumulation of abnormal material in the interstitial tissue may cause structural abnormality in the interstitium without affecting the function of parenchymal cells (eg, increased numbers of fat cells: adiposity). More commonly, however, interstitial abnormalities result in secondary dysfunction of parenchymal cells. Such dysfunction may occur following abnormal accumulation of material in the interstitium (eg, edema, amyloidosis) as well as with changes at the biochemical level (eg, altered electrolyte composition, pH, or temperature).

ACCUMULATION OF EXCESS FLUID (EDEMA)

The accumulation of excessive amounts of fluid in interstitial tissue is called edema. Edema may occur in all tissues but is most easily seen in the skin. The earliest clinical evidence of edema in the skin is the presence of pitting (the ability to produce a depression or pit in the skin by sustained finger pressure). Visible swelling of the skin occurs only when a large amount of excess fluid has collected (see Fig 3–1).

Edema also includes accumulation of fluid in body cavities such as the pleural cavity (hydrothorax, pleural effusion), peritoneal cavity (ascites),

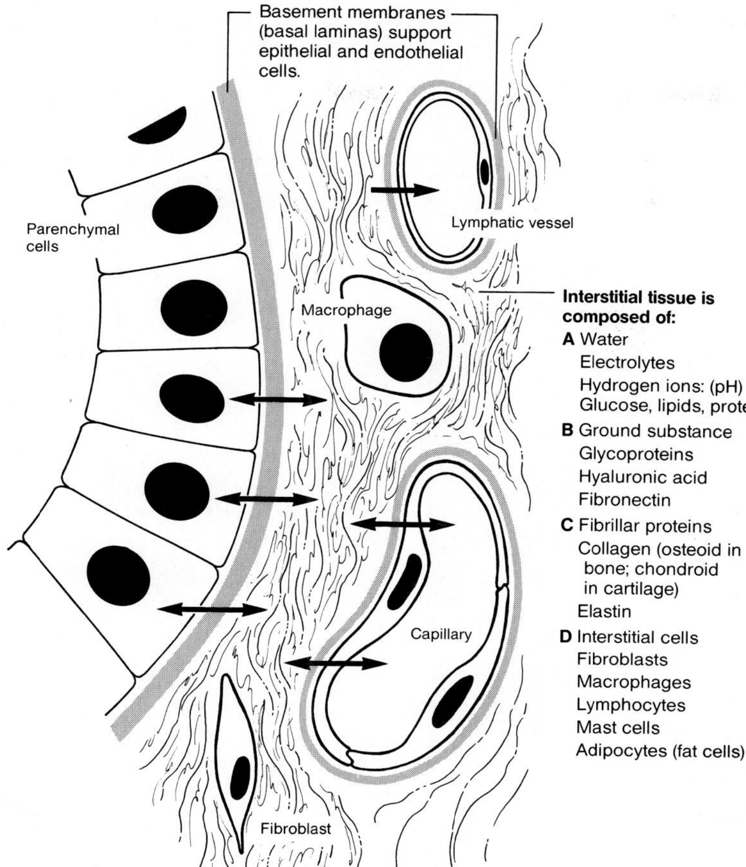

Figure 2-1. Composition of interstitial tissue. The interstitial fluid is in equilibrium with plasma on one hand and parenchymal cell cytoplasm on the other. Movement of water and electrolytes between plasma, interstitium, cells, and lymphatics is shown by arrows.

and pericardial cavity (pericardial effusion). **Anasarca** denotes massive edema of the whole body, including the body cavities.

Edema may be classified as localized (caused by local disturbance of the fluid exchange mechanism in the tissue) or generalized (caused by retention of sodium and water in the body). The distribution of the retained fluid in generalized edema is gravity-dependent, ie, around the ankles in the ambulatory patient and the sacral region in bedridden patients.

Localized Edema

Fluid exchange through the normal capillary wall is governed by the balance of opposing forces: capillary hydrostatic pressure forces fluid out; plasma colloid osmotic pressure draws it in (Fig 2–2). Thus, fluid leaves at the arteriolar end of the capillary (where hydrostatic pressure exceeds colloid osmotic pressure) and enters at the venular end (where colloid osmotic pressure exceeds hydrostatic pressure). Normally, tissue hydrostatic and colloid osmotic pressures are near zero and do not affect this fluid exchange. Fluid passes out of the capillary mainly at the junctions between endothelial cells (pores), which permit only small nonprotein molecules to pass through (ultrafiltration). Protein is retained in the vessel, but a small amount may escape during ultrafiltration and by passage across the endothelial cell (pinocytosis). The small amount of protein that escapes the capillary is rapidly removed by the lymphatics along with any fluid that may not return to the venule. Localized edema occurs if this balance is disturbed (Table 2–1).

A. Inflammatory Edema: Edema is a cardinal sign of acute inflammation (Chapter 3). Inflammatory edema is caused by increased capillary permeability (increased endothelial pore size), which results in exudation of fluid, and increased hydrostatic pressure due to active dilatation of arterioles. The extent of edema is limited by increased lymphatic flow and progressive increase in the hydrostatic pressure in the interstitial tissue as the fluid exudate collects there.

B. Allergic Edema: Acute allergic reactions (Chapter 8) cause local release of vasoactive substances, such as histamine, that cause increased capillary permeability and arteriolar dilatation and result in exudation of fluid and edema.

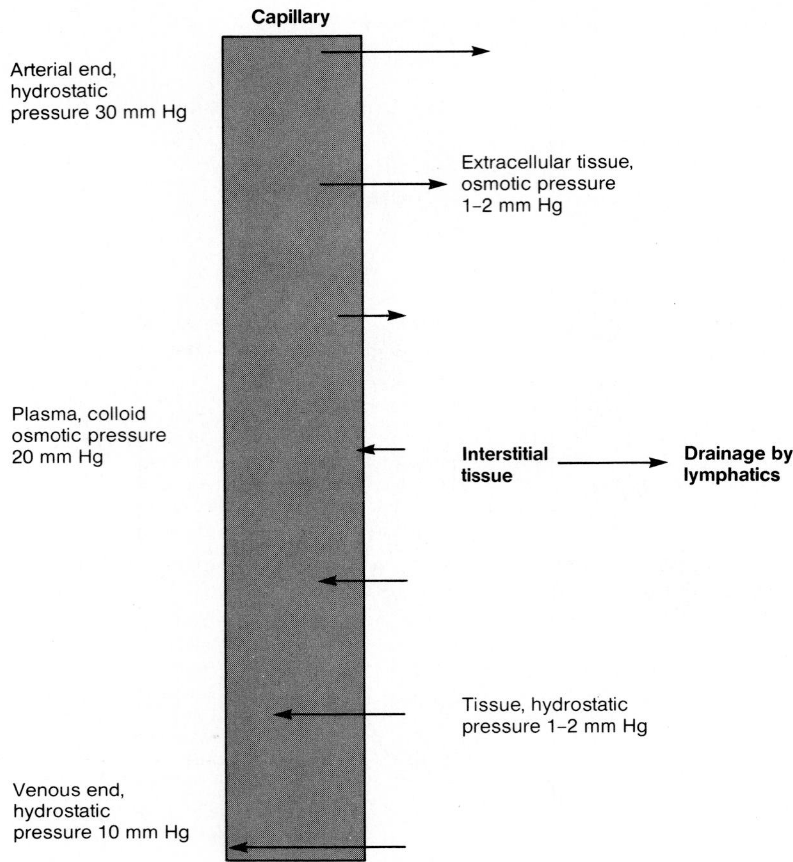

Figure 2–2. Fluid exchange in a normal systemic capillary. Arrows show the net direction of flow of fluid between capillary and interstitium in different parts of the capillary, which reflect the net effect of the factors involved. Excess fluid and any protein molecules are drained by the lymphatics.

Allergic edema is most commonly localized to the skin, where it produces a wheal (**urticaria**, "**hives**"). Rarely, it may involve large areas of skin and affect the larynx and bronchioles, causing respiratory obstruction (**angioneurotic edema**). Though it has a generalized distribution, angioneurotic edema is best considered a form of localized edema, because it is caused by local fluid exchange derangements and not by retention of sodium and water in the body.

C. Edema of Venous Obstruction: The effect of venous obstruction depends on the extent of collateral venous circulation in the area (Chapter 9). When obstruction of a vein leads to complete failure of venous drainage, severe edema and hemorrhage result from increased hydrostatic

Table 2–1. Pathophysiology of localized edema.

Pathologic Condition	Factors Influencing Fluid Accumulation in the Interstitial Space[1]				
	Vascular Permeability	Arteriolar End Hydrostatic Pressure	Venular End Hydrostatic Pressure	Interstitial Tissue Osmotic Pressure	Lymphatic Flow
Acute inflammatory edema	↑	↑	N	N↑	↑
Allergic edema	↑	↑	N	N↑	↑
Edema of venous obstruction	N	N	↑	N	↑
Edema of lymphatic obstruction	N	N	N	N↑[2]	↓↓

[1]In most cases of localized edema, increased lymphatic flow tends to limit fluid accumulation; this obviously cannot occur in lymphatic obstruction. Note that interstitial tissue hydrostatic pressure is not considered; this increases with all causes of edema and tends to limit the degree of edema.
[2]Osmotic pressure rises as a result of failure of lymphatics to remove osmotically active molecules.
(N = normal; ↑ = increased; ↓ = decreased; N↑ = normal or increased.)

pressure and capillary rupture, as occur in the orbit following cavernous sinus thrombosis. When venous drainage is partially impaired, edema is less severe, as occurs in the face in obstruction of the superior vena cava. When veins of the extremities are obstructed, there is often no effect on the tissue, because collateral circulation is sufficient to provide adequate venous drainage.

D. Edema of Lymphatic Obstruction: When lymphatic drainage is obstructed, the small amount of protein that escapes from the capillary by pinocytosis and during ultrafiltration is not removed and accumulates in the interstitial space. Over a long period, the interstitial tissue colloid osmotic pressure increases as the protein accumulates, and edema then develops.

Early lymphatic edema is a pitting edema. Over a prolonged period, however, the edematous tissue undergoes fibrosis, and the affected area becomes firm, thickened, and nonpitting. In the skin, the fibrosis may be associated with marked epidermal thickening, so that the skin comes to resemble that of an elephant (**elephantiasis**).

Generalized Edema

Generalized edema represents the effect of increased total body sodium and water—a result of renal retention. Water retention occurs as a consequence of sodium retention. The latter occurs when the glomerular filtration rate is decreased or when secretion of aldosterone is increased. Sodium balance is a function of the net effect of sodium filtration (loss) in the glomerulus and sodium reabsorption in the proximal and distal convoluted tubules; absorption in the distal convoluted tubule is controlled by the renin-angiotensin-aldosterone system (Fig 2–3).

A. Cardiac Edema: Cardiac failure (Chapter 21) results in diminished left ventricular output, which leads to reflex sympathetic stimulation (to maintain blood pressure), renal vasoconstriction, decreased glomerular filtration pressure, and stimulation of the juxtaglomerular apparatus to secrete renin. Renin in turn induces increased aldosterone production (**secondary aldosteronism**) by the angiotensin mechanism (Fig 2–3), leading to retention of sodium and water and generalized edema.

When there is right ventricular failure, the central venous pressure is increased. This increased hydrostatic pressure is transmitted to the venular end of systemic capillaries and favors the accumulation of fluid in the interstitial space. If left ventricular failure occurs alone, the retained water tends to accumulate in the lungs because of increased pulmonary venous pressure (see Pulmonary Edema, below). These hydrostatic factors play a minor role in the genesis of cardiac edema

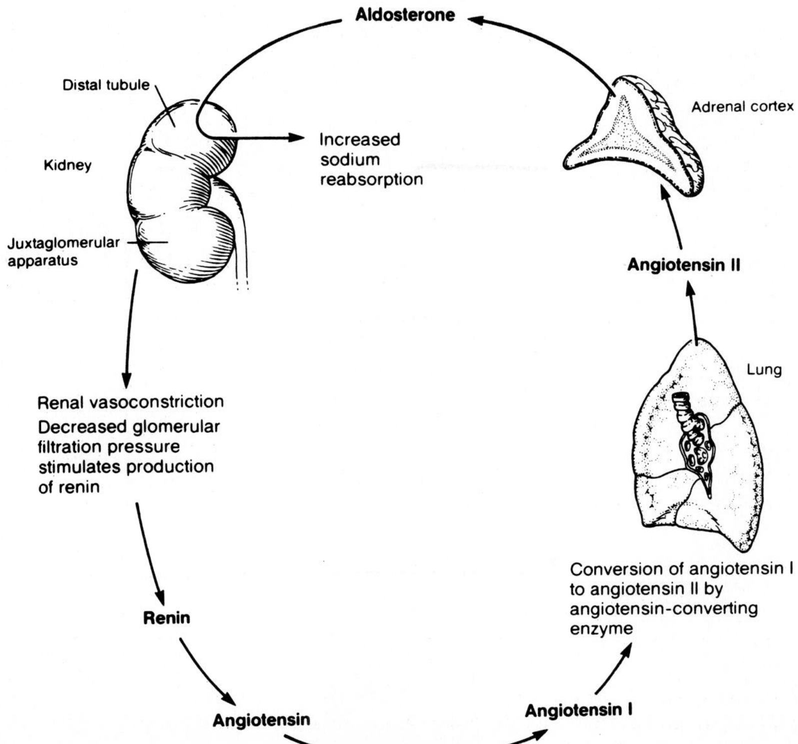

Figure 2–3. The renin-angiotensin-aldosterone mechanism. Aldosterone acts on the distal renal tubule to effect increased reabsorption of sodium.

compared with sodium and water retention in the body, but they are important in determining the distribution of the retained fluid.

B. Edema of Hypoproteinemia: Hypoproteinemia decreases plasma colloid osmotic pressure and alters the forces maintaining fluid balance in systemic capillaries. The resulting loss of fluid from the vascular system and decrease in effective plasma volume cause reflex sympathetic stimulation, renal vasoconstriction, hypersecretion of renin, secondary aldosteronism, sodium and water retention by the kidneys, and generalized edema.

Hypoproteinemia may be caused by insufficient dietary intake of protein (starvation and malnutrition edema), decreased synthesis of albumin in the liver (hepatic edema), or increased loss of protein in the urine (nephrotic syndrome) or from the intestine (protein-losing enteropathy).

There is surprisingly little correlation between plasma albumin levels and extent of edema in different patients. This lack of correlation is thought to be due to variations in the mucopolysaccharides in the interstitial ground substance in different individuals.

C. Renal Edema: Mild edema occurs in acute glomerulonephritis, a condition in which the glomerular filtration rate is markedly diminished, leading to sodium and water retention. Unlike other causes of generalized edema, in which edema fluid is distributed in dependent areas, the edema of acute glomerulonephritis typically occurs in the tissues surrounding the eyes.

Renal diseases associated with protein loss in the urine sufficient to produce hypoproteinemia are characterized by massive edema (nephrotic syndrome). (See Chapter 47.)

Clinical Effects of Edema

Edema occurring in most tissues causes no dysfunction of parenchymal cells. Severe and chronic edema of the skin may be associated with impaired wound healing and increased susceptibility to infection. Edema of internal organs is frequently symptomatic; eg, edema of the liver in acute hepatitis or heart failure is associated with pain, caused by stretching of the liver capsule.

Edema of the following organs is life-threatening:

A. Lungs (Pulmonary Edema): The pulmonary circulation functions at low hydrostatic pressure (< 20 mm Hg for pulmonary artery systolic pressure). Since this is less than plasma colloid osmotic pressure, little fluid escapes from the pulmonary capillaries—a normal phenomenon in view of the pulmonary circulation's main function as a site of gas exchange rather than tissue perfusion. Entry of fluid into the alveoli from the pulmonary capillaries is called pulmonary edema (Fig 2–4). This may interfere with gas exchange in the lungs and, when severe, causes hypoxia and death.

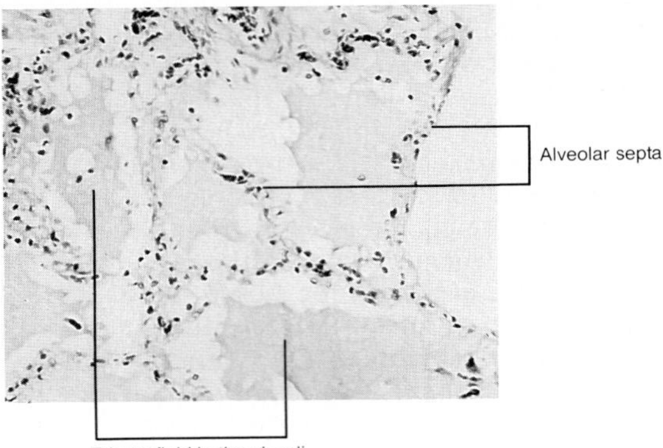

Figure 2–4. Pulmonary edema, characterized by the presence of fluid in the alveoli. The fluid has a frothy appearance resulting from admixture with air.

B. Brain (Cerebral Edema): Cerebral edema occurs in many brain disorders, eg, traumatic lesions, infections, neoplasms, and vascular accidents. The fluid collects mainly in the extracellular space of the white matter.

Edema fluid physically separates neural connections to cause reversible acute cerebral dysfunction. The volume of the accumulated fluid increases intracranial pressure and produces headache and edema of the optic disk (papilledema). A severe increase in pressure may force the temporal lobe down into the tentorial opening (tentorial herniation) or may force the cerebellar tonsil into the foramen magnum (tonsillar herniation) and cause death due to compression of the cardiorespiratory centers in the brain stem (see Chapter 62).

Urgent treatment is required. Infusion of mannitol raises the plasma osmotic pressure and rapidly draws fluid from the brain. Corticosteroids in high doses are also effective in reducing cerebral edema.

C. Serosal Cavities: Accumulation of edema fluid within the pericardial sac and the pleural cavity may interfere with normal cardiac function and expansion of the lung. Fluid accumulation in the peritoneal cavity (ascites) causes abdominal distention but does not usually interfere with normal function of abdominal organs.

CHANGES IN BODY TEMPERATURE

Regulation of Normal Temperature

Body core temperature is a result of balance between heat loss and heat gain and is maintained at around 37 °C (98.4 °F) by the thermoregulatory center in the hypothalamus. Changes in body temperature may result from disordered control mechanisms, as occurs in (1) diseases of the brain stem affecting the thermoregulatory center; (2) any injury associated with either cell necrosis or acute inflammation, since in these processes, pyrogens such as interleukin-1 and prostaglandins are released into the blood and act on the thermoregulatory center; and (3) use of drugs that affect the thermoregulatory center. Changes in body temperature may also result from exposure to extreme environmental conditions.

Interstitial water plays an important role in preventing rapid changes in body core temperature. Because of the large volume (12L) of total interstitial water, a large amount of heat is required to produce even a small change in core body temperature.

Fever & Hypothermia

Fever represents an increase in body core temperature; hypothermia, a decrease. All of the enzyme-dependent cellular biochemical reactions are profoundly affected by changes in temperature. Metabolic rate and therefore energy and oxygen requirements of cells increase with fever. Cardiac output must increase to meet this increased oxygen demand. In patients with cardiac disease, fever can aggravate or precipitate heart failure. At temperatures over 42.2 °C (108 °F), neuronal dysfunction occurs, with delirium. Loss of consciousness and death occur at around 43.3 °C (110 °F).

Cellular metabolic needs decrease with hypothermia. Body core temperatures of 21.1–23.8 °C (70–75 °F) can be tolerated by tissues for short periods without serious effects. During severe hypothermia, circulatory and respiratory needs of tissues are minimal because cellular metabolism is greatly reduced. Induction of hypothermia during surgery enables the surgeon to stop the heart for short periods and permits correction of minor defects in the heart and brain.

ALTERATION IN pH

Maintenance of Normal pH

Cellular enzyme reactions are extremely sensitive to changes in pH. The pH of the cell is in equilibrium with the pH of the interstitial fluid, which in turn is in equilibrium with the pH of plasma. Plasma pH is normally maintained close to 7.4 by a variety of homeostatic mechanisms such as (1) blood buffers, including plasma proteins, hemoglobin, and the bicarbonate-carbonic acid system; (2) renal control of hydrogen ion excretion by the aldosterone-dependent sodium-potassium or sodium-hydrogen pump in the distal renal tubule; and (3) respiratory control of the amount of CO_2 lost during ventilation.

Causes of Abnormal pH (Table 2-2; Fig 2-5)

A. Respiratory Disease (Respiratory Acidosis and Alkalosis): The amount of CO_2 lost from the lungs is directly related to total alveolar ventilation. In respiratory diseases associated with decreased alveolar ventilation, CO_2 is retained and **respiratory acidosis** results. The body compensates by excreting acid (hydrogen ion) in the kidney, causing retention of bicarbonate. Serum pH is decreased, Pa_{CO_2} is increased, and serum bicarbonate is increased.

In conditions where alveolar ventilation is increased, CO_2 is lost, leading to **respiratory alkalosis**. The kidney compensates by excreting bicarbonate to conserve acid (hydrogen ion). Serum pH is increased, Pa_{CO_2} is decreased, and serum bicarbonate is decreased.

Table 2-2. Key changes in several acid-base disorders.

Acid-Base Disorder	Alveolar Ventilation	Pa_{CO_2}	Serum pH	Serum HCO_3^-	Urine pH
Respiratory acidosis	Primary decrease	↑	↓	↑	Acid < 6
Respiratory alkalosis	Primary increase	↓	↑	↓	Alkaline > 7
Metabolic acidosis of renal origin	Compensatory increase	↓	↓	↓	Alkaline > 7 (primary)
Metabolic acidosis of nonrenal origin	Compensatory increase	↓	↓	↓	Acid < 6 (compensatory)
Metabolic alkalosis of renal origin	Compensatory decrease	↑	↑	↑	Acid < 6 (primary)
Metabolic alkalosis of nonrenal origin	Compensatory decrease	↑	↑	↑	Alkaline > 7 (compensatory)

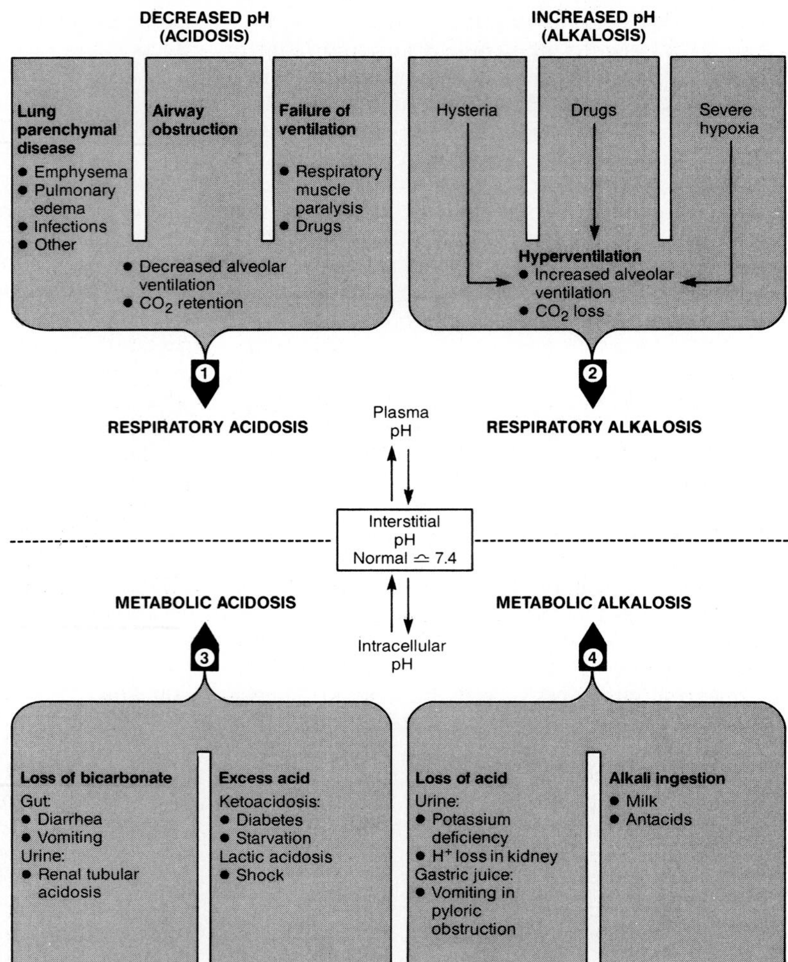

Figure 2-5. Causes of acidosis and alkalosis. Respiratory acidosis **(1)** and alkalosis **(2)** result from abnormalities of alveolar ventilation. Metabolic acidosis **(3)** and alkalosis **(4)** result from a net gain of acid or alkali, either from metabolism or ingestion.

B. Metabolic Disease (Metabolic Acidosis and Alkalosis): Metabolic acidosis occurs as a result of several mechanisms. It may result from (1) failure of the kidney to excrete acid (hydrogen ion) in specific renal tubular defects and in renal failure, (2) loss of alkali due to loss of gastrointestinal fluids in diarrhea and vomiting, or (3) entry of acid (exogenous or endogenous) into the blood. Acidosis stimulates the respiratory center. Increased ventilation washes out CO_2 in the lungs and functions as a compensatory mechanism to remove excess acid from the blood. Serum pH is decreased, $Pa{CO_2}$ is decreased, and serum bicarbonate is decreased. The urine is acid except in patients in whom acidosis is due to renal disease—the urine is then alkaline, since the diseased kidney cannot excrete acid.

Metabolic alkalosis results from (1) excessive renal excretion of acid; (2) loss of gastric acid due to vomiting in pyloric obstruction; or (3) entry of alkali into the blood, typically as a result of ingestion of antacids for the treatment of peptic ulcer. Alkalosis depresses the respiratory center. The resulting decreased ventilation leads to CO_2 retention, which serves to neutralize excess alkali in the blood. Serum pH is increased, $Pa{CO_2}$ is increased, and serum bicarbonate is increased. The urine is alkaline except in patients in whom alkalosis has resulted from renal loss of acid.

Effects of Altered Plasma pH

Changes in plasma pH are reflected in interstitial and intracellular fluid. Even a slight change in cellular pH has a marked impact on enzyme reactions. Reactions associated with energy production are affected first; changes in membrane permeability and electrolyte transfer result from failure of energy production. Changes in pH also cause electrolyte abnormalities. Acidosis causes an efflux of potassium from cells that decreases intracellular potassium and leads to hyperkalemia, whereas alkalosis is associated with hypokalemia. Alkalosis also causes a decrease in ionized calcium levels in the blood that produces changes associated with hypocalcemia.

If pH changes are severe, more enzyme systems fail. Death occurs at a plasma pH above 7.8 or below 6.9.

ELECTROLYTE IMBALANCE (Table 2–3)

Electrolyte abnormalities in extracellular fluid are common. Since intracellular fluid adjusts to changes in extracellular fluid to maintain equilibrium, such electrolyte imbalances often produce cellular changes; eg, changes in potassium and calcium levels impair the function of contractile cells because they affect the cells' ability to generate action potentials. Changes in the plasma sodium level cause severe changes in plasma osmolality that may alter the content of intracellular water and cause cell damage. The main effects of changes in plasma osmolality occur in brain cells and are manifested as confusion and altered level of consciousness; death may occur in severe cases.

DEPOSITION OF CALCIUM (Calcification)

Deposition of calcium in the interstitium is common and takes one of 2 forms.

Metastatic Calcification

Metastatic calcification is due to an increase in serum calcium or phosphorus levels (Table 2–3). Calcification occurs in normal tissues, most commonly the arterial walls, alveolar septa of the lung, and kidneys.

Calcification affecting the renal interstitium (**nephrocalcinosis**) may cause chronic renal failure. Extensive calcification of blood vessels may result in ischemia, particularly in the skin. Rarely, extensive involvement of pulmonary alveoli causes abnormalities in diffusion of gases. Apart from these instances, calcification does not impair function of parenchymal cells in tissues.

Deposition of calcium in tissues is visible radiologically. Microscopically, calcium is intensely basophilic (stains blue with hematoxylin). Deposits of calcium appear granular in the early stages of calcification; larger deposits are amorphous.

Dystrophic Calcification

In dystrophic calcification, calcium and phosphorus metabolism and serum levels are normal, and calcification occurs as a result of local abnormality in tissues (Table 2–4). Functional impairment is uncommon. Dystrophic calcification may provide radiologic markers; eg, a calcified pineal gland accurately points to the midline of the brain.

DEPOSITION OF AMYLOID (Amyloidosis)

The term amyloid denotes a variety of fibrillary proteins deposited in interstitial tissues in certain pathologic conditions. All types of amyloid have the following physicochemical characteristics:

(1) When iodine is added to fresh tissue containing amyloid, a brown color is produced.

(2) In histologic sections, amyloid stains as follows:

(a) With Congo red stain, amyloid appears red with apple-green birefringence when viewed under polarized light.

(b) With hematoxylin and eosin (H&E), it stains homogeneous pink.

(c) With methyl violet, amyloid shows metachromasia, appearing pink. (*Note:* When a substance stain a color that is different from the color of the stain, it is metachromatic.)

(3) On electron microscopy, amyloid appears as nonbranching fibrils 7.5–10 nm wide.

(4) On x-ray diffraction, amyloid exhibits a pleated β-sheet structure. This β-pleated stacking renders the protein very resistant to enzymatic degradation, contributing to its accumulation in tissues.

Chemical Composition

The chemical structure of amyloid protein is quite variable (see Table 2–5, where AL, AA, etc are explained).

A. Amyloid of Immunoglobulin Origin: In AL amyloid, the protein is composed of fragments of the light chains of immunoglobulin molecules. AL is produced by neoplastic plasma cells (myeloma) and B lymphocytes (B cell lymphomas). Amyloid light chains deposited in these diseases resemble the free light chains (Bence Jones proteins) or light chain fragments that are produced by the neoplastic plasma cells or B lymphocytes.

B. Amyloid of Other Origin: The amyloid protein is not part of the immunoglobulin molecule; origins of these types of amyloid are shown in Table 2–5.

Classification

The clinical classification of amyloidosis is based on protein type and tissue distribution.

A. Systemic Amyloidosis:

1. Primary pattern of distribution–(Fig 2–6.) In systemic amyloidosis with a primary distribution, amyloid is found in the heart, gastrointestinal tract, tongue, skin, and nerves. This distribution is seen in primary amyloidosis and neoplasms of B lymphocytes (plasma cell myeloma and B cell

Table 2-3. Electrolyte abnormalities in extracellular fluid.

Electrolyte Imbalance	Disorder	Common Causes	Effects
Increased plasma sodium	Hypernatremia (water loss or relative gain of Na^+)	1. Water privation 2. Water loss from skin (sweating,[1] burns) 3. Renal water loss (diabetes insipidus, diuretics, osmotic diuresis) 4. Adrenal mineralocorticoid excess (Conn's and Cushing's syndromes[2])	1. Increased ECF volume 2. Hypertension 3. Increased ECF osmolality, causing intracellular fluid loss
Decreased plasma sodium	Hyponatremia (water gain or relative loss of Na^+)	1. Water intoxication 2. Adrenal insufficiency (Addison's disease) 3. Inappropriate secretion of antidiuretic hormone (SIADH) 4. Long-term diuretic therapy	1. Hypotension 2. Decreased ECF osmolality, causing intracellular fluid increase
Increased plasma potassium	Hyperkalemia	1. Failure of K^+ excretion (acute and chronic renal failure, adrenal insufficiency, diuretics [spironolactone]) 2. Shift of K^+ from cells (tissue necrosis, acidosis, hyperkalemic periodic paralysis) 3. Excess K^+ intake	Abnormal electrical activity in contractile cells 1. Cardiac arrhythmia 2. High T waves on ECG 3. Muscle weakness and paralysis 4. Cardiac arrest
Decreased plasma potassium	Hypokalemia	1. Intestinal fluid loss (vomiting, diarrhea) 2. Renal K^+ loss (diuretics [most], osmotic diuresis, renal tubular disease) 3. Adrenal mineralocorticoid excess (Conn's and Cushing's syndromes[2]) 4. Shift of K^+ into cells (familial-type periodic paralysis, alkalosis, insulin)	1. Muscle weakness and paralysis 2. Flat, inverted T wave on ECG 3. Renal tubular dysfunction (impaired concentrating ability) 4. Cardiac arrest
Increased serum calcium	Hypercalcemia	1. Primary hyperparathyroidism 2. Secondary hyperparathyroidism 3. Metastatic skeletal lesions 4. Sarcoidosis 5. Vitamin D intoxication 6. Milk-alkali syndrome 7. Parathyroid hormone-like secretions by neoplasms	1. Anorexia, nausea, vomiting 2. Muscle weakness, hypotonia 3. Cerebral dysfunction (confusion, coma) 4. Renal tubular dysfunction 5. Hypertension 6. Shortened QT interval on ECG 7. Metastatic calcification (nephrocalcinosis)
Decreased serum calcium	Hypocalcemia	1. Hypoparathyroidism 2. Intestinal malabsorption 3. Acute pancreatitis 4. Respiratory hyperventilation (decreased ionized calcium) 5. Hypoalbuminemia	1. Tetany, carpopedal spasm, laryngeal stridor, increased irritability of nerves 2. Convulsions, raised intracranial pressure 3. ST interval prolongation on ECG

[1]Sweat is hypotonic; although salt is lost, water is lost more quickly. Sodium depletion (hyponatremia) will occur if fluid loss is replaced with water only.
[2]Conn's syndrome is primary aldosterone excess; Cushing's syndrome is cortisol excess.

Table 2-4. Circumstances in which dystrophic calcification occurs.

Necrotic tissue
- Fat necrosis
- Caseation necrosis in the center of granulomas
- Dead parasites (cysticercosis, hydatid cyst, trichinosis, schistosomiasis, filariasis)

Abnormal blood vessels and heart
- Atheromatous plaques
- Organized thrombi in veins (phleboliths) and arteries
- Abnormal cardiac valves

Aging or damaged tissue
- Pineal gland, choroid plexus, laryngeal cartilage
- Medium-sized arteries (Mönckeberg's medial sclerosis)
- Damaged muscles and tendons

Neoplasms
- Brain tumors (meningioma, craniopharyngioma, oligodendroglioma)
- Papillary thyroid carcinoma, serous tumors of ovary
- Breast carcinoma
- Chondrosarcoma (bone tumor)

Tumoral calcinosis (formation of nodular nonneoplastic calcific masses in subcutaneous tissue)

malignant lymphomas). An underlying plasma cell neoplastic process with a monoclonal immunoglobulin is detectable in serum in more than 90% of patients with primary amyloidosis. In these cases, amyloid is AL. In rheumatoid arthritis, a nonimmunoglobulin amyloid (AA) is deposited in this primary pattern.

2. **Secondary pattern of distribution-**In systemic amyloidosis with a secondary distribution, amyloid is found in the liver, spleen, kidney, adrenals, gastrointestinal tract, and skin. This distribution of amyloidosis occurs in chronic inflammatory diseases such as tuberculosis, lepromatous leprosy, chronic osteomyelitis, chronic pyelonephritis, and inflammatory bowel disease (reactive systemic amyloidosis, secondary amyloidosis). The amyloid protein is AA and is derived from plasma α_1-globulins.

B. Localized Amyloidosis: Localized amyloidosis may take the form of nodular, tumorlike masses that occur rarely in the tongue, bladder, lung, or skin. These amyloid tumors are commonly associated with localized plasma cell neoplasms. In cardiac amyloidosis, amyloid is deposited diffusely in the myocardium and causes cardiac enlargement and heart failure. In cerebral

Table 2-5. Amyloidosis.

Amyloid Protein	Principal Constituent	Associated Diseases	Distribution
AL	Immunoglobulin light chain	Primary amyloidosis Plasma cell myeloma B cell malignant lymphoma	Tongue, heart, gastrointestinal tract, liver, spleen, kidney (primary distribution)
AA	Serum A protein (α_1-globulin)	Rheumatoid arthritis	Tongue, heart, gastrointestinal tract (primary distribution)
AA	Serum A protein (α_1-globulin)	Chronic infections (tuberculosis, leprosy, bronchiectasis, osteomyelitis) Hodgkin's disease Inflammatory bowel disease	Liver, kidney, spleen (secondary distribution)
AA	Serum A protein (α_1-globulin)	Familial Mediterranean fever	Liver, kidney, spleen
AF	Prealbumin	Familial amyloidosis (Portuguese, Swedish, etc)	Peripheral nerves, kidney
AS	Prealbumin	Senile amyloidosis Cardiac amyloidosis Cerebral amyloid angiopathy	Heart, spleen, pancreas Heart Cerebral vessels
AE	Peptide hormone precursors (eg, calcitonin)	Medullary carcinoma of thryoid Pancreatic islet cell adenomas	Locally in the neoplasm
AD	Unknown	Lichen amyloidosis	Skin (dermis)
Alzheimer	A_4 peptide[1]	Alzheimer's disease	Neurofibrillary tangles, plaques, and angiopathy.

[1]A_4 peptide = Alzheimer 4000-MW peptide (derived from a 40,000-MW precursor protein found in serum and cerebrospinal fluid; exact nature unknown).

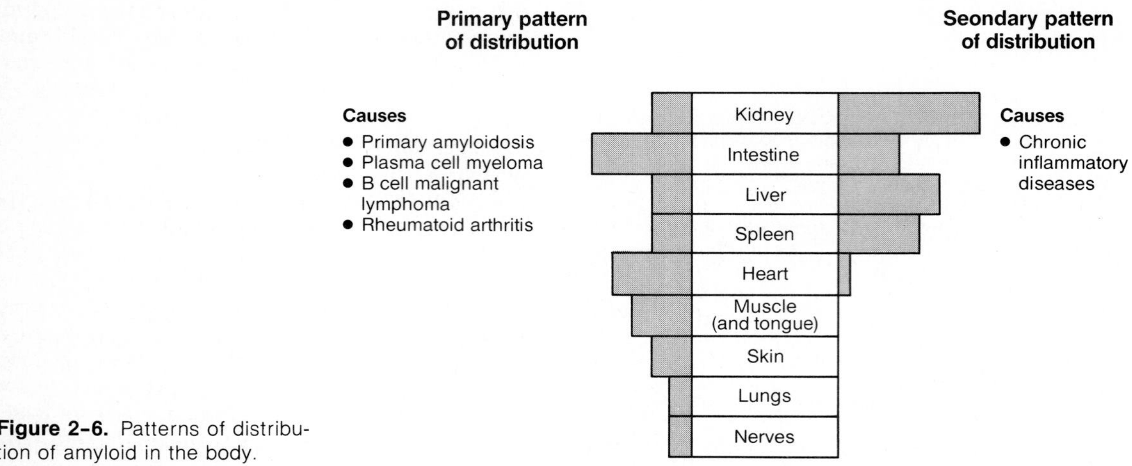

Figure 2–6. Patterns of distribution of amyloid in the body.

amyloid angiopathy, amyloid is deposited only in the blood vessels of the brain; in Alzheimer's disease, deposits of a special form of amyloid occur in the extracellular brain substance (plaques) (see Chapter 64). In lichen amyloidosis, a skin disease characterized by rash, amyloid AD is deposited in the dermis.

C. Amyloid in Neoplasms: Amyloid is present in the stroma of many endocrine neoplasms, eg, medullary carcinoma of the thyroid, pancreatic islet cell neoplasms, and pheochromocytoma (a neoplasm of the adrenal medulla). The amyloid protein is AE, usually derived from precursor molecules of certain peptide hormones (eg, calcitonin).

D. Heredofamilial Amyloidosis: Familial amyloidosis has been reported in only a few families. The amyloid type is AF and is derived from nonimmunoglobulin plasma proteins. Familial amyloidosis is classified as neuropathic, nephropathic, or cardiac, depending on the site of maximal involvement. Amyloidosis (amyloid protein type AA) occurs in familial Mediterranean fever, a disease transmitted by autosomal recessive inheritance characterized by fever and inflammation of joints and serosal membranes.

E. Senile Amyloidosis: Small amounts of amyloid (AS type) are frequently found in the heart, pancreas, and spleen in the elderly. In the late stages of diabetes mellitus, amyloidosis occurs in the abnormal pancreatic islets.

Effects of Amyloid Deposition

Amyloid is deposited in interstitial tissue, commonly in relation to the basement membrane of cells and small blood vessels. Tissues affected by amyloidosis are often enlarged (hepatosplenomegaly, cardiomegaly, thickened peripheral nerves, macroglossia). Affected tissues are also firmer and less flexible or distensible than normal tissues. Therefore, blood vessels affected by amyloidosis do not constrict normally and tend to bleed after injury; diagnostic biopsy may be followed by hemorrhage for this reason. The gross appearance of involved tissue appears pale gray and waxy. Pathologic and clinical effects of amyloidosis are illustrated in Figs 2–7, 2–8 and 2–9.

ACCUMULATION OF MUCOPOLYSACCHARIDES (Myxoid Degeneration)

An increase in the amount of mucopolysaccharides (glycosaminoglycans) in the ground substance of the interstitium is termed myxoid (myxomatous) degeneration. Such alteration is common both in normal individuals and in disease states. Special stains (eg, alcian blue, colloidal iron) are necessary to demonstrate mucopolysaccharides; myxoid degeneration appears on microscopic examination of hematoxylin and eosin-stained sections as loose, weakly basophilic material. Myxoid degeneration of tissues usually does not affect function.

Myxoid degeneration of the interstitium occurs in **hypothyroidism (myxedema)** (see Chapter 58) through an unknown mechanism. Myxoid degeneration is common in joint capsules, where it may lead to formation of a cystic tumor (ganglion) on a tendon or aponeurosis. Myxoid degeneration is common in the stroma of neoplasms such as neurofibromas.

A form of myxoid degeneration may occur in the aorta and cardiac valves, especially the mitral valve. This change is common in Marfan's syndrome, an inherited disease characterized by widespread synthesis of abnormal collagen. When severe, myxoid degeneration may be associated with valvular incompetence and aortic rupture. A similar form of myxoid degeneration—largely confined to the mitral valve leaflets—occurs in other-

Amyloid deposited irregularly in the glomerulus

Amlyoid deposited in wall of afferent arteriole

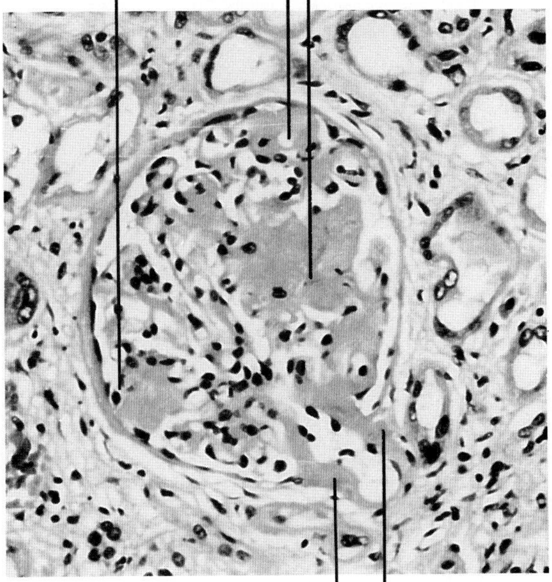

Figure 2–7. Amyloidosis involving a glomerulus. Amyloid appears as a homogeneous acellular material that stains pink with hematoxylin and eosin.

wise normal individuals and is the most common cause of mitral valve incompetence (floppy valve syndrome).

DEPOSITION OF LIPIDS

Pathologic adiposity—the presence of increased numbers of fat cells (adipocytes) in interstitial tissue—occurs in extreme obesity and is most common in the pancreas and myocardium. The fat cells extend between the parenchymal cells of the organ (fatty infiltration). Fatty infiltration occurs in the interstitium—a feature distinguishing this kind of fat accumulation from the more significant fatty change in which triglyceride accumulates in parenchymal cells as a result of cell injury. Although these additional fat cells cause surprisingly few alterations in affected tissue, obesity itself is associated with increased morbidity and mortality because it is often associated with chronic lung disease, hypertension, ischemic heart disease, type II (adult-onset) diabetes mellitus, and osteoarthrosis. Pathologic obesity with hypoventilation is often termed Pickwickian syndrome after a character in Charles Dickens's *The Pickwick Papers.*

INCREASE IN BLOOD & DEPOSITION OF HEMOGLOBIN PIGMENTS

Congestion & Hyperemia

Hyperemia is an increase in the amount of blood within the vessels in a tissue caused by dilatation of the microcirculation and opening of new flow channels due to relaxation of precapillary sphincters. Active dilatation of the microcirculation occurs in acute inflammation (active hyperemia). Passive dilatation of vessels follows obstruction of venous outflow (passive hyperemia, or

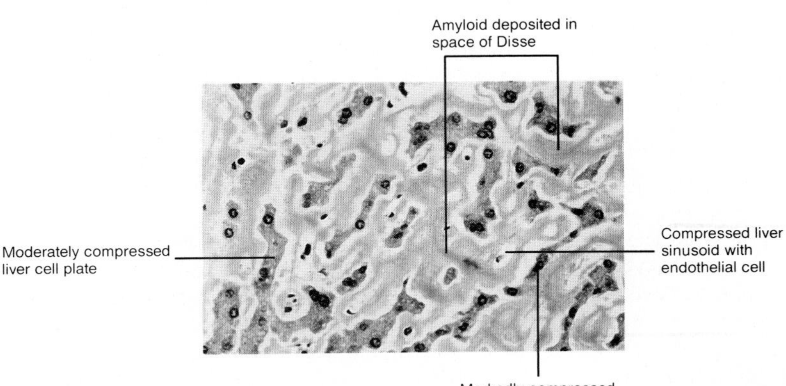

Figure 2–8. Amyloidosis of the liver. Amyloid is deposited in the space of Disse and compresses the liver cell plates.

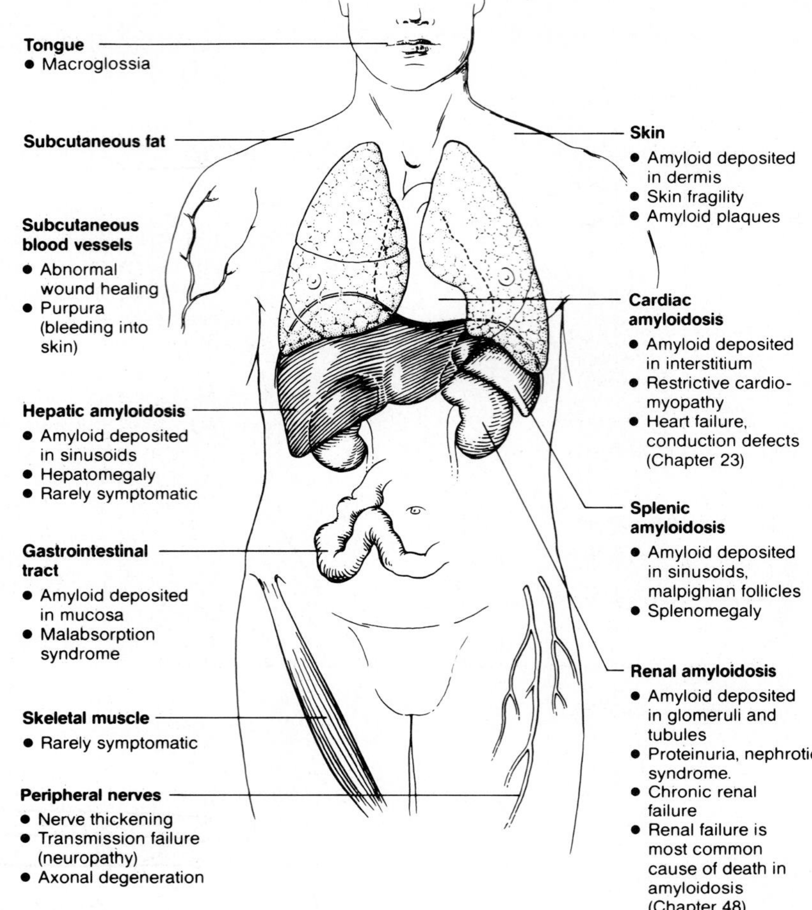

Figure 2-9. Clinical and pathologic effects of amyloidosis.

congestion).The term congestion is used synonymously with hyperemia by some people and with passive hyperemia by others. Hyperemic tissue is red on gross examination; numerous dilated vessels filled with blood are visible on microscopic examination.

Hemorrhage

Hemorrhage is the presence of blood in interstitial tissue outside the blood vessels. Hemorrhage results from escape of erythrocytes across intact vessels (diapedesis; see Chapter 3) or from vascular rupture.

Erythrocytes are rapidly broken down in interstitial tissue, and the iron in hemoglobin molecules is ingested by macrophages in the interstitium and converted to **hemosiderin**, which appears as a brown, granular pigment in the cytoplasm of macrophages. Hemosiderin may spill over from macrophages to be deposited in interstitial connective tissue (localized hemosiderosis). The porphyrin in the hemoglobin molecule is broken down by local macrophages to form bilirubin, which may be absorbed in the blood or deposited in interstitial connective tissue as a golden-yellow, crystalline pigment called **hematoidin**. The chemical composition of hematoidin is similar to that of bilirubin. Neither hemosiderin nor hematoidin deposited in interstitial tissues causes cellular dysfunction.

Accumulation of Hematin

Hematin is a golden—brown granular pigment derived from hemoglobin. It accumulates in reticuloendothelial cells following massive intravascular hemolysis, such as occurs in incompatible blood transfusions and malaria. Though hematin contains iron, the iron is part of an organic complex and is difficult to demonstrate on microscopy (Prussian blue stain for iron is negative). Accumulation of hematin produces no clinical effects.

Section II.
The Host Response to Injury

Evolution of the Response to Injury

The human organism responds to injury in accordance with complex predetermined patterns that, at a tissue level, have their analogues in lower animals. In animal phyla, the first responses to injury to evolve were **phagocytosis** and **regeneration** (present in amebas, hydras, sponges, etc). Phagocytosis, which at the level of these simple organisms is the engulfment of a solid particle by a cell, involves only simple recognition of damage or of "foreignness." The next level of response occurs in larger multicellular animals (invertebrates such as worms, mollusks, insects), in which the existence of a vascular system permits mobilization and transport of specialized inflammatory cells (phagocytes) to the site of injury. This nonspecific **acute inflammatory response** goes beyond simple recognition and phagocytosis to include **chemotaxis** (movement of cells in response to a chemical concentration gradient) and **microcirculatory changes**. In vertebrates, a highly specific

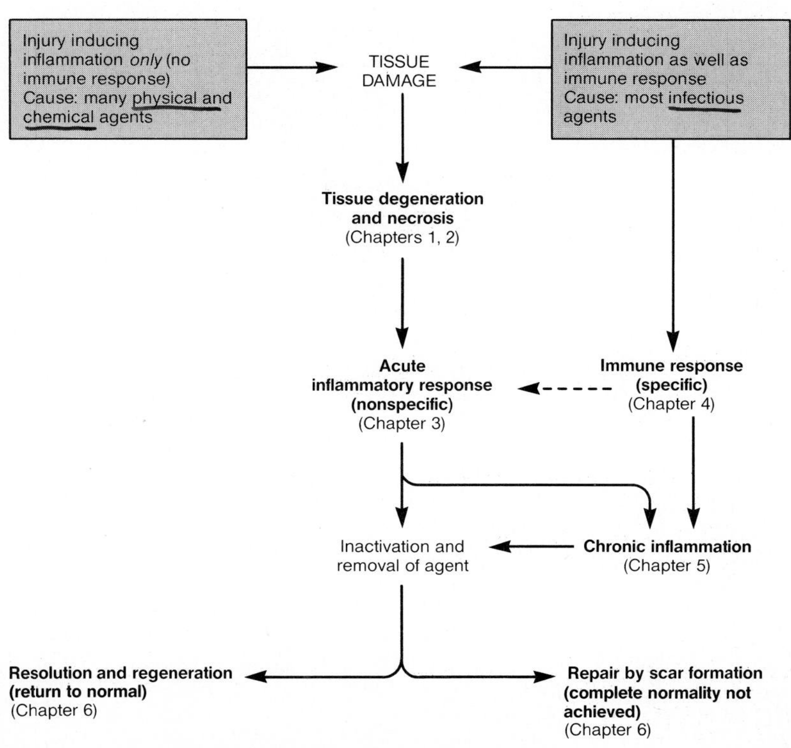

Figure II–1. Host tissue response to injury.

immune response appears that enhances the efficiency of phagocytosis and of the acute inflammatory response to injury. This enhancement is possible because of the presence of cells (lymphocytes) that "remember" an encounter with an injurious agent and produce a greater, more specific, and faster response when they meet that particular agent again. Specificity, memory, and amplification are the features that distinguish the immune response from the acute inflammatory reaction.

Sequence of Host Responses (Fig II-1)

In humans, the first visible tissue change that begins immediately after an injury is the microcirculatory response, which is accompanied by mobilization of phagocytic cells—the **acute inflammatory response** (Chapter 3).

The **immune response** (Chapter 4) is triggered at the time of the injury but takes several days to manifest microscopically visible changes at the site of injury. The term **chronic inflammation** (Chapter 5) is applied to the complex of changes in tissues that represents a combined inflammatory and immune response against an agent that persists in the tissues long enough so that the microscopic changes of the immune response can appear. Chronic inflammation also shows changes associated with tissue damage and repair.

Many texts present acute and chronic inflammation together, with separate discussions of immunity. We choose to follow the sequence acute inflammatory response—immune response—chronic inflammation, because we think it provides a more logical explanation of the sequence of events in injury.

Types of Noxious Agents

Noxious agents causing tissue injury may be classified into 2 broad categories:

(1) Physical or chemical agents and other mechanisms that are not recognized by the immune system. These induce primarily a basic microcirculatory and phagocytic response (inflammation).

(2) Agents that are recognized by the immune system (eg, most infectious agents). These induce a dual response consisting of nonspecific inflammation as well as a specific immune response that enhances the effectiveness of the basic inflammatory reaction.

Function of the Response to Injury

The host response is designed to inactivate and remove the injurious agent, remove any damaged tissue resulting from the injury, and accomplish **repair**. Repair processes are considered in Chapter 6.

Deficiencies of the host responses are discussed in Chapter 7.

The Acute Inflammatory Response 3

Acute inflammation is the early (almost immediate) response of a tissue to injury and is a function of the small blood vessels in the area. It is nonspecific and may be evoked by any injury short of one that is immediately lethal. Acute inflammation may be regarded as the first line of defense against injury. It is dependent on local factors that develop at the site of injury and is characterized by changes in the microcirculation, with exudation of fluid and emigration of leukocytes from blood vessels to the area of injury. Acute inflammation is typically of short duration, occurring before the immune response becomes established, and is aimed primarily at removing the injurious agent. Usually the response is beneficial, but in some cases it produces clinical symptoms that may be dangerous—as in swelling of the brain caused by the acute inflammatory response against a viral infection, in which death due to increased intracranial pressure may occur.

Until the late 18th century, acute inflammation was regarded as a disease. John Hunter (1728–1793, London surgeon and anatomist) was the first to realize that acute inflammation was a response to injury that was generally beneficial to the host: "But if inflammation develops, regardless of the cause, still it is an effort whose purpose is to restore the parts to their natural functions."

• CARDINAL CLINICAL SIGNS

Clinically, acute inflammation is characterized by 5 cardinal signs: **rubor** (redness), **calor** (increased heat), **tumor** (swelling), **dolor** (pain), and **functio laesa** (loss of function) (Fig 3–1). The first 4 were described by Celsus (ca 30 BC—38 AD); the fifth was a later addition by Virchow in the nineteenth century. Redness and heat are due to an increased rate and volume of blood flow to the inflamed area; swelling is due to accumulation of fluid; pain is due to accumulation of chemicals that stimulate nerve endings; and loss of function is due to a combination of factors. These signs are manifested when acute inflammation occurs on the surface of the body, but not all of them will be apparent in acute inflammation of internal organs. Pain occurs only when there are appropriate sensory nerve endings in the inflamed site—for example, acute inflammation of the lung (pneumonia) does not cause pain unless the inflammation involves the parietal pleura, where there are pain-sensitive nerve endings. The increased heat of inflamed skin is due to the entry of a large amount of blood at body core temperature into the normally cooler skin. When inflammation occurs internally—where tissue is normally at body core temperature—no increase in heat is apparent.

• MORPHOLOGIC & FUNCTIONAL CHANGES

The morphologic and functional changes in acute inflammation were described in the late nineteenth century by Cohnheim, who demon-

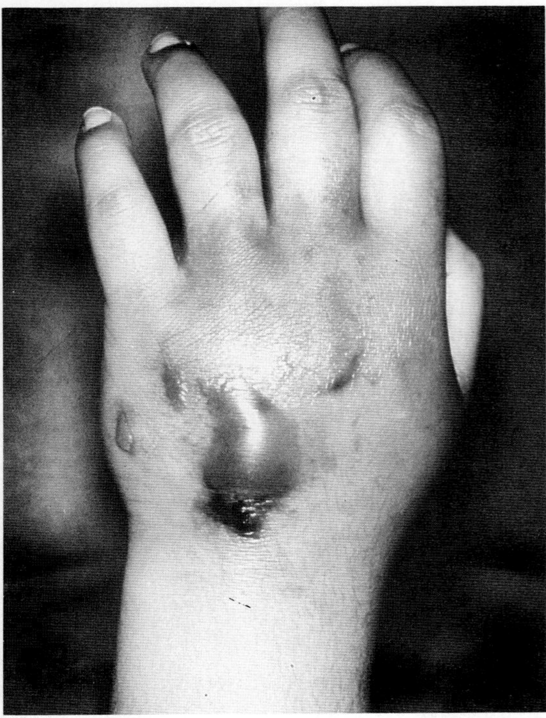

Figure 3–1. Cardinal signs of acute inflammation. Note swelling and redness of the skin around an infected burn. Marked tenderness, increased local temperature, and loss of function were also present.

strated the vascular changes of injury in the vessels of a frog tongue. The 2 main components of the acute inflammatory response are the microcirculatory response and the cellular response.

✓ Microcirculatory Response:

A. Active Vasodilatation (Hyperemia): The first change in the microcirculation is a transient and insignificant vasoconstriction, which is then followed by marked, active dilatation of arterioles, capillaries, and venules. Precapillary sphincters relax, permitting usually closed vascular channels to open. This vasodilatation causes a marked increase in the amount of blood in the area **(hyperemia),** which is one of the typical microscopic features of acute inflammation (Figs 3–2 and 3–3).

B. Increased Permeability: The permeability of capillaries and venules is a function of the intercellular junctions between vascular endothelial cells. These pores normally permit the passage of small molecules (MW < 40,000). Pinocytosis permits selective transfer of larger molecules across the capillary into the interstitium. In normal capillaries, fluid passes out of the microcirculation and into tissues under the influence of capillary hydrostatic pressure—and returns because of plasma colloid osmotic pressure (Chapter 2). Normally, fluid that passes out of the microcirculation is an ultrafiltrate of plasma (Table 3–1).

In acute inflammation, there is an immediate marked increase in the permeability of venules and capillaries due to active contraction of actin filaments in endothelial cells. The effect is separation of intercellular junctions from one another (widening of the pores). Direct damage to the endothelial cells by the noxious agent may also

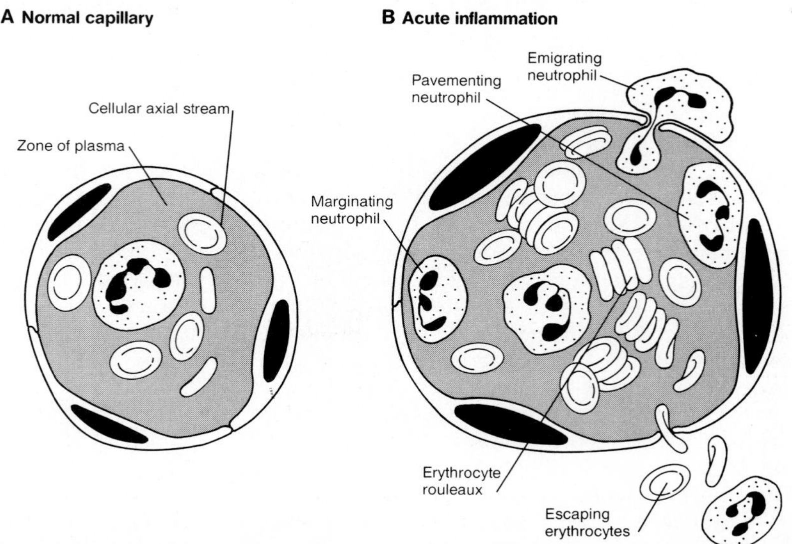

Figure 3–2. Microcirculatory changes in acute inflammation. The capillary in acute inflammation is dilated, has swollen endothelial cells, rouleau formation, and margination and emigration of leukocytes.

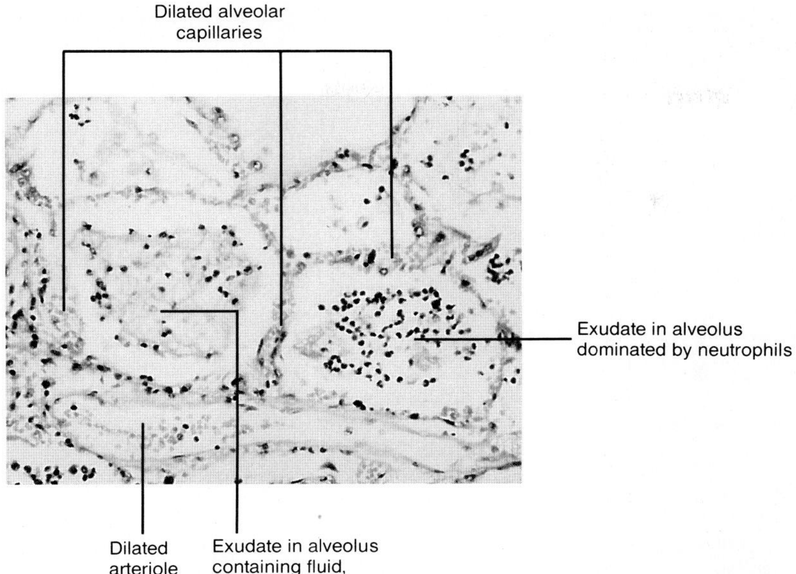

Figure 3-3. Pneumonia (acute inflammation of the lung), showing dilatation of alveolar septal capillaries and an alveolar exudate containing fibrin and neutrophils.

contribute. Increased amounts of fluid and high-molecular-weight proteins are able to pass through these abnormally permeable vessels (see Exudation of Fluid, below).

Increase in permeability in acute inflammation occurs in several different patterns: (1) immediate-transient, (2) immediate-sustained (or prolonged), or (3) delayed-prolonged. The immediate-transient response is mediated mainly by histamine. The mechanism producing the immediate-sustained and delayed-prolonged responses is uncertain and involves other mediators of inflammation besides histamine (Table 3–3, page 43) and differing degrees of endothelial cell damage. These permeability phases typically blend into one another and are seen separately only under controlled experimental conditions.

C. Exudation of Fluid: The passage of a large amount of fluid from the circulation into the interstitial tissue, with associated swelling (inflammatory edema; Chapter 2), is a major feature of acute inflammation. It occurs because of increased capillary permeability and arteriolar dilatation, which increases the hydrostatic pressure in the microcirculation. Increased passage of fluid out of the microcirculation because of increased vascular permeability is termed **exudation**. The composition of an exudate approaches that of plasma (Table 3–1); it is rich in plasma proteins, including immunoglobulins, complement, and fibrinogen, because the abnormally permeable endothelium no longer prevents passage of these large molecules. Fibrinogen in an acute inflammatory exudate is rapidly converted to fibrin by tissue thromboplastins. Fibrin can be recognized microscopically in an exudate as pink strands or clumps (Figs 3–3 and 3–4). Grossly, fibrin is most easily seen on an acutely inflamed serosal surface

Table 3-1. Differences between exudates and transudates.

	Ultrafiltrate of Plasma	Transudate	Exudate	Plasma
Vascular permeability	Normal	Normal	Increased	—
Protein content	Trace	0–1.5 g/dL	1.5–6 g/dL[1]	6–7 g/dL[1]
Protein types	Albumin	Albumin	All[2]	All[2]
Fibrin	No	No	Yes	No (fibrinogen)
Specific gravity	1.010	1.010–1.015	1.015–1.027	1.027
Cells	None	None	Inflammatory	Blood

[1]The protein content of an exudate depends on the plasma protein level. In patients with very low plasma protein levels, an exudate may have a lower protein content than 1.5 g/dL.
[2]All = albumin, globulins, complement, immunoglobulins, proteins of the coagulation and fibrinolytic cascades, etc.

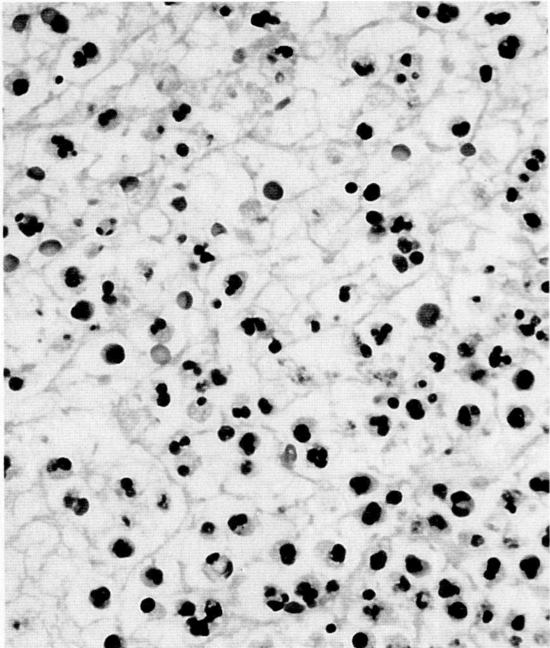

Figure 3-4. An acute inflammatory exudate, showing strands of fibrin and numerous neutrophilic leukocytes. Scattered macrophages are also present.

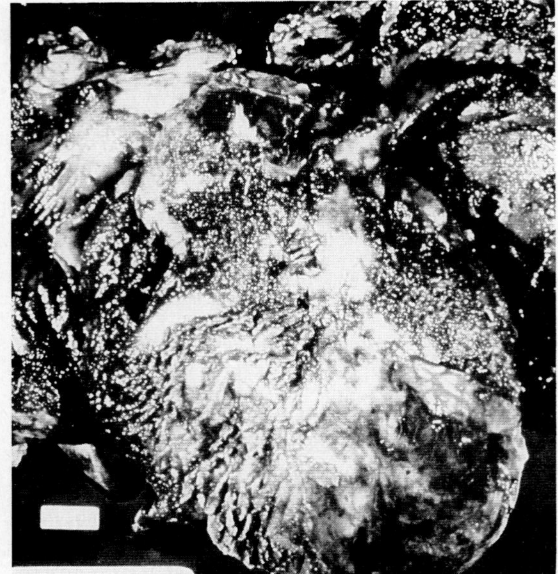

Figure 3-5. Acute fibrinous pericarditis. The normally smooth pericardium has become roughened by the fibrinous exudate ("bread and butter appearance").

that changes from its normal shiny appearance to a rough, yellowish "bread and butter" surface (Fig 3-5).

Exudation must be distinguished from transudation (Table 3-1). **Transudation** denotes increased passage of fluid into tissues through vessels of *normal* permeability. The force that causes outward passage of fluid from the microcirculation into the tissues is either increased hydrostatic pressure or decreased plasma colloid osmotic pressure. A transudate has a composition similar to that of an ultrafiltrate of plasma. In clinical practice, identification of edema fluid as a transudate or an exudate is of considerable diagnostic value, since it provides clues to the cause of the disorder, eg, examination of peritoneal (ascites) fluid (Table 3-2).

Exudation helps combat the offending agent (1) by diluting it; (2) by causing increased lymphatic flow, which removes the agent from the site; and (3) by flooding the area with plasma, which contains numerous defensive proteins such as immunoglobulins and complement.

D. Changes in Blood Flow Rate: Initially, the rate of flow in the dilated blood vessels is greatly increased. As fluid is lost from the vessel by exudation, however, the cellular content of blood increases **(hemoconcentration),** as does blood viscosity. As viscosity increases, the rate of blood flow progressively decreases, sometimes to the point of stasis.

E. Changes in Lymphatic Flow: As fluid collects in the interstitial space, lymphatic flow increases. This is beneficial in that it permits removal of the injurious agent and tissue debris from the site and conveys the noxious agent to the lymph nodes, where it is exposed to the filtering action of phagocytic macrophages. If the agent is antigenic, it then stimulates the specific immune response. Lymphatic drainage may be harmful, however, in that it provides a way for the injurious agent to spread from the site of entry to the rest of the body. In addition, acute inflammation of the lymphatics **(lymphangitis)** and lymph nodes **(lymphadenitis)** may follow the original injury.

Cellular Response

A. Types of Cells Involved: Acute inflammation is characterized by the active emigration of inflammatory cells from the blood into the area of injury. Neutrophils (polymorphonuclear leukocytes) (Fig 3-4) dominate the early phase (first 24 hours). After the first 24-48 hours, phagocytic cells of the macrophage (reticuloendothelial) system—and immunologically active cells such as lymphocytes and plasma cells—enter the area. Neutrophils remain predominant for several days, however.

B. Margination of Neutrophils: In a normal blood vessel, the cellular elements of blood are confined to a central axial stream, separated from

Table 3-2. Selected causes of transudative and exudative peritoneal effusion (ascites).

Transudate	Exudate
Cirrhosis of the liver	Bacterial peritonitis
Portal vein obstruction	Tuberculous peritonitis
Right heart failure	Metastatic neoplasms
Constrictive pericarditis	Mesothelioma (neoplasm of mesothelial cells)
Meigs' syndrome[1]	Connective tissue disease (eg, systemic lupus erthyematosus)
Malnutrition (kwashiorkor)	

[1]Meigs' syndrome is the occurrence of peritoneal and pleural effusion due to transudation of fluid from the surface of an ovarian tumor.

the endothelial surface by a zone of plasma (Fig 3-2). This separation is dependent on a rapid rate of blood flow, which creates physical forces that tend to keep the heaviest cellular particles in the center of the vessel.

As the rate of blood flow in the dilated vessels decreases in acute inflammation, the orderly flow of blood is disturbed. Erythrocytes form heavy aggregates **(rouleaux)** in a phenomenon termed **sludging**. The rouleaux displace the leukocytes from the center of the axial stream. This displacement—coupled with the marked decrease in the amount of plasma because of fluid exudation—forces the leukocytes to the endothelial surface **(margination)**.

C. Pavementing of Neutrophils: Marginated neutrophils adhere to the endothelial surface of blood vessels **(pavementing),** and microscopic examination shows that dilated vessels characteristic of acute inflammation are lined by numerous adherent neutrophils (Fig 3-6). Pavementing is a normal process, but in acute inflammation it is greatly increased as a result of increased adhesiveness of endothelial cells. The cause of this increased adhesiveness is not known for certain but may represent a change in the electrical charge of the cellular surface. Since they both carry negative charges, neutrophils and endothelial cells normally repel each other. A change in surface electrical charge during acute inflammation has not been demonstrated convincingly, however. Another cause is postulated to be the action of chemical mediators that induce chemotaxis, notably com-

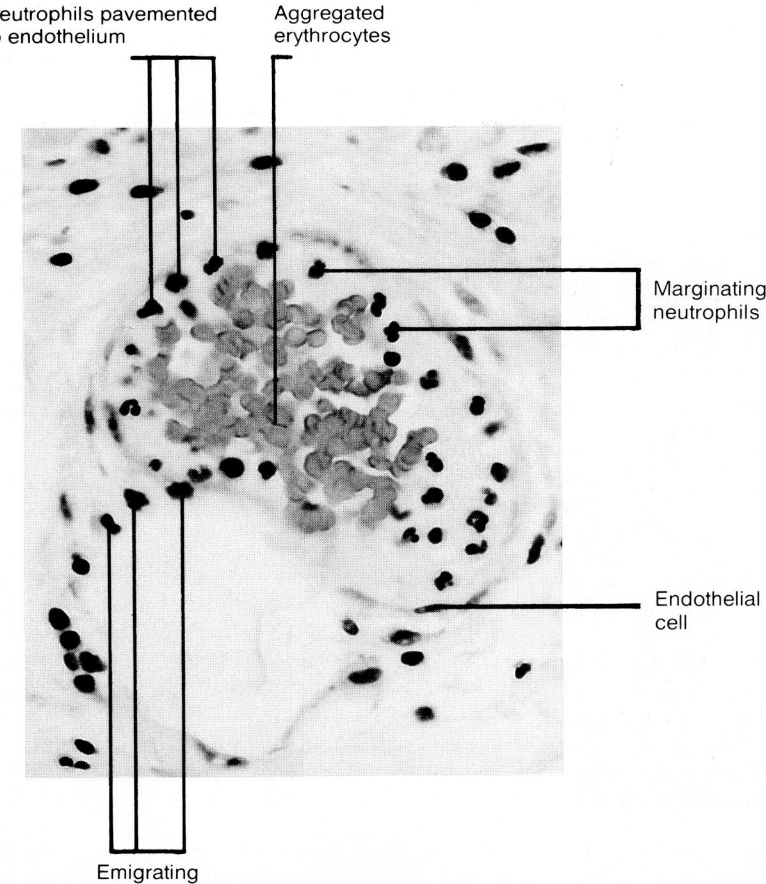

Figure 3-6. Pavementing and emigrating neutrophil leukocytes in a venule in an area of acute inflammation.

plement factor 5a (C5a) and leukotriene B4 (see below). Calcium ions are also believed to increase adhesiveness of endothelial cells in the acute inflammatory response.

D. Emigration of Neutrophils: The adherent neutrophils actively leave the blood vessel (Fig 3–6) by moving along the endothelial surface to an intercellular junction, where they insert a pseudopodiumlike cytoplasmic projection that opens the junction and widens the pore (Fig 3–2). The neutrophils then squeeze their way slowly through the junctions, pass through the basement membrane, and reach the interstitial space **(emigration).** Penetration through the wall takes 2–10 minutes; in interstitial tissue, neutrophils move at a rate of up to 20 μm/min.

E. Chemotactic Factors: The active emigration of neutrophils and the direction in which they move are governed by **chemotactic factors**—including complement factor 5a (C5a), leukotriene B4, and bacterial products—in the inflamed area. Chemotactic factors are those responsible for the movement of cells (in this case, neutrophils) in response to a chemical concentration gradient. Neutrophils have cell surface receptors for these factors, and the interaction between neutrophils and the chemotactic factors causes an influx of calcium ions into the cell. Calcium stimulates contraction of actin filaments in the cell and thereby causes increased cell movement.

F. Movement of Other Cells: Macrophage and lymphocyte emigration is similar to that of neutrophils. Chemotactic factors for macrophages are C5a, leukotriene B4, and other mediators called lymphokines, which are liberated by activated lymphocytes (Chapter 4).

Erythrocytes enter an inflamed area passively—in contrast to the active process of leukocyte emigration. Red blood cells are pushed out of the vessel by hydrostatic pressure through the widened intercellular junctions behind emigrating leukocytes **(diapedesis).** In severe injuries associated with disruption of the microcirculation, large numbers of erythrocytes enter the inflamed area **(hemorrhagic inflammation).**

G. Phagocytosis: (See Fig 3–7.)

1. Recognition-The major mechanism by which neutrophils and macrophages inactivate a noxious agent is phagocytosis. The first step in this process is recognition of the injurious agent by the phagocytic cell, either directly (as occurs with large, inert particles) or after the agent has been coated with immunoglobulin or complement factor 3b (C3b) **(opsonization).** The coating agents are **opsonins.** Opsonin-mediated phagocytosis is the mechanism operating in the immune phagocytosis of microorganisms. Both IgG and C3b are effective opsonins. Immunoglobulin that is specifically reactive with antigens on the injurious agent (specific antibody) is the most effective opsonin. C3b is generated locally by activation of

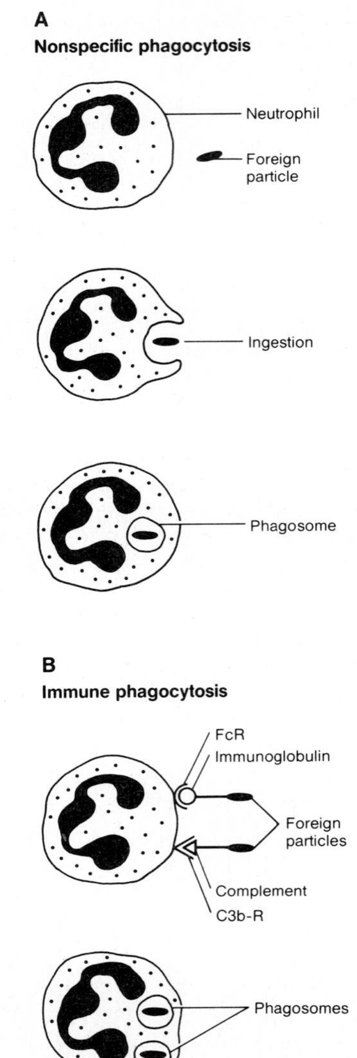

Figure 3–7. Phagocytosis by neutrophil leukocytes. Immune phagocytosis **(B)** is much more efficient than nonspecific phagocytosis **(A).** The presence on the cell membrane of receptors to the Fc fragment of the immunoglobulin molecule (FcR) and C3b component of complement (C3b-R) are important in immune phagocytosis. Note that macrophages have similar phagocytic capability.

the complement cascade. Early in acute inflammation—before the immune response has developed—nonimmune factors dominate, but as immunity develops, they are superseded by the more efficient immune phagocytosis.

2. Engulfment-Once recognized by a neutrophil or macrophage, a foreign particle is engulfed by the phagocytic cell to form a membrane-bound vacuole called a **phagosome,** which fuses with lysosomes to form a **phagolysosome.** Lysosomal enzymes, including lactoferrin and lysozyme (muramidase), then act to degrade the injurious agent. Lysozyme was first discovered in tears by Alexander Fleming, who called it "tear antiseptic." Lysozyme is present in many body fluids and acts by attacking muramic acid linkages in bacterial cell walls.

3. Microbial killing–When the offending agent is a microorganism, it must be killed before degradation can occur. Microbial killing is accomplished through several mechanisms (Fig 3–8).

(1) The **hydrogen peroxide (H_2O_2)-myeloperoxidase-halide system** is the most important microbicidal mechanism and occurs in neutrophils whose cytoplasmic granules contain myeloperoxidase. When a foreign particle is engulfed, the cellular oxidative metabolism is stimulated to form superoxide ion by the action of an oxidase in the plasma membrane. Superoxide is spontaneously transformed to microbicidal H_2O_2 in the lysosome. In addition, myeloperoxidase, in combination with a halide ion (usually chloride), greatly potentiates the microbicidal effect of H_2O_2, probably by forming highly toxic ions such as HOCl.

(2) Other systems operating independently of myeloperoxidase involve toxic oxygen-based radicals, eg, superoxide (O_2^-), hydroxyl ($OH^{\cdot}$), and singlet oxygen, which are produced in all phagocytic cells. Microbial killing resulting from the action of these oxygen-based radicals may be direct or may be mediated by ferric ions present in the phagolysosome. Reaction of superoxide with ferric ion results in the formation of ferrous ion, which reacts with hydrogen peroxide to form hydroxyl radicals. Hydroxyl radicals react with bacterial cell wall phopholipids, resulting in the formation of lipid peroxides, which are unstable, breaking down spontaneously and causing loss of bacterial cell membrane integrity (lipid peroxidation).

(3) Systems dependent on non-oxygen-based toxic radicals, eg, hydrogen ions, enzymes, and other bactericidal substances, also exist within lysosomes.

(4) Immunologic mechanisms such as **macrophage-activating factor,** a lymphokine released by sensitized T lymphocytes, assist microbial killing by macrophages (Chapter 4).

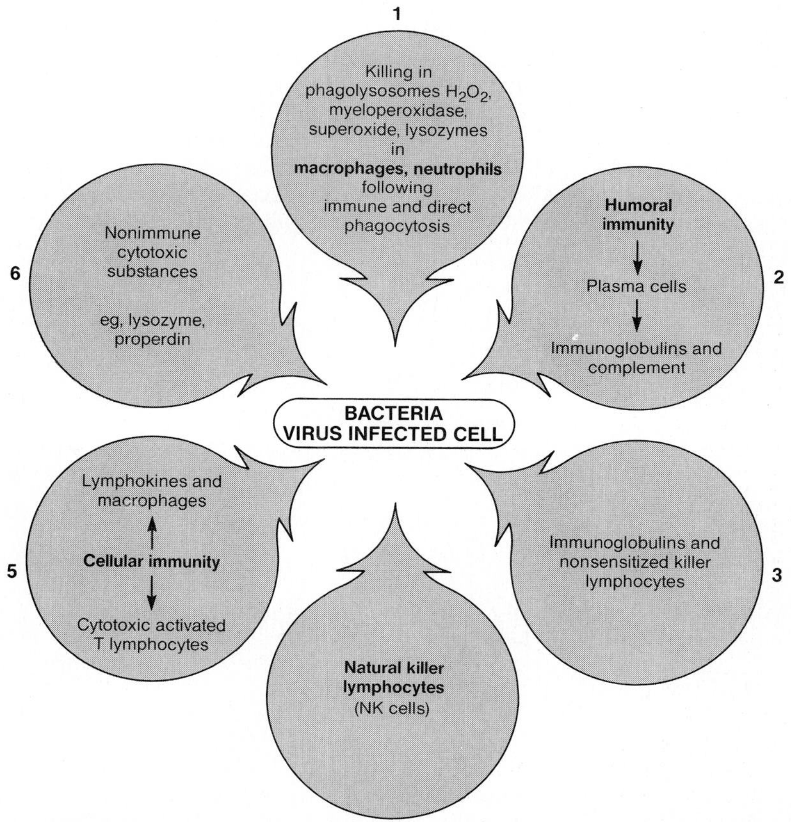

Figure 3–8. Mechanisms of microbial killing.

MEDIATORS OF ACUTE INFLAMMATION

The Triple Response (Fig 3-9)

Sir Thomas Lewis, in a series of elegant and simple experiments in 1927, elucidated the basic factors that mediate acute inflammation. Firmly stroking the forearm with a blunt instrument such as a pencil evokes the **triple response:** (1) Within 1 minute, a red line appears along the line of the stroke as a result of dilatation of arterioles, capillaries, and venules at the site of injury; (2) simultaneously, a red flare develops surrounding this line as a result of vasodilatation in the tissue surrounding the injury; and (3) a wheal forms because of exudation of fluid along the line of injury.

Removal of the nerve supply to the tissue prevents only the occurrence of the flare. Lewis showed that vasodilatation in tissue surrounding the injury—a minor part of the acute inflammatory response—is mediated by a local axon reflex (Fig 3-9). The major components of acute inflammation—the red line and the wheal—were shown to be independent of neural connections in the tissue. Lewis then demonstrated that local injection of histamine (Lewis's "H substance") produced a reaction equivalent to the red line and wheal. This discovery laid the foundation for understanding the role of chemical mediators in acute inflammation.

Specific Mediators (Table 3-3)

In the years since Lewis's experiments, it has become apparent that histamine can account for only a small part of the acute inflammatory response. Many other chemical mediators have been discovered, but the exact role of individual mediators in inflamed tissue is unknown; their actions in vivo can only be postulated on the basis of their demonstrated in vitro activity.

A. Vasoactive Amines: Histamine and **serotonin** are released from mast cells and platelets and can be identified early in the course of acute inflammation. Histamine is more important than serotonin in humans; it acts mainly on venules that have H_1 histamine receptors. Both of these amines cause vasodilatation and increased permeability and are probably the main agents responsible for the immediate-transient phase of the acute inflammatory response. Histamine levels decrease rapidly within an hour after the onset of inflammation and cannot account for the sustained vascular response that occurs in acute inflammation.

B. The Kinin System: Bradykinin, the final product of the kinin system, is formed by the action of **kallikrein** on a precursor plasma protein (high-molecular-weight kininogen). Kallikrein is present in its inactive form prekallikrein in plasma and is activated by activated factor XII (Hageman factor) of the coagulation cascade. Bradykinin causes increased vascular permeability and stimulates pain receptors.

C. The Coagulation Cascade: Coagulation is initiated by activation of factor XII and leads to the production of fibrin. The fibrinopeptides that are also formed in this process cause increased vascular permeability and are chemotactic for neutrophils.

D. The Complement System: (Chapter 4.) C5a and C3a, which are formed in the activation of complement, cause increased vascular permeability by stimulating release of histamine from mast cells. C5a is a powerful chemotactic agent

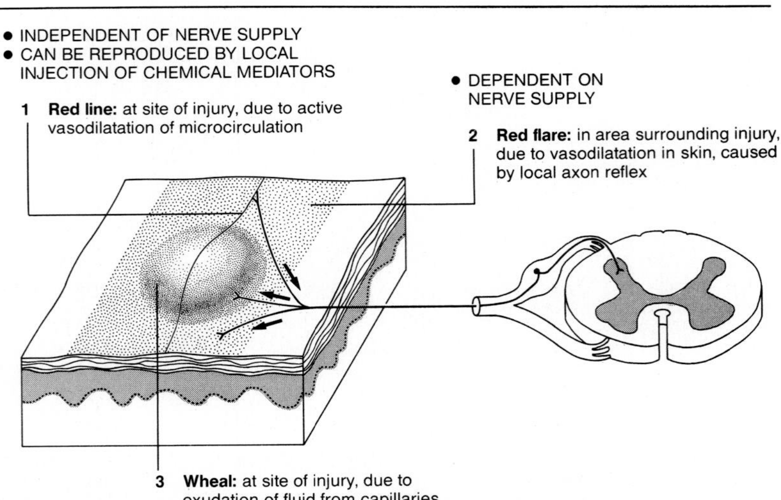

Figure 3-9. Lewis's triple response. The red line and wheal are caused by chemical mediators; the flare is mediated by a local axon reflex and is the only element that is dependent on the nerve supply.

Table 3-3. Mediators of acute inflammation.

Mediator	Vasodilation	Increased Permeability		Chemotaxis	Opsonin	Pain
		Immediate	Sustained			
Histamine	+	+++	–	–	–	–
Serotonin (5-HT)	+	+	–	–	–	–
Bradykinin	+	+	–	–	–	+++
Complement 3a	–	+	–	–	–	–
Complement 3b	–	–	–	–	+++	–
Complement 5a	–	++	–	+++	–	–
Prostaglandins	+++	+	+?	+++	–	+
Leukotrienes	–	+++	+?	+++	–	–
Lysosomal proteases	–	–	++[1]	–	–	–
Oxygen radicals	–	–	++[1]	–	–	–

[1]Proteases and oxygen-based free radicals derived from neutrophils are believed to mediate a sustained increase in permeability by means of their damage to endothelial cells.

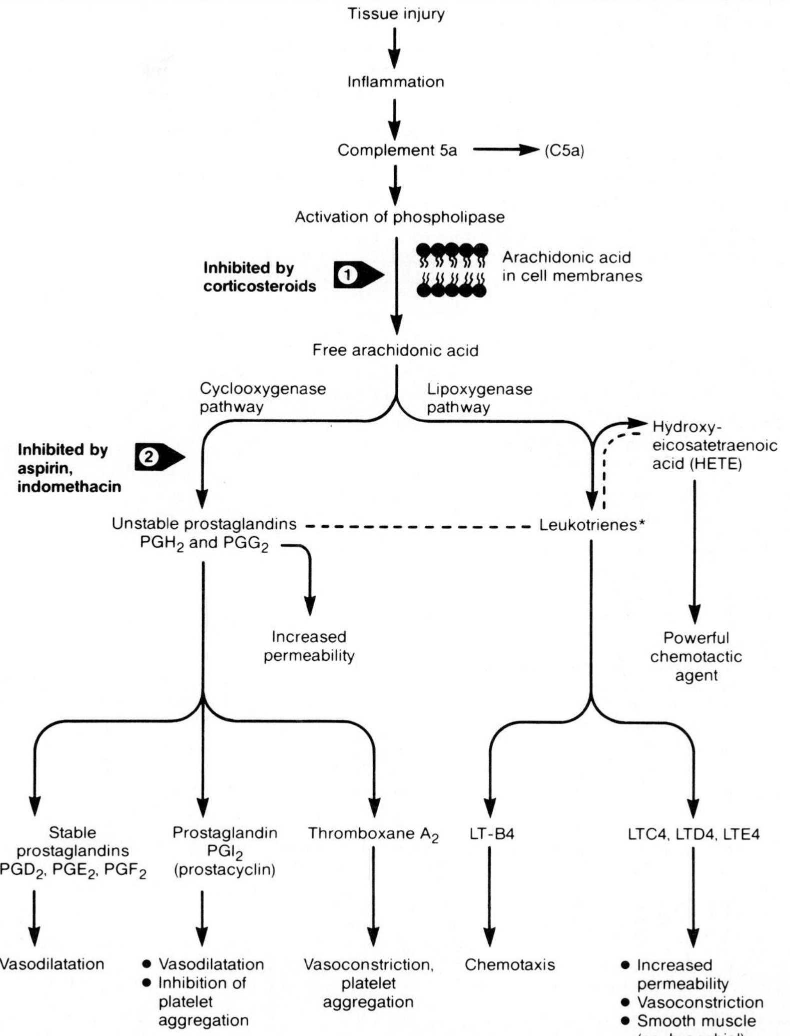

Figure 3-10. Metabolites of arachidonic acid and their influence on the acute inflammatory response.

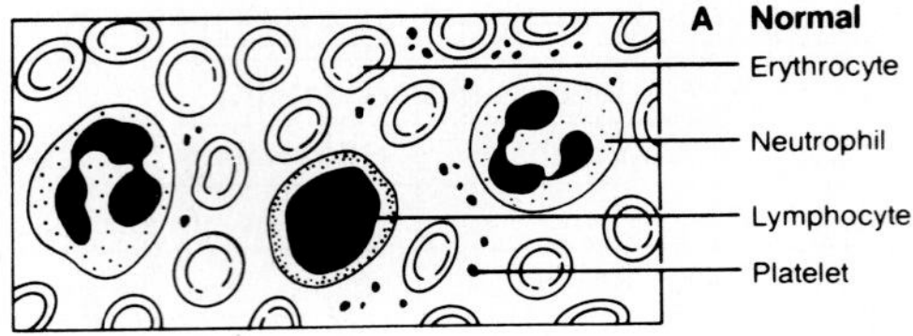

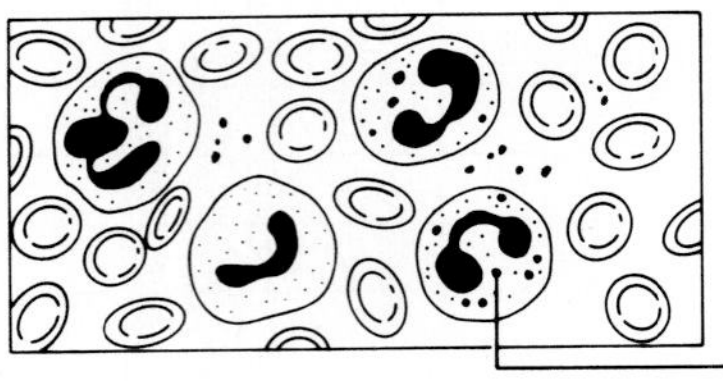

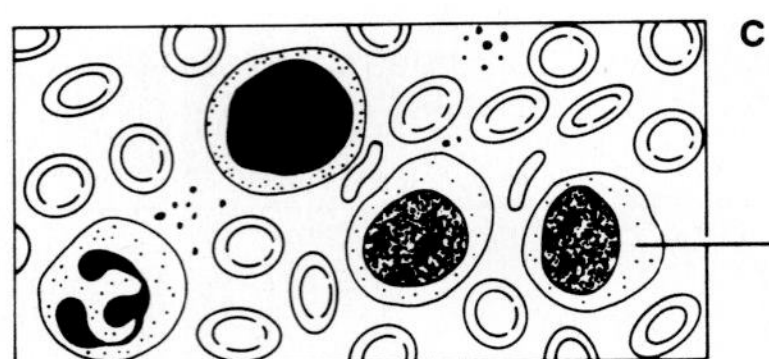

Figure 3-11. Changes in peripheral blood leukocytes in acute inflammation. The exact change observed varies with different causative agents and may give clues to the cause of the disease.

Table 3-4. Types of acute inflammation.

Type	Features	Common Causes
Classic type	Hyperemia; exudation with fibrin and neutrophils; neutrophil leukocytosis in blood.	Bacterial infections; response to cell necrosis of any cause.
Acute inflammation without neutrophils	Paucity of neutrophils in exudate; lymphocytes and plasma cells predominant; neutropenia, lymphocytosis in blood.	Viral and rickettsial infections (immune response contributes).
Allergic acute inflammation	Marked edema and numerous eosinophils; eosinophilia in blood	Certain hypersensitivity immune reactions (see Chapter 8).
Serous inflammation (inflammation in body cavities)	Marked fluid exudation.	Burns; many bacterial infections.
Catarrhal inflammation (inflammation of mucous membranes)	Marked secretion of mucus.	Infections, eg, common cold (rhinovirus); allergy (eg, hay fever).
Fibrinous inflammation	Excess fibrin formation.	Many virulent bacterial infections.
Necrotizing inflammation, hemorrhagic inflammation	Marked tissue necrosis and hemorrhage.	Highly virulent organisms (bacterial, viral, fungal), eg, plague (*Yersinia pestis*), anthrax (*Bacillus anthracis*), herpes simplex encephalitis, mucormycosis.
Membranous (pseudomembranous) inflammation	Necrotizing inflammation involving mucous membranes. The necrotic mucosa and inflammatory exudate form an adherent membrane on the mucosal surface.	Toxigenic bacteria, eg, diphtheria bacillus (*Corynebacterium diphtheriae*) and *Clostridium difficile.*
Suppurative (purulent) inflammation	Exaggerated neutrophil response and liquefactive necrosis of parenchymal cells; pus formation. Marked neutrophil leukocytosis in blood.	Pyogenic bacteria, eg, staphylococci, streptococci, gram-negative bacilli, anaerobes.

for neutrophils and macrophages. C3b is an important opsonin. C5a activates the lipoxygenase pathway of arachidonic acid metabolism (see below).

E. Arachidonic Acid Metabolites: Arachidonic acid is a 20-carbon unsaturated fatty acid found in phospholipids in the cell membranes of neutrophils, mast cells, monocytes, and other cells. Release of arachidonic acid by phospholipases initiates a series of complex and as yet incompletely understood reactions that culminate in the production of prostaglandins, leukotrienes, and other mediators of inflammation (Fig 3–10).

F. Neutrophil Factors: Neutrophils release their myeloperoxidase-containing cytoplasmic granules in the area of inflammation. **Proteases** and toxic oxygen-based free radicals generated by the neutrophil are believed to cause endothelial damage leading to increased vascular permeability. This mechanism is important in the imme-

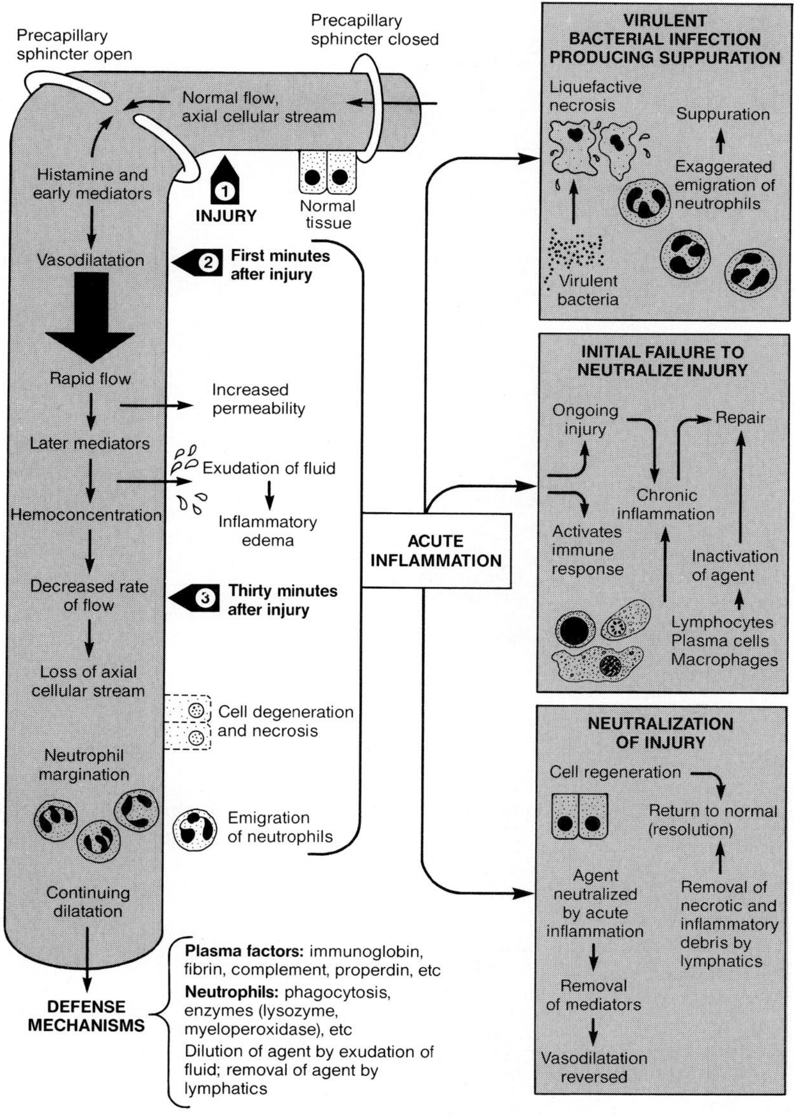

Figure 3–12. Summary diagram to show changes in the first few minutes **(2)** and later **(3)** of an acute inflammation caused by injury **(1).** The possible results of acute inflammation are also shown in the boxes on the right.

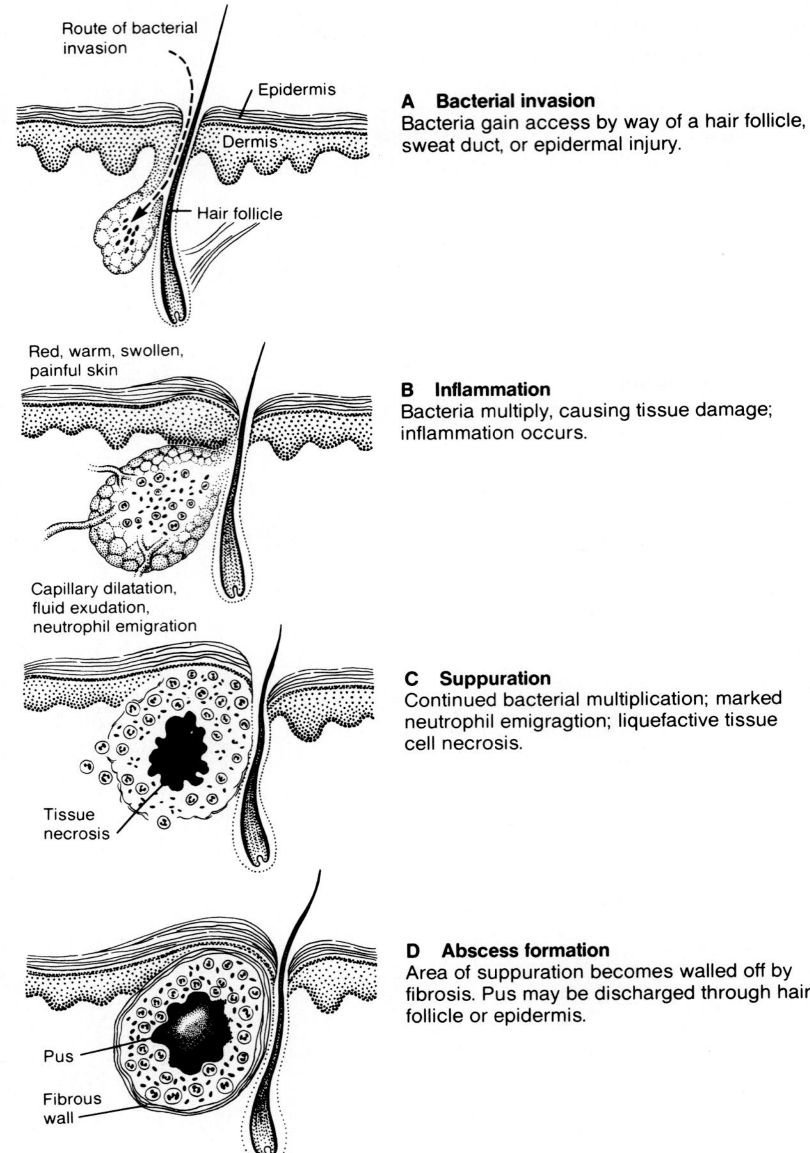

Figure 3–13. Bacterial infection **(A)** of a hair follicle of the skin, resulting in acute inflammation **(B)** followed by liquefactive necrosis **(C)** and abscess formation **(D)**.

diate-sustained and delayed-prolonged phases of the microcirculatory response.

Neutrophils, basophils, and macrophages also release a complex lipid called acetyl glyceryl ether phosphorylcholine (AGEPC; formerly called **platelet-activating factor)** that causes vasodilatation, increased vascular permeability, and leukocyte chemotaxis in vitro. Its role in vivo is uncertain.

G. Other Mediators and Inhibitors: Numerous other chemical mediators of acute inflammation have been described that are ignored here because they play either a minor or a dubious role. Negative feedback (inhibition) of inflammation also occurs but is not well understood; possible inhibitory factors include C1 esterase inhibitor (inhibits the complement cascade) and α_1-antitrypsin (inhibits proteases).

• SYSTEMIC CLINICAL SIGNS

Acute inflammation may be accompanied by systemic features in addition to the local cardinal signs described above.

Fever

Fever may result following the entry of pyrogens and prostaglandins into the circulation at the site of inflammation. These act upon the brain stem to reset body temperature.

Changes in the Peripheral White Blood Cell Count

The total number of neutrophils in the peripheral blood is increased **(neutrophil leukocytosis)**; initially, this is due to accelerated release of neutrophils from bone marrow. Later, neutrophil production in the marrow is increased. Peripheral blood neutrophils tend to be the less mature forms with fewer nuclear lobes (band forms), and they frequently contain large cytoplasmic granules **(toxic granulation)**. The term "shift to the left" signifies this change to an increased number of immature neutrophils in the peripheral blood (see Chapter 26). Viral infections tend to produce neutropenia (decreased number of neutrophils in the blood) and lymphocytosis (excess of normal lymphocytes in the blood). Acute inflammation resulting from viral infection therefore represents an exception in that the microcirculatory changes and fluid exudation are accompanied by a lymphocytic rather than a neutrophil response (Fig 3–11).

Changes in Plasma Protein Levels

Increase of acute phase reactants, including C-reactive protein, α_1-antitrypsin, fibrinogen, haptoglobin, and ceruloplasmin, occurs in acute inflammation. Increased levels of these substances in turn lead to an **increased erythrocyte sedimentation rate**, a simple and useful (though nonspecific) clue to the presence of inflammation.

• TYPES OF ACUTE INFLAMMATION

The preceding description of acute inflammation is that of the classic, most frequently occurring form. It is important to recognize variations from this common type, since they provide clues to the causative agent (Table 3–4).

• COURSE OF ACUTE INFLAMMATION

The acute inflammatory response is aimed at neutralizing or inactivating the agent causing the injury. The response may follow one of several courses (Fig 3–12):

(1) In uncomplicated acute inflammation, tissue returns to normal in a process of **resolution** (Chapter 6), in which the exudate and cellular debris are liquefied and removed by macrophages and lymphatic flow.

(2) When tissue necrosis has occurred before the agent is neutralized, **repair** ensues, and dead cells are either replaced by regeneration or repaired by scar formation (Chapter 6).

(3) In virulent bacterial infections, exaggerated emigration of neutrophils with liquefactive necrosis occurs **(suppurative inflammation)**. The liquefied mass of necrotic tissue and neutrophils is called **pus**. When an area of suppuration becomes walled off, an **abscess** results (Fig 3–13).

(4) When the noxious agent is not neutralized by the acute inflammatory response, the body mounts an **immune response** (Chapter 4), which leads to chronic inflammation (Chapter 5).

Table 3–5. Summary of clinical and laboratory evaluation of acute inflammation.

Systemic features
Fever (usually of acute onset and rapidly rising)
Changes in peripheral white blood cell count
Neutrophil leukocytosis with "shift to the left"
Lymphocytosis and neutropenia in acute viral infections
Changes in plasma proteins
Elevated levels of acute phase reactants (eg, C-reactive protein, alpha$_1$-antitrypsin, haptoglobin)
Increased erythrocyte sedimentation rate
Local features (cardinal clinical signs; seen at site of injury only)
Redness
Swelling
Heat
Pain
Loss of function
Laboratory evaluation
Examination of inflammatory exudate
Characteristic high protein levels and high specific gravity
Presence of acute inflammatory cells (neutrophils; lymphocytes in viral infections)
Biopsy and microscopic examination of tissue
Hyperemia
Edema
Neutrophils
Fibrin
Diagnostic tests
Microbiologic (culture and Gram-stained smear)
Immunologic: Serum antibody levels, complement levels, etc.

• DIAGNOSIS OF ACUTE INFLAMMATION (Table 3-5)

Local cardinal signs of inflammation permit diagnosis of acute inflammation when the process involves surface structures—skin, conjunctiva, mouth, etc. Acute inflammation in internal organs such as the lung and kidney may first manifest with systemic changes such as fever and alterations in the blood (white cell count, proteins, etc). More rarely, it is necessary to examine a fluid exudate or tissue sample (biopsy) to establish the presence of acute inflammation.

4 The Immune Response

The immune response is a complex series of cellular interactions activated by the entry into the body of foreign (nonself) antigenic materials such as infectious agents and a variety of macromolecules. After processing by macrophages, the antigen is presented to lymphocytes, which are the major effector cells of the immune system (Fig 4–1). Lymphocyte activation by antigen results in proliferation and transformation of the lymphocytes, which lead to 2 main types of immune response:

(1) Cell-mediated immunity is a function of T lymphocytes, leading to the production of effector (killer) T cells, which have the ability to destroy antigen-bearing cells by direct toxicity, and of specific products called lymphokines that mediate cell interactions (macrophage, T cell, B cell) in the immune response. Furthermore, 2 subtypes of T cells serve to modulate the immune response: helper T cells enhance it; suppressor T cells have the opposite effect.

(2) Humoral immunity is a function of B cells and is characterized by the transformation of B cells into plasma cells, which secrete immunoglobulins (antibodies) that have specific activity against the inciting antigen.

CHARACTERISTICS OF THE IMMUNE RESPONSE

The immune response is characterized by **(1) specificity** (ie, reactivity is directed toward and restricted to the inducing agent, termed the **antigen**); **(2) amplification** (the ability to develop an enhanced response on repeated exposure to the same antigen); and **(3) memory** (the ability to recognize and mount an enhanced response against the same antigen on subsequent exposure even if the first and subsequent exposures are widely separated in time). These features distinguish the immune response from other nonspecific host responses such as acute inflammation and nonimmune phagocytosis.

Tolerance to Self Antigens

The concepts of self and nonself (foreignness) are central to immunologic reactivity (Fig 4–2). Many molecules in a host individual are antigenic (ie, they induce an immune response) if introduced into another individual but are not recognized as antigens by the host. This failure to re-

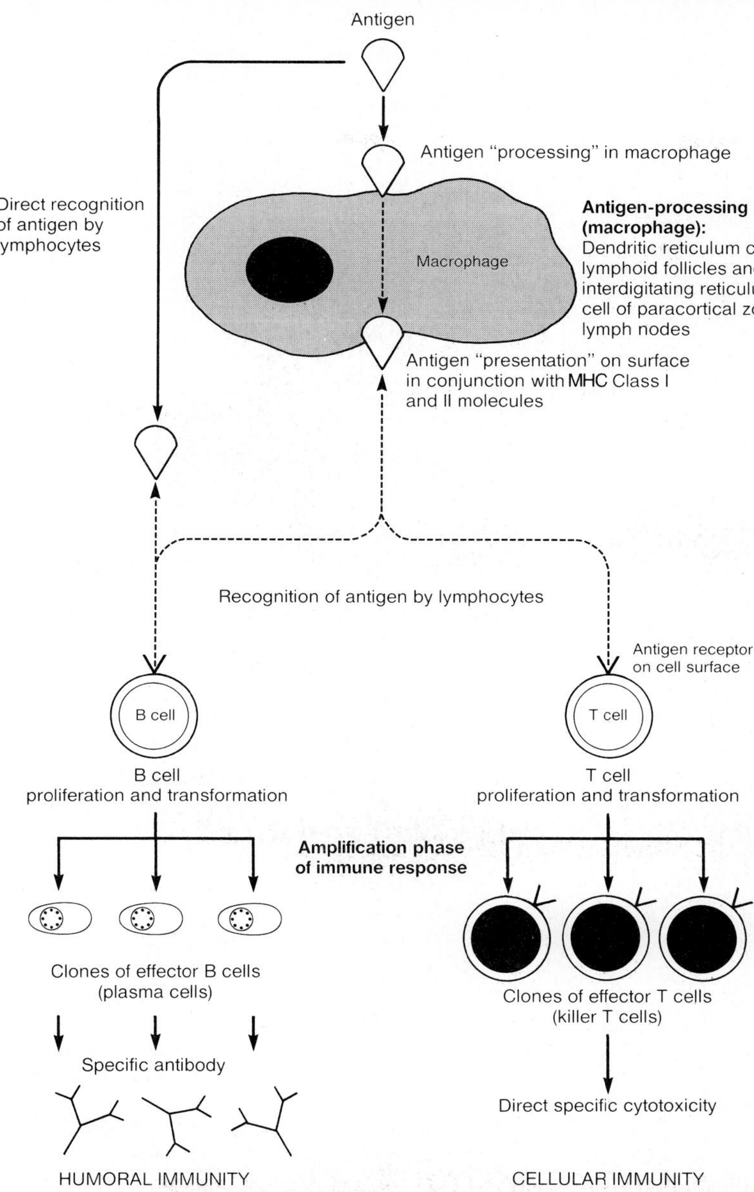

Figure 4–1. Summary of the immune response. Lymphocytes (both B and T) bearing specific antigen receptors are induced to proliferate (amplification phase) after they react with an antigen. The process by which lymphocytes recognize an antigen commonly involves an antigen-processing cell (various types of macrophages). Proliferation produces the effector cells of the immune response. Effector B cells (plasma cells) produce specific antibody, which mediates humoral immunity. Effector T cells exert a direct cytotoxic effect and mediate cellular immunity. Humoral immunity is so called because it can be transferred from an immune individual to a susceptible one by injection of serum containing antibody; cellular immunity can be transferred only by injection of live T cells.

spond to self antigens is **natural tolerance,** and it prevents the immune system from destroying the host's own tissues. Tolerance to self antigens is induced in the embryo and even at that stage demonstrates specificity and memory.

The mechanisms of natural tolerance are not fully understood, and 2 principal theories have been proposed to account for it. Some workers feel that tolerance is due to deletion in embryo of those clones of lymphocytes capable of recognizing self antigens, so that the capacity for self-recognition is in effect destroyed. Others feel that natural tolerance results from the production of specific suppressor cells (lymphocytes) that inhibit an immune response to self antigens (see also Autoimmunity, Chapter 8).

Specificity

The specificity of the immune response is dependent on the ability of the immune system to produce an almost unlimited number of antibodies of differing specificity plus an almost equally diverse repertoire of T lymphocytes bearing specific antigen receptors on their surfaces. An antigen evokes a response from a specific B or T lymphocyte that is preprogrammed to react against it (ie, the lymphocyte bears receptors with appropriate specificity for the antigen). This receptor function is performed by immunoglobulin on B cells and by an immunoglobulinlike molecule on T cells. When challenged by an antigen, the specific lymphocyte (B or T) selectively multiplies into a clone of sensitized effector cells that can

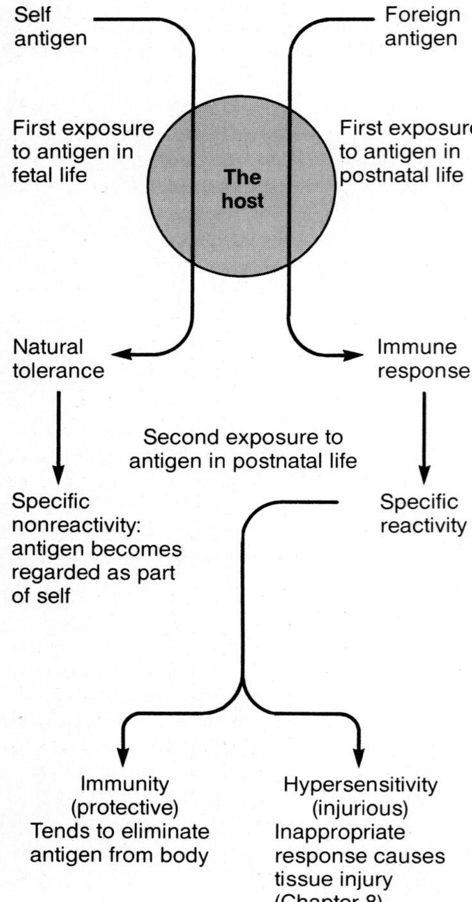

Figure 4-2. Antigens are molecules that induce an immune response in an appropriate recipient (host). From the point of view of an individual organism, antigens can be self (ie, part of the host's own tissues) or foreign. The developing fetal immune system usually encounters only "self" antigens, to which tolerance occurs. After birth, foreign antigens are encountered and the nature of the host response changes to an immune response (Fig 4-1) designed to neutralize and remove the antigen. Note that if a foreign antigen is presented in fetal life, natural tolerance may result. If a self antigen is hidden from the immune system in fetal life and first presented in postnatal life, an immune response may result. Tolerance, then, is an active "decision" by the immune system not to mount an immune response to a specific antigen (specific nonreactivity). By contrast, an immune response is an active "decision" that mobilizes the immune system into a complex response against that antigen (specific reactivity). This immune response usually is protective (immunity) but occasionally may be harmful to the host (hypersensitivity).

mount a highly specific response against that antigen: from B cells, plasma cells that in turn produce immunoglobulin; from T cells, cytotoxic T lymphocytes (Fig 4-1). This specific response usually has a net protective effect **(immunity);** occasionally, adverse reactions develop that cause tissue injury **(hypersensitivity)** (Chapter 8).

ANTIGENS

Antigens are molecules that evoke an immune response when introduced into a host that recognizes them as nonself. They are relatively large "rigid" molecules (typically proteins or polysaccharides) with a molecular weight in excess of 5000. Smaller molecules called **haptens**—including some lipids, carbohydrates, oligopeptides, nucleic acids, and various drugs that are not large enough alone to act as antigens—may be antigenic when combined with larger-molecular-weight "carriers."

Antigenic Determinants (Epitopes)

The exact part of the antigen or hapten that reacts with the immune system is called the antigenic determinant, or epitope. It is usually a small portion of the molecule and is frequently composed of only a few (4–8) amino acids or sugar residues. A single antigenic molecule may bear several different epitopes, each with a characteristic rigid 3-dimensional configuration determined by the primary, secondary, or tertiary structure of the molecule. These different antigenic determinants are recognized separately by the immune system, and antibodies are produced that provide a reciprocal "fit" (ie, they show specificity; see Fig 4-3).

Types of Antigens

A. Extrinsic Antigens: Antigens may be extrinsic, ie, introduced into the body from outside; these include microorganisms, transplanted foreign cells, and foreign particles that may be ingested, inhaled, or injected into the body.

B. Intrinsic Antigens: Intrinsic antigens are derived from molecules in the body so altered—eg, by addition of hapten, partial denaturation of native molecules, or transformation in the development of cancer cells—as to be regarded as foreign, or nonself, by the immune system.

C. Sequestered Antigens: Certain antigens such as lens protein and spermatozoa are anatomically sequestered from the immune system from early embryonic life; consequently, tolerance to these molecules does not develop, and their release into the circulation in later life may result in an immune response. Immunologic reac-

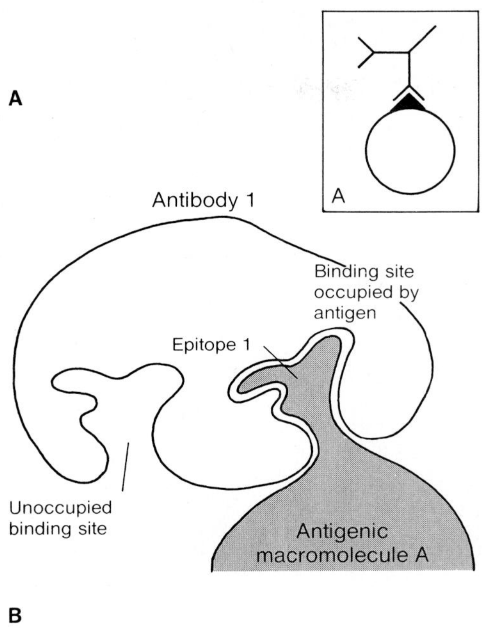

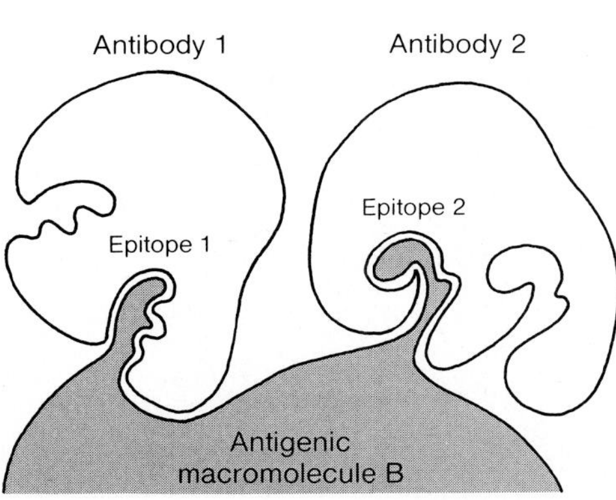

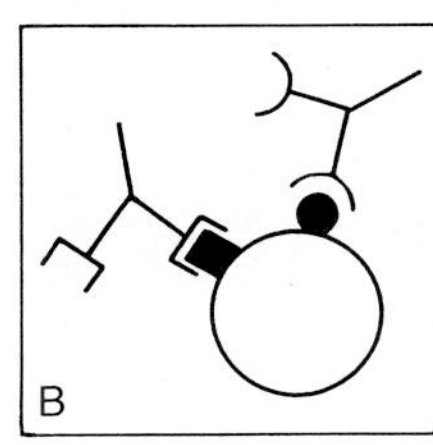

Figure 4-3. Antigen, epitopes, and antibody specificity. In **A,** macromolecule A has a single antigenic determinant site (epitope 1) that has combined with one of 2 identical binding sites on antibody 1. In **B,** macromolecule B has 2 epitopes (1 and 2) that have bound 2 different antibodies (1 and 2). Note that binding sites on the antibodies have different 3-dimensional shapes that correspond exactly to those of the epitopes; ie, they are specific. Inserts show the abbreviated method used in this book for depicting antigen-antibody interactions.

tivity against altered or sequestered self antigens is responsible for some autoimmune diseases (Chapter 8).

Recognition of Antigens

Foreign antigens must be recognized by the immune system before an immune response can develop. The mechanisms by which recognition occurs are uncertain and vary with the nature of the antigen, its route of entry into the body, etc. An optimal immune response to most antigens occurs only after interaction of the antigen with macrophages, T lymphocytes, and B lymphocytes (Fig 4–1). A macrophage acting in this role is termed an **antigen-processing cell**. Dendritic reticulum cells in lymphoid follicles and interdigitating reticulum cells in the paracortical zone of lymph nodes are believed to be specialized macrophages adapted to process antigens for B cells and T cells, respectively (see below). "Processing" appears to involve internalization of antigen by the macrophage, followed by reexpression of antigen on the cell surface in conjunction with MHC (major histocompatibility complex) molecules. Antigen receptors on T cells recognize the combination of antigen-MHC molecules on the macrophage, leading to T cell activation and the release of various lymphokines (Table 4–3). Helper T cells recognize antigen in association with MHC class II molecules; suppressor T cells, with MHC class I molecules. The usual form of B cell activation (T cell-dependent) appears to involve cooperation with both macrophages and T cells. B cells recognize some multivalent antigens directly (T cell-independent antigens).

CELLULAR BASIS OF THE IMMUNE RESPONSE

LYMPHOID TISSUE

Lymphoid tissue is the seat of the immune response.

Central Lymphoid Tissue

The central lymphoid tissue is composed of the thymus (Fig 4–4) and bone marrow, in which primitive lymphoid cells in the fetus are developed and "primed." (**Priming** refers to the early period of lymphocyte development when diversity occurs and tolerance develops. In humans, development of diversity and tolerance is considered essentially complete within a few months after birth.)

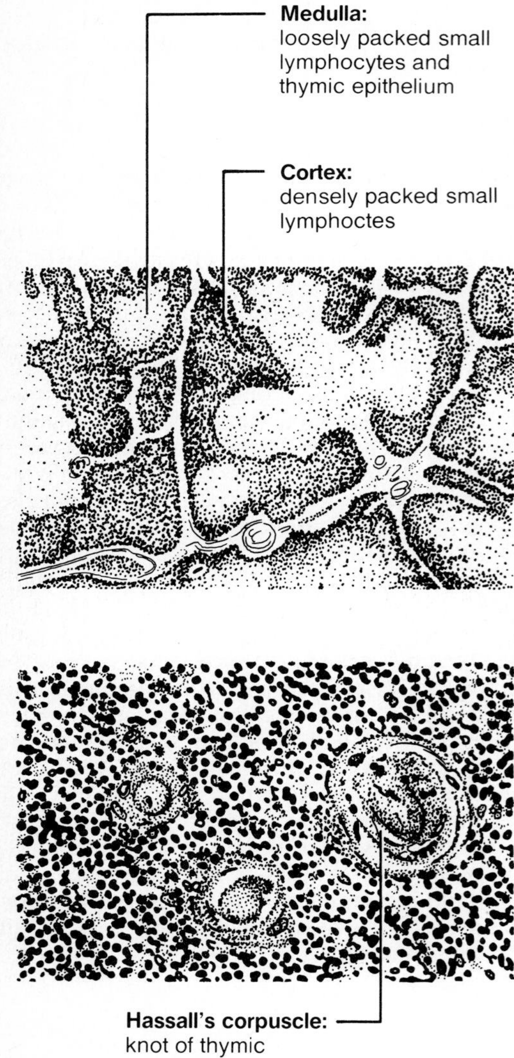

Figure 4-4. Thymus (diagrammatic). The intimate relationship between thymic epithelial cells—derived from the third pharyngeal pouch—and lymphocytes is important for lymphocyte maturation. Thymic epithelial cells release the hormone thymopoietin (thymosin), which induces lymphocyte maturation. They also express major histocompatibility (MHC) antigens that appear to "condition" the T cells to the types of MHC antigens expressed on antigen-processing cells with which T cells interact in the immune response (Fig 4-1). Mature T lymphocytes leave the thymus through the venules to populate the blood and peripheral lymphoid tissues.

Peripheral Lymphoid Tissue

The peripheral lymphoid tissue is composed of **lymph nodes** (Fig 4-5), **spleen** (Fig 4-6), **Waldeyer's ring** (the tonsils) in the oropharynx (Fig 4-7), and **gut-associated lymphoid tissue** in which reside the mature lymphocytes that respond to antigenic stimuli. The **peripheral blood** also contains lymphocytes. Circulating lymphocytes constitute a pool of cells that is being continuously exchanged with cells of the peripheral lymphoid tissue (Fig 4-8).

LYMPHOCYTES

Lymphocytes are derived from **lymphoid stem cells in the bone marrow** and develop in fetal life (Fig 4-9). Lymphocytes may be classified on the basis of their site of development in the fetus: **(1) T (thymus-dependent) lymphocytes** develop in the thymus; and **(2) B lymphocytes** develop independently of the thymus. B lymphocytes develop in the bursa of Fabricius in birds (hence B cells); the functional bursal equivalent in humans is the fetal liver or bone marrow.

Inactive small lymphocytes are about 8–10 μm in diameter, with scanty cytoplasm and a spherical nucleus occupying almost the entire cell. The nucleus has condensed chromatin that is strongly basophilic on routine histologic sections. All resting lymphocyte subpopulations resemble one another morphologically and can be distinguished only by immunologic methods (Table 4–1; see also Figs 4–10 and 4–12).

T Lymphocytes (T Cells)

A. Distribution of T Cells in the Body: T lymphocytes develop in the fetal thymus (Fig 4–10). After maturation, T lymphocytes are distributed by the circulation to the T cell domains of peripheral lymphoid tissue. These areas include **(1)** the **paracortex of the lymph nodes,** between the lymphoid follicles (Fig 4–5; 70% of lymphocytes in lymph nodes are T lymphocytes); and **(2)** the periarterial lymphoid sheath in the **splenic white pulp** (Fig 4–6; 60% of splenic lymphocytes are T cells). T lymphocytes continuously and actively recirculate between the peripheral blood and peripheral lymphoid tissue (Fig 4–8). Eighty to 90 percent of peripheral blood lymphocytes are T cells.

B. T Cell Transformation: Following stimulation (activation) either by specific antigen or by nonspecific agents such as mitogens, eg, phytohemagglutinin (PHA, a plant extract), T lymphocytes transform into large, actively dividing cells known as **transformed T lymphocytes,** or **T immunoblasts,** which then divide to produce effector T cells (Fig 4–11). T immunoblasts are 15–20 μm in diameter, with abundant cytoplasm and a cen-

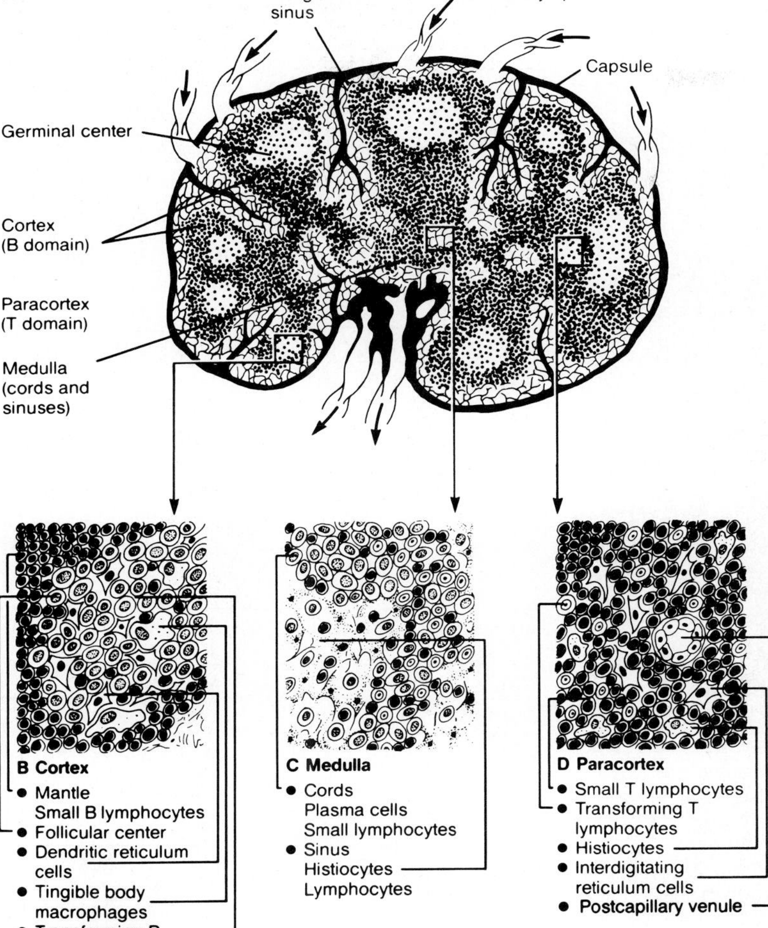

Figure 4-5. Lymph node (diagrammatic). The lymph node is a dynamic tissue. Its histologic appearance is governed by the immune responses occurring at the time of biopsy. Antigen enters through the afferent lymphatics and is processed by dendritic reticulum cells in the cortex or interdigitating reticulum cells in the paracortex **(A)**. Focal B cell proliferation around the dendritic reticulum cells produces collections of transforming B cells—these are the reactive centers **(B).** T celi transformation occurs diffusely in the paracortex in conjunction with interdigitating reticulum cells **(D).** The products of transformation (plasma cells and sensitized T cells) move centrally into the medulla and leave via efferent lymphatics **(C).** Lymphocytes are recruited into the lymph node via the afferent lymphatics and through the postcapillary venules.

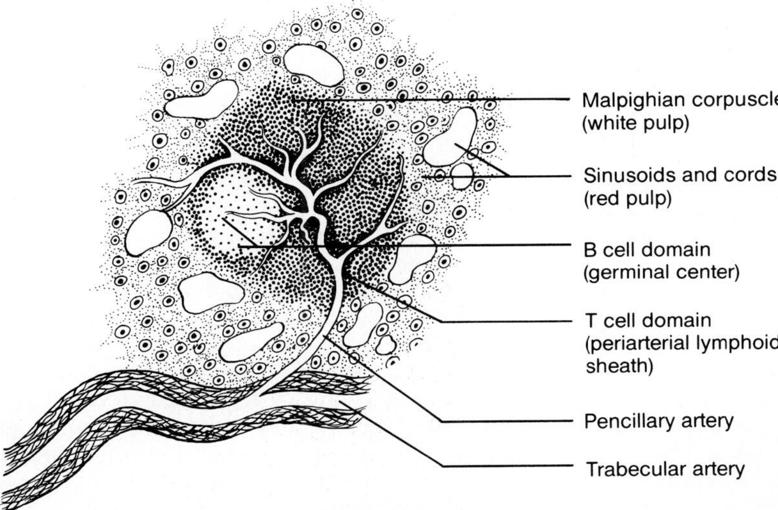

Figure 4-6. Diagrammatic representation of the spleen, showing white pulp and red pulp. The germinal centers have the same basic structure already described for lymph nodes; the T cell domains resemble lymph node paracortex. Antigen is presented to the spleen via the bloodstream, which serves also as the route for entry and egress of lymphocytes.

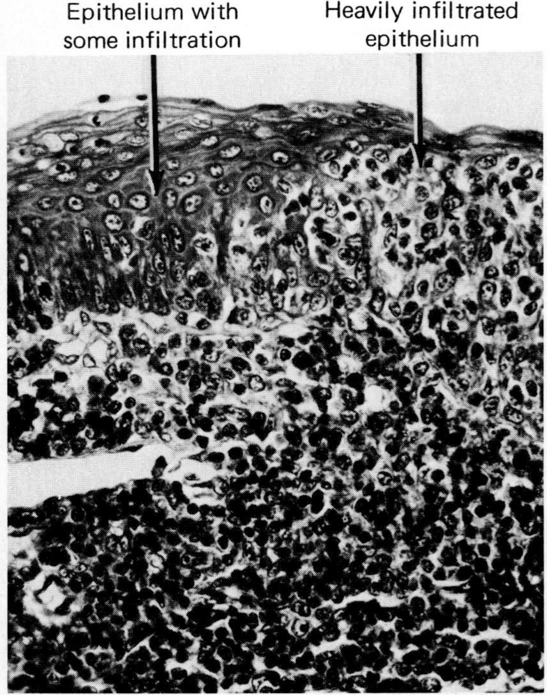

Figure 4-7. Photomicrograph of a palatine tonsil. The stratified squamous epithelium and submucosa is infiltrated by lymphocytes. The tonsil is part of Waldeyer's ring of lymphoid tissue in the oropharynx. In most tonsillectomy specimens, numerous reactive centers will be present—evidence of an active immune response. (Reproduced, with permission, from Junqueira LC, Carneiro J, Kelley RO: *Basic Histology,* 6th ed. Appleton & Lange, 1989.)

tral, irregularly shaped nucleus characterized by folds and grooves, fine chromatin, and a nucleolus. T immunoblasts are difficult to distinguish morphologically from B immunoblasts. Effector T lymphocytes morphologically resemble resting small lymphocytes and are often termed **sensitized, cytotoxic,** or **killer** T cells (Fig 4–11 and Table 4–2).

This process of T cell transformation constitutes the **amplification phase** of the immune response (Fig 4–1), during which the few T cells bearing receptors that recognize the particular antigen form a clone of numerous **effector T cells** reactive against the same antigen because they also have the appropriate receptor. The entire process of T cell activation begins when macrophages intercept an antigen; by some mechanism that is not yet clearly understood, they "process" the antigen and reexpress it at the cell surface in conjunction with MHC molecules before presenting it to the T cell. Recognition occurs if the T cell bears the specific receptor able to recognize the antigen-MHC duplex.

Table 4-1. Selected monoclonal antibodies employed for leukocyte identification and their corresponding CD antigens.[1]

CD Antigen	Corresponding Monoclonal Antibodies	Principal Leukocytes Expressing the Antigen
CD1	OKT6, Leu6	Thymocytes
CD2	OKT11	T cells and NK cells (E rosette receptor)
CD3	OKT3, Leu4	Mature T cells (Pan-T)
CD4	OKT4, Leu3	"Helper-inducer" T cells
CD5	OKT1, Leu1[2]	T cells (Pan-T)[2]
CD8	OKT8, Leu2	"Suppressor-cytotoxic" T cells
CD9	BA-2	Subset of B cells
CD10	CALLA	Cells of common acute lymphoblastic leukemia
CD11	OKM1, Mo-1	Monocytes, granulocytes, NK cells (C3b receptor)
CD15	Leu M1	Monoctyes, granulocytes
CD20	B1	Most B cells
CD24	BA-1	Early B cells
CD45	CLA	Most leukocytes (common leukocyte antigen)
CD57	NK-1, Leu7	Natural killer cells
CD71	OKT9	Monocytes, early lymphoctyes (transferrin receptor)
CD75	LN-1	B cells in follicular center phase
None assigned	PC-1	Plasma cells

[1]The CD (cluster designation) terminology for leukocyte antigens has been recommended by the World Health Organization following a series of international workshops.

[2]Note that as new data become available, it is apparent that expression of many of these antigens is not wholly restricted to a single cell lineage, eg, the Pan-T cell antibodies OKT1 and Leu1 (CD5) also react with a subset of normal B cells and with B cell lymphocytic leukemia.

C. Functions of Effector T Cells: Effector T cells play important roles in 3 functions of the immune system.

1. Cell-mediated immunity-Cell-mediated immunity incorporates 2 main aspects.

a. Cytotoxicity-Cells bearing surface antigens that are recognized by effector T cells are subject to direct cell killing by the T cells (cytotoxic or killer cells). Direct toxicity occurs in immunologic response to antigens on the surface of neoplastic cells, transplanted tissues, and virus-infected cells. Cytotoxic T cells apparently cause lysis by pro-

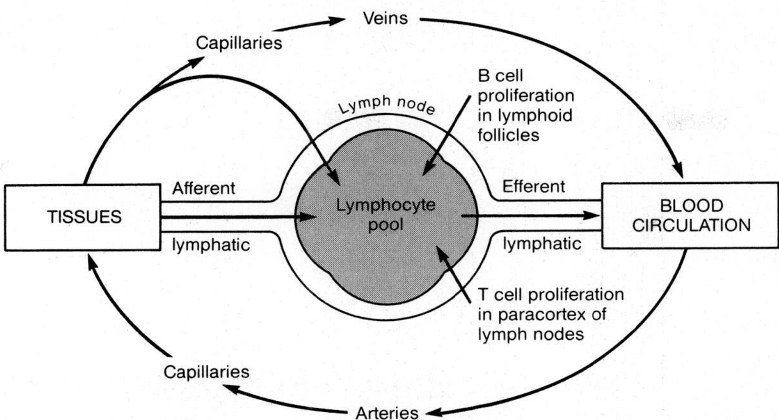

Figure 4-8. Diagrammatic representation of lymphocyte exchange between lymph nodes, tissues, and blood. Lymphocytes enter the node via afferent lymphatics and through specialized postcapillary venules that favor egress of lymphocytes into the node. Lymphocyte proliferation occurs in the lymph node in response to any antigen present, and the progeny leave via efferent lymphatics, thereby disseminating the immune response throughout the body.

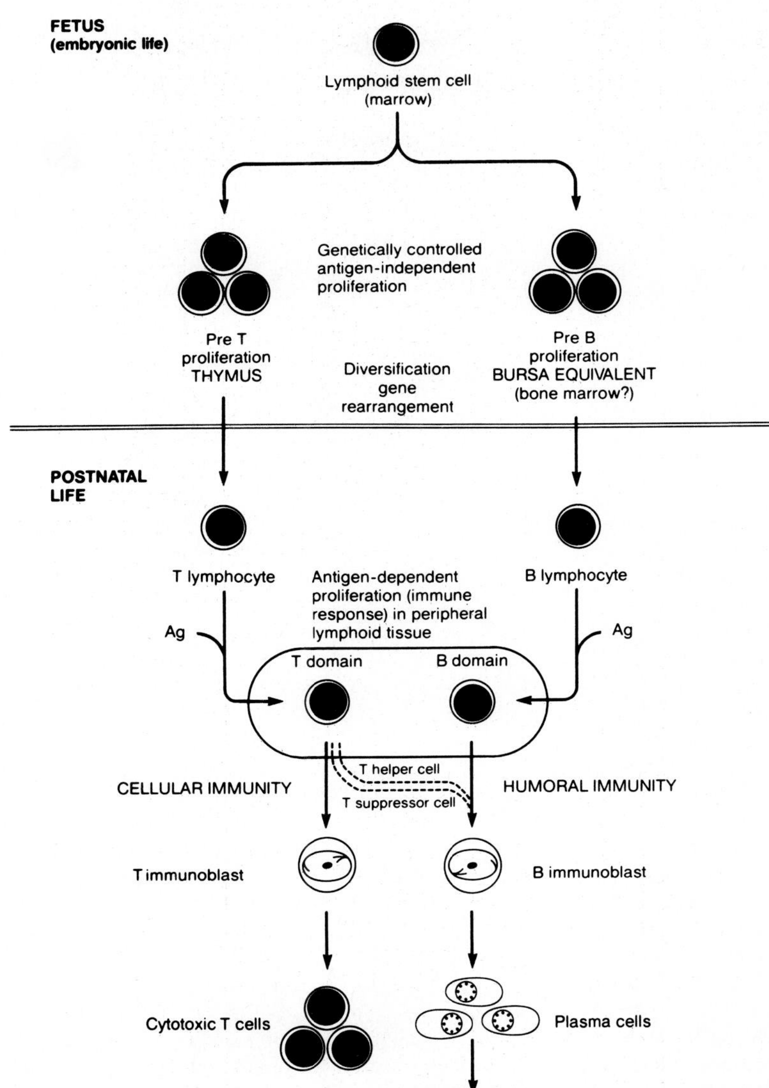

Figure 4-9. Lymphocyte proliferation. Lymphocyte proliferation in the embryo is genetically controlled—a small number of stem cells proliferate to produce the numerous T and B lymphocytes populating the lymphoid tissues at birth. Diversification of antigen receptors (Figs 4-18 and 4-19) takes place at this stage. Lymphocyte proliferation in postnatal life occurs as part of the immune response—only those lymphocytes capable of recognizing a particular antigen respond to produce effector cells which respond to that antigen.

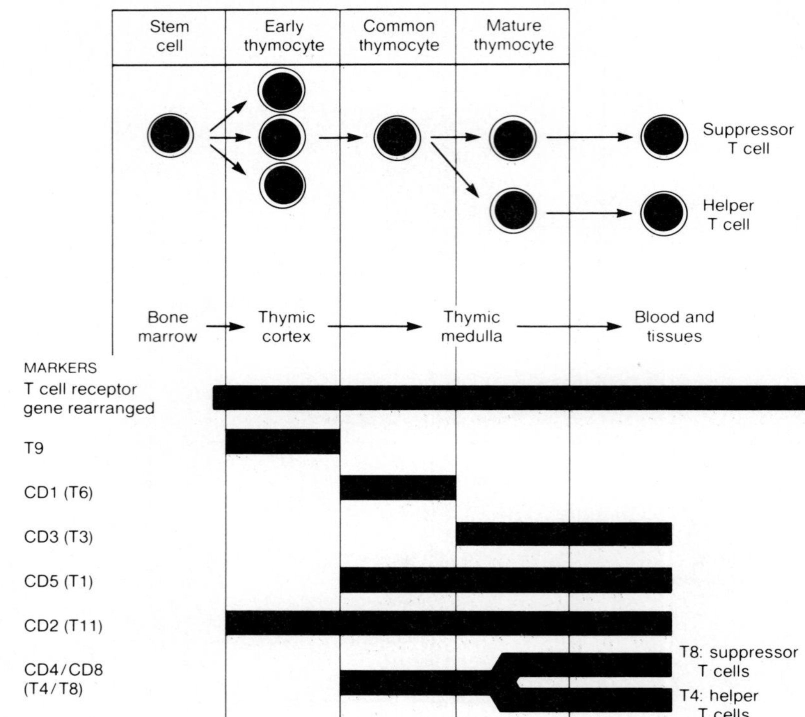

Figure 4-10. T cell development in the human fetal thymus, depicting the appearance and disappearance of T cell phenotypic markers—detected by monoclonal antibodies—during T cell proliferation and maturation.

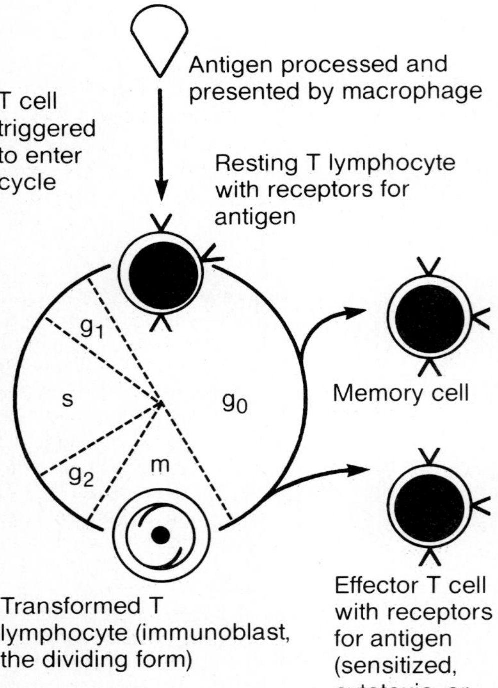

Figure 4-11. T cell transformation in the immune response occurs when T cells are activated by antigen that has been processed by an antigen-processing cell (macrophage). This interaction induces T cell proliferation. The T cell enters the S phase of the cell cycle with RNA and protein synthesis prior to mitotic cell division (M). The daughter cells either reenter the cycle, revert to resting "memory cells," or leave the cycle to mature to effector T cells. In practice, several cycles occur sequentially during the immune response prior to the production of effector cells. G_1 = gap 1; S = synthesis phase; G_2 = gap 2; M = mitosis; G_0 = resting phase.

Table 4–2. Morphologic and functional attributes of lymphoid cells.

Morphology	Name	Functional Groups
	Small lymphocyte	1. Resting lymphocytic stem cells. 2. Resting mature T cells bearing antigen receptors. 3. Resting mature B cells bearing antigen receptors (immunoglobulin). 4. Cytotoxic, sensitized, killer, or effector T cells. 5. B and T memory cells (probably equivalent to resting sensitized B and T cells). 6. Helper and suppressor T cells. 7. Null (or nonmarking) cells (includes NK cells).
	Lymphoblast[1]	1. Actively dividing stem cells. 2. Actively dividing T and B cells in embryonic life.
	Immunoblast[1] (transformed lymphocyte)	1. Dividing, antigenically stimulated T cell (progenitor of sensitized effector T cell). 2. Dividing, antigenically stimulated B cell (progenitor of plasma cell).
	Follicular center cell	Intermediate cell found during antigen-stimulated B cell proliferation in lymphoid follicles. Several morphologic stages (cleaved versus noncleaved; small versus large) are recognized.
	Plasma cell	End stage of B cell differentiation (immunoglobulin-secreting cell).

[1]Although immunoblasts and lymphoblasts are morphologically distinct, some authorities do not make a distinction between them. Both are dividing forms of the lymphocyte and have the primitive-appearing (blast) nucleus of proliferating cells. Lymphoblasts represent the rapidly dividing lymphocytes of the fetus; the name underlines a close morphologic resemblance to the cells of acute lymphoblastic leukemia. The term immunoblast was coined for the dividing lymphocyte that occurs as part of the immune response and gives rise to immunocytes (ie, lymphocytes and plasma cells).

ducing holes in the surface membranes of antigen-positive cells.

b. Production of lymphokines–Effector T cells play a crucial role in regulating the immune response by producing soluble proteins **(lymphokines)** that regulate the functions of certain cells, eg, macrophages and other lymphocytes (Table 4–3).

2. Regulation of B lymphocyte activity–Two important subtypes of T lymphocytes are instrumental in regulating the function of B lymphocytes. **Helper T cells** (CD4 antigen-positive) assist in activation and transformation of B lymphocytes and in immunoglobulin production. **Suppressor T cells** (CD8 antigen-positive) inhibit B cell activation and regulate immunoglobulin synthesis. Helper and suppressor T cells also display similar regulatory effects in cell-mediated immunity. The normal ratio of helper T lymphocytes to suppressor T lymphocytes (CD4/CD8 ratio) in peripheral blood is 0.9–2.7, with some variation in very young or very old people. This ratio may be greatly decreased in certain diseases, including immunodeficiency states and AIDS.

3. Delayed hypersensitivity–See Chapter 8.

D. Identification of T Cell Subpopulations: T lymphocytes and their subsets cannot be distinguished morphologically either from one another or from B lymphocytes and are best characterized by the presence of antigens that are specific for each subpopulation and therefore act as immunologic markers. These antigens are detected by specific monoclonal antibodies that have been developed against different subpopulations of lymphocytes (Fig 4–10 and Table 4–1). Use of these antibodies also permits localization of the various T lymphocyte subpopulations in lymphoid tissue using immunofluorescence or immunoperoxidase methods. Genetic techniques detecting rearrangement of T cell receptor genes are also useful in recognizing T cells. Other markers such as the E rosette test are obsolete.

B Lymphocytes

A. Distribution of B Cells in the Body: B lymphocytes develop in the functional equivalent of the avian bursa of Fabricius (probably the fetal bone marrow in mammals) through a complex

Table 4–3. Lymphokines (cytokines).[1]

Lymphokine	Action	Source
MIF (migration inhibitory factor)	Inhibits random macrophage migration.	T cells
MAF (macrophage-activating factor)	Enhances lytic action of macrophages.	T cells
γ-Interferon	Enhances lytic action of macrophages.	T cells
Fibroblast-activating factor	Induces proliferation of fibroblasts.	T cells
B cell growth factor (BCGF)	Stimulates B cell proliferation.	T cells
B cell differentiation factor (BCDF)	Induces differentiation of B cell progeny to plasma cells	T cells
Interleukin-2 (T cell growth factor)	Stimulates T cell proliferation.	T cells
Interleukin-3 (similar to colony-stimulating factor)	Supports monocyte proliferation.	T cells
Interleukin-1 (endogenous pyrogen)	Promotes immunoglobulin production by B cells and differentiation of T cells; may enhance NK activity plus other cell types affected.	Macrophages[2]
β-Interferon	May inhibit growth of several cell types, including tumor cells.	Macrophages
Angiogenesis factor	Stimulates new capillary formation.	Macrophages

[1]Strictly speaking, only factors released by T lymphocytes can be called lymphokines; however, the term is sometimes used loosely to include the products of macrophages. "Cytokines" is a more general term denoting hormonelike mediators secreted during immune and inflammatory reactions.
[2]Macrophages = monocytes in blood; histiocytes in tissue.

process involving multiplication and diversification (Fig 4–12). B lymphocytes are then distributed by the circulation to the B cell domains of the peripheral lymphoid tissue. These areas include (1) primary and reactive (secondary or germinal) follicles or centers and medullary sinuses of the lymph nodes (Fig 4–5; 30% of lymphocytes in the lymph nodes are B cells); and (2) reactive centers in the malpighian bodies of the splenic white pulp (Fig 4–6; 40% of splenic lymphocytes are B cells). Like T cells, B cells also recirculate between lymphoid tissues and peripheral blood (Fig 4–8), though less actively. Ten to twenty percent of peripheral blood lymphocytes are B cells.

B. B Cell Transformation: Following stimulation by either a specific antigen or a nonspecific mitogen such as pokeweed mitogen, B lymphocytes are transformed through a series of intermediate stages into **plasma cells** (Figs 4–1, 4–13, and 4–16). Plasma cells synthesize immunoglobulins (antibodies) that are specific for the stimulating antigen. The production of circulating antibodies against specific antigens is the cornerstone of the type of acquired immunity called **humoral immunity**.

C. Identification of B Cells: Plasma cells have a distinctive morphologic appearance (Table 4–2). They are 12–15 μm in diameter and have abundant basophilic cytoplasm in which a prominent Golgi zone is visible as a pale area (hof) on one side of the nucleus. (The basophilia is due to the presence of RNA required for synthesis of immunoglobulin.) The nucleus is eccentrically placed, with chromatin distributed in coarse clumps at its periphery ("cartwheel" or "clockface" pattern). Immunoglobulin can be demonstrated in the cytoplasm by immunologic techniques and often accumulates in plasma cells to such an extent that it is visible on light microscopy as eosinophilic globules. (Russell bodies are cytoplasmic accumulations of immunoglobulin; Dutcher bodies are invaginated into the nucleus.)

Whereas plasma cells are easily identified on the basis of their distinctive morphology, other B lymphocytes must be identified by immunologic or genetic techniques (Fig 4–12). Immunofluorescence or immunoperoxidase techniques using antibodies to human immunoglobulin detect the presence of synthesized immunoglobulin. B lymphocytes express immunoglobulin on their surfaces, whereas plasma cells, which are highly differentiated B lymphocytes, contain large amounts of cytoplasmic immunoglobulin but express little surface immunoglobulin. Specific monoclonal antibodies that react to B cells are also used (Table 4–1). Monoclonal antibodies against B cells are at present less well characterized than the corresponding antibodies against T cells. Genetic techniques that detect the presence of rearranged immunoglobulin genes can also help to identify B lymphocytes.

Null Cells (NK Cells & K Cells)

Null cells are a heterogeneous group of lymphocytes defined by an inability to form E rosettes (an immunologic test formerly used to identify T

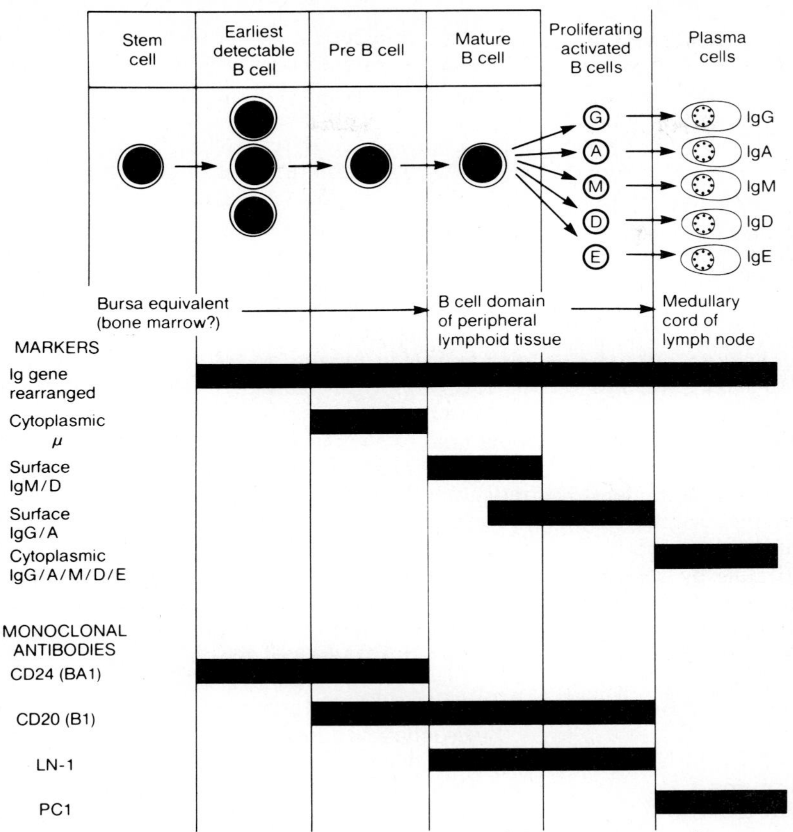

Figure 4–12. B cell development in the embryo and in postnatal life. Like T cell differentiation, B cell differentiation occurs in the embryo and is accompanied by phenotypic changes. Gene rearrangement occurs, involving the immunoglobulin genes, to produce a multiplicity of B cells, each potentially able to produce immunoglobulins of a different specificity (see also Fig 4–16). Expansion of this population gives rise to the B cells present at birth. Exposure to antigens postnatally produces selective proliferation of B cells able to recognize the antigen. The end result is differentiation of plasma cells and production of antibody. Surface immunoglobulins and other phenotypic markers are expressed at various times during this differentiation process.

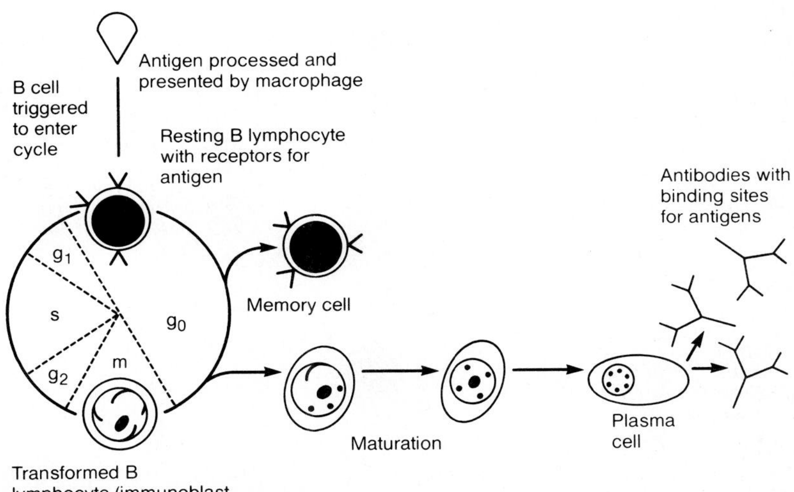

Figure 4–13. B cell transformation in the immune response begins with reaction of an antigen with specific receptors on the surface of the B cell: for most antigens, participation of helper T cells and antigen-processing cells (macrophages) is necessary at this stage. The B cell then enters the cell cycle from the resting stage to begin proliferation. Before mitosis, the activated (transformed) B cell is termed a B immunoblast. After mitosis, the daughter cells either reenter the cell cycle, revert to resting B lymphocytes (memory cells), or leave the cell cycle to mature to plasma cells after passing through intermediate forms termed plasmablasts. Maturation occurs not in a single cycle but over 6–8 successive cycles.

lymphocytes) and by lack of surface immunoglobulin (hence nonmarking or "null" cells). This group includes some cells that are demonstrably T or B cells by recently developed genetic techniques or by monoclonal antibody studies, and the designation should perhaps be abandoned. A proportion of null cells clearly represent cells early in the T or B cell differentiation pathways prior to expression of many surface markers (Figs 4–10 and 4–12). Null cells account for 5–10% of peripheral blood lymphocytes.

Null cells are often naturally cytotoxic and are called **natural killer (NK) cells;** they can lyse some foreign cells even if the organism has never been exposed to the inciting antigen. Some null cells (termed **K cells)** participate in cell destruction with the aid of antibody (antibody-dependent cell-mediated cytotoxicity [ADCC]). There is evidence that NK cell activity and ADCC (K cell) activity may be 2 different functions of the same cell type (Fig 4–14). NK cells are identifiable by use of a monoclonal antibody termed anti-NK-1 (or, more recently, Leu-7). NK cells may have a protective role in cancer, serving to eliminate potentially neoplastic cells.

MACROPHAGES (Monocytes of Blood; Histiocytes of Tissues)

Distribution in the Body

Macrophages are distinct from lymphocytes but also play an important supporting role in the immune response, both as **antigen-processing cells** at the initiation of the response and as **phagocytes** at the effector stage. In blood they are termed monocytes; in tissue, histiocytes or tissue macrophages. Bone marrow reconstitution studies in animals and humans (including bone marrow transplants) provide good evidence that all macrophages are derived from monocyte precursors in bone marrow. Macrophages are found in all tissues of the body as tissue histiocytes but are present in greater numbers in lymph nodes, both diffusely and arranged in subcapsular and medullary sinuses (Fig 4–5). Tissue macrophages also line the sinusoids in the red pulp of the spleen (Fig 4–6). In the liver, macrophages are known as Kupffer cells, and they also appear in lung as alveolar macrophages and in brain tissue as microglial cells. In peripheral blood and bone marrow, they appear as monocytes and their precursors. **Dendritic reticulum cells** in the lymph node follicles and **interdigitating reticulum cells** in the paracortical zone are special antigen-handling cells for B and T lymphocytes, respectively (Fig 4–5): Although their derivation is uncertain, they are thought to be related to the macrophage series. In the older literature, the term reticuloendothelial system was used to encompass all of these cell types.

Identification of Macrophages

Macrophages contain numerous specific cytoplasmic enzymes and may be identified in tissues by histochemical techniques that detect these enzymes. Macrophages show direct histochemical staining for several enzymes (eg, nonspecific esterase) simply by addition of the appropriate substrate, whereas other enzymes, such as muramidase (lysozyme) and chymotrypsin, may be demonstrated by labeled antibody (immunohistochemical) methods using antibodies directed against the enzyme proteins. Monoclonal antibod-

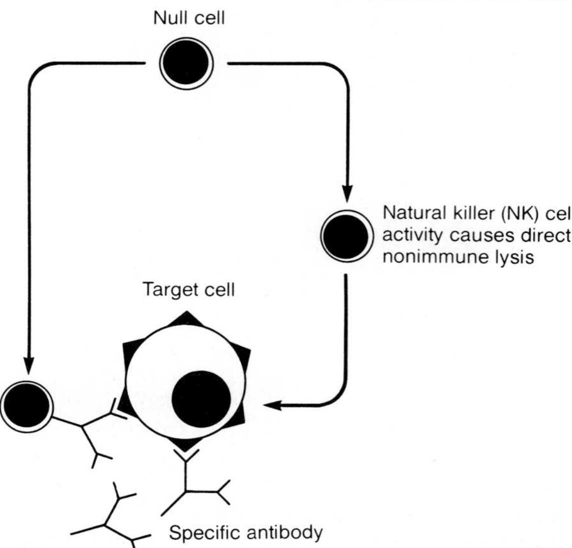

Figure 4–14. NK cell activity and antibody-dependent cell-mediated cytotoxicity (ADCC) may be 2 functional expressions of the same cell (null cell). In antibody-dependent cell-mediated cytotoxicity, the antibody binds to antigenic determinants on the target cell. The K cell then attaches to the target cell with its Fc receptor (which links to the Fc part of the bound antibody), and lysis results. NK cells, on the other hand, cause direct cell lysis that is not mediated by an immune response and does not involve an antigen-antibody interaction.

ies (Leu M1 [CD15], OKM1, Mo-1 [CD11]; see Table 4–1) have also been prepared against monocyte-macrophage antigens, but the significance of macrophage subpopulations identified by these different antigens has not been established.

Functions of Macrophages

Macrophage functions include phagocytosis, antigen processing, and interaction with lymphokines.

A. Phagocytosis:

1. Nonimmune phagocytosis–Macrophages are able to phagocytose foreign particulate matter, microorganisms, and the debris of cellular injury directly, without evoking the immune response. However, microbial phagocytosis and killing by macrophages are greatly facilitated by the presence of specific immunoglobulin and complement and by lymphokines produced by immunologically activated T lymphocytes (Table 4–3).

2. Immune phagocytosis–Macrophages have surface receptors for C3b and the Fc fragment of immunoglobulins. Any particle that is coated with immunoglobulin or complement (ie, opsonization has occurred) is phagocytosed more readily than "naked" particles (see Chapter 3).

B. Processing of Antigens: Macrophages process antigens and present them to B and T lymphocytes in a suitable form (Fig 4–1); this cellular interaction involves simultaneous recognition by lymphocytes of MHC molecules and processed antigens displayed on the surface of macrophages.

C. Interaction With Lymphokines: Macrophages interact with lymphokines produced by T lymphocytes (macrophage-activating factor, macrophage inhibitory factor, gamma-interferon) to defend the body against certain injurious agents. Formation of granulomas is a typical result of such interaction. Macrophages also produce lymphokinelike factors, including interleukin-1, beta-interferon, and T and B cell growth-promoting factors (Table 4–3). The various interactions of lymphocytes and macrophages in the tissues are manifested morphologically as chronic inflammation.

IMMUNOGLOBULINS (Antibodies)

Synthesis of Immunoglobulins

Immunoglobulins are synthesized by plasma cells that differentiate from transformed, antigen-stimulated B lymphocytes (B immunoblasts). All immunoglobulin molecules synthesized by a single plasma cell are identical and have specific reactivity against a single antigenic determinant. Likewise, all plasma cells derived through transformation and proliferation of a single B lymphocyte precursor are identical; ie, they constitute a clone (Fig 4–16). Immunoglobulin molecules synthesized by members of different clones of plasma cells have different amino acid sequences that produce different molecular tertiary structures and impart different specificities to the antibody (ie, they react with different antigens). These differences in amino acid sequences occur in the so-called V (variable) region of the immunoglobulin molecule (Fig 4–15).

Structure of Immunoglobulins (Fig 4–15)

The basic immunoglobulin molecule is composed of 2 heavy (H) chains and 2 light (L) chains connected by disulfide bonds. **Light chains** consist of either 2 κ chains or 2 λ chains. **Heavy chains** may be one of 5 varieties, and it is these variations that define the class of immunoglobulin (IgA, IgG, IgM, IgD, IgE) (Table 4–4). Several subclasses of heavy chains exist. These various immunoglobulin chains are themselves antigenic if injected into animals **(isotypes),** and the antibodies produced against them in animals may be used to recognize and distinguish the different light chain types and heavy chain classes in humans.

Each chain has a constant and a variable part. The **constant part** remains constant in amino acid sequence and antigenicity within an immunoglobulin class; the **variable part,** in contrast, is characterized by widely divergent amino acid sequences. The antigen-combining (binding) sites are in the variable region of the chain. Each IgG molecule consists of 2 paired chains that form 2 binding sites (Fig 4–15). In the variable part of each chain are hypervariable regions—3 in the light chains and 4 in the heavy chains. Amino acid sequence variations in these hypervariable regions determine the specificity of antibody. These hypervariable regions may also serve as antigens **(idiotypes)** if injected into other animals under suitable conditions. The anti-idiotype antibody produced against the hypervariable region has a restricted range of reactivity and combines only with immunoglobulin molecules having that hypervariable region. In essence, the reactivity of an anti-idiotype antibody is restricted to antibody of a particular specificity derived from a single clone. While the above description applies strictly to IgG, the other immunoglobulin classes all show the same basic unitary structure—except that IgM is a pentamer (ie, consists of 5 basic units linked at the Fc ends) and IgA commonly exists as a dimer.

The **constant region** of each immunoglobulin molecule has receptors for complement and is the **Fc fragment** that binds with those cells having Fc receptors (as occurs in antibody-dependent cell-mediated cytotoxicity [Fig 4–14]). Inherited antigenic differences between heavy chains constitute **allotypes.**

Immunoglobulin molecules may be cleaved by various proteolytic enzymes. **Papain digestion**

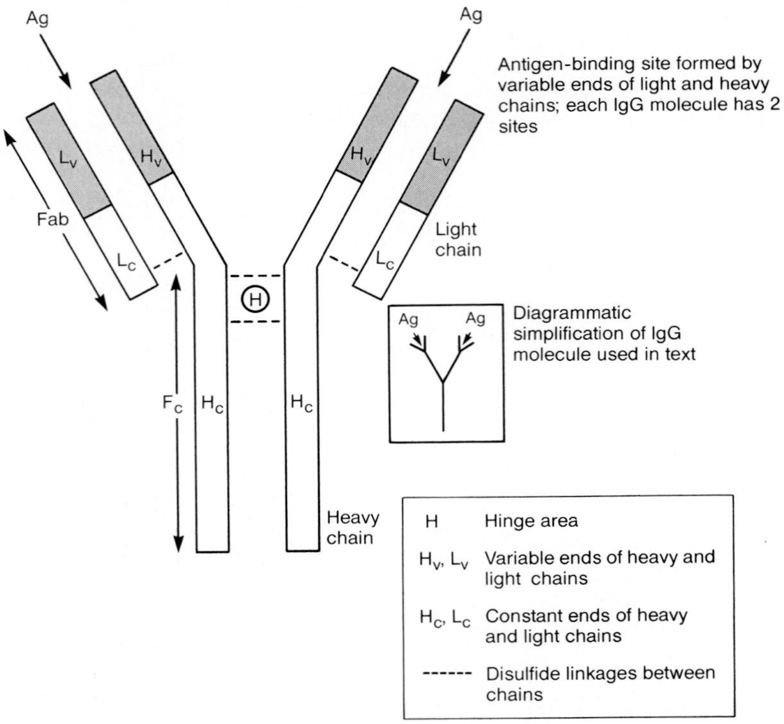

Figure 4–15. Structure of the basic immunoglobulin molecule (IgG). IgD and IgE have a similar structure; secreted IgA is a dimer of this configuration; and IgM is a pentamer. Fab and Fc are fragments produced by enzyme digestion of the immunoglobulin molecule at the hinge region. Fc contains part of both heavy chains; Fab contains a light chain and part of a heavy chain, with one antigen-binding site. $F(ab)'_2$ represents 2 Fab units still conjoined. The structure, as shown, is simplified by omission of polypeptide loops stabilized by disulfide bonds in both heavy and light chains.

Table 4–4. Classes of immunoglobulins.

Property	IgG	IgM	IgA[1]	IgD	IgE
Heavy chain	γ	μ	α	δ	ε
Subclasses	4	2	2	–	–
Light chain	κ or λ	κ or λ	κ or λ	κ or λ	κ or λ
Molecular weight	150,000	900,000	160,000[1]	150,000	190,000
Sedimentation coefficient	7S	19S	7S	7S	7S
Valence[2]	2	10	2	2	2
Complement fixation	+	++	–	–	–
Placental transfer	+	–	–	–	–
Serum concentration (mg/mL)	13–15	0.5	1.9	0.03	0.0003
Half-life (days)	14–21	5	5	3	1

[1]Note that IgA is formed in plasma cells as a monomer (MW 160,000) and is secreted through epithelia as a dimer, a process that involves linkage of two IgA monomers by J chain, then combination with a secretor piece (or secretory component; see Fig 4–17). The final molecular weight is 380,000. Secretory component is produced by epithelial cells and is believed to facilitate secretion of IgA across membranes as well as to protect the molecule from enzymatic digestion.

[2]The number of antigen-binding sites per molecule.

cleaves the molecule at the hinge region (Fig 4–15) into 2 Fab (antibody) fragments and one Fc (crystallizable) fragment. **Pepsin digestion** produces an $F(ab)'_2$ fragment and an Fc fragment. The Fc fragment represents the constant region; the invariability of the amino acid sequence is a major reason why it is crystallizable. The Fab and $F(ab)'_2$ fragments carry one and 2 antigen-binding sites, respectively. The Fc component carries certain antigens, including those that permit immunologic distinction of the 5 major classes. The complement-binding site is also in the Fc portion. Digestion and fragmentation of the immunoglobulin molecule in this way have no physiologic significance; however, this approach was of historical importance in elucidating the structure of immunoglobulins, and it is still valuable in the experimental analysis of immune reactions.

Regulation of Antibody Production

Antibody production is initiated by activation of responsive B cells by antigen. Serum levels peak in 1 or 2 weeks and then begin to decline (Fig 4–22). Continued presence of free antigen tends to sustain the response, while increasing levels of antibody facilitate removal of antigen and thereby reduce B cell stimulation. Other more refined regulatory mechanisms also exist. **Helper T cells** (CD4-positive) play a vital role in initiating the B cell response to many antigens, and their continuing presence augments antibody production. This effect is due, at least in part, to release of lymphokines such as BCGF and BCDF (Table 4–3; B cell growth and differentiation factors, respectively). **Suppressor T cells** (CD8-positive) have the opposite effect, serving to down-regulate the immune response; suppression in its extreme form may be one mechanism underlying tolerance. One additional regulatory mechanism invokes the development of an **anti-idiotype network.** It has been proposed that in an immune response the production of a particular specific antibody inevitably is followed by production of second (anti-idiotype) antibody with specificity against the variable V sequences (idiotype or antigen-binding site) of the first antibody. The anti-idiotype antibody is capable of recognizing the idiotype component of the B cell antigen receptor (which is composed of immunoglobulin identical to the first antibody in terms of idiotype), thereby competing with antigen and serving to inhibit B cell activation.

ANTIGEN RECOGNITION & GENERATION OF ANTIGEN RECEPTOR DIVERSITY

Many different antibodies exist. Collectively, they react with a huge range of antigens. Likewise, a diverse array of T cells recognizes a wide variety of different antigens. The mechanisms responsible for generating recognition diversity have now been elucidated.

Specific antigen recognition is accomplished by lymphocytes that express receptors for antigen on their surfaces. Numerous receptors with differing specificities exist, displaying reactivity for the whole range of known antigens, but each individual lymphocyte expresses receptors for only a single antigen. It follows, therefore, that numerous (about 10^6–10^9) different lymphocytes exist, each expressing a single type of receptor.

The antigen receptor of B lymphocytes is immunoglobulin. A gene-shuffling mechanism (see below) produces diverse immunoglobulin molecules that serve as cell surface antigen receptors and eventually constitute the specific immunoglobulin (antibody) secreted by plasma cells following the immune response. In simplistic terms, the antigen selects lymphocytes that express receptors (ie, surface immunoglobulin of B cells) with reciprocal fit. This interaction induces the B cell to divide and transform, and it eventually produces a clone of plasma cells that secrete an antibody molecule with specific binding sites that are essentially the same as those expressed on the cell surface of the initial antigen-recognizing lymphocyte (Figs 4–1 and 4–16).

T lymphocytes also express antigen receptors, and the T cell population displays a similar degree of diversity. The T cell receptor consists of a pair of polypeptide chains (an alpha and a beta chain), each having a variable and constant region, thereby showing close resemblance to the B cell receptor (which is surface immunoglobulin). The T cell receptor is thus regarded as a member of the "immunoglobulin super family" that includes not only immunoglobulins but also other molecules involved in cell adhesion or cell recognition (Fig 4–17), all of which appear to share a common evolutionary origin. Recognition diversity of the T cell receptor is generated early in embryonic life by a gene-shuffling mechanism very similar to that occurring in the process of immunoglobulin diversification. Also in parallel with B cell activation, antigen selects T cells bearing receptors with the appropriate specificity, thereby inducing proliferation of a specific set of T cells, the net result of which is the generation of numerous effector T cells of identical specificity. Note that antigen recognition by T cells is complex, involving spatial interplay of antigen and MHC molecules on macrophages, with the T cell antigen receptor plus CD3 and CD4 or CD8 molecules on T cells. For helper T cells, MHC class II molecules participate; for suppressor and cytotoxic T cells, MHC class I molecules participate.

T cells bearing a receptor composed of gamma and delta chains have also been described; their function is at present unknown.

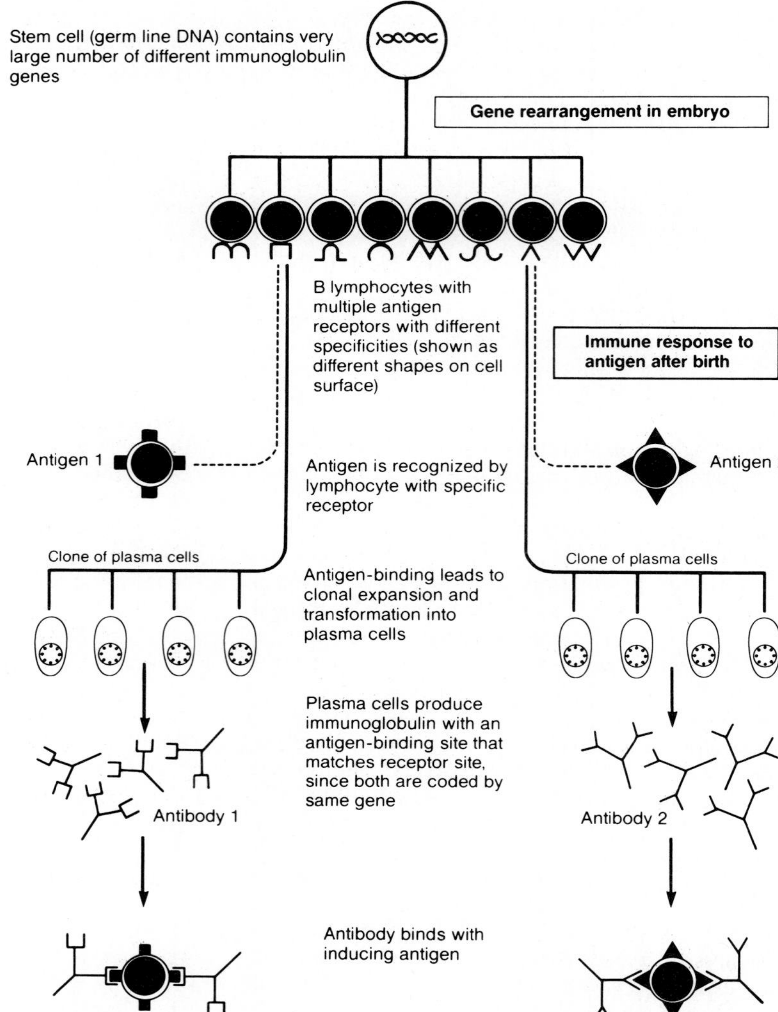

Figure 4–16. The B cell immune response, showing selective induction by antigen (the clonal selection hypothesis). Embryonic immunoglobulin gene rearrangement (Figs 4–18 and 4–19) results in multiple B lymphocytes bearing different surface immunoglobulin molecules that serve as the B cell antigen receptors (diversification). In postnatal life, antigen binds to specific receptors, thereby selecting and stimulating proliferation of the B cell bearing that receptor (clonal expansion). Differentiation to plasma cells follows. ***Note:*** T cell differentiation, selection, and clonal expansion occur in an analogous manner; clones of effector T cells specific for the inducing antigen are generated.

Generation of Diversity: Gene-"Shuffling" Mechanisms

The diversity of antigen receptors on B and T cells is generated at the DNA level during differentiation of lymphoid precursors in embryonic life. The genes involved are situated on chromosomes 2 (κ chain), 22 (λ chain), 8 (heavy chains), 14 (α chain of T cell receptor), and 7 (β chain of T cell receptor). Although each of these genes functions as a "gene unit" to produce a polypeptide chain, each exists in the germ line DNA as a complex "multigene" consisting of many different DNA segments that can be folded or spliced together in multiple arrangements to generate numerous different DNA templates (Figs 4–18 and 4–19). For example, the heavy chain multigene contains as many as 200 different V (variable) segments (V_H), each coding for a particular amino acid sequence that contributes to the binding site for antigen (variable region) of an immunoglobulin heavy chain. The heavy chain gene also contains multiple D (diversity), J (joining), and C (constant region) segments, one for each heavy chain class and subclass (μ, δ, γ_1, γ_2, γ_3, γ_4, α_1, α_2, ϵ). A splicing deletion mechanism brings together one DNA segment from each category to form a VDJC sequence that serves as the functional gene producing an RNA transcript and eventually a complete heavy chain. Light chains are similarly constituted except that they lack D segments. The beta chain T receptor gene also contains multiple V, D, J, and C genes, resembling heavy chain; while the alpha T receptor appears to contain only multiple V and J segments, with a single C region segment.

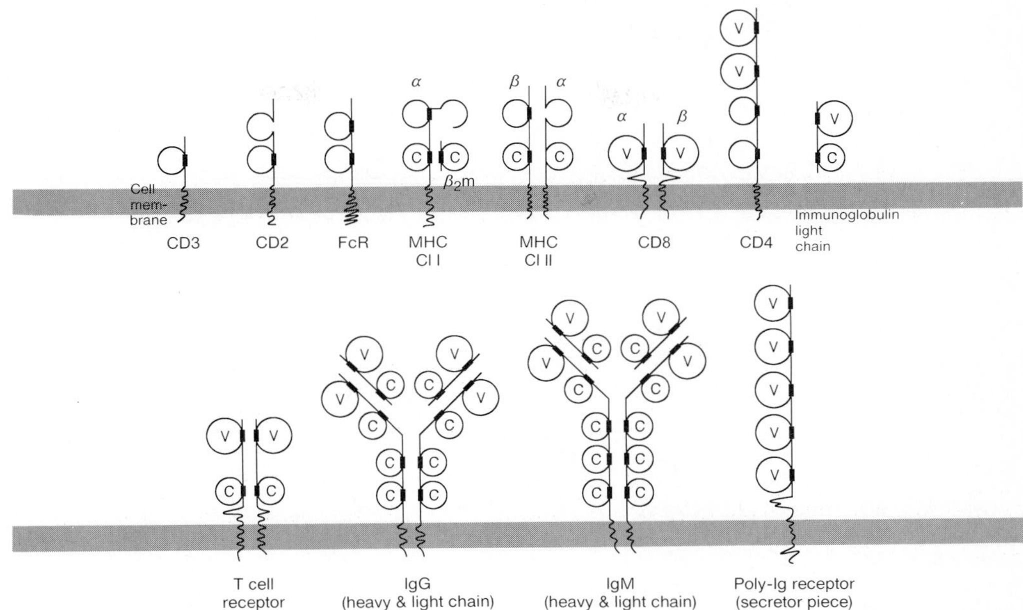

Figure 4–17. The immunoglobulin gene superfamily is defined as a series of genes that appear to share an evolutionary homology (ie, a common ancestry). Gene family members have in common the ability to code for polypeptide chains containing one or more peptide loops stabilized by disulfide bonds. In attempting to understand the complexities of the immune system, it may be helpful to realize that many of the surface molecules that play a part in cell recognition are closely related, including immunoglobulins, T cell antigen receptors, MHC molecules, and the T cell surface antigens CD2, CD3, CD4, and CD8. (See Hunkapiller T, Hood L: Adv Immunol 1989;44:1–63.)

(C) Homology units resembling those in immunoglobin constant region.

(V) Homology units resembling those in immunoglobulin variable region.

Peptide loops, homology not defined, but appearing to resemble primordial homology units.

Intrachain disulfide bridges.

FcR = Fc receptor.
MHC = major histocompatibility complex.
Cl I and Cl II = classes I and II.
Poly-IgR = receptor involved in transport of IgA and IgM across membranes. Secretor piece is that part of the molecule external to the cell surface. It detaches during transport.
β_2M = β_2 microglobulin associates with the MCH class I molecule.

EFFECT OF ANTIGEN-ANTIBODY INTERACTION (Fig 4–20)

Many immunoglobulins (antibodies) exert a direct effect on the antigens with which they specifically react; eg, formation of large aggregates may result in **precipitation** or **agglutination**. When the antigen is a toxin, antigen-antibody interaction may cause **neutralization** of the toxic action.

In some instances, binding of antibody to the surface of an antigenic particle (opsonization) causes it to be recognized by phagocytic cells such as macrophages and neutrophils that have Fc receptors on their surfaces. This process is called **immune phagocytosis.**

Interaction between antigen and antibody may cause structural alterations in the Fc fragment of the immunoglobulin molecule that lead to **activation of complement.**

COMPLEMENT

Activation of Complement

Complement is a system of plasma proteins (C1–C9) that exist in an inactive form and constitute about 10% of serum globulins. Activation of complement may occur in one of 2 ways (Fig 4–21).

A. Classic Pathway: The classic pathway of complement activation is initiated by the interaction of IgM or IgG with an antigen. The antigen-antibody interaction results in fixation of C1 to the Fc part of the antibody molecule. This activates C1q and then proceeds in cascade fashion (Fig 4-21). The early components (C1,4,2) form C3 convertase, which cleaves C3. The final C56789 complex exerts phospholipaselike activity and results in cell membrane lysis (note that the overall sequence is 1,4,2,3,5,6,7,8,9).

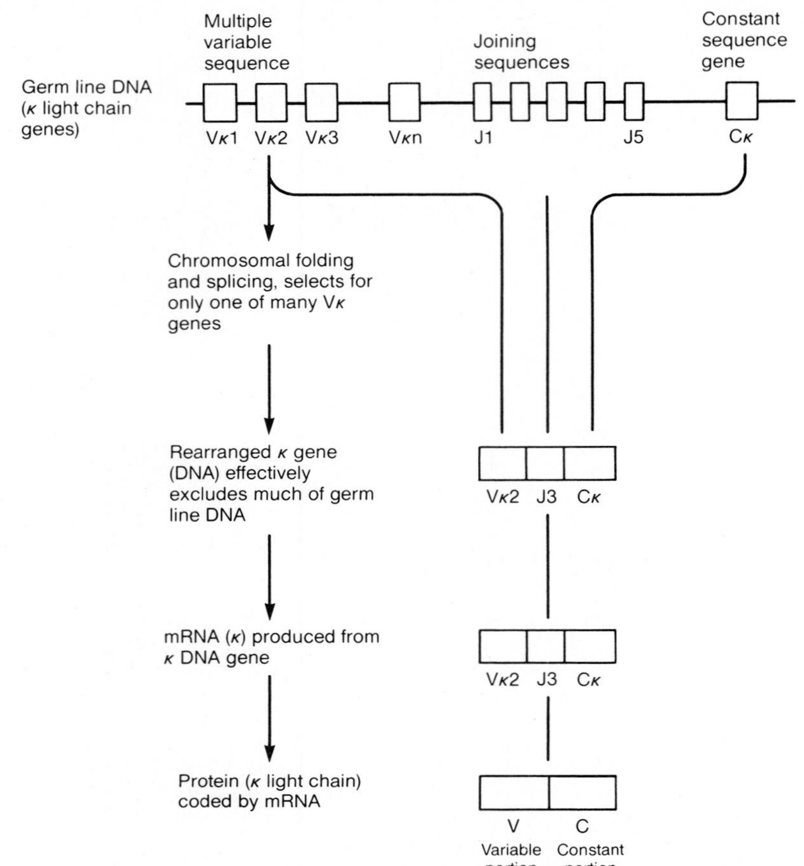

Figure 4-18. Generation of B lymphocyte antigen receptor (immunoglobulin) diversity through rearrangement of germline DNA coding for immunoglobulin. (Only kappa is represented in the figure; a similar process operates for lambda light chain and heavy chain.) This whole process occurs very early in B cell development and is antigen-independent. Detection of rearrangement of the immunoglobulin gene is now considered to be the earliest indication that a cell is committed to B cell differentiation. The T cell receptor gene undergoes an analogous series of rearrangements, thereby generating a diversity of T receptor sites.

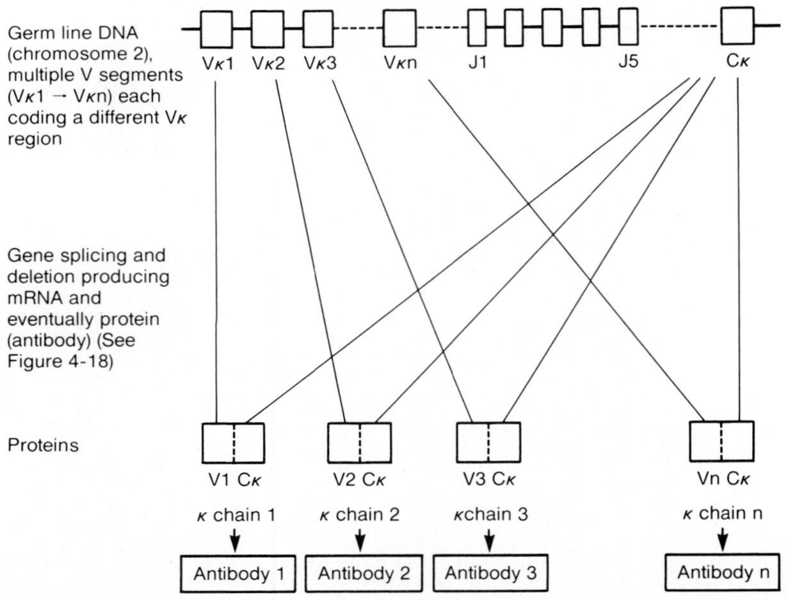

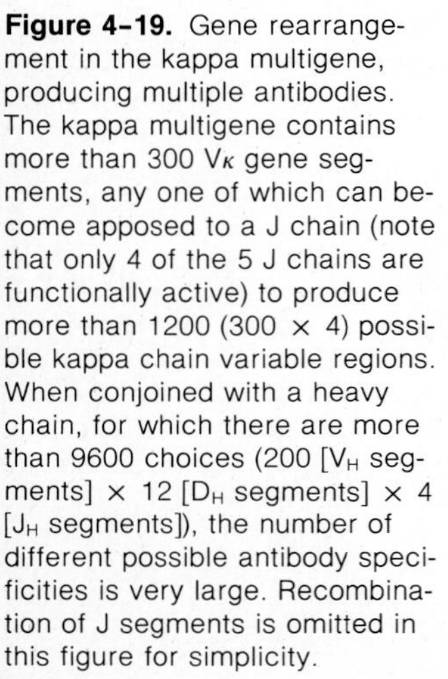

Figure 4-19. Gene rearrangement in the kappa multigene, producing multiple antibodies. The kappa multigene contains more than 300 Vκ gene segments, any one of which can become apposed to a J chain (note that only 4 of the 5 J chains are functionally active) to produce more than 1200 (300 × 4) possible kappa chain variable regions. When conjoined with a heavy chain, for which there are more than 9600 choices (200 [V_H segments] × 12 [D_H segments] × 4 [J_H segments]), the number of different possible antibody specificities is very large. Recombination of J segments is omitted in this figure for simplicity.

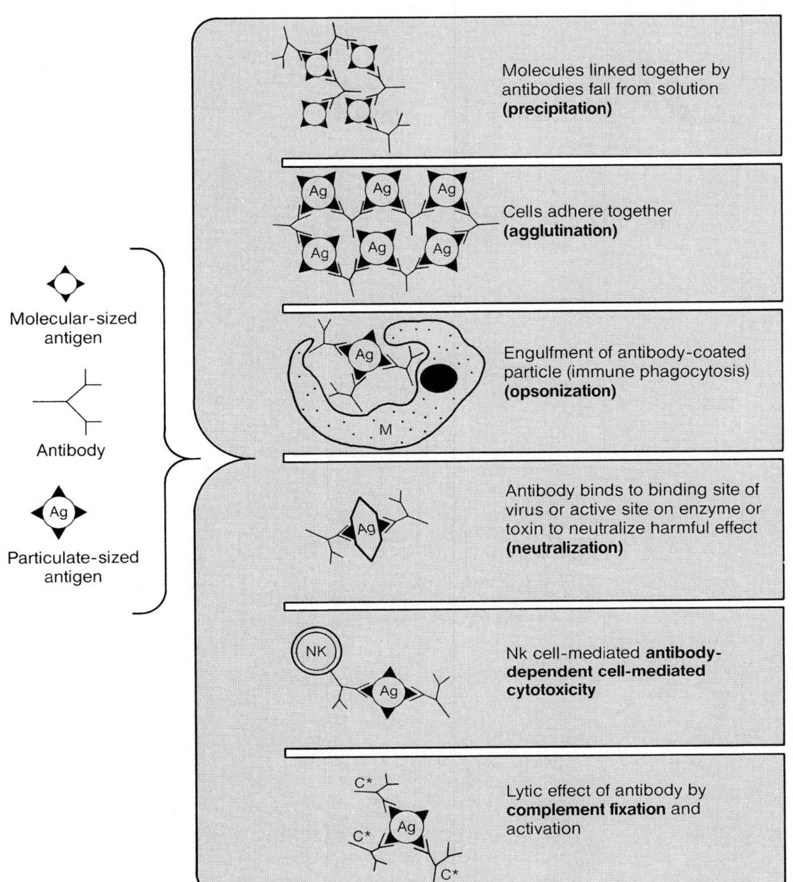

Figure 4-20. Reaction of antibody with antigen. The same or different antibodies acting in the ways depicted in the diagram have often been called precipitins, agglutinins, opsonins, lysins, or neutralizing antibodies, depending on the effect produced. M = macrophage; NK = natural killer cell; C* = complement.

B. Alternative Pathway (Properdin Pathway): The alternative pathway differs from the classic pathway only in its mechanism of activation and its early reactions. Cleavage of C3 in the alternative pathway does not require antigen-antibody interaction or the early (C1,C4,C2) complement factors. The cascade is initiated by aggregated IgG complexes, complex carbohydrates, and bacterial endotoxins. C3 convertase is formed by the interaction of properdin (a serum globulin), 2 other serum factors (B and D), and magnesium ions. The activation sequence after cleavage of C3 is the same as in the classic pathway.

Effects of Complement Activation

Complement activation is associated with an acute inflammatory response characterized by vasodilation, increased vascular permeability, and fluid exudation mediated by anaphylatoxic effects of C3a and C5a. Both C3a and C5a are strongly chemotactic for neutrophils, which enter the area. The antigen is removed by immune phagocytosis induced by the opsonic effect of attached C3b, by neutrophils and macrophages, or by membrane lysis resulting from the final product of the complement cascade.

TYPES OF IMMUNE RESPONSE

Memory is an essential component of the immune response because it facilitates an enhanced, more effective response upon second and subsequent exposure to a particular antigen. Based on whether the immune system has been previously exposed to the antigen or not, 2 types of immune response can be recognized.

The Primary Immune Response

The primary immune response is that which follows the first exposure to a particular antigen. Although antigen is recognized almost as soon as it is introduced into the body, several days elapse be-

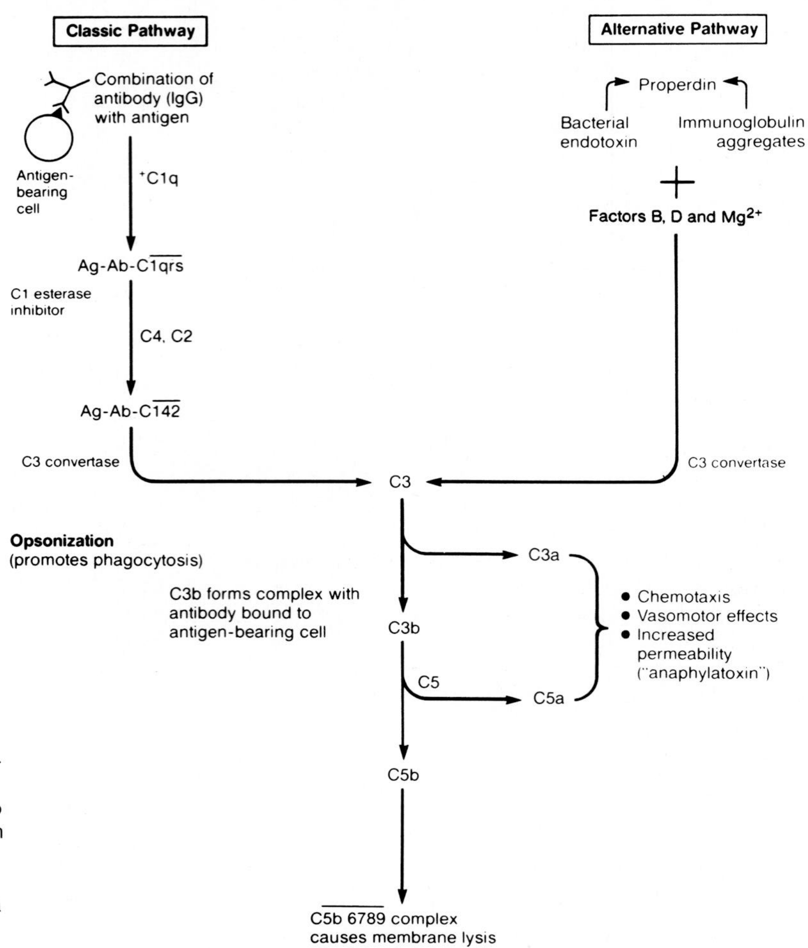

Figure 4-21. Activation of complement. The activated complement factors remain attached to the antigen-antibody complex on the surface of the antigen-bearing cell. Soluble complement fragments such as C3a and C5a are split off and pass into the surrounding interstitial tissue.

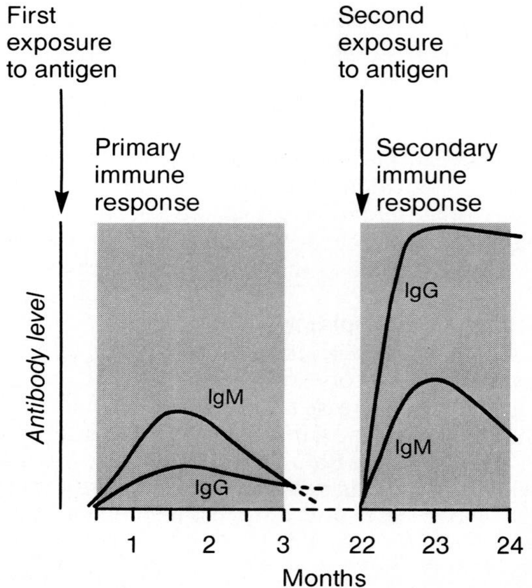

Figure 4-22. Primary and secondary immune responses. In the primary immune response (first exposure), serum antibody levels are detectable in 1–2 weeks and peak at 1–2 months before declining. IgM is the predominant antibody. In the secondary immune response, antibody appears much more rapidly (days), the peak is at a higher level, and antibody levels fall slowly (years). IgG is the predominant antibody.

fore enough immunoglobulin is produced to be detected as an increase in serum immunoglobulin levels (Fig 4–22). During this lag period, those B cells with receptors for that specific antigen undergo 6–8 successive division cycles to produce a large enough clone of antibody-secreting plasma cells. IgM is the first immunoglobulin produced during the primary response; IgG production follows. The change from IgM production to formation of IgG or other immunoglobulins occurs as a normal event in B cell activation and involves switching of the heavy chain genes. Immunoglobulin levels peak and then decline over several days (Fig 4–22).

The Secondary Immune Response

The secondary response follows repeat exposure to an antigen. Recognition again occurs immediately, but production of a detectable increase in serum immunoglobulins occurs much more rapidly (2–3 days) than in the primary response. IgG is the principal immunoglobulin secreted during the secondary response. In addition, peak levels are higher and the decline occurs much more slowly than in the primary response.

The ability to mount a specific secondary response is a function of **immunologic memory.** This specific response should be distinguished from a nonspecific increase in immunoglobulin levels (against antigens other than the inciting antigen) that may occur after antigenic stimulation—the so-called **anamnestic response,** which probably represents incidental stimulation of several B cells by lymphokines generated during the specific response.

Immunologic Memory

The mechanism underlying immunologic memory has not been satisfactorily explained. Following stimulation by antigen, lymphocyte proliferation (clonal expansion) occurs that produces a large number of effector cells (plasma cells in the B cell system; cytotoxic T cells in the T cell system) as well as other small lymphocytes that reenter the cycle and serve to replenish the pool of cells bearing the appropriate receptor (Figs 4–11 and 4–13). It has been argued that because these cells are the product of antigen-induced proliferation, they are capable of an enhanced response if they encounter the antigen again (ie, they act as **mem-**

Table 4–5. Diseases for which immunization is commonly used.

Disease	Immunizing Agent	Mechanism	Comments
Extremely effective; used routinely in USA			
Diphtheria, tetanus	Inactivated toxin[1]	Active	Routinely given in combination (DPT); 3 injections in first 2 years of life.
Pertussis (whooping cough)	Extracted antigen	Active	
Polio	Live attenuated virus	Active	Given orally
Measles, mumps, rubella	Live attenuated[2] virus	Active	Routinely given in combination (MMR) at 18 months; one injection gives lifelong immunity.
Partially effective			
Tuberculosis	Attenuated bacteria (BCG = bacillus Calmette-Guérin)	Active	Used in countries where tuberculosis is endemic; not used in USA routinely.
Effective; used in individuals traveling to endemic areas			
Typhoid	Killed bacteria	Active	Immunity lasts for 2–3 years only.
Cholera	Killed vibrio	Active	
Yellow fever	Live attenuated[2] virus	Active	—
Smallpox[3]	Attenuated[2] viral strain (vaccinia)	Active	Long-lasting immunity.
Effective; use restricted to individuals exposed to disease			
Hepatitis B	Hyperimmune serum	Passive	Short-lived protection: risk of complications.
Hepatitis A	Pooled human serum	Passive	
Tetanus	Antitoxin (horse serum)	Passive	
Rabies	Killed virus	Active	—

[1]Inactivated toxin is called toxoid.
[2]Attenuated; organism grown in culture until nonvirulent.
[3]Smallpox immunization is no longer required as the diseases has been eradicated from the world.

ory cells). In the B cell family, these cells may also have undergone the switch from producing IgM to IgG, and that change may explain the immediate production of IgG during the secondary immune response.

CLINICAL USES OF THE IMMUNE RESPONSE

Serologic Diagnosis of Infection

An understanding of the principles of the 2 types of immune response is helpful in the serologic diagnosis of infectious diseases. Early in the course of an infection, serologic tests for specific immunoglobulins will be negative. (***Caution:*** Negative results of serologic tests do not rule out the possibility of early disease.) After the first week of a primary response, IgM becomes detectable in serum, and levels increase rapidly but decline swiftly during convalescence. (***Note:*** Increased specific IgM indicates active or recent disease.) Rising levels of specific IgM or IgG on paired serum samples drawn several days apart are diagnostic of active infection (if the increase is greater than 4-fold). Note that IgG levels may increase slightly as a nonspecific anamnestic response; this is why a 4-fold increase in antibody levels is required for diagnosis. In contrast to IgM, IgG levels remain high for long periods after infection, so that elevated specific IgG levels may signify only past infection and not necessarily recent or active disease.

Immunization

Immunization represents the practical use of immunologic memory to provide protection against infectious diseases. Two major methods are available (Table 4–5):

(1) Passive immunization—the administration of antibody to an individual exposed to infection. Antibody may consist of pooled human serum (hepatitis A, rubella) or serum from an animal specifically immunized against an antigen (tetanus toxin). Passive immunization is protective only for a short period. A newborn baby has natural passive immunity due to the transplacental transfer of maternal antibodies. This natural passive immunity lasts about 6 months, and during this time the infant is protected against many common infections.

(2) Active immunization—the administration of antigens of the infectious agent, often repeatedly, to stimulate the host's immune response to produce high antibody levels and memory cells. This provides excellent long-term protection, and many childhood vaccines use the principle of active immunization. (***Note:*** The term "vaccination" is derived from Edward Jenner's use of cowpox—vaccinia virus—to prevent smallpox in 1796.)

Chronic Inflammation

5

Chronic inflammation is the sum of the responses mounted by the tissues against a persistent injurious agent: bacterial, viral, chemical, immunologic, etc. The tissues affected by chronic inflammation commonly show evidence of the following pathologic processes:

(1) Immune response: The immune response, both cell-mediated and humoral, is characterized by the presence of lymphocytes, plasma cells, and macrophages (Fig 5–1). Plasma immunoglobulin levels may be elevated. The immune response is directed against antigenic injurious agents.

(2) Phagocytosis: Immune phagocytosis is mediated by macrophages that have been activated by T cell lymphokines and involves antigens that have opsonins (immunoglobulins and complement factors) attached to their surfaces. Nonimmune phagocytosis is directed against foreign nonantigenic particles.

(3) Repair: Repair of tissues damaged by persistent injury is characterized by new blood vessel formation, fibroblastic proliferation, and collagen deposition (fibrosis). Damage to tissues may also result in alteration of self molecules such that they become antigenic and evoke an immune response.

Chronic inflammation may follow an acute inflammatory response that fails to vanquish the agent, or it may occur without a clinically apparent acute phase. Chronic inflammation is recognized and defined by its morphologic features (Table 5–1). It is distinguished from acute inflammation by the absence of cardinal signs such as redness, swelling, pain, and increased temperature. Active hyperemia, fluid exudation, and neutrophil emigration are absent in chronic inflammation. It is distinguished pathologically from acute inflammation by being of a duration that is long enough to permit the tissue manifestations of the immune response and repair. Most agents associated with chronic inflammation cause insidious but progressive and often extensive **tissue necrosis** accompanied by ongoing **repair by fibrosis**. The amount of fibrosis in the tissues is a function of the duration of chronic inflammation.

The specific features of chronic inflammation occurring in response to different noxious stimuli depend on the relative magnitude of each of the processes described above. For example, an agent that evokes a lymphokine-mediated response will produce chronic inflammation characterized by macrophages activated by lymphokines. This would differ from chronic inflammation against an agent that evokes a cytotoxic T lymphocyte response, which is characterized by the presence of T lymphocytes in the affected tissue. Chronic inflammation, therefore, displays a range of tissue changes, and study of these processes is often rewarded by insights about the agent causing the disease. It is from this hopeful perspective that we approach the study of chronic inflammation.

CHRONIC INFLAMMATION IN RESPONSE TO ANTIGENIC INJURIOUS AGENTS

Mechanisms

Chronic inflammation usually occurs in response to an injurious agent that is antigenic, eg, a microorganism. The immune response is triggered when antigen initially enters the body and is reinforced by any subsequent accumulation of antigen, eg, by multiplication of an infectious agent. Local persistence of the antigen leads to accumulation of activated T lymphocytes, plasma cells, and macrophages at the site of injury (Fig 5–1). Because these cells are the prominent cell types in chronic inflammation, effector cells of the immune response are also called **chronic inflammatory cells**. In acute inflammation, on the other hand, although systemic immunity may develop to an antigenic agent, there is no stimulus for cells

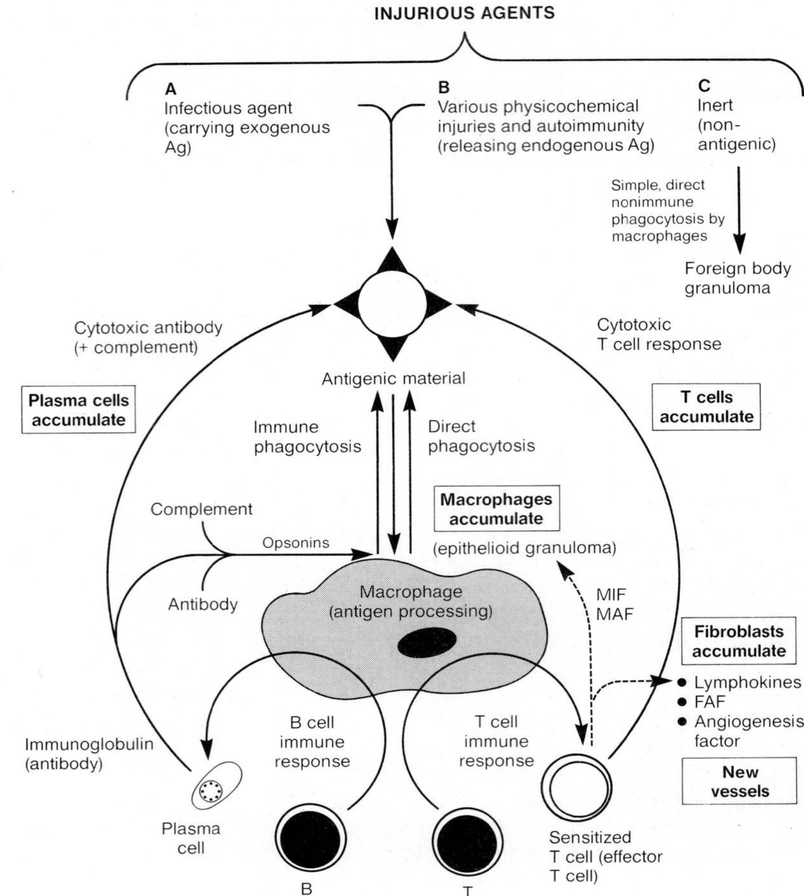

Figure 5-1. Chronic inflammation. Cellular components seen as part of the immune response. In most cases, the persistent injurious agent is antigenic and leads to an immune response involving T cells, B cells, and macrophages. Foreign body granuloma formation, on the other hand, appears to be a direct phagocytic response to inert (ie, nonantigenic) material, and the immune response is not involved. MIF, macrophage-inhibiting factor; MAF = macrophage-activating factor; FAF = fibroblast-activating factor.

associated with the immune response to accumulate at the site of injury, because the antigen typically is rapidly removed.

Although it is triggered at the time of injury, the immune response takes several days to develop because the nonsensitized lymphocytes that initially respond to antigens must pass through several division cycles (Chapter 4) before increased numbers of effector lymphocytes become manifest in the tissues.

Morphologic Types

Differentiation of the various types of chronic inflammation is based on the nature of the inciting agent and the subsequent immune response against it.

A. Granulomatous Chronic Inflammation:

1. Characteristic features–Chronic granulomatous inflammation is characterized by the formation of **epithelioid cell granulomas.*** **Epithelioid cells** are activated macrophages that appear on microscopic examination as large cells with abundant pale, foamy cytoplasm; they are called epithelioid cells because of a superficial resemblance to epithelial cells (Fig 5–2A). An epithelioid cell granuloma is an aggregate of these activated macrophages. Macrophage aggregation is induced by lymphokines produced by activated T cells. Granulomas are usually surrounded by lymphocytes, plasma cells, fibroblasts, and collagen. A typical feature of epithelioid cell granulomas is the formation of **Langhans-type giant cells** that are derived from macrophages and characterized by 10–50 nuclei around the periphery of the cell (Figs 5–2 and 5–3).

2. Causes–Epithelioid cell granulomas form when 2 conditions are satisfied: (1) When macro-

*A granuloma is defined as an aggregate of macrophages. Two types of granuloma are recognized: (1) epithelioid cell granuloma, which represents an immune response in which the macrophages are activated by lymphokines of specifically stimulated T cells; and (2) foreign body granuloma, which represents nonimmune phagocytosis of foreign nonantigenic material by macrophages.

Table 5-1. Differences between acute and chronic inflammation.

	Acute	Chronic
Duration	Short (days)	Long (weeks to months)
Onset	Acute	Insidious
Specificity	Nonspecific	Specific (where immune response is activated)
Inflammatory cells	Neutrophils, macrophages	Lymphocytes, plasma cells, macrophages, fibroblasts
Vascular changes	Active vasodilation, increased permeability	New vessel formation ("granulation tissue")
Fluid exudation and edema	+	−
Cardinal clinical signs (redness, heat, swelling, pain)	+	−
Tissue necrosis	− (Usually) + (Suppurative and necrotizing inflammation)	+
Fibrosis (collagen)	−	+
Operative host responses	Plasma factors: complement, immunoglobulins, properdin, etc; neutrophils, nonimmune phagocytosis	Immune response, phagocytosis, repair
Systemic manifestations	Fever, often high	Low-grade fever, weight loss, anemia
Changes in peripheral blood	Neutrophil leukocytosis; lymphocytosis (in viral infections)	Frequently none; variable white blood cell changes, increased plasma immunoglobulin

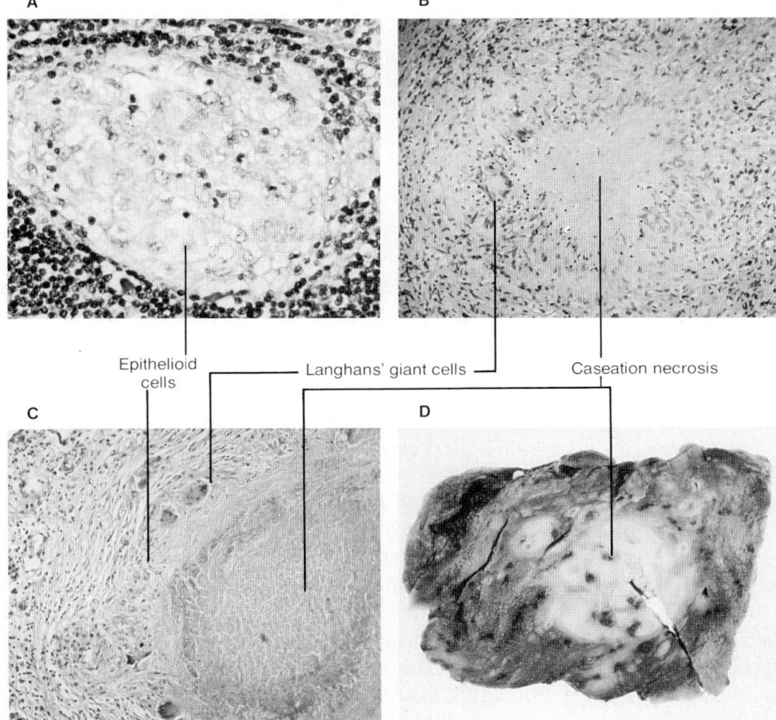

Figure 5-2. Epithelioid cell granuloma (composite). **A:** Early granuloma composed of an aggregate of epithelioid cells with vesicular nuclei, abundant cytoplasm, and indistinct borders. This is surrounded by lymphocytes. **B:** Granuloma with central caseation. Note the presence of a Langhans giant cell. **C:** Large granuloma formed by the coalescence of multiple granulomas. This contains a large central area of caseous necrosis—only a part of the granuloma is shown—which is surrounded by epithelioid cells, Langhans giant cells, and fibrosis. **D:** Fragment of lung showing a caseous granuloma that resembles a tumor. The cut on one side of the tissue was for the purpose of making the section that is shown in **C**.

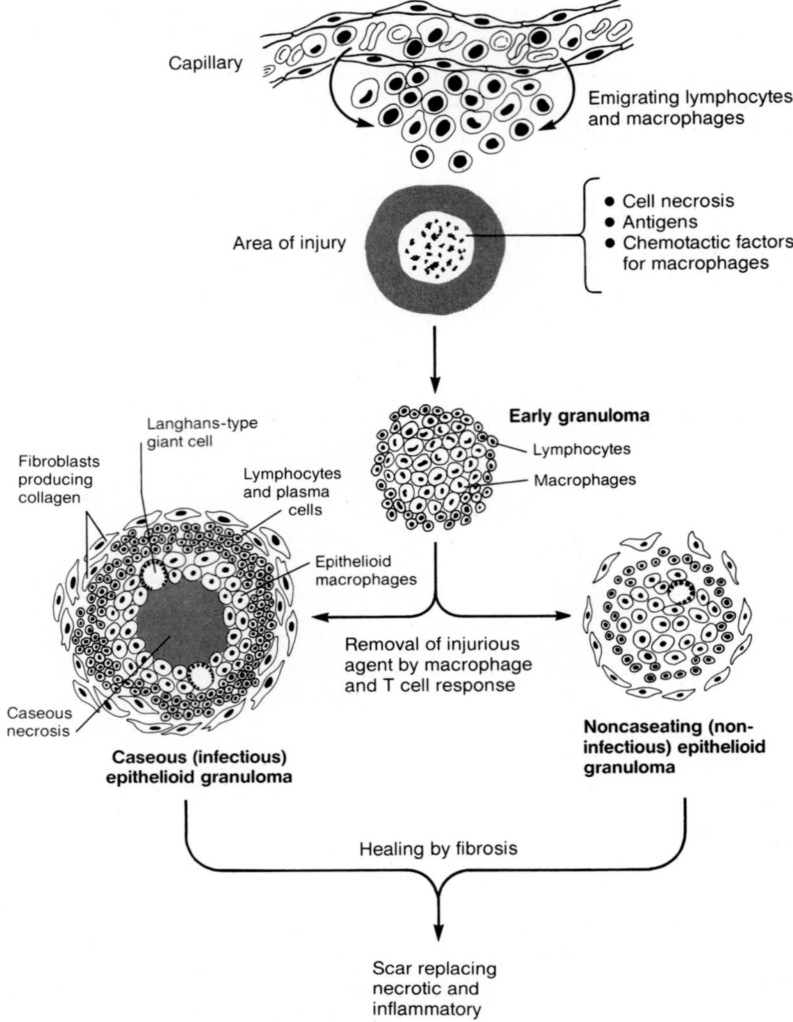

Figure 5-3. Phases in formation of epithelioid granulomas during chronic inflammation. Caseous necrosis occurs especially in those cases in which an infectious agent is responsible for the injury (eg, tuberculosis).

phages have successfully phagocytosed the injurious agent but it survives inside them. The abundant pale, foamy cytoplasm characterizing epithelioid cells probably represents partial digestion of the phagocytosed agent. (2) When an active T lymphocyte-mediated cellular immune response occurs. Lymphokines produced by activated T lymphocytes include **migration-inhibiting factor (MIF),** which inhibits migration of macrophages and causes them to aggregate in the area of injury and form granulomas. **Macrophage-activating factor (MAF),** another lymphokine, increases the ability of macrophages to destroy phagocytosed particles (Fig 5–4).

Epithelioid granulomas occur in several different types of disease states (Table 5–2): (1) Infections due to facultative intracellular organisms (ie, organisms such as mycobacteria and fungi that can grow and multiply both outside and within cells); (2) disorders due to chemical agents such as beryllium (berylliosis) and silica crystals (silicon dioxide) (silicosis); and (3) diseases of uncertain cause, eg, sarcoidosis and Crohn's disease.

3. Changes in affected tissues–Initially microscopic, granulomas expand and fuse with adjacent granulomas over time to form large masses that sometimes resemble cancerous tumors. Parenchymal tissue around the granuloma is lost as a result of necrosis and is replaced by scar tissue when healing occurs.

In most infectious granulomas (ie, those due to a specific microorganism), central **caseous necrosis** is a common feature. On gross examination, caseous material appears yellowish-white and resembles crumbly cheese (Fig 5–2D); on microscopic examination, the center of the granuloma is finely granular, pink, and amorphous (Fig 5–2C). A similar form of necrosis called **gummatous**

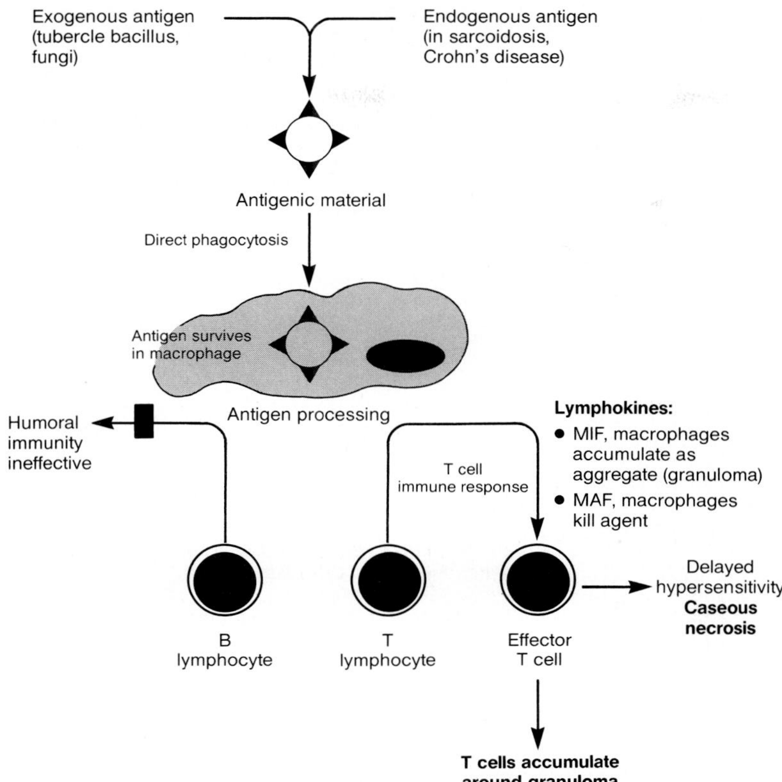

Figure 5-4. Immune mechanism of epithelioid granuloma.

necrosis occurs in syphilis except that the gross characteristics display a more rubbery consistency (hence the term gummatous). Caseous or gummatous necrosis results from a T lymphocyte-mediated hypersensitivity reaction (type IV hypersensitivity [Chapter 8]). Caseation does not occur in noninfectious epithelioid granulomas.

B. Nongranulomatous Chronic Inflammation:

1. Characteristic features-Nongranulomatous chronic inflammation is characterized by the accumulation of sensitized lymphocytes (specifically activated by antigen), plasma cells, and macrophages in the injured area. These cells are scattered diffusely throughout the tissue, however, and do not form granulomas. Tissue necrosis and fibrosis are common.

2. Causes and changes in affected tissues-Nongranulomatous chronic inflammation represents several different types of immune response due to different antigenic agents (Table 5-3).

a. Chronic viral infections-Persistent infection of parenchymal cells by viruses evokes an immune response whose main components are a B cell response and a T cell cytotoxic response (Fig 5-5). The affected tissue shows accumulation of lymphocytes and plasma cells that produce cytotoxic effects on the cell containing the viral antigen, causing cell necrosis (Fig 5-6). This cytotoxic effect is mediated either by killer T lymphocytes or by cytotoxic antibody acting with complement. Ongoing parenchymal cell necrosis is associated with repair characterized by fibroblast proliferation and deposition of collagen.

b. Chronic autoimmune diseases-A similar type of immune response mediated by cytotoxic antibody and killer T cells occurs in several autoimmune diseases. The antigen involved is a host cell molecule that is perceived as foreign by the immune system. The pathologic result is similar to the nongranulomatous chronic inflammation seen in chronic viral infections, with cell necrosis, fibrosis, and lymphocytic and plasma cell infiltration of the tissue (Fig 5-7).

c. Chronic chemical intoxications-Persistent toxic substances such as alcohol produce chronic inflammation, notably in the pancreas and liver. The toxic substance is not antigenic, but by causing cell necrosis it may result in alteration of host molecules so that they become antigenic and evoke an immune response. The features of cell necrosis and repair by fibrosis in such cases dominate the features of the immune response, and in many cases of alcoholic chronic pancreatitis, the lymphocytic and plasma cell infiltration is slight.

Table 5-2. Common causes of epithelioid cell granulomas.

Disease	Antigen	Caseous Necrosis
Infectious diseases		
Tuberculosis	*Mycobacterium tuberculosis*	+ +
Leprosy (tuberculoid type)	*Mycobacterium leprae*	−
Histoplasmosis	*Histoplasma capsulatum*	+ +
Coccidioidomycosis	*Coccidioides immitis*	+ +
Q fever	*Coxiella burnetti* (rickettsial organism)	−
Brucellosis	*Brucella* species	−
Syphilis	*Treponema pallidum*	+ +[1]
Noninfectious diseases		
Sarcoidosis	Unknown	−
Crohn's disease	Unknown	−
Berylliosis	Beryllium (? + protein)	−
Foreign body (eg, in intravenous drug abuse)	Talc, fibers (? + protein)	−

[1]Granuloma formation occurs in late syphilis. The necrosis in syphilitic granulomas resembles caseous necrosis in its pathogenesis and microscopic appearance but differs in its gross appearance, being firm and rubbery rather than "cheesy." This is called gummatous necrosis, and the syphilitic granuloma is called a gumma.

Table 5-3. Common causes of nongranulomatous chronic inflammation associated with injuries where antigens are involved.

Characterized by lymphocytic and plasma cell infiltration of tissue associated with cell necrosis and fibrosis
Chronic viral infections (cytotoxic B and T cell responses)
Chronic viral hepatitis
Chronic viral infections of the central nervous system
Autoimmune diseases (cytotoxic B and T cell responses)
Hashimoto's autoimmune thyroiditis
Chronic autoimmune atrophic gastritis
Rheumatoid arthritis
Chronic ulcerative colitis
Chronic toxic diseases (cell necrosis caused by the toxin results in conversion of cell molecules to antigens)
Chronic alcoholic pancreatitis
Chronic alcoholic liver disease
Characterized by diffuse accumulation of macrophages with numerous intracytoplasmic microorganisms; deficient T cell response
Lepromatous leprosy
Mycobacterium avium-intracellulare infection in patients with AIDS
Rhinoscleroma (*Klebsiella rhinoscleromatis*)
Leishmaniasis
Characterized by the presence of numerous eosinophils in conjunction with other inflammatory cells
Infections with metazoan parasites
Recurrent type I hypersensitivity reactions, eg, bronchial asthma, allergic nasal polyps, atopic dermatitis

d. Chronic nonviral infections-A specific type of nongranulomatous chronic inflammation is seen with certain microorganisms (Table 5-3) that (1) survive and multiply in the cytoplasm of macrophages after direct phagocytosis and (2) evoke a very ineffective T cell response. This type of infection is characterized by the accumulation of large numbers of foamy macrophages in the tissue (Fig 5-8). The macrophages are present diffusely in the tissue without aggregating into granulomas. The ability of the macrophage to kill the organism is limited because of the poor T cell response, permitting the organisms to multiply in the cell. Typically, large numbers of organisms are present in the cytoplasm of the macrophages. The main defense appears to be direct phagocytosis by the macrophages (Fig 5-9). Variable numbers of plasma cells and lymphocytes may be present. Accumulation of infected macrophages in the tissue causes nodular thickening of the affected tissue, a clinical feature that is typical of this type of chronic inflammation.

Leprosy is a good example of how the immune response modulates the type of chronic inflammation that occurs. In patients with a high level of T cell responsiveness against the leprosy bacillus, epithelioid granulomas are formed and the multiplication of the organism is effectively controlled (tuberculoid leprosy). In patients with a low level of T cell responsiveness, the organism multiplies unimpeded in macrophages, which accumulate diffusely in the tissue, leading to a progressive disease (lepromatous leprosy).

e. Chronic metazoan infections-Eosinophils are present in chronic inflammations caused by metazoan parasites. Eosinophils respond chemotactically to a factor released by mast cells and basophils in the presence of IgE (ECF-A; eosinophil chemotactic factor of anaphylaxis) and to the complement fragment C5a. The role of the eosinophil has not been fully elucidated, but there is evidence of Fc receptor-mediated phagocytosis, participation in antibody-dependent cytotoxicity reactions against parasites, control of histamine release by mast cells, and degradation of histamine and leukotrienes.

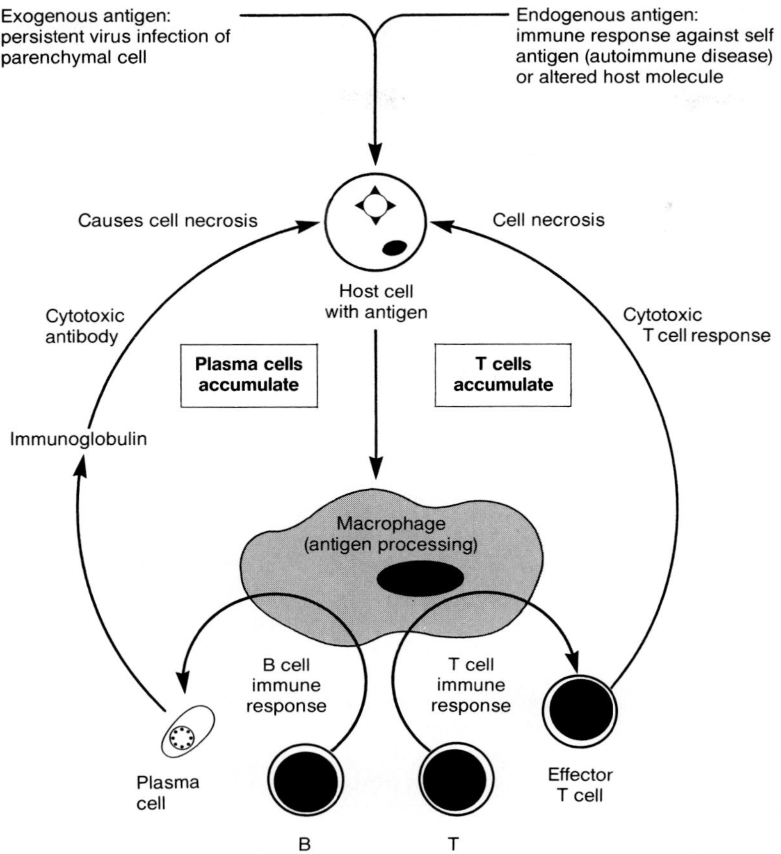

Figure 5-5. Mechanism of chronic nongranulomatous inflammation as seen in chronic viral infections and autoimmune diseases.

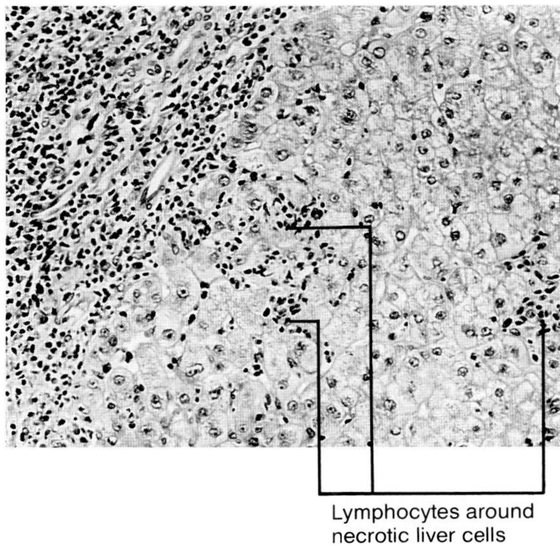

Figure 5-6. Chronic viral hepatitis. The periphery of the liver lobule contains numerous lymphocytes and plasma cells. These cells extend into the lobule and are seen there as aggregates around necrotic liver cells. Hepatitis B virus was demonstrated in the cells by immunologic techniques.

CHRONIC INFLAMMATION IN RESPONSE TO NONANTIGENIC INJURIOUS AGENTS

When foreign material that is large (so large as to preclude phagocytosis by a single macrophage), inert (incites no inflammatory response), and nonantigenic (incites no immune response) enters a tissue and persists there, foreign body granulomas form (Fig 5–1). Nonantigenic material, which includes sutures, talc particles, and inert fibers, is removed by macrophages through nonimmune phagocytosis. Macrophages aggregate around the phagocytosed particles and form granulomas. These frequently contain **foreign body giant cells** characterized by numerous nuclei dispersed throughout the cell (Fig 5–10) rather than arranged around the periphery, as occurs in Langhans-type giant cells. Foreign material is usually identifiable in the center of the granuloma, particularly if viewed under polarized light, when it appears as refractile particles.

Foreign body granuloma is of little clinical significance and indicates only that nondigestible foreign material has been introduced into the tissue; eg, granulomas around talc particles and cot-

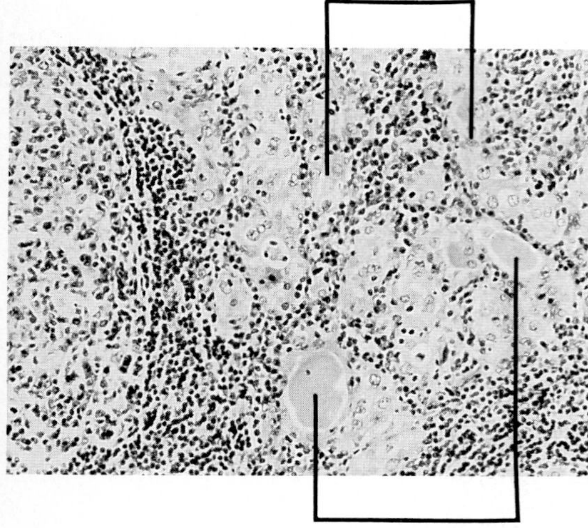

Figure 5-7. Autoimmune chronic thyroiditis (Hashimoto's disease). The thyroid is extensively infiltrated by lymphocytes and plasma cells. There is extensive destruction of thyroid follicular epithelial cells.

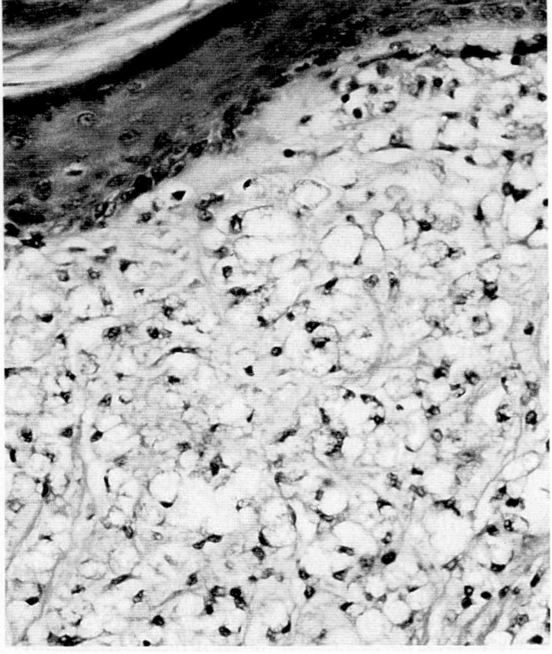

Figure 5-8. Skin in lepromatous leprosy, showing large numbers of foamy macrophages underneath the epidermis. There is no tendency to granuloma formation. Acid-fast staining revealed numerous leprosy bacilli in the cytoplasm of the macrophages.

ton fibers in alveolar septa and portal areas of the liver are good signs of intravenous drug abuse (the talc comes from the impure drug preparation and the cotton from the material used for filtering the drug). Tissue necrosis is not an associated feature.

FUNCTION & RESULT OF CHRONIC INFLAMMATION

Chronic inflammation serves to contain and—over a long period of time—remove an injurious agent that is not easily eradicated by the body. Containment and destruction of the agent are largely dependent on immunologic reactivity, whether these are achieved by (1) direct killing by activated lymphocytes, (2) interaction with antibodies produced by plasma cells, or (3) activation of macrophages by lymphokines produced by T lymphocytes (Fig 5–1; see also Chapter 4).

With the exception of foreign body reactions, chronic inflammation is often associated with **tissue necrosis** and implies serious clinical illness, eg, liver failure in chronic active hepatitis. Chronic inflammation is a feature of many chronic diseases that are characterized either by total lack of recovery or by a long recovery period (months or years).

Associated fibrosis is another serious side effect of chronic inflammation. In certain situations, fibrous scarring itself causes disease—eg, fibrosis of the pericardial sac in chronic pericarditis may restrict cardiac filling and cause heart failure, and pulmonary fibrosis may cause respiratory failure.

When removal or neutralization of the injurious agent is ultimately achieved, the tissue heals, usually by fibrosis. The chronic inflammatory cells disappear, and an acellular fibrous scar marks the site of injury.

MIXED ACUTE & CHRONIC INFLAMMATION

Since acute and chronic inflammation represent different types of host response to injury, features of both types of inflammation may coexist in certain circumstances, as in chronic suppurative inflammation and recurring acute inflammation.

Chronic Suppurative Inflammation

It is difficult to remove the large amounts of pus associated with chronic suppurative inflammation. Infectious agents in pus are basically inaccessible to the actions of antimicrobial drugs and host defense mechanisms, since pus is avascular and lacks a mechanism for penetration by circulating therapeutic drugs or antibodies. Slow proliferation of the causative agent may therefore continue.

The surrounding viable tissue responds with a

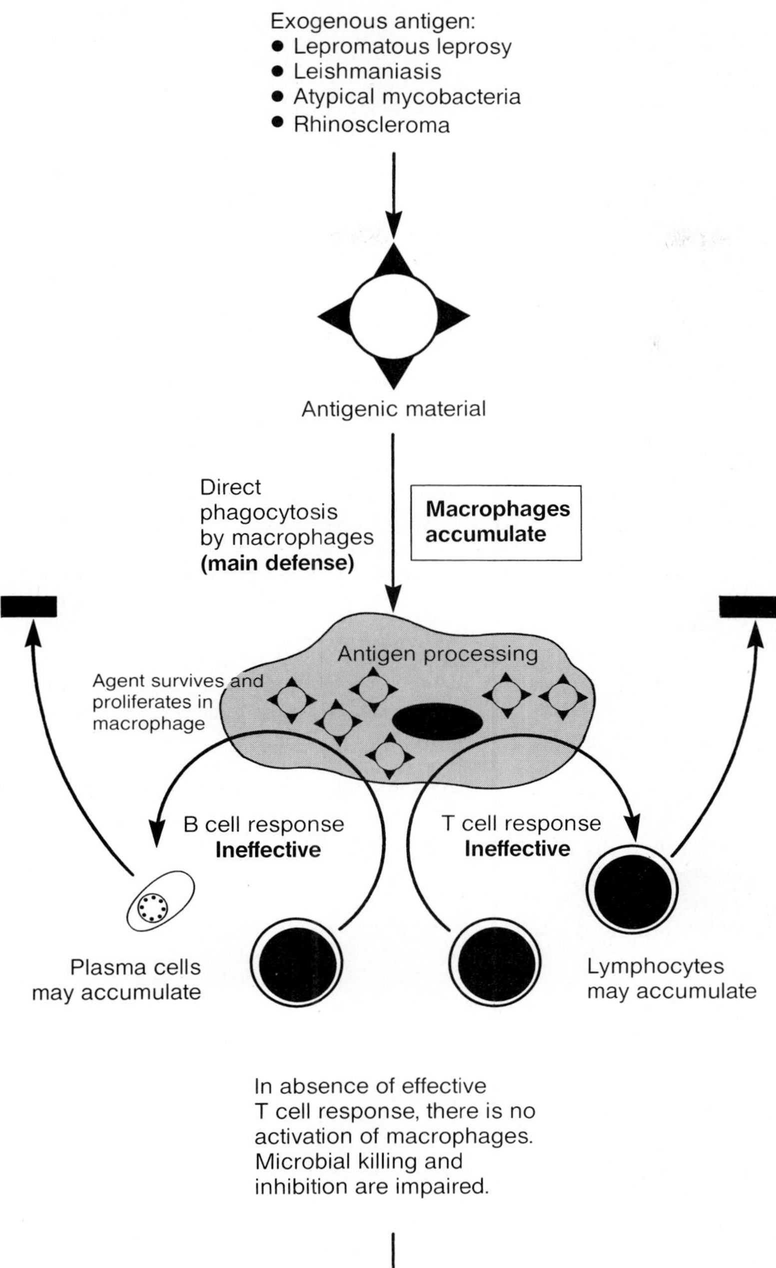

Figure 5–9. Mechanism of chronic nongranulomatous inflammation as seen in chronic nonviral infections.

longstanding inflammatory process in which areas of suppuration (liquefied necrotic tissue and neutrophils) alternate with areas of chronic inflammation (lymphocytes, plasma cells, macrophages) and fibrosis. Such a pattern occurs in chronic suppurative osteomyelitis and pyelonephritis.

If the area of suppuration localizes to an abscess that remains over a long period, a fibrous wall of increasing thickness forms. The difference between an acute and a chronic abscess lies in the thickness of the fibrous wall; both forms are filled with pus.

Recurrent Acute Inflammation

Repeated attacks of acute inflammation may occur if there is a predisposing cause, eg, in the

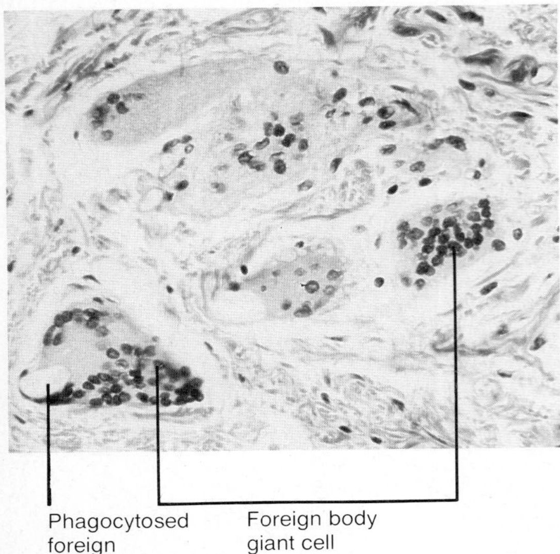

Figure 5-10. Foreign body granuloma, showing macrophages and foreign body giant cells phagocytosing particulate foreign material.

Table 5-4. Summary of clinical and laboratory evaluation of chronic inflammation.

Systemic features
Fever, usually low-grade and of insidious onset
Peripheral white blood cell count
Usually normal
Sometimes lymphocytosis, monocytosis, eosinophilia
Anemia
Weight loss
Changes in plasma proteins
Elevated levels of plasma immunoglobulins
Association with secondary amyloidosis
Increased erythrocyte sedimentation rate
Local features
Cell necrosis slowly progressive, often extensive
Fibrosis
Presence of effector immune cells ("chronic inflammatory cells")
Structural and functional abnormalities due to the above
Laboratory evaluation
Biopsy of lesions
Type of chronic inflammation may provide pointers to etiology
Specific infectious agent may be identified, eg, mycobacteria, fungi
Microbiologic culture examination of tissue for mycobacteria, fungi, etc.
Immunologic studies
Serologic studies for antibodies against syphilis, fungi
Skin tests for tuberculosis, fungi
Serum autoantibody levels for autoimmune disease

gallbladder when there are gallstones. Each attack of acute inflammation is followed by incomplete resolution that leads to a progressively increasing number of chronic inflammatory cells and fibrosis. Depending on the time of examination, the picture may be mainly that of chronic inflammation or of acute superimposed on chronic inflammation. The terms **subacute inflammation** and **acute-on-chronic inflammation** are also used to denote this pattern.

CLINICAL & PATHOLOGIC DIAGNOSIS

Diagnosis of the nature and cause of chronic inflammatory disease is often difficult because of the insidious nature of the process and the lack of defined separate clinical syndromes for many of the infectious agents involved. Precise diagnosis usually requires recourse to a full range of clinical and pathologic studies (Table 5-4).

Healing & Repair

6

Tissue injuries associated with inflammation are eventually followed by some form of healing. Removal of inflammatory and necrotic cellular debris must precede any such healing. Healing occurs rapidly after transitory injury such as a single minor traumatic episode. Healing is also rapid if the injurious agent is quickly inactivated by the host response, whether inflammatory or immune. With persistent low-grade injury, healing occurs concurrently with ongoing chronic inflammation.

The ideal result of healing is to restore the tissue to its normal (preinjury) state, a process termed **resolution**. Removal of debris associated with the inflammatory response is sufficient to restore a tissue to its normal state if injury has been minor (ie, if minimal parenchymal cell necrosis has occurred). After removal of cellular debris, any necrotic parenchymal cells may be replaced by new parenchymal cells of the same type in a process known as **regeneration**.

When resolution and regeneration are not possible, necrotic cells are replaced with collagen; this is termed **organization**, or **repair by scar formation**. In many instances, a combination of healing processes occurs.

The mechanism of healing depends on the type of inflammation, the extent of tissue necrosis, the types of cells involved, and the regenerative ability of damaged parenchymal cells.

RESOLUTION (Fig 6-1)

Resolution is the ideal outcome of healing and occurs in acute inflammatory responses to minor injuries or those with minimal parenchymal cell necrosis. The tissue is in effect restored to the state it was in before injury occurred.

The fibrinous inflammatory exudate and tissue debris derived from the inactivated injurious agent or necrotic host cells (neutrophils, a few parenchymal cells) are liquefied by lysosomal enzymes liberated by neutrophils and then removed by the lymphatics. Any remaining particulate debris is phagocytosed by macrophages that enter the area during the later stages of the inflammatory response.

REGENERATION

Replacement of lost parenchymal cells by division of adjacent surviving parenchymal cells (regeneration) can also restore injured tissue to normal. Whether regeneration occurs depends on (1) the regenerative capacity of involved cells (ie, their ability to divide), (2) the number of surviving viable cells, and (3) the presence of a connective tissue framework that will provide a base for growth of regenerating cells and restoration of normal tissue structure.

Before regeneration can occur, the necrotic cells must be removed. This involves an acute inflammatory response, liquefaction of cells by neutrophil enzymes, and removal of debris by lymphatics and macrophages as described in the preceding section.

The cells of the body can be divided into 3 groups—labile, stable, and permanent—on the basis of their regenerative capacity (Table 6–1).

Labile Cells (Intermitotic Cells)

A. Characteristics: Labile cells normally divide actively throughout life to replace cells that are being continually lost from the body. Labile cells have a short G_0 (resting, or intermitotic) phase (Fig 6–2). Continued loss of mature cells of a given tissue is a continuous stimulus for resting cells to enter the mitotic cell cycle. Examples of

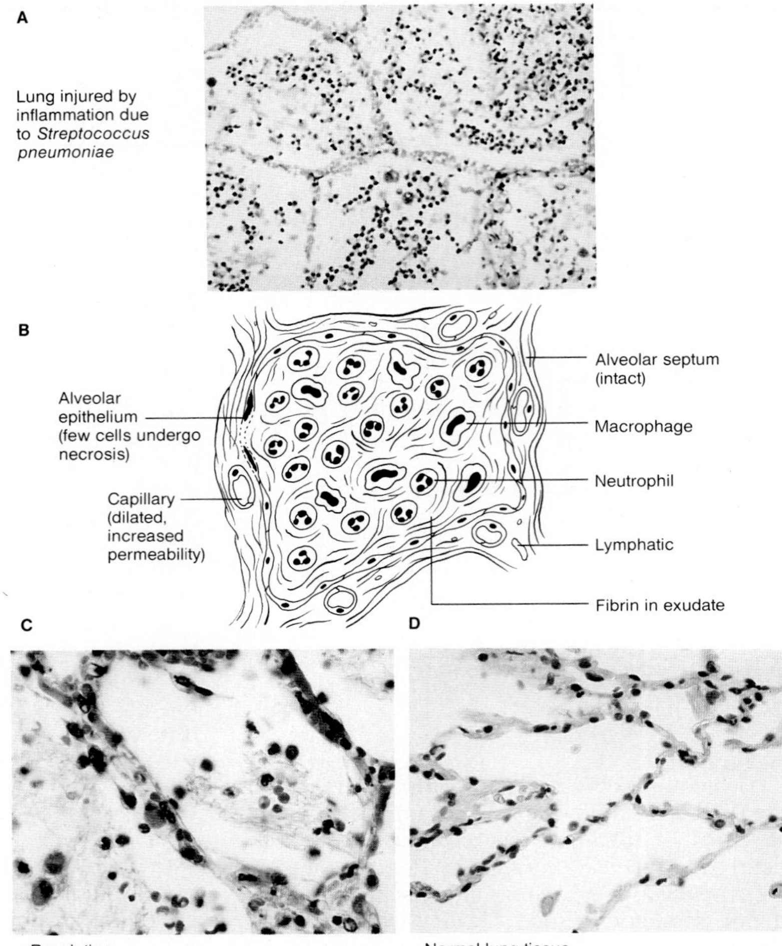

Figure 6–1. Resolution after acute pneumococcal pneumonia. **A and B:** Lung, showing dilated alveolar capillaries and an exudate filling the alveoli. After the bacterium has been killed, resolution occurs by liquefaction of the exudate and phagocytosis by macrophages **(C),** resulting in a normal lung **(D).** Note that any alveolar epithelial cells undergoing necrosis in the acute phase regenerate. The amount of necrosis is small in an uncomplicated case.

labile cells include **basal epithelial cells** of all epithelial linings and **hematopoietic stem cells** in bone marrow (Table 6–1). Mature differentiated cells in these particular tissues cannot divide; their numbers are maintained by division of their parent labile cells.

B. Healing in Tissues With Labile Cells: Injury to a tissue containing labile parenchymal cells is followed by rapid regeneration. For example, surgical removal of the endometrium through curettage or physiologic loss of endometrium during menstruation is followed by complete regeneration of cells from the basal germinative layer within a few days. Similarly, destruction of erythrocytes in peripheral blood (hemolysis) induces hyperplasia of erythroid precursors in bone marrow, with resulting regeneration of destroyed red cells.

Regeneration in tissues with labile cells occurs only when enough labile cells have been spared by injury (Fig 6–3). In the example cited above, overly zealous surgical curettage of the endometrium that removes the entire endometrial lining, including the basal layer, precludes regeneration. Healing occurs by scar formation, which leads to failure of menstruation and infertility (Asherman's syndrome). Likewise, when injury such as that caused by radiation exposure or drugs destroys all of the erythroid precursors in the bone marrow, regeneration cannot occur, and irreversible failure of erythrocyte production follows (aplastic anemia).

Stable Cells (Reversibly Postmitotic Cells)

A. Characteristics: Stable cells typically have a long life span and are therefore characterized by a low rate of division. They remain in the G_0 phase for long periods (often years) but retain the capacity to enter the mitotic cell cycle if the need arises (Fig 6–2). The parenchymal cells of most solid glandular organs (liver, pancreas) and mesenchymal cells (fibroblasts, endothelial cells) are examples of stable cells. Unlike labile cells, which are

Table 6-1. Classification of cells on the basis of their regenerative capacity.

Cell Types	Mitotic Capacity	Examples
Labile (intermitotic)	Short G_0 phase; almost always in mitotic cell cycle	Hematopoietic stem cells Basal cells Epidermis Genitourinary tract Crypt cells of gut mucosa Hair follicle cells Seminiferous germ cells Epithelium of ducts
Stable (reversibly postmitotic)	Long G_0 phase; can divide actively when stimulated	Parenchymal cells Liver Kidney (renal tubules) Lung (alveoli) Pancreas Breast Endocrine glands Mesenchymal cells Osteoblast Chondrocyte Fibroblast Endothelial cell Adipocyte
Permanent (irreversibly postmitotic)	None (cannot divide)	Neurons in central nervous system Ganglion cells in peripheral nervous system Cardiac muscle cells[1] Skeletal muscle cells[1]

[1]Cardiac and skeletal muscle cells demonstrate limited mitotic capability in experimental settings. In humans, they are functionally permanent cells.

undifferentiated cells that divide frequently and must undergo maturation before becoming functional, stable cells are fully differentiated, mature functioning cells that only revert to a dividing mode at need. Although stable cells have a long resting phase, they can divide rapidly upon demand, eg, parenchymal cells of the liver swiftly regenerate after necrosis of hepatocytes.

B. Healing in Tissues With Stable Cells: Regeneration in tissues composed of stable cells requires that enough viable tissue remain to provide a source of parenchymal cells for regeneration and that there is an intact connective tissue framework in the area of necrosis (Fig 6–3). Injuries to the kidney illustrate the need for an adequate connective tissue framework. Selective necrosis of some renal tubular cells (acute renal tubular necrosis) with sparing of the renal tubular framework is rapidly followed by regeneration, and the lost cells are replaced by division of surviving tubular cells. On the other hand, when necrosis of both the parenchyma and the connective tissue framework occurs (renal infarct), no regeneration is possible, and healing occurs by scar formation.

Permanent Cells (Irreversibly Postmitotic Cells)

A. Characteristics: Permanent cells have no capacity for mitotic division in postnatal life. Examples of permanent cells include neurons in the central and peripheral nervous system and cardiac muscle cells.

B. Healing in Tissues With Permanent Cells: Injury to permanent cells is always followed by **scar formation**. No regeneration is possible. Loss of permanent cells is therefore irreversible.

REPAIR BY SCAR FORMATION

A **scar** is a mass of collagen that is the end result of repair by organization and fibrosis. Repair by scar formation occurs (1) when resolution fails to occur in an acute inflammatory process; (2) when there is ongoing tissue necrosis in chronic inflammation; and (3) when parenchymal cell necrosis cannot be repaired by regeneration.

As discussed above, regeneration does not occur when necrotic cells are permanent cells, when the connective tissue framework of a tissue composed of stable cells has been destroyed, or when necrosis is so extensive that no cells are available for regeneration.

The process of repair by scar formation can be divided into several overlapping phases (Fig 6–4).

Preparation

The area of injury is prepared for scar formation by removal of the inflammatory exudate, including fibrin, blood, and any necrotic tissue. This debris is liquefied by lysosomal enzymes derived from neutrophils that have migrated to the area. Liquefied material is removed by lymphatics; any particulate residue is removed by macrophage phagocytosis. This preparatory process is similar to that which occurs in resolution and regeneration.

Ingrowth of Granulation Tissue

Granulation tissue forms and fills the injured area while necrotic debris is being removed. **Granulation tissue** is highly vascularized connective tissue composed of newly formed capillaries, proliferating fibroblasts, and residual inflammatory cells. (*Note:* Granulation tissue must be distinguished from granuloma, which is a tumorlike aggregate of macrophages associated with chronic inflammation.) Capillaries are derived by vascular proliferation in healthy tissue at the periphery of the involved area. Fibroblasts migrate with capil-

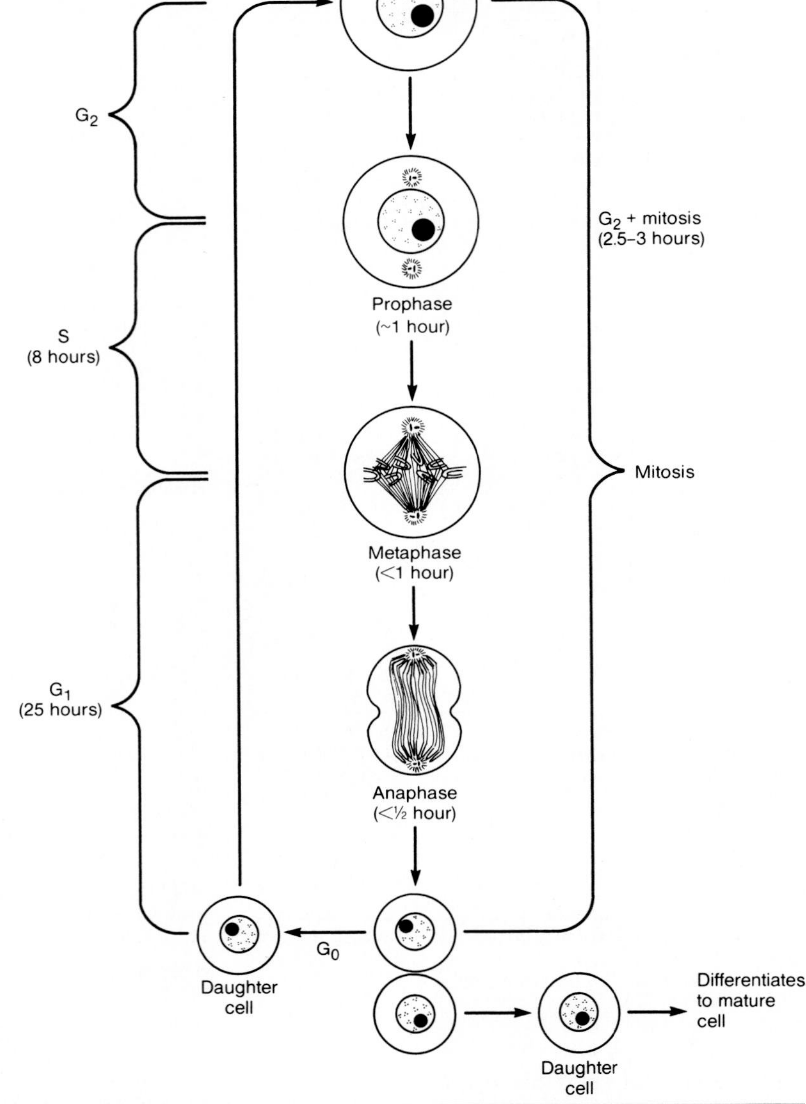

Figure 6–2. The cell cycle. The presynthetic gap (G_1) phase is variable and depends on several factors. In this example of bone cells, it lasts 25 hours. The DNA synthetic (S) phase lasts about 8 hours. The postsynthetic gap (G_2) phase plus mitosis lasts 2.5–3 hours. The G_0 (resting or intermitotic) phase is short in labile cells and long in stable cells. Permanent cells cannot enter the cycle.

laries to the injured area. The proliferation of capillaries, fibroblasts, and other cells in the healing process is controlled by a variety of growth-stimulating and growth-inhibiting factors (Table 6–2).

On gross examination, granulation tissue is soft, fleshy, and deep red because of the numerous capillaries. Microscopic examination shows the thin-walled capillaries lined by endothelium and surrounded by fibroblasts (Figs 6–5A and 6–5B). Both endothelial cells and fibroblasts are metabolically very active, with large nuclei and prominent nucleoli; mitotic figures may be seen. Electron microscopy demonstrates prominent rough endoplasmic reticulum in the cytoplasm of fibroblasts, an indicator of active protein synthesis.

Over time—the duration depends on the extent of injury—the entire area of repair is replaced by ingrowing granulation tissue **(organization).**

Production of Fibronectin

Fibronectin is a glycoprotein that apparently plays a key role in the formation of granulation tissue and is present in large amounts during wound healing. In the early phases of healing, it is derived from plasma, but later it is synthesized by fibroblasts and endothelial cells in granulation tissue. Fibronectin is chemotactic for fibroblasts

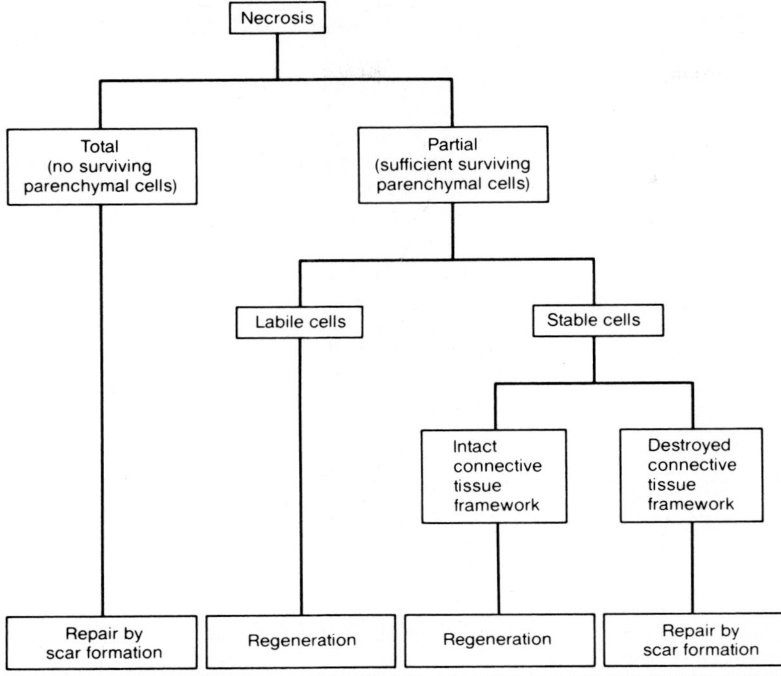

Figure 6–3. Factors influencing regeneration and repair by scar formation after injury to tissues containing labile and stable cells. Note that permanent cells have no capability of regeneration and always heal by scar formation.

and promotes organization of endothelial cells into capillary vessels.

Collagenization

Collagen is the major fibrillary protein of connective tissue. It is synthesized by fibroblasts in the form of a precursor, tropocollagen (procollagen), which has a molecular weight of 285,000 and a long, rodlike shape. Tropocollagen is composed of 3 separate alpha polypeptide chains wrapped together to form a tight triple helix. During or shortly after secretion, final removal of the terminal part of the peptide chain by an enzyme leads to formation of an insoluble molecule of fibrillary collagen. In the extracellular space, these molecules overlap one another by about one-fourth of their length to produce a pattern of gaps and overlapping regions that accounts for the characteristic 67-nm periodicity of the transverse striations seen in collagen fibrils viewed under the electron microscope. Under the light microscope, collagen appears as a fibrillary mass that stains pink with routine hematoxylin and eosin (H&E) stain and green or blue with Masson's and Mallory's trichrome stains. Collagen fibers are flexible but inelastic and are responsible for much of the tensile strength of scar tissue. Fine collagen fibers known as reticulin fibers are present in many tissues. These display slightly different staining characteristics. The terms **fibrous tissue** and **scar tissue** are synonymous with collagen. (*Note:* Fibrin is a molecule derived from plasma fibrinogen and is entirely distinct from collagen; "fibrinous" and "fibrous" are adjectives characterizing unrelated entities.)

Synthesis of tropocollagen by fibroblasts requires hydroxylation of proline by an enzyme whose activity requires ascorbic acid (vitamin C); and hydroxylation and oxidation of lysine, which permit cross-linkage between adjacent polypeptide tropocollagen chains. The detection of hydroxyproline released into the serum or urine by injury to collagen serves as a useful laboratory test in certain diseases of connective tissue.

A. Types of Collagen: At least 5 types of collagen (types I–V) are recognized (Table 6–3) on the basis of minor biochemical variations in the structure of their polypeptide chains. Young fibroblasts in granulation tissue form type III collagen that is later replaced by stronger cross-linked type I collagen.

B. Turnover of Collagen: A fully mature scar is not inactive; continuous slow removal of collagen in the scar by the enzyme collagenase is balanced by synthesis of new collagen by fibroblasts. Even long-established scars may weaken if the normal activity of fibroblasts is impaired, as occurs in vitamin C deficiency or administration of corticosteroids.

Maturation

The collagen content of granulation tissue progressively increases with time. A young scar consists of granulation tissue and abundant collagen

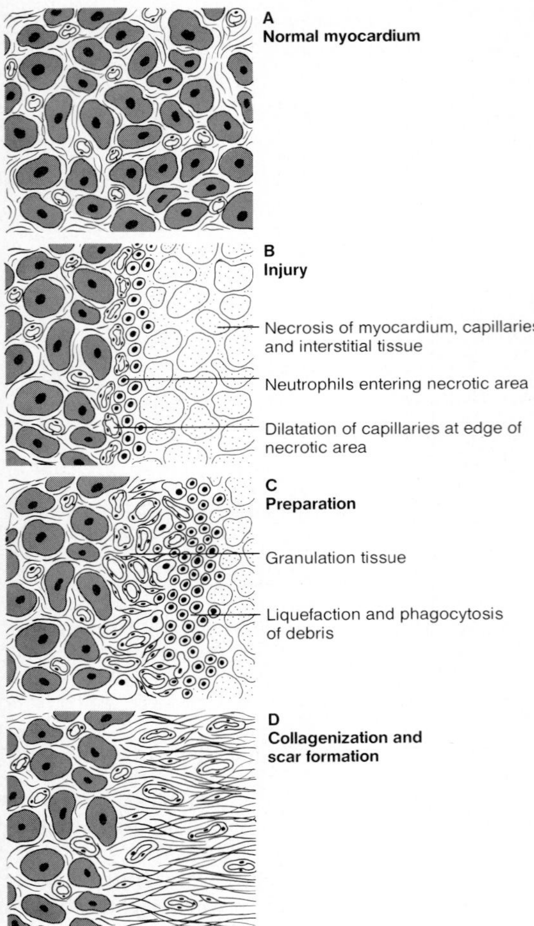

Figure 6–4. Repair of a myocardial infarct by scar formation. A normal myocardium is shown in **A.** The infarct evokes an acute inflammatory response and is invaded from the periphery by neutrophils **(B),** which liquefy the necrotic tissue. This is followed by entry of macrophages and granulation tissue **(C),** which removes the necrotic debris and leads to replacement of the necrotic zone by scar **(D).**

together with a moderate number of capillaries and fibroblasts (Fig 6–5C). It appears pink on gross examination because of the vascularity. As the scar matures, the amount of collagen increases and the scar becomes less cellular and vascular. The mature scar is composed of an avascular, poorly cellular mass of collagen (Fig 6–5D) and is white on gross examination.

Contraction & Strengthening

Contraction and strengthening constitute the final and most important phase of repair by scar formation. Contraction decreases the size of the scar and enables the surviving cells of the organ to function with maximal effectiveness; eg, the conversion of a large myocardial infarct to a small scar permits optimal functioning of the remaining myocardium.

Contraction begins early in the repair process and continues after the scar has matured. Early contraction is due to active contraction of actomyosin filaments in certain specialized myofibril-containing fibroblasts (also called myofibroblasts). Later contraction is a property of the collagen molecule itself.

The **tensile strength** of a scar is dependent on the amount of collagen and progressively increases, from about 10% of normal at the end of the first week to about 80% of normal over several months. The increasing tensile strength is initially due to an increase in the amount of collagen; subsequent increase is thought to be due to a change in the type of collagen produced and an increase in covalent linkages between collagen molecules. The fully formed scar is a firm, inelastic, flexible structure.

HEALING OF SKIN WOUNDS

Understanding the mechanisms involved in the healing of skin wounds provides insight into healing in general. The skin is composed of epidermis, which is made up of stratified squamous epithelium—the basal germinative layer of which is composed of labile cells—and dermis, which is composed of collagen, blood vessels, and skin appendages (adnexa) such as hair follicles, sweat glands, sebaceous glands, and apocrine glands. Stable cells make up the dermal connective tissue and adnexa.

Types of Skin Injury

Skin injuries are classified on the basis of the severity and nature of involvement.

A. Abrasion ("Scrape"): The mildest form of skin injury is characterized by removal of the superficial part of the epidermis. Since the underlying basal germinative layer of labile cells is intact, the epithelium regenerates from below, and the integrity of the epithelium is restored with no scarring.

B. Incision ("Cut") and Laceration ("Tear"): Incisions and lacerations involve the full thickness of the skin (both epidermis and dermis) but with minimal loss of germinative cells. If the skin edges are carefully apposed, as in a sutured surgical incision, only a small gap remains to be repaired. Surgical incisions constitute ideal skin wounds with regard to the healing process, since they do not contain foreign material and are not infected and therefore heal quickly and without incident. This process, in which necrosis and inflammation are minimal, is known as healing by first intention (see below).

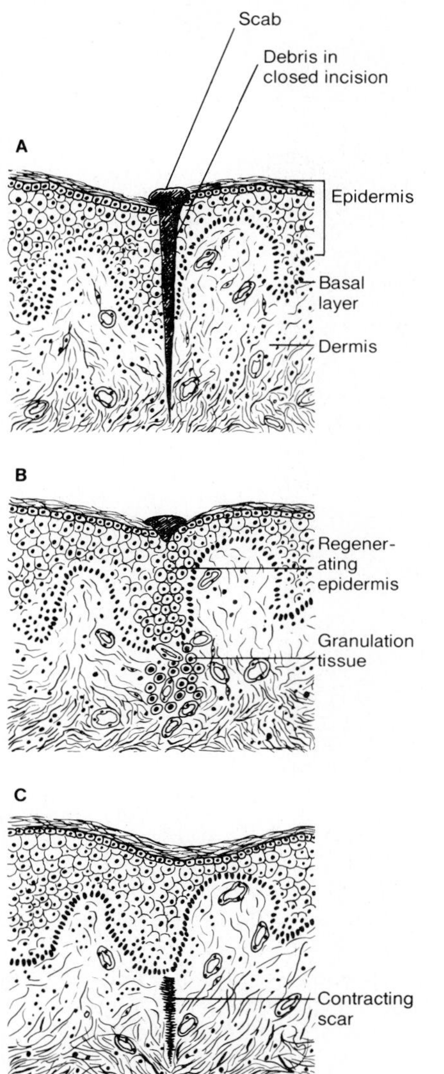

Figure 6-6. Healing of a surgical incision by first intention. **A:** Debris in the narrow gap between apposed skin edges is removed by neutrophils and macrophages. **B:** The epidermis regenerates rapidly, and granulation tissue in the dermal gap becomes collagenized to form a thin dermal scar **(C).**

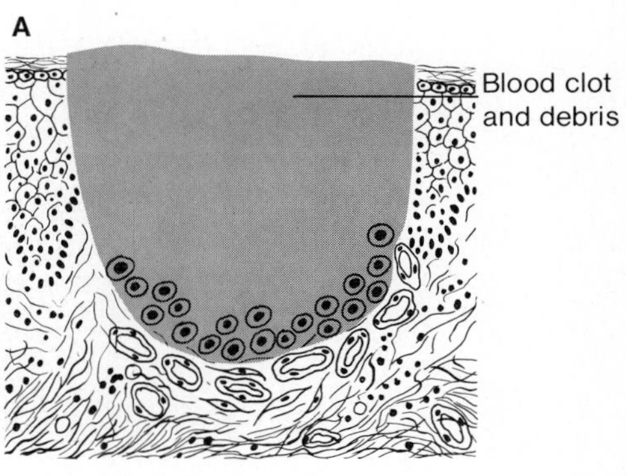

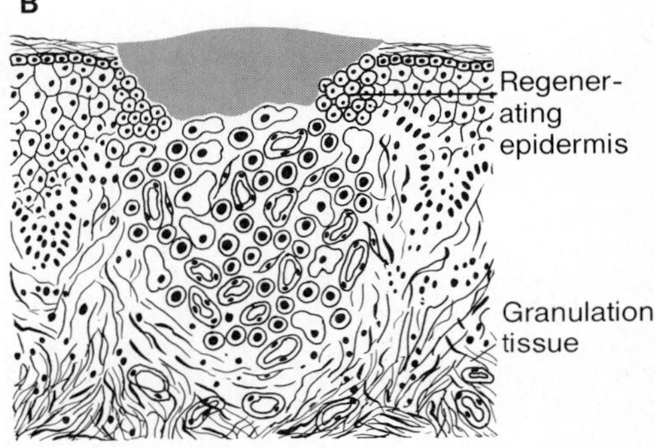

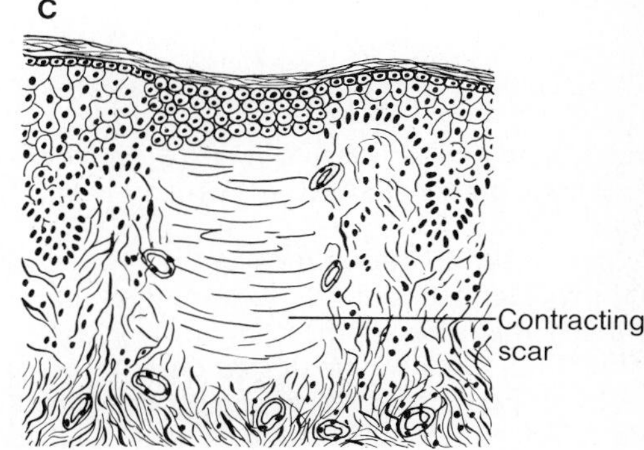

Figure 6-7. Healing by second intention of a large wound with extensive necrosis. **A:** The large area of tissue necrosis evokes acute inflammation with entry of neutrophils from the periphery. Slow liquefaction of debris and ingrowth of granulation tissue from the base **(B)** leads to scar formation **(C).** The epidermis regenerates slowly from the edges.

3. Tensile strength–In the first postoperative week, a surgical incision is artificially held together by sutures, clips, or tape. When the sutures are removed at the end of the first week (leaving them in place longer increases the risk of wound infection), the tensile strength of the young scar is only about 10% that of normal skin. Scar strength increases to about 30–50% of normal skin by 4 weeks and to 80% after several months.

B. Healing by Second Intention (Secondary Union): Wounds that fail to heal by first intention heal by second intention (secondary union [Figs 6–7 and 6–8]).

1. Reasons for failure of primary union–Primary union fails to occur in the following types of wounds: (1) In lacerations characterized by inability to achieve apposition of wound margins and by the presence of foreign material, necrotic tissue, and infection. Such injuries often occur in traffic accidents. (2) In wounds in which infection occurs even though skin edges are apposed. Acute inflammation with suppuration leads to rupture

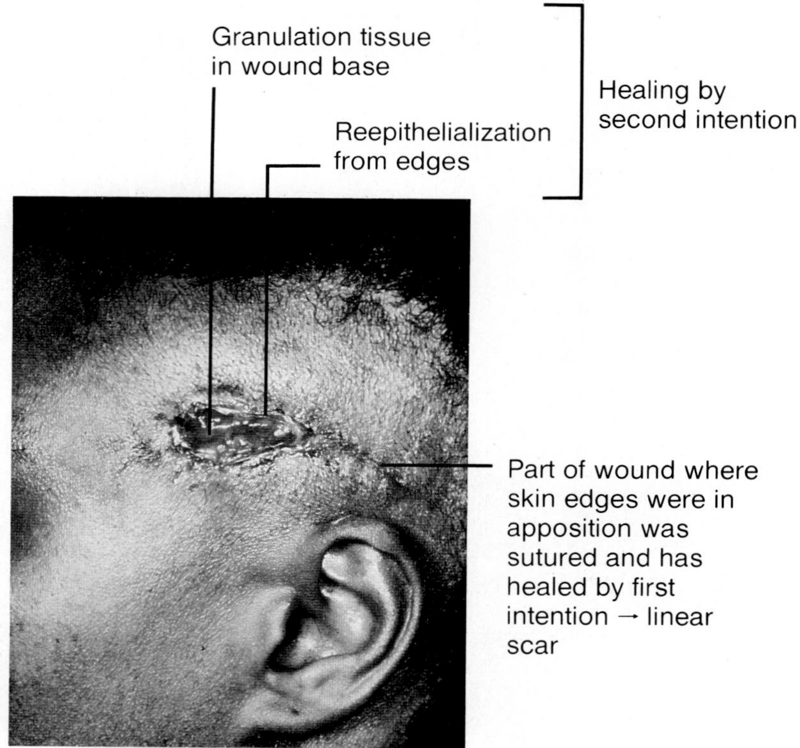

Figure 6–8. Ten-day-old laceration of the face. The posterior part of the wound was sutured and has healed by first intention. The anterior part, which had a large skin defect, was debrided and permitted to heal by second intention. Note the much greater time needed for healing by second intention.

of the wound and drainage of pus. (3) In wounds with large epidermal defects, such as occur in crush injuries and burns.

2. Process of secondary union–The processes involved in healing by second intention are essentially the same as those of healing by first intention but take much longer because of the more extensive damage. Infection is controlled by acute inflammation. The fluid exudate and necrotic tissue are then removed by enzymatic liquefaction, lymphatic drainage, and macrophage phagocytosis. Surgical removal of dead tissue and foreign material from the wound **(debridement)** greatly aids this clearing process. Granulation tissue then grows from the healthy tissue at the base of the wound and displaces the necrotic tissue toward the surface of the skin.

The epidermis regenerates from basal cells at the edges of the wound. Proliferating epidermal cells gradually creep over the granulating surface. In large wounds, reepithelialization may take several weeks. In these situations, surgical transplantation of skin (skin grafting) can help speed healing.

When complete epithelialization of the surface of the wound has occurred, collagenization transforms the underlying granulation tissue to scar tissue. The eventual size of the mature scar is much smaller than that of the original wound as a result of contraction.

Skin appendages such as hair follicles and glands are regenerated if enough residual cells remain to provide a source of proliferating cells. In extensive skin wounds with total destruction of many skin appendages, the resulting dermal scar is typically devoid of these structures.

C. Causes of Defective Wound Healing: (Table 6–4.) Surgeons must recognize the presence

Table 6–4. Factors that adversely affect wound healing.

Local	Systemic
Infection Poor blood supply (ischemia) Presence of foreign material Presence of necrotic tissue Movement in injured area Irradiation Tension in injured area	Advanced age Protein malnutrition Vitamin C deficiency Zinc deficiency Corticosteroid excess Decreased number of neutrophils or macrophages Diabetes mellitus Cytotoxic (anticancer) drugs Severe anemia Bleeding disorders Ehlers-Danlos-syndrome

of any factors that impair healing, since such adverse factors increase the overall risk of surgery and may even contraindicate surgery. If surgery is performed, recovery may take longer, and the risk of wound breakdown (which may be life-threatening) is also increased. More care is required in postoperative management of the incision; eg, sutures may have to remain in place longer than usual.

1. Failure of collagen synthesis–Lack of collagen synthesis is one of the commonest causes of defective wound healing and may result from vitamin C, protein, or zinc deficiency. Preoperative correction of negative protein balance with nutritional supplementation (hyperalimentation) greatly reduces the surgical risk in malnourished patients by improving the chances for uneventful healing.

Ehlers-Danlos syndrome is a group of rare inherited diseases caused by deficiencies of enzymes in the tropocollagen synthetic pathway. In some patients, deficiencies of enzymes causing hydroxylation and oxidation of lysine have been demonstrated, and these patients have abnormal collagen, which leads to various abnormalities, including impaired wound healing, easy bruisability, and fragile skin in some forms of the disease. One interesting effect is hyperextensibility of joints due to laxity of collagen in joint capsules.

2. Excessive collagen production–Synthesis of excessive amounts of collagen in wound healing results in formation of abnormal nodular masses of collagen (keloids) at the sites of skin injury (Fig 6–9A). Keloids often result from minor skin wounds and cause extensive disfigurement. Microscopic examination shows excessive collagen as thick, hyalinized bands (Fig 6–9B). Keloid formation tends to occur more frequently in blacks or darker-skinned individuals and demonstrates a familial tendency but with no single gene inheritance pattern. The cause of excessive collagen synthesis is not known. Excision of a keloid for cosmetic reasons is generally followed by formation of a new keloid.

3. Local factors–Important local factors that cause defective wound healing include the following:

a. Foreign or necrotic tissue or blood–The presence of foreign bodies, necrotic tissue, or excessive blood in the wound impairs healing. At surgery, foreign and necrotic tissue should be completely removed and hemostasis ensured before the incision is closed.

b. Infection–Infection in the wound will result in acute inflammation and (commonly) abscess formation, with breakdown of the wound and delayed healing.

c. Abnormal blood supply–Ischemia due to arterial disease and impaired venous drainage both hinder wound healing.

d. Decreased viability of cells–Irradiation of a tissue or administration of antimitotic drugs in cancer chemotherapy is associated with poor wound healing. These facts have important implications for the management of cancer patients, since the timing of surgery in relation to radiotherapy must be adjusted to minimize the risks associated with defective healing.

A

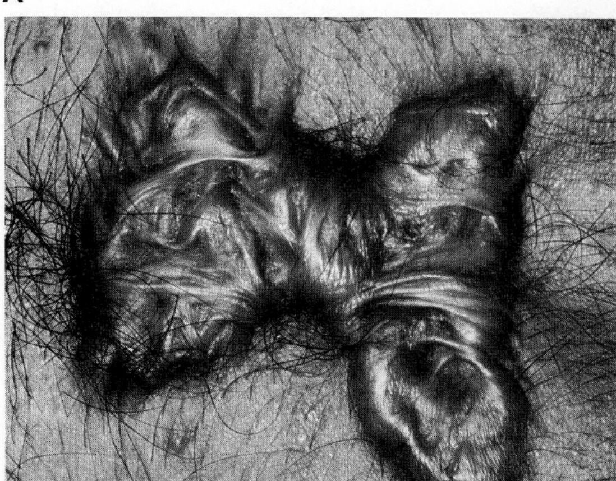

B

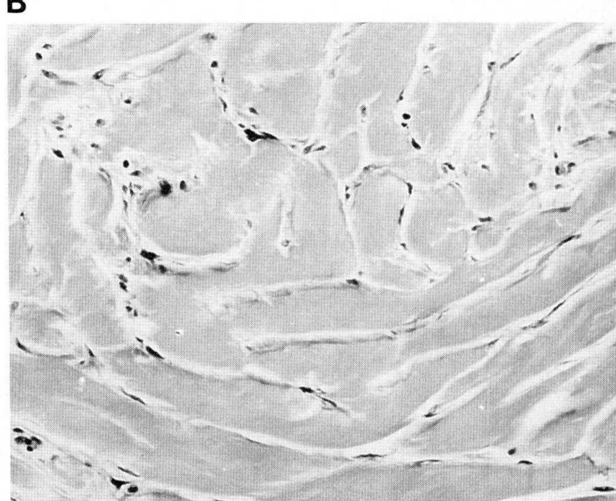

Figure 6–9. Keloid formation. The keloid is an irregularly contracted skin nodule **(A)** composed of thick hyalinized bands of collagen **(B).**

4. Diabetes mellitus–Diabetes mellitus is associated with impaired wound healing. The exact mechanism is unknown but may include deficient local blood supply and increased susceptibility to infection occurring in diabetic patients.

5. Excessive levels of adrenal corticosteroids–Corticosteroid excess, whether due to administration of exogenous corticosteroids or to endogenous adrenal hyperactivity (Cushing's syndrome), is associated with impaired wound healing. Corticosteroids may adversely affect wound healing by interfering with neutrophil and macrophage function.

7 Deficiencies of the Host Response

The nonspecific inflammatory response and the immune response act synergistically in defense against infection. Deficits in either process often result in increased susceptibility to attack by pathogenic microorganisms, manifested clinically as recurrent or intractable infection or as "opportunistic" infection, ie, infection by a pathogen of low virulence that does not cause disease in a normal host.

DEFICIENCIES OF THE INFLAMMATORY RESPONSE

DEFICIENCY OF THE VASCULAR RESPONSE

Diabetes Mellitus

In diabetes mellitus, involvement of small arterioles characterized by thickening of the basement membrane increases susceptibility to infection. These abnormal vessels may fail to dilate and do not show the normal changes in permeability associated with the acute inflammatory response.

Vascular Disease (Ischemia)

Severe arterial narrowing limits the amount of blood entering an injured area during acute inflammation and contributes to the decreased resistance to infection observed in older patients, in whom severe arterial narrowing due to atherosclerosis is common.

ABNORMAL NEUTROPHIL FUNCTION

Quantitative Disorders

Neutropenia (decreased numbers of neutrophils) due to any cause is associated with a defective cellular response in acute inflammation that leads to increased susceptibility to infection. A severe reduction in the peripheral blood neutrophil count ($< 1000/\mu L$) must occur before the risk of infection is significantly increased. The commonest cause of neutropenia in clinical practice is cancer treatment utilizing cytotoxic drugs and radiation therapy (Chapter 26).

Qualitative Disorders

Abnormal neutrophil function may be manifested as disorders of neutrophil motility. Intrinsic abnormalities that affect motility are rare and include **lazy leukocyte syndrome,** in which neutrophil emigration is abnormal; and **Chédiak-Higashi**

syndrome, which is characterized by defective movement and degranulation of neutrophils associated with the presence of large cytoplasmic granular inclusions composed of greatly enlarged lysosomes.

Neutrophil motility may also be rarely impaired by extrinsic factors such as serum inhibitors of leukocyte motility, which are most commonly found in patients with rheumatoid arthritis and elevated serum immunoglobulin levels. Deficiencies of chemotactic factors, notably complement deficiency, may also affect neutrophilic motility.

Disorders of Phagocytosis

Abnormalities of phagocytosis may result from deficiency of opsonins, as occurs in hypogammaglobulinemia and complement factor 3 (C3) deficiency. These conditions are associated with a high incidence of infection. Impaired degranulation occurs in Chédiak-Higashi syndrome and in use of antimalarial drugs and corticosteroids.

Disorders of Microbial Killing

A. Chronic Granulomatous Disease of Childhood: Chronic granulomatous disease of childhood is an X-linked recessive disorder characterized by decreased ability of neutrophils to produce hydrogen peroxide. It is due to a variety of different enzyme deficiencies (NADH oxidase, NADH reductase, cytochrome b) that interfere with energy production at the cellular level.

The disease becomes manifest in the first few years of life, chiefly in males, and is characterized by recurrent infections of skin, lungs, bone, and lymph nodes. Patients are susceptible to diseases caused by organisms such as staphylococci and *Serratia* that produce catalase. The catalase produced by these bacteria destroys the small amount of hydrogen peroxide produced in cells and leads to failure of bacterial killing.

The diagnosis of chronic granulomatous disease may be established by (1) **absent nitroblue tetrazolium dye reduction** by neutrophils in vitro; (2) **decreased bacterial killing curves** by neutrophils in test systems; and (3) histologic examination of involved tissue, which shows **granuloma formation** against bacteria that are normally removed during the acute inflammatory response. The formation of granulomas represents a second line of defense when acute inflammation fails to eliminate injurious organisms.

B. Myeloperoxidase Deficiency: Myeloperoxidase acts with hydrogen peroxidase and halide to effect bacterial killing. Deficiency of myeloperoxidase is a rare cause of clinically significant failure of neutrophil function.

C. Granulocytic Leukemia: Neutrophils, monocytes, or both are increased in number in granulocytic leukemias (cancers of cells of the myeloid series; Chapter 26), but they usually function abnormally. The number of normally functioning noncancerous neutrophils is usually greatly decreased in granulocytic leukemia.

DEFICIENCIES OF THE IMMUNE RESPONSE

CONGENITAL (PRIMARY) IMMUNODEFICIENCY

All types of congenital immunodeficiency are rare.

Severe Combined Immunodeficiency

Severe combined immunodeficiency (SCID) is one of the most severe forms of congenital immunodeficiency. It is characterized by a defect of lymphoid stem cells (① in Fig 7–1) that leads to **failure of development of both T and B lymphocytes.** The thymus fails to descend normally from the neck into the mediastinum and is almost devoid of lymphocytes, as are lymph nodes (Fig 7–2B), spleen, gut-associated lymphoid tissue, and peripheral blood. Immunoglobulins are absent in serum (Table 7–1).

Failure of both cellular and humoral immunity causes a variety of severe infections early in life, with death usually resulting in the first year. Infections due to viral, fungal, bacterial, and protozoal organisms occur (Table 7–2).

Severe combined immunodeficiency probably represents several different inherited diseases, all characterized by failure of differentiation of stem cells. The inheritance pattern is variable. Most patients have the autosomal recessive form (Swiss-type); a few patients have the X-linked recessive form. More than half of patients with the autosomal recessive form lack the enzyme **adenosine deaminase** in cells. Conversion of adenosine to inosine cannot occur and causes accumulation of adenosine and its metabolites, which are lymphotoxic and may interfere with nucleic acid synthesis. The absence of adenosine deaminase in amniotic cells permits prenatal diagnosis of this form of combined immunodeficiency. Treatment consisting of bone marrow transplantation and infusion of cells containing normal amounts of adenosine deaminase has been tried with limited success. A few patients with severe combined immunodeficiency lack nucleoside phosphorylase and inosine phosphorylase, leading to metabolic deficits resembling those present in adenosine deaminase deficiency.

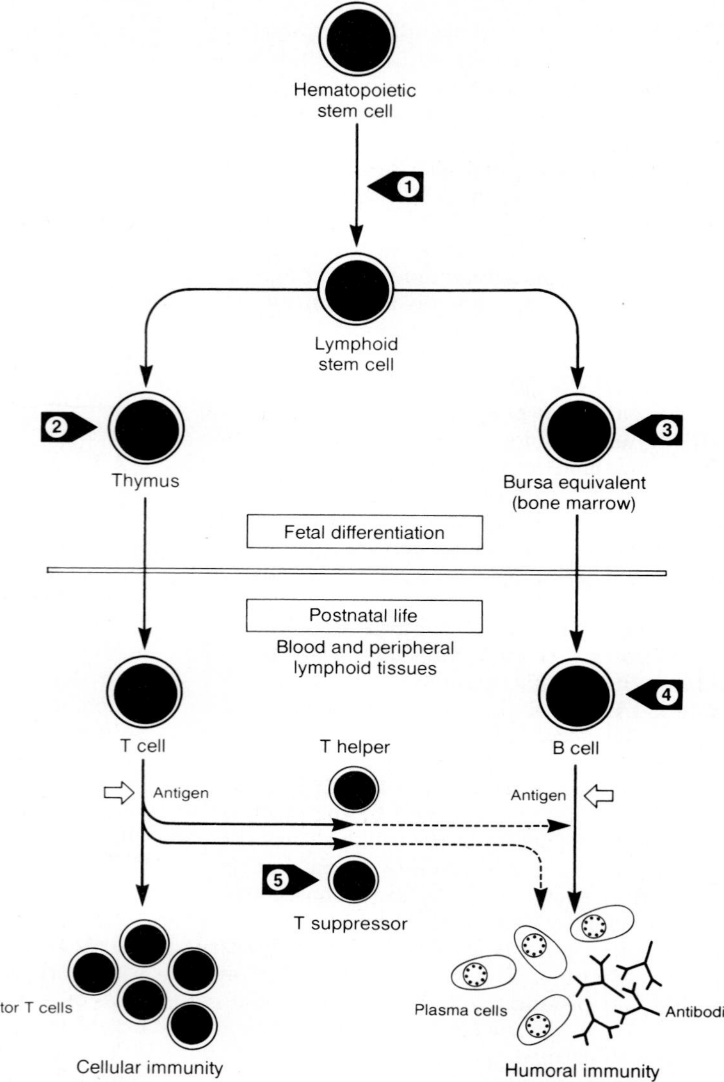

Figure 7–1. Immunodeficiency diseases. Numbers indicate sites of involvement in different disorders and correspond to discussion in text.

Thymic Hypoplasia (DiGeorge Syndrome)

Congenital failure of development of the thymus (② in Fig 7–1) results in lack of T lymphocytes in the blood and T cell areas of lymph nodes (Fig 7–2C) and spleen. The total lymphocyte count in peripheral blood is decreased. Patients show signs of deficient cell-mediated immunity and suffer from severe viral, mycobacterial, and fungal infections in infancy (Table 7–2). B lymphocyte development and number are usually normal. Humoral immunity is abnormal in that T helper cell activity is absent. Serum immunoglobulin levels are usually normal (Table 7–1).

No genetic defect has been identified in thymic hypoplasia. Thymic hypoplasia in DiGeorge syndrome is part of a more severe abnormality of development of the third and fourth pharyngeal pouches. The latter condition is marked by absent parathyroid glands, abnormal aortic arch development, and abnormal facies. When the parathyroids are absent, profound hypocalcemia causes early death. Thymic hypoplasia has been successfully treated with transplantation of human fetal thymus, which restores T cell immunity.

T Lymphopenia (Nezelof's Syndrome)

Nezelof's syndrome represents a cluster of poorly defined deficits of T cell number and function, thought to result from abnormalities of T cell maturation in the thymus, or defects of the thymus itself. DiGeorge syndrome is distinguished from Nezelof's syndrome by its characteristic association with abnormalities of other structures derived from the third and fourth pharyngeal

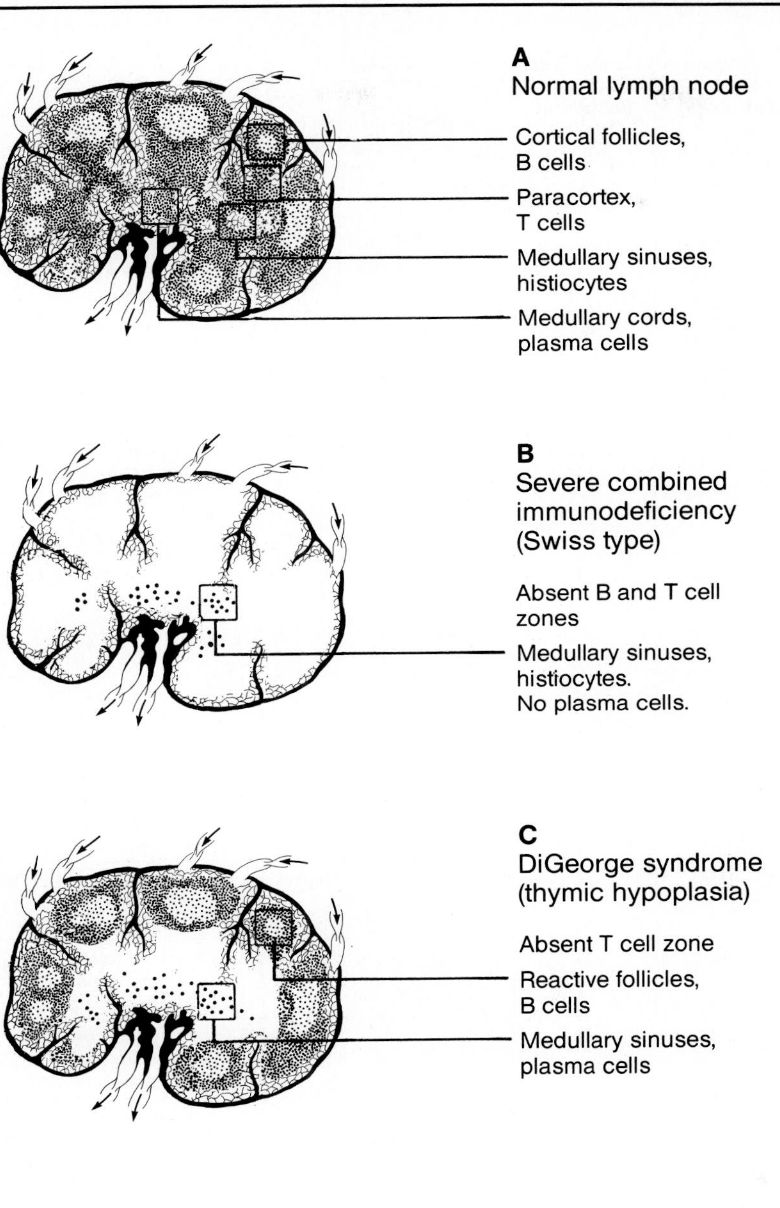

Figure 7-2. Morphologic abnormalities in lymph nodes in congenital immunodeficiency syndromes. **A:** Normal lymph node. **B:** Severe combined immunodeficiency, showing depletion of all lymphocytes. **C:** DiGeorge syndrome showing depletion of T lymphocytes in the paracortex. **D:** Bruton's congenital agammaglobulinemia, showing depletion of B cells in reactive follicles and plasma cells in medullary cords.

Table 7–1. Immunodeficiency diseases.

	Peripheral Blood Lymphocytes	Peripheral Blood T Cells	Peripheral Blood B Cells	Tissue Lymphoid Cells	Serum Immunoglobulin	Other Features
Severe combined immunodeficiency	↓↓	↓↓	↓↓	Absent	↓↓	Lack of adenosine deaminase in 50% of patients with autosomal recessive form of disease.
Thymic aplasia (DiGeorge syndrome)	↓	↓↓	N[1]	T cells depleted in thymus-dependent areas of lymph nodes and spleen	N	Abnormal development of pharyngeal pouches; parathyroids absent.
T lymphopenia (Nezelof's syndrome)	↓	↓↓	N	T cells depleted in thymus-dependent areas of lymph nodes and spleen	N/↓	Heterogeneous group; immunoglobulins may also be decreased.
Bruton's congenital agammaglobulinemia	N	N	↓	Absence of follicles and plasma cells in lymph nodes	↓↓	Neutropenia.
Variable immunodeficiency	N	N	N/↓	Decrease in plasma cells	↓	Associated autoimmune disease; occasionally, lymphadenopathy with follicular hyperplasia.
Selective IgA deficiency	N	N	N	N	↓IgA only	Common (1:1000 general population).
Wiskott-Aldrich syndrome	N/↓	N/↓	N	N	↓(Especially IgM)	Involuted thymus, thrombocytopenia, eczema.
Ataxia-telangiectasia	↓	N/↓	N	Variable	↓(Especially IgA)	Embryonic-type thymus; lymphomas common.
HIV infection (AIDS)	N/↓	↓(Especially helper T cells)	N	Abnormal follicular hyperplasia or lymphocyte depletion	N	Decreased helper:suppressor T cell ratio; Kaposi's sarcoma; B cell lymphomas.
Epithelioid thymoma (Good's syndrome)	↓	↓	N	Decreased or absent plasma cells	N/↓	Decreased eosinophil count; red cell aplasia.

[1]N = normal.

pouches. It appears likely that other entities will be recognized within this group as further data become available.

Bruton's Congenital Agammaglobulinemia

Bruton's agammaglobulinemia is an X-linked recessive disorder seen mostly in male infants and characterized by failure of development of B lymphocytes (③ in Fig 7–1). B lymphocytes are absent in the peripheral blood and B cell domains in lymph nodes and spleen. Reactive follicles and plasma cells are absent in lymph nodes (Fig 7–2D). Serum immunoglobulins are markedly decreased or absent. The thymus and T lymphocytes develop normally. The total lymphocyte count in peripheral blood is normal because T cells, which typically represent 80–90% of blood lymphocytes, are present in normal numbers. Cell-mediated immunity is normal (Table 7–1).

Table 7-2. Infections observed in patients with impaired immunity.[1]

Clinical Setting	Pyogenic Bacteria	Mycobacteria (*M tuberculosis*, Atypical)	Fungi (*Cryptococcus*, *Candida*)	Viruses (CMV, Herpes, Papovavirus[2])	*Pneumocystis Carinii*	*Giardia lamblia*	*Toxoplasma gondii*	*Cryptosporidium, Isospora*
Severe combined immunodeficiency	+	+	+	+	+	–	–	–
Thymic hypoplasia (DiGeorge syndrome)	–	+	+	+	–	–	–	–
Bruton's congenital agammaglobulinemia	+	–	–	–	–	+	–	–
Variable immunodeficiency	+	–	–	–	–	+	–	–
Complement deficiency	+	–	–	–	–	–	–	–
Granulocyte deficiency	+	–	–	–	–	–	–	–
HIV infection (AIDS)	–	+	+	+	+	+	+	+
Immunosuppressive drug therapy	–	+	+	+	+	–	+	–

[1]T cell deficiency results in a susceptibility to fungal, viral, and mycobacterial infections; B cell, complement, and granulocyte deficiency result in susceptibility to infections caused by pyogenic bacteria.
[2]Papovavirus infection of the brain that causes progressive multifocal leukoencephalopathy (PML).

Failure of humoral immunity leads to development of infections in the infant after passively transferred maternal antibody levels decrease, usually in the second half of the first year of life. Recurrent infections of the lungs, meninges, middle ear, and sinuses caused by bacteria such as *Streptococcus pneumoniae, Haemophilus influenzae,* and other gram-negative bacteria are characteristic. Intestinal infestation with *Giardia lamblia* is common (Table 7–2). Treatment with frequent injections of gamma globulin (immunoglobulin concentrate) is effective.

Common Variable Immunodeficiency

Common variable immunodeficiency includes several different diseases characterized by decreased levels of some or all of the immunoglobulin classes. Peripheral blood lymphocytes, including B cell numbers, are usually normal. Plasma cells are usually decreased in lymph nodes in proportion to the immunoglobulin deficiency, suggesting defective B lymphocyte transformation (④ in Fig 7–1). In some cases, an excess of suppressor T cells has been described (⑤ in Fig 7–1), particularly in an acquired form of the disease that develops in adult life. Variable inheritance patterns have been described. The deficient humoral immune response leads to recurrent bacterial infections and giardiasis (Table 7–2). Treatment with prophylactic gamma globulin injections is less satisfactory than in Bruton's agammaglobulinemia.

Isolated IgA Deficiency

Selective deficiency of IgA is the most common immunodeficiency, occurring in about one in 1000 individuals. It is due to a defect in the terminal differentiation of IgA-secreting plasma cells (④ in Fig 7–1); in some patients, it is associated with abnormal suppressor T lymphocytes (⑤ in Fig 7–1).

Most patients with IgA deficiency are asymptomatic. A few demonstrate increased incidence of pulmonary and gastrointestinal infections, since they lack the mucosal IgA that plays a key defensive role in these sites. Most IgA-deficient individuals develop anti-IgA antibodies in their plasma. These antibodies may react with IgA present in transfused blood and cause type I hypersensitivity reactions (Chapter 8). Such allergic transfusion reactions are usually mild (urticarial) but may cause anaphylaxis and death on rare occasions.

Immunodeficiency Associated With Inherited Diseases

A. Wiskott-Aldrich Syndrome: Wiskott-Aldrich syndrome is an X-linked recessive disease characterized by eczema, thrombocytopenia (decreased platelets in blood), and immunodeficiency. T lymphocyte deficiency may develop in the course of the disease, and serum IgM levels are low. Patients develop recurrent viral, fungal, and bacterial infections.

B. Ataxia-Telangiectasia: Ataxia-telangiectasia is an autosomal recessive disease characterized by cerebellar ataxia, skin telangiectasia, and deficiencies of T lymphocytes, IgA, and IgE.

Complement Deficiency

Deficiency of various complement factors has been described; these disorders are all rare. C2 deficiency is the most common. C3 deficiency clinically resembles congenital agammaglobulinemia and is characterized by recurrent bacterial infections in infancy. Deficiency of early complement factors (C1, C4, and C2) is associated with the development of autoimmune diseases, notably systemic lupus erythematosus. Deficiency of the late complement factors (C6, C7, and C8) predisposes to development of recurrent infections caused by *Neisseria.*

SECONDARY & ACQUIRED IMMUNODEFICIENCY

Immunoparesis of varying degree is fairly common. It occurs most often as a secondary phenomenon in various diseases (Table 7–3) and is rarely a primary disease.

Acquired Immune Deficiency Syndrome (AIDS) (Fig 7–3)

A. Incidence: AIDS has become the commonest immunodeficiency disease in the USA since it was first recognized in 1979. By 1988, there were about 60,000 cases of AIDS in the USA alone and as many as 2 million individuals are estimated to be infected with HIV. This increase appears likely to continue, and some sources in the USA predict that by the year 2000 there will be as many as 100 million cases of AIDS worldwide, making it the greatest pandemic of modern times.

B. Definition: AIDS is currently defined by the US Centers for Disease Control (CDC) as the presence of any one of the criteria set forth in Table 7–4. The initial criteria used for case definition were the occurrence of certain indicator diseases such as *Pneumocystis carinii* pneumonia and Kaposi's sarcoma (see Table 7–4 section 1.B for complete list) in a patient without a known cause of immunodeficiency (see Table 7–4 section I.A for list). These criteria were very strict and resulted in considerable underdiagnosis of AIDS. They were modified when testing for the human immunodeficiency virus (HIV), the etiologic agent of AIDS, became widely available. A combination of serum HIV antibody status and the presence of indicator diseases is now used to define AIDS (Table 7–4). Improved diagnosis and more accurate reporting

Table 7-3. Acquired immunodeficiency.

	Mechanism
Primary disease	Rare; usually manifested as hypogammaglobulinemia in adults. Due to increased numbers of suppressor T cells.
Secondary to other diseases	
Protein-calorie malnutrition	Hypogammaglobulinemia.
Iron deficiency	Impaired T cell function.
Postinfectious (measles, leprosy)	Often lymphopenia; usually transient.
Hodgkin's disease	Impaired T cell function.
Multiple myeloma	Impaired immunoglobulin production.
Lymphoma or lymphocytic leukemia	Decreased number of normal lymphocytes.
Advanced cancer	Depressed T cell function, other unknown mechanisms.
Thymic neoplasms	Hypogammaglobulinemia.
Chronic renal failure	Unknown.
Diabetes mellitus	Unknown.
Aging	Decreased number of T cells in some people.
Drug-induced immunodeficiency	Common; caused by corticosteroids, anticancer drugs, radiotherapy, or deliberately induced immunosuppression in transplant patients.
Human immunodeficiency virus (HIV) infection (AIDS)	Reduced number of T cells, mainly helper T cells.

of the disease now permits reliable estimates of its prevalence.

C. Etiology and Pathogenesis: AIDS is caused by an RNA retrovirus called human immunodeficiency virus (HIV)—previously called human T cell lymphotropic virus type III (HTLV III) and lymphadenopathy-associated virus (LAV). The primary targets of attack of HIV are helper (CD4/OKT4-positive) T lymphocytes. The virus uses cell surface receptor molecules for its entry. Other cell types that share common epitopes with the T lymphocyte receptor—eg, macrophages and cells in the central nervous system—are also susceptible to infection with HIV.

The entry of HIV into T lymphocytes may result in (1) acute destruction of the cell, which is the most common effect; or (2) latent infection, with insertion of the proviral genome into the host DNA. Infection of humans with HIV is almost invariably associated with the appearance of anti-HIV antibodies in the serum. These antibodies are not protective, and HIV viremia persists despite their presence. Detection of anti-HIV antibodies and viral isolation from the blood or infected cells are important diagnostic tools (Table 7–5). Anti-HIV antibodies may be detected by **enzyme-linked immunosorbent assay (ELISA)**. The ELISA test is extremely sensitive and specific but is nonetheless associated with a low incidence of both false-positive and false-negative results. It is therefore important to confirm a positive ELISA test with the more specific Immunoblot (Western blot) test.

D. Transmission: HIV infection is transmitted almost exclusively by sexual contact and by direct injection of the agent into the blood through blood transfusion or intravenous drug abuse (Fig 7–3). The risk of transmission by other body fluids such as saliva and tears is very low despite the presence of HIV in such fluids. The risk of infection of health care workers is also low, though a few cases of HIV infection have been reported after accidental blood spills and needle sticks. The risk of infection by casual contact with an infected person is almost nil—and this fact has led to legislation in many communities banning discrimination against victims of AIDS in employment, in education, and in public facilities. The US Army, however, has started using HIV antibody testing to screen out recruits who have been exposed to the virus and might represent a source of infection.

Transmission of HIV during sexual contact occurs at a rate lower than that of gonorrhea or hepatitis B, and current estimates indicate that the risk associated with a single encounter with an HIV-infected partner is less than 5%—compared with 30% in the case of gonorrhea. The use of condoms has been recommended by the Surgeon General of the United States as a means of decreasing HIV transmission during sexual contact. Transmission of HIV by blood transfusion and blood products is highly efficient, with the result that over 90% of individuals transfused with infected blood become infected. Testing for HIV antibody in blood donors has greatly reduced the risk of HIV transmission by transfusion of blood and blood products (eg, factor VIII concentrate that is used to treat hemophilia).

E. Individuals at High Risk for HIV Infection: HIV infection occurs in several high-risk groups: (1) Male homosexuals and bisexuals account for over 70% of cases of AIDS in the USA. (2) Intravenous drug abusers account for about 15%. (3) Central Africans and their sexual partners account for about 5% of cases in the United States, but in some European countries such as Belgium they comprise the largest group. (4) Heterosexual female contacts of male bisexuals and intravenous drug abusers are believed to account for about 3% of cases. (5) Patients transfused with blood products—most importantly hemo-

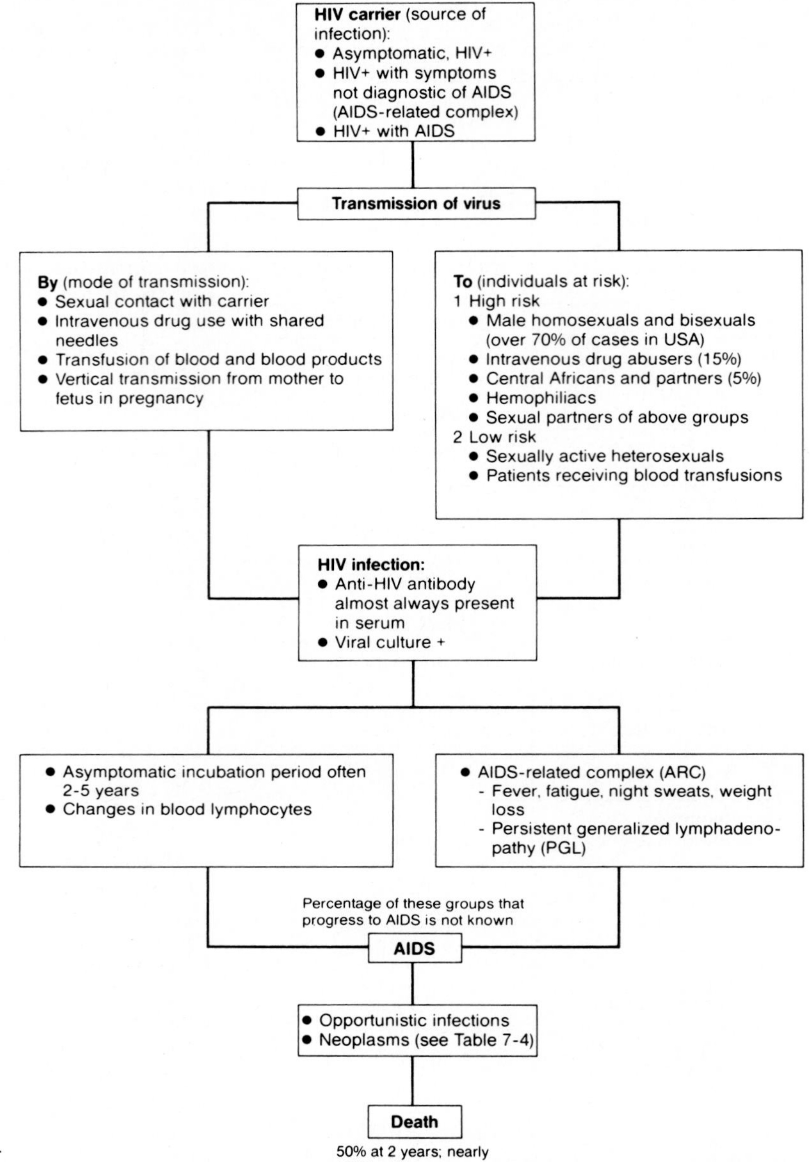

Figure 7-3. Summary of infection with human immunodeficiency virus in humans. Percentages quoted are for the USA.

philiacs and infants—represent an estimated 2% of cases.

Despite the fact that most cases of HIV infection occur in these high-risk groups, the general population may be increasingly at risk. Recovery of HIV from the female genital tract provides the basis for infection of heterosexuals as well as vertical transmission from mother to fetus. In Africa, AIDS occurs frequently in the heterosexual population, and many authorities believe that the incidence in the sexually active heterosexual population will soon increase in the USA.

F. Manifestations and Stages of HIV Infection: (Table 7–6.)

1. Incubation period-The incubation period between HIV infection and the development of AIDS has been calculated in patients infected by blood transfusion—a documented date of inoculation—to be a median of about 4½ years. The incubation period is shorter in young children than in adults (Table 7–6). The longer the individual is infected with HIV, the more likely the development of AIDS. During the incubation period, individuals are positive for HIV antibody and may show changes in the peripheral blood lymphocytes, but they are asymptomatic. The percentage of asymptomatic HIV-positive individuals who go on to develop AIDS is still unknown.

Table 7-4. Definition and diagnosis of AIDS.

I. Without laboratory evidence of HIV infection

If laboratory tests for HIV were not performed or gave indeterminate results and the patient had no other cause of immunodeficiency listed in Section I.A below, then any disease listed in Section I.B indicates AIDS if it was diagnosed by a definitive method.

A. Causes of immunodeficiency that disqualify diseases as indicators of AIDS in the absence of laboratory evidence for HIV infection

1. Any immunosuppressive or cytotoxic therapy within 3 months of the onset of the indicator disease.
2. Any cancer of the lymphoreticular system (other than primary brain lymphoma) diagnosed before or within 3 months after diagnosis of the indicator disease.
3. A congenital immunodeficiency syndrome or an acquired immunodeficiency syndrome atypical of HIV infection, such as one involving hypogammaglobulinemia.

B. Indicator diseases diagnosed definitively

1. Candidiasis of the esophagus, trachea, bronchi, or lungs.
2. Cryptococcosis, extrapulmonary.
3. Cryptosporidiosis with diarrhea persisting for longer than 1 month.
4. Cytomegalovirus infection of an organ other than liver, spleen, or lymph nodes in a patient over 1 month of age.
5. Herpes simplex virus infection causing a mucocutaneous ulcer that persists over 1 month, or bronchitis, pneumonitis, or esophagitis for any duration in a patient over 1 month of age.
6. Kaposi's sarcoma in a patient under 60 years of age.
7. Primary lymphoma of the brain in a patient under 60 years of age.
8. Lymphoid interstitial pneumonia or pulmonary lymphoid hyperplasia in a child under 13 years of age.
9. Disseminated *Mycobacterium avium-intracellulare* complex or *Mycobacterium kansasii* infection (site other than lung, skin, cervical or hilar lymph node).
10. *Pneumocystis carinii* pneumonia.
11. Progressive multifocal leukoencephalopathy.
12. Toxoplasmosis of the brain in a patient over 1 month of age.

II. With laboratory evidence of HIV infection

Regardless of the presence of other causes of immunodeficiency set out in I.A above, in the presence of laboratory evidence for HIV infection, any disease listed in I.B above or II.A or II.B below indicates AIDS.

A. Indicator diseases diagnosed definitively

1. Bacterial infections, multiple or recurrent (more than 2 in a 2-year period), excluding otitis media and skin infections, caused by pyogenic bacteria, in a child under 13 years of age.
2. Disseminated coccidioidomycosis or histoplasmosis (at a site other than lung or cervical or hilar lymph node).
3. Encephalopathy (also called AIDS dementia).
4. Isosporiasis with diarrhea persisting for longer than 1 month.
5. Kaposi's sarcoma at any age.
6. Lymphoma of the brain at any age.
7. Other non-Hodgkin's lymphoma, high-grade, B cell types.
8. Recurrent nontyphoid *Salmonella* septicemia.
9. Any mycobacterial disease other than tuberculosis, disseminated and involving sites other than lung, skin, cervical or hilar lymph nodes.
10. *Mycobacterium tuberculosis* infection, miliary or involving an extrapulmonary site.
11. HIV wasting syndrome ("slim disease").

B. Indicator diseases diagnosed presumptively (ie, clinical diagnosis without pathologic confirmation)

1. Candidiasis of the esophagus.
2. Cytomegalovirus retinitis with loss of vision.
3. Kaposi's sarcoma.
4. Lymphoid interstitial pneumonia in a child under 13 years of age.
5. Mycobacterial disease (positive acid-fast stain without species identification by culture), disseminated and involving sites other than lungs, skin, cervical or hilar lymph nodes.
6. *Pneumocystis carinii* pneumonia.
7. Toxoplasmosis of the brain in a patient over 1 month of age.

III. With evidence against HIV infection

With laboratory test results negative for HIV infection, AIDS is ruled out unless the patient has had:

A. None of the other causes of immunodeficiency listed in Section I.A

AND

B. Either of the following:

1. *Pneumocystis carinii* pneumonia diagnosed by a definitive method

OR

2. Any of the other diseases indicative of AIDS listed in Section I.B diagnosed by a definitive method **and** a T-helper/inducer (CD4) count of less than 400/μL.

Table 7-5. Laboratory tests for HIV infection.

ELISA test[1]: Tests for presence of antibodies to HIV proteins.
Sensitivity: High (99%)
Specificity: High (99.5%)
Predictive value: Limited (because of low prevalence of HIV infection in the population)

Assuming sensitivity is 99%, specificity is 99.5%, and prevalence of HIV-positive individuals is 2%, the predictive value of a positive test is only 80.16%. For example, test 10,000 individuals: if the prevalence is 2%, 200 will be true positives and 9800 will be true negatives. With a 99% sensitivity, 198 of the 200 true positives will give a (true) positive test; with a 99.5% specificity, 49 of the 9800 true negatives will give a (false) positive test. Total number of positive tests is 198 + 49 = 247. Predictive value of a positive test =

$$\frac{\text{True positive}}{\text{Total positive}} \times 100 = \frac{198}{247} \times 100 = 80.16\%$$

Western blot: Detects HIV proteins
Specificity: Very high (test is, however, difficult to interpret)
Use: As a confirmatory test when ELISA is positive

HIV culture: Difficult and time-consuming; requires special test facilities because result is production of live virus.

P24 antigen assay: Detects viral antigen; not available for clinical use.

Polymerase chain reaction for HIV nucleic acid: Amplifies viral nucleic acid sequences up to 1 millionfold, at which point they are readily detectable. Highly specific and extremely sensitive.

[1]ELISA = enzyme-linked immunosorbent assay. HIV viral envelope obtained from culture is bound to a solid phase (eg, small beads). Patient serum is added. Any anti-HIV antibodies in serum bind to the HIV envelope antigen on the beads. Binding of antibody to the beads is then detected by use of an enzyme-labeled antibody directed against human immunogloblin. The intensity of the colored product is proportionate to the titer of HIV antibodies present in the patient's serum.

Table 7-6. Classification of stages of HIV infection: CDC (Centers for Disease Control) staging.

CDC I	Asymptomatic infection (may be brief flulike illness).
CDC II	Conversion to HIV-positive serology (ELISA test).
CDC III	Onset of immunologic defects, generalized lymphadenopathy (also known as ARC [AIDS-related complex]).
CDC IV	Overt AIDS with opportunistic infections and neoplasms.

Mean incubation period (time from infection to overt AIDS):
Children < age 5 years: 2 years
Adults (and older children): 8 years

Adverse prognostic indications include constitutional symptoms (fever, weight loss, diarrhea), low CD4 lymphocytes, low anti-P24 antibody, circulating P24 antigen, persisting viremia.

2. Changes in the immune system-HIV infection leads to a decrease in the number of helper/inducer (CD4/OKT4-positive) T cells in the peripheral blood. This may be accompanied by an increase in the number of suppressor/cytotoxic (CD8/OKT8-positive) T cells, resulting in a decreased helper T cell:suppressor T cell ratio in the peripheral blood. These are of limited value in the diagnosis of AIDS (see Table 7–4, section III). These changes in the immune system lead to functional immunodeficiency. The decreased helper: suppressor T cell ratio is not diagnostic of HIV infection and may occur in several other immunodeficiency states.

3. AIDS-related complex (ARC)-Patients with ARC are HIV-positive and symptomatic but have none of the indicator diseases that are used to define AIDS. ARC patients complain of fatigue, weight loss, night sweats, and diarrhea and have superficial fungal infections of the mouth, fingernails, and toenails. The best-studied components of ARC are the lymph node abnormalities. In the early stages, infected lymph nodes show marked reactive follicular hyperplasia with characteristic histologic features (Chapter 28)—a condition called **persistent generalized lymphadenopathy (PGL).** HIV can be isolated from the lymph nodes of patients with PGL. At a later stage, lymph nodes show lymphocyte depletion. The percentage of patients with ARC who go on to develop AIDS is not known for certain.

4. AIDS-AIDS is the final phase of HIV infection in which the patient develops one of many opportunistic infections or neoplasms that define the disease (Table 7–4 sections I.B and II.A).

Among the opportunistic infections, the following are the most common: *P carinii* pneumonia, esophageal candidiasis, cytomegalovirus infections, atypical mycobacterial infections, toxoplasmosis of the brain, cryptosporidiosis of the intestine, herpes simplex infections, and papovavirus infection of the brain (progressive multifocal leukoencephalopathy).

Kaposi's sarcoma is a malignant vascular neoplasm that affects the skin (Fig 7–4) and many internal organs. It is the neoplasm whose suddenly increased incidence caused AIDS to be first recognized in 1979. Since 1979, these patients have been shown to have also an increased incidence of high-grade non-Hodgkin's malignant B cell lymphomas, particularly of the central nervous system.

G. The Prospects for Prevention: The main method of prevention of AIDS currently available is public education about the methods of transmission of HIV. The use of condoms and "safe

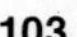

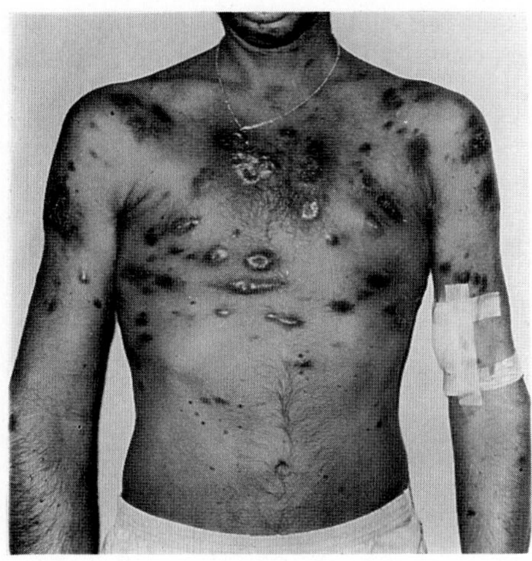

Figure 7-4. Kaposi's sarcoma, disseminated in a patient with AIDS. Note the presence of multiple elevated dark purple skin lesions.

sex'' have been recommended as ways to decrease the risk of infection, but there is little evidence at present that awareness of the risk changes sexual practices significantly.

In some cities, intravenous drug users are provided with sterile needles to decrease the incidence of AIDS transmission by this route. Screening of blood donors for HIV antibody has markedly decreased the incidence of AIDS transmitted by transfusion of blood products. Health care workers, policemen, and firemen routinely take precautions to decrease the risk of becoming infected. None of these measures are expected to significantly reduce the spread of the epidemic.

The 2 main directions of research in AIDS are aimed at developing a vaccine that will prevent infection or a drug that will be effective in treatment. Both a vaccine and an effective drug are still at least several years away.

H. Course and Treatment of AIDS: AIDS is a disease that relentlessly and invariably progresses to death. Almost all patients are dead 5 years after diagnosis, but many die much sooner. Recently introduced drugs such as azidothymidine and ribavirin have been shown to prolong life; however, treated patients continue to develop additional opportunistic infections.

EFFECTS OF IMMUNE DEFICIENCY

The immunocompromised host is susceptible to development of various diseases and disorders.

Infections (Table 7-2)

The development of infections depends on the specific immunodeficiency. T cell deficiency predisposes to infections with viruses, mycobacteria, fungi, and protozoa such as *Pneumocystis carinii* and *Toxoplasma gondii.* B cell deficiency predisposes to pyogenic bacterial infections. These infections reflect the relative importance of cell-mediated and humoral responses in the defense against different microbial agents.

Malignant Neoplasms

Kaposi's sarcoma and malignant B cell lymphomas are the most common malignant neoplasms that develop in immunodeficient individuals. They occur in patients with HIV infection, Wiskott-Aldrich syndrome, and ataxia-telangiectasia and in patients receiving long-term immunosuppressive therapy after renal transplantation. The occurrence of malignant neoplasms may be related to the role of the immune response in removing developing malignant cells that arise in the body (failure of immune surveillance; see Chapter 17), or it may be due to sustained immune stimulation of an inadequate immune system in which the usual controls of cellular proliferation are lacking (eg, leading to B cell lymphoma). In some instances, notably ataxia-telangiectasia, immune deficiency is associated with fragility of chromosomes, which is thought to predispose to neoplasia.

Autoimmune Diseases

Autoimmune diseases are more likely to develop in patients with congenital immunodeficiency (Bruton's agammaglobulinemia, common variable immunodeficiency, selective IgA deficiency, and deficiency of early complement factors). The commonest autoimmune disorders in these patients are rheumatoid arthritis, systemic lupus erythematosus, autoimmune hemolytic anemia, and thrombocytopenia.

Graft-Versus-Host Disease

Graft-versus-host disease is a risk in severely T cell-deficient patients who receive viable ''foreign'' immunocompetent cells in blood transfusions and bone marrow transplants. The absence of host T cell immunity prevents destruction of these foreign cells, which can then proliferate and react against the host. The disease is usually fatal.

DIAGNOSIS OF IMMUNE DEFICIENCY

When immune deficiency is suspected, usually because of recurrent or opportunistic infection, the diagnosis may be confirmed by appropriate immunologic studies (Table 7–1 and 7–5). These include (1) determination of serum immunoglobulin and complement levels; and (2) studies of peripheral blood lymphocytes, including total lymphocyte count, T and B cell number, and identification of lymphocyte subpopulations (eg, helper and suppressor T cells) using monoclonal antibodies. New cytofluorometric techniques facilitate performance of these tests in clinical practice. Other tests such as viral culture and serologic studies (in HIV infection) and enzyme determinations (in severe combined immunodeficiency disease) may be necessary.

Section III. Agents Causing Tissue Injury

This section on specific causes of direct tissue injury is an extension of Section I, in which general mechanisms of tissue injury were described in some detail with only passing reference to specific agents.

Mechanisms of Tissue Injury

Causes of tissue injury act via the general mechanisms described in Section I. The reader may wish to review that section briefly before going on. In this section, tissue injury will be considered from the perspective of the specific agents causing injury, and the pathogenic mechanisms will be explored in greater detail (Fig III–1). The chapters in this section will not emphasize the details of the diseases caused by these agents—that discussion is reserved for the organ system chapters (beginning with Chapter 20), because the clinical consequences of injury are best studied in the context of the impact of the injury on the structure and function of the organ involved.

Tissues may be damaged by deprivation of nutrients or exposure to toxic agents.

A. Lack of Nutrients Essential for Cellular Metabolism: Nutrient deficiency may be generalized, involving the body as a whole (eg, protein-calorie and vitamin deficiency, hypoxia, hypoglycemia), or may involve a single organ as a result of compromise of the blood supply to that organ.

B. Action of Noxious Agents: Noxious agents

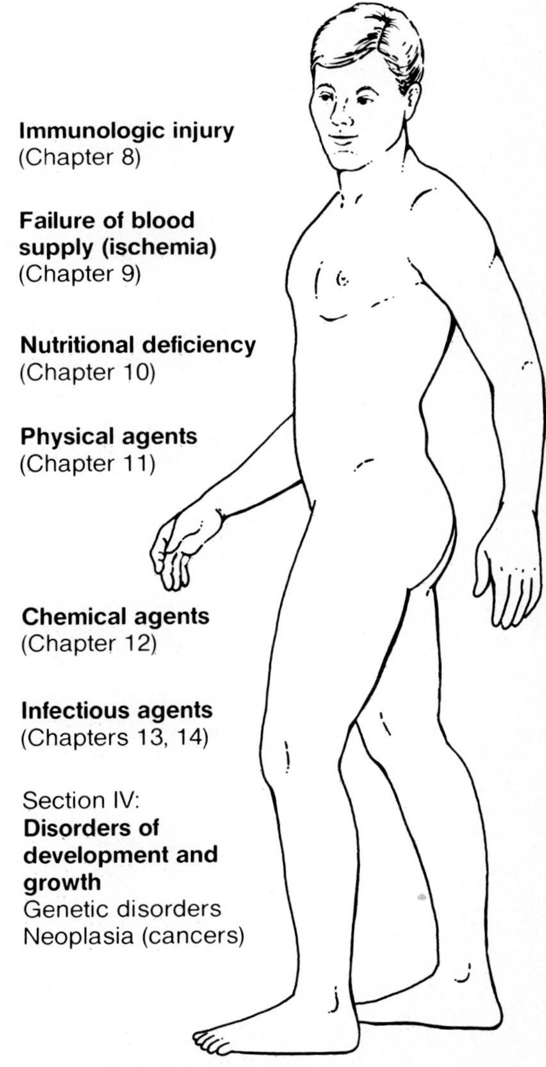

Figure III–1. Principal causes of tissue injury.

include physical agents such as radiation and heat as well as chemical agents (heavy metals, drugs, etc), infectious agents (bacteria, viruses, etc), and endogenous substances that accumulate in the body in inborn errors of metabolism (eg, phenylketonuria) or in failure of organs such as the liver, kidney, and lungs. Immunologic injury occurs when the individual's immune system is inappropriately directed at antigens on host tissues. The production of cytotoxic chemicals (eg, antibodies, complement activation) or cytotoxic cells (eg, effector T lymphocytes) is responsible for immunologic injury.

Immunologic Injury

8

IMMUNOLOGIC HYPERSENSITIVITY

Hypersensitivity is defined as an abnormal exaggerated immune reaction to a foreign agent, with resulting injury to host tissues. Four different mechanisms of hypersensitivity have been elucidated (Table 8–1). All forms except type IV are mediated by humoral mechanisms (ie, by antibodies); type IV hypersensitivity is cell-mediated. In all forms, initial exposure (sensitizing dose) to the antigen involved evokes a primary immune response (**sensitization**). Following a short period (1 or more weeks) during which the immune system is activated, a hypersensitivity response occurs upon any subsequent exposure (challenge dose) to that antigen.

Type I (Immediate) Hypersensitivity (Atopy; Anaphylaxis)

A. Mechanism: (Fig 8–1.) The first exposure to an antigen (allergen) activates the immune system and causes production of **IgE antibodies** (reagins) specifically reactive against the antigen. These become attached to the surface membrane of mast cells and basophils. Production of sufficient antibody to develop clinical hypersensitivity takes 1 or more weeks. When subsequent exposure to the same antigen occurs, an antigen-antibody (IgE) interaction takes place on the surface of the mast cell or basophil and causes degranulation of these cells. The cytoplasmic granules of mast cells release vasoactive substances (histamine, serotonin, leukotrienes [Chapter 3]) that cause vasodilatation, increased vascular permeability, and smooth muscle contraction. The formation of IgE antibodies and release of vasoactive substances are key features of type I hypersensitivity. Mast cells also release factors that are chemotactic for neutrophils and eosinophils; many lesions caused by type I hypersensitivity contain numerous eosinophils in affected tissues and peripheral blood. Eosinophils release arylsulfatase B and histaminase, which serve to cleave leukotrienes and histamine, respectively. Degradation of these vasoactive substances may have an effect in limiting the severity of the hypersensitivity reaction.

B. Disorders Resulting From Type I Hypersensitivity:

1. Localized type I hypersensitivity–Localized expression of a type I hypersensitivity reaction is termed **atopy**. Atopy represents an inherited predisposition to an abnormal response against allergens, and the tendency to develop this form of hypersensitivity is familial. Atopic reactions are common and occur in many organ systems.

a. Skin–In the skin, contact with allergen causes immediate reddening and swelling (some cases of acute dermatitis or eczema). In other cases, swelling and itching predominate (urticaria, or hives). The antigen may come in contact with skin directly or by injection (some insect bites or stings), or it may be ingested, as occurs in some food or drug allergies that produce cutaneous reactions.

b. Nose–In the nasal mucosa, inhalation of the allergen (most commonly pollens) causes vasodilatation and secretion of mucus (allergic rhinitis, or hay fever).

c. Lung–Inhalation of allergens (pollen, dust) leads to contraction of bronchial smooth muscle, resulting in acute airway obstruction and wheezing (allergic bronchial asthma).

d. Intestine–Ingestion of the allergen (eg, nuts, seafood) causes muscle contraction and fluid secretion that produce abdominal cramps and diarrhea (allergic gastroenteritis).

Table 8-1. Hypersensitivity mechanisms.

Type	Antibody	Mechanism	Effect	Examples of Diseases
Type I (immediate, anaphylactic)	IgE	Mast cell or basophil	Edema, bronchospasm	Local (eczema, hay fever, asthma)
			Anaphylaxis	Systemic
Type II (cytotoxic)	IgG or IgM		Lysis, phagocytosis	Transfusion and drug reactions
			Stimulation	Thyrotoxicosis
			Inhibition	Myasthenia gravis
Type III (immune complex)	IgG or IgM		Arthus-type reaction	Local reactions (hypersensitivity pneumonitis)
			Serum sickness-type reaction	Systemic serum sickness (Table 8-4)
Type IV (delayed, cell-mediated)	No antibody		Delayed-type hypersensitivity	Contact dermatitis

▲ antigen; Ag particulate antigen; cell cell bearing hapten or antigen; antibody; C* complement.

2. Systemic type I hypersensitivity reactions–Anaphylaxis is a rare life-threatening systemic type I hypersensitivity reaction. Release of vasoactive amines into the circulation causes smooth muscle contraction, generalized vasodilatation, and increased vascular permeability with leakage of intravascular fluids. The resulting peripheral circulatory failure and shock can lead to death within minutes **(anaphylactic shock)**. In less severe cases, the increased vascular permeability leads to allergic edema throughout the body **(angioneurotic edema)**. Edema of the larynx may cause fatal asphyxia. Systemic anaphylaxis typically results from injected allergens (eg, penicillin, foreign serum, local anesthetics, radiographic contrast dyes). More rarely, anaphylaxis may result from ingested allergens (seafood, egg, berries) or cutaneous allergens (bee and wasp stings). In sensitized individuals, only a small amount of allergen may be required to produce fatal anaphylaxis (eg, the minute dose of penicillin used in a skin test for penicillin hypersensitivity).

Type II Hypersensitivity

A. Mechanism: (Fig 8–2.) Type II hypersensitivity is characterized by an antigen-antibody reaction on the surface of a host cell that causes the destruction of that cell. The antigen involved may be intrinsic to the cell yet perceived by the immune system for some reason as foreign (with resulting autoimmune disease). Alternatively, the antigen may be extrinsic and attached to the cell surface (eg, a drug that serves as a hapten, attaching to a cell membrane protein and inducing an immune response).

Specific antibody, commonly IgG and IgM, is produced against the antigen and interacts with it on the cell surface. This interaction causes cell damage in several ways.

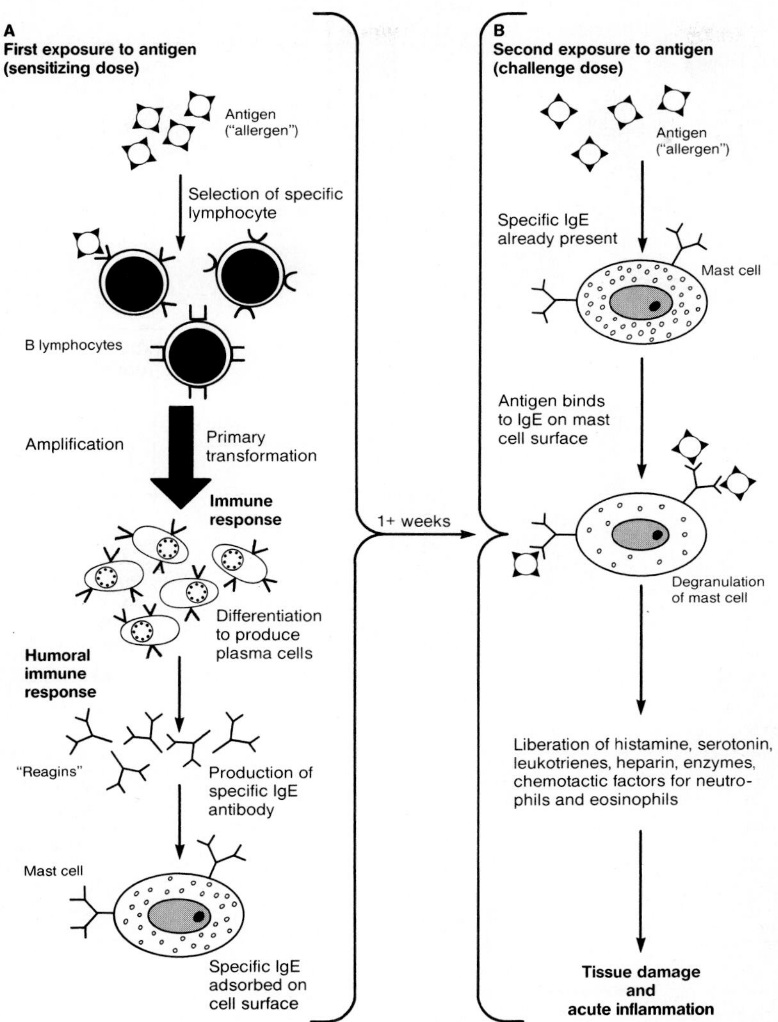

Figure 8-1. Type I hypersensitivity. **A.** The first (sensitizing) dose of antigen results in production of specifically reactive IgE that becomes absorbed on the surface of mast cells. **B.** A second exposure to the antigen results in the antigen-antibody reaction on the mast cell surface, causing rapid release by the mast cell of vasoactive substances responsible for the pathologic changes in the tissue.

1. Lysis–Activation of the complement cascade leads to formation of the C6789 complex and causes lysis of the cell membrane.

2. Phagocytosis–The antigen-bearing cell attaches to phagocytic macrophages that have Fc or C3b receptors which recognize the antigen-antibody complex on the cell. Phagocytosis and cell destruction follow.

3. Antibody-dependent cell-mediated cytotoxicity (ADCC)–The antigen-antibody complex is recognized by nonsensitized null lymphocytes (natural killer [NK] cells) that destroy the cell. This type of hypersensitivity is sometimes classified separately as type VI hypersensitivity.

4. Change in cellular function–Antibody reacts with a cell surface molecule or receptor, causing either increase or inhibition of a cellular metabolic reaction without causing cell necrosis (see Stimulation and Inhibition in Hypersensitivity, below). Some authorities classify this separately as type V hypersensitivity.

B. Disorders Resulting From Type II Hypersensitivity: The manifestation of type II hypersensitivity reactions varies with the type of cell bearing the antigen that triggers antibody formation. Note that blood transfusion reactions are actually normal immune responses against foreign cells (Table 8–2), but since they adversely affect the patient receiving the foreign cells (ie, the transfusion), they usually are included with the hypersensitivity disorders.

1. Antigens on erythrocytes.–

a. Blood transfusion reactions–Antibodies in the patient's serum react against antigens on transfused red cells, causing either complement-mediated intravascular hemolysis or delayed hemolysis due to immune phagocytosis by splenic macrophages. Many erythrocyte antigens may

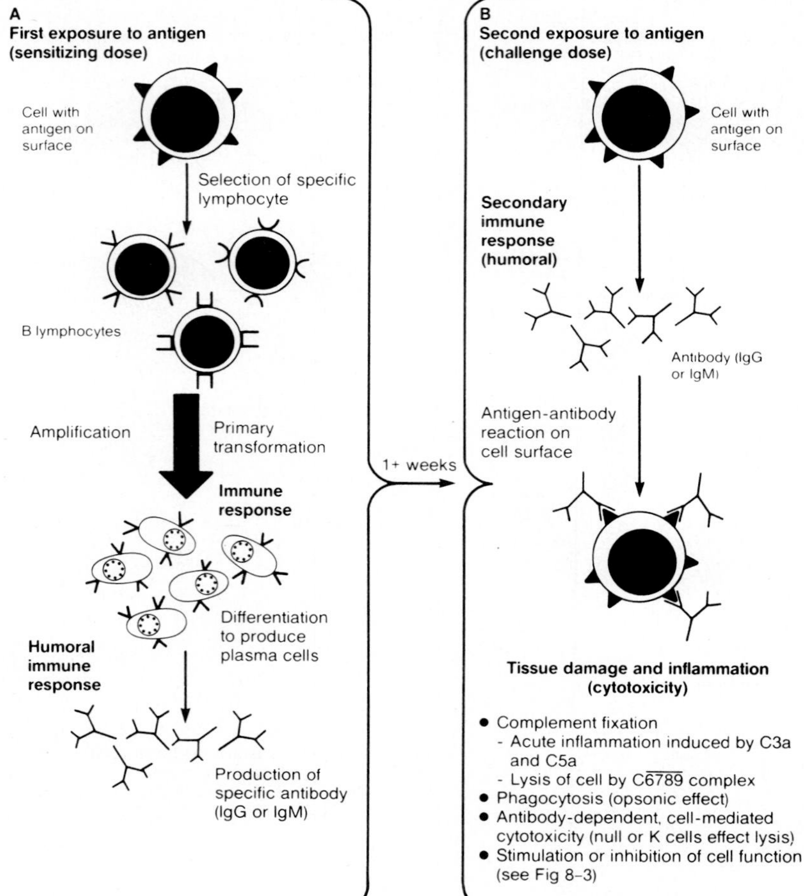

Figure 8-2. Type II (cytotoxic) hypersensitivity. **A.** The first (sensitizing) dose of antigen results in the production of specifically reactive IgG or IgM antibody. **B.** A second exposure to the antigen results in an antigen-antibody reaction that typically occurs on the surface of the cell bearing the antigen and leads to cell necrosis (cytotoxicity) by the several immune mechanisms shown.

Table 8-2A. Blood transfusion reactions caused by nonerythrocyte antigen incompatibilities.

Donor Antigen	Antibody in Recipient Plasma	Mechanism of Damage	Effect
Neutrophil antigens			
HLA antigen	HLA antibodies; especially common in multiply transfused patients	Type II antigen-antibody reaction; complement-mediated lysis; immune phagocytosis.	Destruction of transfused neutrophils; fever, chills, hypotension.
Platelet antigens			
HLA antigens	HLA antibodies	Hypersensitivity type II cytotoxicity	Destruction of transfused platelets; fever.
Platelet antigens	Antiplatelet antibodies		
Plasma proteins			
Protein antigens	Various antibodies to plasma proteins	Release of chemical mediators and pyrogens	Fever.
IgA			
Antigens in the IgA molecule	Anti-IgA present in plasma of IgA-deficient individuals[1]	Type I hypersensitivity	Urticaria; anaphylaxis.

[1]IgA deficiency is present in 0.1% of the population. These individuals frequently have natural anti-IgA antibodies in their plasma.

Table 8–2B. Blood transfusion reactions due to ABO and Rh antigen incompatibilities.[1]

Recipient Blood Types	Antibodies in Recipient Plasma[2]	Compatible Donor Blood Types[3]	Incompatible Blood Types	Mechanism of Damage	Effect
ABO blood group[4]					
A	Anti-B	Group A, group O	Group B	Antigen-antibody reaction on erythrocyte surface	
B	Anti-A	Group B, group O	Group A		
AB[5]	None	Group A, group B, group AB, group O	None	Lysis mediated by C6789	Intravascular hemolysis
O[6]	Anti-A, anti-B	Group O	Group A, group B, group AB	Immune phagocytosis of antibody-coated erythrocytes by splenic macrophages	Extravascular hemolysis
Rh blood type[4]					
Rh−	None unless sensitized by pregnancy or transfusion[7]	Rh−[8]	Rh+ only if the recipient has been sensitized and has anti-Rh antibody in plasma[7]	Antigen-antibody reaction on erythrocyte surface	
				Lysis mediated by C6789	Intravascular hemolysis
				Immune phagocytosis of antibody-coated erythrocytes by splenic macrophages	Extravascular hemolysis
Rh+	None	Either Rh−[8] or Rh+ (does not matter)			

[1]Other uncommon erythrocyte blood group antigens are uncommon causes of transfusion reactions (eg, Lewis, Kidd, Kell systems). The mechanisms are similar to those described above.
[2]In the ABO system, the absence of the erythrocyte antigen is always associated with the presence of the corresponding antibody ("natural antibody") in the plasma, eg, a group O individual will have anti-A and anti-B in the plasma.
[3]Compatibility for blood transfusion *requires* that the donor erythrocytes be compatible with recipient plasma. Antibodies in donor plasma are usually diluted to such an extent that they have no effect on recipient erythrocytes. (They may, however, be significant in massive transfusions.)
[4]The ABO and Rh blood types of an individual are determined by the presence of A, B, and Rh antigen on the erythrocyte membrane.
[5]Group AB individuals (lacking both anti-A and anti-B in plasma) are "universal" recipients.
[6]Group O individuals (lacking both A and B antigens on erythrocytes) are "universal" donors.
[7]Unlike the ABO system, Rh− individuals do not have "natural" anti-Rh antibody in the plasma. Anti-Rh antibodies may be acquired (sensitization) if Rh+ erythrocytes enter the bloodstream of an Rh− individual. This usually occurs during late pregnancy with an Rh+ fetus or when Rh+ blood is transfused.
[8]Transfusion of Rh− blood is safe for both Rh− and Rh+ individuals. Group O (see [6] above) Rh− blood may be used in an extreme emergency before matched blood is made available. (The laboratory can type and cross-match blood in less than 1 hour.)

cause hemolytic transfusion reactions (ABO, Rh, Kell, Kidd, Lewis, etc). In addition, the infused blood itself may contain antibodies that react against host cells, but because the antibodies are greatly diluted in the total blood volume, this reaction is usually of little clinical consequence. Blood typing and cross-matching are effective in preventing such reactions (see Chapter 25).

b. Hemolytic disease of the newborn–In hemolytic disease of the newborn, maternal antibodies that are active against fetal erythrocyte antigens (Rh and ABO) cross the placenta and destroy fetal erythrocytes. Hemolytic disease of the newborn is more common in Rh incompatibility because anti-Rh antibodies in the plasma of the mother are usually IgG and cross the placenta. Anti-A and anti-B are usually IgM and do not cross the placenta.

c. Other hemolytic reactions–Hemolysis may be caused by drugs that act as haptens in combination with erythrocyte membrane proteins, or it may be a result of infections associated with the development of antierythrocyte antigens, eg, infectious mononucleosis, mycoplasmal pneumonia.

2. Antigens on neutrophils–Maternal antibodies to fetal neutrophilic antigens may cause neonatal leukopenia if they cross the placenta. Posttransfusion reactions due to activity of host serum against donor leukocyte HLA system antigens may occur (see Table 8–2A).

3. Antigens on platelets–Neonatal thrombocytopenia and posttransfusion febrile reactions may occur as a result of factors similar to those described for leukocytes. Idiopathic thrombocytopenic purpura is a common autoimmune disease in which antibodies develop against a person's own platelet membrane antigens.

4. Antigens on basement membrane-Antibodies against renal glomerular and pulmonary alveolar basement membrane antigens develop in Goodpasture's syndrome (Chapter 48). Tissue injury results from complement activation.

5. Stimulation and inhibition in hypersensitivity-(Fig 8–3.) Some authors classify inhibition and stimulation associated with hypersensitivity as type V hypersensitivity. In these reactions, antibodies interact with antigens on cells and cause either stimulation or inhibition of the functions of that cell (rather than cell death, as occurs in other forms of type II hypersensitivity). It is the altered cellular function that causes disease; the cell itself may or may not show signs of injury.

a. Stimulation-Graves' disease (primary hyperthyroidism) is caused by stimulatory IgG antibodies that bind to surface antigens on thyroid follicular epithelial cells. This interaction leads to the stimulation of the enzyme adenylate cyclase, which increases cAMP levels in the cell. cAMP is the "internal messenger" that stimulates the thyroid cell to secrete increased amounts of thyroid hormone (Chapter 58).

b. Inhibition-Inhibitory antibodies play a key role in **myasthenia gravis,** a disorder characterized by failure of neuromuscular transmission, with resulting motor weakness. The disease is due to an IgG antibody directed against acetylcholine receptors at the motor end plate. The antibody binds to these receptors and blocks the action of acetylcholine, thereby blocking transmission of the nerve impulse. In **pernicious anemia,** antibodies may bind to intrinsic factor and inhibit absorption of vitamin B_{12}.

Type III Hypersensitivity (Immune Complex Injury)

A. Mechanism: (Fig 8–4.) Interaction of antigen and antibody may result in the formation of

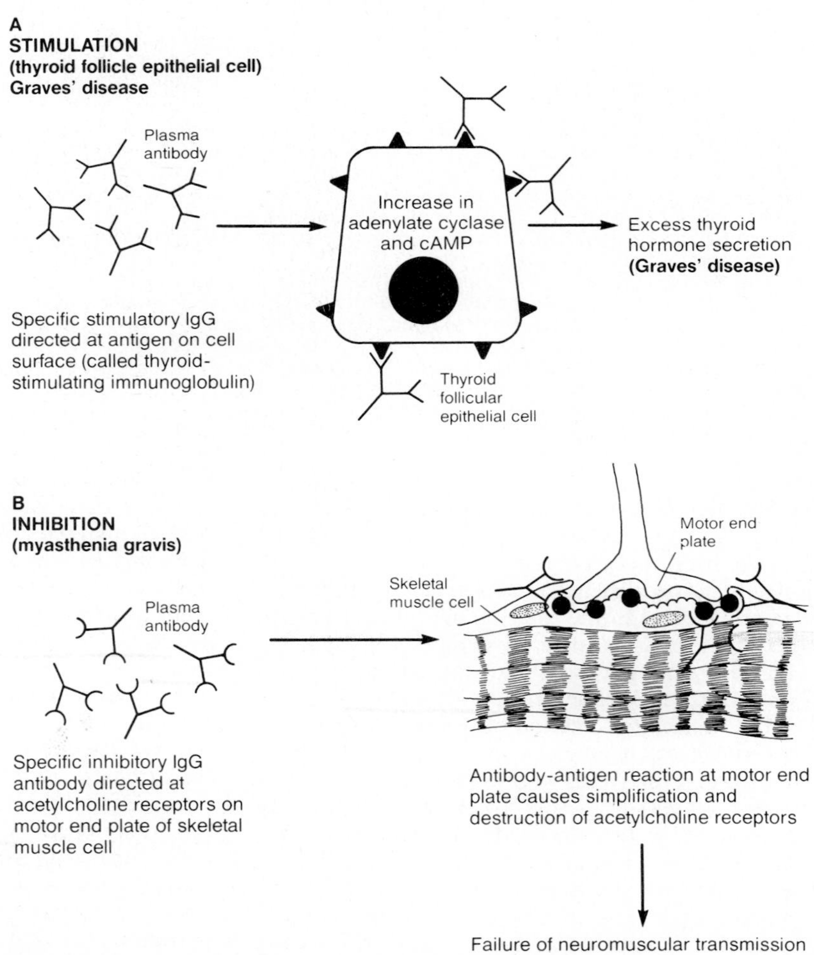

Figure 8-3. Stimulation **(A)** and inhibition **(B)** in type II hypersensitivity. Sensitization takes place as depicted in Fig 8–2, but antibody has a stimulatory or inhibitory effect and is not cytotoxic.

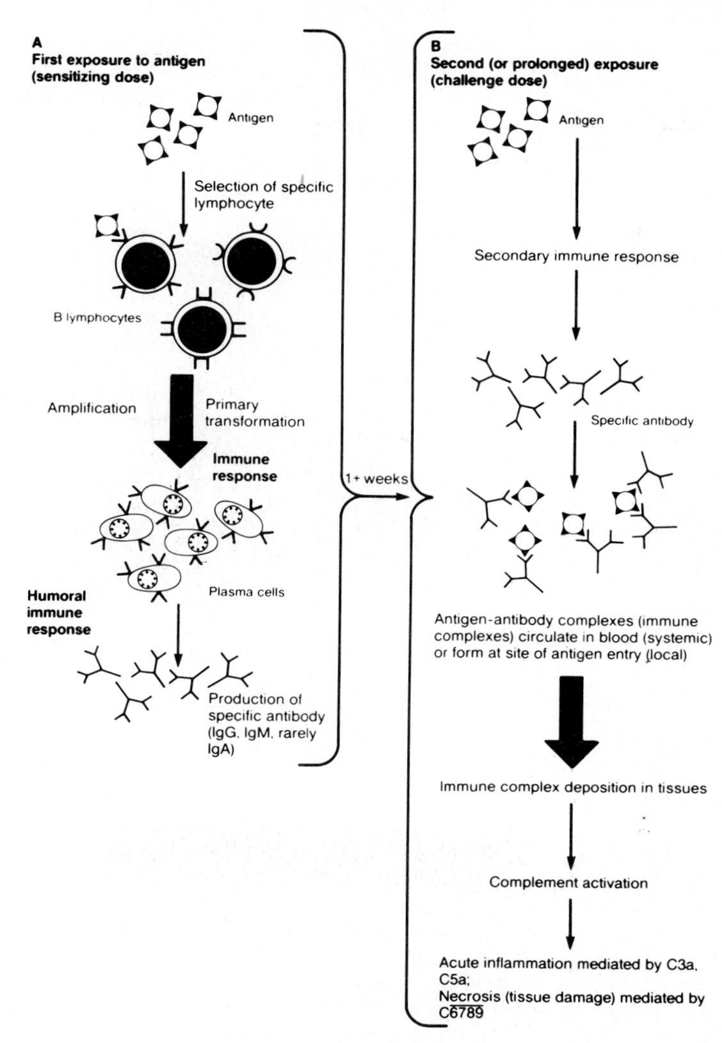

Figure 8-4. Type III hypersensitivity (immune complex disease) results when immune complexes formed by antigen and specific antibody are deposited in tissues. This leads to complement activation, which causes tissue damage and acute inflammation. Immune complex disease may be systemic, caused by circulating complexes (as in serum sickness), or localized, due to formation of immune complexes at the site of entry of antigen (as in the Arthus reaction).

immune complexes, either locally at the site of injury or systemically in the circulation. Deposition of immune complexes at various sites in the body activates complement and causes acute inflammation and injury.

Two types of immune complex injury are recognized.

1. Arthus-type reaction–In the Arthus-type reaction of immune complex injury, tissue necrosis occurs at the site of entry of the antigen. Repeated episodes of antigen exposure result in high levels of precipitating antibody in the serum. Subsequent exposure to the same antigen leads to the formation of large antigen-antibody complexes, which precipitate locally in small blood vessels, where they activate complement and produce a severe local acute inflammatory reaction with hemorrhage and necrosis. This phenomenon is uncommon. It is seen in the skin after repeated injection of antigen (eg, in rabies vaccination, in which multiple injections of vaccine are given). Once high serum levels of precipitating antibody develop, further injection of antigen into the skin produces local inflammation. The severity of inflammation depends on antigen dose. Type III hypersensitivity is believed to be responsible for **hypersensitivity pneumonitis,** a lung disease manifested by cough, dyspnea, and fever 6–8 hours after inhalation of one of several different antigens (Table 8–3). If exposure is sustained, chronic inflammatory granulomatous disease develops. Types I and IV hypersensitivity may coexist with type III.

2. Serum sickness-type reaction–The serum sickness type of immune complex injury is much more common than the Arthus-type reaction. The process is broadly dose-related. Following exposure to a large dose of antigen, such as foreign serum proteins, drugs, and viral and other microbial antigens, immune complexes are formed in

Table 8-3. Different antigens causing hypersensitivity pneumonitis.

Disease	Exposure	Antigen Source
Farmer's lung	Moldy hay	*Micropolyspora faeni*
Bagassosis	Moldy sugar cane	Thermophilic actinomycetes
Air conditioner pneumonitis	Humidifiers, air conditioners	Thermophilic actinomycetes
Redwood, maple, red cedar pneumonitis	Moldy bark, moldy sawdust	Thermophilic actinomycetes, *Cryptostroma corticale,* sawdust
Mushroom worker's lung	Mushrooms, compost	Thermophilic actinomycetes
Cheese worker's lung	Moldy cheese	*Penicillium casei*
Malt worker's lung	Malt dust	*Aspergillus clavatus*
Bird fancier's lung	Bird excreta and serum	Avian serum proteins
Enzyme lung	Enzyme detergents	Alcalase derived from *Bacillus subtilis*
Drug-induced hypersensitivity pneumonitis	Drugs, industrial materials	Nitrofurantoin, cromolyn, hydrochlorothiazide, toluene diisocyanate
"Sauna" lung	Contaminated steam in saunas	*Aspergillus pullulans*

the blood. In the presence of an excess of antigen over antibody, these remain as small, soluble complexes that circulate in the bloodstream. They eventually pass through the endothelial pores of small vessels to be deposited in the vessel wall, where they activate complement and result in complement-mediated necrosis and acute inflammation of the vessel wall (necrotizing vasculitis; Fig 8–5). The vasculitis may be generalized, affecting many organs (eg, in serum sickness due to injection of foreign serum; or in systemic lupus erythematosus, an autoimmune disease), or may affect a single organ (eg, in poststreptococcal glomerulonephritis; see Fig 8–6).

Serum sickness-type immune complex injury may occur in a large number of diseases (Table 8–4). In some of these diseases, including serum sickness, systemic lupus erythematosus, and poststreptococcal glomerulonephritis, the immune complex injury is responsible for the main clinical manifestations of the disease. In others, such as hepatitis B virus infection, infective endocarditis, malaria, and several types of cancer, an immune complex vasculitis occurs as a complication of the

Numerous inflammatory cells (neutrophils and lymphocytes) in vessel wall

Fibrinoid necrosis

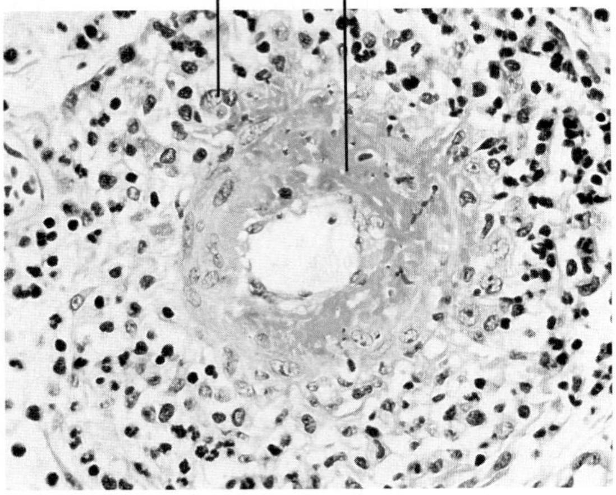

Figure 8–5. Necrotizing vasculitis involving small vessels—typical of immune complex injury. This section was from the intestine of a patient who had systemic (serum sickness-like) immune complex disease caused by an unidentified antigen.

disease. In polyarteritis nodosa, the necrotizing vasculitis that characterizes the disease is associated with hepatitis B virus in some cases; in other cases, no antigen has been identified.

B. Diagnosis of Immune Complex Disease: The diagnosis of immune complex disease may be established by visualization of the immune complexes in tissues by electron microscopy (Fig 8–6B). Rarely, large immune complexes can be seen on light microscopy (eg, in poststreptococcal glomerulonephritis). Immunologic techniques (immunofluorescence or immunoperoxidase staining) use labeled anti-IgG, anti-IgM, or anticomplement antibodies that bind to immunoglobulin or complement in the immune complex. The immune complexes can then be seen because of the label and typically appear as granular ("lumpy") deposits. Circulating immune complexes in the blood can be detected by many techniques (eg, Raji cell assay).

Type IV (Delayed) Hypersensitivity

A. Mechanism: (Fig 8–7.) Unlike other hypersensitivity reactions, delayed hypersensitivity is mediated by cells, not antibody. It is mediated by sensitized T lymphocytes that either are directly cytotoxic or secrete lymphokines that cause tissue changes. Type IV hypersensitivity reactions typically occur 24–72 hours after exposure of a sensitized individual to the offending antigen—in contrast to type I hypersensitivity, which develops within minutes.

A

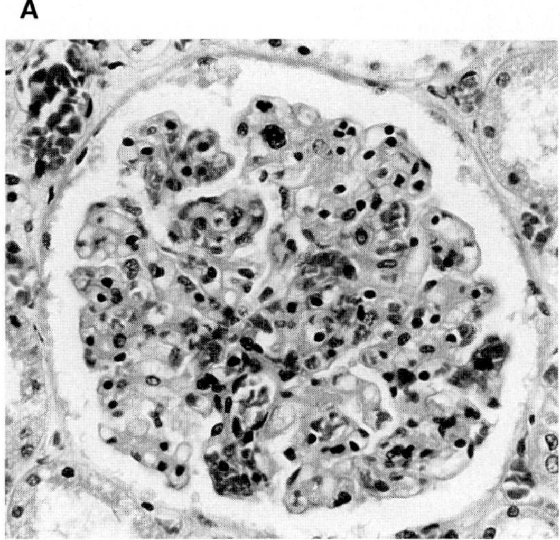

B

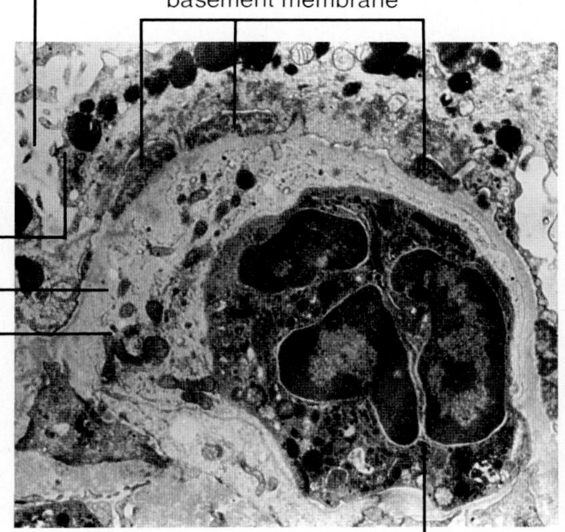

Figure 8-6. A: Poststreptococcal glomerulonephritis. Glomerulus involved diffusely and showing edema and hypercellularity with scattered neutrophils. Immune complexes are not usually seen at the light microscopic level. **B:** Electron micrograph of a small area of a glomerular capillary, showing electron-dense immune complexes deposited in the area between the basement membrane and the epithelial cell. These immune complexes contain antigen (derived in this case from streptococci), IgG, and fixed complement factors. Complement and IgG can be demonstrated by immunofluorescence.

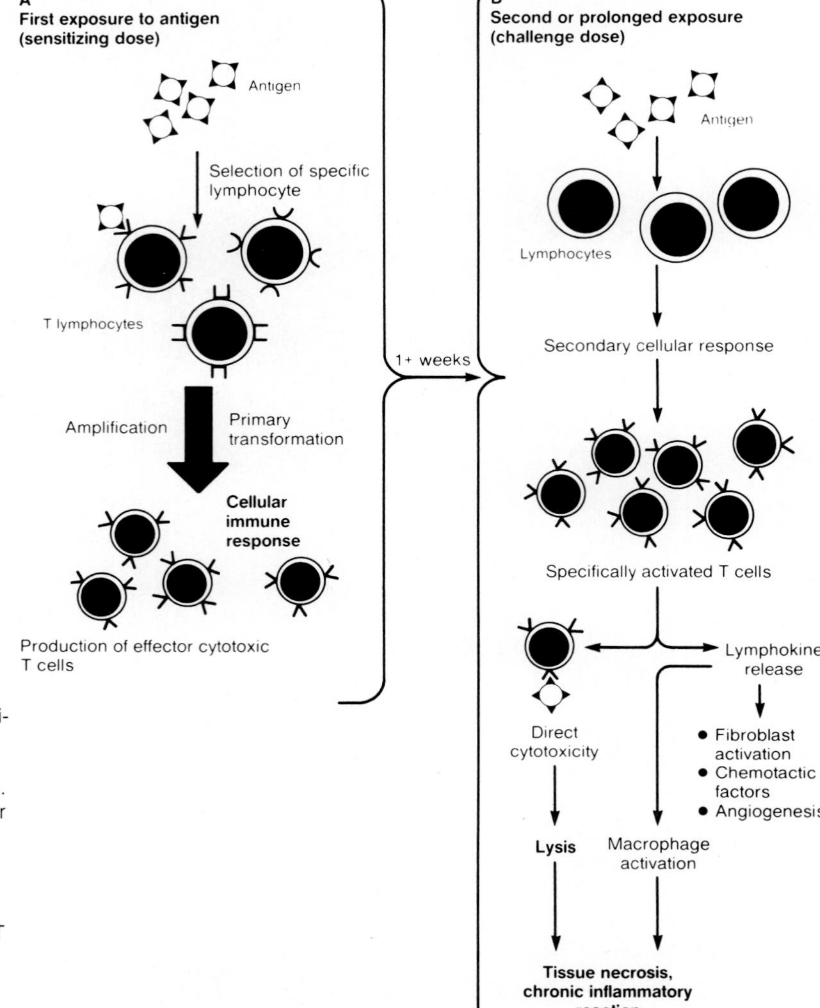

Figure 8-7. Type IV hypersensitivity. **A:** The first (sensitizing) dose of antigen results in a primary cellular immune response. **B:** A second (challenge) dose or prolonged exposure to the antigen invokes a secondary response with production of numerous specifically activated T cells. These may cause direct T cell-mediated cytotoxicity or a lymphokine-mediated granulomatous inflammation with caseous necrosis.

Direct T cell-mediated cytotoxicity, which causes necrosis of the antigen-bearing cells, is believed to be important in contact dermatitis and in the response against cancer cells, virus-infected cells, transplanted cells bearing foreign antigens, and several autoimmune diseases. Histologic examination of tissues affected by direct T cell-mediated cytotoxicity shows necrosis of affected cells and marked lymphocytic infiltration of the tissue (Fig 8–8).

T cell-mediated hypersensitivity is also responsible for caseous necrosis associated with granulomatous inflammation (see Chapter 5). Granulomatous inflammation is the main immune response against mycobacteria and certain fungi and is mainly the result of the action on macrophages of lymphokines secreted by sensitized T cells. The mechanism by which T cell-mediated hypersensitivity causes caseous necrosis is poorly understood. This type of T cell-mediated hypersensitivity is the basis for skin tests used in the diagnosis of infection by mycobacteria (tuberculin and lepromin tests) and fungi (histoplasmin and coccidioidin tests). In these tests, inactivated microbial antigen (eg, tuberculin or purified protein derivative of *Mycobacterium tuberculosis*) is injected intradermally. After 24–72 hours, caseating granulomatous inflammation occurs at the site, causing an indurated nodule that represents a positive test. A positive test indicates the presence of delayed hypersensitivity against the injected antigen and provides evidence for previous exposure to that antigen.

B. Disorders Resulting From Type IV Hypersensitivity: Delayed hypersensitivity occurs in several contexts.

1. Infections-Delayed hypersensitivity occurs in infections caused by facultative intracellular or-

Table 8-4. Diseases in which immune complex formation has been shown to play a role.

Infections
Poststreptococcal glomerulonephritis[1]
Subacute infective endocarditis
Mycoplasma pneumonia
Syphilis
Viral hepatitis (acute and chronic)
Guillain-Barré syndrome
Malaria
Leishmaniasis
Malignant diseases
Lymphocytic leukemias (acute and chronic)
Hodgkin's disease
Various cancers (especially of lung or breast; melanoma)
Autoimmune diseases
Systemic lupus erythematosus[1]
Rheumatoid arthritis
Polyarteritis nodosa[1]
Hashimoto's disease (thyroiditis)
Celiac disease
Henoch-Schönlein purpura
Rheumatic fever
Drug reactions
Serum sickness[1]
Penicillamine toxicity[1]

[1]The main clinical manifestations of these diseases are the result of immune complex deposition in tissues. In the other diseases in this list, immune complexes have been demonstrated but their deposition usually plays a secondary and less important role.

ganisms, eg, mycobacteria and fungi. Tissue necrosis takes the form of caseous necrosis in the center of epithelioid cell granulomas.

2. Autoimmune diseases-In Hashimoto's thyroiditis (Fig 8-8) and autoimmune gastritis associated with pernicious anemia, direct T cell reactivity against antigens on the host cells (thyroid epithelial cells and gastric parietal cells) leads to progressive destruction of these cells.

3. Contact dermatitis-An antigen in direct contact with the skin induces a type IV hypersensitivity response with well-circumscribed lesions, the site of which corresponds precisely to the area of contact (eg, back of a watch, buckle of a suspender, bracelet). Common antigens are nickel, dichromate compounds (in leather), drugs, dyes in clothing, and plants, including poison ivy and poison oak. The existence of sensitization is elicited by patch tests (local application to the skin of the putative irritating antigen). The reaction is eczematous or vesicular and typically pruritic.

4. Graft rejection-See below.

● TRANSPLANT REJECTION

It is often necessary to replace a diseased organ with a healthy one if a patient is to survive or function normally. The frequency of tissue (organ) transplantation has increased dramatically in clinical practice in the past 2 decades. Corneal, skin, and bone grafts are routinely performed. Renal transplantation is performed with a high success rate in most large medical centers. Heart, lung, liver, and bone marrow transplants are still experimental procedures but are being performed with increasing success.

The only absolute limitations upon tissue transplantation are the immunologic reactions against the transplanted cells and the availability of appropriate donor organs. **Autografting**—transplantation of the host's own tissues as **autologous grafts** from one part of the body to another (eg, skin, bone, venous grafts)—does not cause immunologic rejection reactions (Fig 8-9). Exchange of tissue between genetically identical (monozygotic) twins **(isografts)** does not evoke an immune response, since the tissue is perceived as "self."

Before an immune response can occur, antigens

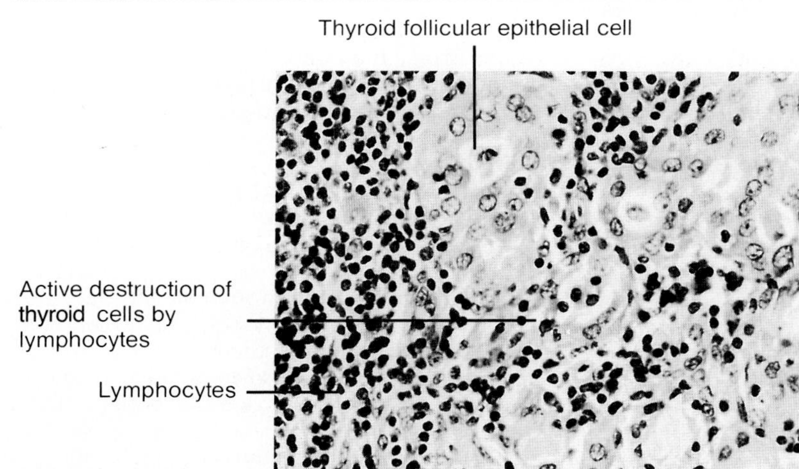

Figure 8-8. Type IV hypersensitivity—direct T cell-mediated cytotoxicity. In this case of autoimmune (Hashimoto's) thyroiditis, the thyroid follicular epithelial cells are being actively destroyed by the diffuse lymphocytic infiltrate.

Autograft (autologous graft)
Self to self, accepted
Isograft
Identical twin to twin, accepted
Allograft
Person to person (not identical twins), variable degree of rejection
Xenograft (heterologous graft)
Species to species, strong rejection

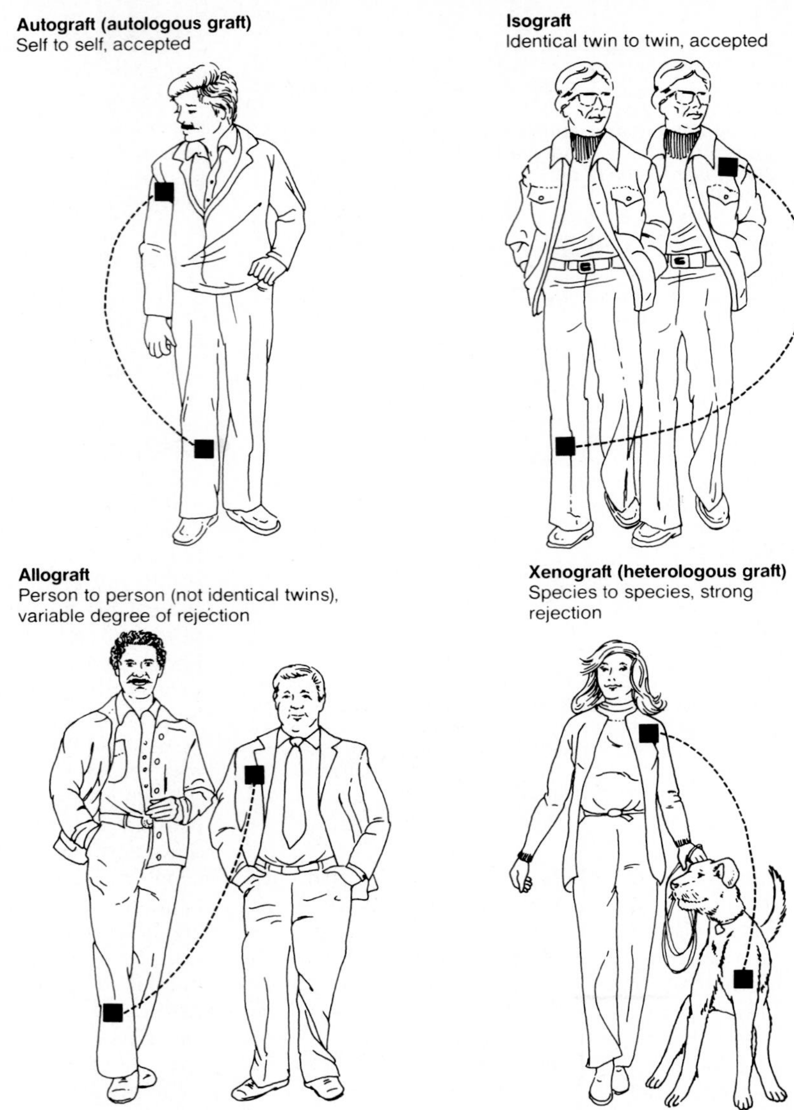

Figure 8–9. Different types of tissue transplants (grafts).

must be exposed to the immune cells in the circulation. Certain avascular grafts (eg, cornea) can thus be performed between different individuals without immunologic rejection, since the absence of a blood circulation prevents immune cells from reaching the graft.

Transplantation of tissue between genetically dissimilar hosts evokes an immunologic response that may lead to **rejection;** the severity of the rejection reaction increases as the genetic differences between host and recipient increase. Currently, almost all organ transplants performed in humans use organs derived from humans. A transplant between genetically dissimilar members of the same species is called an **allograft (allotransplant). Xenografts** (heterologous grafts) are transplants obtained from a species different from the recipient (eg, the baboon heart implanted in an infant a few years ago); such grafts evoke a severe immunologic reaction and are almost never used.

Transplantation (Histocompatibility) Antigens

Immunologic reactivity against transplanted cells is directed against many antigens on the surface membrane of cells.

A. Antigens on Erythrocytes: Although antigens of the ABO, Rh, MNS, and other blood group systems are not histocompatibility antigens per se, compatibility between donor erythrocytes and recipient serum is essential both in blood transfusions and in tissue transplantation. Such compatibility is easily achieved because there are a relatively small number of different groups of clinically significant antigens. Erythrocyte antigen compatibility is determined by typing and cross-matching of erythrocytes.

B. Antigens on the Surface of Nucleated Cells:

1. HLA complex-The antigens of the HLA (human leukocyte antigen) complex are **histocompatibility antigens** (ie, genetically determined isoantigens that elicit an immune response when grafted onto the tissues of an individual with a different genetic makeup). In humans, the major histocompatibility complex (MHC)—the chromosomal site containing the genes that control histocompatibility antigens—is on the short arm of chromosome 6. HLA antigens are surface glycoproteins whose structure is determined by corresponding genetic loci situated close together on the short arm of chromosome 6 (Fig 8–10). Four major loci (HLA-A, HLA-B, HLA-C, and HLA-D) are recognized. A fifth, closely related to the HLA-D locus and called HLA-DR, has also been proposed. Each locus contains 2 alleles (alternative forms of a gene) that code for 2 HLA antigens on the cell. Both antigens are expressed, so that all nucleated cells in the body have 5 pairs of antigens (A, B, C, D, and DR) for a total of at least 10 HLA antigens (Fig 8–11). An individual inherits one allele at each locus from each parent (ie, of the 10 HLA antigens on a cell, 5 are inherited from one parent, and 5 from the other).

The complexity of the HLA antigen system is due to the existence of a large number of different possible alleles for each locus. (At least 23 HLA-A, 49 HLA-B, 8 HLA-C, 19 HLA-D and 16 HLA-DR alleles have been recognized.) These code for a corresponding number of HLA antigens on the cells; ie, in the general population, any two of 23 different antigens may be coded at the A locus, any two of 49 at the B locus, and so forth. The huge number of possible HLA antigen combinations makes it unlikely that any 2 unrelated individuals will share the identical HLA type.

Since the 5 HLA loci are closely linked on chromosome 6, they are usually inherited as a **haplotype** (ie, a maternal group of 5 and a paternal group of 5) (Fig 8–11). Among the offspring of the same 2 parents, there is therefore an approximately 1:4 chance of a complete (2-haplotype) HLA match, a 1:2 chance of a one-haplotype HLA match, and a 1:4 chance of a complete HLA mismatch (Fig 8–11). High degrees of compatibility are seldom achieved among unrelated individuals, so that transplants between siblings have a better chance of survival than those obtained from genetically unrelated sources.

In **HLA typing,** peripheral blood lymphocytes are used to test the compatibility of antigens in donor and recipient cells. HLA-A, HLA-B, HLA-C, and HLA-DR typing is performed by using panels of antisera with antibodies of known HLA

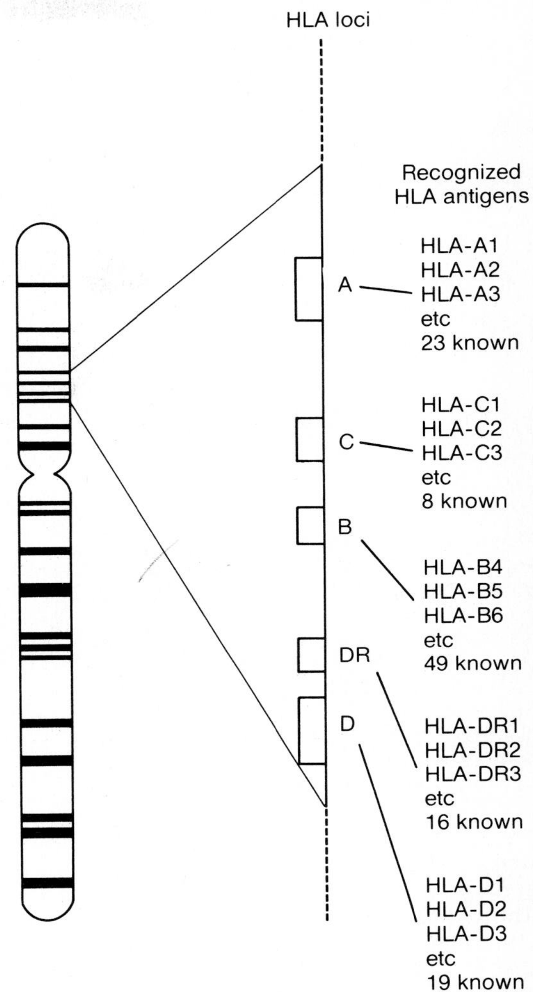

Figure 8–10. HLA genes and antigens (major histocompatibility complex; MHC) on chromosome 6.

specificity; ie, HLA type is serologically determined. HLA-D cannot be determined serologically (appropriate antisera are not available at present) and is typed by the mixed lymphocyte culture technique. The survival of renal allograft is highest when donor and recipient are closely matched for HLA-D and HLA-DR.

2. Histocompatibility antigens other than those of the HLA complex-The fact that an immunologic reaction occurs in a transplant from a sibling who is completely HLA-matched suggests the presence of other active histocompatibility antigens on cells, but these have not yet been characterized. The existence of other antigen systems may explain why a transplant from a totally HLA-unmatched sibling still has a better chance of survival than one from a genetically unrelated donor.

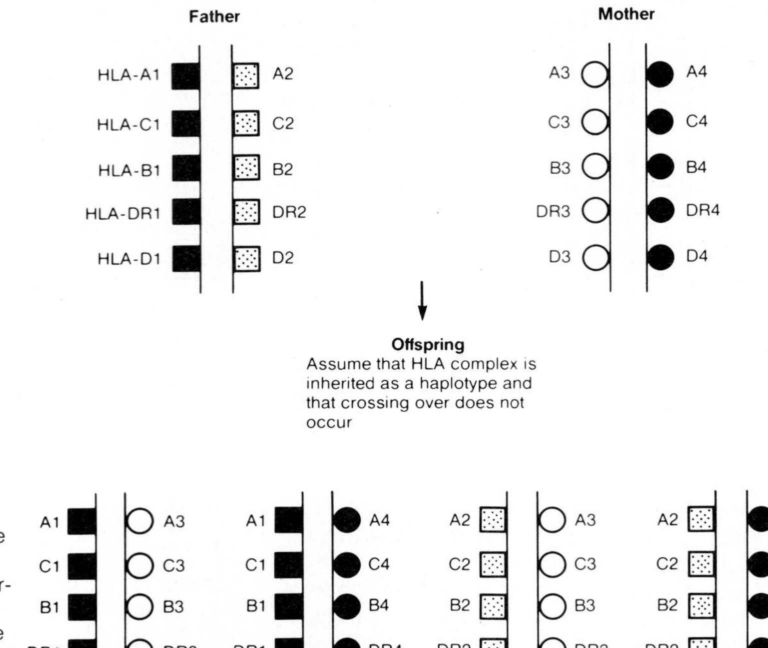

Figure 8–11. Inheritance of the HLA complex as a haplotype. Note that there are only 4 different possible HLA groupings in the offspring. There is therefore a 25% chance that 2 offspring will be HLA-identical (ie, 2-haplotype match) and a 50% chance that they will be HLA-semi-identical (ie, one-haplotype match).

Mechanisms of Transplant Rejection (Table 8–5)

Both humoral and cell-mediated mechanisms play a role in transplant rejection. Although transplant rejection is sometimes considered a hypersensitivity phenomenon because cell injury occurs, it is actually a normal immune response that constitutes an appropriate reaction to foreign antigens.

A. Humoral Mechanisms: Humoral mechanisms are mediated by antibodies against transplanted antigens that may be present in the recipient's serum before transplantation or may develop after the foreign tissue is transplanted. Preoperative testing for preformed antibody against transplanted cells is accomplished by the direct tissue cross-match, which involves an in vitro reaction between donor cells (blood lymphocytes) and recipient serum. Humoral factors injure transplanted tissue through reactions that are equivalent to type II and III hypersensitivity reactions. Antibody-antigen interaction on the surface of transplanted cells result in cell necrosis, and immune complex deposition in blood vessels activates complement and cause injury that is manifested as acute necrotizing vasculitis (Fig 8–12) or chronic intimal fibrosis with narrowing of the vessels. Immunoglobulin and complement in these lesions can be detected by immunologic techniques.

B. Cell-Mediated Mechanisms: Cell-mediated mechanisms involve T lymphocytes that become sensitized to transplanted antigens. These lymphocytes cause cell injury through direct cytotoxicity and secretion of lymphokines. Cell-mediated injury is chacterized by acute (Fig 8–13) and chronic (Fig 8–14) necrosis of parenchymal cells accompanied by lymphocytic infiltration and fibrosis (Fig 8–14). Cellular mechanisms are more important than humoral mechanisms in the rejection process.

Clinical Types of Transplant Rejection

Transplant rejection takes a variety of forms, ranging from a dramatic reaction occurring within minutes after transplantation to one that occurs so slowly that evidence of transplant failure only becomes apparent years after the transplant. The mechanisms involved in these different types of rejection are also different.

A. Hyperacute Rejection: Hyperacute rejection is a fulminant reaction occurring within minutes after transplantation and characterized by severe necrotizing vasculitis (Fig 8–12) with diffuse ischemic damage to the transplanted organ. Deposition of immune complexes and complement activation in the wall of involved vessels can be demonstrated by immunologic techniques.

Hyperacute rejection is due to the presence in

Table 8-5. Immunologic mechanisms involved in transplant rejection.

Active Immunologic Factor in Recipient	Type of Hypersensitivity	Target Sites in Transplant	Pathologic Effect	Type of Clinical Rejection
Preformed antibody against donor transplantation antigens	Type II cytotoxic	Small blood vessels in donor tissue	Fibrinoid necrosis and thrombosis of small vessels; ischemic necrosis of parenchymal cells.	Hyperacute rejection
	Type III immune complex formation (local, Arthus-type)			
Circulating antibody formed due to humoral immune response against donor transplantation antigens	Type II cytotoxic	Parenchymal cells	Acute necrosis of parenchymal cells.	Acute rejection
	Type III immune complex formation (local, Arthus-type)	Small blood vessels	Fibrinoid necrosis and thrombosis in acute phase; intimal fibrosis and narrowing in chronic phase.	Acute rejection, chronic rejection
Activated T cells elicited by cellular immune response against donor transplantation antigens	Type IV	Parenchymal cells	Progressive, slow loss of parenchymal cells.	Chronic rejection

the recipient's serum of high levels of preformed antibodies against antigens on the transplanted cells. The antigen-antibody reaction produces an **Arthus-type immune complex injury** in the vessels of the transplant. Since development of direct tissue cross-matching, hyperacute rejection has become rare.

B. Acute Rejection: Acute rejection is common and may occur within days to months after transplantation. It is "acute" because even though its expression may be delayed until several months after transplantation, it progresses rapidly once it has begun. It is characterized by acute cellular destruction and organ failure (eg, acute myocardial necrosis and failure in a heart transplant).

Both humoral and cell-mediated mechanisms operate in acute rejection. Antibodies developing after transplantation form **immune complexes,** which are deposited in the small vessels of the transplant, activate complement, and cause acute vasculitis, leading to ischemic changes in transplanted tissue. **Cell-mediated immune rejection** is characterized by parenchymal cell necrosis and lymphocytic infiltration of the tissue (Fig 8–14). In renal transplants, acute rejection is manifested as acute renal failure with renal tubular necrosis and marked interstitial lymphocytic infiltration (Fig 8–13). Acute rejection can often be successfully treated with immunosuppressive drugs such as corticosteroids (eg, prednisone) and cyclo-

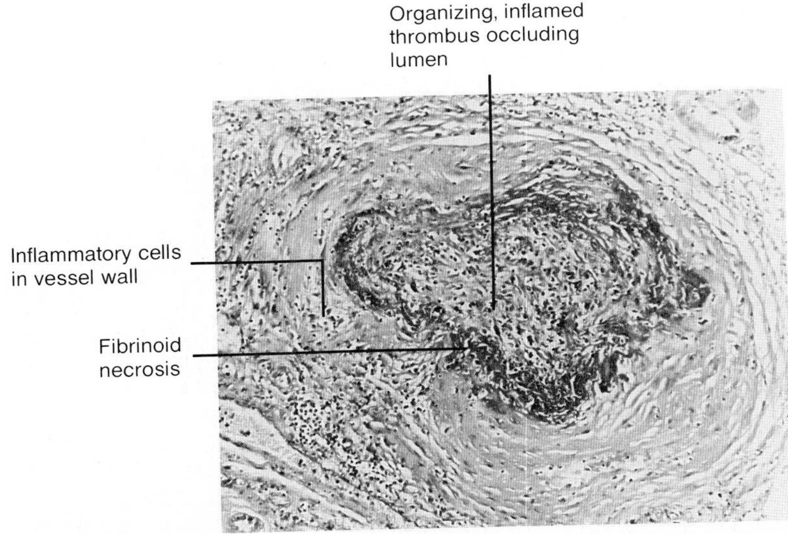

Figure 8–12. Acute rejection of a transplanted kidney showing the effects of immune complex injury in a medium-sized artery. Note the fibrinoid necrosis, vasculitis, and occlusion of the lumen by organizing thrombus. (Compare with Fig 8–5 for similarity.)

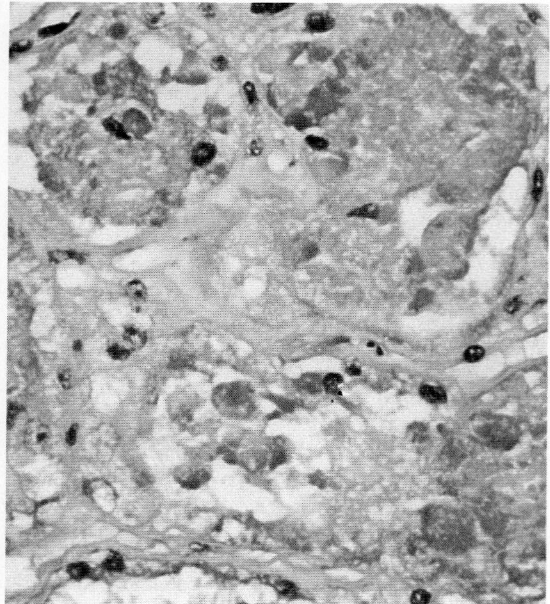

Figure 8-13. Acute renal tubular necrosis in a transplanted kidney 1 week after transplantation. The kidney also showed extensive necrotizing vasculitis that may have contributed to necrosis by causing ischemia. Note that the renal tubular outlines are intact. This patient recovered with aggressive immunosuppressive therapy, the renal tubular epithelium regenerating rapidly.

sporine or with antilymphocyte serum to ablate the patient's T cells.

C. Chronic Rejection: Chronic rejection is present in most transplanted tissues and causes slowly progressive changes with slow deterioration of organ function over a period of several months or years. The patient often has a history of episodes of acute rejection controlled by immunosuppressive therapy.

Cell-mediated immune reaction is the predominant mechanism. It causes slowly progressive destruction of parenchymal cells with increasing fibrosis of the organ. A lymphocytic infiltrate is present. In some patients, the appearance of chronic vasculitis with intimal fibrosis and narrowing of small vessels due to deposition of immunoglobulin and complement represents a chronic humoral response.

Treatment of chronic rejection attempts to achieve a balance between the rate of transplant destruction and the severity of the toxic effects of immunosuppressive drugs used to prevent rejection.

• AUTOIMMUNE DISEASE

Immunologic Tolerance to Self Antigens

The immune system recognizes the body's own antigens as self antigens and does not react against them (natural tolerance [Chapter 4]). Autoimmune diseases occur when a breakdown of this natural tolerance leads to an immune response against a self antigen.

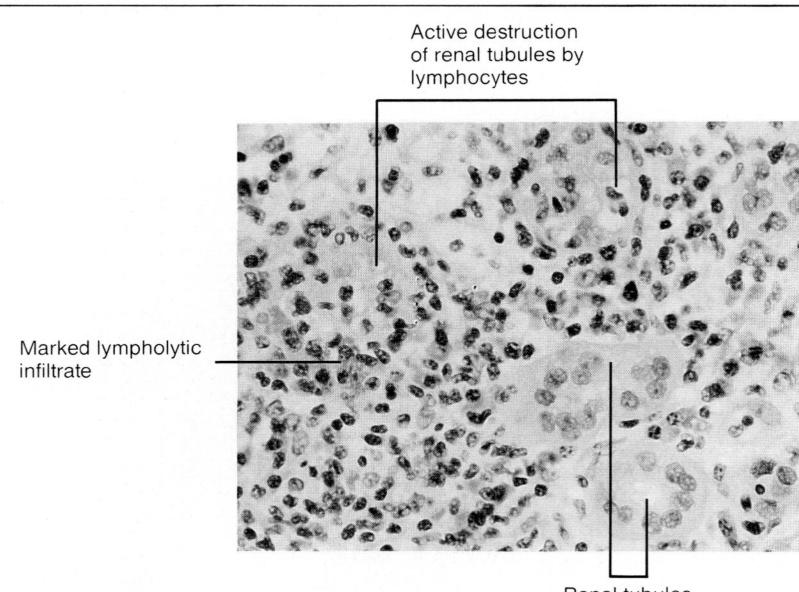

Figure 8-14. Rejection of a transplanted kidney, showing direct T cell-mediated cytotoxicity. The kidney is diffusely infiltrated by lymphocytes that are actively destroying renal tubular cells. Scattered residual renal tubular cells are present.

Natural tolerance to an antigen results when the immune system is presented with that antigen during fetal life. Two principal theories have been proposed to explain the mechanism of natural tolerance.

A. Clonal Deletion Theory: According to Burnet's clonal deletion theory, the lymphocyte clones that have receptors for antigens encountered in fetal life (self antigens) are deleted in the developing organism. Adults should therefore lack self-reactive clones. The subsequent development of autoimmunity is then explained by the emergence of forbidden clones of lymphocytes that are reacting to self antigens, presumably the result of a new B or T cell gene rearrangement at the stem cell level.

B. Specific Cell Suppression Theory: The clonal deletion theory is probably oversimplified, since it has been shown that normal individuals do have lymphocytes with receptors for self antigens. These lymphocytes were obviously not deleted but nevertheless have been suppressed or in some way prevented from reacting. How these lymphocytes are suppressed is not clear, but direct activity of T suppressor cells and the presence of suppressor factors in blood have been proposed as possible mechanisms. The latter include factors that either mask self antigens or, alternatively, bind to the antigen receptors of lymphocytes to preclude the recognition of self antigens. Some of these suppressor factors are believed to be dependent on the production of antibodies by B cells (ie, they are noncytotoxic masking antibodies).

Breakdown of Natural Tolerance (Autoimmunity)

Autoimmunity represents a breakdown of natural tolerance and the subsequent occurrence of a specific humoral or cell-mediated response against the body's own antigens. If the reaction is severe enough, disease results. Cellular injury in autoimmune diseases is caused by both humoral and cell-mediated hypersensitivity (types II, III, and IV). Several different mechanisms for the breakdown of tolerance and the development of autoimmune disease have been proposed (Table 8–6).

Table 8–6. Proposed mechanisms of autoimmune diseases.

Proposed Mechanism	Antigens Involved in Pathogenesis	Reason for or Cause of Mechanism	Resulting Autoimmune Disease
1. Emergence of sequestered antigen	Thyroglobulin (?)	Antigen sequestered in thryoid follicle	Hashimoto's thyroiditis
	Lens protein	Antigen sequestered from bloodstream	Sympathetic ophthalmitis
	Spermatozoal antigens	Antigen developed in adult life	Infertility (male)
2. Alteration of self antigens	Drugs, viruses, other infections	Attachment of hapten, partial degradation	Hemolytic anemias, ?systemic lupus erythematosus, ?rheumatic fever
3. Loss of serum suppressor antibodies	Many types	B cell deficiency; congenital Bruton's agammaglobulinemia	Many types
4. Loss of suppressor T cells	Many types	T cell deficiency; postviral infection	Rare
5. Activation of suppressed lymphocyte clones	Epstein-Barr virus; ?other viruses	B cell stimulation	?Rheumatoid arthritis
6. Emergence of "forbidden" clones	Many types	Neoplastic transformation of lymphocytes; malignant lymphoma and lymphocytic leukemias	Hemolytic anemia, thrombocytopenia
7. Cross-reactivity between self and foreign antigens	Antistreptococcal antibody and myocardial antigens	Antibody against foreign antigen reacts against self antigen	Rheumatic fever
8. Abnormal immune response genes (Ir genes)	Many types	Loss of control of the immune response due to lack of Ir genes.	Many types[1]

[1]Immune response (Ir) genes are closely linked to HLA antigens. Those autoimmune diseases in which Ir gene abnormalities play a part are associated with an increased incidence of certain HLA types (Table 8–8).

Types of Autoimmune Disease

Many diseases are believed to have a basis in autoimmunity (Table 8–7). These are discussed fully in those chapters dealing with the principal involved organ. The antigens involved may be on a specific cell type (**organ-specific** autoimmune disease) or may be universal cellular components such as nucleic acids and nucleoproteins (**systemic**, or non-organ-specific, autoimmune disease). In some organ-specific autoimmune diseases, circulating antibodies against nonspecific cellular elements are present (eg, antimitochondrial antibodies in primary biliary cirrhosis). Some of these are of diagnostic value but do not necessarily play a significant role in the pathogenesis of the disease; formation of autoantibodies may simply reflect release of sequestered antigens as a result of some other type of injury (eg, 30%

Table 8–7. Autoimmune diseases.

Diseases	Autoantibodies[1]
Systemic multiorgan diseases	
Systemic lupus erythematosus	Antinuclear Anti-DNA (double-stranded) Anti-DNA (single-stranded) Anti-Sm Antiribonucleoprotein Others
Mixed connective tissue disease (MCTD)	Antinuclear Antiribonucleoprotein
Progressive systemic sclerosis	Antinuclear Anticentromere
Dermatomyositis	Antinuclear Antimyoglobin
Rheumatoid arthritis (and Sjögren's syndrome)	Anti-immunoglobulin (rheumatoid factor)
Restricted organ-specific diseases	
Myasthenia gravis	Anti-acetylcholine receptor
Hashimoto's thyroiditis	Antithyroglobulin
Graves' disease (toxic goiter)	Thyroid-stimulating immunoglobulin
Insulin-resistant diabetes	Anti-insulin receptor
Juvenile insulin-dependent diabetes	Anti-insulin Anti-islet cell
Goodpasture's syndrome	Anti-lung basement membrane Anti-glomerular basement membrane
Pernicious anemia	Anti-parietal cell Anti-intrinsic factor
Addison's disease	Anti-adrenal cell
Bullous pemphigoid	Anti-skin basement membrane
Pemphigus vulgaris	Anti-skin intercellular matrix
Hypoparathyroidism	Anti-parathyroid cell
Primary biliary cirrhosis	Antimitochondrial
Chronic active hepatitis	Antinuclear Antihepatocyte Anti-smooth muscle
Vitiligo	Antimelanocyte
Infertility (male)	Antispermatozoal
Infertility (female)	Antiovarian (corpus luteum)
Hemolytic anemia	Antierythrocyte
Neutropenia	Antileukocyte
Thrombocytopenia	Antiplatelet

[1]The antibodies named are those typical of each disease state, and not all patients with the disease will demonstrate them. In addition, the presence of these various antibodies is not necessarily limited to a particular disease state (eg, antithyroglobulin antibody is present in Hashimoto's disease [90%], myxedema [70%], Graves' disease [40%], nontoxic goiter and thyroid cancer [30%], pernicious anemia [25%], and normal controls [5–10%]).

of patients with myocardial infarction due to ischemia show circulating antibody to heart muscle after 6 weeks). In normal people, formation of such antibodies is suppressed after a few weeks.

Many autoimmune diseases show an increased familial incidence (eg, systemic lupus erythematosus, Hashimoto's thyroiditis, pernicious anemia), and certain autoimmune diseases also seem to be associated with specific HLA antigens (eg, HLA-D3 with systemic lupus erythematosus [Table 8-8]). A proposed mechanism for many types of autoimmune diseases is the presence of an abnormal Ir (immune response) gene. The close spatial relationship on chromosome 6 of Ir genes and the HLA complex (see Fig 8-10) may explain the association of those autoimmune diseases with certain HLA types.

Mechanisms of Cell Injury in Autoimmune Diseases

The mechanisms involved in producing cell injury in autoimmune diseases include types II, II, and IV hypersensitivity. Type II cytotoxic hypersensitivity is the mechanism responsible for many organ-specific diseases such as autoimmune hemolytic anemia and pemphigus vulgaris. In many of these organ-specific autoimmune diseases, type IV hypersensitivity also plays an important role—eg, in Hashimoto's thyroiditis, T cell-mediated direct cytotoxicity is believed to be the dominant mechanism of cell damage even though antithyroid antibodies are present in the blood and probably contribute to cell necrosis by type II cytotoxic hypersensitivity. Stimulatory type II hypersensitivity is responsible for primary hyperthyroidism (Graves' disease). Inhibitory type II hypersensitivity is responsible for myasthenia gravis, some

Table 8-8. Selected HLA antigens and their association with autoimmune disease.[1]

HLA Antigen	Associated Diseases
DR2	Multiple sclerosis, Goodpasture's syndrome
DR3	Celiac disease, myasthenia gravis, Graves' disease, systemic lupus erythematosus, insulin-dependent diabetes mellitus
DR4	Rheumatoid arthritis, pemphigus vulgaris, IgA nephropathy
DR5	Hashimoto's thyroiditis, pernicious anemia, juvenile rheumatoid arthritis
B27	Ankylosing spondylitis, Reiter's disease, uveitis

[1]The relative increased risk of disease in patients with the associated antigen varies: for ankylosing spondylitis and HLA-B27 it is 90 times higher than in the general population. Expressed another way, among patients with ankylosing spondylitis, 80–90% have HLA-B27, whereas in the general population 8% have this antigen.

Table 8-9. Laboratory tests for immunologic injury.

Hypersensitivity

Type I
- IgE levels (radioimmunoassay or enzyme-linked immunoassay)
- Levels of specific IgE (RAST [*r*adio*a*llergo*s*orbent *t*est] for specific IgE against a panel of selected known allergens)
- Skin tests using panel of selected known allergens (local urticaria indicates positive response)

Type II
- Test for specific antibody to drug or hapten
- Blood typing and cross-matching
  - For agglutinating antibodies
  - For nonagglutinating antibodies (Coombs' test)
- Tissue biopsy studies for bound antibody (immunofluorescence)
- Complement levels and complement utilization[1]

Type III
- Immune complex levels in serum (Raji cell assay)[2]
- Complement levels and complement utilization[1]
- Tissue biopsy studies for bound complexes and complement (immunofluorescence)
- Electron microscopy (dense deposits of immune complexes)

Type IV
- Skin patch tests using known antigens (48-hour exposure elicits delayed reaction)
- Skin tests with intradermal injection of antigens (eg, purified protein derivative [PPD] for tuberculosis)
- Lymphokine release tests (experimental)

Graft rejection
- Preventive testing
  - HLA typing using peripheral blood lymphocytes
    - Serologic typing using anti-HLA antibodies
    - One-way mixed lymphocyte culture (donor and recipient lymphocytes are mixed in culture; if transformation occurs in recipient cells, incompatibility is present)
- Evaluation of rejection or degree of suppression
  - Measurement of T cell levels (monoclonal antibody method)
  - Measurement of level of T cell activation by mitogens

Autoimmunity
- Serum tests for presence of autoreactive immunoglobulin (autoantibody)
- Immune complex assays
- Complement levels and complement utilization[1]
- Tissue biopsy assays
  - For bound antibody or complement (immunofluorescence)
  - For characteristic histologic features (see specific diseases)

[1]Levels of different complement factors show whether the complement cascade has been activated.
[2]Raji cell assay uses Fc receptors on a cell line (Raji B cells) to bind immune complexes.

cases of juvenile diabetes mellitus associated with antibodies against insulin receptors on target cells, and some cases of pernicious anemia associated with the presence of antibodies that inhibit the action of intrinsic factor.

Type III (immune complex) hypersensitivity is responsible for many of the multi-organ autoimmune diseases exemplified by systemic lupus erythematosus. These are characterized by systemic necrotizing vasculitis.

LABORATORY TESTS FOR IMMUNOLOGIC INJURY

Several laboratory tests are available for studying the various types of immunologic injury described in this chapter. Some of the more important and clinically useful ones are summarized in Table 8–9.

Abnormalities of Blood Supply 9

Page 127 to 150

The maintenance of adequate blood circulation is a highly complex process that depends on proper functioning not only of the heart but also of the entire vasculature. Failure of blood supply to a tissue (ischemia) may be localized, due to arterial obstruction or deficient venous drainage, leading to **infarction** (ischemic necrosis of tissue); or generalized, due to severe decrease in cardiac output, leading to a generalized decrease in tissue perfusion **(shock)**.

A CAUSES OF TISSUE ISCHEMIA

• ARTERIAL OBSTRUCTION

Atherosclerosis—the deposition of lipid in the intima of large or medium-sized arteries, with accompanying fibrosis—is the major cause of arterial disease in the United States (Chapter 20). Thrombosis frequently occurs in atherosclerotic arteries and represents the commonest cause of arterial obstruction. Arterial obstruction is also caused by several diseases other than atherosclerosis, and it may affect almost any organ. Atherosclerotic arterial disease is the leading cause of death in the USA. Narrowing or occlusion of the coronary and cerebral arteries is responsible for myocardial infarction (heart attack) and cerebral infarction (stroke), respectively. Over 4 million Americans have clinically evident atherosclerosis; Americans suffer 1.25 million heart attacks and 500,000 strokes each year. Over 800,000 of these episodes are fatal, and they represent 40% of all deaths in the USA. Similar statistics apply to Western Europe; a much lower incidence is seen in developing countries.

Factors Influencing the Effect of Arterial Obstruction

The effect of arterial obstruction on a tissue is governed by the degree of reduction of blood flow to the tissue in relation to its metabolic needs. Tissue changes resulting from arterial obstruction are influenced by several factors.

A. Availability of Collateral Circulation: (Fig 9–1.) Collateral circulation in tissues varies between 2 extremes: In tissues with a rich collateral arterial supply, blood supply is not significantly decreased by occlusion of one artery (Fig 9–1A); eg, radial artery occlusion does not produce ischemia in the hand because the collateral ulnar artery circulation will compensate. In tissues having no collateral arterial supply, obstruction of the end artery supplying the tissue leads to complete cessation of blood flow and infarction (Fig 9–1B), eg, the central artery of the retina or the middle cerebral artery.

When the availability of a collateral arterial circulation falls between these 2 extremes (Fig 9–1C), the result of arterial obstruction depends on other factors discussed in the succeeding paragraphs.

B. Integrity of Collateral Arteries: Narrowing of arteries in the collateral circulation obviously decreases the effectiveness of any available collateral circulation; eg, occlusion of the internal carotid artery in a healthy young adult is usually compensated for by increased flow in the collaterals in the circle of Willis. However, in older

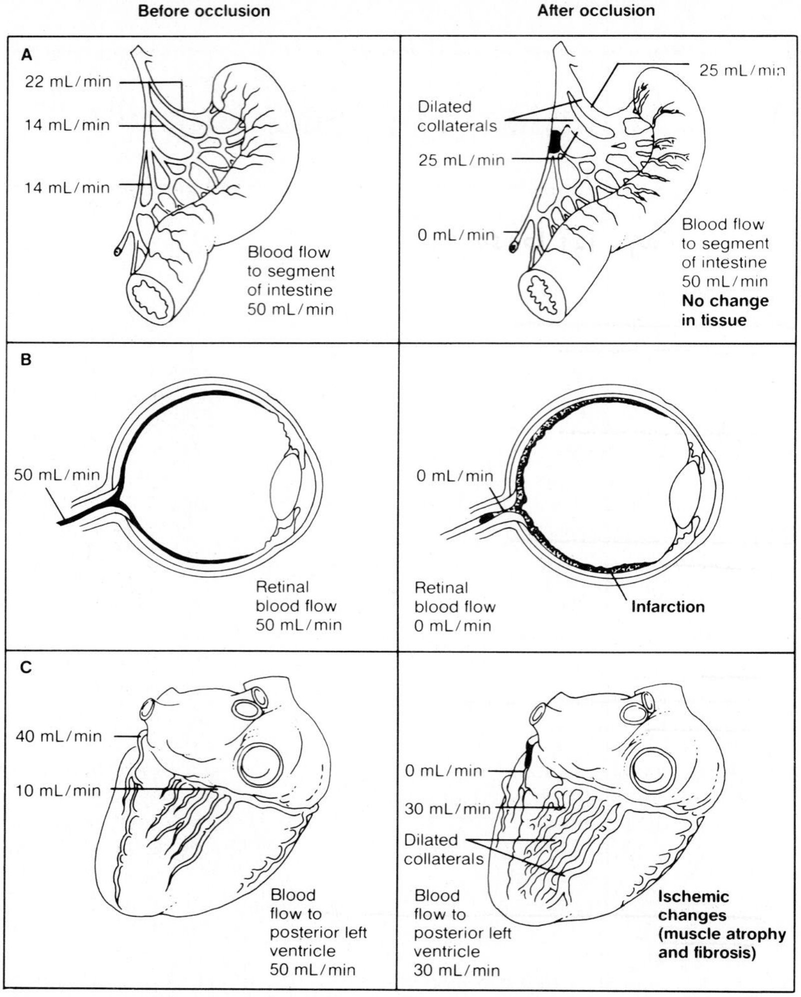

Figure 9–1. Effect of arterial obstruction on tissues. **A:** Loop of intestine supplied by 3 arteries. Obstruction of one supply artery has no effect on the tissue because normal blood flow is maintained by collaterals. **B:** The sole artery of blood supply to the retina is the central retinal artery (which is therefore an end artery), obstruction of which causes retinal infarction. **C:** The posterior wall of the left ventricle is supplied by both left and right coronary arteries. Obstruction of the major supplying artery is partially compensated for by increased flow in collaterals. The exact effect depends on several other factors (see text). In the example shown, the tissue has suffered a reduction in blood flow that has resulted in chronic ischemia with atrophy of myocardial fibers and fibrosis.

people with atherosclerotic narrowing of these collateral arteries, ischemia to the brain frequently occurs when the internal carotid artery is occluded.

Because generalized atherosclerosis occurs mainly in older people, ischemic changes in tissues that normally have an adequate but marginal collateral circulation (eg, intestine and extremities) are much more common in older patients than in younger ones.

C. Rate of Development of Obstruction: Sudden arterial obstruction produces more severe ischemic changes than does gradual occlusion because there is less time for enlargement of potential collateral vessels. For example, sudden occlusion of a previously normal coronary artery leads to myocardial infarction. More gradual occlusion of the same artery produces less ischemic myocardial change because collateral vessels have more time to develop and compensate for reduction in blood flow in the normal vessel.

D. Tissue Susceptibility to Ischemia: Tissues differ in their ability to withstand ischemia. Brain and heart are highly susceptible, and infarction occurs within minutes after arterial occlusion. In contrast, skeletal muscle, bone, and certain other tissues can withstand several hours of ischemia before changes occur. Emergency surgery performed on an occluded brachial or femoral artery can therefore prevent major infarction in an extremity.

E. Tissue Metabolic Rate: Cooling slows the rate of development of ischemic damage because of a general decrease in the tissue's metabolic requirements. This phenomenon is exploited in hypothermia deliberately induced in some types of surgery and in cooling of individual organs that are to be transported for transplantation.

VENOUS OBSTRUCTION

While veins become obstructed frequently, clinically significant venous obstruction is less common than arterial obstruction. This is because of the generally much greater availability of collateral vessels in the venous system than in the arterial system. Venous obstruction causes tissue changes when obstruction involves a very large vein (eg, superior vena cava) or one whose collaterals are not effective in providing an alternative route for venous drainage (eg, central vein of the retina, superior sagittal sinus, renal vein, cavernous sinus).

Effect of Venous Obstruction

Whether venous obstruction has any effect on tissue depends on the presence or absence of adequate collateral venous drainage in the tissue. When collateral venous drainage exists but is marginal, as in the femoral vein in the leg, occlusion may cause mild edema because of increased hydrostatic pressure at the venular end of the capillary (Chapter 2).

As failure of venous drainage after venous obstruction becomes more severe, congestion of the tissue occurs in addition to edema (Fig 9–2), as is seen in the face when the superior vena cava is occluded. In acute severe venous congestion, hydrostatic pressure may rise enough to cause capillary rupture and hemorrhage, eg, orbital congestion and hemorrhage in cavernous sinus occlusion. If venous congestion is extreme, venous infarction may result (see below).

Venous Congestion in Heart Failure

Specific types of venous congestion occur in heart failure, when venous blood backs up in the circulatory system because of failure of the heart to pump all of the venous return.

A. Pulmonary Venous Congestion: Left heart failure causes congestion of the pulmonary circulation. Acute congestion causes dilatation of alveolar capillaries with transudation of fluid into the alveoli (pulmonary edema) (Fig 9–3A). Intra-

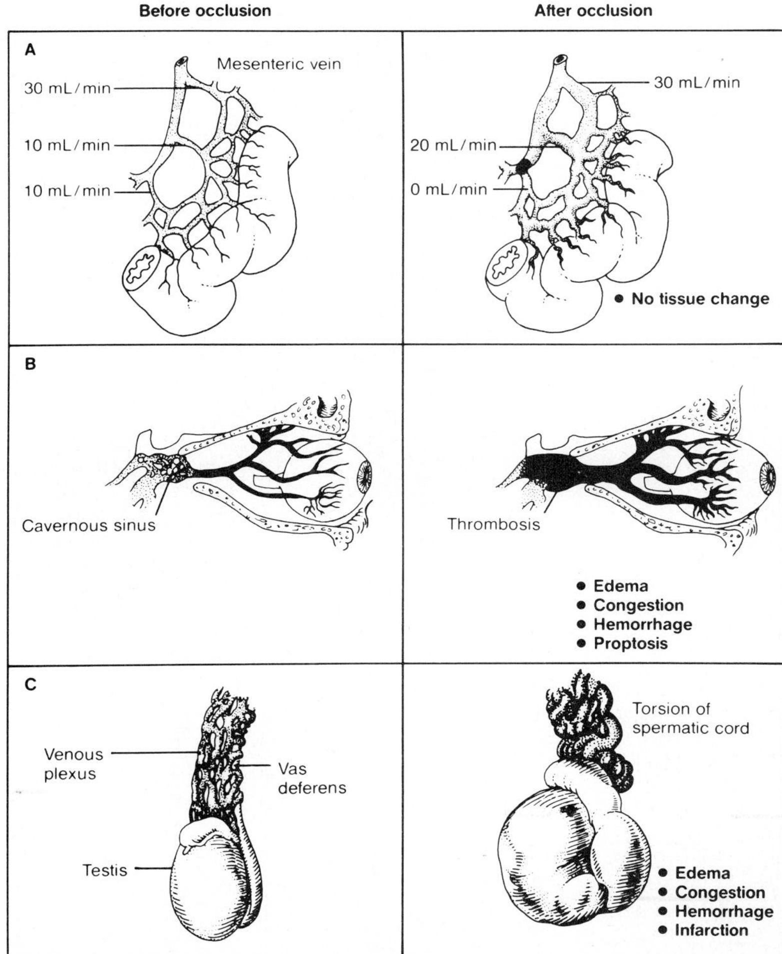

Figure 9–2. Effect of venous obstruction on tissues. **A:** Loop of intestine drained by several veins. Obstruction of the main draining vein causes no change in the tissue because venous drainage is taken over by collaterals. **B:** Venous drainage of the orbit is mainly into the cavernous sinus. Venous collaterals are insufficient to compensate when there is occlusion of the cavernous sinus. Cavernous sinus thrombosis therefore results in edema, congestion, and hemorrhage in the orbit. **C:** The venous drainage of the testis is by numerous veins, all of which pass up the spermatic cord. Twisting (torsion) of the spermatic cord usually obstructs all the veins without initially obstructing the artery. This results in testicular edema, hemorrhage, and venous infarction.

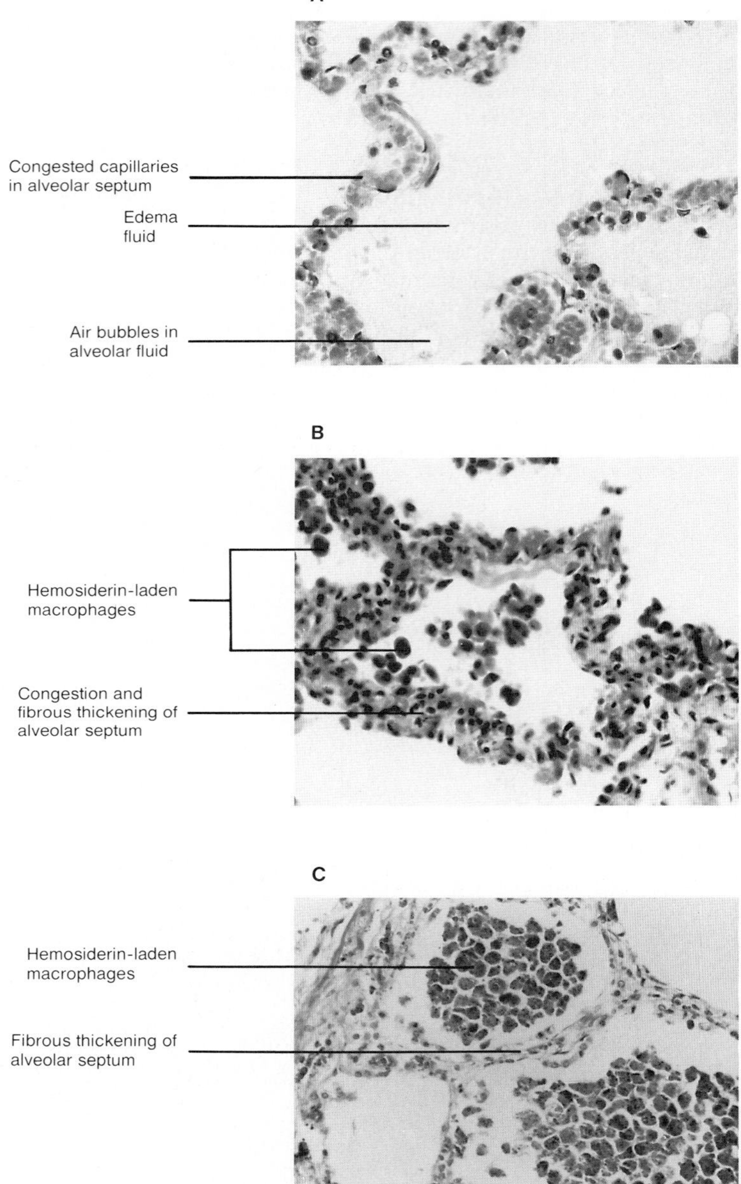

Figure 9–3. A: Acute congestion and edema of the lung in a patient with acute left ventricular failure. The alveolar septa show congestion, and the alveoli are filled with edema fluid. **B:** Chronic venous congestion of the lung. The alveolar septa are thickened by fibrosis, and the alveoli contain scattered hemosiderin-laden macrophages. **C:** Chronic venous congestion of the lung, later stage. The alveolar septa show fibrosis, and there are numerous hemosiderin-laden macrophages in the alveoli.

alveolar hemorrhage may also result. In chronic congestion, the long-standing increase in pulmonary venous pressure stimulates development of fibrosis in alveolar walls (Fig 9–3B). Escape of erythrocytes into alveoli over a long period causes accumulation of hemosiderin-laden macrophages ("heart failure cells") in the alveoli (Fig 9–3C).

B. Hepatic Venous Congestion: Right heart failure causes congestion of the systemic circulation and is first manifested as dilatation of the central hepatic veins and congestion of the sinusoids in the central part of the hepatic lobule (Fig 9–4). These congested, red central areas alternate with the normal paler tissue in peripheral zones and create a mottled effect (so-called "nutmeg liver" because of its resemblance to the cut surface of a nutmeg).

As congestion increases, hypoxia due to re-

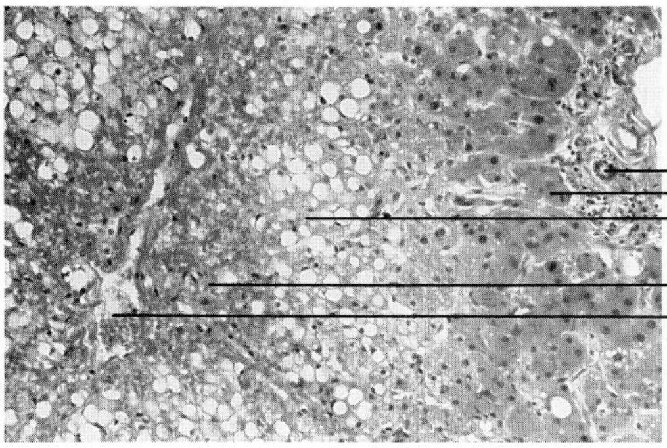

Bile duct in portal area

Normal hepatocytes in periportal area

Fatty change in hepatocytes in midzone of lobule

Congested central zone of lobule with atrophy of hepatocytes

Dilated congested central vein

Figure 9–4. Chronic venous congestion of the liver. The central vein is distended with blood, and the central zone shows congestion and atrophy of liver cells. The midzonal hepatocytes show fatty change.

duced blood flow occurs, with fatty change of liver cells that enhances the mottled appearance. The cells of the central zone of the liver lobule may eventually undergo necrosis; they are then replaced by fibrous tissue. Contraction of the centrizonal fibrous tissue alternating with the surviving peripheral zonal cells may result in a nodular liver (cardiac cirrhosis).

Venous Infarction

Venous infarction results when total occlusion of all venous drainage from a tissue occurs (eg, superior sagittal sinus thrombosis [Fig 9–5], renal vein thrombosis, superior mesenteric vein thrombosis). The result is severe edema, congestion, hemorrhage, and a progressive increase in tissue hydrostatic pressure (Fig 9–2). When tissue hydrostatic pressure increases sufficiently, arterial blood flow into the tissue is obstructed, leading to ischemia and infarction. Venous infarcts are always hemorrhagic (see Classification of Infarcts, below).

Special types of venous infarction occur in **strangulation**, in which constriction of the neck of a hernial sac results in infarction of the contents of the sac; and **torsion**, where twisting of the pedicle of an organ, most commonly the testis, results in venous obstruction and hemorrhagic infarction.

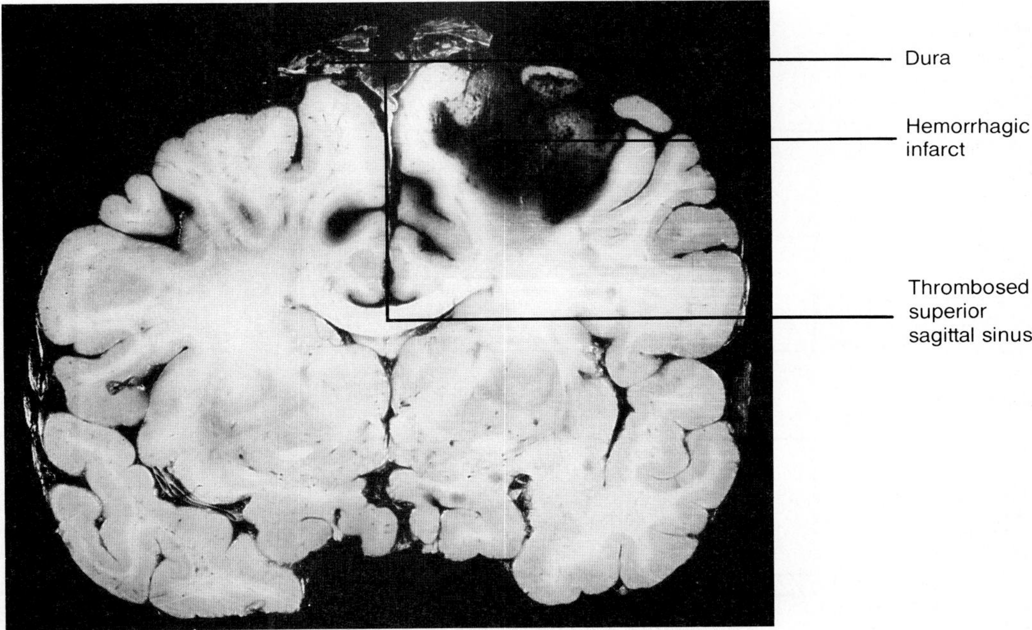

Figure 9–5. Hemorrhagic infarction of the parasagittal region of one cerebral hemisphere secondary to thrombotic occlusion of the superior sagittal sinus. Note that the sinus drains the other cerebral hemisphere as well, but in this patient there must have been an alternative route for venous drainage from the unaffected side.

EFFECTS OF TISSUE ISCHEMIA

INFARCTION

Infarction is the development of an area of localized necrosis in a tissue resulting from sudden reduction of its blood supply (Fig 9–6). Both parenchymal cells and interstitial tissue undergo necrosis. Infarction is most commonly due to arterial obstruction by thrombosis or embolism. More rarely, obstruction of venous drainage results in infarction.

Classification of Infarcts

The appearance of an infarct varies with the site. Various classification schemes are used.

A. Pale Versus Red: Pale (white, anemic) infarcts (Fig 9–6) occur as a result of arterial obstruction in solid organs such as the heart, kidney, spleen, and brain that lack significant collateral circulation. The continuing venous drainage of blood from the ischemic tissue accounts for pallor of such infarcts.

Red (or hemorrhagic) infarcts are found in tissues that have a double blood supply—eg, lung and liver—or in tissues such as intestine that have collateral vessels which permit some continued flow into the area though the amount is not sufficient to prevent infarction. The infarct is red because of extravasation of blood in the infarcted area from necrotic small vessels.

Red infarcts may also occur in tissue if dissolution or fragmentation of the occluding thrombus permits reestablishment of arterial flow to the infarcted area. Venous infarcts are always associated with congestion and hemorrhage and are red infarcts (Fig 9–5).

B. Solid Versus Liquefied: In all tissues other than brain, infarction produces coagulative necrosis of cells, leading to a solid infarct (Chapter 1). In brain, on the other hand, liquefactive necrosis of cells leads to the formation of a fluid mass in the area of infarction. The end result is frequently a cystic cavity (Chapter 1).

C. Sterile Versus Septic: Most infarcts are sterile. Septic infarcts are characterized by secondary bacterial infection of the necrotic tissue. Septic infarcts occur when microorganisms are present in the occluding thrombus or embolus, eg, in emboli derived from vegetations associated with acute infective endocarditis; or when infarction occurs in a tissue (eg, intestine) that normally contains bacteria; or when bacteria from the bloodstream cause secondary infection (this is unusual, since blood is normally sterile). Septic infarcts are characterized by marked acute inflammation that frequently converts the infarct to an abscess. Secondary bacterial infection of an infarct may also result in gangrene (eg, in the intestine).

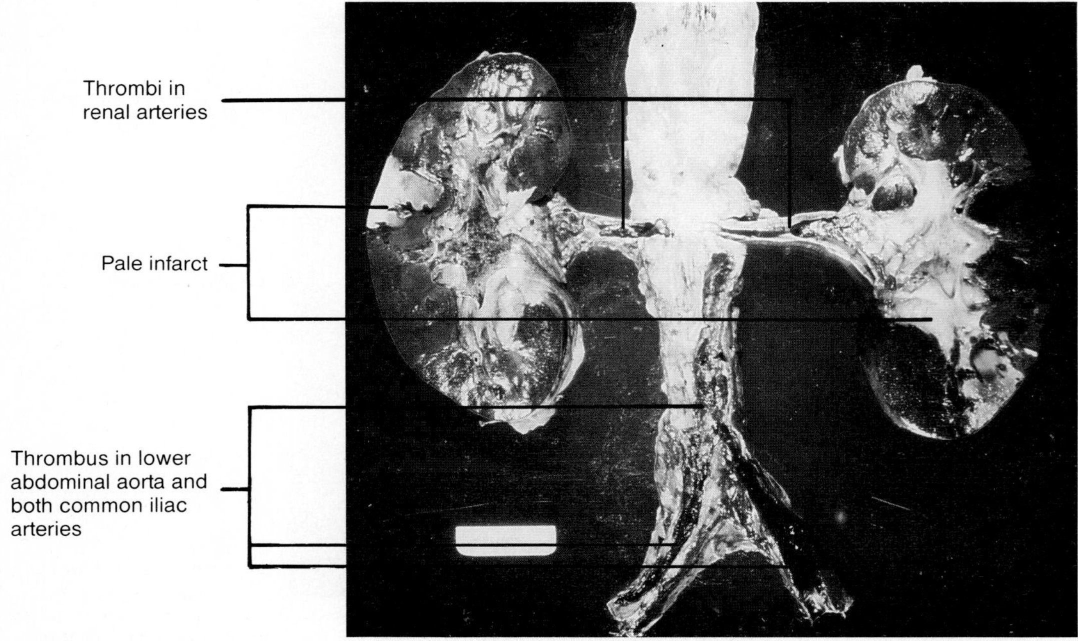

Figure 9–6. Bilateral renal infarction secondary to renal artery thrombosis. The infarcts are pale and wedge-shaped. Note the presence of extensive thrombosis at the bifurcation of the aorta.

Morphology of Infarcts

Infarction occurs in that part of a tissue supplied by an artery which, when occluded, leaves an insufficient collateral blood supply (Fig 9–7). Infarcts in kidney, spleen, and lung are wedge-shaped, with the occluded artery being situated near the apex of the wedge and the base of the infarct on the surface of the organ. The characteristic shape of infarcts in these organs is due to the symmetric dichotomous branching pattern of the arteries supplying them.

The shape of cerebral and myocardial infarcts is irregular and determined by the distribution of the occluded artery and the limits of the collateral arterial supply. In some patients, obstruction of the left anterior descending coronary artery results in infarction of the anterior interventricular septum, apex, and anterolateral left ventricle; in patients who have developed collaterals, the area infarcted may be much smaller. The thickness of the infarct is similarly variable. Intestinal infarcts develop in loops of bowel in accordance with the pattern of the arterial supply. The commonest infarcts of the intestine occur in the small intestine secondary to superior mesenteric artery occlusion.

Evolution of Infarcts (Fig 9–8)

An infarct is an irreversible tissue injury characterized by necrosis of both parenchymal cells and the connective tissue framework. Necrosis induces an acute inflammatory response in the surrounding tissue, with congestion (forming a red rim around a pale infarct in the first few days) and neutrophil emigration (Fig 9–9). Lysosomal enzymes from neutrophils then cause lysis of the infarcted area (heterolysis), and macrophages phagocytose the liquefied debris. Ingrowth of granulation tissue occurs, and acute inflammatory cells are replaced by lymphocytes and macrophages as active necrosis ceases. Lymphocytes and plasma cells probably represent an immune response to the release of endogenous cellular antigens.

Collagen production by fibroblasts in the granulation tissue ultimately leads to **scar formation**. Because of **contraction**, the resulting scar is much smaller than the area of the original infarct. Cytokines released by chronic inflammatory cells are partly responsible for stimulating fibrosis and neovascularization.

Evolution of a **cerebral infarct** differs from the above. Necrotic cells undergo liquefaction because of their enzyme content (autolysis). Neutrophils are less conspicuous than in infarcts of other tissues. Liquefied brain cells are phagocytosed by special macrophages (microglia), which become distended with foamy, pale cytoplasm (Chapter 1). The infarcted area is converted into a fluid-filled cystic cavity that becomes walled off by proliferation of reactive astrocytes (a process termed gliosis, which represents the cerebral analogue of fibrosis).

The rate of evolution of an infarct and the time required for complete healing vary with the size. A small infarct may heal within 1–2 weeks, whereas healing of a larger one may take 6–8 weeks or longer. Evaluation of the gross and mi-

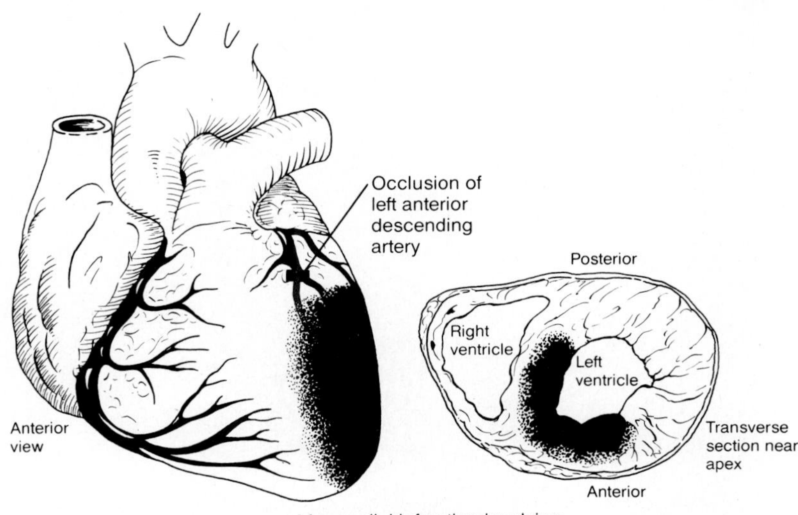

Figure 9–7. Distribution of infarction in the myocardium following acute occlusion of the left anterior descending artery. In cases where collaterals have developed, the infarcted area may be much smaller.

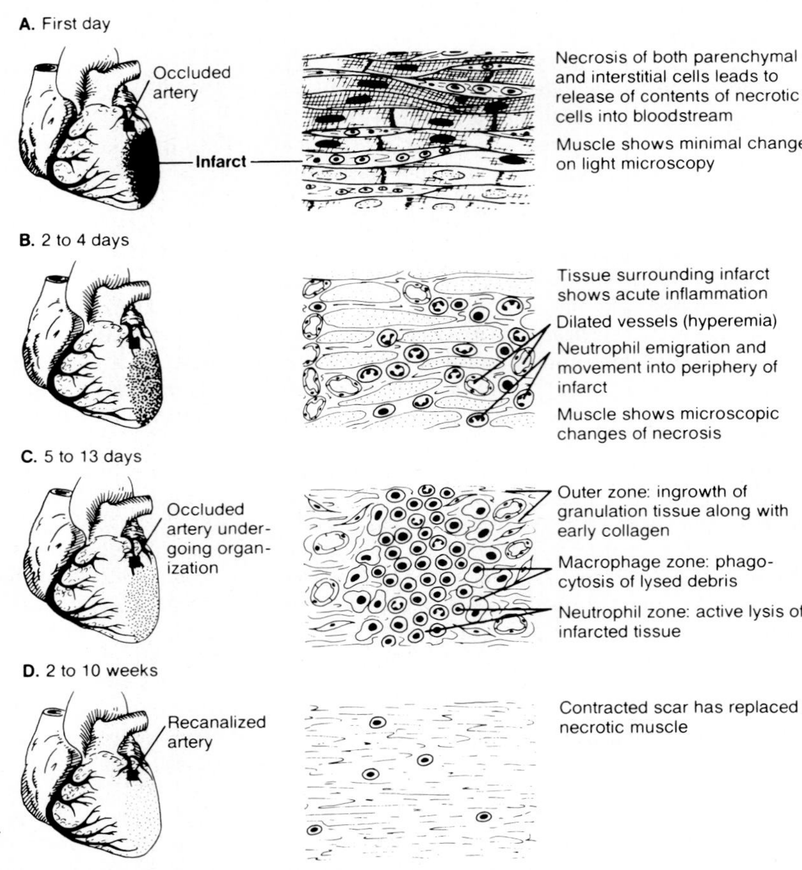

Figure 9-8. Evolution of a myocardial infarct.

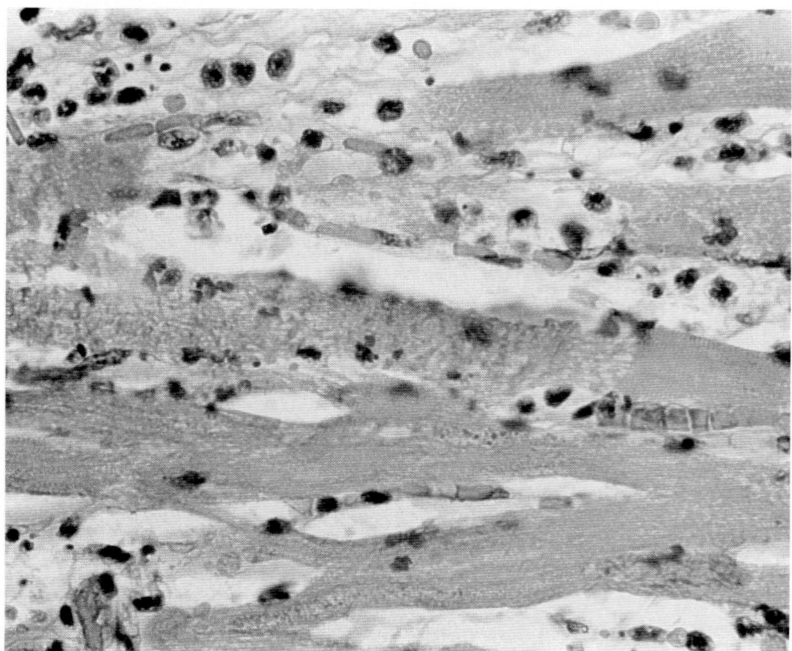

Figure 9-9. Myocardial infarct 2–4 days old, showing infiltration of the infarcted area by neutrophils. Note beginning lysis of the dead muscle fibers.

croscopic changes in an infarcted area enables the pathologist to assess the age of an infarct, which is an important consideration at autopsy in establishing the sequence of events that caused death.

• SHOCK

Shock is a clinical state characterized by a generalized decrease in perfusion of tissues associated with decrease in effective cardiac output.

Causes (Fig 9–10)

A. Hypovolemia (Decreased Blood Volume): Hypovolemia may be due to hemorrhage (either external or internal) or excessive fluid loss, as occurs in diarrhea, vomiting, burns, dehydration, or excessive sweating.

B. Peripheral Vasodilatation: Widespread dilatation of small vessels leads to excessive pooling of blood in peripheral capacitance vessels. The result is reduction of the effective blood volume and therefore a decreased cardiac output (peripheral

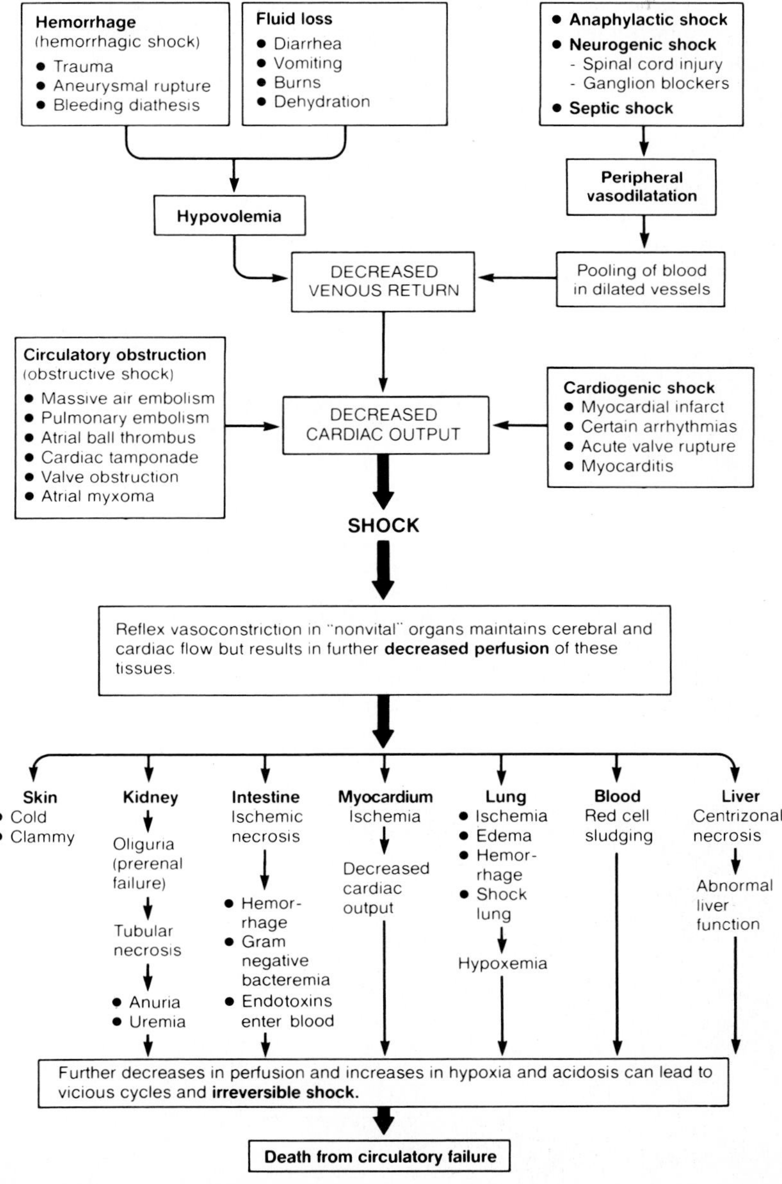

Figure 9–10. Mechanisms causing shock. **Note 1:** In shock resulting from a primary decrease in cardiac output, due either to obstructive or to cardiogenic causes, the jugular venous pressure is elevated. In shock primarily due to decreased venous return, the jugular venous pressure is reduced. **Note 2:** In many instances, decreased perfusion leads to changes that eventually result in a further decrease in perfusion, thus setting up vicious cycles (eg, erythrocyte sludging, myocardial ischemia, shock lung, intestinal ischemia). These contribute to irreversible shock. **Note 3:** Generalized tissue hypoxia leading to progressive acidosis is thought to be a major contributing factor in irreversible shock.

circulatory failure). Peripheral vasodilatation may be due to the action of metabolic, toxic, or humoral factors, eg, **endotoxic shock,** due to gram-negative bacteremia, and **anaphylactic shock;** more rarely, it may be caused by neurogenic stimuli, as occurs during anesthesia or spinal cord injury. Simple fainting is a form of **neurogenic shock;** it is normally self-correcting, because when the patient falls to the ground, the recumbent position increases venous return and thereby restores cardiac output.

C. Cardiogenic Shock: Cardiogenic shock results from a severe reduction in cardiac output due to primary cardiac disease, eg, acute myocardial infarction, acute myocarditis, and certain arrhythmias.

D. Obstructive Shock: Obstruction to blood flow in the heart or main pulmonary artery, as occurs in massive pulmonary embolism or a large left atrial thrombus impacting in the mitral valve orifice, causes obstructive shock. Severely impaired filling of the ventricles, as occurs in cardiac tamponade, produces a significant fall in cardiac output.

Clinicopathologic Features

Shock develops in stages as outlined below.

A. Stage of Compensation: Compensatory mechanisms that are activated by a decrease in cardiac output include reflex sympathetic stimulation, which increases the heart rate (tachycardia) and causes peripheral vasoconstriction that maintains blood pressure in vital organs (brain and myocardium). The earliest clinical evidence of shock is a rapid, low-volume (thready) pulse.

Peripheral vasoconstriction is most marked in less vital tissues. The skin becomes cold and clammy—another early clinical manifestation of shock. Vasoconstriction in renal arterioles decreases the pressure and rate of glomerular filtration, with resulting decreased urine output (oliguria). Oliguria represents a compensatory mechanism to retain fluid. The term **prerenal uremia** is used for this oliguric state resulting from causes outside the kidney; the kidney is normal, and the condition resolves rapidly when cardiac output increases.

B. Stage of Impaired Tissue Perfusion: Prolonged excessive vasoconstriction is harmful, since it impairs tissue perfusion. Decreased hydrostatic pressure in the capillaries prevents normal fluid exchange in the tissues. The slowing of blood flow in the microcirculation causes aggregation of erythrocytes (sludging), which further impairs tissue perfusion.

Impaired tissue perfusion has several adverse effects. It promotes anaerobic glycolysis, leading to production of lactic acid. Lactic acid enters the blood and causes **lactic acidosis,** which is almost always present in shock. Impaired tissue perfusion produces **cell necrosis** in tissues subjected to excessive vasoconstriction. Necrosis is most apparent in the kidney, where acute renal tubular necrosis occurs (Fig 9–11), resulting in acute renal failure. In the lung, hypoxia due to impaired perfusion causes acute alveolar damage with intra-alveolar edema, hemorrhage, and formation of hyaline membranes (**shock lung,** or adult respiratory distress syndrome [ARDS] [Fig 9–12]). In the liver, anoxic necrosis of the central region of hepatic lobules may occur. Ischemic necrosis of the intestine is important because it is frequently associated with hemorrhage that further aggravates the shock state. Damage to the intestinal mucosa also enables bacterial endotoxins to enter the circulation from the gut lumen, with serious effects.

C. Stage of Decompensation: As shock progresses, decompensation occurs. Reflex peripheral vasoconstriction fails, probably as a result of increasing capillary hypoxia and acidosis. Widespread vasodilatation and stasis result and lead to a **progressive fall in blood pressure (hypotension)** until perfusion of brain and myocardium sinks to a critical level. Cerebral hypoxia then causes acute brain dysfunction (loss of consciousness, edema, neuronal degeneration). Myocardial hypoxia leads to further diminution of cardiac output, and death may occur rapidly.

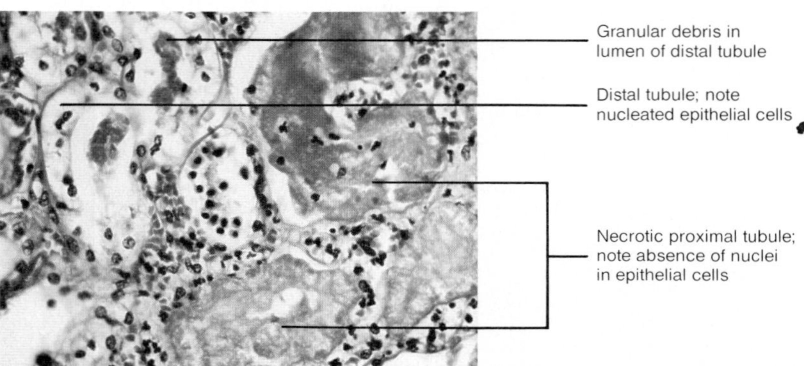

Figure 9–11. Acute renal tubular necrosis involving proximal tubules.

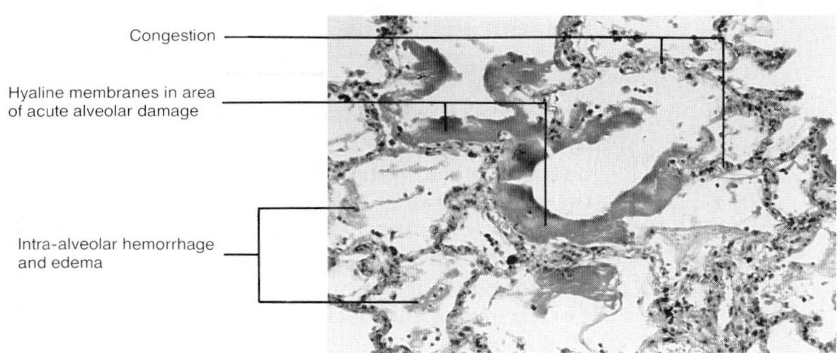

Figure 9-12. Shock lung, showing congestion, intra-alveolar hemorrhage, and edema. Hyaline membrane formation indicates acute alveolar damage.

Prognosis

The prognosis for a patient in shock depends on several factors, the most important of which is the underlying cause. When this can be treated (eg, hypovolemia, which can be corrected by fluid infusion), most patients survive even if they are in an advanced stage of shock when first seen. In patients who recover, necrotic cells—eg, renal tubular cells and alveolar epithelial cells—usually regenerate, and these tissues regain normal function. Patients who die are those in whom the cause of shock cannot easily be treated (eg, massive myocardial infarction) and those for whom treatment is started after lethal tissue injury has occurred **(irreversible shock)**.

CAUSES OF VASCULAR OCCLUSION

There are 4 principal causes of vascular occlusion: (1) **Extramural compression** by fibrosis or a neoplasm, eg, superior vena cava compression by a mediastinal tumor. (2) **Diseases of the vessel wall,** including atherosclerosis and inflammation (vasculitis). (3) **Arterial spasm** is recognized as a rare cause of ischemia in the brain and myocardium. (4) **Thrombosis and embolism** (see below), which occlude the lumen of the vessel, are the most common causes of vessel obstruction.

THROMBOSIS

Thrombosis is the formation of a solid mass from the constituents of blood (platelets, fibrin, and entrapped red and white blood cells) within the heart or vascular system in a living organism. Thrombosis should be distinguished from blood clotting, which occurs in tissue when blood escapes out of a vessel into the surrounding tissue, in vessels after death (postmortem clotting of blood), or in vitro (in a test tube outside the body). A thrombus is composed of layers of aggregated platelets and fibrin, whereas a blood clot contains randomly oriented fibrin with entrapped platelets and red cells.

Normal Hemostasis (Fig 9–13)

Thrombosis is a normal hemostatic mechanism that acts to stop bleeding when a vessel is injured. Under normal conditions, there is a delicate and dynamic balance between thrombus formation and dissolution of thrombus **(fibrinolysis).**

Following trauma, the usual initiating factor in thrombus formation is endothelial injury, which leads to formation of a hemostatic platelet plug and activation of the coagulation and fibrinolytic systems.

A. Formation of Hemostatic Platelet Plug: (Fig 9–14.) Injury to the vascular endothelium exposes subendothelial collagen, which has a strong thrombogenic effect on platelets and results in the **adherence of platelets** at the site. The platelets adhering to the injured endothelium aggregate to form a hemostatic plug, which is the beginning of a thrombus. **Platelet aggregation** in turn activates a mechanism causing **degranulation** of platelets, which releases granules containing serotonin, ADP, ATP, and thromboplastic substances. ADP—itself a powerful platelet aggregator—causes further accumulation of platelets. The layers of platelets alternating with fibrin in a thrombus appear on microscopic examination as pale lines (lines of Zahn) (Fig 9–15).

B. Coagulation of Blood: (Fig 9–14.) Activation of Hageman factor (factor XII in the coagulation cascade) results in the formation of fibrin by activation of the intrinsic coagulation pathway (Chapter 27). Tissue thromboplastins released by injury activate the extrinsic coagulation pathway, which contributes to fibrin formation. Factor XIII acts on fibrin to produce an insoluble fibrillary polymer that—with the platelet plug—makes up the definitive hemostatic plug. Fibrin appears as a pink-staining fibrillary meshwork intermin-

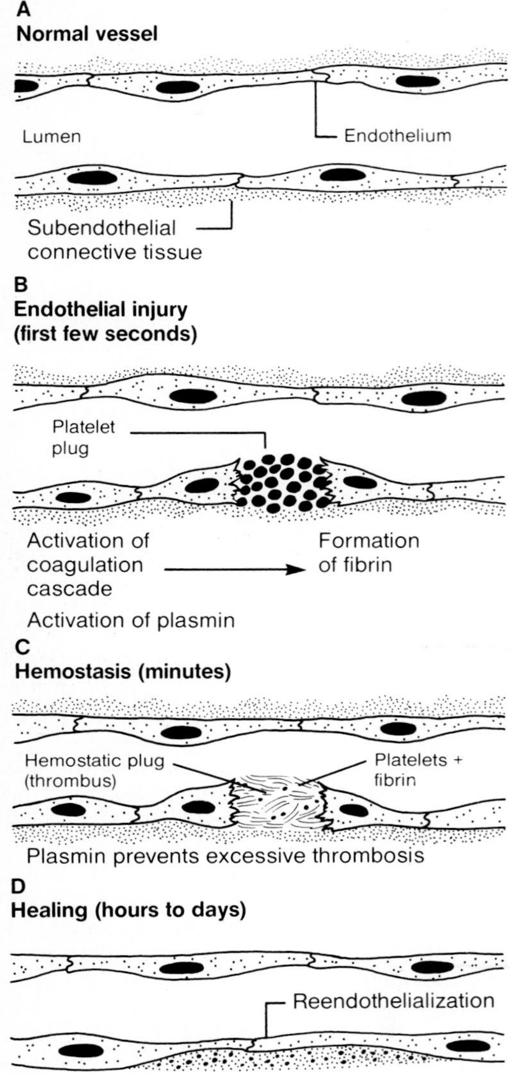

Figure 9-13. Mechanisms of normal hemostasis. **A:** In normal uninjured vessels, subendothelial connective tissue, especially collagen and elastin, is not exposed to the circulating blood. **B:** In the first few seconds after vascular endothelial injury, exposure of subendothelial tissue attracts platelets, which adhere and aggregate at the site of injury. Endothelial injury also activates Hageman factor (factor XII), which in turn activates the intrinsic pathway of the coagulation cascade. Release of tissue thromboplastins activates the extrinsic pathway. **C:** Hemostasis is achieved minutes after injury. Platelet degranulation releases ADP, which stimulates further platelet aggregation and formation of the primary hemostatic platelet plug. Fibrin formed by activation of the coagulation cascade combines with the mass of aggregated platelets to form the definitive hemostatic plug that seals the injury. Plasmin (fibrinolysin) formed by activation of the fibrinolytic pathway prevents excessive fibrin formation. **D:** During healing (hours to days), the thrombus retracts, and organization and fibrosis of the thrombus occur. Reendothelialization of the vessels is the final step.

gled with amorphous pale platelet masses on microscopic examination (Fig 9–15).

Abnormal Hemostasis

The normal balance that exists between thrombus formation and fibrinolysis ensures that just the right amount of thrombus is formed in response to endothelial injury so that hemorrhage from the vessel is prevented. Fibrinolytic activity prevents the formation of excessive thrombus. A disturbance of this balance results in abnormal hemostasis.

Excessive thrombus formation results in narrowing or occlusion of the vessel lumen. This usually occurs as a result of local factors at the site that overwhelm the ability of a normally functioning fibrinolytic system to prevent excess thrombosis. Decreased fibrinolysis alone almost never produces excessive thrombosis.

In contrast, decreased ability to form thrombi results in excessive bleeding and occurs in a variety of bleeding disorders, including decreased platelets in the blood, deficiency of coagulation factors, and increased fibrinolytic activity. These disorders are considered in Chapter 27.

Factors in Thrombus Formation

Endothelial damage, which stimulates both platelet adhesion and activation of the coagulation cascade, is frequently the dominant initiating factor when thrombosis occurs in the arterial circulation. When thrombosis occurs in veins and in the microcirculation, endothelial damage is less conspicuous. **Changes in blood flow** such as a decreased rate of flow and turbulence, and **changes in the blood itself** (eg, increased viscosity, increased fibrinogen levels and platelet numbers) are more important factors in venous thrombosis. The entry of thromboplastic substances into the bloodstream may cause thrombosis. Thromboplastic substances are present in some snake venoms, amniotic fluid, the cytoplasmic granules of neutrophil precursors (promyelocytes), and mucin produced by certain cancer cells.

Types of Thrombi

A thrombus is easily recognized as a solid mass in the lumen of a blood vessel that is often attached to the vessel wall (Fig 9–16). Thrombi in the fast-flowing arterial circulation are composed predominantly of fibrin and platelets, with few entrapped erythrocytes—hence the term **pale thrombi**.

Red thrombi are composed of platelets, fibrin, and large numbers of erythrocytes trapped in the fibrin mesh. Red thrombi typically occur in the venous system, where the slow blood flow encourages entrapment of red cells.

Rarely, **white thrombi** composed almost entirely of aggregated platelet masses form when thrombosis occurs in patients who are receiving

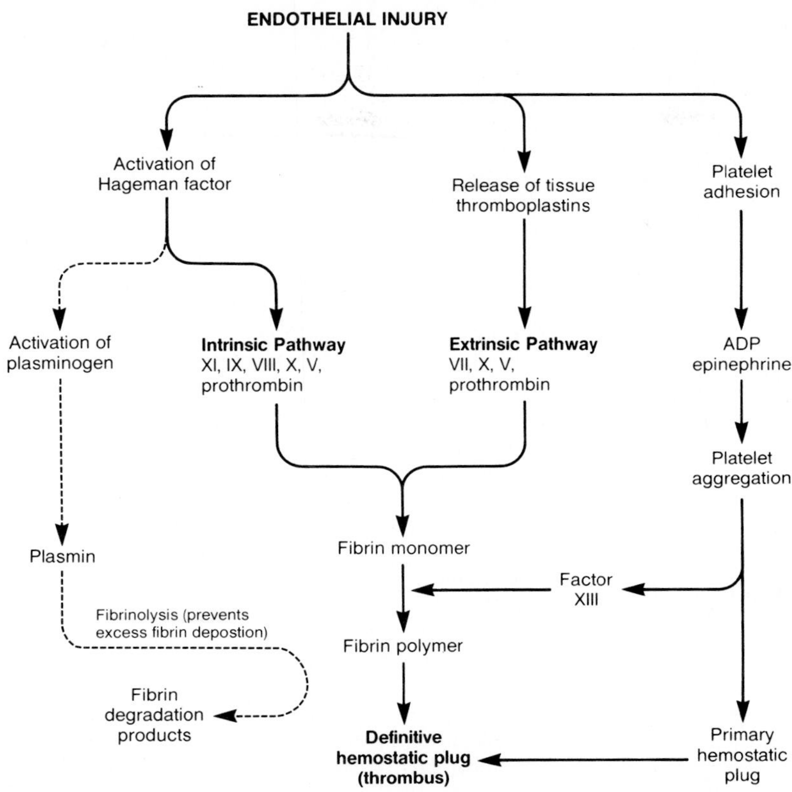

Figure 9-14. Effect of endothelial injury on the coagulation system and platelets, resulting in formation of the definitive hemostatic plug or thrombus. Note that simultaneous activation of the opposing fibrinolytic system provides a degree of control over the extent of thrombus formation.

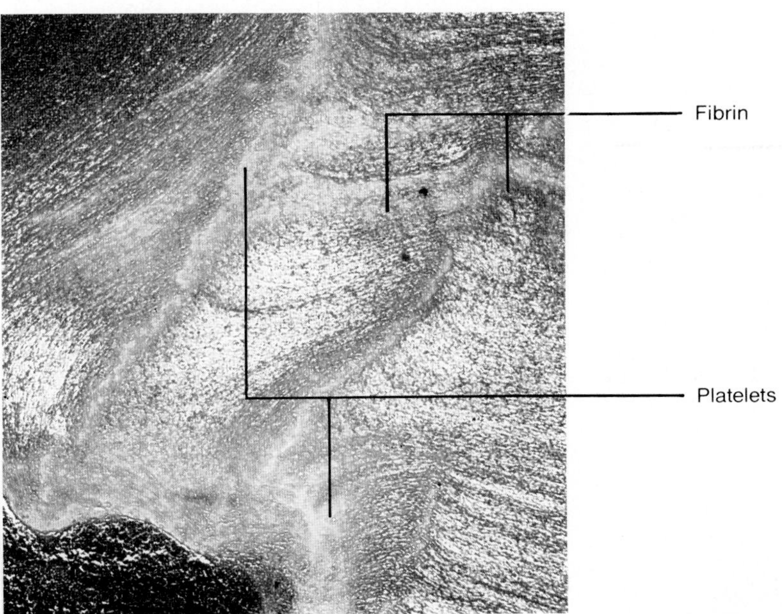

Figure 9-15. Thrombus, showing alternating zones of amorphous platelets (lines of Zahn) and fibrillary fibrin.

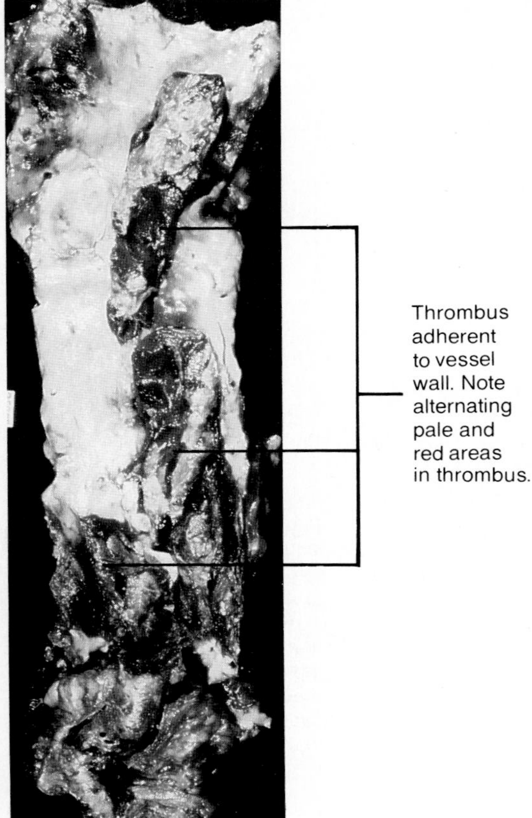

Figure 9-16. Abdominal aorta, showing multiple large thrombi attached to the endothelial surface. The thrombi have alternating pale and red areas.

heparin therapy (the anticoagulant action prevents fibrin formation).

Sites of Thrombosis

A. Arterial Thrombosis: (Figs 9-16 and 9-17.) Arterial thrombosis is common and typically occurs after endothelial damage and local turbulence caused by atherosclerosis (Chapter 20). Large- and medium-sized arteries such as the aorta, carotid arteries, arteries of the circle of Willis, coronary arteries, and arteries of the intestine and limbs are mainly affected.

Less commonly, arterial thrombosis is a complication of arteritis, as occurs in polyarteritis nodosa, giant cell arteritis, thromboangiitis obliterans, and Henoch-Schönlein purpura (Chapter 20). Medium- and small-sized arteries are commonly affected.

B. Cardiac Thrombosis: Thrombi form within the chambers of the heart in the following circumstances.

1. Inflammation of cardiac valves-Endocardial damage occurring in association with inflammation of the cardiac valves (endocarditis, valvulitis) leads to local turbulence and deposition of platelets and fibrin on the valves. These thrombi are called **vegetations** (Fig 9-18). Vegetations are often large and friable (as occurs in infective endocarditis), and fragments of thrombus often break off and are carried in the circulation as emboli (see below).

2. Damage to mural endocardium-Myocardial infarction and ventricular aneurysms are associated with damage to the mural endocardium. Thrombi forming on the walls are often large and may also give rise to emboli.

3. Turbulence and stasis in atrial chambers-Thrombi often form in chambers of the atrium when turbulence and stasis of blood occur, typically in patients with mitral valve stenosis and atrial fibrillation. Thrombi may be so large (ball thrombus) that they obstruct the mitral valve orifice. Fragments of atrial thrombi may become detached and form emboli.

C. Venous Thrombosis: (Fig 9-19.)

1. Thrombophlebitis-Thrombophlebitis denotes venous thrombosis occurring secondary to acute inflammation of the vein. Thrombophlebitis is a common phenomenon in infected wounds or ulcers and characteristically involves the superficial veins of the extremities. The affected vein is firm and cordlike and shows signs of acute inflammation (pain, redness, warmth, swelling). This type of thrombus tends to be firmly attached to the vessel wall, and fragments rarely become detached.

Rarely, thrombophlebitis occurs in multiple superficial leg veins (thrombophlebitis migrans) in patients with visceral cancers, most commonly pancreatic and gastric cancer (Trousseau's sign). Mucins and other cancer cell products have been shown to possess thromboplastinlike activity.

2. Phlebothrombosis-Phlebothrombosis denotes venous thrombosis occurring in the absence of obvious inflammation. Phlebothrombosis occurs mostly in the deep veins of the leg (deep vein thrombosis). Less commonly, veins of the pelvic venous plexus are involved. Deep vein thrombosis is common and has important medical implications because the large thrombi that form in these veins are only loosely attached to the vessel wall and are often easily detached. They travel in the circulation to the heart and lung and lodge in the pulmonary arteries (pulmonary embolism [Fig 9-20]).

a. Causes-Factors causing deep vein phlebothrombosis are those typical of thrombosis in general. Endothelial injury is usually minimal and difficult to demonstrate. Sluggish blood flow is an important causative factor. In the venous plexus of the calf muscles, blood flow is normally maintained by calf muscle contraction (the muscle pump). Paralysis or prolonged immobilization in bed therefore favors stasis of blood and thrombo-

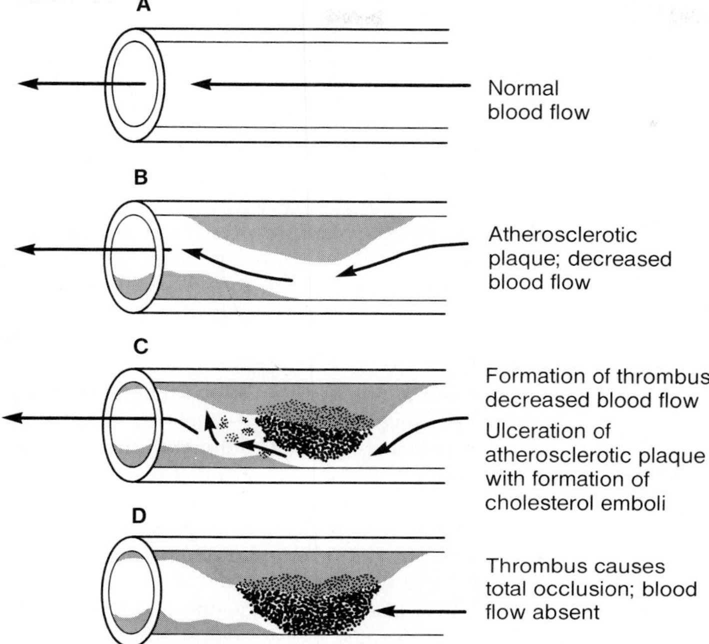

Figure 9–17. Thrombosis is an atherosclerotic artery. **A:** Normal artery, showing typical laminar blood flow. **B:** Atherosclerotic artery, showing atherosclerotic plaques. The endothelium is intact, but the vessel lumen is narrowed. Decreased blood flow and increased turbulence are present. **C:** Ulcerated atherosclerotic plaque from which fragments of the plaque have become detached and passed distally as cholesterol emboli (see Fig 9–28). Blood flow is further decreased and turbulence increased. Thrombosis has occurred over the ulcerated area. **D:** Extension of thrombosis has caused total occlusion of the artery, and there is no blood flow in the vessel.

sis. Awareness of this relationship and the routine use of physical therapy, compressive stockings, and early ambulation after surgery have considerably decreased the incidence of postoperative deep vein thrombosis. Sluggish blood flow also occurs in cardiac failure. Changes in the composition of blood in postoperative or postpartum patients result in an increased tendency toward platelet adhesion and aggregation as well as an increased tendency toward coagulation because of increased levels of some coagulation factors (fibrinogen and factors VII and VIII). Oral contraceptives—particularly those with high estrogen levels—may cause increased blood coagulability. In some patients, several of these causative factors may be responsible for deep vein thrombosis.

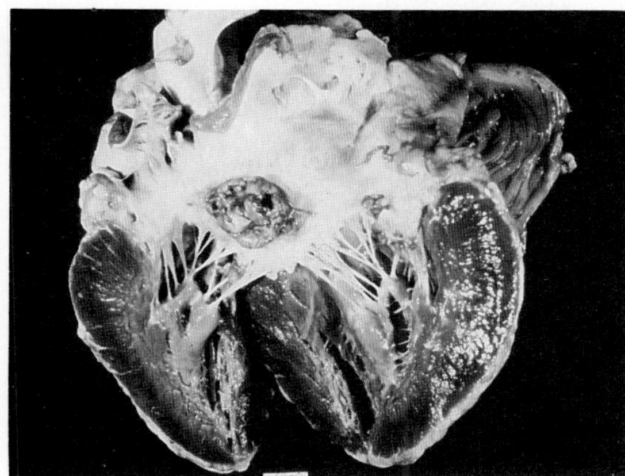

Figure 9–18. Vegetation (= thrombus) on mitral valve in subacute infective endocarditis.

b. Clinical findings–Deep vein thrombosis of the legs typically causes few or no clinical symptoms. Mild edema of the ankles and calf pain when the ankle is dorsiflexed (Homans' sign) are helpful diagnostic features. In many patients, pulmonary embolism is the first clinical manifestation of phlebothrombosis. Deep vein thrombosis can be detected by venography, ultrasonography, and special radiologic techniques using radioisotope markers.

Evolution of Thrombi

Thrombus formation evokes a host response that is designed to remove the thrombus and repair the injured blood vessel. Several outcomes are possible.

A. Fibrinolysis: Lysis of the thrombus (fibrinolysis) accompanied by reestablishment of the lumen is the ideal end result. The fibrin constituting the thrombus is dissolved by **plasmin,** which is activated by Hageman factor (factor XII) whenever the intrinsic coagulation pathway is activated (ie, the fibrinolytic system is activated at the same

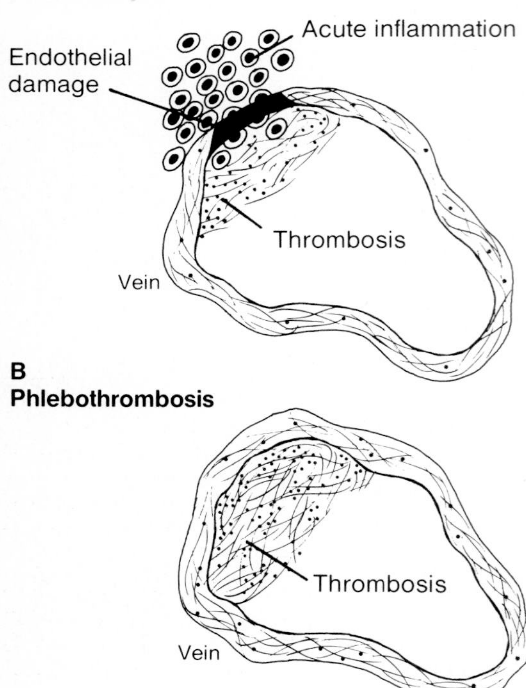

Figure 9–19. Venous thrombosis. **A:** In thrombophlebitis, acute inflammation of the venous wall leads to endothelial damage and thrombosis. The thrombus is adherent to the vein wall, and embolism is rare. **B:** In phlebothrombosis, inflammation and venous endothelial damage are typically minimal. Sluggish blood flow and altered blood coagulability play an important role in thrombus formation. The thrombus is loosely attached to the vein wall and commonly becomes detached to cause embolism.

time as the clotting sequence; this mechanism for clot lysis is a built-in control function that normally prevents excessive thrombosis) (Fig 9–14). Under normal conditions, plasmin prevents excessive deposition of fibrin during physiologic hemostasis. Fibrinolysis is effective in dissolving small thrombi; eg, in disseminated intravascular coagulation, which is characterized by multiple small thrombi, the thrombi are rapidly lysed by fibrinolysis and are often impossible to demonstrate in the microcirculation at autopsy. Fibrinolysis is much less effective in dissolving large thrombi occurring in arteries, veins, or the heart itself. Drugs such as streptokinase and tissue plasminogen activator (TPA), which activate the fibrinolytic system, are effective, when used immediately after thrombosis, in causing lysis of the thrombus and reestablishing perfusion. They have been used with some success in the treatment of acute myocardial infarction, deep vein thrombosis, and acute peripheral arterial thrombosis.

B. Organization and Recanalization: Organization and recanalization commonly occur in large thrombi. Slow liquefaction and phagocytosis of the thrombus are followed by ingrowth of granulation tissue and collagenization (organization). The vessels in the granulation tissue frequently enlarge and may establish new channels across the thrombus (recanalization) (Fig 9–21) through which some blood flow may be restored. Recanalization occurs slowly over several weeks, and although it does not prevent the acute effects of thrombosis, it may slightly improve tissue perfusion over the long term.

C. Thromboembolism: Sometimes a fragment of thrombus is detached and carried in the

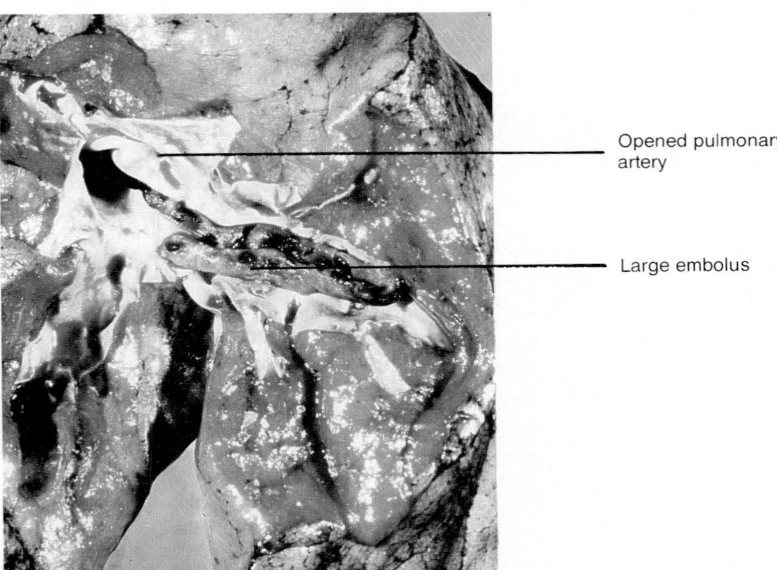

Figure 9–20. Pulmonary embolism. The pulmonary artery has been opened to reveal a large thromboembolus within it. Note the branching of the embolus, probably corresponding to the configuration of the vein it originated in.

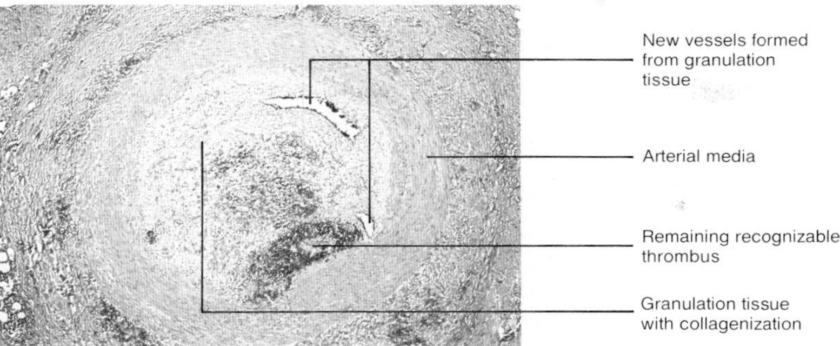

Figure 9-21. Early organization and recanalization of a thrombosed vessel. As the process progresses, the thrombus is completely replaced by collagen, and the vascular channels in the granulation tissue dilate.

circulation to lodge at a distant site—a process termed thromboembolism.

DISSEMINATED INTRAVASCULAR COAGULATION (DIC)

Disseminated intravascular coagulation is the widespread development of small thrombi in the microcirculation throughout the body (Fig 9-22). It is a serious and often fatal complication of numerous diseases and requires early recognition and treatment.

Causes (Table 9-1 and Fig 9-23)

In many cases, the cause of disseminated intravascular coagulation is unknown. Diffuse endothelial injury, as occurs in infections due to gram-negative bacteria (gram-negative sepsis, endotoxic shock), is a common cause. Viral and rickettsial infections may result in direct infection and damage to endothelial cells. Immunologic injury to the endothelium, as occurs in type II and type III hypersensitivity, may also precipitate DIC. Disseminated intravascular coagulation may occur when thromboplastic substances enter the circulation, as occurs in amniotic fluid embolism (amniotic fluid contains thromboplastin, which has procoagulant activity), snakebite (particularly Russell's viper), promyelocytic leukemia (the promyelocytes contain thromboplastic substances), and any condition associated with extensive tissue necrosis.

Effects (Fig 9-23)

A. Decreased Tissue Perfusion: The multiple occlusions of the microcirculation in disseminated intravascular coagulation result in wide-

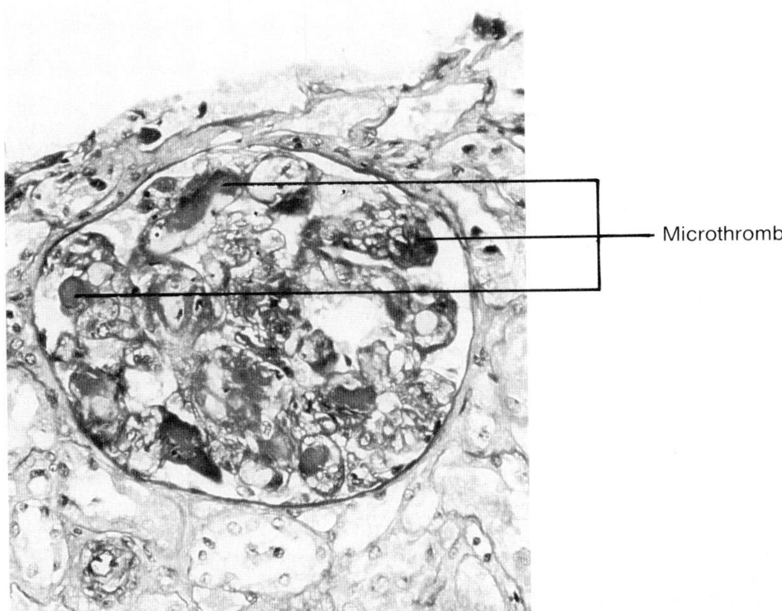

Figure 9-22. Disseminated intravascular coagulation. Numerous microthrombi are seen in glomerular capillaries.

Table 9-1. Disorders associated with disseminated intravascular coagulation.

Infectious diseases
Gram-negative bacteremia
Meningococcal sepsis
Gram-positive bacteremia
Disseminated fungal infections
Rickettsial infections
Severe viremias (eg, hemorrhagic fevers)
Plasmodium falciparum malaria
Neonatal and intrauterine infections
Obstetric disorders
Amniotic fluid embolism
Retained dead fetus
Abruptio placentae
Liver diseases
Massive liver cell necrosis
Cirrhosis of the liver
Malignant diseases
Acute promyelocytic leukemia
Metastatic carcinoma, mainly adenocarcinoma
Miscellaneous disorders
Small vessel vasculitides
Massive trauma
Burns
Heat stroke
Surgery with extracorporeal circulation
Snakebite (Russell's viper)
Severe shock
Intravascular hemolysis

spread impaired tissue perfusion, leading to shock, accumulation of lactic acid, and microinfarction in many organs.

B. Bleeding: Disseminated thrombosis also results in the consumption of coagulation factors in the blood (consumption coagulopathy). Thrombocytopenia combined with the decreased levels of fibrinogen and other coagulation factors leads to failure of coagulation. The resulting bleeding tendency is aggravated by excessive activation of the fibrinolytic system (activation of Hageman factor XII, which initiates the intrinsic coagulation pathway, also leads to conversion of plasminogen to plasmin), which dissolves fibrin in thrombi and thereby promotes bleeding. Fibrin degradation products resulting from the action of plasmin on fibrin also have anticoagulant properties, further aggravating the bleeding tendency. In many patients with disseminated intravascular coagulation, the predominant clinical effect is hemorrhage.

Treatment

Treatment includes heparin to inhibit the formation of thrombi as well as administration of platelets and plasma to restore the depleted coagulation factors. Monitoring the levels of fibrin degradation products, fibrinogen, and platelets aids diagnosis and assesses the effectiveness of therapy.

EMBOLISM

Embolism is the occlusion or obstruction of a vessel by an abnormal mass (solid, liquid, or gaseous) transported from a different site by the circulation. Most emboli are detached fragments of thrombi that are carried in the bloodstream to their sites of lodgment (**thromboembolism**). Numerous other substances such as fat, amniotic fluid, bone marrow, tumor cells, parasites, debris from atheromatous plaques, and foreign particulate matter are less common causes of embolism.

Origin of Emboli

The site of embolism is mostly governed by the point of origin and size of the embolus.

A. Origin in Systemic Veins: Emboli that originate in systemic veins (as a result of venous thrombosis) and the right side of the heart (eg, infective endocarditis affecting the tricuspid valve) lodge in the pulmonary arterial system unless they are so small (eg, fat globules, tumor cells) that they can pass through the pulmonary capillaries. The point of lodgment in the pulmonary arterial circulation depends on the size of the embolus (see below). Rarely, an embolus originating in a systemic vein passes across a defect in the cardiac interatrial or interventricular septum (thus bypassing the lungs) to lodge in a systemic artery (**paradoxic embolism**).

Emboli that originate in branches of the portal vein lodge in the liver, eg, cancer cells from colonic or pancreatic cancer.

B. Origin in Heart and Systemic Arteries: Emboli originating in the left side of the heart and systemic arteries (as a result of cardiac or arterial thrombosis) lodge in a distal systemic artery in sites such as the brain, heart, kidney, extremity, intestine, etc.

Types & Sites of Embolism (Table 9-2)

A. Thromboembolism: Detached fragments of thrombi that lodge in organs situated distally in the circulation are the most common cause of clinically significant embolism.

1. Pulmonary embolism–

a. Causes and incidence–The most serious form of thromboembolism is pulmonary embolism, which may cause sudden death. About 600,000 patients per year develop clinically evident pulmonary embolism in the USA; about 100,000 of them die. *Over 90% of pulmonary emboli originate in the deep veins of the leg (phlebothrombosis).* More rarely, thrombi in pelvic venous plexuses are the source. Pulmonary embolism is therefore common in the following states or conditions that predispose to the development of phlebothrombosis: (1) The immediate postoperative period. About 30–50% of patients show evidence of deep vein thrombosis after ma-

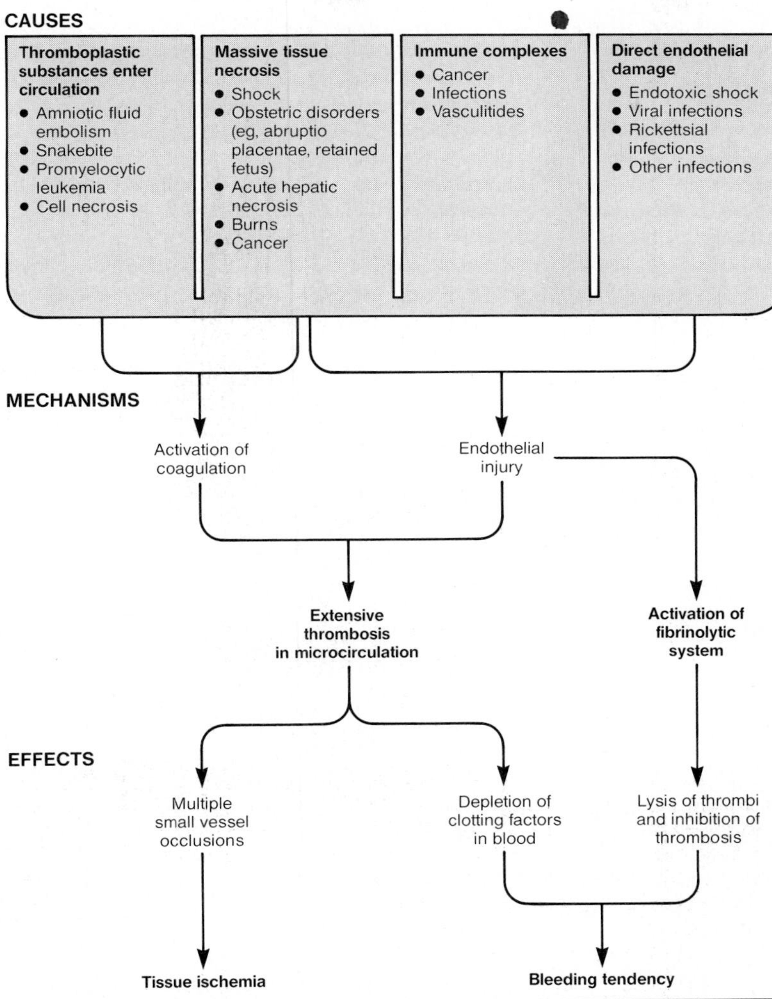

Figure 9-23. Initiating factors and mechanisms in disseminated intravascular coagulation (DIC). A key difference between DIC and normal thrombus formation is that in DIC both coagulation and fibrinolysis occur diffusely throughout the microcirculation—in contrast to the more localized nature of normal thrombosis. In some instances, thrombosis predominates, resulting in ischemic effects; in others, fibrinolysis predominates, resulting in hemorrhage.

jor surgery if they are carefully examined. Only a small number of these patients develop clinically significant pulmonary embolism. (2) The immediate postpartum period. (3) Lengthy immobilization in bed. (4) Cardiac failure. (5) Use of oral contraceptives.

b. Clinical effects-(Fig 9–24.) The size of the embolus is the factor most influencing the clinical effects of pulmonary embolism.

(1) Massive emboli-Large emboli (several centimeters long and of the same diameter as the femoral vein) may lodge in the outflow tract of the right ventricle or in the main pulmonary artery, where they cause circulatory obstruction and **sudden death** (Fig 9–25). Large emboli lodging in a large branch of the pulmonary artery may also cause sudden death, probably as a result of severe vasoconstriction of the entire pulmonary arterial circulation induced reflexly by lodgment of the embolus (Fig 9–20).

(2) Medium-sized emboli-Moderate-sized emboli often lodge in a major branch of the pulmonary artery. In healthy individuals, the bronchial artery supplies blood (and oxygen) to the lung, and the function of the pulmonary artery is mainly gas exchange (not local tissue oxygenation). In a normal person, therefore, a moderate-sized pulmonary embolus creates an area of lung that is ventilated but not perfused with regard to gas exchange. This results in abnormal gas exchange and hypoxemia, but infarction of the lung does not occur. In a patient with chronic left heart failure or pulmonary vascular disease, however, the bronchial arterial circulation is impaired, and the lung is therefore dependent on the pulmonary artery for perfusion of tissue as well as gas exchange. In these patients, obstruction of a pulmonary artery by a moderate-sized embolus results in **pulmonary infarction**.

(3) Small emboli-Small emboli lodge in minor

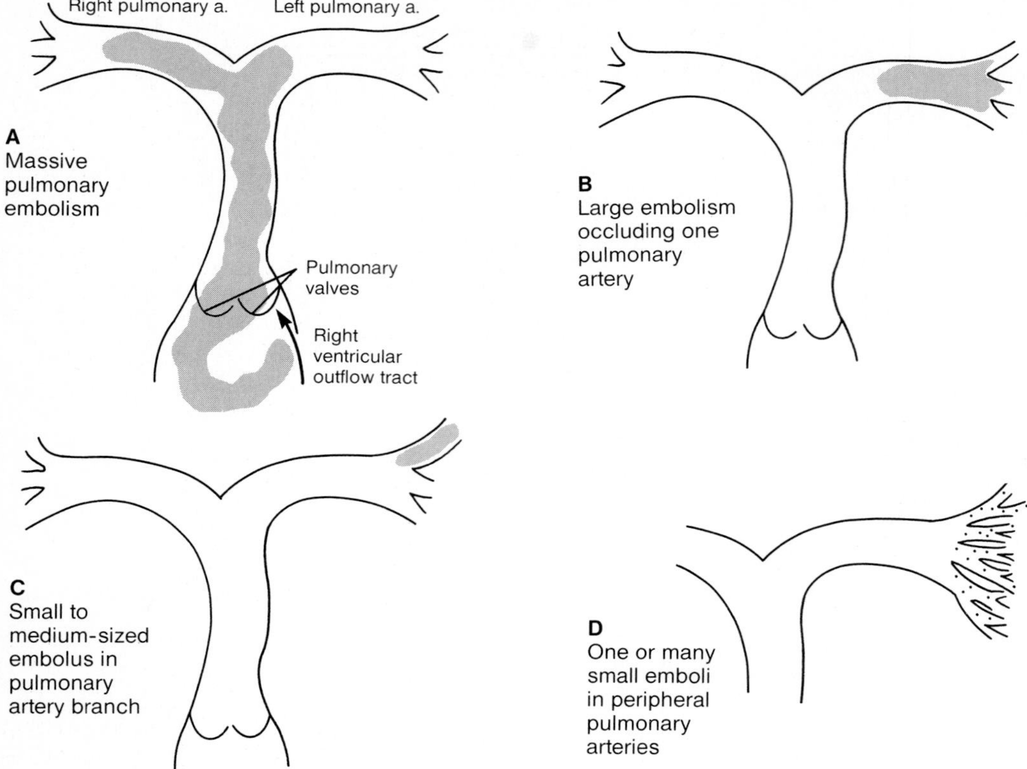

Figure 9-24. Clinical effects of pulmonary embolism. **A:** Massive pulmonary embolism causes circulatory arrest and sudden death (Fig 9–25). **B:** A large embolism occluding one pulmonary artery may cause pulmonary infarction or sudden death due to the reflex vasoconstriction of the pulmonary circulation (see Fig 9–20). Some healthy individuals may show no ill effects, but this is unusual with a large embolus. **C:** A small to medium-sized embolus in a pulmonary arterial branch typically has no effect in healthy individuals. Pulmonary infarction may occur if the bronchial circulation is compromised, as in patients with left heart failure and pulmonary hypertension. **D:** Small emboli have no effect unless they are numerous, in which case they may cause pulmonary hypertension.

emboli either fragment soon after lodgment or dissolve during fibrinolysis, in which case clinical effects are minimal. If numerous small emboli occur over a long period, however, the pulmonary microcirculation may be so severely compromised that **pulmonary hypertension** results.

2. Systemic arterial embolism–

a. Causes–Thromboembolism occurs in systemic arteries when the detached thrombus originates in the left side of the heart or a large artery. Systemic arterial thromboembolism commonly occurs (1) in patients who have infective endocarditis with vegetations on the mitral and aortic valves; (2) in patients who have suffered myocardial infarction in which mural thrombosis has occurred; (3) in patients with mitral stenosis and atrial fibrillation due to left atrial thrombosis; and (4) in patients with aortic and ventricular aneurysms, which often contain mural thrombi. Thromboemboli from any of these locations pass distally to lodge in an artery of some other organ. Because of the anatomy of the aorta, cardiac emboli tend to pass more frequently into the lower extremities or into the circulation derived from the right internal carotid artery than into other systemic arteries.

b. Clinical effects–The clinical effects of systemic thromboembolism are governed by the size of the obstructed vessel, the availability of collateral arterial circulation, and the susceptibility of the tissue to ischemia (see Factors Influencing the Effect of Arterial Obstruction, above). Infarction is common when emboli lodge in the arteries of the brain, heart, kidney, and spleen. Infarction occurs in the intestine and lower extremities only when large arteries are occluded or when the collateral circulation in these tissues is compromised.

B. Air Embolism: Air embolism occurs when enough air bubbles enter the vascular system to produce clinical symptoms; about 150 mL of air causes death. The condition is rare.

1. Causes–

a. Surgery of or trauma to internal jugular vein–In injuries to the internal jugular vein incurred as a result of surgery or other trauma, the negative pressure in the thorax tends to suck air into the jugular vein. This phenomenon does not occur in injuries to other systemic veins because

Table 9-2. Types of embolism.

Origin and Type of Embolism	Circulatory System Involved	Clinical Effect
Thrombi in right side of heart and systemic veins Deep vein thrombosis Right-sided infective endocarditis	Pulmonary	Circulatory arrest, lung infarction, pulmonary hypertension
Thrombi in left side of heart and systemic arteries Cardiac valvular vegetations Cardiac mural thrombus Cardiac atrial thrombus Cardiac aneurysmal thrombus Aortic aneurysmal thrombus	Systemic	Infarction in brain, kidney, intestine, peripheral arteries
Air embolism Puncture of jugular vein Childbirth or abortion Blood transfusion using positive pressure Pneumothorax	Pulmonary (right ventricle)	Total obstruction of pulmonary flow causes sudden death
Nitrogen gas embolism Decompression sickness	Pulmonary and systemic	Ischemia in lung, brain, nerves
Fat embolism Trauma (ie, serious fractures of large bones)	Mostly pulmonary; some fat globules pass to systemic	Microinfarcts and hemorrhages in lung, brain, skin
Bone marrow embolism Trauma	Pulmonary	No clinical significance
Atheromatous embolism Ulcerated atheromatous plaque	Systemic	Microinfarction in brain, retina, kidney
Amniotic fluid embolism Childbirth	Pulmonary	Disseminated intravascular coagulation
Tumor embolism	Depends on location of tumor	Metastasis

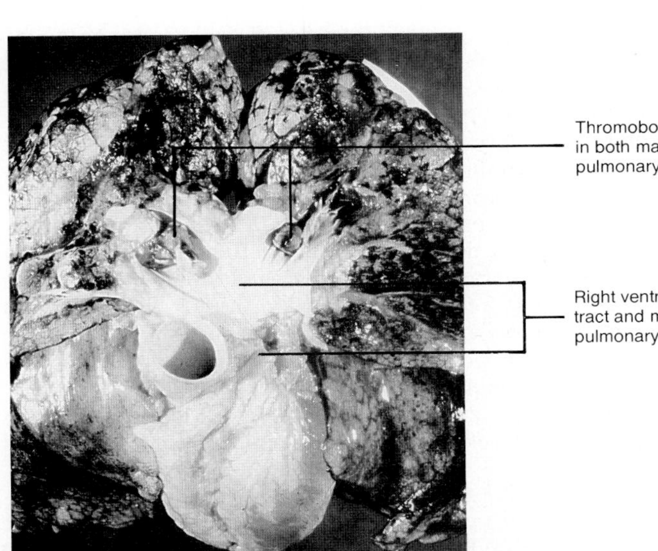

Figure 9-25. Massive pulmonary embolism. The main pulmonary artery has been opened and shows impacted thromboemboli at the orifices of both right and left main pulmonary arteries. This led to sudden death from circulatory obstruction. **Note:** When the pulmonary arteries were further opened, the emboli were seen to be very large. Only their tips are shown here.

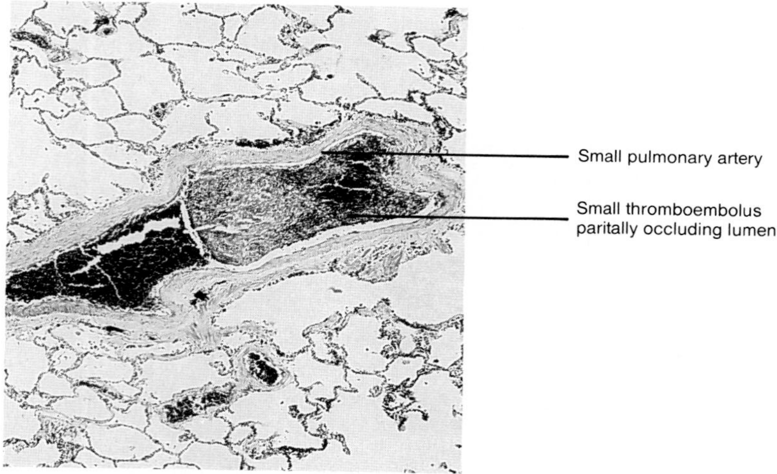

Figure 9-26. Pulmonary thromboembolism partially occluding a small branch of the pulmonary artery in the lung. This has no immediate effect, but pulmonary hypertension may result if recurrent and numerous emboli occur.

they are separated by valves from the negative pressure in the chest.

b. Childbirth or abortion-Air embolism may occur during childbirth or abortion, when air may be forced into ruptured placental venous sinuses by the forceful contractions of the uterus.

c. Blood transfusions-Air embolism during blood transfusions occurs only if positive pressure is used to transfuse the blood and only if the transfusion is inadvertently not discontinued at its completion. Air embolism due to transfusion occurs only if glass bottles have been used to hold blood; the use of collapsible plastic packs for blood transfusion, which is now almost universal, has greatly reduced the risk of this catastrophe.

d. Therapeutic pneumothorax-During therapeutic induction of pneumothorax, air embolism will occur if air is accidentally introduced into a blood vessel instead of the pleural cavity. This procedure was formerly a common method of treating pulmonary tuberculosis.

e. Uterotubal insufflation-The uterus and tubes were formerly insufflated with air to investigate the cause of infertility. CO_2 has replaced air in this procedure and has removed the risk of air embolism, since CO_2 goes rapidly into solution. This procedure is rarely used today.

2. Clinical effects-When air enters the bloodstream, it passes into the right ventricle and accumulates there. The pumping action of the heart churns the air with blood to create a frothy mass in the right ventricle that effectively obstructs the circulation and causes death. More rarely, the frothy air-blood mixture obstructs a pulmonary artery.

C. Nitrogen Gas Embolism (Decompression Sickness):

1. Cause-Decompression sickness is a form of embolism that occurs in caisson workers and undersea divers if they ascend too rapidly after being submerged for long periods (Fig 9-27). The disorder is also called **"the bends"** or **caisson disease** (caissons are high-pressure underwater chambers used for deep water construction work). When air is breathed under high underwater pressure, an increased volume of air, mainly oxygen and nitrogen, goes into solution in the blood and equilibrates with the tissues. Nitrogen is selectively soluble in fat and is incorporated mainly in adipose tissue and in the lipids of the central and peripheral nervous system.

If decompression to sea level is too rapid, the gases that have equilibrated in the tissues come out of solution and escape from tissues as external pressure decreases. Oxygen is rapidly absorbed into the blood, but nitrogen gas coming out of solution cannot be absorbed rapidly enough and forms bubbles in the tissues and bloodstream that act as emboli.

Decompression sickness is uncommon today because the training of undersea divers stresses the importance of regulated decompression during ascent. Professional deep sea divers are slowly decompressed during a carefully graded ascent that permits nitrogen to escape from the tissues without forming gas bubbles. Scuba divers breathing high-pressure compressed air who ascend rapidly from depths as shallow as 10 m may also develop decompression sickness, and those who engage in this recreational activity should be taught and cautioned to ascend slowly.

Decompression sickness can also occur in unpressurized aircraft if they ascend too rapidly to high altitudes (above 2000 m). Mountain climbers who climb too rapidly to high altitudes are also at risk.

2. Clinical effects-Platelets adhere to nitrogen gas bubbles in the circulation and activate the coagulation cascade. The resulting disseminated intravascular thrombosis aggravates the ischemic

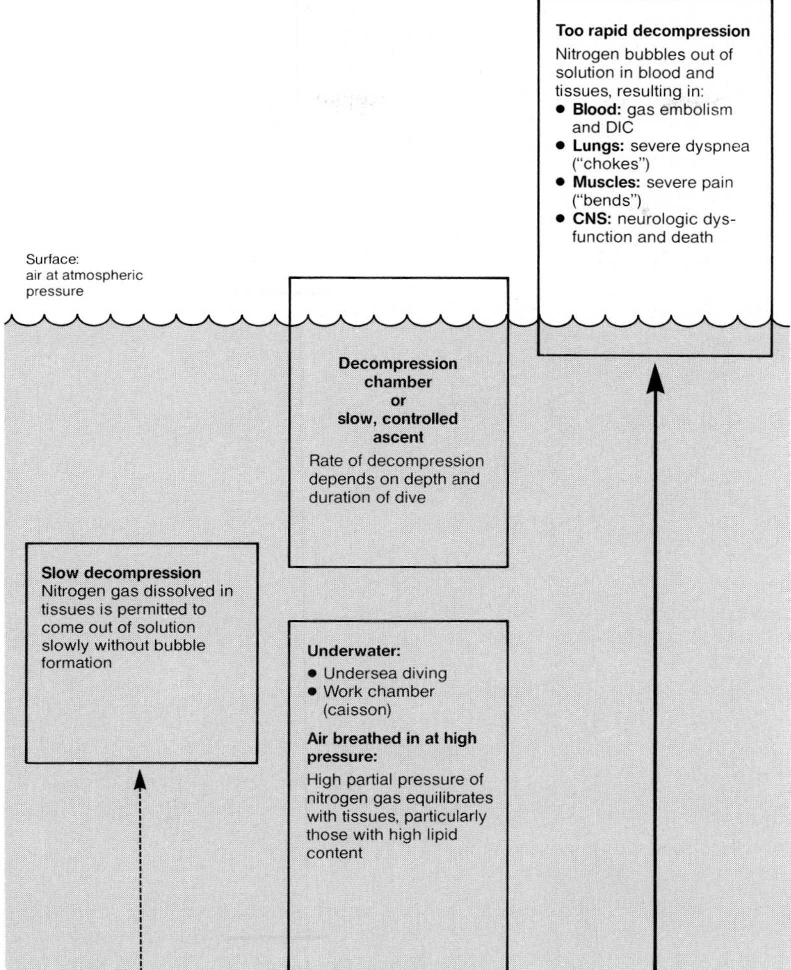

Figure 9-27. Pathogenesis of decompression sickness and its prevention.

state caused by impaction of gas bubbles in capillaries. Involvement of the brain in severe cases may cause extensive necrosis and death. In less severe cases, nerve and muscle involvement causes severe muscle contractions with intense pain ("the bends"). Nitrogen gas emboli in the lungs cause severe difficulty in breathing ("the chokes") that is associated with alveolar edema and hemorrhage.

D. Fat Embolism:

1. Causes-Fat embolism occurs when globules of fat enter the bloodstream, typically after fractures of large bones (eg, femur) have exposed the fatty bone marrow. Rarely, extensive injury to subcutaneous adipose tissue causes fat embolism. Although fat globules can be found in the circulation in as many as 90% of patients who have sustained serious fractures, few patients demonstrate clinically significant signs of fat embolism.

Although simple mechanical rupture of fat cells at trauma sites may explain how fat globules can enter the circulation, other factors are probably involved. It has been shown that fat globules enlarge once they are in the circulation, which explains why small globules that bypass lung capillaries may later become obstructed in systemic capillaries. It is thought that release of catecholamines due to the stress of trauma mobilizes free fatty acids, which coalesce to form progressively enlarging fat globules. Adhesion of platelets to fat globules further increases their size and causes thrombosis. When this process is extensive, it is equivalent to disseminated intravascular coagulation.

2. Clinical effects-Circulating fat globules first encounter the capillary network of the lung. Larger fat globules ($> 20\ \mu m$) are arrested in the lung and cause respiratory distress (dyspnea and abnormal gas exchange). Smaller fat globules escape the lung capillaries and pass into the systemic circulation, where they may obstruct small systemic arteries. Typical clinical features of fat em-

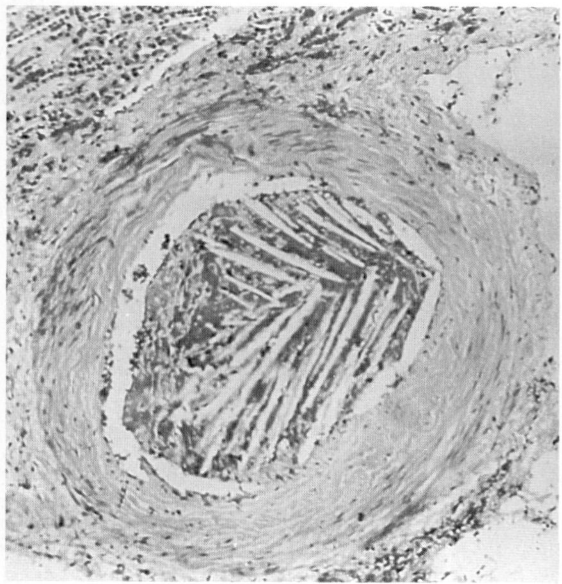

Figure 9-28. Cholesterol embolus derived from an ulcerated atheromatous plaque lodged in a branch of the renal artery.

bolism include a hemorrhagic skin rash and brain involvement manifested as acute diffuse neurologic dysfunction.

The possibility of fat embolism must be considered if respiratory distress, cerebral dysfunction, and a hemorrhagic rash occurs 1–3 days after major trauma. The diagnosis can be confirmed by demonstrating fat globules in urine and sputum. About 10% of patients with clinical fat embolism die. At autopsy, fat globules can be demonstrated by special techniques (frozen sections and special fat stains) in many organs.

E. Bone Marrow Embolism: Fragments of bone marrow containing fat and hematopoietic cells may enter the circulation after traumatic injury of bone marrow. Fragments of bone marrow are commonly found in the pulmonary arteries at autopsy in patients who have suffered rib fractures during cardiopulmonary resuscitative efforts. Bone marrow embolism is of no clinical significance.

F. Atheromatous (Cholesterol) Embolism: Large ulcerated atheromatous plaques often release cholesterol and other atheromatous material into the circulation (Fig 9–28). Emboli are carried distally to lodge in small systemic arteries. Such embolization in brain produces **transient ischemic attacks,** characterized by reversible acute episodes of neurologic dysfunction.

G. Amniotic Fluid Embolism: The contents of the amniotic sac may rarely (1:80,000 pregnancies) enter ruptured uterine venous sinuses during tumultuous labor in childbirth. Though rare, amniotic fluid embolism is associated with a mortality rate of about 80% and is a significant cause of maternal deaths in the USA.

Amniotic fluid is rich in thromboplastic substances that induce disseminated intravascular coagulation, which is the main mechanism by which the disorder is manifested clinically. Amniotic fluid also contains fetal squamous epithelium (desquamated from the skin), fetal hair, fetal fat, mucin, and meconium, all of which may undergo embolization and become lodged in the pulmonary capillaries. Although the emboli in the vessels may not be responsible for the clinical symptoms, their presence in the pulmonary vasculature is useful in making an autopsy diagnosis of amniotic fluid embolism (Fig 9–29).

H. Tumor Embolism: Cancer cells often enter the circulation during metastasis of malignant tumors (see Chapter 17). Typically, these solitary cells or small clumps of cells are too small to obstruct the vasculature. Occasionally, larger fragments of tumor break off and constitute significant emboli—with renal carcinoma, especially in the inferior vena cava; and with hepatic carcinoma, especially in the hepatic veins.

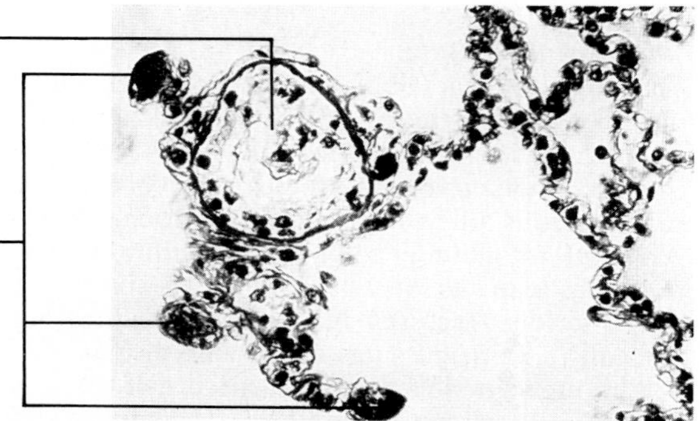

Figure 9-29. Amniotic fluid embolism of lung.

Nutritional Disease 10

ESSENTIAL NUTRIENTS

Humans are dependent on their diet for certain essential nutrients that cannot be synthesized in the body. An adequate diet must provide sufficient total proteins, sufficient total calories, essential amino acids, essential fatty acids, vitamins, and minerals. A deficiency of any of these dietary factors leads to disordered cellular metabolism and cellular injury with recognizable symptoms and signs of nutritional deficiency. Although specific deficiency diseases have not been identified in humans for all of the essential dietary elements (eg, individual essential amino acids and fatty acids), nutritional diseases arising from total protein-calorie deficiency and various vitamin and mineral deficiencies are well-recognized (Table 10–1).

NUTRITIONAL DEFICIENCY

Deficiency of an essential nutrient may arise in a variety of ways.

Primary Nutritional Deficiency

Nutritional deficiency resulting from inadequate food intake (primary malnutrition) is common in developing nations but also occurs rarely in developed countries in inner city slum areas, among the elderly, among individuals consuming fad diets, and in some mentally retarded and alcoholic individuals.

Secondary Nutritional Deficiency

Malnutrition occurring in the presence of adequate food consumption is termed secondary malnutrition.

A. Failure of Intestinal Absorption: Nutritional deficiency may result from a general malabsorptive state or a defect of absorption of a specific substance, eg, failure of vitamin B_{12} absorption in pernicious anemia.

B. Increased Metabolic Demand: Increased demand for specific dietary substances—eg, the increased folic acid requirement in pregnancy—may cause relative insufficiency and evidence of disease.

C. Antagonists: The presence of antagonists to essential dietary substances—eg, folic acid antagonists such as methotrexate used in cancer chemotherapy—may induce symptoms of nutritional deficiency.

NUTRITIONAL EXCESS

At the other extreme of nutritional disease, excessive intake of food results in obesity. Obesity is an important problem in many developed countries and is responsible for considerable clinical illness. Excessive intake of particular food groups may also contribute to the development of certain diseases; eg, cholesterol and saturated fats predispose to atherosclerosis. More rarely, clinical disease occurs with excessive intake of specific food substances, eg, vitamins A and D and iron (Table 10–1).

Table 10-1. Principal human nutrients and disorders resulting from nutritional deficiency or excess.

Nutrient	Physiologic Importance	Deficiency	Excess
Protein	Numerous.	Marasmus; kwashiorkor; growth retardation.	None.
Calories	Numerous.	Marasmus; kwashiorkor; growth retardation.	Obesity.
Fat-soluble vitamins[1]			
Vitamin A	Retinol is constituent of retinal rod pigment rhodopsin. Maintain epithelia.	Loss of night vision; increased thickness of squamous epithelia; Bitot's spots; xerophthalmia, keratomalacia (eyes); follicular hyperkeratosis (skin).	Bleeding; hepatosplenomegaly[2] (rare).
Vitamin D (cholecalciferol)	1,25-Dihydroxycholecalciferol activates calcium absorption in intestine and causes bone mineralization.	Rickets (children); osteomalacia (adults).	Hypercalcemia leading to metastatic calcification and renal damage[2] (rare).
Vitamin K	Required for synthesis of prothrombin and clotting factors, VII, IX, and X.	Hypoprothrombinemia resulting in bleeding tendency.	Hemolytic anemia[2] (rare).
Water-soluble vitamins[1]			
Vitamin C (ascorbic acid)	Required for synthesis of collagen and osteoid.	Scurvy; impaired wound healing.	Minimal—possibly urinary calculi.
Thiamine (vitamin B_1)	Coenzyme in decarboxylase systems; required for synthesis of acetylcholine.	Beriberi (wet and dry); Wernicke's encephalopathy; Korsakoff's syndrome.	None.
Riboflavin (vitamin B_2)	Constituent of flavoproteins.	Cheilosis, glossitis, angular stomatitis; corneal vascularization.	None.
Niacin	Constituent of NAD and NADP.	Pellagra.	Flushing due to vasodilation occurs with intravenous injection (rare).
Pyridoxine (vitamin B_6)	Coenzyme for decarboxylase and transaminase systems.	Glossitis; blepharitis; dermatitis; cheilosis; peripheral neuropathy; sideroblastic anemia.	None.
Folic acid[3]	Required for nucleic acid synthesis.	Megaloblastic anemia.	None.
Vitamin B_{12}[3]	Required for nucleic acid synthesis.	Megaloblastic anemia; subacute combined degeneration of spinal cord; peripheral neuropathy.	None.
Minerals			
Iron[3]	Constituent of hemoglobin and myoglobin.	Hypochromic anemia; loss of mucosal integrity.	Hemochromatosis.

[1]The fat-soluble vitamins are present especially in fatty foods (milk, butter, etc) and may be deficient when there is fat malabsorption for any reason. Water-soluble vitamins are widely distributed in fruits, vegetables, and animal products, with the exception of vitamin B_{12}, which is found almost exclusively in meat. Water-soluble vitamins are less affected by generalized malabsorption states; specific malabsorption of vitamin B_{12} occurs in pernicious anemia.
[2]Note that excess amounts of fat-soluble vitamins accumulate in body fat stores and may lead to toxicity; toxicity of water-soluble vitamins in much rarer, probably because of rapid excretion of any excess in the urine.
[3]Deficiency results in various types of anemia.

PROTEINS & CALORIES

PROTEIN-CALORIE MALNUTRITION (Marasmus; Kwashiorkor)

Causes

The general malnutrition occurring in developing countries is commonly a deficiency of total calorie and protein intake, mainly due to economic factors. Young children tend to be most affected because they have increased metabolic demands for nutrients during the rapid early growth phase and because they often do not fare well in the struggle for access to limited food resources.

Marasmus and kwashiorkor are part of a clinical spectrum of protein-calorie malnutrition, kwashiorkor being the more extreme disorder. Early concepts of marasmus as a purely caloric deficiency and kwashiorkor as a purely protein deficiency are now questioned.

Protein-calorie malnutrition affects about 400 million children in the world, making it a major health problem.

Clinical Features (Fig 10-1)

A. Developmental Effects:

1. Growth retardation–Comparison of the weight and height of a child with the norms for age provides the most accurate estimate of protein-calorie malnutrition. However, establishment of such normal values in itself poses a problem. If weight and height norms for the USA are used for nonindustrialized societies, about 80% of children will be deemed to be growth-retarded. The theory that genetic differences between races account for some of the observed differences has been widely accepted, and norms have been established in that way for individual countries.

This view may be based on a faulty premise, however. The offspring of immigrants to the USA who are small in height and weight apparently because of their genetic endowment have descendants who attain heights and weights comparable to those of their American age mates if they consume a similar diet. Such data suggest that a subtle but pervasive form of malnutrition may actually cause entire populations to suffer from mild growth retardation.

2. Intellectual impairment–Whether protein-calorie malnutrition causes impaired intellectual development is controversial, though evidence is increasing that malnutrition in the first 2 years of life does cause permanent deficits.

3. Immunologic deficiency–Severe protein-calorie malnutrition is associated with defects in both humoral and cellular immunity that result in a high incidence of serious infections. It is probable that less severe immunodeficiency occurs with milder degrees of malnutrition and that it is responsible in part for the high incidence of respiratory and gastrointestinal infections—and the high associated mortality rates—in severely malnourished children in developing societies.

B. Marasmus: Marasmus represents the compensated phase of protein-calorie malnutrition, in which the dietary deficiencies are compensated for by catabolism of the body's "expendable" tissues, adipose tissue and skeletal muscle. The calories and amino acids derived from tissue catabolism are used to maintain normal cellular metabolism.

The catabolism of adipose tissue and muscle leads to extreme wasting, which is the hallmark of marasmus. Because of muscle wasting and loss of subcutaneous fat, the marasmic child has only skin and bone in the extremities, and wasting of facial muscles and fat causes the typical drawn and wizened facial appearance (Fig 10–2).

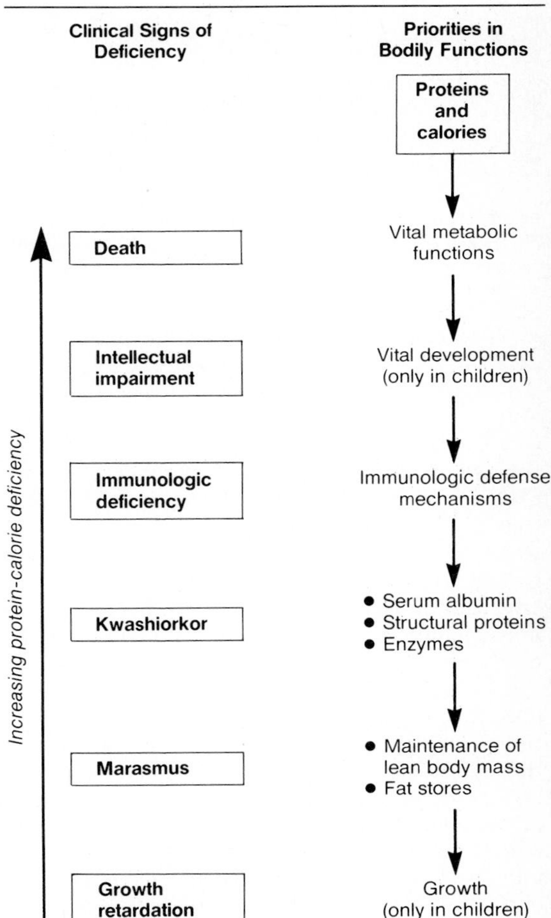

Figure 10–1. Protein and calorie priorities with regard to bodily functions. Increasing protein-calorie deficiency results in clinical features in the reverse order of priorities.

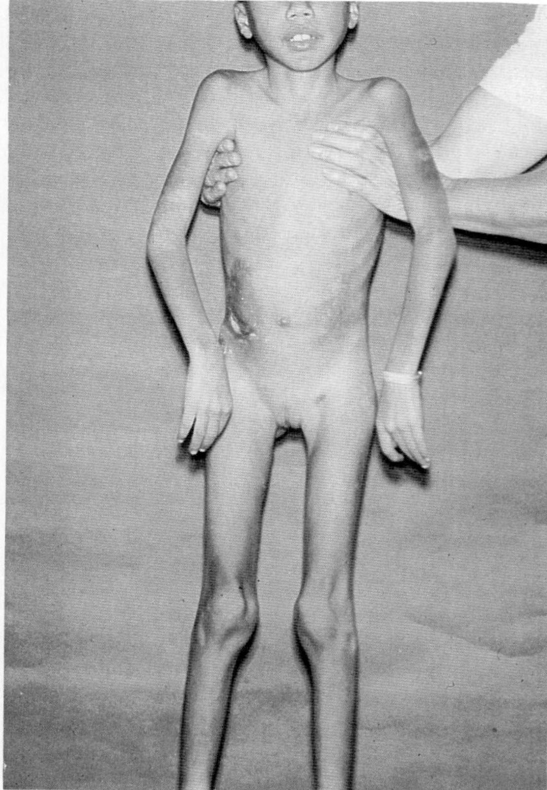

Figure 10-2. Marasmus. Note the extreme loss of subcutaneous fat and wasting of skeletal muscles.

Normal serum albumin levels are maintained, and there is no edema. Adequate synthesis of structural proteins and enzymes also continues. Sufficient glucose is available from gluconeogenesis of protein to maintain cellular metabolism. Marasmic children are alert and will eat ravenously when given food. Since gastrointestinal tract digestive enzymes are secreted in the normal way, any food that is eaten is digested and absorbed normally. Marasmus is therefore relatively easy to treat—simply providing food while ensuring adequate fluid and electrolyte balance is sufficient.

C. Kwashiorkor: Kwashiorkor represents the decompensated phase of protein-calorie malnutrition in which utilization of endogenous protein through tissue catabolism can no longer compensate for dietary lack of protein. As compensatory mechanisms fail, decreased synthesis of enzymes and structural proteins occurs, and serum albumin levels fall. Failure of cellular metabolism occurs and is manifested in the brain, where it causes lethargy and somnolence. Children with kwashiorkor are difficult to feed because of extreme apathy and anorexia. Deficient digestive enzyme production in the intestine and atrophy of small intestinal villi result in failure to absorb ingested food. For these reasons, kwashiorkor is much more difficult to treat than marasmus, and hospitalization is usually required.

Decreased serum albumin levels result in generalized edema. Ascites produces the protuberant abdomen that is characteristic of kwashiorkor. Abnormal fat metabolism causes **fatty liver** with hepatomegaly, which may be associated with development of a nodular liver with fibrosis **(nutritional cirrhosis)**. Changes also occur in the hair, which becomes fine and brittle. Normal pigmentation of the hair is lost, and alternating light and dark bands may be seen (flag sign). Hair is easily pulled out, and, in severe cases, patches of baldness (alopecia) occur. The skin shows abnormal pigmentation and increased desquamation (''flaky paint'' dermatosis). Kwashiorkor is also associated with nutritional anemia due to deficient intake of iron and folic acid and deficient erythropoietin production.

• EATING DISORDERS

Eating disorders resulting from psychiatric disturbances are a common cause of nutritional disturbance. Anorexia nervosa and bulimia are the 2 most common eating disorders.

Anorexia Nervosa

Anorexia nervosa occurs chiefly in teenage girls and results from a distorted perception of body image and size that makes the patient believe she is much fatter than she is. This causes severe restriction of food intake, leading to protein-calorie malnutrition, similar in many ways to marasmus (Fig 10–3).

In addition to marked weight loss and muscle wasting, these patients show abnormal hypothalamic-pituitary function that is believed to be an adaptive mechanism to chronic starvation. Gonadotropin (follicle-stimulating hormone and luteinizing hormone) secretion is decreased, leading to failure of ovulation and amenorrhea. Decreased corticotropin and thyrotropin secretion leads to decreased plasma levels of cortisol and thyroxine. Thermoregulation and secretion of antidiuretic hormone are also frequently abnormal. Death may ensue in extreme cases.

Bulimia

Bulimia occurs chiefly in young women. Fifteen to 20 percent of women under 30 years of age in the USA are believed to suffer from bulimia.

Bulimia is characterized by episodes of overeating (binges) followed by efforts to avoid the threatened weight gain by induced vomiting, laxative abuse, excessive physical activity, and fasting (binge-purge cycles). Bulimics usually have normal body weight. The pathologic effects of bu-

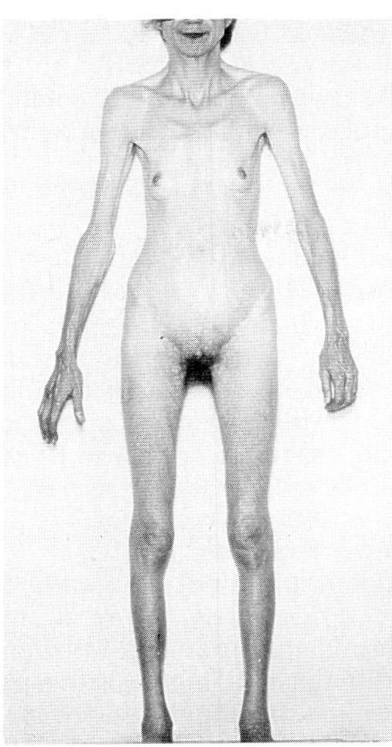

Figure 10-3. Anorexia nervosa, showing extreme emaciation and muscle wasting.

limia are the consequences of induced vomiting, eg, mucosal tears of the esophagus, with bleeding (Mallory-Weiss syndrome) and aspiration pneumonitis; and laxative abuse—commonly resulting in alkalosis and hypokalemia, the latter sometimes severe enough to precipitate cardiac arrhythmias.

OBESITY

Ideal weights are established on the basis of height, sex, and body frame, and obesity is usually defined as a **body weight 20% greater than ideal weight**. However, in a population in which as many as 25% of middle-aged individuals are obese, "normal" weights derived from population studies may constitute a false baseline.

Other definitions of obesity include a 20% increase in weight beyond one's weight at age 25 years and an increase in thickness of subcutaneous tissue measured as skinfold thickness over the triceps. In the latter instance, obesity is present if one can "pinch an inch"—normal skinfold thickness for males is less than 23 mm.

Cause

Obesity is caused by long-term caloric intake in excess of what is required for the maintenance of body functions. The excess calories are converted into stored adipose tissue—mainly subcutaneous fat—but fatty tissue is also distributed in internal organs such as the heart, pancreas, and omentum. The presence of an increased number of fat cells in the interstitium of internal organs (pathologic adiposity) does not usually cause any abnormality of cell function or clinical disease.

In the USA, obesity affects 20% of middle-aged men and 40% of middle-aged women. The incidence of obesity peaks at about age 50 years—an indication that a smaller percentage of obese people survive past this age compared with nonobese individuals.

Clinical Features

A man who is 30% overweight has an increased mortality risk of 42% compared with a man of ideal weight. The increased risk for a similarly overweight woman is 30%. Although a statistical association between obesity and an increased risk of death has been established, the mechanisms are unclear.

A. Hypoventilation Syndrome: Even extreme ("morbid") obesity is rarely an immediate cause of death. Hypoventilation syndrome resulting from obesity (pickwickian syndrome; Fig 10-4) is

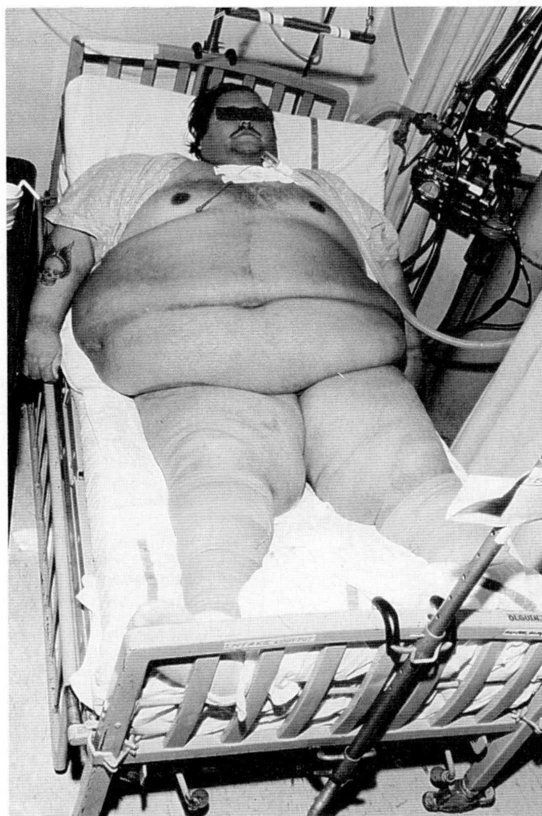

Figure 10-4. Extreme obesity. This patient showed evidence of respiratory insufficiency (pickwickian syndrome).

due to increased fat in the chest wall, which causes decreased alveolar ventilation and consequent chronic CO_2 retention, daytime somnolence, and apneic attacks. If severe, death may result. Although the full-blown syndrome occurs only in gross obesity, milder degrees may account for the increased risk associated with surgery and general anesthesia in obese patients.

B. Diseases Associated With Obesity: The main causes of the increased mortality rate associated with obesity are diseases occurring with greatly increased incidence in the obese (Table 10–2 and Fig 10–5).

VITAMINS

Vitamins are complex organic substances required as coenzymes for many metabolic processes necessary to sustain life. With few exceptions, vitamins are not synthesized in the body and must be provided in the diet. Vitamins are classified as (1) fat-soluble: A, D, E, and K; and (2) water-soluble: B vitamins and vitamin C. The B group of vitamins includes thiamine, riboflavin, nicotinamide, pyridoxine, folic acid, and cyanocobalamin.

VITAMIN A

Vitamin A is a group of compounds that includes vitamin A alcohol (retinol) and the provitamin A carotenes. Dietary vitamin A is absorbed along with fat and is transported to the liver for storage. Retinol in liver stores enters the blood and is complexed with plasma proteins for transport to tissues.

Vitamin A Deficiency (Hypovitaminosis A)

A. Causes: Dietary sources of vitamin A are liver, dairy products (which contain stored or secreted retinol), and carotene-containing leafy green and yellow vegetables. Dietary deficiency of vitamin A is still prevalent among children in underdeveloped areas, mainly in Southeast Asia and India. Sporadic cases are seen in the USA as a result of chronic fat malabsorptive states.

B. Clinical Features:

1. Visual impairment–The earliest effect of vitamin A deficiency is failure of night vision **(nyctalopia).** Night vision is a function of retinal rods and rhodopsin, a light-sensitive pigment. On exposure to light, rhodopsin dissociates, generating a nerve impulse. In vitamin A deficiency, regeneration of rhodopsin in rods fails. In severe deficiency, vision in bright light, which is dependent on retinal cones (which contain iodopsin, a pigment containing vitamin A), also fails.

2. Abnormal maturation of squamous epithelium–Squamous epithelium undergoes thickening owing to hyperplasia and excessive keratinization. This development causes changes in other structures: (1) The conjunctiva becomes muddy, dry **(xerophthalmia),** and wrinkled. **Bitot's spots** (elevated white plaques composed of keratinaceous debris) develop. (2) The cornea opacifies, and erosions develop **(keratomalacia),** which commonly become infected or perforated, causing

Table 10–2. Diseases associated with obesity.

Disease	Mechanism	Clinical Effects
Adult-onset diabetes mellitus	Obesity leads to increased resistance to insulin action, which leads to glucose intolerance. Diabetes mellitus occurs in genetically susceptible individuals.	B cell (pancreatic islet) hyperplasia followed by atrophy. Complications of diabetes mellitus (eg, retinopathy, neuropathy). Risk factor for atherosclerosis.
Hypertension	Statistical association with obesity but no clear mechanism elucidated. Increased secretion of adrenal glucocorticoids is a minor factor.	Risk factor for atherosclerosis. Cerebral hemorrhage (stroke).
Hyperlipidemia	Increased fat mobilization from adipose stores results in increased lipoprotein synthesis in liver.	Risk factor for atherosclerosis. Hypertriglyceridemia, hypercholesterolemia, increased very low density lipoprotein (VLDL).
Atherosclerotic arterial disease	Statistical association with obesity along with other risk factors (diabetes, hypertension, hyperlipidemia).	Myocardial infarction (ischemic heart disease) (heart attack); cerebral thrombosis and infarction (stroke).
Cholelithiasis (gallstones)	Increased cholesterol excretion in bile.	Acute and chronic cholecystitis.
Osteoarthrosis	Increased body weight causes cartilage degeneration in weight-bearing joints.	Lumbar spine, hips, and knees most commonly affected.

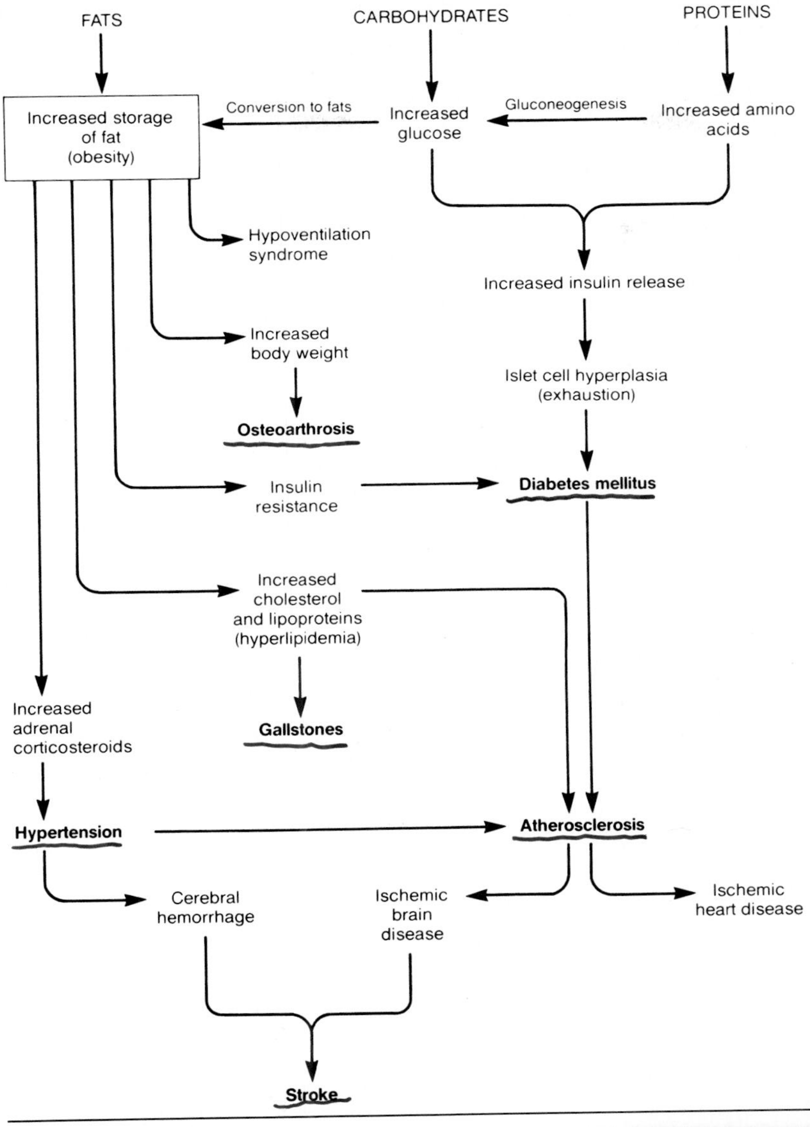

FATS

CARBOHYDRATES

PROTEINS

Increased storage of fat (obesity)

Conversion to fats

Increased glucose

Gluconeogenesis

Increased amino acids

Hypoventilation syndrome

Increased insulin release

Increased body weight

Islet cell hyperplasia (exhaustion)

Osteoarthrosis

Insulin resistance

Diabetes mellitus

Increased cholesterol and lipoproteins (hyperlipidemia)

Increased adrenal corticosteroids

Gallstones

Hypertension

Atherosclerosis

Cerebral hemorrhage

Ischemic brain disease

Ischemic heart disease

Stroke

Figure 10–5. Effects of excessive food intake.

blindness (Fig 10–6). Vitamin A deficiency is one of the commonest causes of blindness in Asia. (3) The skin becomes hyperkeratotic. Hair follicles become elevated and cause a fine papular rash **(follicular hyperkeratosis).** (4) Glandular epithelium in the body, such as in the bronchial mucosa, undergoes squamous metaplasia. (5) Increased susceptibility to respiratory tract and enteric infections may be partly attributable to epithelial changes. Such infections are a major cause of the morbidity associated with vitamin A deficiency.

The effect of vitamin A on squamous epithelial maturation and proliferation led to research into the possible role of vitamin A deficiency as a causative agent in squamous carcinomas. There are no convincing data for a role for vitamin A in caus-

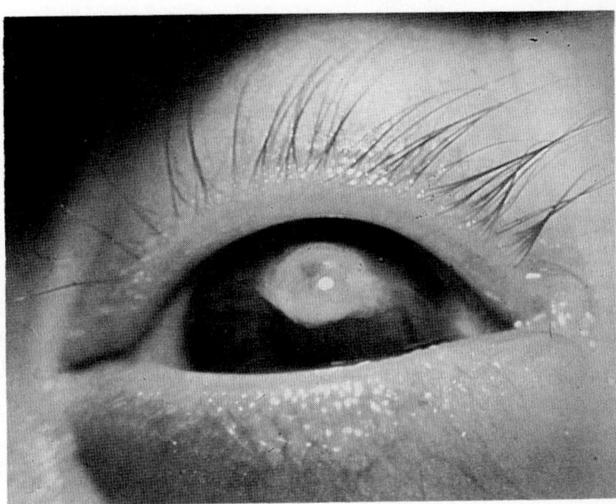

Figure 10–6. Keratomalacia caused by vitamin A deficiency in a 5-month-old child.

ing cancer, but an unexpected side effect of this research was the development of retinoids (vitamin A analogues), which are effective in the treatment of many skin diseases.

Vitamin A Toxicity (Hypervitaminosis A)

Excessive intake of vitamin A produces cerebral dysfunction, raised intracranial pressure, liver enlargement, and bone changes. Chronic toxicity results in mental changes that simulate psychiatric diseases such as depression and schizophrenia.

VITAMIN D

Vitamin D (cholecalciferol) is derived in 2 ways, from the diet and from the skin. In the diet, vitamin D is absorbed in the small intestine with other fats and transported to the liver for storage. In the skin, 7-dehydrocholesterol (an endogenous steroid) is converted to cholecalciferol by the action of ultraviolet rays in sunlight.

The active form of vitamin D is 1,25 dihydrocholecalciferol, which is produced from cholecalciferol by 2 sequential hydroxylation steps (Fig 10–7).

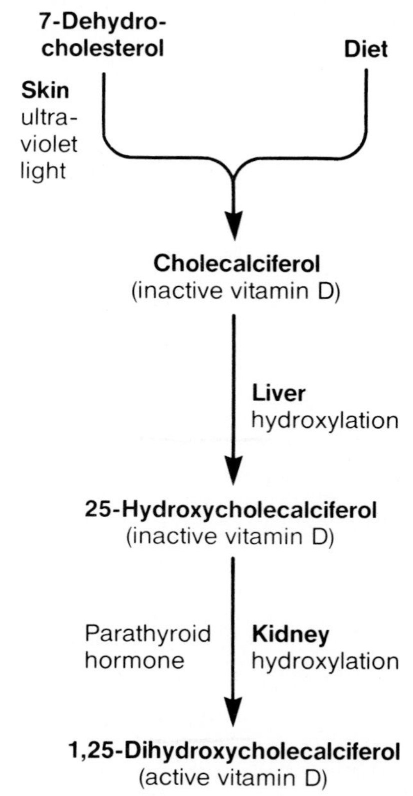

Figure 10–7. Metabolism of vitamin D.

Vitamin D Deficiency

A. Causes: Dietary deficiency of vitamin D is now uncommon in developed areas. It usually occurs when malnutrition coexists with minimal exposure to sunlight. In most industrialized countries, vitamin D fortification of milk has eradicated dietary deficiency, but deficiency may still occur in elderly people taking restricted diets who live indoors and are not exposed to sunlight and in strict vegetarians who eat no dairy products.

Secondary vitamin deficiency may occur in intestinal malabsorption, chronic renal disease (failure of α-hydroxylation of 25-cholecalciferol at the 1 position), or, very rarely, in liver failure (failure of α-hydroxylation at the 25 position).

B. Clinical Features:

1. Pathophysiology–The main effect of vitamin D deficiency is reduced intestinal absorption of calcium. Normally, vitamin D stimulates a calcium carrier protein at the brush border of the intestinal cell that transfers calcium from the intestinal lumen across the cell into the blood. Hypovitaminosis D results in a negative calcium balance with failure of normal calcification of osteoid in bone. Deficient mineralization of bone causes **rickets** (in children with growing bones) or **osteomalacia** (in adults after epiphyseal closure).

2. Rickets–Rickets is a disease of children characterized by failure of mineralization of osteoid in bone with abnormalities of bone growth. Failure of mineralization occurs when the plasma level of either calcium or phosphate is decreased over a prolonged period.

a. Causes and principal clinical types–(Table 10–3.)

(1) Nutritional deficiency–Most cases of rickets in developing countries are caused by dietary deficiency of vitamin D. In developed countries, other causes—notably chronic renal disease, malabsorption syndromes, and X-linked dominant vitamin D-resistant rickets—are more common than nutritional deficiency.

(2) Vitamin D-resistant rickets–This form of rickets is refractory to treatment with vitamin D. It is inherited as an X-linked dominant trait and is characterized by increased phosphate loss in the renal tubules, leading to phosphaturia and hypophosphatemia (hypophosphatemic rickets). Plasma levels of 1,25-dihydrocholecalciferol are normal.

(3) End-organ insensitivity to vitamin D–This is a very rare inherited disease in which the target cell receptors are insensitive to the action of 1,25-dihydrocholecalciferol. Failure of calcium absorption occurs, causing rickets. This condition is also resistant to treatment with vitamin D.

(4) Vitamin D-sensitive rickets–All conditions in which rickets is caused by deficiency of 1,25-dihydrocholecalciferol (Table 10–3) will respond to treatment with exogenous 1,25-dihydrocholecalciferol (calcitriol). An inherited form of vitamin

Table 10-3. Causes of rickets.

Calcium deficiency
Dietary deficiency of calcium
Dietary deficiency of vitamin D
Fat malabsorption syndromes (failure of vitamin D absorption)
Failure of 25α-hydroxylation in liver
Chronic liver disease
Drugs: phenytoin, phenobarbital
Failure of 1α-hydroxylation in kidney
Chronic renal failure
Genetic absence of renal hydroxylase (hereditary vitamin D-sensitive rickets)
Hypoparathyroidism and pseudohypoparathyroidism
Genetic end-organ insensitivity to 1,25-dihydroxycholecalciferol
Phosphate deficiency
Dietary phosphate deficiency
Renal tubular phosphate loss
Fanconi syndrome
Renal tubular acidosis
X-linked dominant vitamin D resistance
Other rickets-osteomalacia syndromes (rare)
Hypophosphatasia (deficient alkaline phosphatase in bone)
Tumor osteomalacia (interference with vitamin D metabolism)
Defects in bone matrix formation
Aluminum toxicity

D-sensitive rickets is caused by partial deficiency of the renal hydrolase enzyme required for 1,25-dihydrocholecalciferol synthesis.

b. Clinical features-Rickets occurs in children, in whom failure of mineralization disrupts new bone formation at the epiphyses (growing regions of bone), causing growth retardation (Fig 10–8). The epiphyseal region of bones affected by rickets shows a mass of disorganized cartilage, uncalcified osteoid, and abnormal calcification of trabeculae on microscopic examination.

Clinically, rickets is characterized by widening of the epiphyses of bones of the wrists and knees; masses of osteoid that develop at the costochondral junctions produce a row of small bumps on either side of the sternum ("rachitic rosary").

The poorly mineralized bones of rickets are much softer than normal bones, so that various deformities result. Bending of weight-bearing bones occurs, eg, bowing of the tibias and abnormal curvatures in vertebrae and the pelvis. Protuberances appear on bones at points of muscle action. Thoracic abnormalities may occur as a result of the pull of the contracting diaphragm on the ribs; a transverse line appears in the lower rib cage (Harrison's sulcus). The inward pulling of ribs by the intercostal muscles and forward protrusion of the sternum (pigeon breast) are characteristic of rickets. Softening of the cranial bones (craniotabes) also occurs.

3. Osteomalacia-Osteomalacia is the disorder resulting from failure of bone mineralization in adults. Most cases are due to either dietary deficiency or abnormal metabolism of vitamin D. Since bone growth is complete, growth retardation does not occur. Normal adult bone continually turns over by a process of osteoclastic resorption of the trabeculae that is balanced by osteoblastic bone formation. Normally, bone trabeculae have only a thin seam (12–15 μm thick) of uncalcified osteoid on the osteoblastic side of the trabecula. In osteomalacia, because of defective mineralization of osteoid, the uncalcified osteoid seams widen (usually $>$ 20 μm thick), producing a characteristic appearance on histologic sections. Furthermore, the surface area of bony trabeculae that is covered by uncalcified osteoid increases from the normal 1–3% to over 20%.

Osteomalacia causes bone pain, but gross skeletal deformities are rare. Subtle radiologic changes such as alteration in bony contours and fine fractures help to establish the diagnosis.

The diagnosis of rickets or osteomalacia is based upon a combination of clinical features, radiographic findings, and laboratory findings, including normal or low serum calcium and phosphate, normal or high alkaline phosphatase, and low vitamin D levels by immunoassay. Urinary calcium is low. Urinary hydroxyproline is elevated as a result of collagen catabolism in bone.

Vitamin D Toxicity (Hypervitaminosis D)

Vitamin D toxicity occurs only with extreme overdose. Increased calcium absorption and bone resorption cause hypercalcemia, which leads to metastatic calcification, nephrocalcinosis, and chronic renal failure.

• VITAMIN K

Vitamin K is a necessary cofactor for a carboxylase that is involved in the synthesis of blood coagulation factors II (prothrombin), VII, IX, and X in the liver. The main source of vitamin K in humans is the intestinal bacterial flora, which synthesizes some but not enough of the vitamin to meet all needs. A small amount must therefore be provided in the diet.

Vitamin K Deficiency

A. Causes: Dietary deficiency of vitamin K is rare because the vitamin is widespread in different kinds of foods. Common causes of vitamin K deficiency include intestinal malabsorption of fat; a lack of intestinal bacterial flora, as occurs in newborns before the intestine is colonized by bacteria (hemorrhagic disease of the newborn), or after prolonged broad-spectrum antibiotic therapy; and the presence of vitamin K antagonists, eg, coumarin derivatives, which exert an anticoagulant effect because they antagonize vitamin K. Many rat poisons are also vitamin K antagonists.

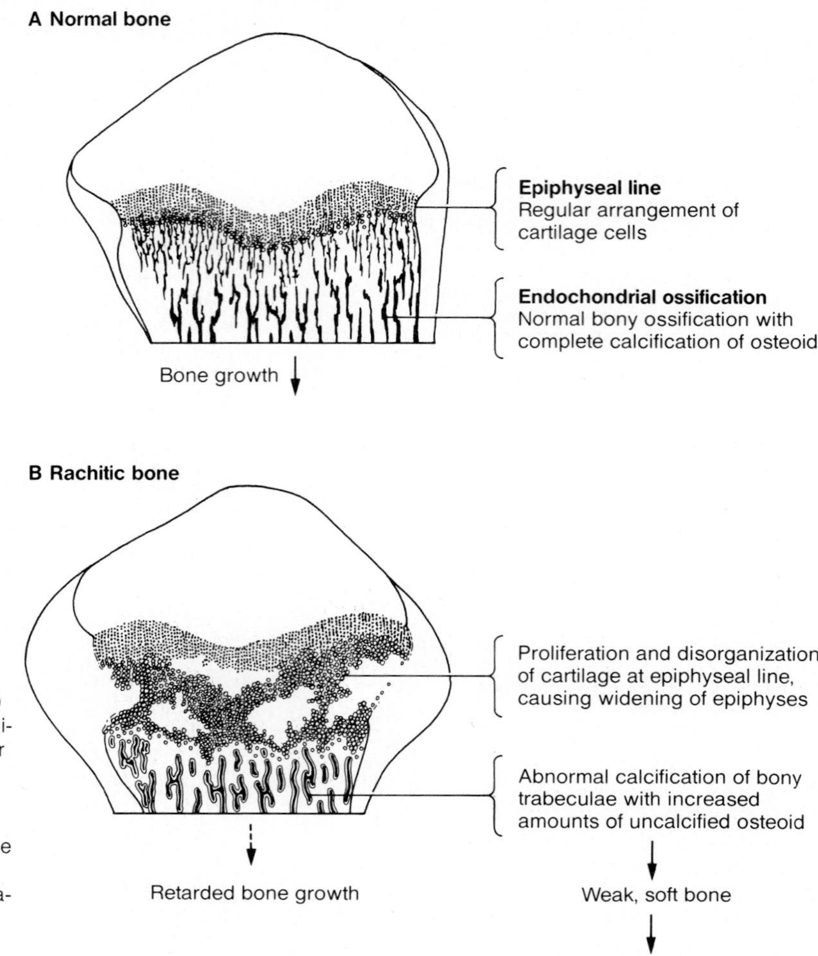

Figure 10-8. Changes in the growing end of bone (epiphysis) in normal **(A)** compared to rachitic bone **(B)**. The normal regular linear arrangement of cartilage cells is replaced in rickets by masses of abnormal, proliferating, disorganized cartilage at the epiphyseal line. Bone growth is retarded, and failure of calcification results in soft trabeculae with increased amounts of uncalcified osteoid.

B. Clinical Features: Vitamin K deficiency is characterized by decreased plasma levels of blood coagulation factors II (hypoprothrombinemia), VII, IX, and X. The resulting bleeding tendency is manifested as bruises in the skin, gastrointestinal tract hemorrhage (usually melena), and hematuria. Blood coagulation studies reveal an increased prothrombin time.

Vitamin K Toxicity

Vitamin K toxicity is rare. In the few reported cases, acute hemolytic anemia has been the major manifestation.

VITAMIN E

Vitamin E (tocopherol) acts as an antioxidant in cells, protecting organelles from the noxious action of free radicals and peroxides produced in the cell. Vitamin E is present in a wide variety of foods, and dietary deficiency is rare. It is absorbed with fats, and low serum vitamin E levels occur in patients with severe chronic fat malabsorption.

Vitamin E produces several deficiency diseases in animals, including brain and skeletal muscle dysfunction, sterility in male rats, and hemolytic anemia. In adult humans, however, no specific deficiency disease has been identified. Volunteers chronically deprived of vitamin E demonstrated decreased serum levels of vitamin E and an increased susceptibility of erythrocytes to lysis by hydrogen peroxide in vitro; there was no evidence of hemolytic anemia in vivo. Recently, acute hemolytic anemia has been reported to occur in vitamin E-deficient premature infants.

VITAMIN C

Vitamin C (ascorbic acid) is a water-soluble vitamin present in fresh fruit and leafy vegetables. It is required for the synthesis of collagen, ground substance, and osteoid and acts as a cofactor in the hydroxylation of proline and lysine and in the aggregation of polypeptide chains into the triple helix of tropocollagen. In vitamin C deficiency, fibroblasts secrete abnormal tropocollagen molecules that cannot form normal collagen fibers, leading to impaired wound healing and abnormal synthesis of connective tissue and bone matrix protein. Vitamin C may also play an unknown role in iron metabolism and neutrophil function.

Vitamin C Deficiency

A. Causes: Deficiency of vitamin C causes **scurvy,** almost always the result of dietary inadequacy. Vitamin C deficiency was common in the past when seamen on long voyages subsisted on a diet that included no fresh fruits or vegetables (Table 10–4).* Today, scurvy occurs in infants fed certain powdered milks deficient in vitamin C and in elderly people whose diets lack fresh fruit or vegetables. Scurvy also occurs in developing countries where malnutrition is prevalent.

Vitamin C is rapidly absorbed in the jejunum, and deficiency due to malabsorption is uncommon.

B. Clinical Features: In vitamin C deficiency, the collagen types with the highest hydroxyproline content (eg, those in blood vessels) are most severely affected. One of the early clinical features of deficiency is therefore an increased tendency to hemorrhage, probably due to increased fragility of capillaries. Skin petechiae and ecchymoses due to vascular rupture, bleeding gums, and hemorrhages into nails, joints, and subperiosteal tissues occur in severe deficiency.

Wound healing is also abnormal. The tensile strength of scar tissue is reduced, and scars have a greater tendency to reopen. The granulation tissue that forms is normal initially but later appears abnormal because of the accumulation of an amorphous mass of abnormal protein in place of fibrillary collagen.

The gums become swollen and bleed easily. The teeth become loose, probably because of loss of collagen support in the tooth socket. There is an increased tendency to gum infections.

Abnormalities in bone formation are the result of abnormal synthesis of osteoid, the bone matrix protein. Bone growth at the epiphysis is impaired, leading to growth retardation. The gross changes may resemble those of rickets, but the 2 conditions are easily distinguished on microscopic examination. Rickets is characterized by the presence of excess osteoid and lack of calcification, whereas scurvy is associated with deficient osteoid and much calcified cartilage. Scorbutic bone is weak and liable to become deformed under the stress of weight bearing and muscle action.

Vitamin C Toxicity

Large doses of vitamin C are commonly ingested to treat or prevent the common cold or sometimes as a prophylactic measure against cancer, though the value of these practices is unproved. High doses of vitamin C have been shown to predispose to arsenic toxicity by converting inactive organic arsenicals in food to toxic arsenic compounds. Megadoses of vitamin C may also increase the incidence of urinary calculi.

Table 10–4. Scurvy—a "controlled clinical trial."[1]

On the 20th of May 1747, being on board the Salisbury at sea, he [Dr James Lind] took twelve scorbutic patients under his care. They had putrid gums, spots and lassitude with weakness of the knees. These were put on the following regimens, in addition to normal diet:

Number of Patients	Regimen
2	1 quart of cider/day
2	25 drops of elixir of vitriol
2	6 spoonfuls of vinegar
2	1 pint of sea water
2	A purgative of garlic, balsam of Peru and mustard seed
2	2 oranges and a lemon

The oranges and the lemon had the best effect; one of those who had taken them was fit for duty at the end of six days; the other being more recovered than the other patients was appointed to look after them. Next to the oranges the cider had the best effect. . . .

[1]Narrative and data reconstructed by the author from an article in the first edition of *Encyclopaedia Britannica* (1771).

*"Limey" is a slang term for Englishman that originated with the British practice of carrying limes on long voyages to prevent scurvy once the association was recognized.

THIAMINE (Vitamin B_1)

Thiamine is required as a coenzyme in the decarboxylation of pyruvate and α-ketoglutarate, which produces acetyl-CoA. Because this is an essential step in glucose metabolism in the citric acid cycle, thiamine deficiency results in impaired energy production within the cell. Blood pyruvate levels are elevated in thiamine deficiency. Thiamine is also a cofactor for the enzyme transketolase, and a decrease in erythrocyte ketolase activity is used as a test for thiamine deficiency. In addition, thiamine is required for synthesis of the neurotransmitter acetylcholine, deficiency of which may lead to neurologic abnormalities. Thiamine excess is not toxic.

Thiamine Deficiency

A. Causes: In industrialized areas, thiamine deficiency is rare and is seen mainly in chronic alcoholics in association with poor nutrition. In developing countries, thiamine deficiency is uncommon because the vitamin is distributed widely in food, particularly cereals. However, deficiencies do occur in Southeast Asia in populations that eat highly polished rice (thiamine is present in the outer part of the rice seed, which is removed in polishing) and in Africa and South America in populations that subsist on cassava, which lacks thiamine.

B. Clinical Features:

1. Wet beriberi–Wet beriberi is characterized by cardiac failure, which produces massive peripheral edema, from which the term "wet" is derived. The heart is enlarged and flabby. Histologic changes are nonspecific, consisting of interstitial edema, swelling of myocardial fibers, and fatty change. The biochemical basis of cardiac dysfunction is uncertain but may represent failure of energy production in the cell.

2. Dry beriberi–Dry beriberi is characterized mainly by changes in the nervous system. Segmental demyelination of peripheral nerves is common and causes **peripheral neuropathy**. Neuronal loss in the cerebral cortex, brain stem, and cerebellum leads to a clinically characteristic psychotic state known as **Korsakoff's syndrome,** characterized by memory failure and confabulation (fabrication of imaginary experiences). Another important manifestation of thiamine deficiency in the brain is **Wernicke's encephalopathy,** which involves the mamillary bodies and periventricular region of the brain stem. Petechial hemorrhages in the acute phase are followed by atrophy and brownish pigmentation arising from deposition of hemosiderin (Fig 10–9). The oculomotor nuclei in the periaqueductal region are typically involved, causing abnormalities in eye movements. Wernicke's encephalopathy frequently coexists with Korsakoff's syndrome, and both disorders are seen mainly in alcoholics. This interrelationship has important implications for treatment of alcoholics, who should be given thiamine before a loading dose of glucose; otherwise, acute depletion of thiamine stores to maintain glucose metabolism may occur and precipitate encephalopathy.

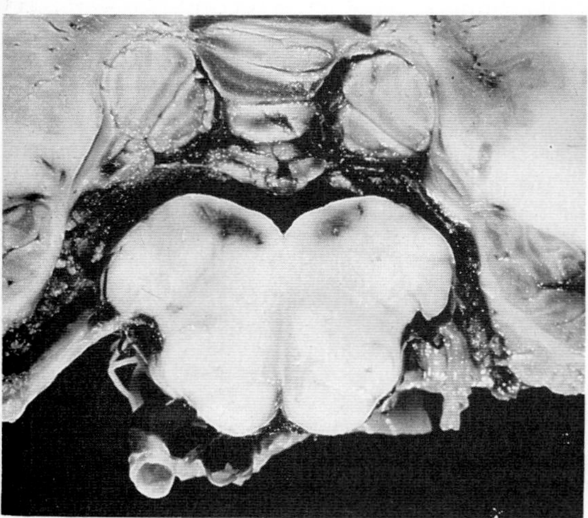

Figure 10-9. Medulla oblongata in Wernicke's encephalopathy, showing bilateral hemorrhages in its dorsal aspect in the floor of the fourth ventricle.

RIBOFLAVIN (Vitamin B_2)

Riboflavin is an important constituent of flavoproteins, which participate in electron transfer in the respiratory chain. Riboflavin deficiency may theoretically impair cellular energy production, although this does not explain the clinical features of deficiency.

Riboflavin is widely distributed in both animal and plant foods. Deficiency is usually caused by inadequate dietary intake and is common only in developing countries. Excessive intake of riboflavin causes no ill effects.

Clinical manifestations of riboflavin deficiency include inflammation and fissuring of the lips **(cheilosis),** which is most marked at the angles of the mouth **(angular stomatitis)**. The tongue is inflamed, with atrophy of the mucous membrane, so that it becomes smooth and deep purplish red (magenta) (Fig 10–10). Vascularization of the cornea is the most characteristic feature of riboflavin deficiency. It may be followed by corneal opacities, ulceration, and blindness. A scaly rash affecting the face and genitalia may occur.

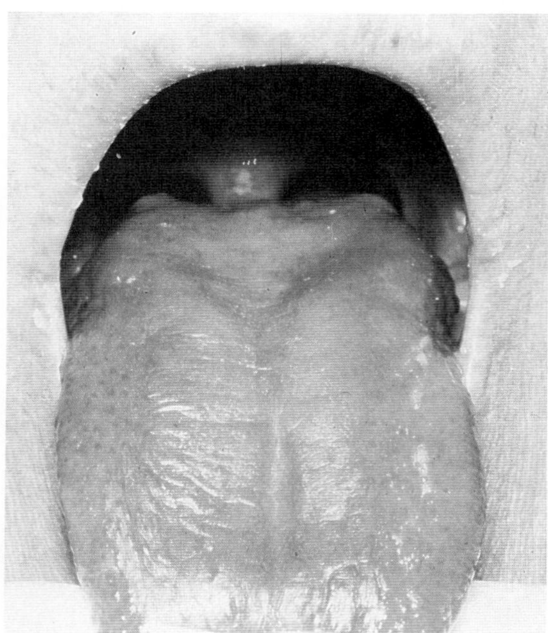

Figure 10-10. Riboflavin deficiency, showing inflamed tongue. Note also early fissuring at the angles of the mouth.

NICOTINIC ACID (Niacin) & NICOTINAMIDE (Niacinamide)

Niacin is an integral part of nicotinamide adenine dinucleotide (NAD) and NAD phosphate (NADP), which are coenzymes participating in most oxidation-reduction reactions in the cell.

Niacin Deficiency

A. Causes: Niacin is present in many foods, including cereals, meat, and vegetables. It is also synthesized in the body from tryptophan. Niacin deficiency occurs when there is a severe combined deficiency of both niacin and protein, as occurs in developing countries; it is rare in industrialized societies, where it occurs mainly in chronic alcoholics. Niacin deficiency may rarely occur in patients with carcinoid tumors, because these tumors use large amounts of tryptophan to synthesize serotonin (5-hydroxytryptamine).

B. Clinical Features: Niacin deficiency causes **pellagra,** which is characterized clinically by dermatitis, diarrhea, and dementia ("the 3 D's"). These clinical abnormalities cannot be easily explained on the basis of the known physiologic actions of niacin.

1. Dermatitis-The characteristic dermatitis involves mainly sun-exposed skin. Affected skin is reddened because of increased dermal vascularity, darker because of increased melanin pigmentation, and rough because of excessive keratinization (Fig 10–11). In the later stages, the skin thickens as a result of dermal fibrosis. Involvement of the neck produces a characteristic "necklace" of affected skin.

2. Diarrhea-The mucosa of the mouth, tongue, and gastrointestinal tract also shows nonspecific inflammatory changes and mucosal atrophy. The tongue becomes swollen, red, and shiny. The mucous membrane changes in the intestine lead to diarrhea.

3. Dementia-Dementia results from a progressive degeneration of neurons in the cerebral cortex.

Niacin Toxicity

Excessive dietary intake of niacin causes no ill effects. Administration of large doses intravenously causes vasodilatation, which may produce a burning sensation in the face and head. The phenomenon is temporary and produces no persistent abnormality.

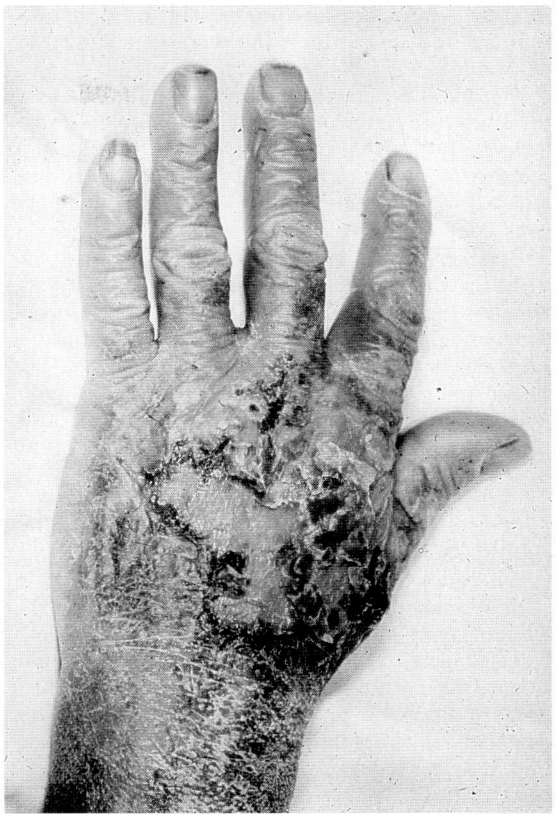

Figure 10–11. Dermatitis in pellagra.

PYRIDOXINE (Vitamin B_6)

Pyridoxine is converted in the body to pyridoxal 5-phosphate, a coenzyme involved in numerous cellular enzyme systems. Pyridoxine is found in virtually all foods, and pure dietary deficiency is rare even in developing countries.

Pyridoxine Deficiency

A. Causes: Pyridoxine deficiency is manifested under certain circumstances. Infants who are fed poor-quality processed milk preparations deficient in pyridoxine develop convulsions that respond to the administration of pyridoxine. Deficiency may occur in pregnancy, when there is an increased metabolic demand for pyridoxine. Infants breast-fed by a pyridoxine-deficient mother may in turn show signs of deficiency. By far the commonest cause of clinical pyridoxine deficiency is the ingestion of drugs that are pyridoxine antagonists. These include isoniazid (INH, an antituberculosis drug), oral contraceptives containing estrogen, methyldopa (an antihypertensive drug), and levodopa (used in the treatment of Parkinson's disease).

B. Clinical Features: Common clinical manifestations of pyridoxine deficiency include minor changes in skin (seborrheic dermatitis), eyes (blepharitis), and mouth, including inflammation of the lips (cheilosis) and tongue (glossitis) with fissuring of the angles of the mouth (angular stomatitis). These signs are not clearly accounted for by what is known about the metabolic functions of pyridoxine.

Pyridoxal 5-phosphate plays a role in the synthesis of the neurotransmitter gamma-aminobutyric acid (GABA). Neurologic manifestations of pyridoxine deficiency—eg, convulsions in infants and peripheral neuropathy in adults—may be caused by deficient synthesis of GABA.

Pyridoxal 5-phosphate is an important coenzyme in the synthesis of δ-aminolevulinic acid, which is the precursor of the porphyrin portion of the hemoglobin molecule. Abnormal hemoglobin synthesis in pyridoxine deficiency may lead to hypochromic and sideroblastic anemia. Patients with some forms of idiopathic sideroblastic anemia may demonstrate a clinical response to high doses of pyridoxine.

FOLIC ACID & VITAMIN B_{12}

Folic acid and vitamin B_{12} (cyanocobalamin) deficiencies are among the commonest vitamin deficiencies in industrialized societies. In their active forms, these vitamins are coenzymes in several reactions involving the synthesis of nucleic acids. The main clinical manifestation of folate and vitamin B_{12} deficiency is megaloblastic anemia. The cause, detailed effects, and diagnosis of folic acid and vitamin B_{12} deficiency are discussed in Chapter 24.

MINERALS

The body requires many trace minerals in addition to iron, calcium, magnesium, and phosphate. Trace minerals needed for adequate functioning include zinc, copper, selenium, iodine, fluoride, manganese, cobalt, molybdenum, vanadium, chromium, and nickel. Although a physiologic role has been identified for most of these elements, specific clinical deficiency states have been documented only for zinc, copper, iodine, and selenium.

IRON

Iron deficiency due to inadequate intake, impaired absorption, or blood loss is one of the commonest deficiency states in humans. Iron is required mainly as a constituent of hemoglobin, and iron deficiency causes a decrease in the amount of hemoglobin in erythrocytes **(hypochromic anemia)** (Chapter 24). The thinning of mucosal epithelium in the mouth, pharynx, and stomach and the occasional formation of mucosal webs in the esophagus associated with iron deficiency remain unexplained.

Iron excess causes increased storage of iron in the body **(hemochromatosis)** (Chapters 1 and 43).

TRACE ELEMENTS

Iodine

Iodine forms an integral part of the thyroid hormone molecule. Iodine deficiency causes a decrease in thyroid hormone output, thereby stimulating pituitary thyroid-stimulating hormone (TSH) production and causing thyroid hyperplasia and enlargement (goiter) (Chapter 58).

Fluoride

Fluoride is incorporated into the structure of teeth and bone and helps to provide strength and hardness. Fluoride deficiency is closely associated with development of dental caries. In areas where natural water is deficient in fluoride, the high incidence of dental caries can be reduced by the use of toothpastes containing fluoride or adding fluoride to the water supply. Excess fluoride intake causes mottling of tooth enamel.

Calcium & Phosphate

Calcium and phosphate are major components of bone. Calcium and phosphate levels in blood and their absorption from the intestine are regulated by parathyroid hormone and vitamin D. Most abnormalities of calcium and phosphate metabolism result from parathyroid disease or vitamin D-related disease (eg, rickets, osteomalacia). Rarely, excessive intake of calcium—**milk-alkali syndrome,** due to chronic ingestion of milk and antacids (containing alkali in the form of bicarbonate by patients with peptic ulcers in an effort to relieve pain)—causes hypercalcemia, which may lead to acute neurologic dysfunction and death.

Hypocalcemia in **malabsorption syndrome** is attributable partly to deficient absorption of vitamin D and partly to formation of insoluble calcium soaps (complex fatty acids) in the gut. The effects of calcium excess and deficiency are discussed in Chapter 2.

Magnesium

Magnesium deficiency results in tetany similar to that seen with hypocalcemia. Magnesium deficiency in humans occurs in malabsorption syndromes and kwashiorkor and in patients receiving diuretic therapy or magnesium-deficient parenteral nutrition products.

Zinc

Zinc deficiency has been described in populations whose diets contain a large amount of unrefined cereal. The phytic acid in the outer layers of cereals binds with dietary zinc and prevents absorption. Clinical manifestations of zinc deficiency include anemia, growth retardation, and gonadal atrophy. Diarrhea and skin rashes also occur. Zinc deficiency has also been reported to cause impaired wound healing in trauma victims.

Copper

Copper is necessary for proper functioning of various enzyme systems in the body. Deficiency of copper is rare and manifested clinically as decreased hematopoiesis (causing anemia and neutropenia), decreased bone production (leading to osteoporosis), and neurologic abnormalities caused by demyelination and faulty synthesis of neurotransmitters.

Selenium

Selenium deficiency has been implicated as a cause of congestive cardiomyopathy. This type of cardiomyopathy has been described in China (Keshan disease) and rarely elsewhere in patients with severe malabsorption who have been receiving parenteral nutrition.

11 Disorders Due to Physical Agents

- Mechanical Trauma
  - Abrasion (Scrape)
  - Contusion (Bruise)
  - Laceration and Incision (Tearing and Cutting)
  - Fracture
- Pressure Injuries
  - Increase in Atmospheric Pressure
  - Decrease in Atmospheric Pressure
- Injuries Due to Heat and Cold
  - Localized Cold Injury
  - Generalized Cold Injury (Hypothermia)
  - Localized Heat Injury (Burns)
  - Generalized Heat Injury
- Electrical Injuries
- Ionizing Radiation Injury
  - Exposure of Humans to Ionizing Radiation
  - Mechanism of Radiation Injury
  - Effects of Radiation Injury
  - Total Body Irradiation
  - Localized Irradiation
  - Ultraviolet Radiation
- Other Radiation

• MECHANICAL TRAUMA

Management of trauma (eg, from motor vehicle or other accidents, penetrating gunshot wounds) makes up a large part of modern medical practice. Specialized trauma centers have been established in most large city hospitals, and they are often the busiest part of the hospital. In many industrialized societies, trauma is the leading cause of death in children and young adults.

The type of tissue injury incurred varies with the type and severity of trauma (eg, blunt trauma, crush injury, gunshot wound) and the structures involved. Several broad categories of tissue injury are recognized.

Abrasion (Scrape) (Fig 11–1)

Abrasions are the most minor type of injury and occur in the skin; the superficial layers of the epidermis are scraped away. Healing is rapidly achieved by regeneration of epidermal cells from the remaining deeper basal epidermal layers, and there is no scarring.

Contusion (Bruise)

Contusions usually result from blunt trauma. Vascular damage occurs, with extravasation of blood into the tissue. The bleeding is usually rapidly controlled by hemostatic mechanisms. The red blood cells present in the injured tissue are then slowly degraded. The various pigments derived from the breakdown of hemoglobin are responsible for the change in color from red through purple, black, green, and brown. The presence of hemosiderin-laden macrophages on microscopic examination of the region signifies that hemorrhage has occurred there. In more severe injuries, sufficient blood may collect in the tissues to produce a distinct lump (hematoma).

Contusions most commonly occur in the skin, but they may also occur in internal organs, where they can cause significant malfunction. Myocardial contusion may lead to cardiac arrhythmias and acute cardiac failure. In the brain, contusions are common in the inferior frontal lobe because of movement of the brain against protuberances of the base of the skull in the anterior cranial fossa (Fig 11–2). Cerebral lesions represent foci for possible development of epileptic seizures.

Contusions are dangerous in patients with bleeding disorders such as hemophilia. In these patients, bleeding is not controlled by hemostatic mechanisms, and minor vascular injury often leads to massive bleeding (hematoma) in soft tissue, muscle, and joints with devastating results.

Laceration & Incision (Tearing & Cutting) (Fig 11–1)

Lacerations and incisions are characterized by anatomic discontinuity of the involved structures. Bleeding due to disruption of small and large blood vessels is much more severe than in a contusion. Depending on which structures are injured, other effects may be manifested. For example, spinal cord transection causes complete motor and sensory failure below the level of injury, and laceration of a major artery results not only in severe hemorrhage but also in ischemia in the tissues supplied by the artery. Extreme laceration associated with tearing away of tissue is called avulsion.

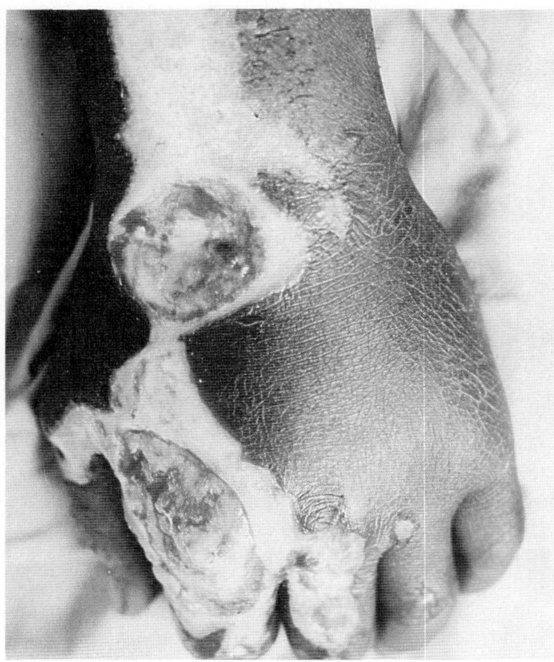

Figure 11-1. Hand injured in a traffic accident, showing skin defects caused by tearing away (avulsion) surrounded by extensive abrasion.

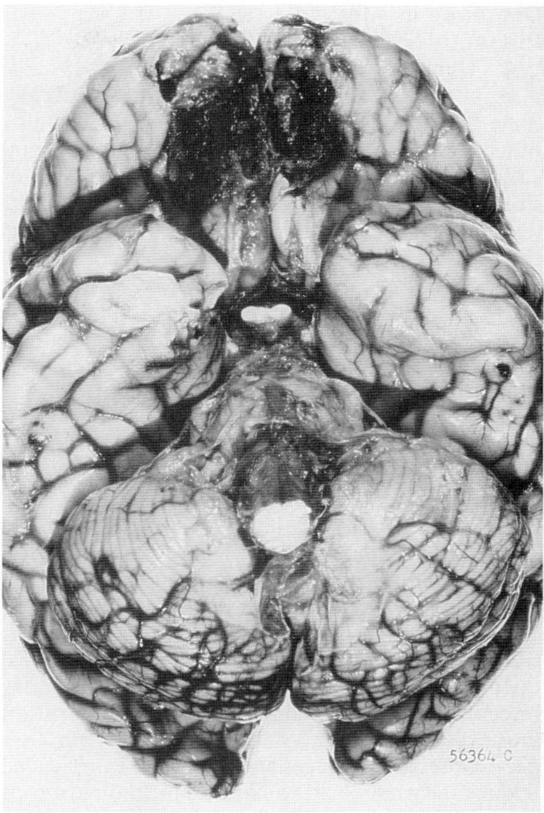

Figure 11-2. Contusions of inferior frontal lobe. These result from movement of the brain against the irregular bony surface of the floor of the anterior cranial fossa as a consequence of relative movement between brain and skull in head injuries.

Fracture

Fracture denotes a break or rupture of bone in which normal continuity is lost. Rarely, the term fracture is used to denote laceration of solid organs, as in fracture of the liver.

• PRESSURE INJURIES

Injuries resulting from sudden changes in atmospheric pressure are common in wartime because of the blast effects of bombs, grenades, and other weapons. Blast injuries are being encountered more frequently in civilian medicine as well. Industrial accidents (such as occur in the petrochemical industry) may also result in major blast injuries.

Increase in Atmospheric Pressure

A. Blast Injuries: Explosions produce pressure waves that act on the body in one of 2 ways: (1) Pressure waves may enter the body through any orifice (eg, mouth or anus) and cause a sudden increase in the intraluminal pressure of gas-filled structures such as the lung and intestine. Rupture of alveoli, lung laceration and hemorrhage, or intestinal perforation may occur. (2) Pressure waves acting on the surface of the body may compress the thorax and abdomen and increase the intracavitary pressure. This may cause laceration and rupture of the diaphragm and solid viscera such as the liver and spleen.

The severity of pressure injuries is determined by the force of the pressure waves, the distance from the explosion, and whether water or air is the transmitting medium.

B. Undersea Diving: Less violent increases in ambient pressure, as occur in undersea diving, may also cause injury. When air is breathed at high partial pressures (as it is in caissons or when breathing from scuba diving tanks), the oxygen and nitrogen in the air equilibrate at this high partial pressure with body tissues. Sudden decompression caused by rapid ascent to the surface may cause the dissolved nitrogen gas to come out of solution and form bubbles that cause severe tissue damage (see Nitrogen Gas Embolism in Chapter 9).

Decrease in Atmospheric Pressure

A. Hypoxia: A sudden severe decrease in atmospheric pressure may occur in pressurized aircraft if cabin decompression occurs at high altitudes. This phenomenon is unlikely under normal conditions but can be caused by on-board explosions, as has occurred with terrorist hijacking attempts. Injuries are due to the decrease in the partial pressure of oxygen, which causes hypoxia and rapid loss of consciousness. When decompression is less rapid or less severe, as occurs in high mountain climbing (> 4500 m), breathing oxygen-enriched air compensates for the decreased partial pressure of oxygen.

B. Middle Ear Pressure Changes: Minor changes in atmospheric pressure—as in mountain climbing or rapid altitude changes in an aircraft—may cause discomfort in the middle ear if the pressure there fails to equilibrate with atmospheric pressure through the auditory (eustachian) tubes. (Most pressurized aircraft cabins are stabilized at a pressure equivalent to that at about 1500 m.) Swallowing or yawning may facilitate equilibration of pressure. Obstruction of the pharyngeal opening of the auditory tubes due to respiratory infection or allergic rhinitis makes equilibration more difficult and may lead to severe pain. Repeated pressure changes such as those experienced by air crews may lead to chronic inflammation of the middle ear (barotitis). Sudden extreme pressure changes in the atmosphere, as with explosions, may rupture the tympanic membrane.

C. Mood Changes: Normal atmospheric pressure is 760 mm Hg, with weather-related changes varying from 745 mm Hg (low pressure) to 785 mm Hg (high pressure). Some have claimed that even these minimal changes may have psychologic consequences. More suicides occur during periods of low atmospheric pressure.

INJURIES DUE TO HEAT & COLD

Localized Cold Injury

The severity of local injury due to cold depends on the temperature, the rate of chilling, and the duration of exposure. Two distinct conditions are recognized:

A. Immersion Foot (Trench Foot): Trench foot was recognized as a common complication of trench warfare during World War I. Trench foot is the result of long, continued exposure of an extremity to mud or water at cold but **nonfreezing temperatures**. Similar changes occur in any part of the body that is similarly exposed.

The initial response of tissue to cold water is vasoconstriction. Prolonged vasoconstriction causes ischemic damage to muscle and nerve. After several hours of continued immersion, vasomotor paralysis occurs, leading to fixed vasodilatation and damage to the microcirculation. The involved area becomes swollen and blue and is often extensively blistered. Thrombosis ultimately occurs, often after several days' exposure, leading to gangrene.

B. Frostbite: Frostbite occurs more rapidly than trench foot and develops when a part of the body is exposed to **freezing temperatures**. Frostbite is not uncommon in temperate zones during the winter months, when individuals are caught unprepared in snowstorms or snow-related accidents. Vasoconstriction, dilatation, and occlusion of vessels by agglutinated cells and thrombi occur, causing ischemic necrosis of the exposed area, often within a few hours.

Generalized Cold Injury (Hypothermia)

A. Mechanism of Injury: Generalized hypothermia occurs when the entire body is exposed to low temperatures. It is most common in elderly individuals during the winter months, particularly in the homeless. Exposure to cold causes generalized vasoconstriction in skin vessels—a reflex response that acts to conserve body heat. Vasoconstriction in internal organs occurs only when body core temperature falls. When the body core temperature is lowered, vasoconstriction is not harmful over the short term because decreased cellular metabolism decreases the need for oxygen.

After a varying period of exposure, reflex vasoconstriction in the skin vessels fails, and there is widespread sustained vasodilatation. Local changes in the skin occur that are similar to those described for localized cold injury, but the changes occur throughout the body. Vasodilatation in the skin also causes a rapid decrease in body core temperature that hinders cellular metabolism and leads to pooling of blood in the peripheral vessels. Effective plasma volume is decreased, and circulatory failure results.

B. Clinical Features: The exact changes that occur are determined by the temperature and duration of exposure. With exposure to extreme cold, death may be rapid, and there are few visible tissue changes at autopsy. Death in these cases is caused by failure of cellular metabolism due to decreased body core temperature. When cold is not as severe, longer exposure is necessary to cause death, in which case extensive skin changes resembling those of frostbite are seen at autopsy.

C. Therapeutic Use of Hypothermia: The decreased level of tissue metabolism resulting from hypothermia is sometimes used to advantage in cardiovascular and brain surgery. The circulation to these organs can be arrested for a few minutes if metabolic needs have been reduced by hypothermia, permitting simple repairs such as clipping of aneurysms and mitral valvotomy. The use of refrigeration is also important in blood banks, where storing blood at 4 °C (39.2 °F) slows the metabolism of erythrocytes enough so that they can be kept for several weeks.

Rarely, the slowing of metabolism induced by cold may be lifesaving, as in accidental submersion of a child in very cold water, when the lethal effects of drowning may be delayed for 10 minutes or more.

Localized Heat Injury (Burns)

A. Incidence: Burns are a major cause of death in the USA. Most large hospitals have specialized burn units designed to address the specific problems arising in the management of burned patients.

B. Evaluation of Burns: The severity of a burn is determined by several factors.

1. Depth–(Fig 11–3.) The most minor burn causes erythema and edema in the epidermis, with focal necrosis of epidermal cells **(first-degree burn** [Fig 11–3]).

Second-degree burns involve the full thickness of the epidermis, with more extensive epidermal necrosis and part of the dermis but sparing the adnexa of the skin (hair follicles, etc). Second-degree burns show vesiculation (blister formation) in addition to erythema and edema.

First- and second-degree burns are also called **partial-thickness burns** (Fig 11–4).

Full-thickness (third-degree) burns (Fig 11–5) involve the entire epidermis and dermis, including adnexal structures. When epidermis is lost, a protein-rich exudate oozes from the surface, and there is a high risk of infection.

First-degree burns heal rapidly without scarring, the surviving epidermal cells regenerating rapidly to replace lost cells. Second-degree burns also heal rapidly because surviving epithelial cells in the basal region of the epidermis and adnexal structures are a source of germinative cells for regeneration. Dermal scarring, however, occurs in most second-degree burns. Third-degree burns

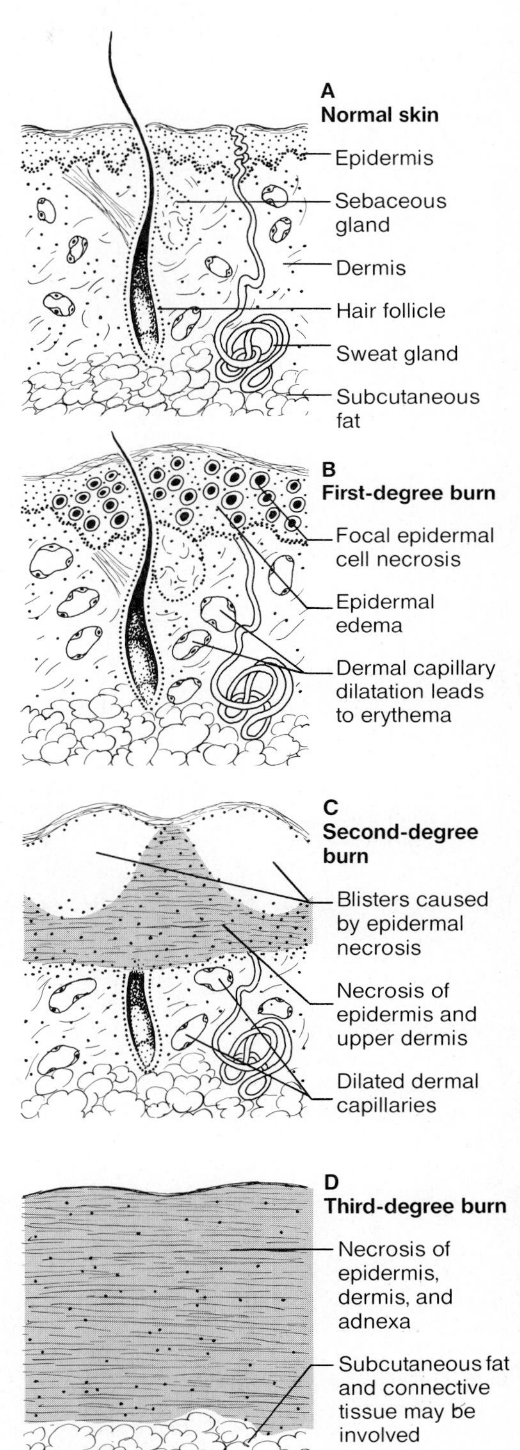

Figure 11–3. Classification of burns according to depth of necrosis. **A:** Normal skin and adnexa. **B:** First-degree burns are associated with focal epidermal necrosis but no blistering. Dilatation of dermal capillaries leads to erythema. Healing is uneventful, with epidermal regeneration occurring from the basal layer. There is no scarring. **C:** In second-degree burns, necrosis of both the epidermis and the upper dermis occurs, with blistering and erythema. The residual adnexal structures in the deep dermis are spared. Healing occurs by regeneration of epidermis from the edge of the wound and from residual adnexal epithelium. Dermal scarring occurs. **D:** Third-degree burns are associated with necrosis of the epidermis, dermis, and adnexal structures. Subcutaneous fat or connective tissue may or may not be injured. Healing occurs by regeneration of epidermis from the edge of the wound only. Dermal scarring occurs.

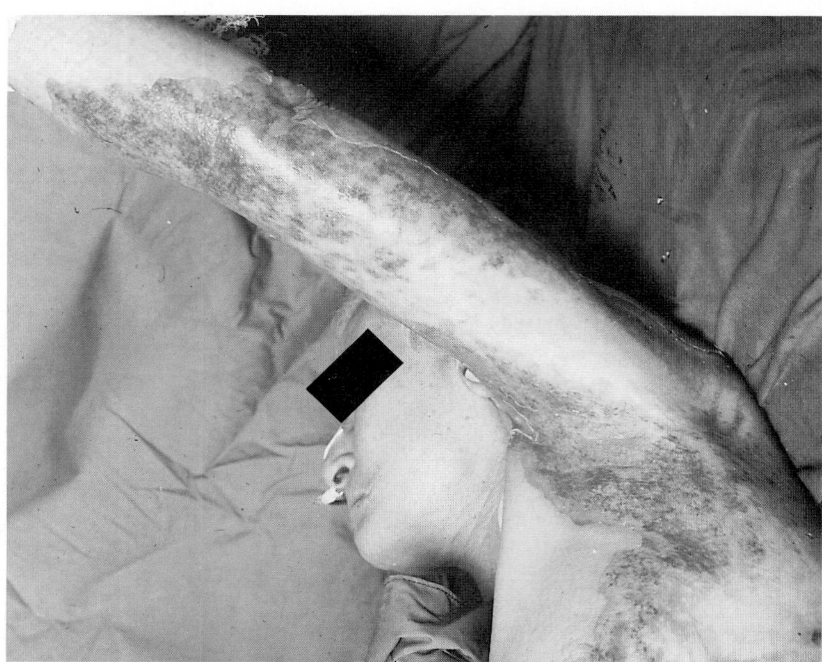

Figure 11-4. Partial-thickness burn involving the arm, axilla, and lateral chest wall.

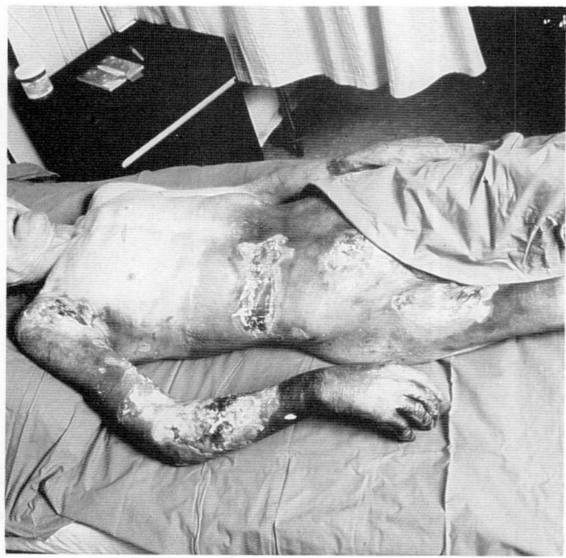

Figure 11-5. Severe burns involving the right arm, leg, and abdomen. Many areas show complete loss of skin with ulceration (full-thickness burns). These are surrounded by burns of lesser degree. The chest and neck are spared.

heal very slowly by regeneration of epithelium from the unburned skin at the edges. Dermal scarring is usually severe.

2. Surface area-(Fig 11-6.) The severity of burn injury is dependent mainly on the body surface area involved (Table 11-1). When more than 10% of body surface area is covered with full-thickness burns, the loss of protein-rich fluid from the surface of the burn may be so great that hypoproteinemia and hypovolemia occur; these may lead to shock. Treatment in burn centers has improved survival rates dramatically, and in the best centers even patients with burns over 75% of their bodies may recover.

3. Site-Burns in clean areas that can be immobilized heal better than similar burns in more difficult or contaminated areas (eg, perineal and groin burns, which are difficult to treat).

4. Smoke inhalation-Most deaths in fires result from smoke inhalation and not actual burning. Inhalation of hot gases and smoke devoid of oxygen causes death due to hypoxia. Extensive thermal damage of the lungs leads to alveolar necrosis, hemorrhage, and edema. Actual burning of the body usually occurs after death. At autopsy, examination of the air passages in fire victims shows carbon (soot) particles, an important finding in forensic pathology, since an individual who is first murdered and then burned will not show evidence of smoke inhalation. In airplane crashes and home fires, toxic fumes from burning plastics have proved to be an important lethal factor. In burns that are not associated with fires,

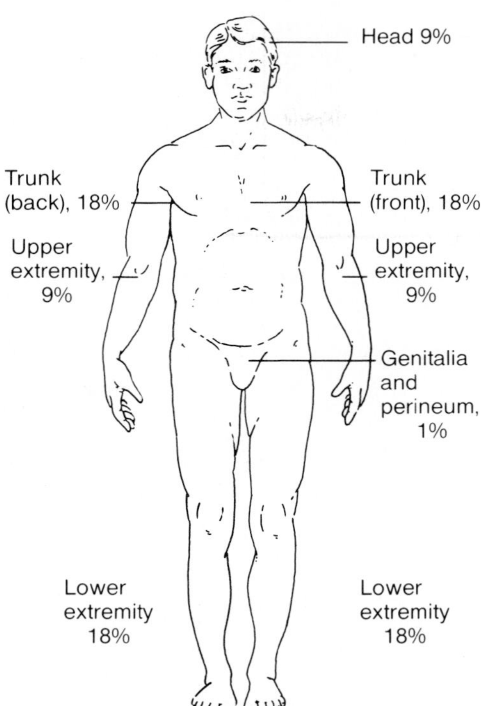

Figure 11-6. Rule of nines for estimating percentage of body surface area involved in burns.

Table 11-1. Classification of burns according to severity.[1]

Major burns
Second-degree, > 25% body surface area in adults
Second-degree, > 20% body surface area in children
Third-degree, > 10% body surface area
Burns involving hands, face, eyes, ears, feet, perineum[2]
Burns associated with smoke inhalation, electrical injury, and other major trauma
Burns in patients at poor risk (elderly, very young children)
Moderate burns
Second-degree, 15–25% body surface area in adults
Second-degree, 10–20% body surface area in children
Third-degree, 2–10% body surface area
Minor burns
First-degree, burn of any surface area
Second-degree, < 15% body surface area in adults
Second-degree, < 10% body surface area in children
Third-degree, < 2% body surface area

[1]Modified and reproduced, with permission, from Mills J et al (editors): *Current Emergency Diagnosis & Treatment,* 2nd ed. Lange, 1985.
[2]This category does not by itself threaten life, but it threatens vital structures and therefore requires special management.

such as burns with hot liquids and acids, smoke inhalation is not a factor.

C. Complications:

1. Hypovolemia-Hypovolemia may result from fluid exudation on the surface of the burn. The severity of hypovolemia correlates directly with the surface area involved. Urgent fluid replacement is required to prevent shock and acute renal failure.

2. Necrosis of erythrocytes-Thermal necrosis of burned erythrocytes occurs in burned blood vessels, and free hemoglobin and red cell stroma enter the plasma. Entry of hemoglobin and red cell stroma into the plasma is occasionally severe enough to cause acute renal failure.

3. Necrosis of epidermis and dermis-Coagulative necrosis of epidermis and dermis forms a black eschar (crust) on the burned area. The eschar hardens and contracts over the first few days; when a circumferential burn of a limb has occurred, contraction of the eschar may prevent blood flow (somewhat in the manner of a tourniquet) and cause ischemia. Incision of an encircling eschar (escharotomy) is often necessary in such cases.

4. Infection-Burned skin no longer serves as a barrier to infection and actually promotes the growth of microorganisms. Surface infection of the necrotic zone with bacteria (and sometimes fungi) is almost inevitable. Infection may occasionally invade the underlying viable tissue and blood vessels and lead to systemic infection. Numerous bacteria, including staphylococci and *Pseudomonas* species, and fungi such as *Candida albicans* and *Aspergillus* are common offenders. Biopsy of a suspect area with demonstration of organisms in viable tissue and blood vessels is necessary to detect such infection at an early stage.

5. Peptic ulcers-Acute peptic ulcers of the stomach and duodenum (Curling's ulcer) may occur following major burn injury and cause severe gastrointestinal bleeding. The pathogenesis of these ulcers is not well understood, but excessive adrenal corticosteroid secretion induced by the acute stress of the burn has been implicated.

6. Scarring-When large areas of the body are burned, severe scarring occurs during healing and often requires extensive cosmetic plastic surgery. Scars may also cause contractures that interfere with function. Burn scars are also associated with an increased risk of developing squamous carcinoma many years later.

Generalized Heat Injury

Generalized heat injury is common and results from exposure to a hot environment, eg, during heat waves, in the desert, in closed vehicles, or during strenuous exercise on a hot day. Sweating is an extremely effective mechanism that usually prevents increase in body core temperature in these circumstances. Diseases associated with generalized heat injury—in order of increasing severity—are heat cramps, heat exhaustion, and heat pyrexia (heat stroke). Malignant hyperthermia is an inherited disorder of skeletal muscle characterized by hyperpyrexia in response to induction of general anesthesia; it is not caused by exposure to a hot environment.

A. Heat Cramps: Loss of water and salt in sweat—particularly during exercise in hot weather—may cause painful spasms of voluntary muscles, especially of the extremities. Heat cramps can be prevented and treated by salt replacement.

B. Heat Exhaustion: Heat exhaustion is characterized by weakness, headache, nausea, and vertigo, followed by collapse, which is usually brief. This is due to hemoconcentration resulting from water and electrolyte loss in sweat and to peripheral vasodilatation, which occurs as a compensatory mechanism. The latter causes venous pooling, decreased effective plasma volume, and decreased cardiac output. The skin is gray and wet, and blood pressure may be low. The body temperature is usually normal. Heat exhaustion is not dangerous, and most patients recover when removed to a cool area. Rarely, intravenous fluid replacement is necessary.

C. Heat Pyrexia (Heat Stroke): Heat stroke is a severe life-threatening condition caused by heat exposure. Elderly patients and those with existing chronic diseases such as diabetes mellitus, alcoholism, and atherosclerosis are most vulnerable. Heat pyrexia represents failure of heat regulation by the body due to unknown causes and is usually preceded by cessation of sweating. Hyperpyrexia with body temperatures of 41 °C (106 °F) are common, and temperatures as high as 45 °C (113 °F) have been reported.

Heat stroke is accompanied by confusion, delirium, and loss of consciousness. Peripheral vasodilatation causes peripheral circulatory failure and shock. The combination of increased metabolic rate resulting from increased body temperature and circulatory failure causes ischemic necrosis of many tissues, including the myocardium, kidney, and liver.

Heat pyrexia has a high mortality rate. Treatment consists of dissipating body heat as quickly as possible by any means available—most effectively by immersing the patient in an ice water bath.

D. Malignant Hyperthermia: Malignant hyperthermia is an inherited disease of skeletal muscle characterized by the development of hyperpyrexia upon administration of certain drugs used in anesthesiology, eg, halothane and muscle relaxants. These drugs cause an influx of calcium into the muscle cell that leads to ATPase stimulation, increased catabolism, and heat production. Myofibrillary disruption may occur, releasing potassium and myoglobin into the plasma and leading to hyperkalemia and acute renal failure, respectively. Treatment with procainamide and correction of electrolyte imbalance is usually successful. In the absence of exposure to anesthetic agents, these patients are essentially normal. Note that malignant hyperthermia is not caused by exposure to a hot external environment.

ELECTRICAL INJURIES

Approximately 1000 deaths occur annually in the United States as a result of electrocution, and another 200 deaths result from lightning strikes. Electrical injuries occur mainly among utility company and construction workers exposed to high-voltage wires, but accidents associated with electrical appliances in the home and workplace are responsible for about 30% of all electrical injuries severe enough to warrant hospital admission.

Electric current can only flow in a closed circuit that is characterized by a difference in potential or voltage between 2 points in the circuit. Injury occurs when the human body becomes a part of this circuit. In most cases, one part of the body is in contact with a live wire and another part with the ground. The severity of electrical injury is directly related to the amount of current that flows through the body. Current flow is related directly to the voltage difference and inversely to the electrical resistance. Severe electrical injuries are therefore more common in countries that use a 220- to 240-volt domestic supply (eg, England) than those that use a 110-volt supply (eg, USA, continental Europe). Electrical injuries caused by lightning and contact with high-voltage wires, which carry several thousand volts of electrical energy, are very severe. The amount of current flowing through the body depends on the amount of resistance at the points of entry and exit—eg, wet skin, which has a much lower resistance than dry skin, predisposes to more severe electrical injury.

The severity of tissue damage resulting from the passage of an electric current through the body is dependent on the following factors: (1) The electrical resistance of the tissue to the flow of current. This is inversely related to the water content of the tissue. Dry skin and bone have high resistance, whereas blood, nerve, and muscle are good conductors. (2) The exact path taken by the current through the body and the organs in the pathway. For example, if earth is the exit point, a current that enters the body in the leg and leaves through the foot will be much less harmful than one which enters the hand, since in the latter instance cardiac arrhythmias may develop as the current passes across the heart. (3) The duration of contact with the source of current. Alternating current (AC) is more dangerous than direct current (DC) because it causes tetanic contraction of muscles that may prevent the victim from letting go of the contact source.

The passage of electric current through the body has 2 main effects:

(1) The current interferes with the functioning of tissues that depend on the generation of electrical action potentials. Current passing through the respiratory and cardiac centers in the brain stem disrupts nerve impulses and leads to cardiorespiratory arrest, a common cause of death; paralysis of the conducting system of the heart causes arrhythmias and heart block, leading to cardiac arrest and acute heart failure; and stimulation of skeletal muscle may cause contractions so violent that they may cause bone fractures.

(2) The passage of current also generates heat, the amount depending on the strength of the current, the electrical resistance of individual tissues, and the duration of contact. The skin has high electrical resistance and commonly shows thermal burns at the entry and exit points of the current (Fig 11–7). In injuries due to extremely high voltage, linear burn marks may appear all over the skin (lightning marks). Current of very high voltage (eg, lightning) may produce enough heat in skin to cause charring (flash burns) and in tissues to convert water into steam, causing soft tissues to explode and bones to fracture. Heat generated in blood vessels in the path of the current results in thrombosis, sometimes at sites far distant from the obviously injured area.

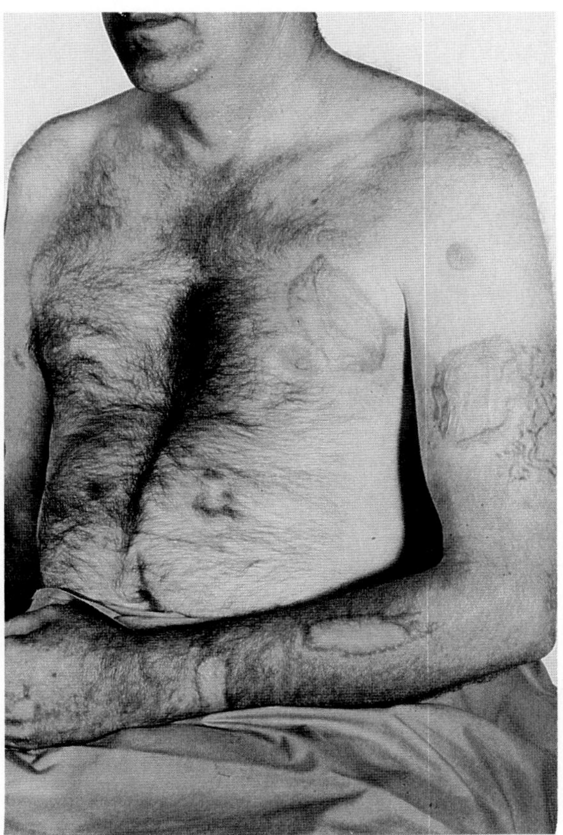

Figure 11–7. Multiple electrical burns of the skin of the left arm and the left side of the chest.

IONIZING RADIATION INJURY

Exposure of Humans to Ionizing Radiation

Ionizing radiation includes that part of the electromagnetic wave spectrum comprising x-rays and gamma rays (Fig 11–8) and certain types of particulate radiation (alpha and beta particles, neutrons, protons, and deuterons [Table 11–2]). All of these different types of radiation, which are derived from different sources, have in common the ability to produce ionization within tissues exposed to them. **Natural radiation** is derived from radioactive elements in the environment and cosmic rays. In addition, humans have developed the ability to generate radioactive substances for use in nuclear medicine, nuclear power plants, nuclear weapons, and nuclear propulsion. Modern nuclear bombs are immensely more destructive than the original atomic bombs, releasing energy in the form of blast or shock waves, heat, and ionizing radiation, both immediate and delayed (''fallout'').

Ionizing radiation is used in medicine for diagnostic and therapeutic purposes. Radiology is a branch of medicine that uses x-rays to visualize internal structures of the body and provide valuable diagnostic information. Nuclear medicine uses various radioisotopes for diagnosis—eg, administration of radioactive iodine enables the physician to detect uptake of iodine in tissues, mainly in the thyroid gland; and abnormal patterns of uptake provide information about possible disease of the thyroid gland. Such diagnostic tests use very small doses of radiation that are generally not harmful. Higher doses of radiation are used in the treatment of cancer **(radiotherapy),** because many types of cancer cells are more susceptible to radiation than are normal tissues. Such radiation treatment often includes use of x-rays in high doses directed at the tumor and isotopes that emit alpha and beta particles implanted directly in the tumor. Treatment may damage normal tissues included in the field of radiation.

The unit used to measure the radiation absorbed by tissues is the gray (Gy)—formerly the rad; 1 Gy = 100 cGy = 100 rads. (See Table 11–3.) The overall effect of radiation is determined not only by the dose but also by the amount of tissue exposed to that dose—eg, the effect of 10 Gy (1000 rads) to the whole body is different from that of 10 Gy limited to the axillary lymph nodes.

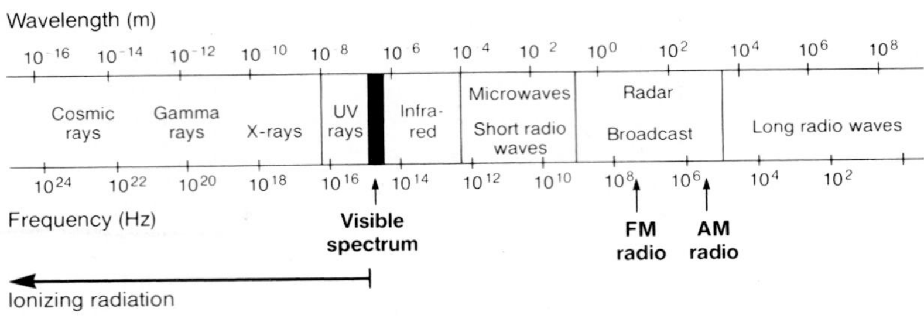

Figure 11-8. The electromagnetic wave spectrum. The shaded area between the infrared and ultraviolet regions is the visible spectrum. Longer x-rays penetrate poorly (so-called "soft" x-rays); shorter, higher-energy x-rays penetrate readily. Gamma rays resemble x-rays but are derived from natural sources (radioisotope decay); x-rays are artificially generated.

Mechanism of Radiation Injury

Ionizing radiation—by definition—has enough energy to displace electrons from the outer shell of atoms to produce ions (ionization). These charged particles react with one another to form neutral free radicals (atoms or molecules that are highly reactive because they carry unpaired electrons in their outer shells). Free radicals interact with adjacent molecules to produce alterations of these molecules and subsequent cell injury.

Two principal mechanisms of cell damage caused by radiation are recognized (Fig 11–9):

A. Direct Action: High-energy radiation directly alters or inactivates vital molecules in the cell, eg, DNA, RNA, and proteins.

B. Indirect Action: Radiation causes ionization of intracellular water, producing high-energy particles, eg, H_2O^+ and H_2O^-. These immediately dissociate and interact to form toxic free radicals such as $H^\cdot$, $OH^\cdot$, and $H_2O^\cdot$, which are highly unstable particles that rapidly dissipate their energy by reacting with adjacent vital cellular molecules such as DNA, RNA, and proteins to cause cell injury. The intermediate interactions between radiation and water occur in a few microseconds.

Effects of Radiation Injury

DNA represents the main target of action of radiation. After high doses of radiation, extensive DNA injury leads to cellular necrosis. With

Table 11-2. Ionizing radiation.

Type of Radiation		Description	Features
Particulate radiation			
Alpha particle	(+)(○)(○)(+) in circle	Nature: helium nucleus Charge: +2 Mass number: 4	Shallow penetration in tissue; causes dense ionization and damage. Causes little harm externally but dangerous if used internally as an alpha particle-emitting isotope.
Beta particle	⊖	Nature: electron Charge: −1 Mass number: negligible mass	Penetrates up to 1 cm of soft tissue. Dense ionization. Used to treat skin cancer; dangerous if used internally.
Neutron	○	Nature: neutron Charge: no charge Mass number: 1	Exists in low- and high-energy forms; the latter penetrates tissues and causes dense ionization.
Proton	⊕	Nature: proton Charge: +1 Mass number: 1	Not used routinely in medicine.
Deuteron	(+)(○) in circle	Nature: deuterium (heavy hydrogen) nucleus Charge: +1 Mass number: 2	Can be used for radiolabeling of compounds.
Waveform radiation			
X-rays Gamma rays		Waves of varying lengths. Behave as photons (discrete units of radiant energy) in tissue. No mass or charge.	Deep penetration of tissues; low density of ionization, so tissue damage is minimal compared with alpha and beta particles.

Table 11-3. Radiation terminology.

Term	Definition
Rad	Unit of absorbed dose for any type of radiation (energy absorbed per unit mass); 1 rad is an absorbed dose of 100 ergs per gram of tissue.
Roentgen (R)	Unit of exposure (ionization per unit volume of air); 1 R is the amount of radiation that produces ionization equivalent to a charge of 1 electrostatic unit in 1 mL of air; international unit of x-ray and gamma radiation.
Relative biologic effectiveness (RBE)	Expression of biologic effect of different types of radiation. The RBE of alpha particles is 20 times greater than that of beta particles; ie, they are 20 times more damaging to tissues.[1]
Rem (roentgen equivalent man)	Unit of dose of any type of radiation that has the same biologic effect in humans as 1 R of x-rays or gamma rays; 1 rem = RBE × 1 rad.
Gray (Gy)	SI unit of measure superseding the term rad; 1 Gy = 100 rads.

[1]The RBE for alpha particles is 20; for beta particles, x-rays, and gamma rays, it is 1 (ie, the last 3 forms of radiation produce about the same amount of damage).

smaller doses, less severe abnormalities result that cause varying structural and functional abnormalities of DNA; eg, the cell's ability to undergo normal mitosis may be affected. These DNA changes are permanent and may be associated with the later development of cancer in radiated cells; leukemia (cancer of white blood cells) developed in many Hiroshima survivors several years after the dropping of the atomic bomb.

The effects of radiation on cells appear to be cumulative. For this reason, the maximum dose that a single target site can receive is fairly limited if multiple doses of radiation are anticipated—even if there is a significant interval between treatments.

The severity of tissue damage produced by radiation depends on several factors.

A. Dose: Large doses of radiation obviously cause more damage than small ones.

B. Penetration: The depth of penetration of tissue varies with the different types of radiation. Alpha particles have a limited ability to penetrate tissues, and their energy is dissipated in a small area surrounding the point of entry. The smaller beta particles (electrons) penetrate more deeply, and their energy dissipates over a larger area. Because the amount of radiation per unit volume of tissue is greater for alpha than for beta particles, the degree of radiation damage is greater with the former. X-rays and gamma rays penetrate deeply, often passing through the body with little dissipation of energy. These types of radiation are well suited to diagnostic tests because they can be detected on the body surface (with x-ray film or gamma counters) and cause little tissue damage.

C. Sensitivity of Tissues: Different tissues are affected to varying degrees by radiation (Table 11-4).

D. Duration of Exposure: Effects differ with the duration of exposure.

Total Body Irradiation

A. Causes: Total body irradiation occurs as a result of nuclear fallout from explosion of a nuclear weapon or following a nuclear accident.

B. Effects: The effect of total body irradiation is dose-dependent (Table 11-5). A dose of radiation greater than 10 Gy (1000 rads) to the whole body is invariably fatal, and one in excess of 2 Gy (200 rads) will cause death in a significant number of exposed individuals. These doses are not large when one considers that doses of 50-70 Gy (5000-7000 rads) are often delivered to a localized area of the body in the treatment of cancer. In a nuclear explosion, the dose received by an individual depends on the size of the explosion, the type of radiation emitted, and the distance from the source. Several well-defined syndromes are recognized with varying dosage levels.

1. **Vaporization**-Vaporization of all body tissues occurs if the victim is in the immediate vicinity of a nuclear explosion.

2. **Cerebral syndrome**-The cerebral syndrome appears after radiation doses in excess of 10 Gy (1000 rads). It is invariably fatal, either instantaneously or within a few days. In the latter event, the brain shows diffuse hemorrhagic necrosis (Fig 11-10). Symptoms of cerebral dysfunction do not occur with doses under 10 Gy (1000 rads).

3. **Gastrointestinal syndrome**-The gastrointestinal syndrome occurs with radiation doses in the range of 3-10 Gy (300-1000 rads). It is characterized by extensive necrosis of the intestinal mucosa, leading to nausea, vomiting, and diarrhea that begin a few hours after exposure. With doses above 5 Gy (500 rads), diarrhea is severe, and death commonly occurs within a few days from fluid and electrolyte loss. With doses in the range of 3-5 Gy (300-500 rads), symptoms are less severe but may persist for a long time. Death may occur as late as a month after exposure. Patients who survive recover slowly, and return of the intestine to normal may take over 6 months. Patients who recover from a nonlethal gastrointestinal syndrome commonly succumb to the hematopoietic syndrome.

4. **Hematopoietic syndrome**-Hematopoietic syndrome occurs after radiation doses of 2-6 Gy (200-600 rads) and is commonly associated with the gastrointestinal syndrome. The first change is

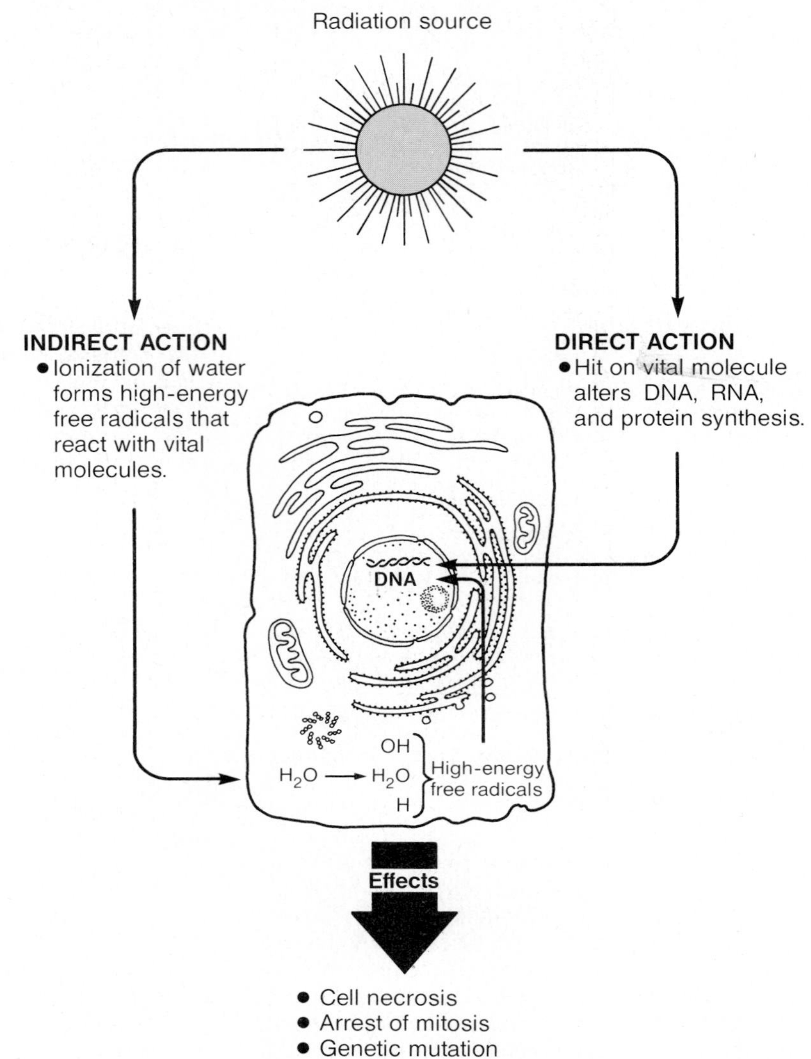

Figure 11-9. Effects of radiation on cells.

Table 11-4. Radiosensitivity of cells.[1]

	Permanent Cells (No or Very Low Mitotic Activity)	**Stable Cells (Little Mitotic Activity)**	**Labile Cells (Rapidly Proliferating Tissues)**
Degree of Radiosensitivity	Radioresistant	Intermediate radiosensitivity	Radiosensitive
Normal cells and tissues	Adult neurons	Muscle Connective tissue Liver Endocrine organs Glial cells	Bone marrow Intestinal epithelium Hair follicles Gonads Skin
Tumors	Ganglioneuroma (tumor of neurons) Benign neoplasms of connective tissue	Sarcoma (cancer of connective tissue cells) Glioma (tumor of glial cells) Liver cell cancer	Leukemia and lymphoma (of marrow and lymphocytes) Germinoma (neoplasm of gonads)

[1]Radiosensitivity correlates with the degree of mitotic activity of the tissue or tumor. Radioresistant and radiosensitive are relative terms, since all tissues are radiosensitive if the dose is high enough. Sensitivity also varies in different species: cockroaches can survive doses of several thousand rads; bacteria, doses of 10,000 rads or more.

Table 11-5. Effect of total body irradiation.

Dose (Gy)	Syndrome	Latent Period	Clinical Features	Mortality Rate
0–0.5 Gy (0–50 rads)	None[1]	—	—	—
0.5–2 Gy (50–200 rads)	Acute radiation syndrome	Weeks–months	Fatigue, nausea, vomiting	0%
2–6 Gy (200–600 rads)	Hematopoietic syndrome	1–2 weeks	Leukopenia, thrombocytopenia	20–50%
3–10 Gy (300–1000 rads)	Gastrointestinal syndrome	1 day–2 weeks	Mucosal necrosis, diarrhea, fluid and electrolyte loss	50–100%[2]
10+ Gy (1000+ rads)	Cerebral syndrome	Hours–2 days	Ataxia, convulsions, delirium, coma	100%

[1]Though there are no immediate effects, low-level exposure of an individual to radiation is associated with an increased long-term incidence of cancer and low-level exposure of a population produces an increased mutation rate, with the possibility of birth defects.
[2]The mortality rate associated with gastrointestinal syndrome is almost 100% at doses over 6 Gy (600 rads). With exposure to lower doses (between 3 and 6 Gy [300–600 rads]), patients have features of both the gastrointestinal and hematopoietic syndromes and the mortality rate is lower.

a decrease in the number of peripheral blood lymphocytes (lymphopenia), which occurs as early as 24 hours after exposure and is also associated with depletion of lymphocytes in the lymph nodes and spleen. Bone marrow hypoplasia follows (Fig 11-11), leading to decreased production of granulocytes, erythrocytes, and platelets. Death occurs in 20–50% of patients with this syndrome; infection is a major cause of death.

5. **Acute radiation syndrome (systemic radiation sickness)**–Radiation sickness occurs after radiation doses of 0.5–2 Gy (50–200 rads). It is nonlethal and characterized by varying periods of listlessness, fatigue, vomiting, and anorexia. A transient reduction in peripheral blood lymphocytes and granulocytes is common (mild hematopoietic syndrome). Variations of systemic radiation sickness may also occur in patients receiving

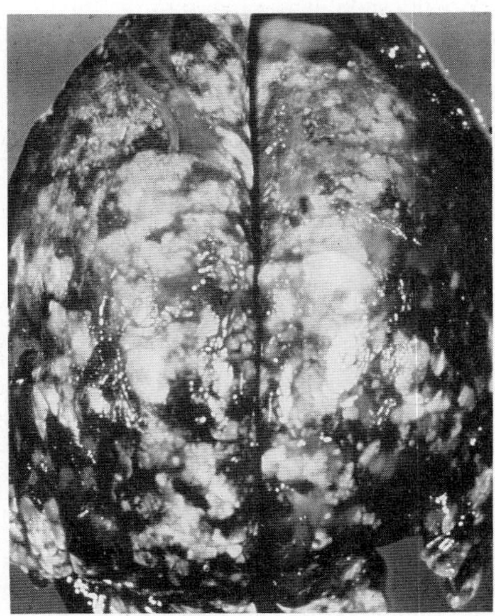

Figure 11-10. Brain of mouse that received a high dose of radiation to the whole body. Shows extensive hemorrhagic necrosis.

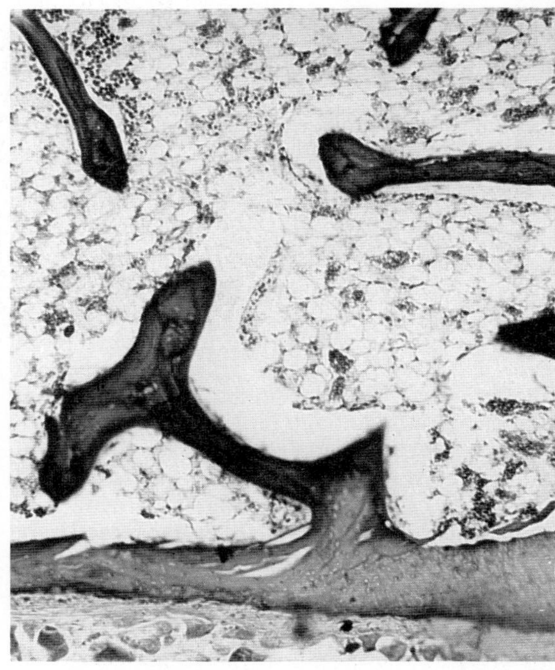

Figure 11-11. Effect of radiation on bone marrow, showing marked depletion of hematopoietic cells. Low magnification.

much higher doses (> 20 Gy [2000 rads]) to localized areas as part of cancer therapy.

6. Long-term effects-Survivors of radiation exposure—even those who have been exposed to low levels—demonstrate abnormalities of one kind or another. Detailed study of survivors of Hiroshima and Nagasaki has shown an increased incidence of cancer (particularly leukemia), cataracts, infertility, and bone marrow aplasia. These changes appeared long after exposure, and even the offspring of exposed individuals appear to be at increased risk for development of abnormalities.

The lower limits of safe exposure to radiation are unknown, though various federal and international standards have established "safe" dose limits for individuals and populations. The only absolutely safe dose of radiation is zero, but this cannot be achieved because of background radiation from natural sources (decay of naturally occurring radioisotopes, cosmic rays, etc). To place the risk of radiation exposure in perspective, a routine diagnostic x-ray delivers a much smaller dose than is received from natural sources in a year or even from a single transatlantic flight at 30,000 feet.

Localized Irradiation

Localized irradiation to a limited area of the body is used in the treatment of cancer. The rationale behind such treatment is that cancer cells (which are rapidly proliferating) are more sensitive to radiation than are the normal (nonproliferating or slowly proliferating) cells surrounding them, so that a radiation dose can be selected and focused to achieve death of tumor cells with a lesser degree of damage to normal structures. The radiation can also be focused on the cancer by a variety of different techniques so that the surrounding normal tissue will receive a minimum amount of radiation.

A. Sensitivity of Tissues:

1. Cancer cells (malignant neoplasms)- Cancers may be classified on the basis of their response to radiation into radiocurable, radiosensitive, and radioresistant neoplasms. Predictions about tumor response to radiation must take several factors into account: (1) Experience with radiation therapy as a form of treatment. Most types of tumors have undergone a trial of radiation, and the results of such treatment are recorded in the medical literature. (2) Type of tissue (Table 11-4). (3) Rate of proliferation of cancer cells. Cancers of cells that have a high rate of division, eg, acute leukemias (cancers of blood cells) and germinomas (cancers of gonadal germ cells), are generally radiosensitive. Cancers arising from cells that have a low turnover rate, eg, sarcomas (cancers of mesenchymal cells) and liver cell cancer, are more radioresistant. Benign neoplasms of connective tissue with a lower mitotic rate than their malignant counterparts are even more radioresistant.

a. Radiocurable neoplasms-Occasionally, neoplasms are so sensitive to radiation that they can be cured by radiation therapy.

b. Radiosensitive neoplasms-Radiosensitive neoplasms show a major reduction in tumor size after radiation therapy, but they are not eradicated (ie, a percentage of malignant cells survives and proliferates), eg, many sarcomas, glial neoplasms of the brain, and breast cancer.

c. Radioresistant neoplasms-Tumors that show little or no reduction in size after radiation therapy are radioresistant. Most cancers show some response, particular if dosage level is very high.

2. Normal tissues-When localized irradiation is used, every effort is made to shield normal tissues and focus the radiation on the tumor mass; because such techniques are imperfect, the surrounding normal tissues invariably receive some radiation. The amount of radiation that may be given to a tumor is limited mainly by its toxic effect on normal tissue; eg, the local radiation dose to brain tumors cannot exceed 60 Gy (6000 rads) because necrosis of surrounding normal brain occurs with higher doses. The effect of radiation on normal tissues can be predicted on the basis of (1) accumulated clinical experience with radiotherapy and (2) the turnover rate of cells. The rate of complications associated with radiotherapy given to various body sites will have been documented in the medical literature. Labile cells with a high turnover rate, eg, hematopoietic cells, intestinal mucosal cells, and testicular germ cells are highly sensitive to the effects of radiation. Stable cells of solid organs such as the liver and kidney are less sensitive. Permanent cells such as muscle and nerve are radioresistant (Table 11-4).

B. Radiation Damage of Normal Tissues: Tissues that have been exposed to radiation demonstrate various abnormalities. In all tissues, collagenous connective tissue is partially broken down and shows a unique hyalinization. Blood vessel changes vary from the development of abnormal telangiectatic vessels to thickening and hyalinization of the walls. Fibroblasts and endothelial cells are enlarged and demonstrate nuclear abnormalities, including hyperchromatism and abnormal chromatin clumping. Karyotypic analysis shows aneuploidy and polyploidy with various chromosomal abnormalities. In addition to these general changes, specific changes occur in various organs.

1. Skin-In the first 2-6 weeks after radiation exposure, erythema, swelling, and epidermal desquamation (acute radiodermatitis) are seen. Later, chronic radiodermatitis occurs, characterized by epidermal atrophy with atypical cytologic features in the cells, dermal fibrosis, and the development of telangiectasias and hyalinized vessels. The skin becomes blotchy and atrophic, has an irregular surface, and, in severe cases, is ulcerated (Fig 11–12). Loss of pigmentation and hair also occurs. Chronic radiodermatitis persists for years and is difficult to treat. Cancer of the squamous epithelium may occur many years after exposure.

2. Bone marrow–Marked hypoplasia of bone marrow may occur within hours after radiation exposure (Fig 11–11). The degree of hypoplasia of the marrow depends on the dose of radiation received. If a significant percentage of active marrow has been irradiated, a decrease in blood granulocyte levels may occur at about the end of the first week, and anemia may develop after 2–3 weeks. Regeneration of bone marrow is rapid if stem cells survive elsewhere in the marrow. Radiation of the entire bone marrow is sometimes used in the treatment of certain types of leukemia and lymphoma. After radiation has caused necrosis of the entire bone marrow (normal and cancer cells), it is repopulated by transplanted bone marrow (Fig 11–13). Although it is relatively radioresistant, bone itself may show periosteal loss and necrosis at higher doses (radio-osteonecrosis). Irradiation of epiphyses in children halts bone growth.

3. Lymphoid tissues–Lymphoid tissues are extremely radiosensitive and are rapidly depleted if exposed to radiation. Irradiation of large lymph nodes may cause a transient decline in the peripheral blood lymphocyte count and increased susceptibility to infection.

4. Lung–The lung is quite radioresistant, and changes appear only after high doses. When a large area of lung is affected, radiation pneumonitis can be fatal. In the acute phase, which occurs in the first few weeks, acute endothelial swelling and increased permeability of alveolar capillaries lead to pulmonary edema and formation of hyaline membranes due to diffuse alveolar epithelial damage. Chronic changes include interstitial fibrosis, which causes failure of diffusion that may lead to incapacitating dyspnea and even death.

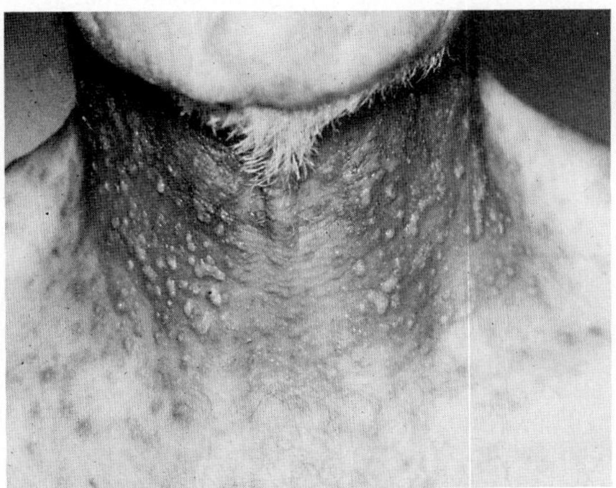

Figure 11–12. Radiation dermatitis. Note discoloration and epidermal irregularity. Patient received radiation to the neck as treatment for cancer.

5. Intestine–The mucosa of the intestine is radiosensitive and shows changes during abdominal and pelvic irradiation. In the acute phase, hyperemia and ulceration are seen; later, chronic mucosal atrophy may lead to malabsorption. In the colon, radiation colitis causes diarrhea with blood and mucus, which may be severe and debilitating. When the rectum is involved, severe pain may occur. Mucosal telangiectasia, atypical epithelial cells, atrophy, and fibrosis are the usual histologic findings.

6. Long-term effects–Two important long-term effects of radiation exposure are difficult to predict with accuracy.

a. Carcinogenic effect–The carcinogenic effect of radiation exposure is an important and well-known risk factor. The later development of radiation-induced neoplasms in patients who have been successfully treated for cancer is an increasingly common problem.

b. Genetic effect–Exposure to radiation causes an increased number of genetic abnormalities (mutations) that may be passed to subsequent generations.

C. Methods to Minimize Injury of Normal Tissues: During cancer treatment using localized irradiation, many techniques are used to increase the dose delivered to the tumor and decrease the amount of radiation reaching surrounding normal tissue. The balance between benefit (reduction of tumor mass) and harm (injury to normal tissue) is achieved by adjusting the radiation dose as well as the ports through which radiation is delivered.

1. Shielding–Lead shields permit radiation to enter the body only through predetermined ports, or windows; eg, the lungs are shielded when the mediastinum is being irradiated.

2. Radioisotope implants–Implants containing radioactive isotopes are inserted into neoplasms for local release of radiation; if alpha-particle radiation is used, a high dose is delivered locally to the tumor with little penetration into normal tissue.

3. Selective uptake–Use of a radioactive isotope of a substance that is selectively taken up by cancer cells permits more selective radiation of the cancer cells, eg, the administration of radioactive iodine in the treatment of well-differentiated thyroid carcinoma. The thyroid cancer cells take up the iodine like normal thyroid cells. Again, an isotope that emits alpha particles provides the maximum benefit.

4. Monoclonal antibodies–A promising approach uses monoclonal antibodies targeted against specific tumor-associated antigens to carry small amounts of radioactive isotopes to the tumor site.

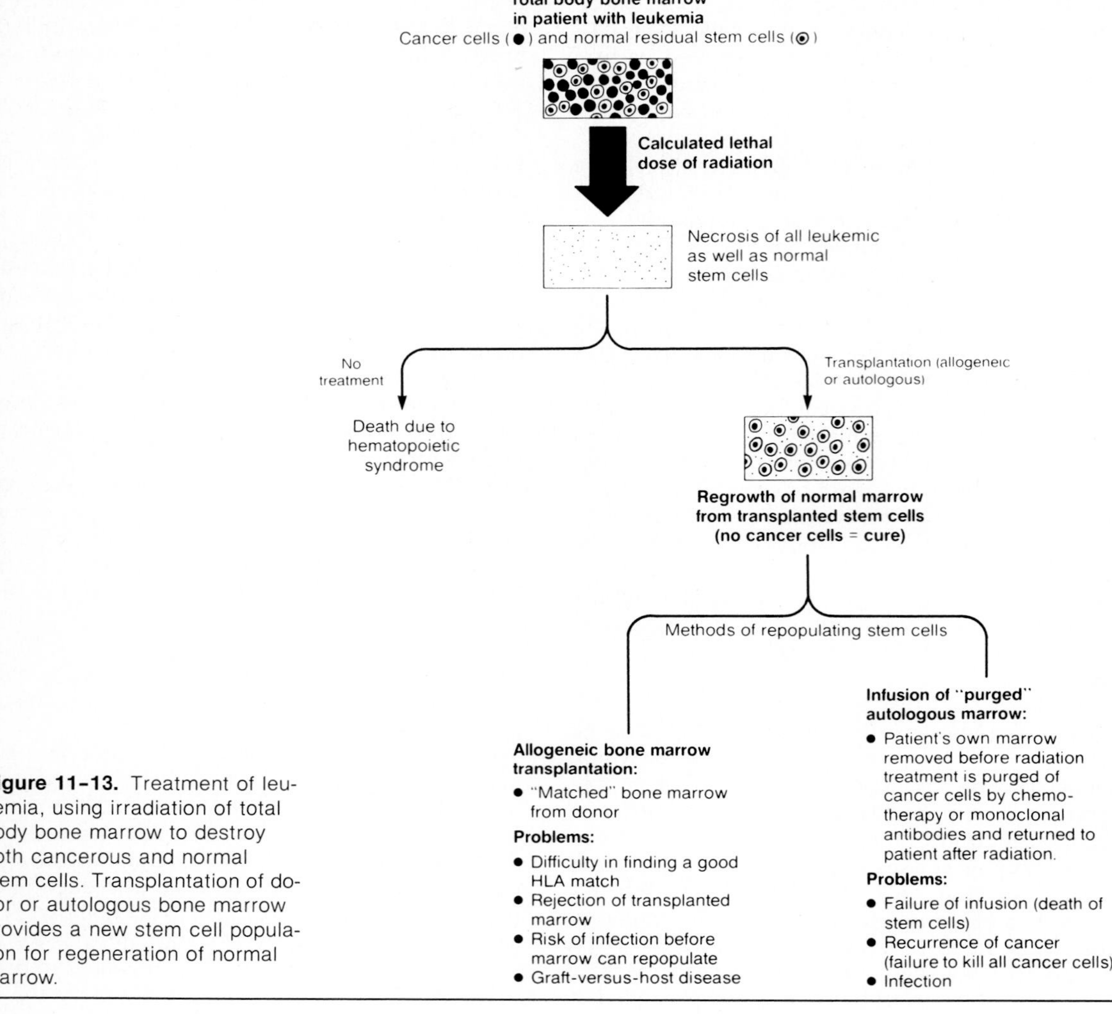

Figure 11-13. Treatment of leukemia, using irradiation of total body bone marrow to destroy both cancerous and normal stem cells. Transplantation of donor or autologous bone marrow provides a new stem cell population for regeneration of normal marrow.

5. Fractionated doses–The total radiation dose is divided into multiple graded doses that are administered over time to permit normal cells to recover in the interval between doses.

Ultraviolet Radiation

Ultraviolet rays are present in sunlight. They have very low penetrating capability and are rapidly absorbed by many types of clothing, sunscreens, and melanin. Dark-skinned individuals are protected almost completely by melanin skin pigment from the effect of ultraviolet radiation. Light-skinned individuals who are exposed to bright sunlight for long periods are at risk for radiation-induced injury. Farmers, other outdoor workers, and sunbathers in Australia and parts of southwestern USA are at greatest risk.

Ultraviolet radiation penetrates the superficial layer of the skin, causing damage to the epidermis and dermis. It causes direct cell injury. Acute overexposure to ultraviolet light causes thermal damage and inflammation of the skin. This is characterized by erythema and severe pain (sunburn). More chronic exposure leads to changes in the DNA of epidermal cells, characterized by abnormal dimeric linkage of pyrimidine bases. These changes predispose to various types of cancer of the skin, particularly basal cell carcinoma, squamous carcinoma, and malignant melanoma.

OTHER RADIATION

Many different types of nonionizing radiation have medical as well as commercial uses.

Lasers

Lasers are highly concentrated beams of light that are being increasingly used to treat a variety of disorders, eg, retinal disease, atherosclerotic plaques in arteries, dysplasia of the uterine cervix, and brain tumors. The destructive effect of lasers is due to production of intense heat at the site of application. Because the laser beam is coherent—

ie, composed of wavelengths of the same frequency and phase that are all traveling in the same direction—it can be accurately focused on minute areas of abnormal tissue to destroy or coagulate them.

Ultrasound Waves

Ultrasonography is used for diagnostic purposes, particularly in obstetrics for fetal and placental localization. Numerous studies have shown that ultrasound waves do not cause tissue damage, and their use is considered safe.

Microwaves

Microwaves are used in food preparation and in the communications industry. The mechanism of injury is heat production. Normal household use is not associated with any harmful effects, and strict standards exist for shielding of microwave appliances.

Ionizing Radiation

Ionizing radiation is used to sterilize various products such as medical instruments (eg, syringes) and, most recently, meat processed for human consumption. Numerous studies have shown that use and ingestion of irradiated products and foods are not harmful, since the products are not thereby rendered radioactive and no radiation is delivered to the user.

12 Disorders Due to Chemical Agents

- Classification of Chemicals Causing Injury
    - Chemicals of Abuse
    - Therapeutic Drugs
    - Industrial and Agricultural Chemicals
- Mechanisms of Human Exposure
- Ethyl Alcohol Abuse (Alcoholism)
- Cigarette Smoking
- Psychotropic Drug Abuse
- Metals
    - Lead Poisoning
    - Mercury Poisoning
    - Aluminum Poisoning
    - Arsenic Poisoning
- Insecticides and Herbicides
    - Chlorinated Hydrocarbons
    - Organophosphates
    - Paraquat
- Industrial Chemicals
    - Methyl Alcohol (Methanol)
    - Ethylene Glycol
    - Carbon Tetrachloride
    - Carbon Monoxide
    - Cyanide
- Therapeutic Agents (Drugs)
    - Prescription Drugs
    - Commonly Used Drugs

CLASSIFICATION OF CHEMICALS CAUSING INJURY

Several groups of chemicals have been implicated as causes of disease.

Chemicals of Abuse

Ethyl alcohol, tobacco, and psychotropic drugs such as narcotics, cocaine, amphetamines, sedatives, marihuana, and so forth are common drugs of abuse. Drug abuse is an age-old problem (Table 12–1) and represents the commonest type of chemical injury. The list of drugs of abuse grows as so-called designer drugs are developed in an attempt to increase the magnitude and range of psychotropic effects provided by other licit and illicit drugs.

Therapeutic Drugs

Prescribed drugs may also cause injury through adverse side effects or drug interactions, overdosage, improper use, etc.

Industrial & Agricultural Chemicals

Metals, insecticides, herbicides, and many chemicals produced as by-products of industrial processes and disposed of at toxic waste sites constitute a major public health hazard. Toxic waste has contaminated groundwater supplies and fauna in some areas. Various toxic chemicals are also present as constituents of common household products such as insecticides, cleaners, and detergents.

MECHANISMS OF HUMAN EXPOSURE

Voluntary Abuse

Addicts voluntarily use habituating substances because of physiologic or psychologic dependence. Psychotropic drugs are also used sporadically by many otherwise normal individuals as a means of either escaping reality or experiencing unusual sensory phenomena.

Suicide or Homicide

Drugs may be taken or surreptitiously administered with suicidal or homicidal intent. The types of drugs used for these purposes vary with locale as well as with time—eg, arsenic was commonly used for murder and suicide in Roman times, whereas insecticides, cyanide, carbon monoxide, sedatives, and acetaminophen are more commonly used today.

Accidental Ingestion

Toxic chemicals, particularly household products, may be accidentally ingested by young children, and such incidents are an important cause of death in this age group. Accidental ingestion may occur in any age group if containers of toxic substances or the substances themselves are inadvertently switched or mislabeled.

Occupational Exposure

Exposure to toxic chemicals is common in agricultural and industrial workers. Although various safety guidelines have been developed to protect workers, some exposure is inevitable. Pathologists, for example, handle specimens that have been fixed with formalin; the formaldehyde va-

Table 12-1. Drug abuse in religion and ritual.

Mushrooms	
Amanita muscaria (fly agaric)	Siberia 6000 BC; later ritual drinks of ancient Hindus (soma) and Zoroastrians (hoama).
Psilocybin mexicana	Aztecs (coronation of Montezuma 1502); South and Central American Indians.
Other plants	
Poppy (opium, morphine; heroin is synthetic derivative)	Sumerians, Greeks, Mesopotamia 3000 BC; spread to China and East by 7th century; opium dens, opium pipes 18th century, opium wars 19th century.
Cannabis (marihuana, bhang, hashish, Kif, charas)	Scythians 500 BC; Assassins (Arabic = "hashish users") 1100–1300 AD, a fanatical Islam sect dedicated to murder of enemies.
Peyote cactus (mescal, mescaline, peyotl)	Long-term use in South and Central America (peyotl = "divine messenger").
Choboa, yopo, parica from *Piptadenia* tree	Snuff, reported by Columbus in West Indies.
Coca (cocaine)	Long-term use in Peru, Incas; increase energy, relieve fatigue and hunger.
Kava (from species of pepper)	Social and ritual drink in South Pacific.
Datura (jimson weed)	Medicinal, ritual use in North and South America.
Grains (alcohol)	Ancient Egyptians, Greeks, Romans, Chinese, witchcraft, Roman Catholic Church; widespread social use; fraternity house rituals.
Chemicals	
Amphetamines, LSD, synthetic hallucinogens	Recent social use; some modern "rituals."

pors emanating from such specimens have been shown to be toxic. Low-level exposure to formaldehyde is therefore an occupational hazard for pathologists.

Incidental Unrecognized Inadvertent Exposure

Exposure to trace levels of toxic chemicals in food (eg, nitrites used as preservatives in meats), drinking water (toxic pollutants in ground water supplies), and air (ozone, oxides of nitrogen in smog, and "passive smoking") is a major potential cause of disease. Further studies are needed to define the extent of this threat.

• ETHYL ALCOHOL ABUSE (Alcoholism)

Incidence

The recreational use of alcohol is an almost universally accepted social practice (Table 12–2), and many different alcoholic beverages are produced from sources such as fermented milk, fruit, or grain. Abuse of alcohol is a major worldwide health problem and has been estimated to affect the lives of about 10% of people in the USA. Alcoholism is difficult to define in terms of amount of alcohol consumed but can be recognized when the habit adversely affects the life of the individual in some way. Alcoholism results in impairment of social and occupational functioning, increasing tolerance to the effects of alcohol, and physiologic dependence.

Clinical Syndromes

A. Acute Alcoholic Intoxication:

1. Blood alcohol concentration-Acute intoxication due to alcohol correlates with the blood alcohol concentration (BAC). Clinical evidence of intoxication appears at a BAC of about 100 mg/dL, which has been accepted as establishing a legal presumption of impaired driving ability in many jurisdictions worldwide—in some, the legal presumption is lower (80 or even 50 mg/dL). Alcoholic coma usually occurs when the BAC reaches 300–500 mg/dL. The clinical effects resulting from specific blood alcohol levels may be masked in chronic alcoholics who have developed a tolerance to the drug. In such individuals, there may be little outward evidence of intoxication at levels considerably higher than 100 mg/dL. Conversely, alcohol intoxication may be enhanced in the presence of other drugs, notably sedatives and tranquilizers, with actions additive to that of alcohol.

The measured BAC following ingestion of alcoholic beverages is dependent on so many factors, some of them unpredictable, that estimations based on the amount consumed and the rate of consumption are unreliable. Figs 12–1 and 12–2 are useful as guides or for forensic purposes, but for the driver interested in road safety the only rule that works is, "Do not drink and drive!"

The following factors influence BAC after consumption of alcoholic beverages.

a. The type of alcoholic beverage-The alcohol content of different beverages varies between beer (3–8%), wine (8–15%), fortified wines such as sherry and port (15–23%), and spirits such as whisky, gin, and vodka (40–60%). The alcoholic content is expressed as "proof," which is the percentage content times 2 (eg, 100 proof whisky is 50% alcohol). US proof is different from British proof: 87.6 proof on the British scale equals 100 proof on the US scale.

Table 12-2. Alcoholic beverages (numerous others exist).[1]

Country of Origin	Substrate	Fermented Alcohol	Distilled "Hard" Liquor
Asia, eastern Europe	Mare's milk, cow's milk	Koumiss Kefir	Skhou Arika
United Kingdom	Honey Apples	Mead Cider	Distilled mead Cider
China	Rice, millet	Tchoo	Sautchoo
Sri Lanka, India	Rice, molasses, palm sap	Toddy	Arrack
France, Italy	Grapes	Wine	Brandy, cognac
Ireland, Scotland	Oats, barley malt, rye, corn	Beer	Usquebaugh, aqua vitae, whiskey[2]
Japan	Rice	Sake	Sochu
West Indies	Sugar cane	...	Rum
Russia	Grain or potato	...	Vodka
Netherlands, United Kingdom	Grain (and juniper berries)	...	Gin
Mexico	Agave, tequila cactus	...	Tequila

[1]Almost any sugar or starch source can be used to produce alcohol.
[2]Usquebaugh, aqua vitae = "water of life."

b. The rate of ingestion-BAC varies with the rate of ingestion of alcohol. Formulas can be worked out relating expected BAC to numbers of drinks ingested over a period of time, and BAC levels can be controlled by pacing of alcohol ingestion. In individuals who drink heavily, BAC levels rise rapidly and cause alcoholic coma, which prevents further intake. Vomiting due to gastric irritation also limits intake. Death from alcoholic intake is rare but has occurred with forced intake of large amounts of alcohol in fraternity initiation rites.

c. The rate of absorption-Absorption of alcohol occurs rapidly through the gastric and upper small intestinal mucosa. The rate of absorption is greatest when the stomach is empty and decreases as the amount of gastric contents available to dilute the alcohol increases. The presence of fat in the stomach decreases the rate of alcohol absorption.

d. The rate of tissue distribution-Alcohol is distributed in the body, particularly in adipose tissue, resulting in a dilutional effect. This is related to body weight, which is why obese persons have lower blood levels than lean ones for the same amount of alcohol consumed.

e. The rate of metabolism-Alcohol is metabolized in the liver by alcohol dehydrogenase, an enzyme whose activity varies greatly from one individual to the next. An average person metabolizes about 150 mg/kg/h of alcohol. This amounts to about 10 g or 20 mL of alcohol per hour for a 70-kg individual—equivalent to one 12-oz (360-mL) can of beer, one shot (35 mL) of whisky, or one 4-oz (120-mL) glass of wine. The rate may vary considerably from these average values.

f. The rate of excretion-The excretion of alcohol in urine and exhaled air is usually a small but constant amount that correlates with BAC. This is the principle underlying the forensic use of urine and breath testing as alternatives to blood testing.

2. Clinical features-Ethyl alcohol (ethanol) is a central nervous system depressant. The highest cortical brain centers are affected first, so that inhibitions are relaxed. Socially unacceptable and even criminal behavior may result. Destruction of family life, spouse and child abuse, and impaired work performance are associated with alcoholism.

At relatively low blood levels (about 50 mg/dL), alcohol impairs fine judgment, fine motor skills, and reaction time. Alcohol has been implicated as a contributing cause in about 50% of fatal traffic accidents.

Acute alcohol ingestion may also be associated with acute liver injury characterized by focal liver cell necrosis (Chapter 43), accompanied by fever, jaundice, and painful enlargement of the liver. Acute alcoholic liver disease may be accompanied by hemolytic anemia (Zieve's syndrome). Death due to acute alcohol intoxication is rare because lethal blood levels (> 500 mg/dL) are difficult to achieve: rapid ingestion of alcohol usually induces vomiting, and slower drinking leads to alcoholic stupor or coma at lower blood alcohol levels.

3. Assessment of blood alcohol concentrations-Assessment of BAC has important legal implications in cases of driving "under the influence." In most states in the USA, a person is deemed to have impaired driving ability if the BAC is over 100 mg/dL. Alcohol is excreted in the urine and on the breath. Breath analyzer devices

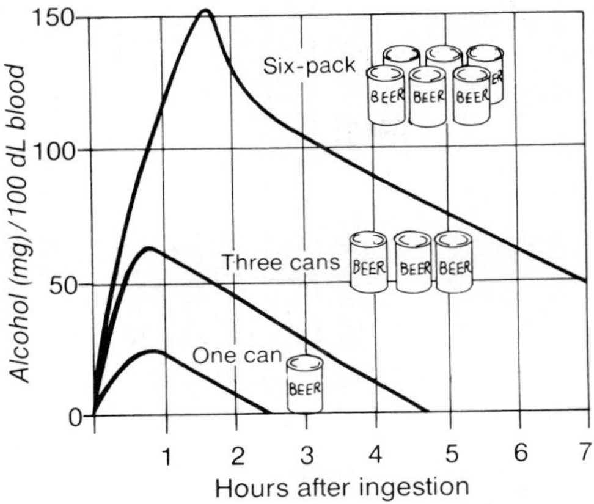

Equivalents	Alcohol content
Can of beer 360 mL	3–8%
Measure of spirits 35 mL	40–60%
Glass of wine 120 mL	8–15%
Glass of sherry or port 80 mL	15–23%

Figure 12–1. Approximation of blood alcohol concentrations following alcohol ingestion for a 70-kg individual.

enable law enforcement officers to assess BAC on the basis of ethanol concentration in expired air.

B. Chronic Alcoholic Intoxication: Chronic ingestion of alcohol produces toxic effects in many organs.

1. Chronic alcoholic liver disease-(Chapter 43.) Chronic liver disease (cirrhosis of the liver) is a common cause of death in alcoholics.

2. Chronic pancreatitis-(Chapter 45.) Pain and pancreatic dysfunction accompany chronic pancreatitis.

3. Alcoholic cardiomyopathy-Alcoholic cardiomyopathy is uncommon but may lead to cardiac dilatation and congestive cardiac failure. Cardiomyopathy has been noted most commonly in individuals drinking beer with a high cobalt content; cobalt and alcohol have additive toxic effects on myocardial cells.

4. Nervous system abnormalities-Peripheral neuropathy is a prominent manifestation of nervous system abnormalities associated with alcohol abuse.

5. Associated malnutrition-Malnutrition is common in chronic alcoholics owing to inadequate intake of food; since alcohol depresses the appetite, alcoholics tend to forego food in favor of drink. Vitamin deficiency is common and includes deficiencies of thiamine **(Wernicke's encephalopathy, Korsakoff's psychosis),** folic acid **(megaloblastic anemia),** and pyridoxine **(sideroblastic anemia).**

Not all chronic alcoholics develop these complications, and there is no direct correlation with the extent of abuse. Only 10–20% of heavy drinkers develop clinically significant chronic liver disease, and over half show no signs of liver disease. Most patients with chronic alcoholic liver disease give a history of intake of about 200 g of alcohol (about half of a 1-L bottle of 80-proof whiskey or ten 12-oz cans of beer) daily for over 10 years. A significant risk of chronic liver disease exists with intake of 50 g/d.

C. Fetal Alcohol Syndrome: Alcohol ingestion during pregnancy causes dose-related fetal growth retardation and increased infant perinatal mortality rates. Heavy drinking may lead to fetal mental retardation.

D. Alcohol Withdrawal Syndrome: Chronic alcoholism is a true addiction, with both psychologic and physical dependence on ethanol. Withdrawal of alcohol in such a patient causes delirium tremens, a life-threatening condition characterized by delirium, dehydration, tremors, and visual and tactile hallucinations (eg, seeing "pink elephants" and formication—a feeling that ants are crawling on the skin). Dehydration, electrolyte imbalance, excitability, and autonomic nervous system hyperactivity require urgent treatment and strong nursing care.

CIGARETTE SMOKING

Cigarette smoking increases the overall risk of death by as much as 70% compared to nonsmokers, and smokers die 5–8 years earlier than nonsmokers. Smoking is the single most important environmental factor contributing to premature death in the USA and the United Kingdom (Table 12-3). Smoking low-tar and low-nicotine cigarettes decreases this risk by only a small amount. Pipe and cigar smoking are less dangerous, probably because less inhalation occurs. Chewing tobacco and snuff was a popular habit in the United States until about 1940. Babe Ruth of baseball fame was a heavy user of chewing tobacco. A major advertising effort in the late 1970s has led to the resurgence of oral snuff and tobacco chewing, particularly among young male athletes.

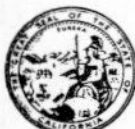

BLOOD ALCOHOL CONCENTRATION (BAC) CHARTS

DRINKING UNDER 21 YEARS OF AGE IS ILLEGAL.

(Drivers under 18 years old with a BAC of .05-.09 can be cited for violation of Section 23140 CVC.)

IF YOU DRINK, DON'T DRIVE!

Prepared by the Department of Motor Vehicles in cooperation with the California Highway Patrol, The Office of Traffic Safety, the Department of Alcohol and Drug Programs and the Department of Justice.

There is no safe way to drive after drinking. These charts show that a few drinks can make you an unsafe driver. They show that drinking affects your **BLOOD ALCOHOL CONCENTRATION (BAC).** The **BAC** zones for various numbers of drinks and time periods are printed in white, grey, and black.

HOW TO USE THESE CHARTS: First, find the chart that includes your weight. For example, if you weigh 160 lbs., use the "150 to 169" chart. Then look under "Total Drinks" at the "2" on this "150 to 169" chart. Now look below the "2" drinks, in the row for 1 hour. You'll see your **BAC** is in the grey shaded zone. This means that if you drive after 2 drinks in 1 hour, you could be arrested. In the grey zone, your chances of having an accident are 5 times higher than if you had no drinks. But, if you had 4 drinks in 1 hour, your **BAC** would be in the black shaded area. . .and your chances of having an accident 25 times higher. What's more, it is **ILLEGAL** to drive at this **BAC** (.10% or greater). After 3 drinks in 1 hour, the chart shows you would need 3 more hours—with no more drinks—to reach the white **BAC** zone again.

REMEMBER: "One drink" is a 12-ounce beer, or a 4-ounce glass of wine, or 1¼-ounce shot of 80-proof liquor (even if it's mixed with non-alcoholic drinks). If you have larger or stronger drinks, or drink on an empty stomach, or if you are tired, sick, upset, or have taken medicines or drugs, you can be **UNSAFE WITH FEWER DRINKS.**

TECHNICAL NOTE: These charts are intended to be guides and are not legal evidence of the actual blood alcohol concentration. Although it is possible for anyone to exceed the designated limits, the charts have been constructed so that fewer than 5 persons in 100 will exceed these limits when drinking the stated amounts on an empty stomach. Actual values can vary by bodytype, sex, health status, and other factors.

DL 606 (REV. 3/88)

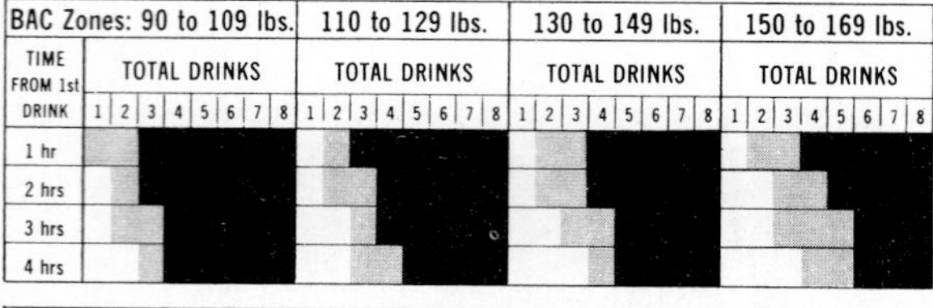

SHADINGS IN THE CHARTS ABOVE MEAN:

☐ (.01%-.04%) Seldom illegal ☐ (.05%-.09%) May be illegal ■ (.10% Up) Definitely illegal

☐ (.05%-.09%) Illegal if under 18 yrs. old

Figure 12–2. California Department of Motor Vehicles chart of blood alcohol concentration after ingestion of various amounts of alcohol. Note: Recently California decreased the legal BAC limit for driving from 0.1% to 0.08 %.

Table 12–3. Pharmacology and pathology of cigarette smoking.[1]

Pharmacology	
Active ingredient:	Nicotine ($C_{10}H_{14}N_2$)
Addictive agent:	Nicotine
Dose per inhalation:	50–150 μg
Dose per cigarette:	1–2 mg
Lethal dose:	50 mg
Absorption:	From lungs (instantaneous); more slowly from buccal mucosa
Half-life:	Levels fall rapidly, requiring new dose every 30–40 minutes in addicts
Other toxic substances:	Numerous carcinogens
Diseases of increased incidence and severity in smokers[2]	
Cancer of the lung (X 10)	
Chronic obstructive pulmonary disease (X 10) (chronic bronchitis and emphysema)	
Atheroslerotic arterial disease (X 2)	
Ischemic heart disease (angina and infarction)	
Cerebral thrombosis and infarction	
Thromboangiitis obliterans (Buerger's disease) (X 100)	
Chronic peptic ulcer (X 2–3)	
Cancer of the oral cavity and tongue (X 5)	
Cancer of the urinary bladder (X 5)	
Cancer of the larynx and pharynx (X 5)	
Cancer of the esophagus (X 5)	

[1]Modified from Christen AG, Cooper KH: Strategic withdrawal from cigarette smoking. *CA* 1979; **29**:96.

[2]Figures in parentheses = increased risk compared to the nonsmoking population.

Oral snuff and tobacco contain nicotine, which is absorbed through the oral mucosa into the bloodstream. Addiction results with regular use. Oral snuff and tobacco increase the risk of oral cancer and cause regression of the gums. It is of interest that Ruth died of oropharyngeal cancer at age 52.

Inhalation of cigarette smoke causes toxic effects in the upper respiratory tract and lungs; damage to distant organs occurs through absorption of toxic constituents into the bloodstream or their excretion in the urine. Most of the associations between smoking and disease have been established by statistical evidence. The exact mechanisms by which smoking causes these diseases are not known.

Cigarette smoking has been directly implicated as a cause of **chronic bronchitis** and **emphysema,** which constitute **chronic obstructive pulmonary disease (COPD).** Smoking is also an important contributory cause of **lung cancer,** particularly squamous carcinoma and small-cell undifferentiated (or oat cell) carcinoma. Although definite statistical associations have been established, the mechanisms involved and the specific compound associated with these 2 kinds of lung injury are still uncertain.

Cigarette smoking has also been statistically associated with the incidence of several **other cancers,** notably those of the bladder, oral cavity, larynx, and esophagus. Smoking is also a major risk factor for the development of **atherosclerotic vascular disease,** which leads to ischemic heart disease and cerebrovascular disease. Pipe smoking and tobacco chewing are associated with oral and gastric cancers.

PSYCHOTROPIC DRUG ABUSE

Types of Drugs Abused

Drug abuse is a major problem worldwide. The types of drugs abused include (1) stimulants such as cocaine and amphetamines; (2) depressants such as heroin, barbiturates, and benzodiazepines (eg, diazepam); and (3) hallucinogens such as marihuana, lysergic acid diethylamide (LSD), and phencyclidine (PCP). These drugs may be ingested, smoked, sniffed, injected into the skin ("skin-popping"), or injected intravenously (mainlining).

Effects

Drug abuse injures the body either directly or indirectly as a result of contaminated preparations, needles, etc.

A. Direct Effects: All of the psychotropic drugs have effects on the nervous system. The danger of overdose is exacerbated by the fact that different preparations of drugs available in the street contain unknown and variable concentrations of active drug. For example, some recent deaths in the USA have been attributed to the availability of a higher grade of cocaine, so that addicts ingesting what they thought was a customary dose in effect died of an overdose. Cocaine is particularly dangerous because it increases myocardial excitability and may cause ventricular fibrillation at relatively low blood levels.

The alteration in mental function often associated with psychotropic drugs such as cocaine, heroin, and PCP increases the risk of traffic accidents, criminal behavior, and acts of violence, including suicide, during states of acute intoxication. Habitual use of these drugs leads to emotional and physical dependence and severe withdrawal symptoms, which may include convulsions, if the drug is suddenly withheld.

B. Indirect Effects: Street drugs are not pure; the active principle is mixed with a variety of crystalline substances such as talc and sugar, and the agents used to "cut" (dilute) the drug frequently contain impurities such as cotton fibers. When contaminated preparations are injected, foreign body granulomas form around talc and cotton fibers that are deposited in tissues. For the pathologist, the presence of such lesions in the skin, alveolar septa, and portal triads in the liver on microscopic examination provides evidence of intravenous drug abuse.

Infection may be transmitted by unsterile needles shared by intravenous drug abusers. Causative organisms include staphylococci, which may cause local abscesses and cellulitis at sites of infection, bacteremia, and bacterial endocarditis; hepatitis B virus; and human immunodeficiency virus (HIV, the cause of AIDS). Fifteen to 20 percent of cases of AIDS in the USA have occurred in intravenous drug abusers.

C. Long-Term Effects: The chronic toxic effects of psychotropic drug abuse are not known with certainty. **Marihuana** smoking is believed to cause chronic bronchitis and abnormalities in bronchial epithelium. Although marihuana contains more carcinogens by weight than do cigarettes, it has not yet been shown to cause lung cancer. Changes in reproductive function have been reported with chronic marihuana abuse but have not been confirmed. **Cocaine** sniffing may cause atrophic changes in the nasal mucosa and perforation of the nasal septum. Chronic **heroin** usage may rarely be associated with focal glomerulonephritis. Although various abnormalities have been reported with chronic use of LSD and heroin, none have been conclusively established. Physicians who have become addicted to heroin and have abused pure heroin stolen from hospitals in the past have shown no chronic adverse changes even after prolonged use. The dangers of drug abuse therefore appear to center around acute overdose, dependence, and the effects of contaminants.

METALS

Lead Poisoning

A. Causes: Lead is used in the manufacture of batteries, paints of all types, and as a gasoline additive. Lead is a pervasive environmental pollutant. In 1979, an estimated 731,000 tons of lead were used in the USA, and a total in excess of 7 million tons have been used as gasoline additives in the USA. Much of this lead has been deposited on the ground. Unpolluted earth has an average of 15 mg/kg of lead. In comparison, surface soils in many large cities may contain over 500 mg/kg of lead; and house dust may contain up to 7.5 g/kg of lead—particularly in homes built before 1940, when lead-based paints were used. Lead in fumes generated from burning painted wood, newspapers, and magazines causes an increase in lead content of urban air. The levels in most cities are still far below toxic levels.

When absorbed by ingestion and inhalation, lead is deposited in tissues such as bone and kidney and accumulates there. Chronic toxicity occurs if there is more than 0.5 mg/d of lead intake. The MLD of absorbed lead is 0.5 g.

Toxic exposure to lead more commonly occurs (1) in workers in industries concerned with the processing or manufacturing of lead, batteries, paints, and gasoline; and (2) in young children, especially those living in poor socioeconomic conditions. The problem is widespread in nonindustrialized societies but also exists in the USA, where one study revealed elevated blood lead levels in nearly 20% of black children under 5 years of age living in poor urban areas. Children are exposed to lead in soil, paint, and water. Acute lead poisoning may occur in children who ingest large amounts of soil (this phenomenon, called pica, occurs in malnutrition, certain neurologic diseases, and rarely in otherwise normal children).

B. Effects: Acute lead poisoning is rare. Lead is typically ingested in small doses over a long period and accumulates to toxic levels that cause changes in many tissues of the body.

1. Erythrocytes–Lead inhibits several enzymes in the hemoglobin synthetic pathway, notably ferrochelatase, which brings about iron chelation to protoporphyrin. Serum free erythrocyte protoporphyrin, urinary coproporphyrin III, and δ-aminolevulinic acid levels are increased, providing useful tests for chronic lead poisoning. Impairment of hemoglobin synthesis leads to **anemia**. Red cells show decreased hemoglobin (hypochromia) and prominent basophilic stippling—the latter due to clumps of RNA resulting from inhibition of pyrimidine 5-nucleotidase, which permits accumulation of pyrimidine nucleotides and subsequently impairs degradation of RNA.

2. Nervous system–Involvement of the nervous system is the most significant toxic effect and occurs mainly in children. **Lead encephalopathy** is characterized by necrosis of neurons, edema, demyelination of white matter, and reactive proliferation of astrocytes. If severe, as in acute poisoning, convulsions may occur, leading to coma and death. In very young children, mental development is impaired. In adults, demyelination of motor peripheral nerves typically causes a motor neuropathy characterized by footdrop and wristdrop.

3. Kidney–Damage to the proximal renal tubular cells causes aminoaciduria and glycosuria. On histologic examination, injured tubular epithelial cells are characterized by diagnostic pink intranuclear inclusions composed of complexes of lead and protein.

4. Gastrointestinal tract–Lead produces severe contraction of the smooth muscle of the intestinal wall, which causes intense colicky pain and abdominal rigidity **(lead colic, "painter's cramps")**. This condition may mimic an acute surgical emergency of the abdomen.

5. Other affected areas–Deposition of lead in the gums causes a blue line to appear along the margins of the gums. Deposition in the epiphyseal region of growing bones in children produces dense areas on radiographs that are diagnostic of lead poisoning.

Mercury Poisoning

Although mercury is a common industrial waste product and the element is present in low concentration in seawater all over the world, mercury poisoning is rare. Ingestion of small amounts of mercury is not as dangerous as exposure to lead, because most of the mercury is excreted and does not accumulate in the body like lead. Mercury causes tissue damage by combining with sulfhydryl groups of various enzymes and interfering with mitochondrial ATP production.

A. Acute Mercury Poisoning: Acute poisoning commonly results from ingestion of mercuric chloride with suicidal intent or inhalation of metallic mercury vapor in industry. Mercury is also an ingredient in some insecticides and fungicides and contributes to the toxic effect if the substance is ingested, either directly from the container or indirectly as a contaminant of grain. Proximal renal tubular cells are the main target of acute mercury poisoning. Acute renal tubular necrosis causes profound renal failure. Ulcerations of the mouth, stomach, and colon—which may cause gastrointestinal bleeding—are additional findings.

B. Chronic Mercury Poisoning: Chronic poisoning occurs mainly in coastal areas affected by industrial pollution and in workers exposed to metallic mercury vapor in industry. Fish in polluted coastal areas become contaminated, and eating them may lead to chronic mercury poisoning. The best-known outbreak occurred in Minamata, Japan (Minamata disease). Mercury was previously used in the manufacture of hats, and workers frequently showed signs of poisoning. Neurologic manifestations are the predominant signs of chronic poisoning. Loss of neurons causes cerebral and cerebellar atrophy with dementia, emotional instability ("mad as a hatter"), failure of coordination, and visual and auditory disturbances.

Chronic toxicity is commonly manifested in the kidney as proteinuria and nephrotic syndrome due to glomerular abnormalities. Thickening of the basement membrane and proliferative changes in the glomerular cells have been described.

Aluminum Poisoning

Aluminum toxicity has been reported in hemodialysis patients using dialysates containing aluminum and in patients receiving long-term total parenteral nutrition with aluminum-containing casein hydrolysate. Aluminum is deposited in bone and causes osteomalacia by blocking normal calcification. Aluminum is also toxic to neurons and may lead to cerebral dysfunction (dementia).

Arsenic Poisoning

Arsenic was widely used as a poison by the Romans and others (eg, the Borgias in Renaissance Italy). Today, arsenic is a constituent of many agricultural pesticides (it is an effective rat poison), and chronic poisoning may occur in farm workers. Arsenic binds to sulfhydryl groups in proteins, leading to dysfunction of many enzymes involved in metabolism.

Acute poisoning is rare and almost always due to pesticide ingestion with suicidal intent. Large doses cause rapid death (often within a few hours) due to circulatory failure and derangement of vital energy-producing enzyme systems. Agonizingly severe abdominal pain and renal tubular necrosis often precede death.

Chronic ingestion of small amounts of arsenic leads to its accumulation in hair, skin, and nails, and examination of hair and nail samples for arsenic content is a sensitive diagnostic technique. The diagnosis of arsenic poisoning is confirmed by demonstration of high arsenic levels in urine. Chronic poisoning leads to changes in many tissues. (1) The skin shows increased pigmentation and focal thickening due to increased keratin formation (arsenical keratosis; Fig 12–3). Epidermal cells show abnormalities (dysplasia) such as increased size of nuclei, irregular clumping of chromatin, and variation in cell size. These changes predispose to the development of skin cancer (squamous carcinoma). (2) Nails show abnormal transverse ridges (Mees' lines). (3) Peripheral nerves demonstrate demyelinating neuropathy. (4) There is a higher incidence of hepatic angiosarcoma, a rare liver tumor.

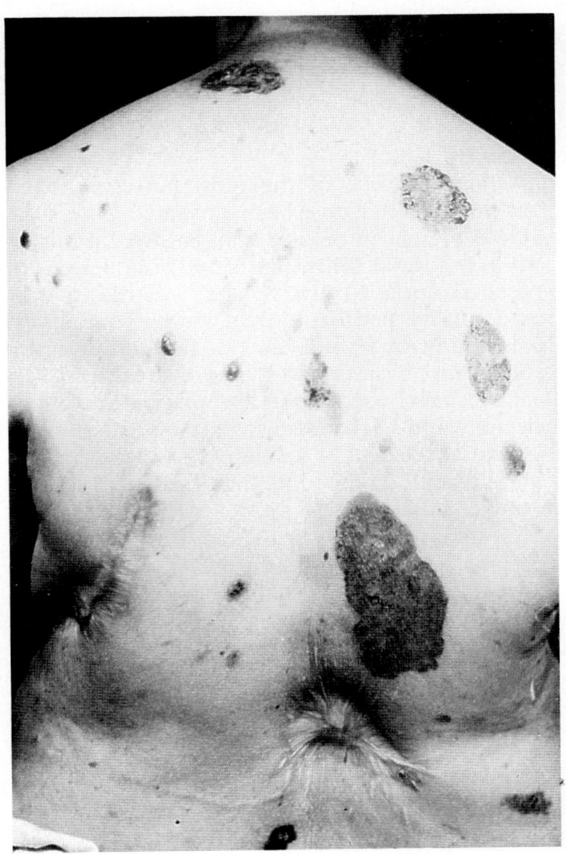

Figure 12–3. Arsenical keratosis. The largest lesion proved to be an infiltrating squamous carcinoma on biopsy.

INSECTICIDES & HERBICIDES

Insecticides are widely available in agriculture and in pesticides sold for home use. They are thus often used in suicide attempts and may contaminate the environment and food sources, eg, fish. Because of constant exposure to these agents, farm workers are at high risk. Accidental ingestion by children is common.

Insecticides may be absorbed into the blood from the skin (direct contact), lungs (inhalation), or intestine (ingestion). Small doses accumulate in the body and may lead to chronic poisoning.

The effects on tissues depend on the nature of the insecticide.

Chlorinated Hydrocarbons

Chlorinated hydrocarbon insecticides such as DDT and dieldrin are widely used. Acute ingestion of large doses causes mostly neurologic effects. An initial phase of stimulation characterized by delirium and convulsions is followed by neuronal damage leading to coma and death. Chronic exposure leads to accumulation in the liver, with fatty change; the long-term effect on the liver is unknown.

Organophosphates

Organophosphate insecticides such as malathion are acetylcholinesterase inhibitors that were originally developed for military use as nerve gases. Malathion is widely used in developing countries to control mosquitoes. Malathion spraying of large areas of populated land was recently carried out in California to control fruit fly infestation. Acute poisoning due to ingestion of large doses is rapidly fatal, because the anticholinesterase effect prevents transmission of neuromuscular impulses, with resulting muscular paralysis. Pupillary constriction and blurring of vision occur early. Abdominal cramps, diarrhea, salivation, sweating, and bronchoconstriction occur as a result of autonomic nerve dysfunction. The long-term effects of chronic low-level exposure are unknown.

Paraquat

Paraquat is a herbicide that is used less frequently than other similar preparations but is extremely dangerous if ingested. Within a few days after ingestion, acute illness develops that is characterized by ulceration of the oral mucosa, necrosis of the liver, renal tubular cells, and lung. Respiratory effects are the most serious and are due at least in part to interference with the action of pulmonary surfactant. In the acute phase, diffuse alveolar damage with hyaline membrane formation, pulmonary hemorrhage, and edema are noted. The acute phase rapidly progresses to diffuse pulmonary fibrosis and death, and the mortality rate is high.

• INDUSTRIAL CHEMICALS

A few of the more common industrial toxins are discussed below.

Methyl Alcohol (Methanol)

Methyl alcohol is widely used in some countries as a solvent and is added to laboratory-grade ethyl alcohol to make it undrinkable. Methyl alcohol is highly toxic, and a dose of 20 mL may be fatal. After absorption, it is metabolized by alcohol dehydrogenase to formaldehyde and formic acid, both of which are highly toxic and cause profound **metabolic acidosis**. With high doses, death occurs from various neurotoxic effects. With lower doses, the primary targets are the retina and optic nerve, which undergo irreversible degeneration by the direct toxic effect of formaldehyde that leads to blindness. Treatment of methyl alcohol toxicity is directed toward preventing conversion of methanol to formaldehyde. Ethyl alcohol is administered intravenously because it is metabolized in preference to methyl alcohol by alcohol dehydrogenase; this effectively blocks further metabolism of methyl alcohol.

Ethylene Glycol

Ethylene glycol is a common ingredient of antifreeze products. About 50 deaths a year occur in the USA as a result of ingestion of antifreeze by alcoholics. Ingestion causes severe **metabolic acidosis** that may lead to convulsions, coma, respiratory failure due to pulmonary edema, and death. Ethylene glycol is metabolized to calcium oxalate, which is deposited as crystals in many tissues. Deposition in the renal interstitium causes acute renal failure.

Carbon Tetrachloride

Carbon tetrachloride was at one time widely used as a solvent and dry-cleaning fluid and now has a more limited use in industry. It is absorbed into the bloodstream through inhalation or ingestion and has toxic effects in the brain (convulsions, coma), liver (necrosis of the central zone of the hepatic lobule with toxic hepatitis), and proximal renal tubular cells (acute renal failure).

Carbon Monoxide

Carbon monoxide is an inert gas that is a component of automobile exhaust fumes and a constituent of natural gas (coal gas) used for heating in some parts of the world. Carbon monoxide is frequently produced by improper combustion in household gas and paraffin heaters; inadequate ventilation may lead to accumulation of fatal levels in ambient air—and consequently in the bloodstream. Carbon monoxide poisoning is responsible for several hundred deaths annually in the USA. Cigarette smokers show higher than normal levels of carbon monoxide in the blood, which may be a contributory factor to the adverse effects of smoking.

Carbon monoxide combines with hemoglobin to form carboxyhemoglobin, which cannot carry oxygen, and tissue hypoxia results. Because carbon monoxide has an affinity for hemoglobin that is over 200 times that of oxygen, exposure to even small amounts of carbon monoxide rapidly depletes the oxygen-carrying capacity of the blood. Symptoms of hypoxia appear when 20% of blood hemoglobin has been converted to carboxyhemoglobin; death occurs when 70% of hemoglobin is affected. The manifestations of carbon monoxide poisoning are those of acute hypoxia involving the brain, eg, headache, confusion, visual disturbances, dizziness, convulsions, and coma. Cerebral edema may result from increased permeability of the hypoxic vessels. Poisoning can be recognized clinically by the cherry-red color of the blood, skin, and mucous membranes due to the presence of carboxyhemoglobin, which has a bright red color. In many cases, however, skin color is normal. The diagnosis of carbon monoxide poisoning is confirmed by the demonstration of carboxyhemoglobin in the blood.

Cyanide

Cyanide is one of the most powerful toxins known, the lethal dose being around 0.1 mg. Cyanide is present in organic combined form (amygdalin) in several fruits, particularly in the seeds of peaches, apricots, and berries. Laetrile, a drug used outside the USA to treat cancer, contains cyanide derivatives, and cases of fatal cyanide poisoning have occurred after Laetrile treatment. Cyanide is also used for electroplating and metal cleaning and in the manufacture of batteries. An industrial accident in India in 1984 released fumes of a cyanide compound that caused over 2000 deaths.

Cyanide combines with and inactivates cytochrome oxidase, the final enzyme in the respiratory chain, thereby blocking cellular energy production. Acute poisoning causes rapid death due to failure of cellular oxidative and respiratory processes.

• THERAPEUTIC AGENTS (Drugs)

Prescription Drugs

No drug is free from adverse effects, and the risk of toxicity must always be weighed against the drug's intended benefit.

A. Dose-Related Toxic Effects: Toxic effects are often dose-related. This relationship may be used to therapeutic advantage; eg, cytotoxic drugs are predictably toxic at certain known dosages. Drugs that kill cancerous cells also kill rapidly multiplying bone marrow cells; the decreased production of granulocytes increases the susceptibility to infection, but this risk is worth the benefit derived from killing the cancerous cells. Doxorubicin (Adriamycin), a powerful anticancer drug, causes myocardial toxicity, and the dosage must be carefully monitored to prevent cardiac failure. Chloramphenicol, an antibiotic, causes bone marrow depression at high dosage that is corrected when the drug is withdrawn.

B. Idiosyncratic Side Effects: With some drugs, toxicity may occur but is not predictable. Such toxicity is much more dangerous than dose-related toxicity, since it occurs unexpectedly and may arise with only small doses. Adverse effects, which may be irreversible and are often fatal, include the following: (1) Massive liver cell necrosis with use of halothane (a general anesthetic) or isoniazid (an antituberculous drug). (2) Acute interstitial renal disease and renal failure with use of methicillin, sulfonamides, and other drugs. (3) Bone marrow suppression (aplastic anemia) with use of chloramphenicol, phenylbutazone, and gold salts (used in treatment of rheumatoid arthritis). It should be noted that aplastic anemia resulting from an idiosyncratic reaction to chloramphenicol is more profound and less reversible than the dose-related bone marrow suppression that also occurs with this drug. (4) Lung fibrosis with use of anticancer drugs such as bleomycin and methotrexate and with nitrofurantoin (a urinary antiseptic). (5) Acute cardiac dysfunction with use of local anesthetic agents such as procaine.

C. Allergic or Hypersensitivity Reactions: Allergic reactions are often unpredictable, though a history of sensitization may sometimes be elicited. The mechanisms of sensitization are described in Chapter 8. Clinical manifestations are diverse. **Anaphylaxis** is the most serious reaction and occurs most commonly with use of penicillin and foreign serum. **Rashes** are the most common adverse reaction and take a variety of forms, often urticarial or eczematous. Rarely, skin involvement may be so severe that extensive skin necrosis occurs (Stevens-Johnson syndrome). This may result from numerous drugs, including penicillin and sulfonamides. **Hemolytic anemia, thrombocytopenia, glomerulonephritis,** and various other autoimmune diseases may also be due to drug hypersensitivity.

Commonly Used Drugs

Many drugs are sold without prescription, ie, over-the-counter. These include **analgesics** and mild **antihistamines** for use in the treatment of headaches, common colds, and allergies. Although these drugs are safe for ordinary use, they can be dangerous, and toxic effects have been recognized with use of some of them. Other drugs, such as oral contraceptive agents, though they are prescription drugs, are freely used by a large number of people.

A. Aspirin: Aspirin (and other salicylates) are consumed in large amounts worldwide. At therapeutic dosage levels, aspirin is safe, but overdoses can be fatal. Deaths of young children who consumed 10–12 adult-dose (325 mg) tablets were instrumental in spurring the development of childproof packaging. The fatal dose for an adult is 15 g.

Aspirin stimulates respiration and produces an initial **respiratory alkalosis**. As aspirin accumulates in the bloodstream, it overwhelms the acid-buffering capacity of the circulation and causes **metabolic acidosis**. Aspirin also alters platelet function to produce a bleeding tendency. Erosive acute gastritis is common and may cause severe hemorrhage. Recently, aspirin use in children following viral infections such as chickenpox and influenza has been linked to the occurrence of **Reye's syndrome,** characterized by acute fatty change of the liver with liver failure and encephalopathy, and associated with a high mortality rare.

B. Abuse of Phenacetin-Containing Analgesics: Chronic abuse of analgesics containing a mixture of aspirin and phenacetin (formerly popular worldwide) has been associated with renal papillary damage. In the acute phase, renal papillary necrosis may cause acute renal failure. With chronic ingestion, interstitial fibrosis and calcification of renal papillae occur and may result in chronic renal failure. Phenacetin has been removed from many proprietary analgesic preparations in the USA.

C. Acetaminophen (Paracetamol): Acetaminophen (known as paracetamol outside the USA) is a drug widely used for alleviation of minor pains and fever. Overdosage causes massive dose-related hepatic necrosis that is often fatal. Acetaminophen is metabolized in the liver by a glutathione-dependent enzyme system. High doses of acetaminophen exhaust the supply of glutathione and result in production of toxic metabolites that cause liver cell necrosis; the actual toxic dose is determined by the amount of glutathione available. In alcoholics, the toxic dose is lower than in normal individuals and may not be much higher than the therapeutic dose.

D. Oral Contraceptives: Though oral contraceptives are prescription drugs, they are freely available. Early preparations contained high levels of estrogen that were later acknowledged to cause several adverse effects, including (1) an increased incidence of thrombotic complications, including arterial and venous thrombosis and pulmonary embolism; (2) liver lesions, including focal nodular hyperplasia, liver cell adenoma, and (rarely) liver cell carcinoma; and (3) an increased incidence of gallstone disease with gallstone formation due to cholesterol supersaturation of bile induced by estrogens.

Modern oral contraceptives have low levels of estrogen, which may result in a greatly lowered risk of these adverse effects. There was great concern in the past about whether contraceptives containing female sex hormones would increase hormone-induced or hormone-dependent cancers. It now appears that women taking oral contraceptives have no increased risk of endometrial and ovarian cancer. The relationship between breast cancer and oral contraceptive use is still controversial, but present evidence is not ominous.

Infectious Diseases: I. Mechanisms of Tissue Changes in Infection

13

Infection is the entry and multiplication of a parasitic agent in a host. **Infectious disease** results when tissue damage occurs or when host inflammatory and immune responses are evoked. The outcome of an infection is influenced by 2 opposing factors: the ability of the agent to overcome host defenses and the ability of the host to resist infection (Fig 13–1).

Specific infectious diseases are considered in detail in the organ system chapters, which explain the functional changes arising from infection in these organs. This chapter discusses the various classes of infectious agents and the manifestations of disease occurring in tissues infected by them. Tables 13–6 and 13–7 together correlate specific agents, their reproductive characteristics, the diseases they cause, and common sites of infection with the various manifestations of tissue injury and the body's response to infection.

CLASSIFICATION OF INFECTIOUS AGENTS

Classification According to Structure

Infectious agents can be arranged in order of increasing structural complexity, beginning with viruses and proceeding through rickettsiae, chlamydiae, mycoplasmas, bacteria, fungi, algae, and protozoa to metazoa (Table 13–1). Protozoa and metazoa are sometimes collectively termed parasites, though the designation parasite is sometimes also used more generally to describe all infectious agents. The major groups of agents that cause human disease are summarized in this chapter. Individual agents are discussed in the appropriate organ system chapter and cross-referenced in Table 13–7.

Each group of infectious agents can be further subdivided on the basis of several additional classification criteria (Table 13–1). For example, **viruses** are classified as RNA and DNA viruses on the basis of the type of nucleic acid in their genomes. **Bacteria** are divided into cocci, rods (bacilli), spirochetes, and vibrios on the basis of their shape; they are termed gram-positive or gram-negative on the basis of their reaction on Gram staining; and they are called aerobic or anaerobic on the basis of their oxygen requirement for growth. **Rickettsiae** and **chlamydiae** are small bacteria that are obligate intracellular parasites. **Fungi** may be yeasts, molds (mycelial fungi), or dimorphic fungi (having both yeast and mold forms). **Protozoa** and **metazoa** are classified into genera and species according to structural criteria.

Classification According to Pathogenicity

The ability of an infectious agent to establish itself in tissues is called **infectivity,** and its ability to cause disease is called **pathogenicity**. Pathogenic agents can be classified as low-grade or high-grade pathogens; the latter are said to be **virulent**. The distinction is important, because although virulent organisms may readily cause dis-

Table 13-1. Infectious agents of humans, classified according to structure.

Group	Cellular Complexity	Type of Nucleic Acid	Additional Classification Criteria	Major Pathogenic Types	Growth Characteristics	Culture Requirements
Viruses	Virion	Either DNA or RNA	DNA or RNA Size Morphology Immunologic	Adenovirus, herpesvirus, poxvirus, papovavirus, arbovirus, myxovirus, retrovirus, picornavirus, etc	Obligate intracellular	Grow only in tissue culture.
Rickettsiae	Simple cells (prokaryotes)	Both DNA and RNA	Immunologic	*Rickettsia prowazekii, Rickettsia tsutsugamushi, Rickettsia rickettsii, Coxiella burnetii*	Obligate intracellular	Grow only in tissue culture.
Chlamydiae	Simple cells (prokaryotes)	Both DNA and RNA	Immunologic	*Chlamydia psittaci, Chlamydia trachomatis*	Obligate intracellular	Grow only in tissue culture.
Bacteria (including mycoplasmas, spirochetes, vibrios)	Simple cells (prokaryotes)	Both DNA and RNA	Morphology (cocci, bacilli, spirochetes, etc) Gram stain Oxygen requirement Biochemical reactions Immunologic	*Staphylococcus, Streptococcus, Neisseria, Clostridium, Corynebacterium,* enterobacteria, *Brucella, Haemophilus, Yersinia, Salmonella, Mycobacterium, Bacteroides, Vibrio, Mycoplasma,* etc	Some are intracellular; some are extracellular.	Most grow on artificial media.

Fungi	Complex cells (eukaryotes)	Both DNA and RNA	Morphology Type of spores	Dermatophytes, *Aspergillus, Mucor, Candida, Coccidioides, Histoplasma, Cryptococcus, Blastomyces*	Some are intracellular; some are extracellular	Most grow on artificial media.
Algae	Complex cells (eukaryotes)	Both DNA and RNA		Rarely infect humans		Not routinely cultured; many cannot be cultured.
Protozoa	Complex cells (eukaryotes)	Both DNA and RNA	Morphology Sexual cycle	Amebas, *Giardia, Trichomonas, Trypanosoma, Leishmania, Toxoplasma, Plasmodium, Pneumocystis, Cryptosporidium, Isospora*	Some are intracellular; some are extracellular	Not routinely cultured; a few cannot be cultured.
Metazoa Helminths and flukes	Multicellular parasites	Both DNA and RNA	Morphology (flat and round worms)	*Taenia, Ascaris, Enterobius, Trichuris, Necator, Strongyloides, Echinococcus, Trichinella, Clonorchis, Schistosoma, Wuchereria, Brugia*	Extracellular	Cannot be cultured.
Insecta, Arachnida	Multicellular parasites	Both DNA and RNA	Morphology	*Sarcoptes scabiei*, fleas, and ticks	Extracellular	Cannot be cultured.

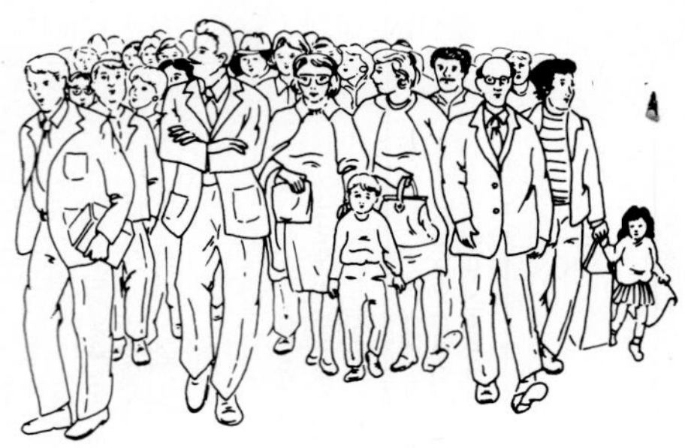

Factors related to the infectious agent

- Succesful transmission to host
- Site of attack
- Number of organisms
- Pathogenicity
  - Ability to invade tissues
  - Toxin production
  - Multiplication
  - Resistance to host defense mechanisms
  - Ability to cause necrosis
  - Enzyme release

Factors related to the host

- General factors
  - Age[1]
  - Racial factors[2]
  - Nutritional status
  - Diseases predisposing to infections: diabetes mellitus, chronic renal failure
- Natural defenses
  - Integrity of skin and mucosa
  - Mucus, ciliary action, normal flow of mucus, urine, etc
  - Normal microbial flora (broad-spectrum antibiotics may lead to resistant infections)
- Inflammation
  - Leukocytes
  - Effectiveness of phagocytosis and microbial killing
- Immune status
  - Immunization (or lack of) against organism in question
  - Lymphocytes (immune deficiency diseases)
  - Complement

Figure 13–1. The outcome of infection of a host by an infectious agent depends on the interrelationships of many factors related to both the agent and the host. **Note 1:** Age is an important factor. Although children contract many infections, this is because they more frequently encounter organisms that are "new" to them. **Note 2:** Racial factors may reflect exposure of a population to an infectious agent during evolution; eg, Pacific Islanders and Native Americans succumbed to measles and tuberculosis when first exposed, probably because of lack of previous encounters with organisms causing these diseases. Sometimes, the relationship is more complex; individuals in areas endemic for *Plasmodium falciparum,* a malarial parasite, have an increased incidence of deficiency of glucose-6-phosphatase in their erythrocytes, presumably because this has given them an advantage in their interaction with the parasite.

ease in normal people, low-grade pathogens cause disease only in immunocompromised hosts **(opportunistic infections)**. Such individuals lack resistance to various agents that typically do not cause illness in immunocompetent people.

Classification According to Site of Multiplication

The ability of infectious agents to multiply inside or outside cells can be used as a basis for classification (Table 13–2). This scheme is useful in understanding the host response to infection, because the types of inflammatory and immune responses elicited by infection are largely determined by the site of multiplication of the agent.

A. Obligate Intracellular Organisms: Obligate intracellular organisms can grow and multiply only in host cells and require the metabolic apparatus of the host cell for growth. They infect parenchymal cells in particular. Culture of such organisms requires living cell systems, eg, embryonated eggs, tissue cell culture, or laboratory animals.

B. Facultative Intracellular Organisms: Facultative intracellular organisms are capable of both extracellular and intracellular growth and multiplication. Intracellular growth usually occurs in macrophages. The multiplication pattern in these organisms ranges from that of *Mycobacterium leprae,* which almost never multiplies outside cells, to that of *Actinomyces israelii,* which rarely multiplies intracellularly. Most of the agents in this group can be cultured on artificial media; an exception is *M leprae,* which cannot be grown on artificial media or in cell culture.

C. Extracellular Organisms: As the name implies, extracellular organisms multiply outside cells. Except for the larger parasites, which cannot be cultured at all, extracellular organisms can be cultured on artificial media. *Treponema pallidum,* the spirochete that causes syphilis, also cannot be cultured.

TISSUE CHANGES IN INFECTION

When a tissue is infected, pathologic changes (and disease) may result from the combined effects of cellular damage induced by the infectious agent, the host inflammatory response, and the

Table 13-2. Classification of infectious agents according to site of multiplication in tissues.

Obligate Intracellular Organisms	Facultative Intracellular Organisms	Extracellular Organisms
All viruses All rickettsiae All chlamydiae Protozoa[1]	Mycobacteria *Mycobacterium leprae* *Mycobacterium tuberculosis* Atypical mycobacteria *Brucella* species *Actinomyces; Nocardia* species *Kelbsiella rhinoscleromatis* *Francisella tularensis* *Pseudomonas mallei* and *Pseudomonas pseudomallei* *Salmonella typhi* Fungi *Coccidioides immitis* *Histoplasma capsulatum* *Cryptococcus neoformans* *Blastomyces dermatitidis* *Paracoccidioides brasiliensis* *Sporothrix schenckii* Protozoa[1]	*Mycoplasma* All bacteria except those listed as facultative intracellular organisms Fungi *Candida albicans* *Aspergillus* species *Mucor* species Other mycelial fungi Protozoa except those listed in footnote[1] All metazoan parasites

[1]*Leishmania, Trypanosoma, Plasmodium,* and *Toxoplasma* are difficult to classify as either obligate or facultative intracellular organisms. In humans, they typically reproduce intracellularly; *Trypanosoma* and *Plasmodium* multiply in parenchymal cells and *Leishmania* and *Toxoplasma* in macrophages.

host immune response (Fig 13–2). Infection does not necessarily cause disease, however. In **latent infections,** the causative agent, often a virus, remains dormant in infected cells without causing any cell damage. At a later date—often years after the primary infection—evidence of disease may appear as a result of reactivation of the infectious agent.

Tissue Damage Caused by Infectious Agents

Direct tissue damage produced by infectious agents is an important cause of pathologic changes. The extent of direct damage is a function of the agent's virulence; highly virulent organisms such as *Yersinia pestis* (the etiologic agent of plague) cause rapid, extensive tissue necrosis. The mechanisms producing tissue damage differ with the various infectious agents.

A. Obligate Intracellular Organisms: When viruses infect cells, they cause various changes, as shown in Fig 13–3. Rickettsiae and chlamydiae also replicate in cells, causing many of the changes seen in viral infections.

1. Cell necrosis–Infection of a cell by an obligate intracellular agent results in acute necrosis when replication of the agent is accompanied by a lethal abnormality in cell function. Different pathogenic agents have affinity for different parenchymal cells (organotropism). Even when an agent infects many different cell types, damage may occur only in some cell types; eg, in poliovirus infection, the main site of infection and viral replication is the intestinal mucosa, whereas the clinical picture is dominated by damage to motor neurons in the spinal cord and brain stem. The various manifestations of clinical disease arise from the different cell types injured in viral infections (Table 13–3). Similar diseases may be produced by different agents causing acute necrosis of one particular cell type; thus, acute hepatitis may be caused by any of several different types of viruses, but the clinical presentation is similar for all of the agents.

In obligate intracellular infections associated with acute cell necrosis, patients may die in the acute phase of illness (eg, due to encephalitis, myocarditis, or massive liver cell necrosis), or they may recover. Recovery is due mainly to an effective immune response that neutralizes the virus. Return to normal function occurs unless necrotic cells are unable to regenerate, as occurs in encephalitis, in which loss of neurons leads to a residual neurologic deficit.

Less frequently, viral infection (or the immune response against the virus) causes slow cell necrosis over a long period, sometimes years. These **persistent viral infections** occur in the liver (chronic persistent and chronic active viral hepatitis, which may be caused by hepatitis B and hepatitis non-A, non-B viruses) and in the brain, where they are characterized by slowly progressive loss of neurons. These so-called **slow virus infections** include subacute sclerosing panencephalitis

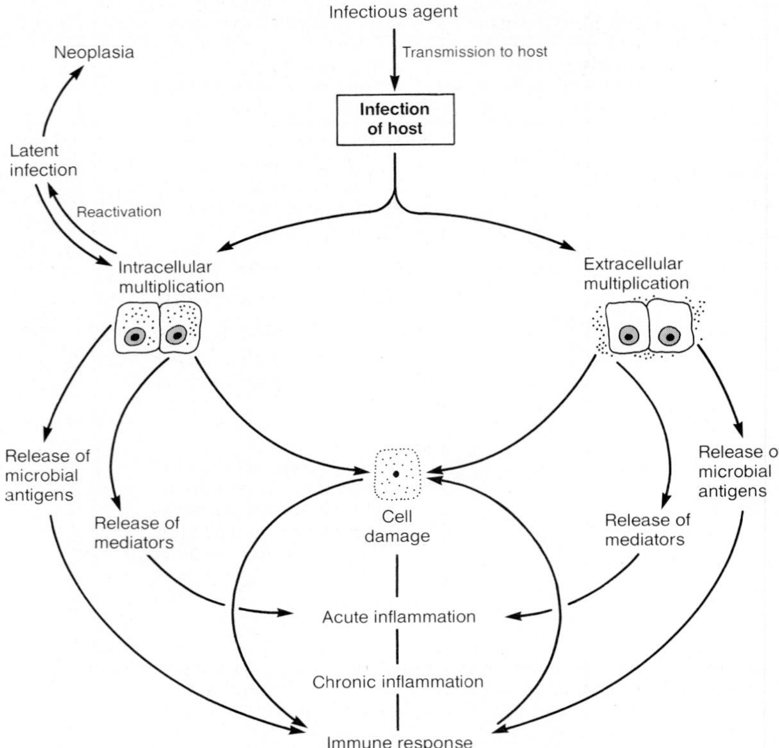

Figure 13-2. Mechanisms of cell damage and disease causation in infectious diseases. Note that the protective effects of inflammation and the immune response are not shown in this diagram.

Table 13-3. Organotropism of obligate intracellular organisms.

Tissue Injured	Disease	Commonly Associated Obligate Intracellular Agents
Nervous system		
Brain (diffusely)	Acute encephalitis	Arboviruses (several types) Herpes simplex, cytomegalovirus[1]
	Subacute sclerosing panencephalitis	Measles virus
Hippocampal gyrus	Rabies	Rabies virus
Motor neurons of brain stem and spinal cord	Poliomyelitis	Poliovirus
White matter	Progressive multifocal leukoencephalopathy	Human papovavirus[1]
Leptomeninges	Acute viral meningitis	Mumps virus Poliovirus Lymphocytic choriomeningitis virus
Skin and mucous membranes		
Epidermis (vesicular rashes)	Chickenpox, shingles	Varicella-zoster virus
	Smallpox	Variola virus
	Vaccinia	Vaccinia virus
	Common wart	Human papillomavirus
	Molluscum contagiosum	Molluscum contagiosum virus

Table 13-3. Organotropism of obligate intracellular organisms. **Cont'd.**

Tissue Injured	Disease	Commonly Associated Obligate Intracellular Agents
Oropharynx	Herpetic stomatitis	Herpes simplex type 1
	Herpangina	Coxsackievirus type A
Upper respiratory tract	Coryza (common cold)	Rhinovirus
	Viral pharyngotonsillitis	Influenza and parainfluenza viruses Adenovirus Epstein-Barr virus
External genitalia	Herpes genitalis	Herpes simplex type 2
	Nongonococcal urethritis	*Chlamydia trachomatis* (types D–K)
	Lymphogranuloma venereum	*C trachomatis* (types L1–L3)
	Condyloma acuminatum (genital wart)	Human papillomavirus
Conjunctiva	Acute conjunctivitis	Herpesviruses Adenovirus Enteroviruses *C trachomatis* (types D–K)
	Trachoma	*C trachomatis* (types A–C)
Dermis	Measles (rubeola)	Measles virus
	Rubella (German measles)	Rubella virus
Parotid salivary gland	Acute parotitis	Mumps virus
Lower respiratory tract Bronchioles Alveoli	Acute bronchiolitis Viral pneumonitis	Influenza and parainfluenza viruses Adenovirus Respiratory syncytial virus Cytomegalovirus[1]
	Psittacosis	*Chlamydia psittaci*
	Q fever	*Coxiella burnetii*
Pleura, chest wall	Pleurodynia	Coxsackievirus
Gastrointestinal tract, liver, pancreas Intestinal mucosa	Viral gastroenteritis	Rotavirus
Liver	Acute viral hepatitis	Hepatitis A, B, non-A, non-B viruses Delta agent Cytomegalovirus (neonatal hepatitis) Yellow fever
	Q fever	*C burnetii*
	Chronic viral hepatitis	Hepatitis B virus Hepatitis non-A, non-B virus
Lymphoid system B lymphocyte	Infectious mononucleosis	Epstein-Barr virus
T lymphocyte	Japanese T cell lymphoma	Human T cell lymphotropic virus type I
	HIV infection (AIDS, AIDS-related complex)	Human immunodeficiency virus
Cardiovascular system Myocardium	Acute myocarditis	Coxsackievirus type B
Pericardium	Acute viral pericarditis	Coxsackieviruses
Small vessel endothelium	Hemorrhagic fevers	Arboviruses
	Typhus fever	Rickettsiae

[1]In immunocompromised hosts.

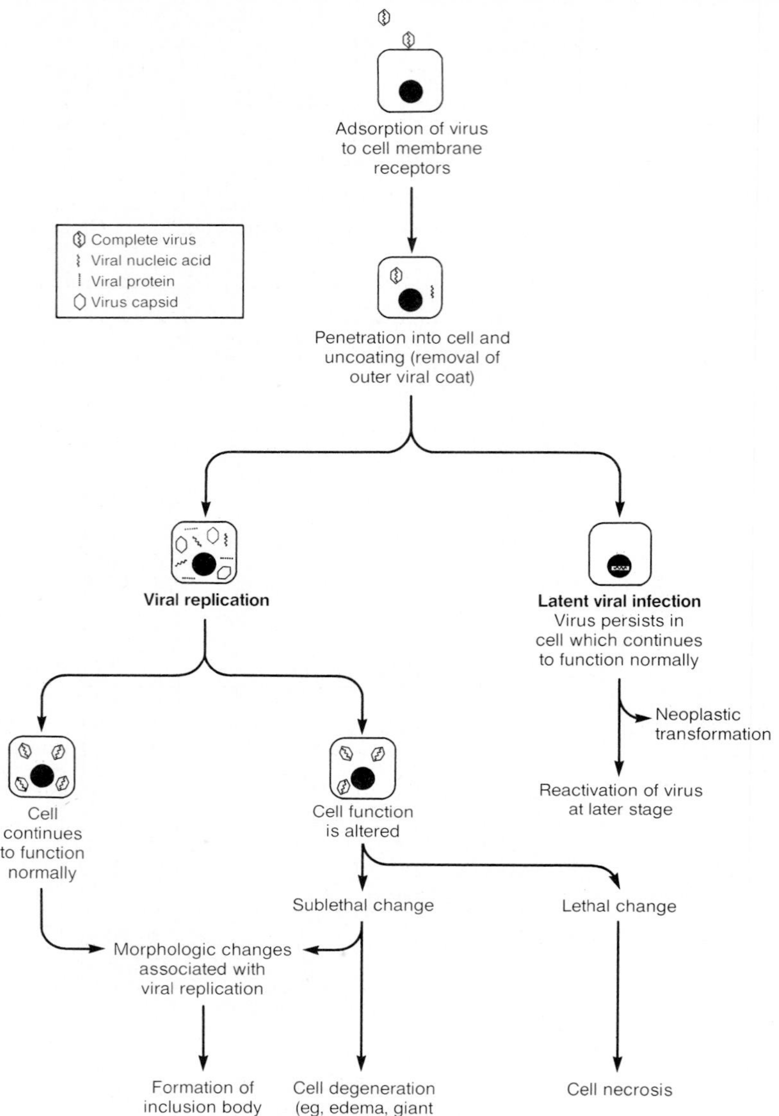

Figure 13-3. Some possible pathologic consequences of infection of a cell by a virus.

(caused by measles virus), kuru, and Creutzfeldt-Jakob disease.

2. Cell swelling-Sublethal injury caused by obligate intracellular agents leads to various types of cellular degeneration, most commonly swelling. For example, diffuse swelling of surviving hepatocytes accompanies cell necrosis in acute viral hepatitis. Rickettsiae tend to grow in endothelial cells and cause endothelial cell swelling that may lead to thrombosis and hemorrhage.

3. Inclusion body formation-Inclusion bodies are sometimes formed during viral and chlamydial replication in cells. They are visible on light microscopy and represent somewhat crude evidence of the presence of infection by obligate intracellular agents. They are composed either of assembled viral particles or of remnants of viral nucleic acid synthesis. Inclusion bodies occur in the nucleus or the cytoplasm and aid in the diagnosis of specific viral infections in histologic examination of tissues (Table 13-4; Figs 13-4, 13-5, and 13-6). In hepatitis B virus infection, the cytoplasm of infected hepatocytes has a ground-glass appearance (Fig 13-7A) and shows positive staining with orcein (Shikata) stain (Fig 13-7B) and with anti-hepatitis B antibodies when immunologic techniques are used. Immunologic techniques (eg, immunoperoxidase staining; Fig 13-8) that detect viral antigens and molecular biology techniques such as the use of DNA or RNA probes that recognize specific viral nucleic acid sequences are more sensitive methods of detecting

Table 13-4. Characteristic histologic changes produced in cells infected by obligate intracellular agents.

Infectious Agents	Histologic Features
Cytomegalovirus (Figs 13-4, 13-8)	Enlargement of cell (cytomegaly). Eosinophilic, large intranuclear inclusion surrounded by a halo.[1] Small, multiple, granular, basophilic cytoplasmic inclusions.
Herpes simplex virus (Fig 13-5) and varicella-zoster virus	Large, eosinophilic intranuclear inclusion surrounded by a halo.[1] Nuclei with ground-glass appearance. Multinucleated (3-8 nuclei) giant cells.
Variola (smallpox) virus	Multiple, granular, round, eosinophilic cytoplasmic inclusions (Guarnieri bodies).
Rabies virus	Round, 2-10 μm, eosinophilic cytoplasmic inclusions (Negri bodies).
Hepatitis B virus (Fig. 13-7)	Cytoplasm with ground-glass appearance.
Measles virus (Fig 13-9)	Multinucleated (10-50 nuclei) Warthin-Finkeldey giant cells. Small eosinophilic intranuclear inclusions.
Molluscum contagiosum virus	Homogeneous eosinophilic cytoplasmic inclusion that fills the cell, pushing the nucleus aside.
Chlamydia (Fig 13-6)	Small, multiple, eosinophilic cytoplasmic inclusions.

[1]Also called Cowdry A inclusions. Though most commonly seen in herpesvirus infections, Cowdry A inclusions are not pathognomonic for herpesviruses; they may occasionally be produced by other viruses.

virus in infected cells. These methods are useful in the diagnosis of viral infections when light microscopy fails to show diagnostic features.

4. Giant cell formation–The formation of multinucleated giant cells occurs in some viral infections. Measles virus produces massively enlarged cells (Warthin-Finkeldey giant cells) that contain 20–100 small uniform nuclei (Fig 13–9). These cells may be seen in any tissue infected by the measles virus, commonly the lung and lymphoid tissues of the appendix and tonsil. Herpes simplex and varicella-zoster infections produce giant cells in infected stratified squamous epithelial cells (skin, mouth, external genitalia, and esophagus). These cells have 3–8 nuclei that either have a glassy appearance or contain Cowdry A inclusions (Fig 13–5).

5. Latent viral infection–Many viruses can remain latent in the infected cell, often for the lifetime of the host. Reactivation of latent infection may occur at any time, however.

a. Reactivation–Herpes simplex and varicella-zoster viruses tend to remain latent in sensory ganglia that have been infected during the primary infection. Repeated reactivation may occur for various reasons (stress, trauma, coexistent disease, immunodeficiency); virus then migrates via the nerves to the skin or mucosa, where cell necrosis occurs and blisters form. Viral reactivation in herpes simplex type 1 infection causes ulcerating blisters (cold sores or fever blisters) that typically occur around the lips. Following an attack of chickenpox in childhood, varicella-zoster virus may remain dormant in dorsal ganglia, to become manifest as zoster (shingles) as late as 40 years after the childhood disease.

b. Oncogenesis (production of neoplasms)–(See Chapter 19.) Some viruses are thought to cause neoplasms in animals (eg, Rous sarcoma virus, mouse mammary tumor virus) and humans. Epstein-Barr virus has been implicated as a cause

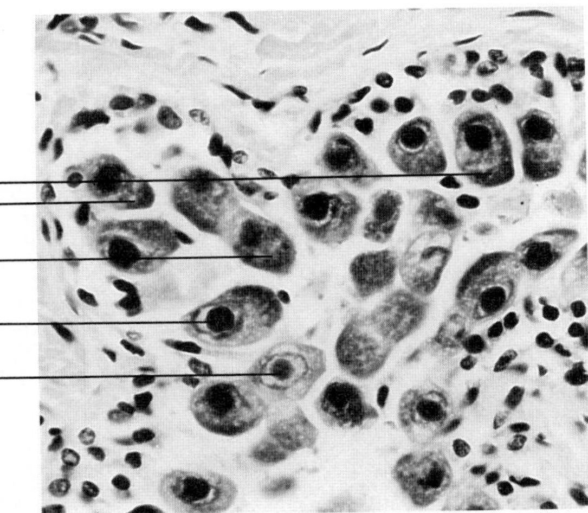

Figure 13-4. Prostate epithelial cells, showing infection with cytomegalovirus. Nearly all of the cells are infected and show marked enlargement. Many cells show small, granular cytoplasmic inclusions as well as large intranuclear inclusions surrounded by a halo.

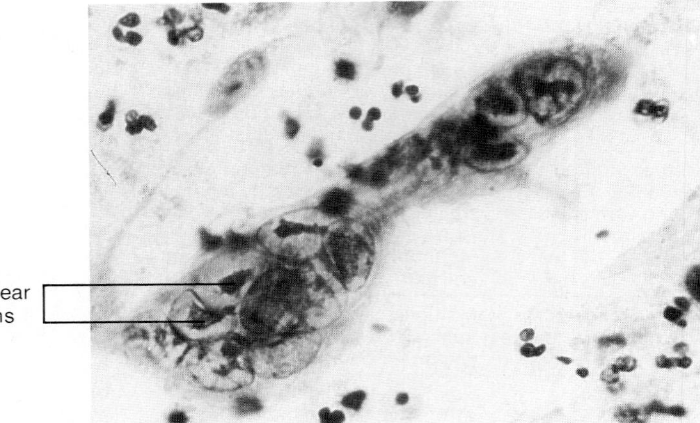

Figure 13-5. Papanicolaou smear from the uterine cervix, showing infection of epithelial cells by herpes simplex virus. Note the multinucleated giant cell and the large intranuclear (Cowdry A) inclusions.

of Burkitt's lymphoma and nasopharyngeal carcinoma; the retrovirus human T cell lymphotropic virus type I (HTLV-I) is thought to cause Japanese T cell lymphoma.

B. Facultative Intracellular Organisms: Facultative intracellular organisms such as mycobacteria and fungi frequently cause tissue damage and undoubtedly possess mechanisms that give them the capability of causing cell damage. These mechanisms are not well understood. Much of the tissue effects of facultative intracellular organisms are attributed to the inflammatory (commonly granuloma formation), immune (delayed hypersensitivity responsible for caseous necrosis), and healing (fibrosis) responses to these infections.

B. Extracellular Organisms: Extracellular organisms such as bacteria, fungi, and protozoa cause cell injury in one of several ways (Fig 13–10).

1. Release of locally acting enzymes-As they multiply, virulent organisms produce many enzymes that are liberated into the tissues, where they break down various substrate molecules. The specific enzymes that cause pathologic changes are not defined in many bacterial infections. In others, information derived from in vitro studies of bacteria may be used to explain tissue changes resulting from infection.

Staphylococcus aureus produces coagulase, which converts fibrinogen to fibrin. Coagulase production is closely linked to virulence, and coag-

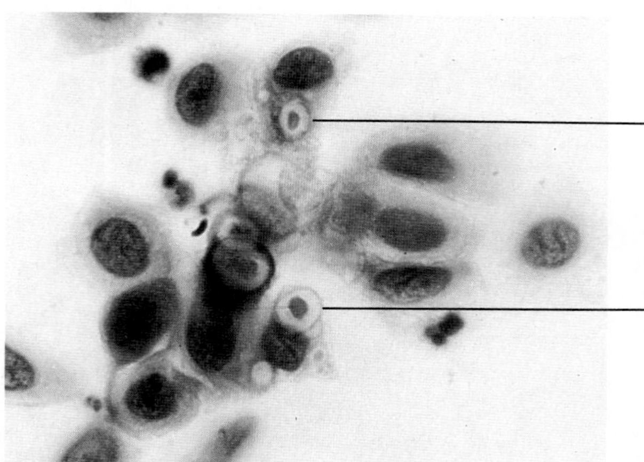

Figure 13-6. Papanicolaou smear from uterine cervix, showing infection of epithelial cells by *Chlamydia trachomatis*. Note the presence of intracytoplasmic inclusions in the infected cells.

A

Ground-glass cells

B

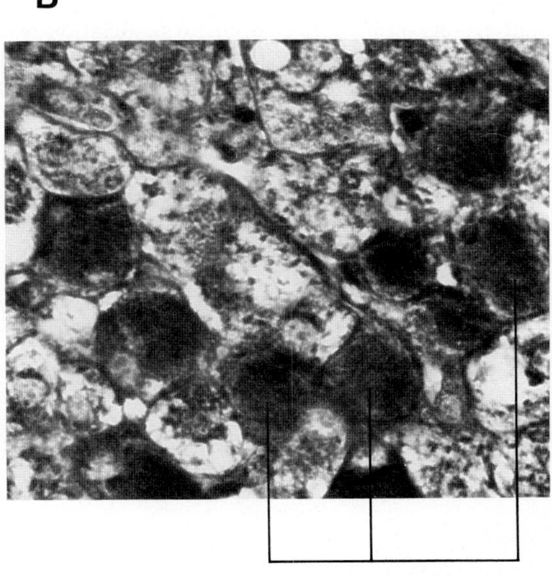

Figure 13–7. A: Hepatitis B virus infection of the liver, showing typical ground-glass change in cytoplasm. **B:** Hepatitis B virus infection of liver, showing positive cytoplasmic staining with orcein (Shikata) stain. Immunocytochemical methods may also be used to demonstrate the presence of virus.

ulase-negative staphylococci (eg, *Staphylococcus epidermidis*) have low virulence. In vivo, coagulase is believed to cause the bacterium to become coated with a layer of fibrin that may increase its ability to resist phagocytosis. This resistance to phagocytosis may be linked not only to the virulence of staphylococci but also to their tendency to cause suppurative inflammation with tissue necrosis.

Streptococcus pyogenes produces hyaluronidase, which degrades hyaluronic acid in ground substance and facilitates the spread of infection; streptokinase, which activates plasminogen and promotes breakdown of fibrin; and several hemolysins that hemolyze erythrocytes. These enzymes are responsible for the spreading nature characteristic of streptococcal infections and the thin, blood-stained exudate that may occur.

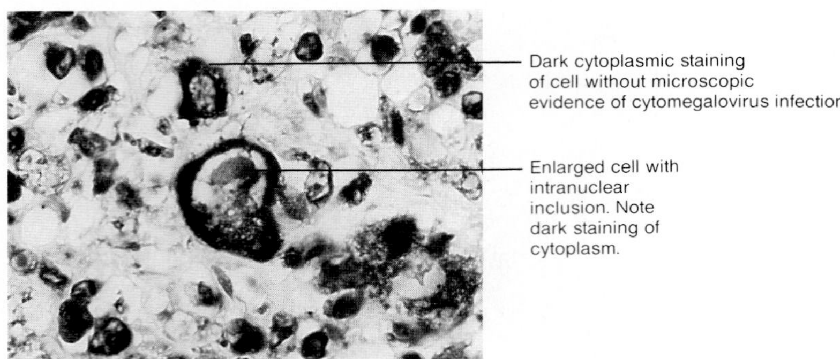

Figure 13-8. Cytomegalovirus infection revealed by an immunocytochemical (immunoperoxidase) method using antibody against cytomegalovirus. Positive (dark) staining of viral antigen is seen in many cells, including some that do not have morphologic evidence of infection.

Clostridium perfringens, which causes gas gangrene, produces many enzymes, including lecithinase, which breaks down cell membrane lipid and causes cell necrosis; hyaluronidase; collagenase, which degrades collagen; and hemolysins. These enzymes are largely responsible for the severe spreading necrotizing inflammation that characterizes gas gangrene. Gas production in tissues is the result of fermentation of sugars during growth of the bacterium.

2. Production of local vasculitis-Highly virulent organisms—eg, anthrax bacillus *(Bacillus anthracis), Aspergillus,* and *Mucor*—may infect and cause thrombosis of local small vessels and cause ischemic necrosis in and around the area of infection.

3. Production of remotely acting toxins- Some bacteria produce toxins that are carried in the circulation to cause cell injury far removed from the point of infection.

a. Endotoxins-Endotoxins are lipopolysaccharide components of the cell walls of gram-negative bacteria that are released into the bloodstream after the death and lysis of bacteria. In the blood, endotoxins act on small blood vessels to cause generalized peripheral vasodilatation (leading to circulatory failure and shock), endothelial cell damage, and activation of the coagulation cascade (resulting in disseminated intravascular coagulation). Endotoxins also cause fever and activate the complement system. Endotoxic (gram-negative) shock most commonly follows severe urinary tract infections or intestinal surgery, but it may occur in association with any gram-negative infection.

b. Exotoxins-Exotoxins are substances (often proteins) actively secreted by living bacteria that are released into the environment surrounding the organism and often exert their toxic effects at a site distant from their origin after distribution by

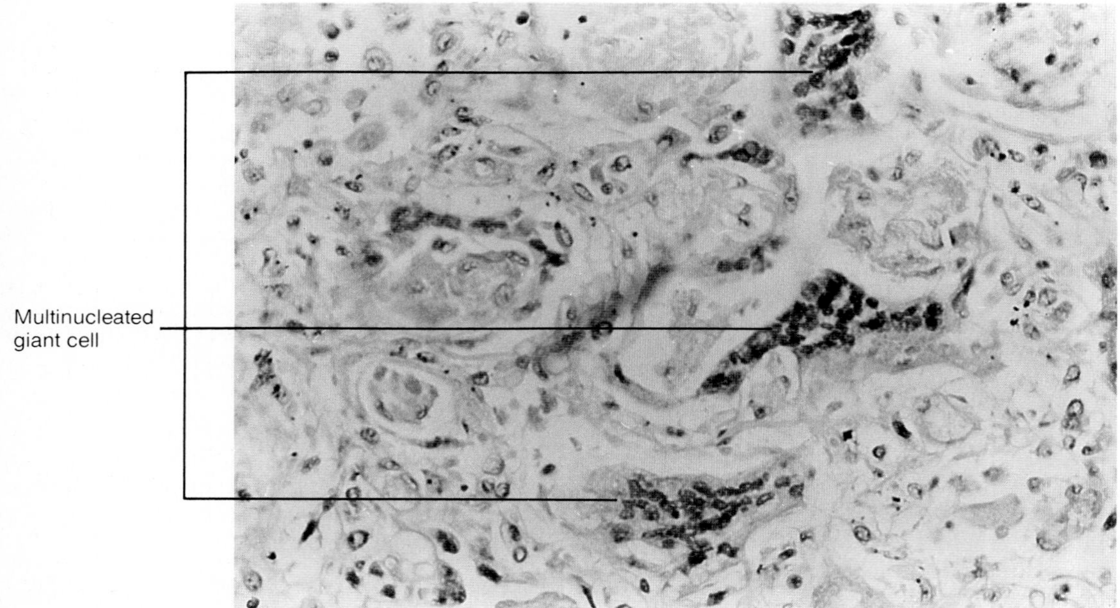

Figure 13-9. Measles pneumonia, showing multinucleated giant cells.

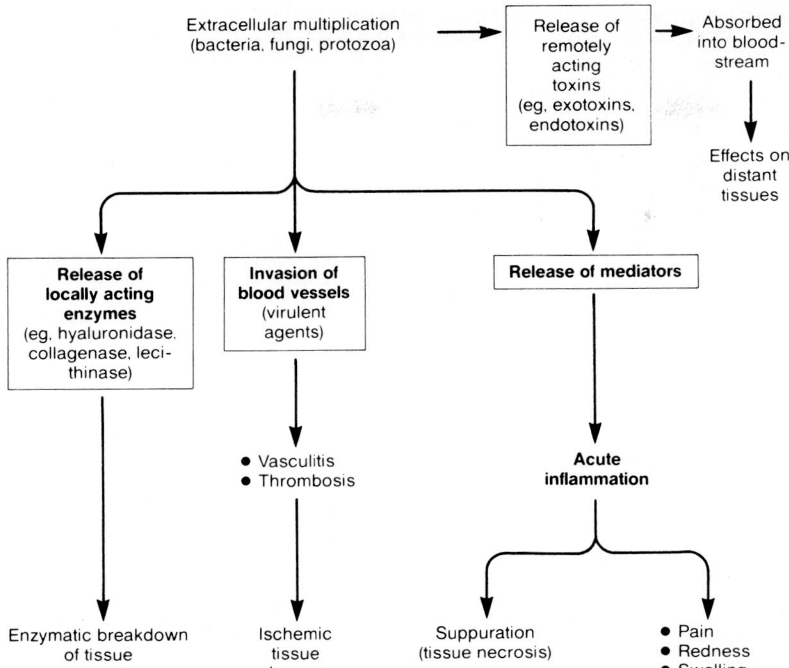

Figure 13–10. Mechanisms of tissue damage in infections with extracellular organisms.

the bloodstream. Their actions cause many diseases (Table 13–5) that are relatively specific for the exotoxin and organisms involved. Exotoxins are highly antigenic, inducing the formation of specific antibodies (antitoxins). Exotoxins usually are heat-labile and are destroyed by cooking or heating to above 60 °C. (By contrast, endotoxins are relatively heat-stable.)

c. Enterotoxins–Enterotoxins are exotoxins that act on intestinal mucosal cells. They are elaborated during bacterial multiplication either within the intestinal lumen (eg, *Vibrio cholerae*) or outside the body in foods that are subsequently eaten (eg, *Staphylococcus aureus*). The toxins attach to surface receptors on intestinal mucosal cells and cause either structural damage (eg, *Clostridium difficile* enterotoxin) or functional alteration (eg, *V cholerae* enterotoxin).

Tissue Changes Caused by the Host Response to Infection (Fig 13–11)

As noted previously (Fig 13–2), the multiplication of an infectious agent in tissues evokes both inflammatory and immune responses (Chapters 3, 4, and 5) whose functions are to inactivate or neutralize the agent, thereby protecting the host.

The host response frequently causes many of the clinical symptoms associated with the infection and may sometimes cause tissue damage and even death; eg, the accumulation of an inflammatory exudate in acute pericarditis may interfere with cardiac function and cause death.

The exact nature of the host response depends on various factors, including the site of multiplication of the agent in tissues (Table 13–6). Identification of the type of cellular response to infection provides clues to the causative organism; eg, neutrophils in the cerebrospinal fluid of a patient with meningitis suggest bacterial meningitis; increased numbers of lymphocytes point to viral or tuberculous meningitis. Relative changes in the proportions of various leukocyte types in peripheral blood are also helpful in this respect.

When information derived from a study of the host response is combined with knowledge of the frequency with which different agents infect specific tissues, the identity of the infecting agent may be narrowed further (Table 13–7). For example, in an adult patient presenting with clinical evidence of acute meningitis (fever, headache, neck stiffness), the presence of numerous neutrophils in the cerebrospinal fluid suggests infection with an extracellular agent. Within this group, *Neisseria meningitidis* is the most common cause of bacterial meningitis in adults and is therefore the most likely causative agent.

A. Acute Inflammation: Pain, redness, warmth, and swelling associated with many infections are the result of acute inflammation. **Fever** is a complex response mediated by exogenous pyrogens (factors released by the organisms) or endogenous

Table 13-5. Diseases caused by bacterial toxins.

Bacterium	Disease	Toxin	Mechanism of Disease
Staphylococcus aureus	Staphylococcal gastroenteritis	Enterotoxin	Toxin preformed in food outside body; probably acts on neural receptors in intestine to stimulate vomiting. Self-limited illness; low mortality rate.
	Toxic shock syndrome	Hemolysin (exotoxin [TSST-1])	Toxin produced in tampons, infected wounds; causes diffuse erythematous skin rash. Serious disease with high mortality rate.
	Neonatal bullous impetigo	Exfoliatin (epidermolysin)	Toxin causes epidermal necrosis ("scalded skin syndrome"). Serious disease with high mortality rate.
Streptococcus pyogenes	Scarlet fever	Erythrogenic toxin	Toxin causes erythemic diffuse skin rash; associated with streptococcal pharyngitis; low mortality rate.
Corynebacterium diphtheriae	Diphtheria	Diphtheria toxin	Exotoxin absorbed into blood from site of bacterial multiplication in upper respiratory tract. Inhibits polypeptide synthesis in cells; causes myocarditis and peripheral neuritis; high mortality rate.
Clostridium tetani	Tetanus	Tetanus toxin	Exotoxin produced in wound is absorbed into bloodstream and nerves; blocks release of an inhibitory mediator in spinal neurons and thereby leads to muscle spasm and seizures; binds to gangliosides in the central nervous system; high mortality rate.
Clostridium botulinum	Botulism	Botulinus toxin	Toxin preformed in food; interferes with acetylcholine release at neuromuscular end plate to produce muscle paralysis. High mortality rate.
Vibrio cholerae	Cholera	Enterotoxin	Enterotoxin produced by multiplying vibrios in intestinal lumen attaches to mucosal cell receptors, causing activation of adenyl cyclase, increased cyclic AMP production, and secretion of electrolytes and water by the cell. Severe secretory diarrhea. High mortality rate.
Clostridium difficile	Pseudomembranous enterocolitis	*C difficile* toxin	Broad-spectrum antibiotics (especially clindamycin) favor overgrowth of *C difficile* in gut lumen. Toxin produced causes necrosis of epithelial cells. High mortality rate; good response to vancomycin.
Clostridium perfringens	Gastroenteritis	Enterotoxin	Toxin has unknown mechanism; causes secretory diarrhea; self-limited disease with low mortality rate.
Toxigenic *Escherichia coli*	Traveler's diarrhea	Enterotoxins	Several toxins described; one has action similar to that of *V cholerae.* Self-limited mild disease with low mortality rate.

Table 13-5. Diseases caused by bacterial toxins. **Cont'd.**

Bacterium	Disease	Toxin	Mechanism of Disease
Shigella dysenteriae type 1	Dysentery	Exotoxin	Affects central nervous system, leading to coma. May affect endothelial cells and cause disseminated intravascular coagulation. These changes complicate acute colitis caused by direct infection.
Neisseria menigitidis Gram-negative bacilli	Meningococcemia Gram-negative bacteremia	Endotoxin	Endotoxins are cell wall constituents of gram-negative bacteria. In the blood they cause fever; activate complement; activate factor XII (Hageman factor), leading to disseminated intravascular coagulation; and have vasoactive effects leading to shock.

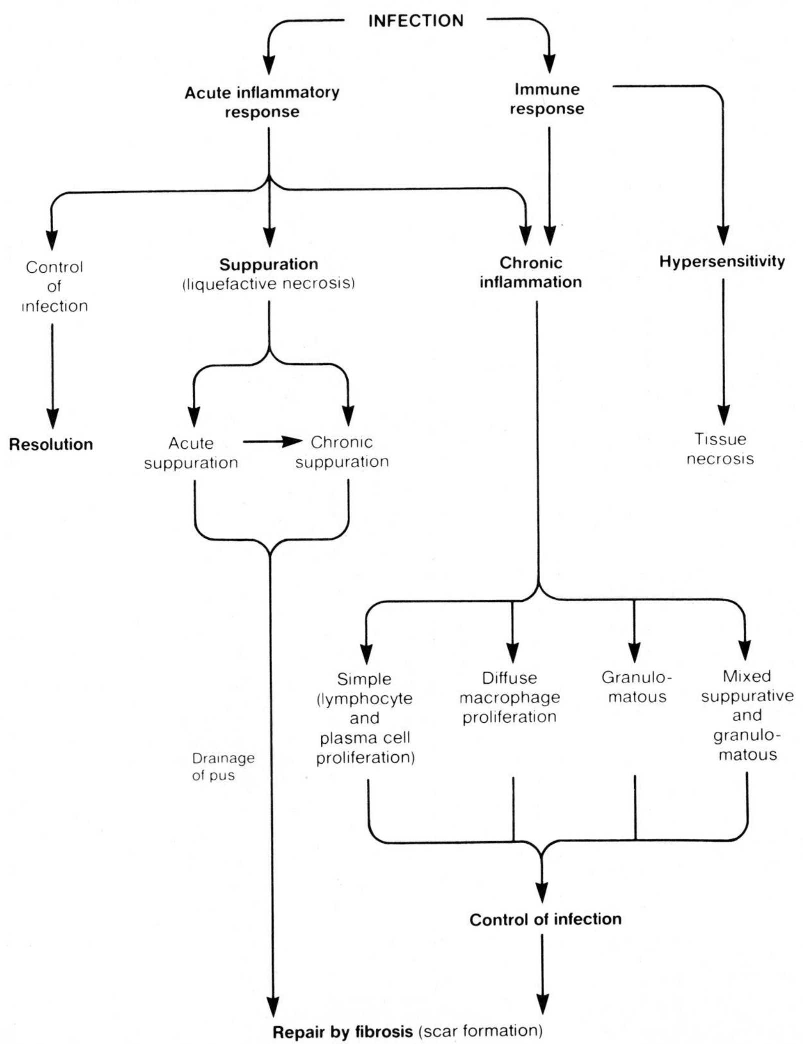

Figure 13-11. Tissue changes caused by host response to infection.

Table 13-6. Characteristics of inflammatory and immune responses according to the site of multiplication of the infecting organism.

	Site of Multiplication		
	Extracellular	**Intracellular (in Macrophages)**	**Intracellular (in Parenchymal Cells)**
Class of organism	Extracellular. Facultative intracellular.	Facultative intracellular.	Obligate intracellular.
Acute inflammation	Common. Numerous neutrophils. Suppuration may occur, eg, bacterial pneumonia.	Uncommon. Usually few neutrophils. Acute macrophage proliferation, eg, *Salmonella typhi* (typhoid fever).	Common. Few neutrophils. Lymphocytes and plasma cells, eg, viral meningitis.
Chronic inflammation	Common; follows unresolved acute inflammation. Chronic suppuration; chronic abscess. Occasionally chronic from outset, eg, actinomycosis. Neutrophils still numerous, eg, chronic lung abscess	Common. Macrophage proliferation with or without granulomas. Caseous necrosis may develop as a result of type IV hypersensitivity, eg, tuberculosis.	Common. Lymphocytes and plasma cells. Variable cell necrosis, eg, chronic hepatitis.
Predominant immune response	Humoral (with complement).	Cell-mediated (lymphokine-mediated).	Both humoral and cell-mediated.
Duration of immunity after exposure	Short-lived	Intermediate; may be associated with delayed hypersensitivity (as shown on skin tests).	Often lifelong in many viral infections, eg, mumps, smallpox.

pryrogens, including the lymphokine interleukin-1. Acute inflammation caused by one infectious agent cannot be clinically distinguished from that caused by another.

Extracellular organisms (most bacteria) typically induce a host response characterized by the appearance of large numbers of neutrophils (Fig 13–12). The neutrophils are attracted by chemotactic factors released at the site of infection. There is an associated neutrophil leukocytosis in the peripheral blood.

Facultative intracellular organisms rarely evoke an acute inflammatory response, and when they do (eg, in typhoid fever caused by *Salmonella typhi*) they are characterized by a cellular infiltrate dominated by macrophages with few neutrophils. Peripheral blood neutropenia is also a feature of typhoid fever.

Obligate intracellular organisms (mainly viruses and rickettsiae) induce an acute cellular response characterized by the appearance of lymphocytes, plasma cells, and macrophages but few neutrophils (reflecting absence of factors chemotactic for neutrophils and a more prominent immune response) (Fig 13–13). The peripheral blood may show an increase in lymphocytes but not neutrophils.

B. Suppurative Inflammation: Suppuration (pus formation) complicating acute inflammation is characterized by liquefactive necrosis; an **abscess** is a walled-off area of suppuration (Chapter 3).

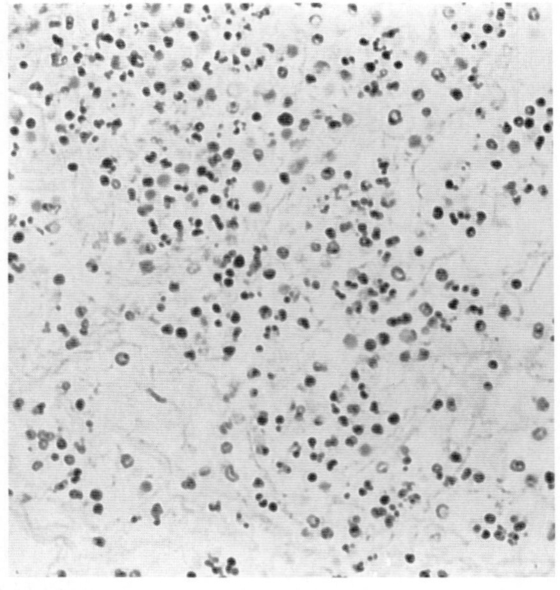

Figure 13–12. Acute bacterial meningitis, showing the acute inflammatory exudate on the meningeal surface. The exudate is characterized by large numbers of neutrophils.

Table 13-7. Infectious agents classified according to the tissues they commonly infect and according to whether they are obligate intracellular, facultative intracellular, or extracellular organisms. Note that when this information is used in conjunction with Table 13-6, one can derive the type of inflammation, immune response, and basic disease process caused by any agent. A complete discussion of individual infectious diseases is postponed for the systemic pathology section (cross-referenced in first column).

Site of Infection	Obligate Intracellular Organisms	Facultative Intracellular Organisms	Extracellular Organisms
Blood (Section VI)	Malaria (erythrocytes)[1]		Bacteria (bacteremia)
Lymphoid system (Section VI)	Cytomegalovirus Infectious mononucleosis Human immunodeficiency virus	*Mycobacterium tuberculosis* Atypical mycobacteria Dimorphic fungi[2] *Pseudomonas mallei* (glanders) *Pseudomonas pseudomallei* (melioidosis) *Francisella tularensis* *Brucella* species *Toxoplasma gondii*[1]	*Yersinia pestis* Pyogenic bacteria
Heart (Section V)	Coxsackievirus (myocarditis) Coxsackievirus (pericarditis)	*Trypanosoma cruzi*[1] *T gondii*[1]	(Endocarditis due to) Viridans streptococci, *Streptococcus faecalis, Candida* sp. *Staphylococcus aureus* *Trichinella spiralis*
Blood vessels and lymphatics (Section V)	Rickettsiae (endothelium)		Filarial worms (lymphatics)
Upper respiratory tract (Section VII)	Viruses causing common cold Viruses causing pharyngitis	*Mycobacterium leprae* *Klebsiella rhinoscleromatis* *Actinomyces israelii* *Leishmania braziliensis*[1]	*Streptococcus pyogenes* *Mycoplasma pneumoniae* *Corynebacterium diphtheriae* *Haemophilus influenzae* *Mucor* species *Candida* species
Lung (Section VIII)	Influenza virus Adenovirus Respiratory syncytial virus *Coxiella burnetii* (Q fever) *Chlamydia psittaci*	*M tuberculosis* Atypical mycobacteria Dimorphic fungi[2] *Cryptococcus neoformans*	*M pneumoniae* *Streptococcus pneumoniae* *S aureus* *Legionella pneumophila* *Klebsiella pneumoniae* *Aspergillus* species *Y pestis* *Bacillus anthracis* *Pneumocystis carinii*
Eye (Section VII)	Adenovirus *Chlamydia trachomatis* Cytomegalovirus	*T gondii*[1]	*Haemophilus aegyptius* *Neisseria gonorrhoeae* *Acanthamoeba* species *Onchocerca volvulus* *Loa loa*
Gastrointestinal tract (Section IX)	Rotaviruses Cytomegalovirus	*M tuberculosis* Atypical mycobacteria *Salmonella typhi*	*Salmonella* species (other than *S typhi*) *Shigella* species *Escherichia coli* *Campylobacter* *Yersinia* species *Vibrio cholerae* *Clostridium difficile* *Entamoeba histolytica* *Giardia lamblia* *Cryptosporidium* *Isospora* Intestinal helminths
Liver (Section X)	Hepatitis A, B, non-A, non-B viruses; delta agent Yellow fever virus Cytomegalovirus *C burnetii*		Pyogenic bacteria *E histolytica* *Echinococcus granulosus*
Urinary tract (Section XI)		*M tuberculosis*	Coliform bacteria *S faecalis* *Leptospira* species

continued

Table 13-7. Infectious agents classified according to the tissues they commonly infect and according to whether they are obligate intracellular, facultative intracellular, or extracellular organisms. **Cont'd.**

Site of Infection	Obligate Intracellular Organisms	Facultative Intracellular Organisms	Extracellular Organisms
External genitalia (Section XII)	Herpes simplex *C trachomatis*		*N gonorrhoeae* *Haemophilus ducreyi* *Calymmatobacterium granulomatis* *Candida* species *Trichomonas vaginalis* *Treponema pallidum*
Bone (Section XVI)		*M tuberculosis* Dimorphic fungi[2]	Pyogenic bacteria *E granulosus*
Nervous system (Section XV) Brain substance	Herpes simplex Arboviruses Measles virus Poliovirus Rabies virus Cytomegalovirus Papovavirus	*M tuberculosis* Dimorphic fungi[2] *C neoformans*	Pyogenic bacteria *Taenia solium* (cysticercosis)
Leptomeninges	Viruses causing menigitis (mumps, polio)	*M tuberculosis* *C neoformans* Dimorphic fungi[2]	*Neisseria meningitidis* *S pneumoniae* *H influenzae* *Listeria monocytogenes* *E coli* *Streptococcus agalactiae* *Leptospira* species *T pallidum*
Skin (Section XIV)	Herpes simplex Varicella-zoster Smallpox virus Measles virus Rubella virus Papillomavirus	*M leprae* Atypical mycobacteria Dimorphic fungi[2] *Leishmania tropica*	*S aureus* *S pyogenes* *B anthracis* Dermatophyte infections Wound infections *O volvulus*

[1]*Toxoplasma, Plasmodium, Trypanosoma,* and *Leishmania* species are difficult to classify as either strictly obligate or facultative intracellular organisms and have been placed in this table somewhat arbitrarily.
[2]Dimorphic fungi include all those listed as facultative intracellular organisms in Table 13–2.

Suppuration occurs when organisms (usually bacteria or fungi) multiply in the extracellular space. It is more likely to develop when anatomic abnormalities in a tissue interfere with resolution of acute inflammation. Obstruction of the lumen of the bronchi, urinary tract, or appendix is frequently complicated by suppurative inflammation. The causative bacteria in these situations vary; infection with multiple anaerobes (polymicrobial infection) is common.

1. Acute suppuration–This type of suppuration occurs in infections due to certain kinds of bacteria that are relatively resistant to phagocytosis, eg, *S aureus,* encapsulated gram-negative bacilli such as *Klebsiella, Pseudomonas,* and *Escherichia* species, and type 3 pneumococci. The thickness of the pneumococcal capsule is directly related to the organism's ability to resist phagocytic killing. Pneumococci types 1 and 2, which have thin capsules, cause acute pneumonia without suppuration—in contrast to type 3 pneumococcus, which has a thick mucoid capsule and causes suppurative pneumonia.

2. Chronic suppuration–Chronic suppuration represents either persistent acute suppurative inflammation (eg, chronic osteomyelitis) or a primary phenomenon due to infection with filamentous bacteria (*Actinomyces* and *Nocardia* species) or certain mycelial fungi (eg, *Madurella* and *Streptomyces* species). These infections are characterized by progressive tissue destruction, fibrosis, and multiple abscesses (Fig 13–14). The abscesses frequently form draining sinuses in the skin that discharge pus containing small yellow colonies of organisms (sulfur granules). **Actinomycosis,** caused by *Actinomyces* species, occurs in the jaw, lungs, and cecal region. **Mycetoma** is a more general term for this type of chronic suppurative inflammation. Mycetoma involving the foot **(Madura foot)** may be caused by any of these organisms.

C. Chronic Inflammation: Chronic inflammation is best regarded as the visible evidence of an immune response occurring in infected tissue. The inciting antigens are mostly derived from the infectious agent but may include antigens released by damaged host tissues. Chronic inflammation may follow an acute response (as in chronic suppuration, described above), or it may occur de novo if the initial phase of infection causes little

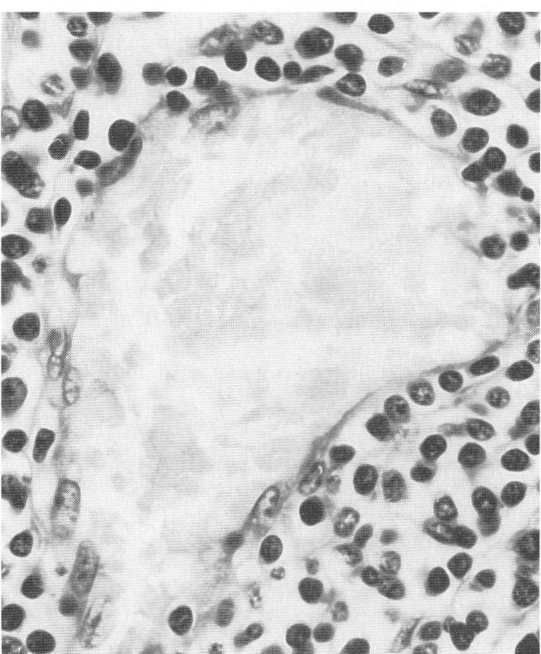

Figure 13-13. Acute viral encephalitis, showing the lymphocytic infiltrate around a cerebral blood vessel. Note the absence of neutrophils in this acute inflammatory process.

cellular damage and fails to excite an acute inflammatory response (as occurs in infections due to certain viruses and intracellular bacteria).

The term chronic inflammation encompasses several different kinds of cellular immune responses.

1. Chronic granulomatous inflammation- (Chapter 5.) Epithelioid cell granulomas represent a specific host response to infections that are caused by the multiplication of facultative intracellular agents in macrophages. The response is T cell-mediated and associated with type IV hypersensitivity. Activated T lymphocytes produce lymphokines that cause accumulation and activation of macrophages. The delayed hypersensitivity associated with this response leads to caseous necrosis. Granulomatous inflammation is always chronic, and it may be associated with extensive tissue necrosis. Repair is by fibrosis and usually occurs concurrently with ongoing necrosis.

Agents that cause epithelioid cell granulomas include (1) mycobacteria (*Mycobacterium tuberculosis, M leprae,* atypical mycobacteria), (2) fungi that grow as nonmycelial forms in tissues (*Coccidioides immitis* [Fig 13-15], *Histoplasma capsulatum, Cryptococcus neoformans, Blastomyces dermatitidis, Sporothrix schenckii,* and *Paracoccidioides brasiliensis*), (3) *Brucella* species, and (4) *T pallidum,* which also causes necrotizing granulomas (gummas) late in the disease. *T pallidum* is an extracellular organism and is an exception. It is rarely identified in granulomas, which are probably the result of an abnormal immunologic response to treponemal antigens.

Identification of the specific agent causing granulomatous inflammation is most effectively achieved by culture. Histologic examination is also useful (Fig 13-15), because the agent can sometimes be identified with special stains for mycobacteria (acid-fast stain) or fungi (methenamine silver stain). In a significant number of cases, no organism can be demonstrated in histologic sections, and culture is essential.

2. Chronic inflammation with diffuse proliferation of macrophages- (Fig 13-16.) In this form of chronic inflammation, there is a deficient cell-mediated immune response and T cell lymphokines are absent. Macrophages do not aggregate to form granulomas but infiltrate infected

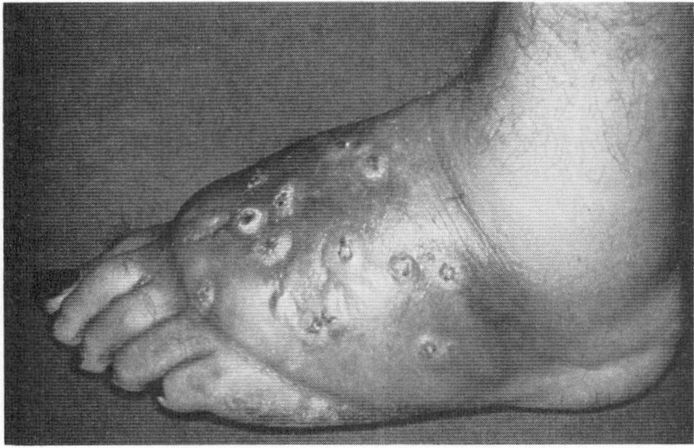

Figure 13-14. Madura foot (a form of mycetoma), showing swelling of the foot with multiple sinuses opening on the skin and draining pus. The severe induration to palpation is due to the fibrosis. Mycetoma is a chronic suppurative inflammation caused by filamentous bacteria or fungi such as *Madurella* species.

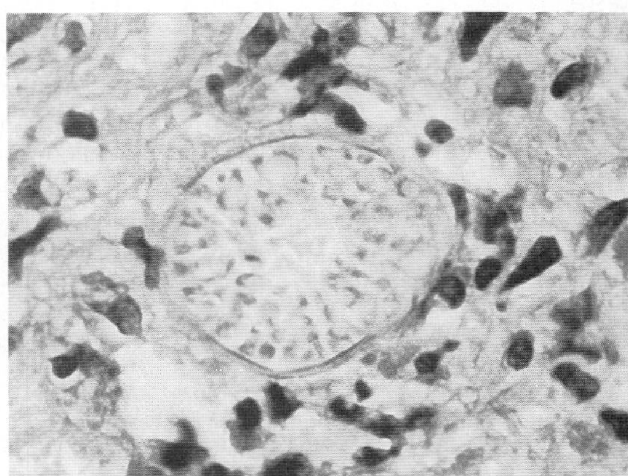

Figure 13-15. *Coccidioides immitis* granuloma, showing a mature spherule with endospores in the center.

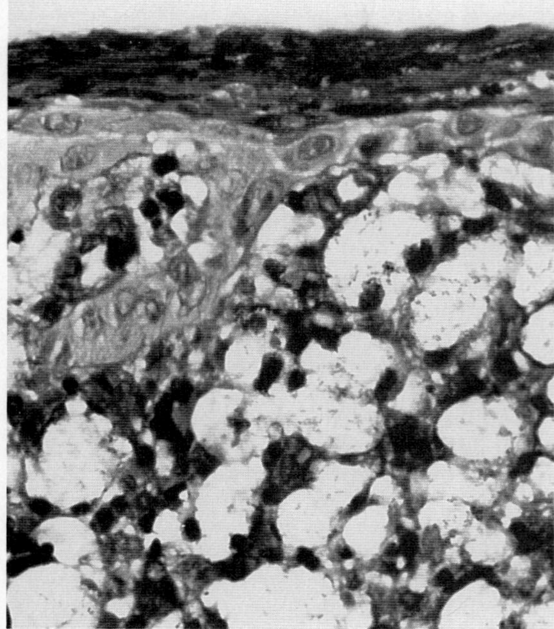

Figure 13–16. Infection of the nasal submucosa by *Klebsiella rhinoscleromatis,* a facultative intracellular organism that causes chronic inflammation with diffuse proliferation of macrophages. Note the presence of numerous bacilli in the macrophages. Identification of the specific organism can be achieved by immunologic techniques.

tissues diffusely. Macrophages have foamy cytoplasm containing numerous organisms; they do not become epithelioid cells. No caseous necrosis occurs, because there is no delayed hypersensitivity.

Chronic inflammation with diffuse proliferation of macrophages occurs in response to infection caused by facultative intracellular organisms. Such organisms include (1) mycobacteria, including *M leprae, M tuberculosis,* and atypical mycobacteria, when disease (eg, lepromatous leprosy, tuberculosis in the elderly, and atypical mycobacteriosis in AIDS) occurs in immunodeficient patients. Note that when these same infections occur in individuals with active T lymphocyte function, they elicit granulomatous inflammation. (2) *Klebsiella rhinoscleromatis,* occurring in the nasal cavity (rhinoscleroma [Fig 13–16]). (3) *Leishmania* species, protozoal parasites that cause infection in skin, mucous membranes, and viscera.

In these infections, the main defense against the invading microorganism appears to be nonimmune phagocytosis by macrophages. Nonimmune phagocytosis by macrophages is relatively ineffective in killing the organisms, which continue to proliferate in the cell. A common feature of all these infections is the presence of numerous organisms in the macrophages. Proliferation of macrophages frequently causes a marked degree of clinically detectable enlargement of affected tissues.

3. Chronic inflammation with lymphocytes and plasma cells–This type of inflammation typically occurs in response to persistent infection caused by obligate intracellular organisms (eg, viruses causing chronic viral hepatitis and chronic viral infections of the brain). It represents a combined humoral and cell-mediated immune response. The associated cell necrosis is followed by fibrosis.

D. Combined Suppurative and Granulomatous Inflammation: A combination of suppuration and granulomatous inflammation is commonly seen in deep fungal infections; it is probably due to multiplication of the causative organisms both within macrophages and outside the cell.

A less common but distinctive lesion in which there is a combined suppurative and granulomatous inflammation is the **stellate granuloma,** in which neutrophils are present in the center of an irregular star-shaped (stellate) epithelioid cell granuloma. Stellate granulomas may be seen in the following infections: (1) lymphogranuloma venereum (LGV), caused by *Chlamydia trachomatis* (types L1–L3) and characterized by genital ulceration and lymph node involvement (lymphadenitis); (2) cat-scratch disease, characterized by fever and lymph node enlargement and caused by a small gram-negative bacterium (not yet characterized) that stains positively with silver stains; (3) tularemia (caused by *Francisella tularensis*), (4) glanders (caused by *Pseudomonas mallei*), and (5) melioidosis (caused by *Pseudomonas pseudomallei*).

All of these agents are facultative intracellular organisms except *Chlamydia trachomatis,* which is an obligate intracellular agent. The specific diagnosis of these infectious diseases depends on culture or immunologic tests.

Infectious Diseases: II. Mechanisms of Infection

14

INCIDENCE OF INFECTIOUS DISEASES

The great variation in the incidence of infectious diseases throughout the world largely reflects differences in geographic and socioeconomic conditions and the impact of modern public health measures and medical care. Highly effective public health measures include immunization, health education, sanitation, and vector control. In developed countries, health care has a high priority, and large sums are spent to maintain adequate standards of housing and sanitation. In developing countries, in contrast, limited resources may result in crowded living conditions, poor sanitation, lack of hospital facilities, and lower standards of health care.

Infectious Disease in the USA

A. In Hospital Practice: (Table 14–1.) Infectious diseases are a common problem in the USA, with approximately 5 million cases seen in hospitals annually throughout the country. About 40% of infections in hospitals are acquired in the hospital itself **(nosocomial infections)**. The genitourinary tract, surgical wounds, and lungs are the most common sites of nosocomial infection. Most nosocomial infections are caused by bacteria and fungi; viruses, protozoa, and metazoa rarely cause such infections. **Hospital-acquired pneumonia** is the most serious such infection, with a mortality rate of 20%. Disseminated infections caused by bacteria and fungi, mainly in immunocompromised patients, also account for a significant number of nosocomial infections. In newborn nurseries, hospital-acquired epidemic diarrhea is a common problem.

The high incidence of hospital-acquired infections is due to the following factors:

1. Increased susceptibility–Hospitalized patients demonstrate increased susceptibility to infection by virtue of concurrent illness and immunosuppressive drugs.

2. Use of invasive procedures–Invasive surgical, diagnostic (eg, lumbar puncture, phlebotomy), and therapeutic procedures (eg, bladder catheterization, indwelling intravascular catheters) provide infectious agents with a portal of entry. The materials used in these procedures are themselves sometimes fomites (eg, contaminated intravenous fluids, tubing, respirators).

3. Numerous sources of infection–Hospitals harbor numerous sources of infection—mainly other patients with infectious diseases. Organisms or spores in the environment (eg, dust, hospital linen) are less important sources.

4. Use of antibiotics–Widespread use of antibiotics promotes overgrowth of antibiotic-resistant strains of gram-negative enteric bacilli (eg, *Escherichia coli, Pseudomonas aeruginosa, Proteus* species, *Klebsiella* species, and *Serratia* species) and *Staphylococcus aureus.* These organisms are often resistant to many antibiotics and therefore pose serious problems in treatment.

B. In Community Practice: Viral infections of the upper respiratory tract (eg, coryza, influenza) and the gastrointestinal tract (eg, viral gastroenteritis) are the infections most commonly encountered by physicians in general practice in a community setting. These illnesses are self-limited, and patients typically do not consult a physician. Hospitalization is required only when illness is severe (eg, rare cases of influenza, especially in

Table 14-1. Common infections seen in hospitals in the USA.[1]

Infection	Community-Acquired	Hospital-Acquired
Number of cases/year	**3 Million**	**2 Million**
Breakdown according to type of infectious agent (%)		
Bacteria	93	90
Viruses	6	Rare
Fungi	<1	10
Parasites (ie, protozoa, metazoa)	<1	Rare
Breakdown according to site (%)		
Genitourinary tract[2]	38	41
Lung	20	12
Upper respiratory tract	8	<1
Gastrointestinal tract	3	<1
Central nervous system	<1	<1
Disseminated infection[3]	<1	9
Others	29[4]	37[5]

[1]Note that this table represents only those infections serious enough to warrant hospitalization. The pattern of infectious diseases encountered in general medical practice outside hospitals differs greatly, with mild viral infections of the upper respiratory and gastrointestinal tracts accounting for a great number and percentage of cases.

[2]Common genitourinary tract infections in the community include sexually transmitted infections such as gonorrhea.

[3]Disseminated infections, commonly caused by bacteria and fungi, occur in immunocompromised patients, usually those being treated for cancer.

[4]Includes a wide variety of other sites.

[5]Includes infections of surgical wounds which are responsible for a majority of this group of hospital-acquired infections.

the elderly). Acquired immunodeficiency syndrome (AIDS), though still relatively uncommon, is a sexually transmitted viral infection that is of growing importance not only because of its increasing incidence but also because of its high (near 100%) mortality rate.

Community-acquired bacterial infections have a somewhat different distribution and generally are associated with a lower mortality rate than hospital-acquired infections both because the host is better able to respond to the infection and because the infectious agents are usually susceptible to antibiotic therapy. Sexually transmitted diseases (eg, gonorrhea, syphilis), urinary infections in young women, and respiratory infections (eg, streptococcal pharyngitis, sinusitis, otitis, pneumonia) represent the most common bacterial infections.

Infectious Disease in Developing Countries (Table 14-2)

Along with malnutrition, infection represents the major health care problem in developing countries, and many deaths result from these conditions. The total number of cases dwarfs the corresponding figures from developed countries. It is estimated that there are about 5 billion cases of infectious diarrhea in Asia, Africa, and Latin America every year; of this number, there are 5–10 million deaths, mainly in young children. Protozoal and helminthic infections are also prevalent in developing nations; about 1 billion individuals are estimated to harbor the roundworm *Ascaris lumbricoides* in the gut, and hookworm infestation is the commonest cause of iron deficiency anemia in these regions.

Problems associated with infections occurring in developing countries fall into broad groups: (1) Lack of appropriate means or facilities for treatment, so that relatively minor infections such as viral gastroenteritis are associated with a disproportionately high mortality rate. (2) Lack of childhood immunization, so that diseases such as mea-

Table 14-2. Annual incidence of major infections in Asia, Africa, and Latin America.[1]

Disease	Number of Cases per Year	Number of Deaths per Year
Diarrhea	5 billion	5–10 million[2]
Malaria	150 million[3]	1–2 million
Measles	80 million	900,000
Schistosomiasis	20 million[3]	750,000
Tuberculosis	7 million	400,000
Whooping cough	20 million	250,000
Amebiasis	1.5 million	30,000
Typhoid	500,000	25,000
Hookworm	1.5 million[3]	50,000
Ascariasis	1 million[3]	20,000
Filariasis	3 million[3]	. . .

[1]These are estimates based on available statistics, which are inexact.

[2]Most deaths from diarrhea occur in young children, in whom fluid and electrolyte loss has serious effects. The cause of diarrhea is frequently a self-limiting rotavirus infection.

[3]The prevalence of these infections is much higher: 1 billion people are believed to harbor *Ascaris* without symptoms; 900 million have hookworm, 800 million have malaria, 250 million have filariasis, and 200 million have schistosomiasis.

sles and whooping cough are widespread. (3) Lack of basic public health programs such as health education, vector control, and sanitation, so that malaria, amebiasis, typhoid, cholera, and intestinal helminth infestation more easily gain a foothold in the community. Malnutrition, which is a common problem, increases the susceptibility to infection and therefore its incidence. The fact that infection is no longer the most common cause of death in developed nations attests to the increasing effectiveness of modern public health and hygiene measures. Likewise, the dramatic change in disease patterns from medieval times (Table 14–3) can largely be attributed to improved sanitation and living conditions. However, while many infectious diseases have been successfully controlled, the only one that has been eradicated from the world is smallpox.

Table 14–3. Causes of death, 1665, London, England.[1]

Cause	Deaths	Cause	Deaths
Abortive and Stilborne	617	Headmouldshot & Mouldfallen	14
Aged	1545	**Jaundies**	110
Ague and Feaver[2]	5257	Impostume	227
Appoplex and Suddenly	116	Kild by several accidents	46
Bedrid	10	**Kings Evill**[6]	86
Blasted	5	Leprosie	2
Bleeding	16	Lethargy	14
Bloudy Flux, Scowring & Flux	185	Livergrowne	20
Burnt and Scalded	8	Meagrom and Headach	12
Calenture	3	Measles	7
Cancer, Gangrene and Fistula	56	Murthered, and Shot	9
Canker, and Thrush	111	Overlaid and Starved	45
Childbed	625	Palsie	30
Chrisomes and Infants	1258	**Plague**	68596
Cold and Cough	68	Plannet	6
Collick and Winde	134	Plurisie	15
Consumption and Tissick[3]	4808	Poysoned	1
Convulsion and Mother	2036	Quinsie	35
Distracted	5	Rickets	557
Dropsie and Timpany	1478	Rising of the Lights	397
Drowned	50	Rupture	34
Executed	21	Scurvy	105
Flox and Smal Pox	655	Shingles and Swine pox	2
Found dead in streets, fields, etc.	20	Sores, Ulcers, broken and bruised Limbes	82
French Pox[4]	86	Spleen	14
Frighted	23	**Spotted Feaver and Purples**[7]	1929
Gout and Sciatica	27	Stopping of the Stomack	332
Grief	46	Stone and Strangury	98
Griping in the Guts[5]	1288	Surfet	1251
Hangd & made away themselves	7	**Teeth and Worms**	2614
		Vomiting	51
		Wenn	1

[1]Reproduced, with permission, from Gale AM: *Epidemic Diseases.* Pelican, 1959. 1665 was the year of the great plague epidemic that killed more than 10% of the total population of the city in 1 year. Note also the importance of other infectious diseases (bold print) as a cause of death.
[2]Ague: includes malaria.
[3]Consumption and Tissick: cavitary pulmonary tuberculosis.
[4]French Pox: syphilis.
[5]Griping in the Guts: ?infectious diarrheas.
[6]Kings Evill: scrofula or tuberculosis of lymph nodes.
[7]Spotted feaver and purples: ?Scarlet fever, ?other infections with rashes.

METHODS & PATHWAYS OF INFECTION

In general, microorganisms must enter the host's tissues and proliferate there to cause disease (Fig 14–1). Those organisms that produce exotoxins are sometimes notable exceptions to this rule; eg, *Clostridium botulinum* may cause death without ever entering the host (see Table 13–5).

Humans encounter many microorganisms every day, but few enter the tissues, and most that do are rapidly destroyed by the host's defense mechanisms. Other organisms, usually of low pathogenicity, colonize the skin, upper respiratory tract, genitourinary tract, and gastrointestinal tract in large numbers as normal resident (commensal) flora. These organisms help prevent infection by competing with more virulent organisms for growth factors. The incidence and expression of infectious disease associated with a given agent vary with specific factors in both the agent and the host (Table 14–4).

Portals of Entry of Infectious Agents (Table 14–5)

Infectious agents gain access to the body either through the skin or through tissues that communicate with the environment outside the body. The respiratory tract, gastrointestinal tract, and genitourinary tract are common portals of entry for infectious agents (Fig 14–2) and frequently become the site of infection. Internal organs such as the brain, bones, and heart have no communication with the outside except through the bloodstream or lymphatics, and infectious diseases of these structures are usually the result of vascular spread of an agent that enters the body at one of the portals of entry. An understanding of the portals of entry of an infectious agent permits development of rational strategies to prevent transmission of infection; eg, the incidence of infections due to agents that enter through the intestine (infectious diarrheas, poliomyelitis, hepatitis A infection, etc) decreases dramatically when fecal contamination of food and water is reduced through improved sanitation.

Portals of entry have well-developed specific defense mechanisms to prevent entry of pathogens. Infection represents either a breakdown of

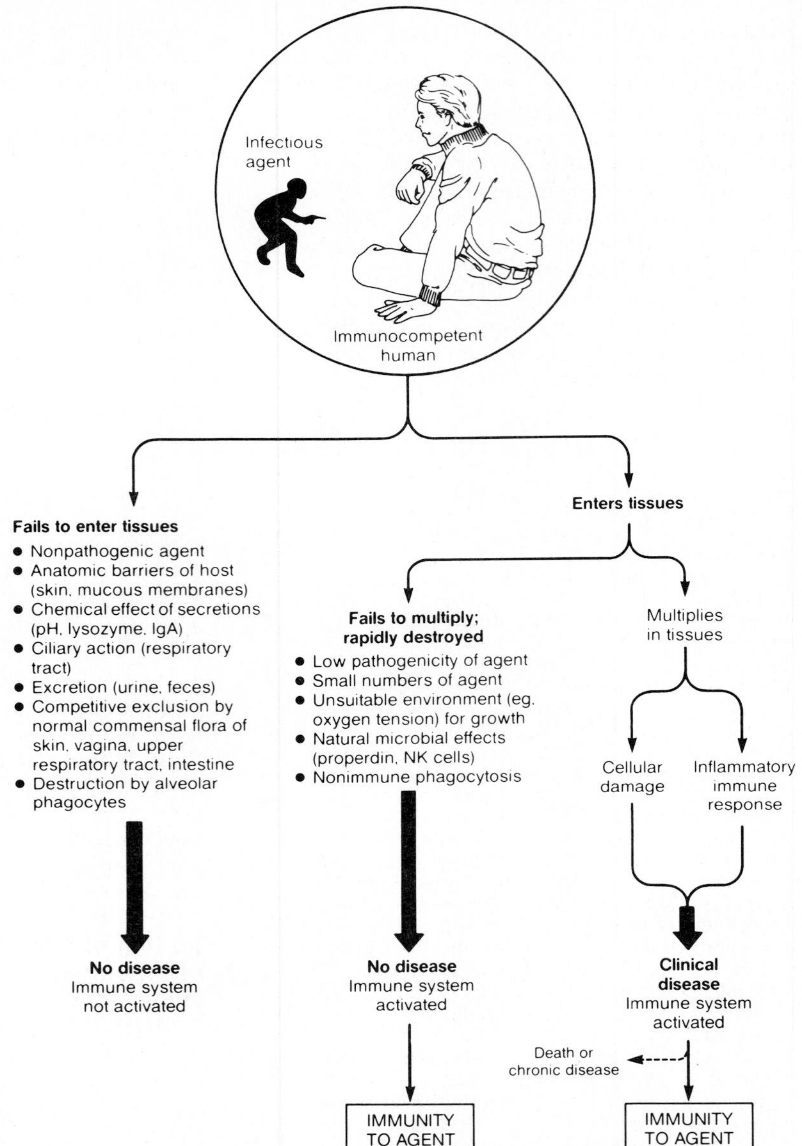

Figure 14–1. Possible results of an encounter with an infectious agent.

these defenses or invasion by a highly virulent organism. Infection of the site of entry may be followed by dissemination of the agent via blood vessels or lymphatics. In many cases, the infectious agent enters the bloodstream without causing visible changes at the portal of entry.

A. Skin: The outer layer of the skin is composed of keratinized stratified squamous epithelium that forms a highly effective physical barrier to infection. Secretions of adnexal glands (eg, sweat and sebum) provide an additional chemical barrier. Abnormal skin, including chronically wet and macerated, burned, or ischemic skin, is not as effective a barrier and may be associated with an increased incidence of infection.

Infection of the skin may occur in several different ways.

1. Direct contact–A few skin infections are acquired by direct physical contact with an infected individual, eg, herpes simplex infections, dermatophyte fungal infections (tinea or ringworm), or impetigo caused by *Staphylococcus aureus* or *Streptococcus pyogenes.*

2. Wound infections–Many infectious agents enter the skin through wounds, including many pyogenic bacteria that cause wound infections with abscess formation and cellulitis (acute inflammation of subcutaneous tissue) and also spread to other parts of the body via the lymphatics and blood vessels. *Clostridium perfringens*

Table 14-4. Effects of *candida albicans* infection in different kinds of hosts.[1]

Host	Result
Healthy normal adult male	*Candida* may be present as normal commensal flora in mouth and upper respiratory tract. Infection is rare.
Sexually active normal female	Same as above; *Candida* vaginitis (surface infection) may result if vaginal pH is not acid and normal flora is suppressed.
Neonates	Increased incidence of surface infection (oral cavity, skin).
Patient receiving broad-spectrum antibiotic therapy	Surface infection of the oral mucosa (oral thrush); *Candida,* which is resistant to antibiotics, proliferates when normal flora is suppressed by the antibiotic.
Patient with diabetes mellitus	Increased incidence of surface infection (oral mucosa) caused by *Candida;* due to failure of some defense mechanism (unknown).
Patient with burns	Infection of burned surface; in severe burns, infection may invade blood vessels and be disseminated in bloodstream.
Patient with prosthetic cardiac valve or arterial graft	*Candida* endocarditis or graft infection may develop. Focus of *Candida* infection at primary access site may or may not be present.
Intravenous drug abuser	*Candida* in injected material enters bloodstream directly and causes endocarditis (cardiac valves are highly susceptible to overgrowth with *Candida*).
Patient with indwelling vascular catheter	Increased incidence of disseminated *Candida* infection (organism gains access via catheter).
Patient with acquired immune deficiency syndrome (AIDS)	Surface infection of oral cavity (thrush) or esophagus common; disseminated infection uncommon.
Patient receiving cancer chemotherapy (severe immunodeficiency)	Disseminated candidiasis.

[1]Similar tables can be drawn up for virtually every infectious agent.

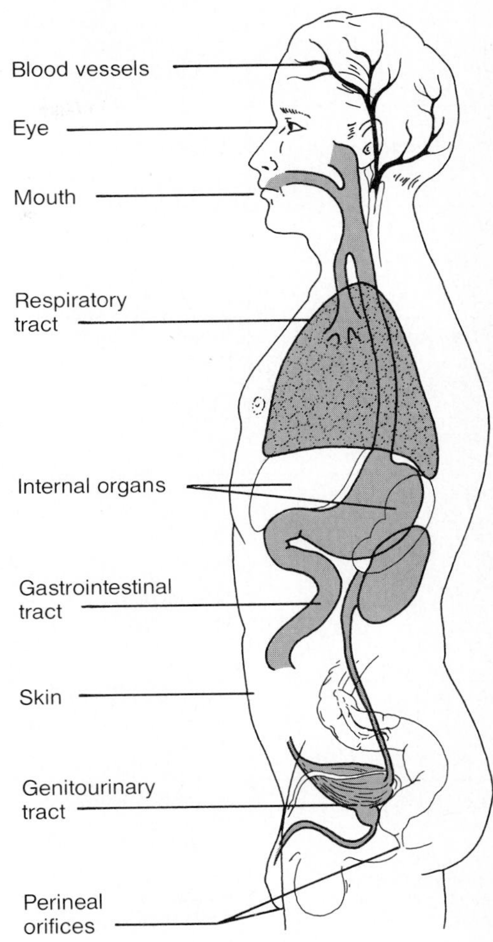

Figure 14-2. Diagrammatic representation of portals of entry of infectious agents in humans. The chief portals of entry are the skin, gastrointestinal tract, respiratory tract, and genitourinary tract, which communicate with the outside either directly or through orifices. Internal organs such as the heart, brain, and adrenals become infected only when the infectious agent is transmitted via the bloodstream (except in infections secondary to trauma).

(one of the causes of gas gangrene) and *Clostridium tetani* (which causes tetanus) multiply in deep puncture wounds that contain necrotic and foreign material and favor the anaerobic growth of these organisms. Sporotrichosis is a fungal infection due to *Sporothrix schenckii* and is commonly acquired by gardeners who prick themselves with infected thorns or handle contaminated sphagnum moss.

3. Injection by vectors–The skin sometimes becomes infected as a result of penetration by an arthropod vector carrying an infectious agent. The skin lesions of leishmaniasis, the chagoma associated with Chagas' disease, the chancre associated with African trypanosomiasis (sleeping sickness), and the eschar of scrub typhus are examples. The vector may act as a simple carrier of the infectious agent or may be an integral part of the life cycle of the agent (Table 14–6).

Viruses transmitted by arthropod vectors are called **arboviruses** (arthropod-borne viruses). In most arbovirus infections, the agent enters cutaneous lymphatics or blood vessels and is transported to other parts of the body without causing a significant skin lesion at the site of entry.

Table 14–5. Portals of entry of representative infectious agents.

Site of Entry	Obligate Intracellular Organisms	Facultative Intracellular Organisms	Extracellular Organisms
Skin			
Direct contact	Papillomavirus	*Mycobacterium leprae* *Sporothrix schenckii*	*Staphylococcus aureus* *Streptococcus pyogenes* *Bacillus anthracis*
Wound infection			Pyogenic bacteria *Clostridium* species
Vectors[1]	Arboviruses *Plasmodium* (malaria)	*Leishmania* species *Trypanosoma* species	*Yersinia pestis*
Intravenous needles[1]	Hepatitis B virus Human immunodeficiency virus (HIV, AIDS virus) Cytomegalovirus		Pyogenic bacteria *Treponema pallidum*
Penetration			Helminth larvae (eg, *Schistosoma*)
Respiratory tract	Herpes simplex Varicella-zoster virus (chickenpox) Measles virus, rubella virus Cytomegalovirus Mumps virus Epstein-Barr virus *Coxiella burnetii*	*Mycobacterium tuberculosis* Dimorphic fungi *Cryptococcus neoformans* Atypical mycobacteria *Nocardia asteroides* *Candida* species *M leprae*	*Streptococcus viridans* Pneumococcus Meningococcus *Corynebacterium diphtheriae* *Y pestis* *Listeria monocytogenes*
Intestine	Hepatitis A virus Poliovirus; other enteroviruses		*Salmonella* species *Shigella* species *Entamoeba histolytica* *Trichinella spiralis*
Genital tract	Herpes simplex HIV *Chlamydia trachomatis*		*Neisseria gonorrhoeae* *Calymmatobacterium granulomatis* *T pallidum*
Placenta (in congenital infection)	Rubella virus Cytomegalovirus HIV	*Toxoplasma gondii* *M tuberculosis*	*L monocytogenes* *T pallidum*

[1]Intravenous injection and many vectors introduce the organism directly into the bloodstream.

4. Injection by humans–Transfusion of infected blood and blood products may result in the direct intravenous injection of human immunodeficiency virus (HIV), hepatitis B virus, hepatitis non-A, non-B virus, cytomegalovirus, plasmodia (malarial parasites), and *Treponema pallidum.* Screening of donors, blood, and blood products has greatly decreased the incidence of transfusion-induced hepatitis B, malaria, syphilis, and HIV infection. In all of these infections, the skin acts merely as the portal of entry and shows no evidence of disease.

Contaminated needles used by drug abusers for intradermal or intravenous injection provide another method of entry of infection through the skin. Intravenous drug users demonstrate an increased incidence of both local pyogenic bacterial skin infections and systemic infections, including bacteremias, hepatitis B, cytomegalovirus infection, and HIV infection.

5. Active larval penetration–The larvae of a few helminthic parasites can penetrate intact skin to gain entry to the body (eg, hookworm larvae, cercariae of *Schistosoma* species, larvae of *Strongyloides stercoralis*). The entry point of the larvae may be marked by a transient skin lesion.

B. Respiratory Tract: The respiratory tract consists of upper and lower divisions, separated by the vocal cords. The upper respiratory tract and the larger air passages are continually exposed to inhaled infectious agents, which are usually trapped by mucus secreted by the mucous membrane. The mucus is continuously wafted upward by the beating action of the ciliary epithelium from the bronchi toward the pharynx. Mucus contains protective chemicals such as lysozyme (in nasal passages, derived from tears), and IgA (in the respiratory passages). The normal commensal bacterial flora of the upper respiratory tract competitively inhibits the growth of infectious agents. The pharynx contains a rich collection of submucosal lymphoid tissue (Waldeyer's ring) that provides a local immunologic barrier. The lower respiratory tract is relatively sterile. Aspiration of

Table 14-6. Arthropod vectors of human infections.

Disease	Infectious Agent	Vector
Simple transmission by vector		
Plague	*Yersinia pestis*	Fleas (rarely ticks, lice)
Relapsing fever	*Borrelia recurrentis*	Lice, ticks
Lyme disease	*Borrelia burgdorferi*	Ixodid ticks
Typhus, spotted fever	*Rickettsia* species	Fleas, ticks, mites, lice
Epidemic encephalitides	Togaviruses, bunyaviruses	Mosquitoes, ticks
Yellow fever	Togavirus group B	Mosquitoes
Dengue fever	Togavirus group B	Mosquitoes
Hemorrhagic fevers	Bunyaviruses	Mosquitoes, ticks
Colorado tick fever	Reovirus (genus *Orbivirus*)	Ticks
Vector is intrinsic part of parasite life cycle		
Malaria	*Plasmodium* species	*Anopheles* mosquitoes
Leishmaniasis	*Leishmania* species	Sandflies (*Phlebotomus* in Old World; *Lutzomyia* and *Psychodopygus* in New World)
Sleeping sickness	*Trypanosoma* species	Tsetse flies (*Glossina*)
Chagas' disease	*Trypanosoma cruzi*	Reduviid bugs
Babesiosis	*Babesia microti*	Ticks
Filariasis	*Wuchereria, Brugia* species	Mosquitoes
Onchocerciasis	*Onchocerca volvulus*	*Simulium* flies
Loiasis	*Loa loa*	*Chrysops* flies

pharyngeal secretions into the larynx is prevented by the cough reflex. More distally, the alveoli in the lung contain active phagocytic macrophages.

Inhalation of infectious agents, usually in the form of infected droplets, is responsible for most respiratory infections. Many viruses infect the upper respiratory tract (see Table 13–3). Bacterial infections of the upper respiratory tract are less common and include streptococcal pharyngotonsillitis, epiglottitis caused by *Haemophilus influenzae,* and diphtheria. The upper respiratory tract may also serve as a portal of entry for agents such as measles, rubella, varicella-zoster (chickenpox), and mumps viruses and *Neisseria meningitidis.*

Entry of pathogenic organisms into the lower respiratory tract is facilitated by deficiencies in local defense mechanisms: (1) Depression of the cough reflex, as occurs with use of narcotic drugs, in general anesthesia, and in coma secondary to diabetic ketoacidosis, epilepsy, or alcohol intoxication. (2) Interference with ciliary transport, as occurs with heavy alcohol use and cold. (3) Loss of ciliated cells, as occurs in squamous metaplasia due to smoking. (4) Bronchial obstruction that causes accumulation of secretions distal to the obstruction and increases the likelihood of infection.

Most infectious agents that reach the lung parenchyma cause disease there (see Table 13–7). In many of these infections—including infections due to *Mycobacterium tuberculosis, Streptococcus pneumoniae, Coxiella burnetii,* and several fungi—the agent enters the bloodstream and is disseminated to other organs.

C. The Gastrointestinal Tract: Food and drink may be contaminated with pathogenic infectious agents that are ingested and thereby gain access to the intestine. Many of these diseases (eg, rotavirus gastroenteritis, amebiasis, giardiasis, salmonellosis, and shigellosis) are transmitted by fecal contamination of food and water. Several agents, including hepatitis A virus and poliovirus, are transmitted in a similar manner but do not cause significant intestinal disease, since the intestine is involved merely as a portal of entry.

Important defense mechanisms of the intestine are as follows: (1) The mucosal lining, which is an effective physical barrier. (2) The acidity of the stomach. (3) The continuous flow of the contents of the intestinal lumen. Stagnation, as occurs in diverticula and intestinal obstruction, leads to bacterial overgrowth. (4) The mucus secreted by the intestine, which contains IgA. Patients with IgA deficiency are susceptible to development of enteric infections. (5) The submucosal lymphoid tissue, which provides an immediate immunologic barrier. (6) Commensal intestinal flora (particularly in the colon) that competitively excludes many pathogens.

Broad-spectrum antibiotics that destroy the commensal flora may lead to infection of the gut by pathogenic organisms (eg, *Clostridium difficile* enterocolitis).

D. Genitourinary Tract: The urinary tract is normally sterile except for a few millimeters at the external urethral meatus. The excretion of urine is believed to have a protective flushing effect. Obstruction of urinary flow results in an increased risk of urinary tract infection. Likewise, alteration in the normal vaginal flora may predispose to development of infection (eg, candidal vaginitis following administration of broad-spectrum antibiotics). The urinary tract serves as a portal of entry for infectious agents (usually commensal bacteria of the intestine) that ascend from the perineum. Ascending urinary tract infections are much more common in females than in males because of the short urethra and the proximity of the urethra to the anus.

The genital tract also acts as a portal of entry for agents that cause sexually transmitted infections. Local diseases of the external genitalia include syphilis, gonorrhea, genital herpes, and lymphogranuloma venereum. Infectious agents may also enter the bloodstream and lymphatics via the genital tract to cause sexually transmitted disease elsewhere in the body, eg, syphilis, gonorrhea, hepatitis B, and HIV infection.

Infection of the Bloodstream

Infectious agents that overcome defenses at the portals of entry may multiply locally, causing infection at the site of entry, eg, pneumococcal pneumonia. The organism may then enter the lymphatics and the bloodstream from this infected site. On the other hand, the organism may enter the lymphatics or bloodstream *without* producing signs of infection at the site of entry; eg, in meningococcal bacteremia, the respiratory tract (which serves as the portal of entry) is usually normal.

The presence of microorganisms in the blood (bacteremia, viremia, parasitemia, fungemia) is always abnormal and usually of clinical significance. The diagnosis of bacteremia, viremia, and fungemia is established by blood cultures. Parasitemia can frequently be diagnosed by identifying the parasite in blood smears (eg, malaria). Most bacteremias in clinical practice fall between the extremes of a transient bacteremia and septicemia (severe bacteremia).

A. Transient Bacteremia: In transient bacteremia, microorganisms are present in small numbers in the bloodstream and do not multiply there, since they are rapidly removed by the body's defense mechanisms. This condition is relatively common—as in persons with infected teeth and gums, who may often liberate small numbers of pathogenic agents into the blood during mastication and while brushing the teeth—and does not produce clinical symptoms.

Transient bacteremia may produce disease in the following clinical situations: (1) In immunocompromised hosts whose immune systems are unable to neutralize the organisms, which may therefore multiply and produce severe disseminated infections. (2) In patients with chronic cardiac valve disease or cardiac prostheses. The organisms are able to grow in damaged or prosthetic valves, and in such patients bacteremia may be complicated by infective endocarditis. (3) In otherwise normal individuals, when organisms become established in an internal organ and cause infection, eg, viral encephalitis. Why only some individuals develop such infections is unknown.

B. Severe Bacteremia (Septicemia): Septicemia is often used synonymously with severe bacteremia to denote a serious infection in which large and increasing numbers of microorganisms have overwhelmed the body's defense systems and are actively multiplying in the bloodstream. Severe bacteremia is associated with toxemia (presence in the blood of bacterial toxins) and is manifested clinically by high fever, chills, tachycardia, and hypotension. Death may result.

TRANSMISSION OF INFECTION

Successful parasitism requires not only the ability to infect a host and multiply but also the ability to be transmitted to an appropriate host or from one host to another. Transmission is an integral part of the life cycle of all parasites, and understanding how an agent is transmitted enables us to take appropriate action to prevent disease, eg, eradication of the mosquito vector makes control of malaria possible. Most simple infectious agents have straightforward means of transmission. Protozoa and more complex agents have complex life cycles that often require different kinds of intermediate hosts.

Transmission of Agents With Simple Life Cycles (Fig 14–3)

Microorganisms such as viruses, chlamydiae, rickettsiae, mycoplasmas, and bacteria are simple organisms that require no developmental stage during transmission. Transfer of such agents from one host to another may be accomplished by physical contact, as in skin infections and sexually transmitted diseases, or by inhalation, injection, or ingestion of contaminated droplet nuclei, food, water, feces, and other substances. Arthropod vectors may also transmit such agents (Table 14–6).

A few bacteria (*Clostridium tetani, Bacillus anthracis*), many fungi, some protozoa (eg, *Entamoeba histolytica* and *Giardia lamblia*), and some metazoa (eg, intestinal helminths, schistosomes) produce specialized structures (spores, cysts, and ova) that can withstand adverse environmental conditions and increase chances of survival when a suitable host is not immediately available. Such spores may lie dormant in soil or water and become reactivated under favorable conditions (eg, tetanus spores multiply in a deep puncture wound that favors anaerobic growth). When these infective structures are not formed in the host, the disease cannot be directly transmitted from one person to another. For example, in infection with *Coccidioides immitis,* the infective arthrospore is formed in the soil and not usually in the patient.

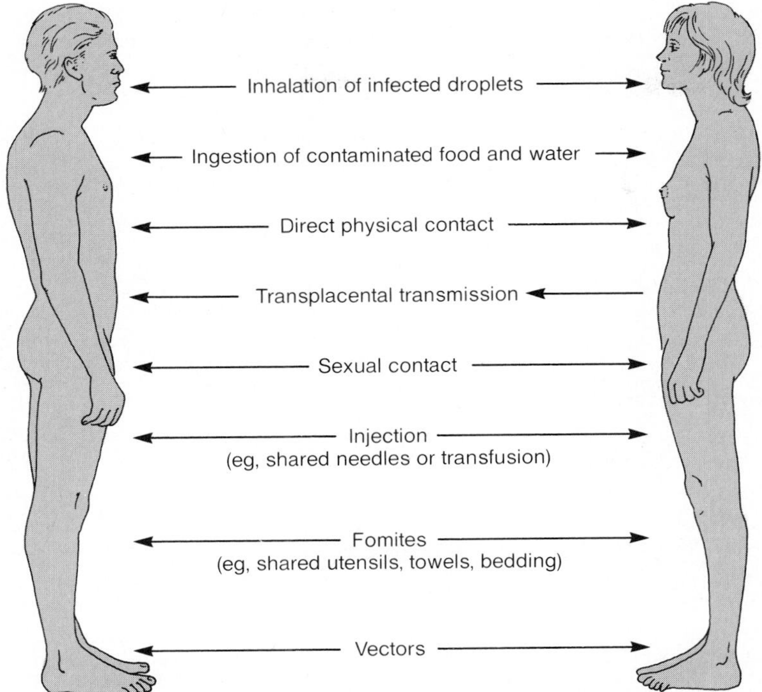

Figure 14-3. Simple cycles of infection (human to human). Simple organisms that require no developmental stage during transmission (eg, viruses, bacteria) are transmitted in this manner.

A patient with coccidioidomycosis is therefore not infectious.

Viruses, though viewed as the simplest life forms, may have complex patterns of transmission that are sometimes described as either **horizontal,** denoting transmission from one host to another—directly or by vectors—or **vertical,** in which viral nucleic acid is transmitted in genetic material from parent to offspring. Vertical transmission is difficult to establish in many cases because it is difficult to distinguish intrinsic genes from the incorporated viral genome.

Transmission of Agents With Complex Life Cycles

Some protozoa and all metazoal parasites have highly complex life cycles, frequently with a sexual as well as a nonsexual (or vegetative) cycle of multiplication, often in different hosts. When more than one cycle exists, the host in which the sexual cycle takes place is the **definitive host;** the vegetative cycle occurs in the **intermediate host.** In the case of *Schistosoma* species (Fig 14–4), which has one of the most complex life cycles, the definitive host is usually a human (exceptions include baboons for *Schistosoma mansoni* and many domesticated animals for *Schistosoma japonicum*), and the intermediate host is the snail. Understanding these life cycles is helpful in developing a rational strategy to control these agents and prevent human disease. Table 14–7 summarizes the method of transmission of selected protozoal and metazoal parasites. Many infections due to these agents are considered in greater detail in the organ system chapters.

Humans may sometimes be infected with metazoal parasites whose natural host is an animal and not humans (Table 14–8). These are accidental human infections, and infection of a human host represents the end of the cycle, since there is no further transmission from humans to another host for these agents (Fig 14–5). These animal parasites generally produce more severe disease when they infect humans than do those parasites for whom humans are the natural host.

Reservoirs of Infection

Human infection often derives from a reservoir of infection, ie, an alternative host or passive carrier that harbors but is not affected by a pathogenic parasite. Most human infectious diseases are caused by infectious agents that selectively parasitize humans. Such infections must be acquired from a human source: either an infected individual or an asymptomatic carrier of the infectious agent.

A few diseases are acquired from animal reservoirs (Table 14–9). In such cases, a history of exposure to the animal reservoir is required to confirm the diagnosis. This exposure may take several forms: consuming the flesh or other products of an infected animal (eg, clonorchiasis, trichinosis);

Table 14-7. Protozoan and metazoan infections of humans.

Disease	Organism	Tissues Involved	Transmission
Protozoa			
Amebiasis	*Entamoeba histolytica*	Colon, liver	Fecal-oral route
Amebic meningoencephalitis	*Naegleria fowleri* *Acanthamoeba* sp	Brain, meninges	Swimming in infested waters
Amebic keratoconjunctivitis	*Acanthamoeba castellani*	Cornea, conjunctiva	Contaminated contact lenses
Balantidiasis	*Balantidium coli*	Colon	Fecal-oral route
Trichomonal vaginitis	*Trichomonas vaginalis*	Vagina, cervix	Sexual intercourse
Cutaneous leishmaniasis	*Leishmania tropica*	Skin	Sandfly bite
Mucocutaneous leishmaniasis	*Leishmania braziliensis*	Nasal and oral mucosa	Sandfly bite
Kala-azar (visceral leishmaniasis)	*Leishmania donovani*	Liver, spleen	Sandfly bite
Chagas' disease	*Trypanosoma cruzi*	Heart, gastrointestinal muscle	Reduviid bug bite
Sleeping sickness	*Trypanosoma* species	Brain	Tsetse fly bite
Malaria	*Plasmodium* species	Erythrocyte, liver	Mosquito bite
Toxoplasmosis	*Toxoplasma gondii*	Brain, lymph nodes, heart, retina	Contact with feces of infected cats; transplacental
Babesiosis	*Babesia microti*	Erythrocyte	Tick bite
Cryptosporidiosis	*Cryptosporidium* species	Intestine	Fecal-oral route
Isosporiasis (coccidiosis)	*Isospora belli*	Small intestine	Fecal-oral route
Pneumocystis pneumonia	*Pneumocystis carinii*	Lung	Inhalation
Metazoan parasites			
Pinworm infestation	*Enterobius vermicularis*	Large intestine	Fecal-oral route
Roundworm infestation	*Ascaris lumbricoides*	Small intestine, lung	Fecal-oral route
Whipworm infestation	*Trichuris trichiura*	Large intestine	Fecal-oral route
Hookworm infestation	*Necator americanus*	Small intestine	Infested soil
	Ancylostoma duodenale	Small intestine	Infested soil
Strongyloidiasis	*Strongyloides stercoralis*	Small intestine, lung	Infested soil
Filariasis	*Wuchereria bancrofti*	Lymphatics, lung	Mosquito bite
	Brugia malayi	Lymphatics, lung	Mosquito bite
Onchocerciasis	*Onchocerca volvulus*	Skin, eye	*Simulium* fly
Loiasis	*Loa loa*	Skin, eye	*Chrysops* fly
Pork tapeworm infestation	*Taenia solium*	Small intestine	Infected pork
Beef tapeworm infestation	*Taenia saginata*	Small intestine	Infected beef
Fish tapeworm infestation	*Diphyllobothrium latum*	Small intestine	Infected fish
Schistosomiasis	*Schistosoma* species	Bladder, intestine	Exposure to snail-infested water
Clonorchiasis	*Clonorchis sinensis*	Bile ducts	Infected fish
Liver fluke infestation	*Fasciola hepatica*	Bile ducts	Infected aquatic vegetation (eg, watercress)
Lung fluke infestation	*Paragonimus westermani*	Lung	Infected crab

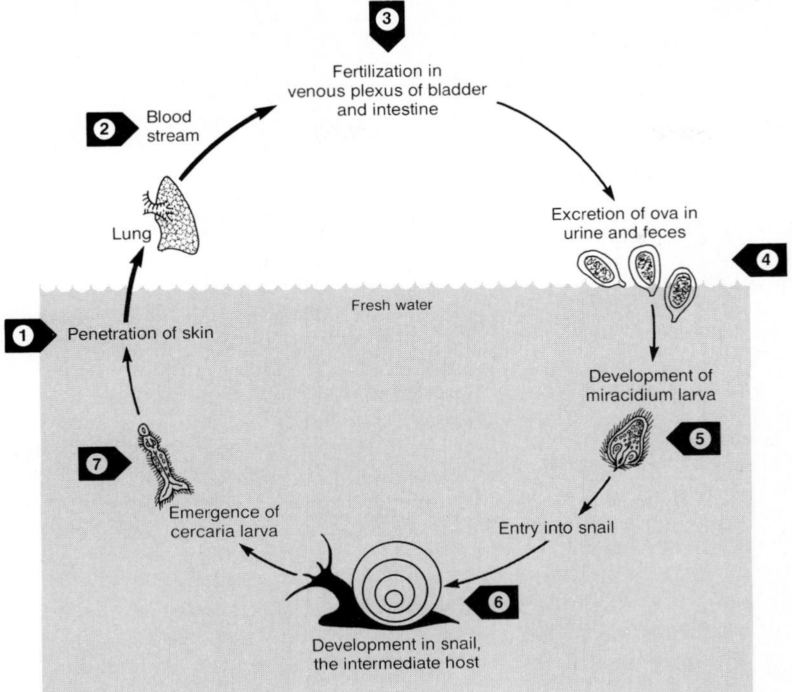

Figure 14-4. Life cycle of *Schistosoma* species. The infective cercarial larva **(7)** penetrates the skin of the human host **(1),** migrates in the blood **(2),** and settles in the venous plexus of the bladder *(S haematobium),* colon *(S mansoni),* or small intestine *(S japonicum)* **(3),** where they mature into adult worms. These produce ova that penetrate the bladder or intestinal wall and are excreted in the urine or feces **(4).** In the soil, they develop into miracidium larvae **(5)** that must undergo a phase of development in a snail intermediate host **(6)** before the infective cercarial larva is produced.

Table 14-8. Parasites with animals as natural host.[1]

Disease	Parasite	Natural Hosts	Transmission to Human	Tissues Involved
Hydatid cyst (echinococcosis)	*Echinococcus granulosus*	Sheep, dog	Ingestion of infected dog feces	Liver, bone, lung
Trichinosis	*Trichinella spiralis*	Pig, bear, etc	Ingestion of undercooked pork or other meat	Muscle, heart, brain
Cysticercosis	*Taenia solium*	Pig, human[2]	Ingestion of infected human feces	Brain, muscle, skin
Cutaneous larva migrans (creeping eruption)	*Ancylostoma braziliensis* (dog and cat hookworm)	Dog, cat	Ingestion of infected animal feces	Skin
Visceral larva migrans	*Toxocara canis, Toxocara catis, Ascaris suum* (dog and cat roundworm)	Dog, cat	Ingestion of infected animal feces	Liver, eye, lung
Dirofilariasis	*Dirofilaria immitis* (heartworm)	Dog	Mosquito bite	Lung (infarction)

[1]Humans are accidental hosts and represent a dead end in the life cycle of these parasites, since there is no transmission from humans to another host.
[2]*T solium* is the tapeworm whose adult form infests the human intestine. In the parasite's normal life cycle, ova passed in human feces are ingested by pigs, which are the normal intermediate hosts. The infective larval form (cysticercus) develops in pig muscle. Human tapeworm infection results when undercooked infected pork is eaten. In human cysticercosis, humans take the place of pigs in the cycle.

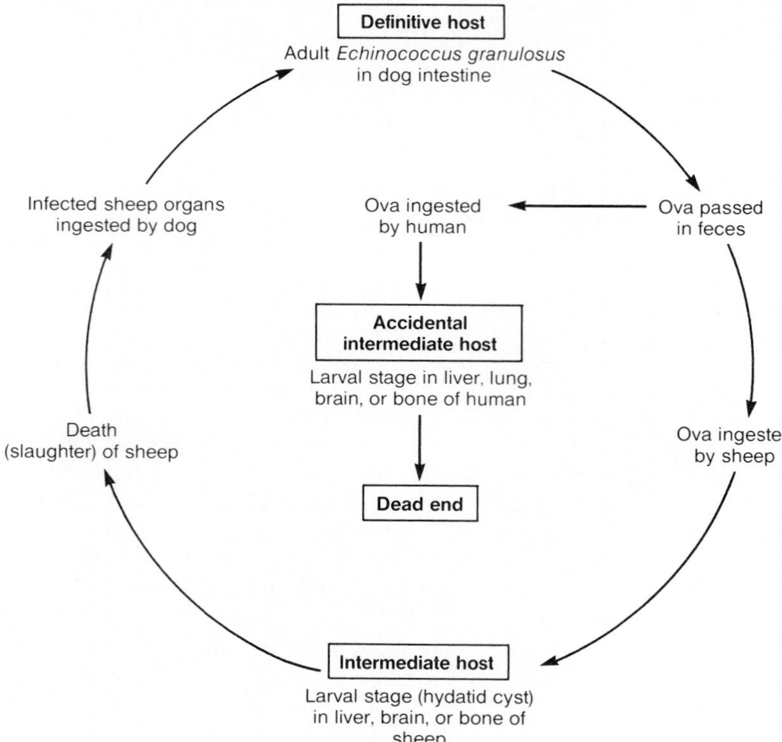

Figure 14-5. Life cycle of *Echinococcus granulosus.* Humans are accidental intermediate hosts and not part of the natural life cycle of the parasite.

handling the hides or carcasses of infected animals (eg, anthrax); handling, inhaling, or ingesting the excreta of an infected animal (eg, leptospirosis, brucellosis); being bitten or scratched by an infected animal (eg, cat-scratch disease, rabies); inhaling or ingesting the infectious agent directly (eg, human glanders); or being bitten by an arthropod vector that has bitten an infected animal (eg, plague, arbovirus encephalitis).

Diseases transmitted from an animal reservoir tend to have a restricted geographic distribution that is dependent on the prevalence of infected reservoirs in different areas; eg, *Echinococcus granulosus* infection (hydatid cyst disease) occurs much more commonly in sheep-farming countries such as Australia.

DIAGNOSIS OF INFECTIOUS DISEASE

The aim of diagnosis in infectious diseases is (1) to recognize that a sick patient is ill with an infectious disease; and (2) to identify the specific agent responsible for the disease so as to be able to decide on the most appropriate treatment, since the susceptibility of most agents to selected antimicrobial agents is known.

Identification of the infectious agent may be achieved in several ways.

Clinical Examination

A few infectious agents produce highly characteristic clinical illnesses, eg, herpes zoster, malaria. In these cases, recognition of the specific agent may be achieved by clinical examination alone. In most infectious diseases, however, clinical examination suggests a range of possible etiologic agents, and specific diagnosis requires stepwise refinement of the possibilities through laboratory tests, culture, or immunologic studies (Table 14–10).

Microbiologic Examination

Demonstration of the agent—either by microscopic examination or culture of tissues and fluids removed from the patient—is the most common means of providing an etiologic diagnosis of infectious disease. With few exceptions (eg, *T pallidum, Mycobacterium leprae*), microorganisms can be isolated in culture. Living cell systems are

Table 14–9. Infections having animal reservoirs.

Disease	Infectious Agent	Animal Reservoir
Plague	*Yersinia pestis*	Wild rats, ground squirrels, chipmunks
Tularemia	*Francisella tularensis*	Rabbits, ground squirrels
Anthrax	*Bacillus anthracis*	Cattle, sheep
Glanders	*Pseudomonas mallei*	Horses, mules, donkeys
Leptospirosis	*Leptospira* species	Rats, dogs, pigs, cattle
Brucellosis	*Brucella* species	Cattle, goats, pigs
Cat-scratch disease	Unknown bacteria	Cats
Psittacosis	*Chlamydia psittaci*	Birds
Encephalitis	Arboviruses	Horses, wild primates
Rabies	Rabies virus	Dogs, cats, bats, foxes, skunks, raccoons
Cryptococcosis	*Cryptococcus neoformans*	Birds
Toxoplasmosis	*Toxoplasma gondii*	Cats
Larva migrans (visceral and cutaneous)	Animal helminths	Cats, dogs
Hydatid cyst (echinococcosis)	*Echinococcus granulosus*	Cattle, sheep
Trichinosis	*Trichinella spiralis*	Carnivores (pigs, bears)
Beef or pork tapeworm	*Taenia* species	Pigs, cattle
Fish tapeworm	*Diphyllobothrium latum*	Fish
Schistosomiasis	*Schistosoma* species	Snails (particular species)
Clonorchiasis	*Clonorchis sinensis*	Fish

necessary for growth of obligate intracellular agents; artificial culture media usually suffice for extracellular and facultative intracellular agents. Larger parasites, including protozoa and metazoa, are not usually cultured, but because of their large size they or their larvae or ova are usually recognizable on direct examination of tissues and smears of infected material.

Culture of an organism is also important when antimicrobial sensitivity of that agent varies, eg, in many bacterial infections. Although antibiotics are often chosen on the basis of existing clinical findings and treatment is started empirically after specimens have been obtained for culture, in vitro antibiotic sensitivity of the cultured organism is used to guide appropriate antibiotic therapy.

Immunologic Techniques

A sharp (4-fold) increase in antibody titers against a specific agent is diagnostic of acute infection by that agent. In general, immunologic diagnosis requires paired serum samples, one obtained early in the disease and one during convalescence 2–3 weeks later. High antibody titers in a single specimen are of less significance than high levels in multiple samples. In general, IgM levels rise first, peak in 2–3 months, and then fall progressively; IgG levels rise after IgM in a primary immune response. A nonspecific (anamnestic) rise in IgG antibodies of a wide range of specificities may occur in many infections. Such nonspecific responses do not involve IgM antibodies. An increased IgM level of a specific antibody is therefore of greater diagnostic value than an increased IgG level.

Immunologic markers—specific antibody labeled with fluorescent dyes—are being employed more frequently to detect infectious agents in tissues and smears; eg, fluorescent-labeled antibody against *Legionella pneumophila* is used to demonstrate the organisms in sputum samples and thereby permit specific diagnosis of legionnaires' disease in a patient with pneumonia. Development of DNA probes with high levels of specificity against cytomegalovirus and Epstein-Barr virus has provided a means of identifying these viral genomes in infected cells.

Histologic Examination

Larger infectious agents such as fungi, protozoa, and metazoal parasites can often be identified in tissue sections on the basis of distinctive structures such as ova, cysts, yeast, spherules, or hyphae. A few bacteria can be identified or at least partially characterized in tissues. Silver stains permit identification of spirochetes and *Legionella pneumophila;* acid-fast stains demonstrate mycobacteria; and the morphologic features of *Actinomyces* and *Nocardia* on tissue Gram stain are fairly typical. Some viruses (eg, cytomegalovirus, herpes simplex virus, and measles virus) may be specifically identified by the changes produced in cells, eg, inclusions, giant cells (Chapter 13). Immunohistologic techniques provide the most specific means of recognizing microbes in tissue sections and are becoming available for a growing list of microbial agents.

It should be stressed that precise culture and immunologic techniques vary for different organisms. It is vital for the physician to direct the lab-

Table 14-10. Diagnosis of acute meningitis: Example of steps commonly followed in the diagnosis of infectious disease.

Clinical or Laboratory Finding	Interpretation
Acute illness with fever, headache, and neck stiffness	**Possible acute meningitis** Initial study: Obtain cerebrospinal fluid.
Abnormal cerebrospinal fluid with inflammatory cells	**Acute meningitis** Possible agents: Pyogenic bacteria (meningococcus, pneumococcus, *Haemophilus influenzae, Streptococcus agalactiae, Listeria monocytogenes, Escherichia coli*), *Leptospira* species, *Mycobacterium tuberculosis;* many viruses; *Cryptococcus neoformans,* other fungi; amebas (*Acanthamoeba, Naegleria species).*
Purulent cerebrospinal fluid with numerous neutrophils	**Extracellular agent** Possible agents: Pyogenic bacteria, *Leptospira,* fungi, amebas Further study: 1. Identify agent in cerebrospinal fluid (Gram stain for bacteria, sediment for amebas, India ink preparation for *Cryptococcus,* darkfield illumination for *Leptospira*). 2. Culture cerebrospinal fluid and blood. 3. Obtain serum for antibody titers. 4. Perform latex agglutination test or immunoelectrophoresis on cerebrospinal fluid and blood to detect possible cryptococcal antigen.
Clear cerebrospinal fluid with mononuclear cells	**Obligate intracellular agent** Possible agents: Viruses Further study: 1. Culture cerebrospinal fluid for viruses. 2. Obtain serum for viral serologic tests.
Clear cerebrospinal fluid with neutrophils and mononuclear cells	**Extracellular or facultative intracellular agent** Possible agents: Pyogenic bacteria (partially treated or chronic disease); mycobacteria; fungi. Further study: 1. Perform Gram and acid-fast stains of cerebrospinal fluid. 2. Culture cerebrospinal fluid and blood. 3. Obtain serum for antibody titers. 4. Perform skin tests.

oratory to seek a *range* of organisms that may be causing disease. Too long a list of possible etiologic organisms will lead to unnecessary and expensive laboratory work; too short a list may result in failure to identify the infectious agent. For example, when an unknown lung mass is removed, the possibility that it may be a granuloma must be recognized and tissue sent for mycobacterial and fungal culture. Failure to do so may result in less than optimal treatment because of inability to identify the agent.

Section IV. Disorders of Development & Growth

This section deals with abnormalities that occur in cellular growth and development of the individual from conception to death. Chapter 15 describes abnormalities occurring during fetal development, abnormalities of postnatal development, abnormalities of sexual development, and aging.

In addition, throughout life, cells grow, undergo mitotic division, differentiate, and die in a controlled fashion that maintains the normal size and structure of tissues. Abnormalities in these processes are described in Chapters 16–19, with special emphasis on neoplasia (Chapters 17–19).

15 Disorders of Development

NORMAL FETAL DEVELOPMENT

The initial divisions of the fertilized ovum (zygote) (Fig 15-1) create a mass of cells (blastocyst) consisting of an inner cell mass (the embryonic disk) surrounded by an outer layer (the trophoblast). The cells of the trophoblast actively penetrate the endometrium and form the placenta.

The cells of the embryonic disk are totipotential (ie, they have the capacity to produce all cells of the body) and eventually give rise to the embryo. Initial differentiation into the 3 primary germ layers—ectoderm, mesoderm, and entoderm—ultimately gives rise to the organs of the body through repeated division, organization, and further differentiation. The mass of primitive cells from which an organ develops is known as the **anlage**. The fully developed organ is composed of highly differentiated cells committed to the performance of particular functions and having limited residual capacity for division and differentiation. Most human organs are fully formed and functional at birth. Organs such as the heart complete development earlier in fetal life than others such as the lung, which reaches full maturity after the thirty-fourth week. The brain shows considerable development after birth, attaining maturity at about age 7 years. Sexual development occurs during puberty.

ABNORMAL FETAL DEVELOPMENT

Definitions (Fig 15-2)

A. Agenesis: Failure of development of primitive organ anlagen in the embryo results in agenesis—complete absence of the organ. Agenesis of a vital organ such as the heart or brain is incompatible with survival, and the fetus dies in utero. If the tissue is not vital or is one of a pair of or-

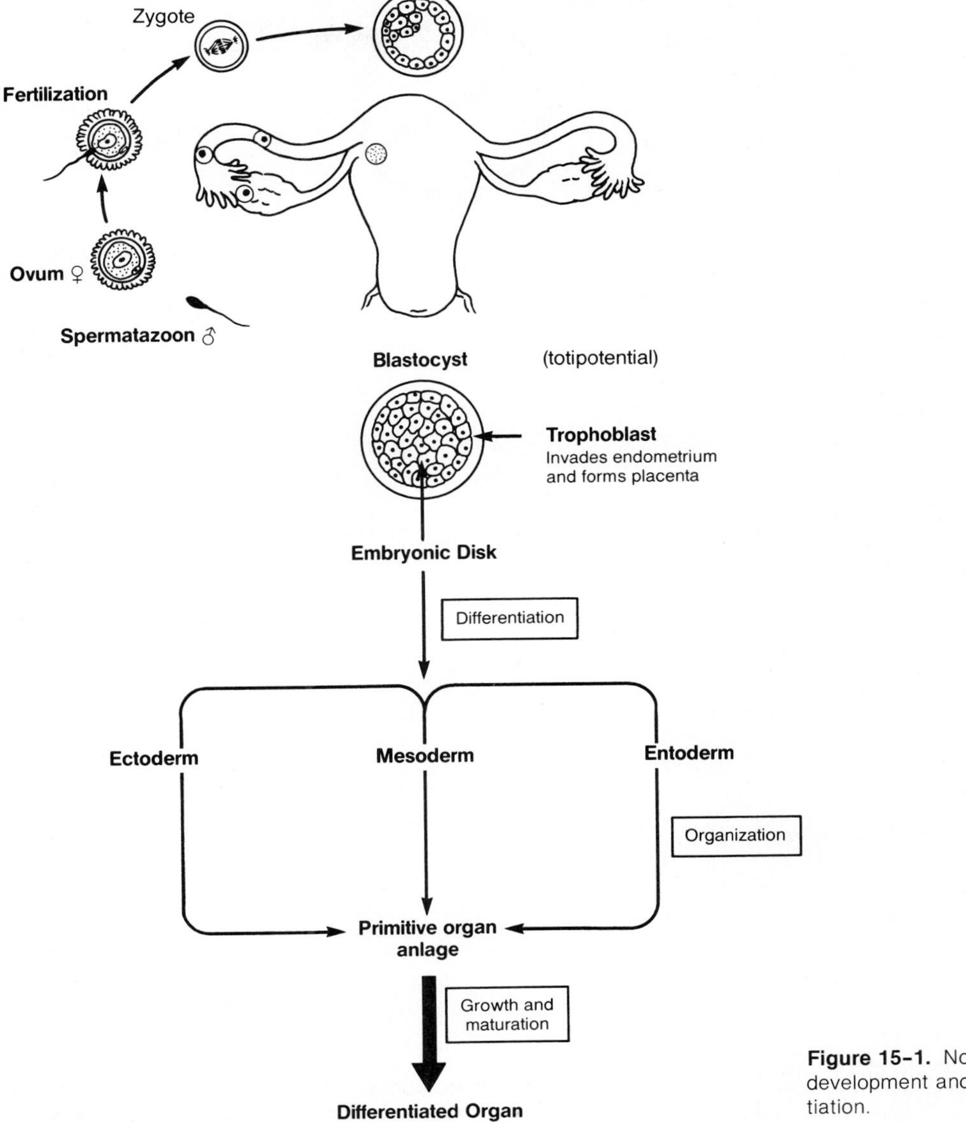

Figure 15–1. Normal embryonic development and organ differentiation.

gans, such as a kidney, the remainder of the embryo may develop normally.

B. Dysgenesis: Abnormal differentiation of the anlage leads to a structurally abnormal organ. For example, in renal dysgenesis, a mass of tissue composed of abnormal epithelium-lined cysts and mesenchymal tissues such as cartilage is found instead of a normal kidney (Fig 15–3). Dysgenesis sometimes affects only part of an organ.

C. Hypoplasia and Aplasia: When the anlage differentiates normally but growth or development ends prematurely, a structurally normal but small organ results (hypoplasia). In aplasia, the organ is completely absent. Aplasia can be distinguished from agenesis only if an undeveloped anlage or its vascular connections can be identified. In agenesis, there is no anlage or vascular pedicle.

Causes of Fetal Abnormalities

In most instances, the exact cause of fetal abnormalities is unknown. Known causes fall into 2 major groups: those affecting the genome and those acting mainly on the proliferating cells of the embryo or fetus. Almost any cause of injury to a child or adult (Fig III–1) may also act on the fetus. Although the fetus is in a sheltered environment, it is particularly susceptible to injury during

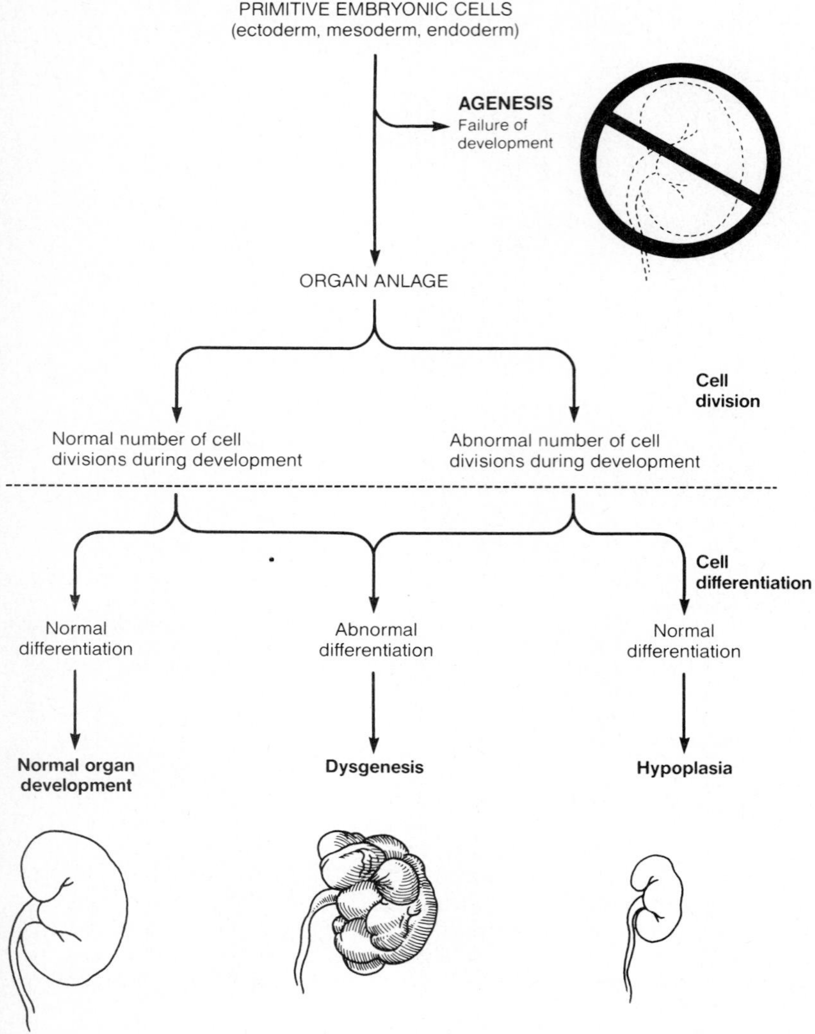

Figure 15-2. Abnormal organ development.

times of rapid cell multiplication and primary differentiation of organs. In addition, normal growth of the fetus is critically dependent upon normal expression of genetic information and the integrity of the placenta and maternal blood flow, abnormalities of which may lead to fetal abnormality (Table 15-1). The most severe fetal abnormality is death, termed spontaneous abortion in the first 14 weeks and intrauterine death thereafter.

FETAL ABNORMALITIES CAUSED BY GENETIC DISORDERS

The term "mutation" denotes any stable heritable genetic change, whether or not it is associated with detectable structural abnormalities of the chromosomes.

Chromosomal Aberrations

• **A. Normal Chromosomal Complement:** The normal human cell has 46 chromosomes: 22 pairs of autosomes and 2 sex chromosomes (Fig 15-4). One of each of these homologous pairs of chromosomes is derived from each parent.

The chromosomal structure of cells can be determined by examination of peripheral blood lymphocytes or skin fibroblasts. Mitotic division of the cells is stimulated and then arrested at metaphase with colchicine; the chromosomes that have separated at metaphase can then be counted and identified individually using special staining techniques ("banding"). The accurate identification and placement of an individual's chromosomes in their proper sequence is known as his or her **karyotype**. The karyotype of a normal male is 46,XY; for a normal female, 46,XX. Abnormal karyotypes (eg, 45,X) are variations of these pat-

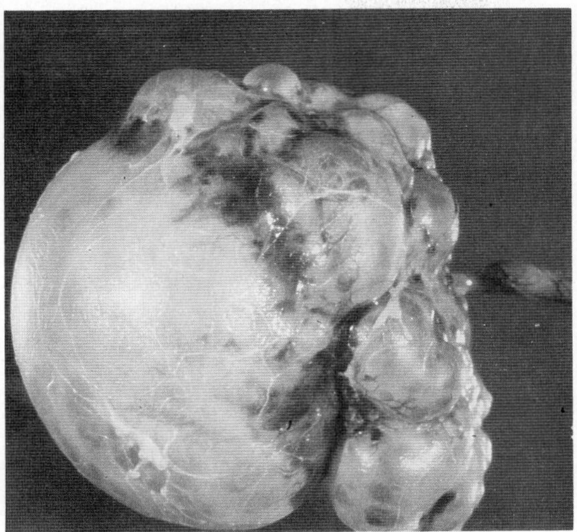

Figure 15-3. Renal dysgenesis. The kidney is grossly abnormal and shows multiple cysts. (The nodular structures seen on this surface view were filled with fluid when cut open.)

Table 15-1. Factors causing fetal (congenital) abnormalities or injury.

Genetic disorders
Chromosomal aberrations[1]
Single gene abnormalities
Polygenic abnormalities
External agents (teratogens)
Ionizing radiation
Infection (eg, rubella, cytomegalovirus, toxoplasmosis, syphilis)[1]
Drugs and poisons
Alcohol and smoking
Mechanical trauma
Abnormalities of placentation (Chapter 55)
Vascular insufficiency[1]
Placental separation[1]
Maternal-fetal transfer of IgG antibodies
Hemolytic disease of the newborn (Chapter 25)[1]
Neonatal myasthenia gravis (Chapter 66)
Neonatal thyrotoxicosis (Chapter 58)
Other associated factors
Nutritional deficiency
Diabetes mellitus[1]
Socioeconomic status
Maternal and paternal age
Premature delivery[1]

[1]Common causes of fetal death. Spontaneous abortion occurs in 20–25% of all conceptions; lethal congenital abnormalities occur in 1–2% of all births; and nonlethal abnormalities (which may become manifest in later life) occur in 2% of all live births.

terns. **Cytogenetics** is the study of chromosomal structure and chromosomal aberrations in cells.

The **autosomes** are divided into 7 groups (A–G) on the basis of the size and position of the centromeres (Fig 15–4).

The **sex chromosomes** are a pair of X chromosomes in the female and an X and a Y chromosome in the male. The genetic sex of an individual may be ascertained by examination of the karyotype, which is very accurate, or by examination of cells for the presence of a Barr body. When two X chromosomes are present in a cell, as in a normal female, one of them—the Barr body—becomes inactivated and condensed on the nuclear membrane. Absence of Barr bodies indicates that the cell has only one X chromosome (normal male: XY; Turner's syndrome: XO). Barr bodies are most easily seen in a smear of squamous epithelial cells obtained by scraping the buccal mucosa. The Y chromosome can be identified in interphase nu-

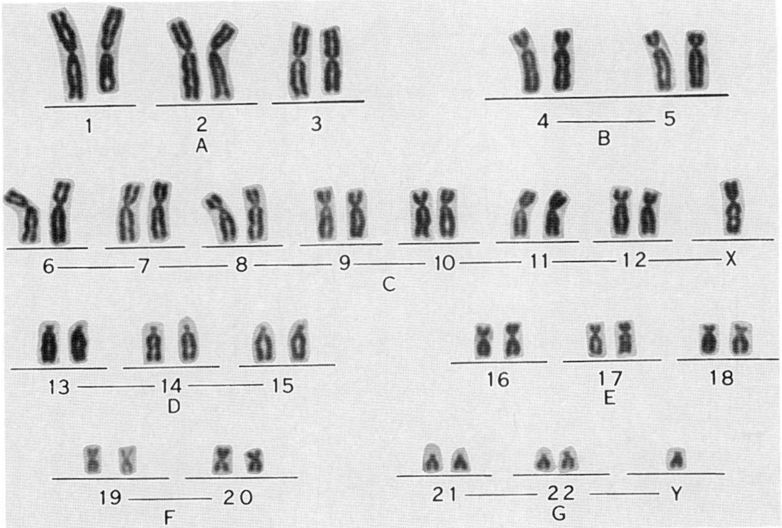

Figure 15-4. Chromosomes of normal human male (46,XY). These consist of the sex chromosomes (XY) plus 22 pairs of autosomes that by convention are classified as follows: Groups A and F are large and small metacentric chromosomes (ie, the centromeres are located near the center of the chromosome); groups B, C, and E are large, medium, and small submetacentric chromosomes (eccentrically located centromeres); and groups D and G are medium and small acrocentric chromosomes (centromeres located near the end). In a human female (46,XX), the Y chromosome is replaced by a second X chromosome.

clei by its strong fluorescence in ultraviolet light after it has been stained with quinacrine, and this is another means of establishing genetic sex.

B. Mechanisms of Chromosomal Aberrations:

1. Nondisjunction in meiosis–Nondisjunction is failure of paired homologous chromosomes to separate during the first meiotic division that leads to the production of gametes (ova and spermatozoa) in the gonads (Fig 15–5A). Thus, some gametes receive 2 and others receive none of the involved chromosome pair. After the second meiotic division, the resulting gametes will have 24 and 22 chromosomes. Such gametes are **aneuploid** (the number of their chromosomes is not an exact multiple of 23, the haploid chromosome number for humans).

Union of an aneuploid gamete with a normal

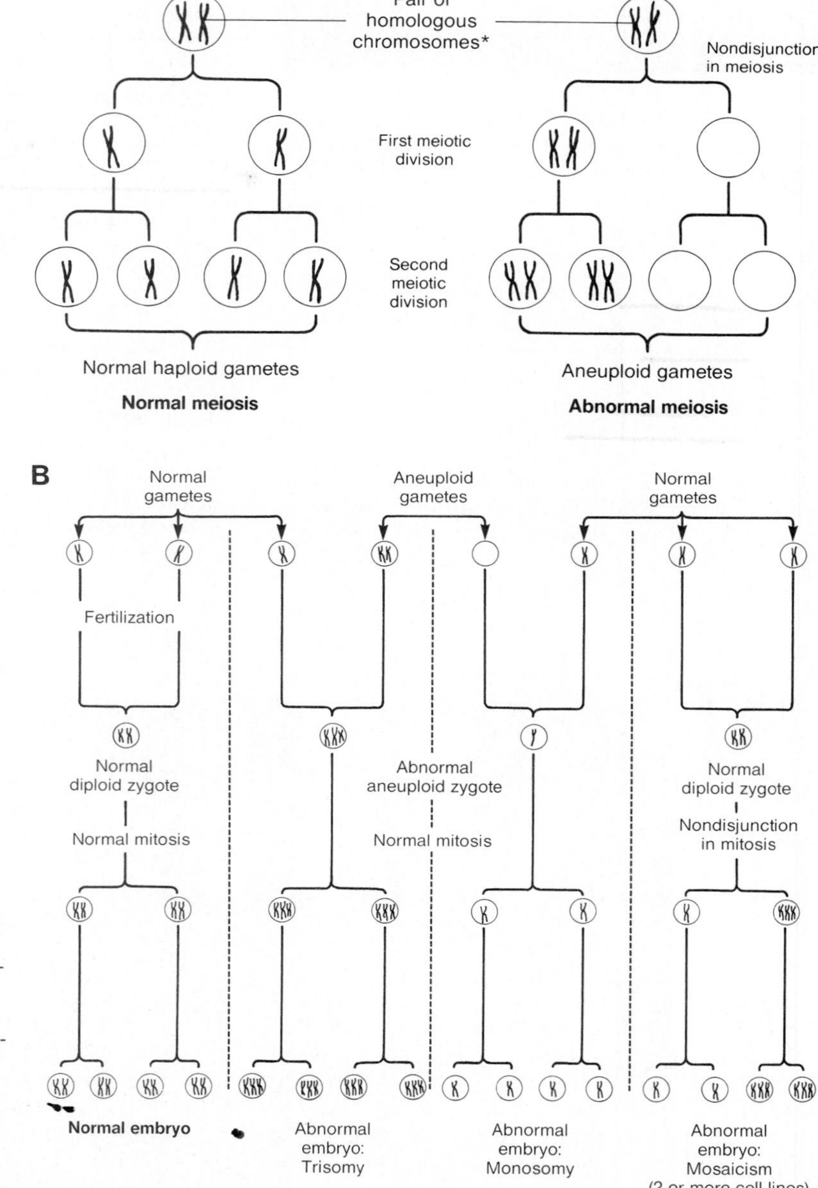

Figure 15–5. A: Nondisjunction in meiosis compared with normal meiosis (one pair of homologous chromosomes is represented). **B:** Fertilization between normal haploid and aneuploid gametes, resulting in normal and abnormal zygotes. Nondisjunction may also occur during early mitotic divisions of a normal zygote, leading to 2 different cell lines in the body (mosaicism).

gamete leads to an aneuploid zygote that has either 3 of the involved chromosomes **(trisomy)** or only one **(monosomy)** (Fig 15–5B).

Trisomy and monosomy involving the sex chromosomes are generally compatible with life, eg, Klinefelter's syndrome (XXY), Turner's syndrome (XO), and others (XXX, XYY). These disorders are associated with relatively minor structural abnormalities; however, there are major abnormalities of gonadal development.

Autosomal monosomy, on the other hand, is usually associated with a profound loss of genetic material and is incompatible with life. A few autosomal trisomies (21, 13, and 18) are compatible with survival but are associated with severe abnormalities.

2. Nondisjunction in mitosis–Nondisjunction of the early zygote during mitotic division produces **mosaicism:** the presence in an individual of 2 or more genetically different cell populations (Fig 15–5B). In this type of nondisjunction (which may also occur during the second meiotic division), the 2 chromatids of a chromosome fail to divide. Mosaicism commonly affects sex chromosomes; autosomal mosaicism that is compatible with life is rare. Mosaic individuals manifest phenotypic abnormalities that are intermediate between those associated with the 2 cell populations; eg, 45,X/46,XX is a Turner syndrome mosaic karyotype, and the individual's appearance will be somewhere between that of a normal female and those of classic Turner's syndrome (45,XO).

3. Deletion–Deletion is loss of part of a chromosome after chromosomal breakage. Most deletions are lethal, because a great deal of genetic material is lost. Deletions of the short arms of chromosomes 4 and 5 produce well-defined clinical syndromes (Wolf's syndrome and cri du chat syndrome, respectively). Chromosomal deletion is common in malignant neoplastic cells such as leukemic cells.

4. Translocation–Translocation is the transfer of a broken segment of one chromosome to another chromosome. In **balanced translocations,** all genetic material is present and functional, and the individual is phenotypically normal.

The commonest balanced translocation is transfer of the entire 21 chromosome to chromosome 14. Such an individual has 45 chromosomes, with absence of one each of chromosomes 14 and 21 and the presence of an abnormal large chromosome containing the material of both chromosomes 14 and 21; assuming the patient is male, the karyotypic designation is 45,XY,t(14,21). The gametes produced by such an individual may be abnormal (Fig 15–6); offspring with monosomy 21 (incompatible with life) and translocation-type Down's syndrome may result.

Other balanced translocations are being recognized as an important cause of habitual or repeated abortion.

A specific balanced translocation in which translocations of some chromosomal material from chromosome 22 to chromosome 9 occurs in about 90% of patients with chronic granulocytic leukemia. The abnormally small 22 chromosome that remains is called the Philadelphia chromosome (Ph^1).

5. Other chromosomal rearrangements–Inversion, isochromosome formation (an isochromosome has identical genetic material on either side of the centromere), and ring chromosome formation may occur after breakage or abnormal division of the centromere. These may produce clinical syndromes; eg, an isochromosome of the long arm of the X chromosome produces a syndrome similar to Turner's syndrome. In addition, single changes (additions or deletions) in the composition of DNA bases result in misreading of the triplet code but cause no detectable structural changes in the chromosomes. These abnormalities constitute single gene disorders and are considered in a later section.

C. Causes of Chromosomal Aberrations: Most chromosomal defects occur at random without known cause, but in some cases a cause can be identified.

1. Increasing maternal age–Nondisjunction is associated with increasing maternal age, as i clearly shown in **trisomy 21** (Down's syndrome). The risk of trisomy 21, which is 1:2000 live births in women under 30 years of age, increases to 1:50 for women over 45 years of age. For this reason, routine chromosomal analysis of fetal cells obtained by amniocentesis is recommended for pregnancies occurring in women older than age 35 years. Increasing maternal age is also associated with other nondisjunction syndromes, eg, Klinefelter's syndrome.

2. Ionizing radiation–The incidence of chromosomal abnormalities is high in the survivors of the Nagasaki and Hiroshima atomic blasts. A "safe" low dose of ionizing radiation has not been established. For this reason, diagnostic abdominal x-rays should be avoided whenever possible in pregnant women.

3. Drugs–Drugs and other chemical agents are an uncommon cause of structural chromosomal abnormalities. When used in early pregnancy, anticancer agents that interfere with DNA synthesis may cause chromosomal abnormalities that lead to fetal death. The use of these agents in the treatment of cancer in the mother is perceived as a problem of medical ethics. Many commonly used drugs, including aspirin, have been shown to cause karyotypic abnormalities in tissue cultures; whether these drugs have this effect in vivo is unknown. LSD also produces chromosomal abnormalities in rats.

D. Common Autosomal Abnormalities:

1. Down's syndrome (trisomy 21)–Down's syndrome is the most common autosomal disor-

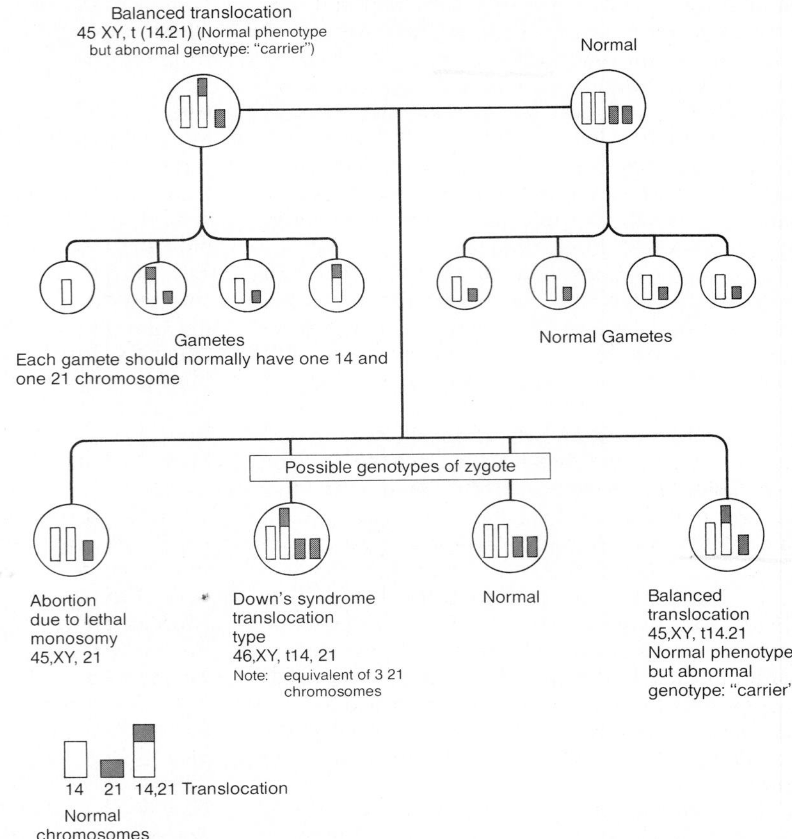

Figure 15-6. Zygote formation in a patient with balanced translocation.

der. It results from the presence of 3 chromosome 21s, producing a characteristic clinical appearance (Fig 15-7). The infant has oblique palpebral fissures with a flat profile, upward-slanting eyes, and prominent epicanthal folds (a purported resemblance to Asian facial features, accounting for the older term "mongolism"). Severe mental retardation is a constant feature. Thirty percent of patients have congenital heart anomalies, most commonly ventricular septal defect. These children also have an increased susceptibility to infections, duodenal ulcers, and acute leukemia.

About half of children with Down's syndrome die by age 10 years. Survival to adulthood is becoming more frequent with improved management and development of specialized care centers. Men with Down's syndrome are generally infertile; women with the disease have borne children. The offspring of mothers with Down's syndrome may be normal, because the extra 21 chromosome is not transmitted to all gametes.

Three types of Down's syndrome are recognized:

a. Nondisjunction Down's syndrome-Most cases (95%) of Down's syndrome are due to this

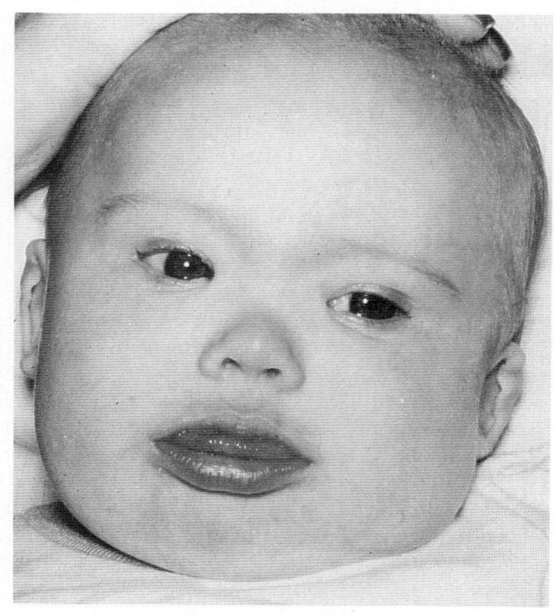

Figure 15-7. Down's syndrome, showing upward-slanting eyes, a flat profile, and protuberant tongue.

mechanism. These cases are associated with increasing maternal age and occur chiefly in babies born to women over age 35 years. The child has an extra 21 chromosome (47,XX,+21 or 47, XY,+21); the parents have normal karyotypes.

b. Translocation Down's syndrome–A few cases of Down's syndrome (5%) are due to inheritance of a balanced translocation from one of the parents—commonly a 14,21 translocation (Fig 15–6), more rarely a 21,22 translocation. One parent carries the abnormal chromosome. The infant with Down's syndrome has 46 chromosomes, one of which has the genetic material of both chromosomes 14 and 21. Translocation Down's syndrome is not associated with increased maternal age but carries with it an increased risk that the carrier parent will produce further offspring with Down's syndrome (familial Down's syndrome).

c. Mosaic Down's syndrome–In this very rare type of Down's syndrome, only one of 2 cell lines in the body shows trisomy for chromosome 21.•

2. Edwards' syndrome (trisomy 18)–Trisomy 18 (47,XX/XY,+18) is rare. It produces severe defects, and few children survive beyond 1 year of age. Clinically, failure to thrive and severe mental retardation are accompanied by characteristic physical abnormalities such as "rocker bottom" feet and clenched hands with overlapping fingers.

3. Patau's syndrome (trisomy 13)–Trisomy 13 (47,XX/XY,+13) is also rare. Most affected infants die soon after birth. Trisomy 13 is characterized by abnormal development of the forebrain (absent olfactory bulbs, fused frontal lobes, single ventricle) and midline facial structures (cleft lip, cleft palate, nasal defects, single central eye [cyclops]).

4. Cri du chat (cat cry) syndrome–This disorder is caused by deletion of the short arm of chromosome 5. A mewing, catlike cry is typical. Severe mental retardation and cardiac anomalies are common. Survival rates are slightly higher than those of patients with trisomy 18 or 13.

5. Acquired chromosomal abnormalities–These occur quite commonly as somatic mutations in children and adults and are associated with a variety of neoplasms (Chapter 18). The germ cells are usually not involved, and these anomalies are therefore not heritable. ••

• E. Common Sex Chromosomal Abnormalities:

1. Klinefelter's syndrome (testicular dysgenesis)–Klinefelter's syndrome is common, with an incidence of 1:600 live male births. It is usually caused by nondisjunction of the X chromosome in the mother of the affected male child, resulting in an extra X chromosome (47,XXY) (Figs 15–8 and 15–9). More rarely, patients with Klinefelter's syndrome have more than two X chromosomes (48,XXXY or 49,XXXXY).

The Y chromosome dictates testicular differentiation of the primitive gonad that results in a male phenotype. No abnormality is usually noted until puberty. The extra X chromosome interferes with normal development of the testis at puberty in some unknown manner. The testes remain small and do not produce spermatozoa. Seminiferous tubules contain mainly Sertoli cells with few spermatogonia, and the tubules undergo progressive atrophy (Fig 15–10). Patients are usually infertile. Testosterone levels are low, leading to failure of development of male secondary sexual characteristics. Patients tend to be tall (testosterone induces fusion of epiphyses) and of eunuchoid habitus with a high-pitched voice, small penis, and female distribution of hair (Fig 15–11). Gynecomastia (enlargement of breasts) may occur. Intelligence is usually not affected.

The diagnosis of Klinefelter's syndrome may be made by finding Barr bodies in a buccal scraping of a phenotypic male or by performing karyotypic analysis, which should always be done to confirm the diagnosis (Fig 15–10).

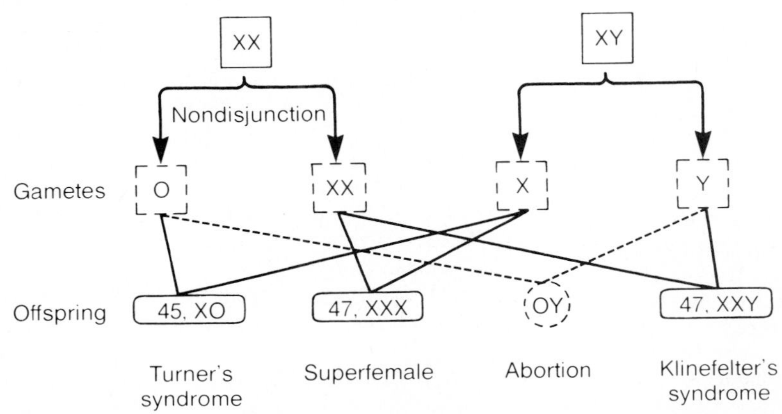

Figure 15–8. Nondisjunction of sex chromosomes, leading to offspring with Turner's syndrome, Klinefelter's syndrome, and "superfemale" or XXX syndrome.

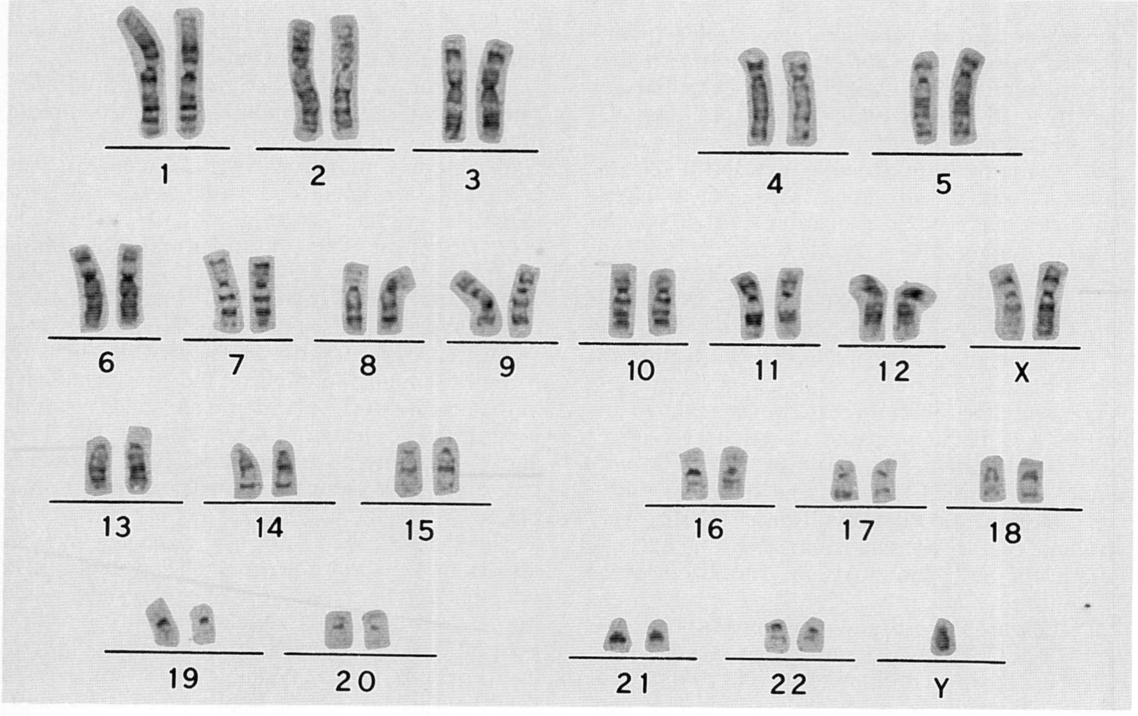

Figure 15–9. Karyotype of a male with Klinefelter's syndrome (47,XXY).

2. Turner's syndrome (ovarian dysgenesis)– Turner's syndrome is less common than Klinefelter's syndrome, occurring in 1:2500 live female births. It is caused by nondisjunction of the X chromosome in either parent of an affected female, leading to absence of one X chromosome (45,XO; Fig 15–8). About half of patients with Turner's syndrome show mosaicism (45,X/46,XX) owing to nondisjunction occurring in a postzygotic mitotic division.

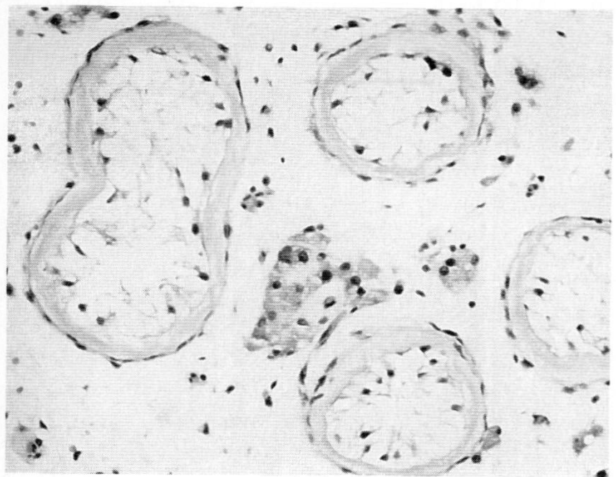

Figure 15–10. Testis in Klinefelter's syndrome. The seminiferous tubules show absent spermatogenesis, containing only Sertoli cells. The basement membrane of the tubules is greatly thickened. A cluster of interstitial cells is present. High magnification.

Loss of the second X chromosome frequently causes fetal death, and many affected fetuses are aborted. Liveborn infants show lymphedema of the neck that persists into adulthood as a characteristic webbing of the neck (Fig 15–12). Congenital cardiac anomalies (most commonly coarctation of the aorta), short stature, obesity, and skeletal abnormalities (most typically an increase in the carrying angle of the forearm) are common. Intelligence is usually not affected.

In the presence of one X chromosome (and no Y chromosome), the primitive gonad develops as an ovary, and the baby with Turner's syndrome is phenotypically female. The absence of the second X chromosome causes failure of ovarian development at puberty. The ovaries remain small and lack primordial follicles ("streak ovaries"). Failure of estrogen secretion causes failure of the endometrial cycle (amenorrhea) and poor development of female secondary sex characteristics, including the breasts.

The diagnosis may be established by absence of Barr bodies in the buccal smear of a female and by karyotypic analysis.

3. XXX syndrome ("superfemale")– The presence of a third X chromosome in a female causes the triple X disorder. Most patients are normal. A few show mental retardation, menstrual problems, and decreased fertility.

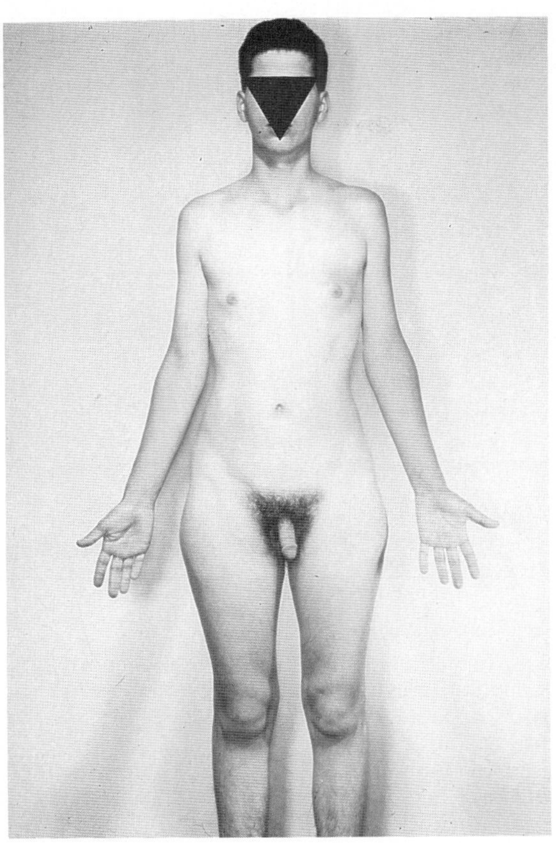

Figure 15–11. Klinefelter's syndrome. The individual is tall, with female fat and hair distribution. Gynecomastia is present. The testes (not seen) were very small.

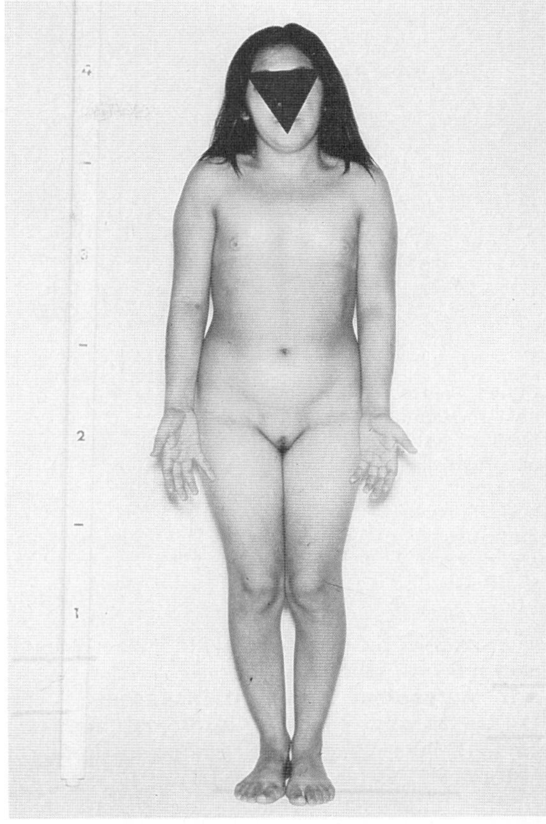

Figure 15–12. Turner's syndrome. Note short stature, poor development of breasts and pubic hair, and webbing of the neck.

4. XYY syndrome–The presence of an extra Y chromosome in a male causes XYY syndrome. Most patients are normal. Initial studies suggesting that 47,XYY individuals were more common in prison populations and that the chromosomal abnormality in some way produced antisocial behavior have not been confirmed.

Single-Gene (Mendelian) Disorders

A. Dominant and Recessive Genes: Diseases caused by a single abnormal gene are inherited in a manner predicted by mendelian laws. The pattern of inheritance depends on whether the abnormal gene is on a sex chromosome or an autosome and whether it is dominant or recessive.

If a gene has 2 alleles (alternative forms of the gene) A and a, 3 genotypes (AA, Aa, and aa) are possible. In **homozygous** genotypes (AA and aa) the 2 alleles are identical. In **heterozygous** genotypes (Aa), the alleles are different. The terms "dominant" and "recessive" denote the degree of expression of a gene. The mode of inheritance is **dominant** if only one abnormal allele is required for phenotypic expression of the disease (genotypes Aa, AA; Fig 15–13). A **recessive** trait, on the other hand, requires the presence of *two* abnormal alleles for expression of disease (genotype aa; Fig 15–14).

Analysis of the family history (pedigree) of an individual affected with a single-gene disease (proband; propositus or index case) is helpful in establishing the inheritance pattern of the disease.

1. Dominant inheritance–If the A allele is abnormal, the disease is expressed in both the AA and the Aa genotypes (Fig 15–13). In many instances, the presence of 2 abnormal genes (AA genotype) is incompatible with life. In diseases with dominant inheritance patterns, the aa genotype is normal.

2. Recessive inheritance–If the a allele is abnormal, however, the disease will occur only in the aa genotype (Fig 15–14). The person who is an Aa heterozygote for a recessive trait carries the gene but does not express the disease (**heterozygous carrier of the trait**). If the gene products of both the A and the a alleles can be detected in the Aa

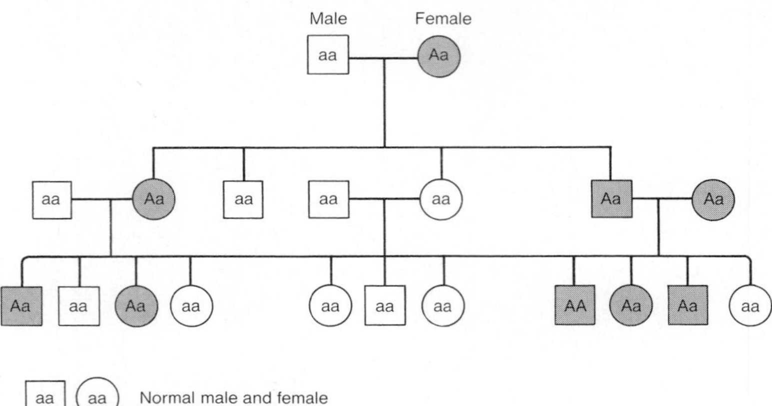

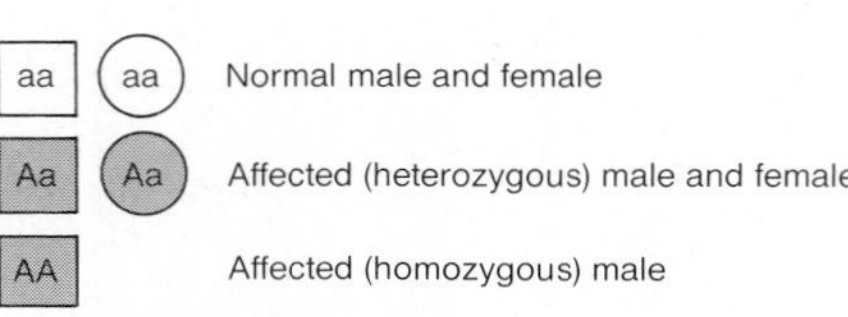

Figure 15-13. Autosomal dominant inheritance. Circles denote females; squares are males. The abnormal allele is A. The presence of the abnormal allele in one chromosome is sufficient for expression of the disease.

heterozygote, the disease is said to have a **codominant** mode of inheritance.

• **B. Autosomal Dominant Diseases:** (Table 15-2.) Diseases with an autosomal dominant mode of inheritance have a characteristic family history (Fig 15-13; Table 15-3).

Most autosomal dominant diseases are mild, and heterozygotes survive to adult life. Transmission of the abnormal gene to the next generation only occurs following reproduction by affected individuals.

A characteristic of many autosomal dominant disorders is the variation in frequency with which the abnormal gene is manifested clinically as a disease (penetrance) and the degree of abnormality seen in different individuals (expressivity). In neurofibromatosis (von Recklinghausen's disease), for example, complete expression of the gene leads to innumerable neurofibromas throughout the body and early death. At the other extreme, a patient with the abnormal gene may be asymptomatic, displaying only a few areas of abnormal skin pigmentation (café au lait spots). A person with minimal clinical signs of disease may have offspring who have more complete expression of the abnormal gene. The cause of such variable penetrance and expressivity of abnormal genes is unknown.

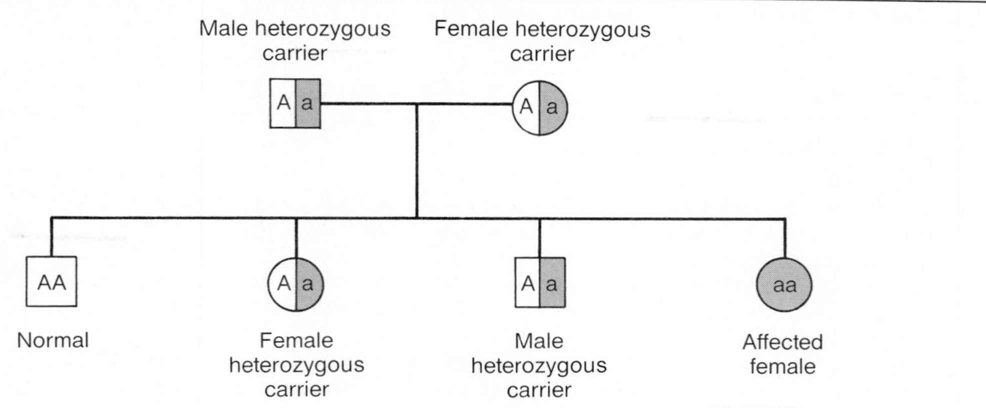

Figure 15-14. Autosomal recessive inheritance. Circles denote females; squares are males. The abnormal allele is a. An individual must have the abnormal allele in both homologous chromosomes for expression of the disease. When only one allele is present, the individual is a carrier.

Table 15-2. Common autosomal disorders.[1]

Autosomal Dominant	Autosomal Recessive
Achondroplasia (dwarfism)	Cystic fibrosis (mucoviscidosis)
Marfan's syndrome	Alpha$_1$-antitrypsin deficiency
Neurofibromatosis	Phenylketonuria
Von Willebrand's disease	Wilson's disease
Hereditary hemorrhagic telangiectasia	Tay-Sachs disease
Osteogenesis imperfecta	Sickle cell anemia
Acute intermittent porphyria	Glycogen storage diseases
Huntington's chorea	Galactosemia
Hereditary spherocytosis	
Adult renal polycystic disease	
Hereditary angioedema	
Familial hypercholesterolemia	

[1]Approximately 750 autosomal dominant disorders have been described.

Table 15-3. Features of autosomal dominant and recessive inherited diseases.

Autosomal Dominant	Autosomal Recessive
1. A = abnormal dominant gene.	1. a = Abnormal recessive gene.
2. Patient with disease is Aa heterozygote; AA homozygote is usually not compatible with life.	2. Patient with disease is aa homozygote. AA is normal; Aa is symptomless carrier.
3. Males and females are equally affected.	3. Males and females are equally affected.
4. At least one parent (Aa) shows overt disease.	4. Both parents are symptomless carriers (Aa); neither parent shows overt disease.
5. Overt disease is present in every generation.	5. Disease skips generations.
6. Higher incidence of overt disease among siblings; 50% chance of disease in children when one parent is affected.	6. Lower incidence of overt disease among siblings; 25% chance of disease in children of 2 symptomless carriers.
7. Cannot be transmitted by an individual without disease.	7. Can be transmitted by an individual without disease (carrier); offspring of a parent with overt disease (aa) and of a normal individual will all be carriers.
8. No association with consanguineous marriages.	8. Associated with consanguineous marriages.

C. Autosomal Recessive Diseases: (Table 15-2.) Diseases with an autosomal recessive mode of inheritance also have a characteristic family history (Fig 15-14; Table 15-3).

Most autosomal recessive traits are characterized by enzyme deficiency leading to biochemical disorders that have come to be called **inborn errors of metabolism**. The diseases are usually fatal in early life, though with treatment some patients survive to adult life; eg, people with phenylketonuria can lead normal lives if phenylalanine is removed from the diet.

Autosomal recessive traits are rare, and there is little chance of encountering the gene in an asymptomatic carrier in the general population. Many autosomal recessive diseases occur with greatest frequency in societies that discourage interracial mating. Tay-Sachs disease, for example, is virtually restricted to those of Ashkenazic Jewish ancestry. Very rare autosomal recessive diseases tend to occur in offspring of consanguineous matings when the parents have a common ancestor who carried the abnormal gene.

D. Sex Chromosome-Linked Diseases: (Table 15-4.) All sex chromosome-linked diseases are linked to the X chromosome and are characterized by an unequal incidence of the disease in the 2 sexes, in contrast to diseases linked to autosomes.

X-linked recessive diseases are common. The abnormal gene is usually expressed only in the male, who has only one X chromosome (Fig 15-15). In the female, disease is expressed only in an individual who is homozygous for the abnormal gene—a rare occurrence. X-linked recessive disorders are transmitted by asymptomatic female heterozygous carriers of the abnormal gene. Half of the male offspring of a mating between a carrier female and a normal male will manifest the disease. If an affected male mates with a normal female, all of the daughters will be carriers and the sons will be unaffected. If an affected male mates with a heterozygous carrier female, half of the sons and half of the daughters will be affected. X-linked recessive diseases are often severe and com-

Table 15-4. Common sex-linked disorders.

X-linked recessive
Hemophilia A
Christmas disease (hemophilia B)
Bruton's agammaglobulinemia
G6PD deficiency
Testicular feminization
Duchenne muscular dystrophy
Chronic granulomatous disease
Red-green color blindness[1]
X-linked dominant
Hypophosphatemic (vitamin D-resistant) rickets
Y-linked
None known

[1]Total color blindness is autosomal recessive and very rare.

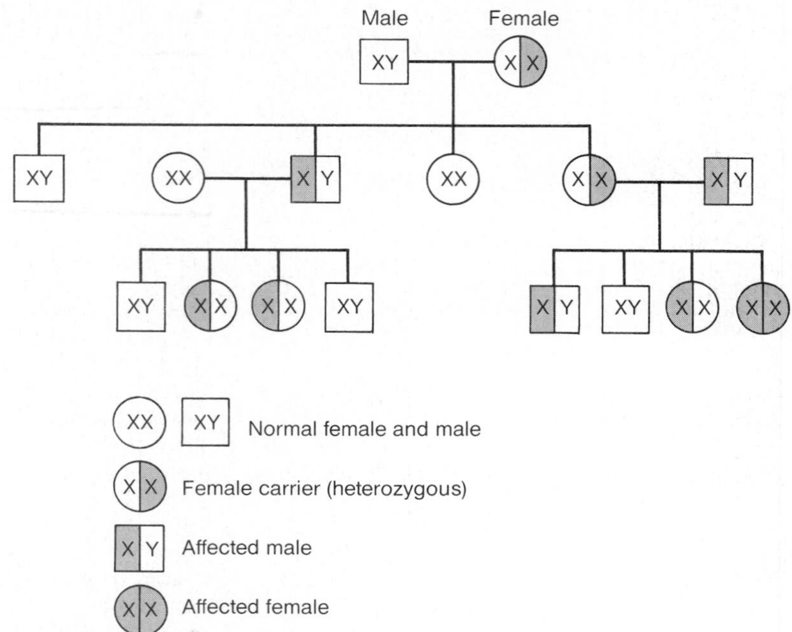

Figure 15-15. X-linked recessive mode of inheritance. The circles denote females; squares are males. The abnormal allele is the X in the shaded area.

monly cause death early in life. Modern treatment, such as is available for hemophilia, has permitted survival of affected individuals to adult reproductive life.

X-linked dominant diseases are uncommon. Pseudohypoparathyroidism and hypophosphatemic rickets are the main examples. Since females have two X chromosomes, X-linked dominant diseases are more common in females. An affected heterozygous female transmits the disease to 50% of her sons and 50% of her daughters. An affected male will transmit the disease to all of his daughters but to none of his sons (Fig 15-16).

E. Inborn Errors of Metabolism: These diseases are caused by an inherited single-gene abnormality that causes failure of synthesis of an enzyme and a subsequent block in a metabolic pathway. Enzyme deficiency results in abnormal amino acid, lipid, carbohydrate, or mucopolysaccharide metabolism and accumulation of the substrate and deficiency of the product of the enzymatic reaction. Cell damage may result from either mechanism. These diseases are all rare; most have an autosomal recessive mode of inheritance; a few are inherited as X-linked recessive diseases.

1. Abnormal amino acid metabolism-(Table 15-5.) The inherited diseases associated with deficiency of enzymes involved in phenylalanine and tyrosine metabolism are good examples of inborn errors of metabolism (Fig 15-17). In **phenylketonuria,** the absence of phenylalanine hydroxylase prevents conversion of phenylalanine to tyrosine. This produces a tyrosine deficiency in the cell (with deficient melanin production and lack of pigmentation), as well as accumulation of phenylalanine and its metabolites, which are toxic to nerve cells (producing mental retardation). Phenylketonuria is an example of a biochemical abnormality that produces no specific morphologic change in affected cells. Diagnosis is made by detection of high levels of phenylalanine in the urine or serum.

2. Abnormal lipid metabolism (lipid storage diseases)-(Table 15-6.) Several inherited deficiencies of enzymes involved in the metabolism of complex lipids have been identified. These deficiencies cause metabolic blocks that lead to accumulation of abnormal amounts of complex lipids in cells. Most of these enzymes are lysosomal, and abnormal lipid storage occurs within secondary lysosomes—hence the term **lysosomal storage diseases**. Except for Fabry's disease, which has an X-linked recessive inheritance pattern, these diseases are autosomal recessive in inheritance.

Storage of lipid occurs in different cells in the various diseases. Involvement of parenchymal cells causes degeneration and necrosis of these cells. When neurons are involved, as in **Tay-Sachs disease** and the infantile forms of **Gaucher's disease** and **Niemann-Pick disease,** severe mental retardation and death occur. Kidney failure occurs with renal involvement in Fabry's disease. In the milder adult forms of Gaucher's disease and Niemann-Pick disease, accumulation of lipid occurs in reticuloendothelial cells, producing enlargement of liver and spleen.

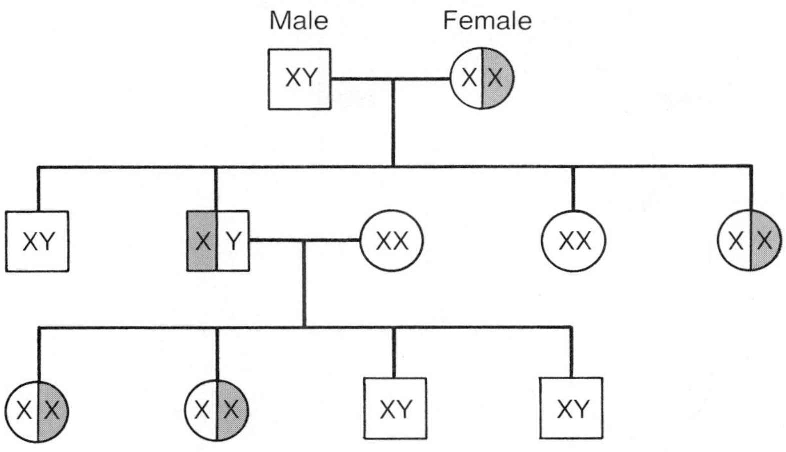

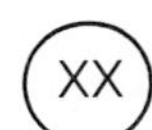

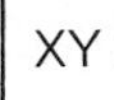

Normal female and male

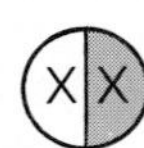

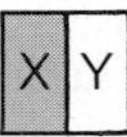

Affected female and male

Figure 15-16. X-linked dominant mode of inheritance. Circles denote females; squares are males. The abnormal allele is the X in the shaded area.

a. Diagnosis-The diagnosis can be made in several ways.

(1) Clinical features-In Tay-Sachs disease, lipid deposition in the macula of the retina produces a cherry-red spot visible on ophthalmoscopy. Diffuse skin lesions occur in Fabry's disease. Hepatosplenomegaly occurs in Gaucher's disease.

(2) Microscopic examination-Light microscopic examination of affected tissues such as brain, bone marrow, liver, and spleen (Fig 15-18) permits identification of the abnormal, lipid-distended cells. The affected cells in Tay-Sachs and Niemann-Pick disease have foamy cytoplasm. Gaucher's cells have a characteristic fibrillary ("crinkled paper") cytoplasm.

Characteristic inclusions in the greatly distended lysosomes are demonstrated on electron microscopy. In Tay-Sachs disease, these are whorled; in Niemann-Pick disease, they appear as

Table 15-5. Examples of inherited enzyme deficiency causing abnormal amino acid metabolism.

Disease	Amino Acids Affected	Enzyme Deficiency	Inheritance Pattern	Clinical Features
Phenylketonuria	Phenylalanine	Phenylalanine hydroxylase	AR[1]	Mental retardation; musty or mousy odor; eczema; increased plasma phenylalanine levels.
Hereditary tyrosinemia	Tyrosine	Hydroxyphenylpyruvic acid oxidase	AR	Hepatic cirrhosis, renal tubular dysfunction; elevated plasma tyrosine levels.
Histidinemia	Histidine	Histidase	AR	Mental retardation; speech defect.
Maple syrup urine disease (branched-chain ketoaciduria; ketoaminoacidemia)	Leucine, valine, isoleucine	Branched-chain ketoacid oxidase	AR	Postnatal collapse; mental retardation; characteristic "maple syrup" odor in urine.
Homocystinuria	Methionine, homocystine	Cystathionine synthase	AR	Mental retardation; thromboembolic phenomena; ectopia lentis.

[1]AR = autosomal recessive.

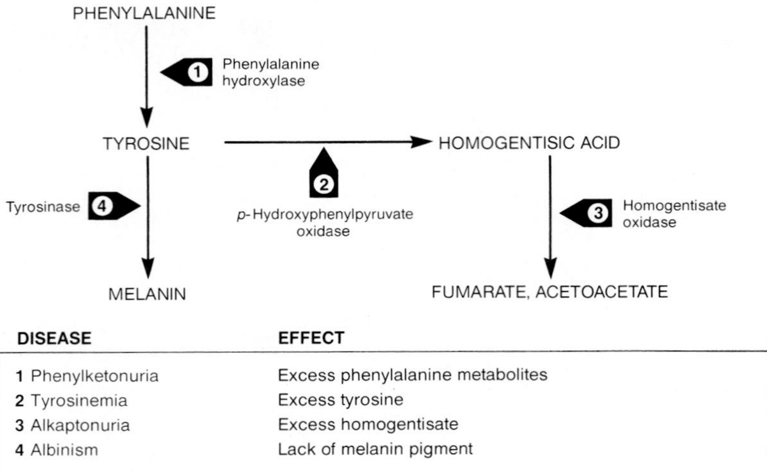

Figure 15-17. Pathway of metabolism of phenylalanine and tyrosine. The numbers relate to recognized deficiency states.

parallel lamellas ("zebra bodies"); and in Gaucher's disease the stored lipid is arranged in linear stacks.

(3) Demonstration of the enzyme deficiency- The definitive diagnostic test is demonstration of the enzyme deficiency in cultured skin fibroblasts.

b. Prevention and treatment-Lipid storage diseases have no treatment. Prevention is achieved by genetic counseling and amniocentesis.

(1) Genetic counseling-Heterozygous carriers of Tay-Sachs disease can be identified by serum enzyme assay. Screening of high-risk populations such as Ashkenazi Jews, with a carrier rate of 1:30 for the abnormal Tay-Sachs gene, enables identification of heterozygous carriers at risk for producing affected children.

(2) Amniocentesis-In high-risk pregnancies, amniocentesis permits identification of affected fetuses by demonstrating the enzyme deficiency in fetal fibroblasts cultured from amniotic fluid. Therapeutic abortion may then be undertaken if desired.

3. Abnormal glycogen metabolism (Glycogen storage disease)-(Table 15-7.) Glycogen storage diseases are caused by deficiency of an enzyme involved in the metabolism of glycogen. Most of these diseases have an autosomal recessive mode of inheritance, with onset of disease in infancy or childhood. Interference with glycogen metabolism produces a variety of effects.

a. Accumulation of glycogen-Glycogen accumulates in the cytoplasm and appears as granules that can be recognized on electron microscopy; tissues in which glycogen is stored become distended. In routinely fixed tissues, glycogen is dissolved by the aqueous formalin fixative; affected cells in routine slides appear distended and empty on examination by light microscopy (Fig 15-19). Demonstration of glycogen in cells requires fixation in nonaqueous absolute alcohol and staining with Best's carmine or periodic acid-Schiff (PAS) reagent.

b. Dysfunction of involved cells-Hepatic involvement causes hepatomegaly, fibrosis, and liver failure; myocardial involvement causes heart failure.

c. Abnormal glucose delivery-With liver involvement (eg, type I), **hypoglycemia** occurs because breakdown of liver glycogen is the main source of blood glucose. With skeletal muscle involvement, lack of glucose in the cell causes muscle cramps and weakness.

Table 15-6. Inborn errors of lipid metabolism: Lysosomal (or lipid) storage diseases.

Disease	Enzyme Defect	Accumulated Lipid	Tissues Involved
Tay-Sachs disease	Hexosaminidase A	G_{M2} ganglioside	Brain, retina
Gaucher's disease	β-Glucosidase (glucocerebrosidase)	Glucocerebroside	Liver, spleen, bone marrow, brain
Neimann-Pick disease	Sphingomyelinase	Sphingomyelin	Brain, liver, spleen
Metachromatic leukodystrophy	Arylsulfatase A	Sulfatide	Brain, kidney, liver, peripheral nerves
Fabry's disease	α-Galactosidase	Ceramide trihexoside	Skin, kidney
Krabbe's disease	Galactosylceramidase	Galactocerebroside	Brain

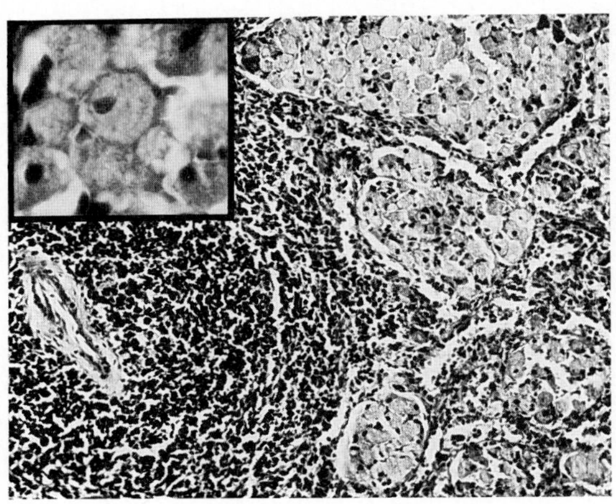

Figure 15–18. The spleen in Gaucher's disease. Aggregations of foamy histiocytes are seen (shown at high magnification in the inset) in the red pulp (right half of picture). Part of a splenic lymphoid follicle is shown on the left.

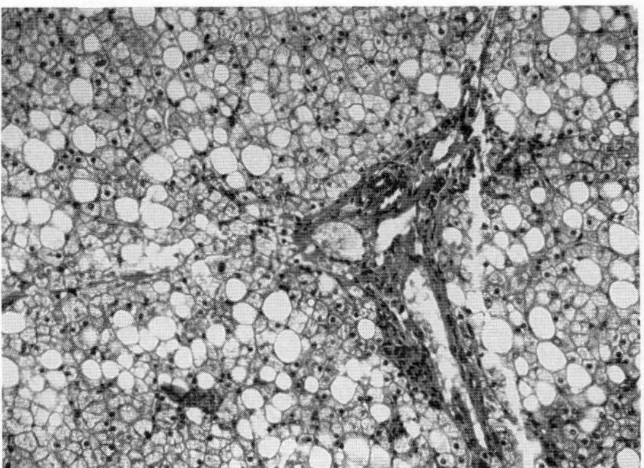

Figure 15–19. The liver in glycogen storage disease. Involved liver cells appear as empty cells because the glycogen has been dissolved by the aqueous formalin fixative. A normal portal area is seen in the center.

4. **Abnormal mucopolysaccharide metabolism (mucopolysaccharidoses)–**(Table 15–8.) The mucopolysaccharidoses are rare inherited lysosomal storage diseases in which deficiency of a lysosomal enzyme leads to the accumulation of mucopolysaccharides (glycosaminoglycans) in lysosomes in a variety of cells. All have an autosomal recessive pattern of inheritance except Hunter's syndrome, which is an X-linked recessive disease.

Accumulation of glycosaminoglycans in cells results in great enlargement of affected cells. Involvement of macrophages and endothelial cells leads to hepatosplenomegaly and deformities due to changes in skin and bones. Grotesque facial deformities occur (gargoylism is the alternative name for Hurler's syndrome). Affected cells are distended and, in routine preparations, demonstrate clear cytoplasm (balloon cells). Peripheral blood cells show glycosaminoglycan deposits as large purple cytoplasmic granules (Alder-Reilly bodies).

Dysfunction of affected parenchymal cells also occurs. Degeneration of involved neurons causes mental retardation; myocardial involvement causes heart failure.

• **F. Detection of Heterozygous Carrier State in Recessive Traits:** Heterozygous carriers of a recessive trait, whether autosomal or X-linked, do not show evidence of clinical disease. In many disorders, however, partial expression of the abnormal gene occurs in heterozygous carriers, and a biochemical abnormality is produced. This abnormality acts as a marker and permits detection of the heterozygous carrier, which in turn makes possible genetic counseling and early diagnosis of affected offspring.

Hemophilia A, which is due to deficiency of coagulation factor VIII resulting from an abnormal recessive gene linked to the X chromosome, is a

Table 15–7. Glycogen storage diseases.

Type	Enzyme Defect	Severity of Disease	Involved Tissues
I (von Gierke's disease)	Glucose-6-phosphatase	Severe	Liver, kidney, gut
II (Pompe's disease)	α-1,4-Glucosidase	Lethal	Systemic distribution but heart most affected
III (Cori's disease)	Amylo-1,6-Glucosidase (debranching enzyme)	Mild	Systemic distribution; liver commonly affected
IV (Andersen's disease)	Amylo-1,4→1,6-transglucosidase (branching enzyme)	Lethal	Systemic distribution but liver most affected
V (McArdle's disease)	Muscle phosphorylase	Mild	Skeletal muscle
VI (Hers' disease)	Liver phosphorylase	Mild	Liver
VII–XII	Extremely rare diseases	Variable	Variable

Table 15-8. Mucopolysaccharidoses (MPS syndromes).

Type	Enzyme Defect	Accumulated Mucopoly-saccharide	Tissues Involved	Mode of Inheritance[1]	Severity
I (Hurler's syndrome)	α-L-Iduronidase	Heparan sulfate, dermatan sulfate	Skin, cornea, bone, heart, brain, liver, spleen	AR	Severe
II (Hunter's syndrome)	L-Iduronosulfate sulfatase	Heparan sulfate, dermatan sulfate	Skin, bone, heart, ear, retina	XR	Moderate
III (Sanfilippo's syndrome)	Many types	Heparan sulfate	Brain, skin	AR	Moderate
IV (Morquio's syndrome)	*N*-Acetylgalactos-amine 6-sulfatase	Keratan sulfate, chondroitin sulfate	Skin, bone, heart, eye	AR	Mild
V–VII	Rare diseases characterized by many types of enzyme defects	Variable	Variable	AR	Mild

[1]AR = autosomal recessive; XR = X-linked recessive.

good example of how heterozygous carriers are detected. Patients with hemophilia have low levels of factor VIII in the plasma. Female heterozygous carriers have plasma levels of factor VIII that fall between those of normal and hemophiliac patients. The ratio between factor VIII clotting activity (low in hemophilia A) and factor VIII-related antigen (normal in hemophilia A) permits detection of over 90% of heterozygous carriers (see Chapter 27).

Carrier detection is now possible in a large number of autosomal recessive diseases. Screening of populations for carriers is cost-effective only in families known to have the abnormal gene and in ethnic groups with a high incidence of the disease, eg, Tay-Sachs disease in individuals of Jewish ancestry.

Polygenic (Multifactorial) Inheritance

Familial diseases such as high blood pressure and diabetes mellitus are believed to be due at least in part to the presence of several abnormal genes. It is thought that this inherited predisposition for development of disease has an additive effect on environmental factors. Apart from statistical data relating to the familial incidence of these diseases, however, inheritance is not predictable on the basis of genetic laws.

FETAL ABNORMALITIES CAUSED BY EXTERNAL AGENTS (Teratogens)

Congenital anomalies (Table 15–9) due to abnormal development of the fetus affect about 2% of newborns and represent an important cause of neonatal morbidity and death. Most anomalies have no detectable chromosomal abnormality and are not inherited. Although a few teratogenic ("monster-producing") agents have been identified, the cause of most congenital anomalies is unknown.

Ionizing Radiation

In addition to its action on DNA and the genetic apparatus of the cell, ionizing radiation has direct toxic effects on other components of the developing fetus, and various congenital anomalies have been reported following irradiation in pregnancy. Because it is not known whether there is a "safe" low dose of radiation during pregnancy, abdominal x-rays should be avoided except when essential for diagnosis of diseases threatening the life of the mother or fetus.

Teratogenic Viral Infections

Rubella is the best-recognized teratogenic virus, ie, one that causes developmental defects. Transplacental infection of the fetus by the virus during the first trimester of pregnancy, when the fetal organs are developing, is associated with a high incidence of congenital anomalies. The risk is greatest (about 70%) in the first 8 weeks of pregnancy. Rubella virus interferes with protein synthesis in tis-

Table 15-9. Common congenital anomalies.

Congenital heart disease
Neural tube defects (eg, meningomyelocele)
Cleft lip and palate
Congenital pyloric stenosis
Intestinal atresia
Tracheoesophageal fistula
Imperforate anus
Clubfoot (talipes equinovarus)
Congenital dislocation of hip

sue culture. **Rubella syndrome** denotes the triad of congenital heart disease, deafness, and cataracts that is common in affected infants. Many other anomalies, including microcephaly, mental retardation, and microphthalmia, have been reported. The risk of rubella infection of fetuses has decreased dramatically since the introduction of rubella antibody testing and immunization.

The teratogenic effect of other viral infections in early pregnancy is uncertain. Congenital anomalies have been reported following many infections, including influenza, mumps, and varicella, but whether this is incidental or represents a teratogenic effect of these viruses is unknown. If these viruses have a teratogenic effect, it is much less than that of rubella virus.

Drugs

As with irradiation, the use of drugs of any sort during pregnancy should be discouraged except to save the life of the mother or when the benefits outweigh the risk to the fetus. No drug can be considered totally safe, especially during early pregnancy, and well-established drugs are preferred to newer ones. Although all drugs approved for use in the USA have undergone rigorous testing in pregnant animals, their safety in humans can be established only after many years of use, as exemplified by thalidomide and diethylstilbestrol.

A. Thalidomide: Thalidomide is a mild sedative that was commonly used in Europe in the 1960s until it was shown by epidemiologic evidence to cause a distinctive fetal anomaly (phocomelia) when used in pregnancy. Failure of development of the limbs results in hands and feet that resemble the flippers of seals—short stumps closely attached to the trunk.

B. Diethylstilbestrol (DES): Diethylstilbestrol is a synthetic estrogen used extensively between 1950 and 1960 to treat threatened abortion in the mistaken belief that estrogens prevent abortion. Female offspring of women who have taken DES in pregnancy develop epithelial abnormalities of the vagina, including collections of mucous glands (vaginal adenosis) and, more seriously, clear cell adenocarcinoma, a characteristic vaginal cancer.

Alcohol (Fetal Alcohol Syndrome)

Exposure of the fetus to alcohol during organogenesis in early pregnancy leads to congenital abnormalities, the extent of which correlates with the amount of alcohol consumed by the mother, who may not even know she is pregnant. Fetal alcohol syndrome occurs in one of every 1000 live births in the USA and in 30–50% of infants born to women who consume over 125 g of alcohol (about 450 mL of whisky) per day. Fetal alcohol syndrome is characterized by growth retardation, a characteristic abnormal facial appearance (short palpebral fissures, epicanthal folds, micrognathia, a thin upper lip), cardiac defects (commonly septal defects), vertebral anomalies (including spina bifida), and mental retardation with microcephaly and brain malformation.

Cigarette Smoking

Heavy smoking during pregnancy is associated with fetal growth retardation. To date, no teratogenic effects have been reported.

POSTNATAL DEVELOPMENT

NORMAL POSTNATAL DEVELOPMENT

The organs of the body vary considerably in degree of development and maturity at birth. Postnatal growth and development is a remarkably trouble-free process.

Most tissues (eg, skeletal muscle, bone, skin, gastrointestinal tract, endocrine glands) are fully developed and functional at birth and show growth during childhood (Fig 15–20). Liver and kidney are immature but sufficiently developed to function adequately after delivery, though many newborn infants develop transient mild jaundice as a result of immaturity of liver enzyme systems.

The **lungs** mature late in fetal life and are immature in premature infants—especially those born before 34 weeks of gestation. Maturity of the lungs is critical for survival in premature infants. Lung maturity of the fetus may be assessed by estimating the lecithin, sphingomyelin, and phosphatidylglycerol levels in amniotic fluid. As the lung matures—normally after 34 weeks—lecithin and phosphatidylglycerol appear in increasing amounts in amniotic fluid. Problems related to lung immaturity rarely occur if the amniotic fluid lecithin:sphingomyelin ratio is over 2:1 or when significant amounts of phosphatidylglycerol are present.

The **brain** shows rapid growth and development after delivery, reaching full size and development in early childhood (Fig 15–20). Brain development after birth includes migration of primitive neuroectodermal cells and myelination in the central nervous system.

Lymphoid tissues show maximum growth during childhood, after which involution occurs.

Genital tissues (gonads, reproductive organs, and secondary sexual characteristics) develop during puberty.

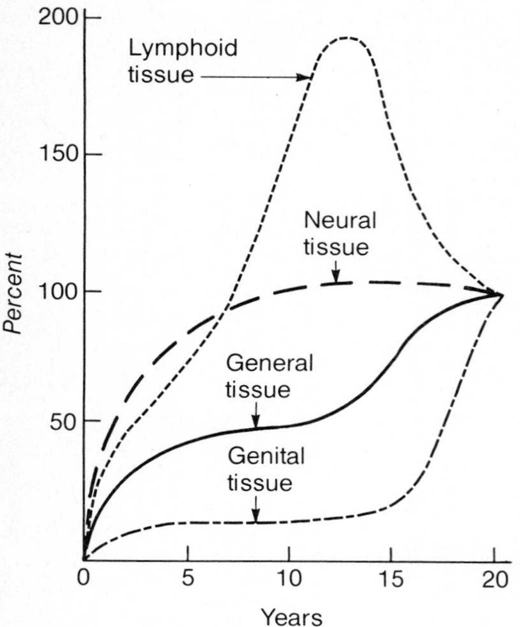

Figure 15-20. Graph showing major types of postnatal growth and development of various organs. **General tissues** (eg, muscle, skeleton, respiratory and digestive organs, skin, kidney, etc) are fully developed and functional at birth and show growth during childhood. **Neural tissues** (eg, brain) show rapid development to full capacity in early childhood. **Lymphoid tissues** show maximum development in childhood, after which involution occurs. **Genital tissues** (gonads, reproductive organs, secondary sexual characteristics) develop during puberty.

Table 15-10. Leading causes of death during childhood; USA, 1980.

Neonatal period; 6.4 deaths per 1000 live births
Complications of prematurity
Respiratory distress syndrome
Intracranial hemorrhage
Necrotizing enterocolitis
Birth trauma
Birth asphyxia
Neonatal infections
Hemolytic disease of the newborn
Congenital anomalies
First year
Congenital anomalies
Sudden infant death syndrome
Infectious diseases
Accidents
Neurologic diseases
Malignant neoplasms
Age 1–4 years
Accidents
Congenital anomalies
Malignant neoplasms (including leukemia)
Infectious diseases
Age 5–14 years
Accidents
Malignant neoplasms (including leukemia)

DISEASES OF INFANCY & CHILDHOOD

Postnatal growth and development may, however, be interrupted by many disease processes. The frequency and nature of these diseases vary greatly in the first 4 weeks (neonatal period), the first year (infancy), ages 1–4 years, and ages 5–14 years. The risk of death is greatest during the neonatal period, with a mortality rate of 6.4 per 1000 live births in the United States (1980 data). Neonatal deaths result chiefly from complications of pregnancy and labor (Table 15–10). Neonatal deaths account for 50% of all infant deaths in the United States, the infant mortality rate being 12.8 per 1000 population. The infant mortality rate is regarded as a sensitive indicator of the quality of the health care system and is much higher in developing countries than developed ones. The lowest infant mortality rates in the world are in the Scandinavian countries and the Netherlands.

The risk of death falls dramatically after the first year. The death rate in the age group from 1 to 4 years is about 0.6 per 1000 population, and that in the 5- to 14-year age group is about 0.3 per 1000. Forty percent of deaths in the 1- to 4-year age group and 50% of deaths in the 5- to 14-year age group are caused by accidents, further emphasizing the low risk of death from natural causes in the childhood years.

Disorders Associated With Low Birth Weight

Normal infants at term weigh 2700–3900 g. A premature infant is defined as one with a birth weight of less than 2500 g regardless of gestational age. Term infants (ie, those born between 38 and 42 weeks of gestation) weighing less than 2500 g are called small-for-gestational age (SGA) infants. Preterm infants (ie, those born before 38 weeks of gestation) may be appropriate-for-gestational age (AGA) or SGA. SGA status may result from congenital anomalies, fetal infections, placental insufficiency from vascular lesions and infections, or maternal hypertension, heavy smoking, narcotic and cocaine abuse, and alcohol abuse.

Disorders associated with low birth weight are the result of immaturity of organs. They occur in the following infants (in decreasing order of frequency): (1) those born before 34 weeks of gestation, the risks increasing as gestational age decreases; (2) those born between 34 and 38 weeks who are SGA; (3) preterm infants under 2500 g who are AGA; and (4) term infants under 2500 g. The mortality rate for infants under 1000 g is 90%. The survival rate improves rapidly when infants achieve a weight of 1500 g.

The chances for survival of a newborn correlate well with its Apgar score. Apgar testing assesses 5 parameters (heart rate, respiratory effort, muscle tone, skin color, and response to a catheter in the nostril) at 1 and 5 minutes after delivery. Each factor receives a score of 0–2, and a score of 10 obviously reflects optimal condition. Infants with a 5-minute Apgar score of 0 or 1 have a mortality rate in the neonatal period of 50%. The rate drops to 20% when the score is 4 and to almost zero when the score is over 7.

A. Respiratory Distress Syndrome (RDS): RDS causes the deaths of about 7000 infants a year in the USA. It most commonly affects infants under 34 weeks of gestational age and is caused by immaturity of type II pneumocytes, which fail to secrete adequate surfactant. Surfactant is a surface tension-reducing agent that performs the vital function of keeping alveoli expanded. Deficiency of surfactant causes alveolar collapse in the first hour after delivery following reasonably normal initial expansion of the lung, because the alveoli cannot remain expanded without the surface tension-reducing factor. Progressive respiratory distress, hypoxemia, and cyanosis occur. Alveolar collapse is associated with hypoxic necrosis of alveolar epithelium and exudation of protein-rich fluid into dilated alveolar ducts. This fluid forms eosinophilic hyaline membranes—a microscopic hallmark of the disease (see Chapter 34). RDS is also called hyaline membrane disease.

Treatment with artificial ventilation and oxygen has improved survival in RDS, but the overall mortality rate remains around 30%. Prolonged high-concentration oxygen therapy must be used with extreme caution because it is toxic to the lung (permanent interstitial fibrosis) and eyes (retrolental fibroplasia and blindness).

B. Intraventricular Hemorrhage: Intraventricular hemorrhage may occur in preterm infants with or without RDS. Hemorrhage begins in the periventricular region of the cerebral hemispheres and extends into the ventricular cavity in most cases. The cause is unknown, but immaturity of the brain, poor support of the fragile vessels in this region by the subependymal tissue, increased fibrinolytic activity, and hypoxia are believed to contribute. Severe intraventricular hemorrhage carries a mortality rate of about 75%.

C. Necrotizing Enterocolitis: This is a dangerous complication of premature infants treated in neonatal intensive care units. It is characterized by extensive mucosal necrosis and ulceration involving the ileum and colon. The cause is unknown, though hypoxia and bacterial infection—notably *Escherichia coli*—probably contribute. Treatment commonly includes surgical resection of the involved intestine. The mortality rate is high.

Perinatal Infections

In contrast to teratogenic infections such as rubella, which occur in early pregnancy, perinatal infections are caused by transplacental infection in late pregnancy or infection of the fetus by contagion during delivery. They present as infectious diseases in the neonatal period. TORCHS complex is a general term for infections acquired in this way and is an acronym for toxoplasmosis, other (viruses), rubella, cytomegalovirus, herpes simplex, and syphilis.

A. *Toxoplasma gondii* and Cytomegalovirus Infections: These third-trimester fetal infections involve chiefly the brain and eyes. Extensive necrosis of the brain, most prominent in the periventricular region, is accompanied by dystrophic calcification and leads to microcephaly and mental retardation in survivors. The eyes show chorioretinitis, frequently associated with visual impairment.

B. *Treponema pallidum* Infection (Congenital Syphilis): Syphilis is also a third-trimester transplacental infection of the fetus born to a mother with early active syphilis. When infection is severe, intrauterine death occurs. With lesser infections, congenital syphilis occurs, manifested in infancy by fever, skin rashes, mucosal lesions, osteochondritis, and lymph node enlargement—or later in childhood with abnormal permanent teeth (Hutchinson's teeth, Moon's teeth), bone defects, nerve deafness, and blindness due to interstitial keratitis.

C. Rubella Virus Infection: Rubella infection in late pregnancy leads to severe infection of the fetus characterized by fever, petechial skin rash, and liver enlargement. The infantile immune system responds poorly to the virus, and affected infants frequently have prolonged infection with excretion of virus for several months after delivery.

D. Infections Acquired in the Birth Canal: Herpes simplex represents the most significant birth canal infection and occurs when the mother has active infection at the time of delivery. Fetal infection results either in severe viremia or encephalitis. The mortality rate is very high. Infants who recover commonly have severe permanent neurologic deficits due to irreversible necrosis of the brain during the acute phase of infection. Active genital herpes infection of the mother is an absolute indication for cesarean section.

Other infections acquired during passage through an infected birth canal include gonorrhea and lymphogranuloma venereum, both of which cause severe conjunctivitis.

Sudden Infant Death Syndrome (SIDS; "Crib Death")

SIDS is a common disease that causes about 10,000 deaths a year in the USA. It is the sudden and unexpected death of a previously well infant in whom no cause of death is found at autopsy. SIDS occurs predominantly during sleep and has a maximum incidence in the age group from 2 to 4 months. The cause is unknown. An abnormality of the respiratory center that causes cessation of respiration during sleep appears the most likely cause. However, a variety of other causes, including botulism, have been suggested.

Congenital Anomalies, Inborn Errors of Metabolism, & Hemolytic Disease of the Newborn

These are common problems during early childhood. The first 2 have been considered earlier in this chapter. Hemolytic disease of the newborn is discussed in Chapter 25.

Malignant Neoplasms

Malignant neoplasms, though much less common overall in children than in adults, account for over 10% of deaths in the age group from 5 to 14 years and 7% of deaths in children 1–4 years of age. Malignant neoplasms in children are those of the lymphoid and hematopoietic cells (lymphomas and leukemias), mesenchymal cells (sarcomas, most commonly osteosarcoma and embryonal rhabdomyosarcoma), and the central nervous system (Table 15–11). Infants tend to develop tumors in primitive embryonic cells, which commonly have the suffix *-blastoma:* in the kidney (nephroblastoma), adrenal gland (neuroblastoma), retina (retinoblastoma), cerebellum (medulloblastoma), and liver (hepatoblastoma). All of these neoplasms in children are highly malignant, with a tendency to early spread throughout the body. Many of them respond well to chemotherapy (eg, leukemia, embryonal rhabdomyosarcoma), and a few can be cured (eg, leukemia, nephroblastoma). In general, however, malignant neoplasms of childhood have high mortality rates.

Table 15–11. Common malignant neoplasms of infancy and childhood.

Neoplasm	0–5 Years	5–18 Years
Acute lymphoblastic leukemia	+++	++
Acute granulocytic leukemia	+	++
Malignant lymphoma	+	++
Neuroblastoma	+++	+
Nephroblastoma (Wilms's tumor)	+++	+
Embryonal rhabdomyosarcoma	++	+
Retinoblastoma	++	+
Medulloblastoma	++	+
Cerebellar astrocytoma	+	++
Hepatoblastoma	+	–
Osteosarcoma	–	++
Thyroid carcinoma	–	++

SEXUAL DEVELOPMENT

NORMAL SEXUAL DEVELOPMENT

Primary Sexual Development

The development of the gonads and genital organs in the embryo is directed by the sex chromosomes (Fig 15–21). Normal sexual development requires sequential interactions of chromosomes, genes, gonads, hormones, and receptors, with an associated "sexual imprinting" of the central nervous system, which governs subsequent sexual development.

A. Male: When a Y chromosome (specifically, a Y modulator gene on the short arm of the Y chromosome) is present, as in a normal male, the primitive gonad differentiates into a testis. The developing testis elaborates a hormonal factor that causes local regression of the müllerian duct; it also produces androgens that lead to development of the male reproductive organs (Chapter 51).

B. Female: In the absence of a Y chromosome, as in the normal female, the primitive gonad develops as an ovary. The müllerian duct continues to develop and forms the female internal reproductive organs (Chapters 52–54).

Secondary Sexual Development

The development of secondary sexual characteristics and the production of gametes at puberty are initiated by the hypothalamic-pituitary axis. Gonadotropic hormones secreted by the pituitary stimulate development of the gonads. The testes produce spermatozoa and testosterone. The ovaries begin cyclic ovulation and secrete estrogen and progesterone. The sex hormones are responsible for development of secondary sexual characteristics such as hair and body fat distribution, breast development, and voice changes. In the female, menstruation signifies the onset of reproductive capability (Chapter 52).

ABNORMAL SEXUAL DEVELOPMENT

Abnormal primary sexual development leads to **ambiguous genitalia ("intersex")** in infants. Abnormal secondary sexual development results in failure of production of gametes and sex hormones at puberty, with subsequent abnormalities of secondary sex characteristics. The principal types of abnormal sexual development are set forth in Table 15–12.

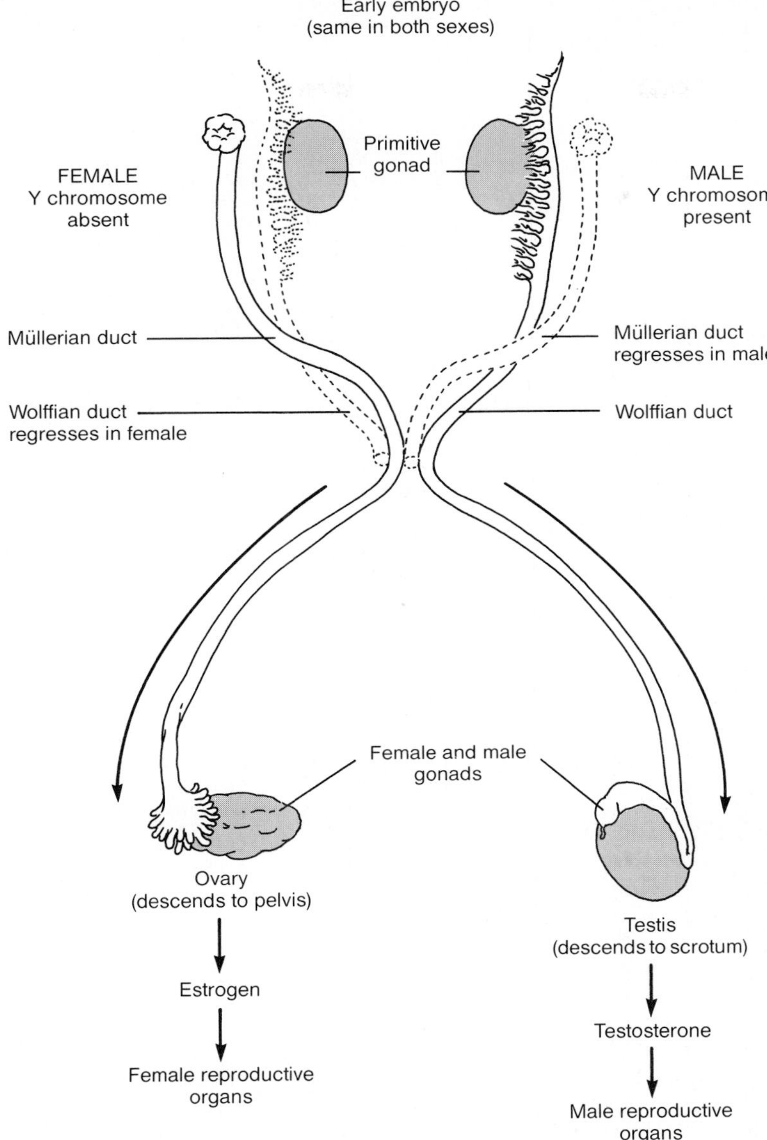

Figure 15-21. Normal sexual development. The primitive gonads in the embryo develop into testes when a Y chromosome is present. The testis produces a müllerian duct-regressing hormone and androgens that result in development of the male reproductive organs from the wolffian duct. In the absence of a Y chromosome, the gonads develop into ovaries and the female reproductive organs develop from the müllerian duct.

True Hermaphroditism

The term hermaphroditism is derived from Greek mythology—Hermes was a male messenger of the gods and Aphrodite the goddess of love. True hermaphroditism is a rare condition in which both testicular and ovarian tissue develops in the same individual. The genetic makeup of true hermaphrodites varies; many individuals are 46,XX or 46,XY, but some show mosaicism: 46,XX/46,XY. The exact mechanism underlying hermaphroditism is uncertain, but the disorder may be associated with transfer to another chromosome of that part of the Y modulator gene that dictates testicular development.

Pseudohermaphroditism

Pseudohermaphroditism is relatively common. In pseudohermaphroditic individuals, the gonads correspond to the genetic sex, but abnormal development of the external genitalia causes difficulty in determining the sex. Classification as a male or female pseudohermaphrodite is based on the individual's genetic sex.

The penis of a male with extreme hypospadias (opening of the urethra on the ventral aspect of the penis [Chapter 51]) may resemble a female urethra and clitoris. Failure of testicular descent, when associated with failure of fusion of the scro-

Table 15-12. Abnormalities of sexual development.

Syndrome	Karyotype	Barr Bodies	Gonads	External Genitalia
True hermaphroditism	Variable; 46XX, 46XY, mosaicism	+ or −	Both ovarian and testicular tissue are present.	Variable; male or female or both.
Sex chromosome defects				
Klinefelter's syndrome	47,XXY	+	Dysgenetic testes	Male (eunuchoid; poorly developed secondary sex characteristics; infertile).
Turner's syndrome	45, XO	−	Dysgenetic (streak) ovaries	Female (poorly developed secondary sex characteristics; infertile; amenorrhea).
Male pseudohermaphroditism				
Testicular feminization	46, XY	−	Testes (immature)	Female; end-organ failure to androgen action; no uterus (infertile, amenorrhea); secondary sex characteristics well developed and female because of presence of adrenal estrogens.
Failure of development of external genitalia	46, XY	−	Testes	Male; ambiguity caused by undescended testes, bifid scrotum, hypospadias, poor penile development.
Bilateral cryptorchidism	46, XY	−	Testes	Failure of testicular development; infertility.
Female pseudohermaphroditism				
Primary (idiopathic)	46, XX	+	Ovaries	Male (unknown cause).
Androgens in utero	46, XX	+	Ovaries	Female; variable masculinization at birth.
Adrenogenital syndromes	46, XX	+	Ovaries	Female: masculinization at birth due to excess adrenal androgenic hormones.

tum in a male, may result in an appearance that resembles the female external genitalia.

Ambiguous genitalia may occur in females with congenital adrenal hyperplasia (see Chapter 60). Congenital absence of an enzyme in the synthetic pathway for adrenal steroids leads to overproduction of adrenal androgenic hormones. In the female, this may cause clitoral hypertrophy so marked that the clitoris is mistaken for a penis. A female with this disorder may resemble a male with undescended testes and hypospadias, and there may be confusion about the person's sex.

Testicular Feminization Syndrome

An individual with testicular feminization syndrome is a genetic male (46,XY) but phenotypically a female. This syndrome is caused by an inherited (X-linked recessive) absence of receptors for androgens on the cells of the end-organs of androgen action **(end-organ insensitivity)**. Failure of androgen action leads to failure of testicular descent, with formation of female external genitalia, including a vagina. At puberty, individuals develop female secondary sex characteristics because of the unopposed action of adrenal estrogenic hormones, and they appear to be normal young females. They are able to engage in sexual intercourse and may marry. The absence of the uterus—an organ derived from the müllerian duct, which regresses under the influence of müllerian duct regression factor, which is secreted and acts normally in patients with testicular feminization—results in failure of menstruation and infertility and brings these patients to medical attention. They also lack body hair in either the typical female or typical male distribution.

Chromosomal analysis (which shows a normal male karyotype) is diagnostic. It is important in the treatment of these patients to remove the pelvic testes, which have an increased incidence of malignant neoplasms, and to permit the patient to lead her life as a female, which she is in all respects other than genetically and in the absence of the internal reproductive organs derived from the müllerian duct.

Klinefelter's Syndrome (47,XXY)

The patient is phenotypically male. The presence of an additional X chromosome leads to failure of testicular development at puberty; the seminiferous tubules undergo fibrosis and hyalinization. The testes remain atrophic, and male secondary sex characteristics fail to develop (Figs 15–9, 15–10, and 15–11). Gynecomastia is common.

Turner's Syndrome (45,X)

In the absence of a Y chromosome, patients with Turner's syndrome develop as phenotypic females. The absence of a second X chromosome causes failure of normal ovarian development, and ovaries remain as streaks of ovarian stroma without follicles (streak gonads). Lack of ovulation results in infertility and failure of menstruation. The absence of a second sex chromosome also results in physical deformities (Fig 15–12).

AGING

Aging is the final phase of human development and may be defined as the aggregate of structural changes that occur with the passage of time; it is characterized by progressive inability to sustain vital functions, with death the eventual result. The life expectancy of humans varies from country to country (it is high in industrialized countries with well-developed systems of medicine and health care delivery, as in the Scandinavian countries, and lower in developing nations). It is generally higher in females than males. In the USA, the average male life expectancy at birth is between 70 and 75 years; for females, between 75 and 80 years.

There is a steady loss of function in various critical organs with age. Extrapolation from such observations would indicate that humans have a finite biologic life span of 90–110 years, so that even if cardiovascular diseases and cancer were eradicated, the current average life expectancy would increase by only a few years.

THEORIES OF AGING

Several different theories have been proposed to explain aging, but no one of them is entirely satisfactory, and it is probable that aging is due to a combination of several processes.

Programmed Aging Theory

According to this theory, the genome of every cell is programmed at conception to cease mitotic division after a certain time. This has been demonstrated by normal fibroblasts and other cells in tissue culture, which undergo a finite number (40–60) of divisions. Epithelial and lymphoid cells appear to have a greater capacity than fibroblasts to divide in culture, though it is debatable whether these cultured cells still reflect the behavior of normal cells in vivo. Programmed cessation of mitotic division does not explain the attrition in permanent (irreversibly postmitotic) cells such as neurons and muscle cells. To explain loss of these cells, proponents of this theory suggest that such cells are also programmed to make errors in transcription of nucleic acid that lead to cell death.

Much evidence supporting the theory of programmed aging derives from rare diseases that are characterized by acceleration of the aging process. These include infantile and adult **progeria**, in which affected individuals exhibit rapid aging independently of environmental factors or other disease processes. In infantile progeria, a young child resembles a wizened old person, with loss of hair, fusion of epiphyses, atherosclerosis, and arterial calcification. The life span in progeria is variable but always greatly shortened, and early demise cannot be prevented by treating associated diseases.

DNA Damage Theory

According to this theory, aging is the result of DNA damage, due either to somatic mutations or to failure of DNA repair mechanisms in aging cells. DNA changes lead to errors in RNA transcription and in that way cause defects in cellular synthesis of protein. Although these changes undoubtedly occur in aging cells, they could just as easily be the result of the aging process rather than the cause.

Neuroendocrine Theory

This theory holds that the aging process is programmed into brain cells at birth and that these cells direct the process by means of hormonal and neural influences. Proponents of this theory point to the control of puberty, which is initiated by the hypothalamus via pituitary hormones, as evidence that the brain can be programmed to function in this manner. Experiments in rats provide some supportive evidence in that removal of the pituitary increases life span. However, no hormones have yet been identified in humans or animals that can produce changes associated with aging.

Immune Theory

A decline in immunologic reactivity occurs with increasing age, which predisposes to development of infections, autoimmune diseases, and neoplasia in elderly persons. This theory postulates that such progressive immunologic dysfunction is inevitable and that it is responsible for limitations on life span. In experimental animals, immunologic manipulations such as thymic transplants have been shown to increase life span. On the other hand, if they are kept in a microbe-free environment, mice with thymic aplasia and marked immune deficiency live as long as normal mice do.

Although immune dysfunction may influence the life span of the individual, it clearly plays little part in many of the morphologic abnormalities associated with aging.

Free Radical Theory

Aging is accompanied by the accumulation of lipofuscin in cells—mainly in the heart, liver, and brain. Lipofuscin is derived from the action of oxygen-based free radicals on plasma membranes of cellular organelles by lipid peroxidation. While lipofuscin itself is harmless, it provides evidence for a general increase in free radical injury of cells as the individual ages. This is due probably to decreased activity of enzymes such as superoxide dismutase that normally inactivate free radicals. Because free radicals can cause cell death, increasing free radical injury with age may contribute to increasing cell loss and the aging process.

Cumulative Injury Theory

It has been suggested that aging may merely represent the aggregate effect of pathologic insults sustained during the life of the individual and that it is not an independent process at all. If this were true, eradication of disease would lead to an increase in life expectancy and perhaps even to "living forever." All available evidence suggests, however, that it is not true. The concept that the human species has a finite life span implies that the aging process operates independently of environmental disease-causing factors. In the quest for immortality, humans must therefore seek not simply the eradication of disease but rather an actual reversal of the aging process.

CHANGES ASSOCIATED WITH AGING (Table 15-13)

Morphologic Changes

As life expectancy increases, the study of aging (gerontology) becomes increasingly important. It is crucial to distinguish changes that are part of the aging process from diseases that are common in older individuals. Changes associated with aging must be accepted as inevitable; on the other hand, diseases associated with aging should be aggressively treated to permit the individual to function at the highest possible level.

A. Cellular Changes:

1. Cell loss-Many cellular metabolic functions are altered with increased age and lead to decreased cell size and number and to atrophy of organs. Cell loss occurs in all tissues but is most evident in organs composed of permanent (irreversibly postmitotic) cells such as the brain and heart, in which replacement of lost cells does not occur. Cell loss in the brain is selective, with the greatest loss occurring in the basal ganglia, substantia nigra, and hippocampus.

2. Organelle changes-The endoplasmic reticulum of aged cells is often disorganized, and its usual close relationship with ribosomes is lost. Free ribosomes are present in the cytoplasm in greater numbers than normal, with resulting abnormalities of protein synthesis. The activity of many enzymes is decreased in aged cells.

Mitochondria of aged cells show abnormalities in size, shape, and cristae. These, coupled with decreased levels of cytochrome C reductase, decrease the efficiency of energy production.

An increased rate of organelle breakdown in aged cells is associated with the presence of increased numbers of phagolysosomal vacuoles in the cells and the deposition of **lipofuscin** (Chapter 1)—a brown pigment believed to be derived from degraded organelle membranes—which is evident in elderly individuals in many organs such as the heart, brain, and liver.

Specialized cytoplasmic structures are often abnormal in aged cells. Myofibrils in muscle cells show decreased contractility. Nerve cells show decreased synthesis of acetylcholine. Poor functioning of cytoskeletal microfilaments in macrophages leads to decreased efficiency of phagocytosis. Hormone receptors on the cell surface become abnormal, resulting in inefficient action of hormones such as insulin.

3. DNA abnormalities-DNA abnormalities are common in aged cells and are mainly the result of a progressive failure of cellular DNA repair mechanisms. DNA abnormalities also occur frequently in normal cells, however, and their repair is a vital requirement for maintenance of a healthy cell. Failure of DNA repair can potentially affect any cellular function and frequently leads to cell death.

B. Connective Tissue Changes: Changes in connective tissue are often used to gauge the progress of aging. Weakening of fibrous tissues, in association with intermittent muscle spasm, may increase the incidence of diverticula in the colon. Weakening of the abdominal and pelvic walls leads to abdominal hernias (inguinal, umbilical, diaphragmatic) and prolapse of organs (uterus, rectum) through the pelvic floor.

Deposition of abnormal substances in connec-

Table 15-13. Tissue changes and disorders associated with aging.

Tissue	Aging Changes	Diseases Occurring More Commonly in the Elderly[1]
Skin	Atrophy, dermal elastosis, loss of elasticity, dryness	Actinic keratosis, seborrheic keratosis, carcinoma, melanoma
Heart	Myocardial atrophy, amyloidosis, lipofuscin deposition, valve calcification, endocardial fibrosis	Ischemic heart disease, aortic valve stenosis
Arteries	Medial calcification, loss of elastic fibers	Atherosclerosis, hypertension
Lungs	Senile emphysema, decreased bronchial ciliary activity	Bronchogenic carcinoma
Brain	Cortical atrophy, lipofuscin deposition, amyloidosis	Subdural hematoma, Alzheimer's disease, Parkinson's disease; cerebrovascular disease
Bone	Osteoporosis	Fractures, vertebral collapse
Joints	Cartilage degeneration	Osteoarthritis
Kidneys	Thickening of glomerular basement membrane, amyloidosis	Glomerular sclerosis
Prostate	Hyperplasia	Urinary obstruction, carcinoma
Testis	Atrophy	. . .
Ovary	Atrophy	Carcinoma
Uterus	Endometrial atrophy; endometrial and endocervical polyps	Endometrial carcinoma; uterine prolapse
Vagina	Atrophy and drying of epithelium	. . .
Breast	Atrophy, fibrosis, duct ectasia	Fibrocystic changes, carcinoma
Gastrointestinal tract	. . .	Diverticulosis of colon, colonic adenoma, carcinoma of stomach and colon
Pancreas	Atrophy, fibrosis	Carcinoma, diabetes mellitus
Eyes	Presbyopia	Cataract
Ears	. . .	Otosclerosis

[1]These diseases are considered in the systemic pathology section.

tive tissue is common in old age and makes the line between disease and simple aging difficult to define. Calcification of the media of muscular arteries is common and usually without clinical significance. Deposition of amyloid (senile amyloidosis) may occur in the heart, brain, and many other organs; clinical disease may result.

1. Elastic tissue changes-Changes in elastic tissue of the body result in loss of elasticity and wrinkling of the skin. This occurs first in the sun-exposed regions of the body—mainly the face—suggesting that aging changes in elastic fibers are accelerated by sunlight. Loss of elasticity in large arteries such as the aorta leads to decreased distensibility. The systolic pressure increases with age because of the aorta's decreased ability to accommodate cardiac output. Loss of elastic tissue in the lungs is associated with destruction and dilatation of alveoli (senile emphysema). This change is usually not severe enough to cause pulmonary dysfunction.

2. Ground substance changes-Changes in the ground substance of tissues results in various abnormalities. In the lens, for example, these changes are associated with the development of opacities (cataracts), which usually impair vision. Cataract formation may be accelerated by disease, eg, diabetes mellitus. The lens also loses its accommodative power with age, so that visual changes—most commonly presbyopia (far-sightedness)—occur, and the individual cannot see objects in the near distance.

3. Cartilage and bone changes-Changes in articular cartilage lead to erosions and fibrillations. The end result is **osteoarthrosis** (Chapter 68). Osteoarthrosis is most common in weight-bearing joints of the spine and the lower extremities, suggesting that wear and tear is an aggravating factor.

Loss of bone (**osteoporosis**) is also a manifestation of aging, perhaps indirectly due to reduction in muscle activity. It is characterized by loss of both bone matrix and mineral, with resulting thinning of bones. Compression of vertebrae causes a decrease in total height. If collapse of vertebral bodies occurs, abnormal curvature (**kyphosis**) results. Old people are therefore often represented in caricature as short and bent over. Osteoporosis in the long bones predisposes to fractures, particularly in the neck of the femur. Although osteoporosis is a common sign of aging, it does not occur uniformly in all elderly people, so that other factors besides age are implicated. Osteoporosis is much more common in postmenopausal women than in other people because of lack of the anabolic effects of estrogens, and estrogen replacement therapy delays onset of the disease. Lack of physical exercise accelerates the onset and progression of osteoporosis.

C. Hair Changes: In old people, the hair becomes thin and sparse and loses its pigment. These characteristic changes are due to progressive failure of hair follicles to produce both keratinlike hair protein and pigment. Gray hair may develop in some people in their 20s or 30s.

D. Reproductive System Changes: **Menopause** is the cessation of menses, which signifies the end of reproductive life in women. Cessation of ovulation results in decreased ovarian hormone levels, endometrial atrophy, cessation of menses, atrophy of the reproductive system, and increased secretion of pituitary gonadotropins by removal of feedback inhibition. Increased FSH levels are thought to be responsible for some menopausal symptoms, eg, hot flushes. Menopause usually occurs between age 40 and 50 years.

Although testicular function declines with age, the existence of a corresponding climacteric in men (so-called male menopause) is controversial.

Changes in Host Defense Mechanisms

The thymus begins to atrophy even in childhood. Some authorities maintain that this is the earliest form of aging or even a direct cause of aging—a belief that may account for the use of injections of embryonic thymus extracts in an attempt to retard the aging process.

Abnormal immune function in the elderly predisposes to development of infections (Fig 15–22). Viral infections of the respiratory tract and bacterial infections of the respiratory and urinary tracts

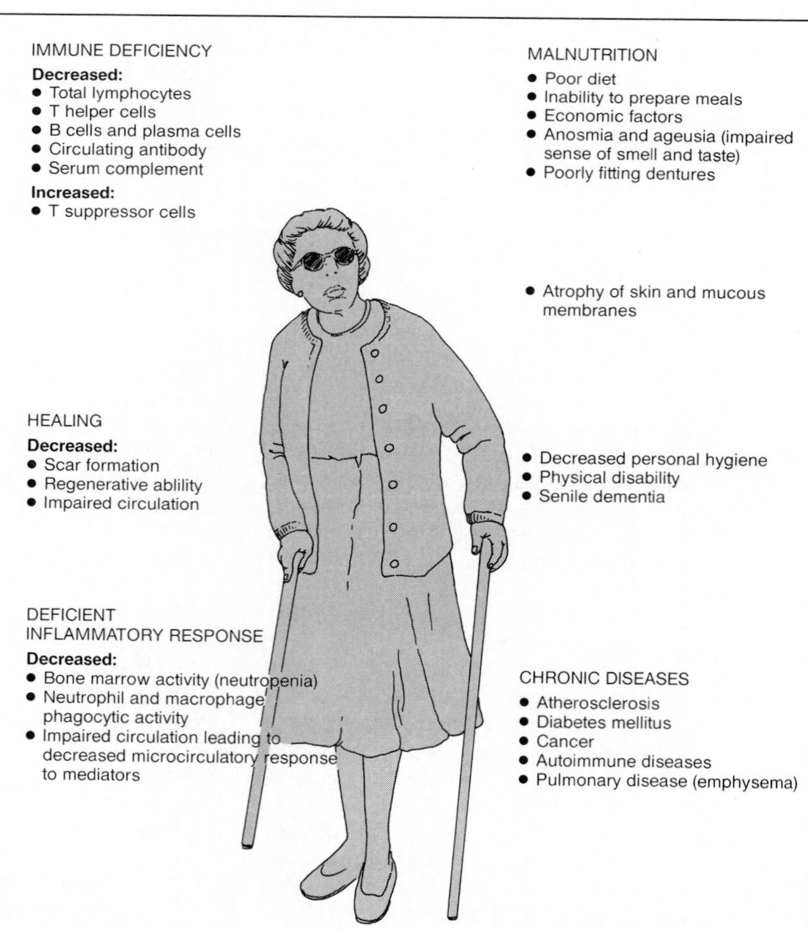

Figure 15–22. Factors leading to an increased incidence of infection in the elderly.

and skin are common. The incidence of tuberculosis is increased and the disease is more virulent in the elderly. Pneumonia is a common cause of death. Older individuals frequently develop autoantibodies and show an increased incidence of autoimmune diseases such as pernicious anemia, Hashimoto's thyroiditis, and Addison's disease. Neoplasms are also more common in the elderly. Cancer is predominantly a disease of older individuals and may in part be related to the decreased ability of the immune system to rid the body of cancer cells. . .

DISEASES ASSOCIATED WITH AGING

Older individuals are susceptible to many different diseases that affect virtually every organ of the body (Table 15–13). It is important to identify diseases responsible for clinical symptoms in elderly patients, because treatment can produce dramatic improvement. Treatment is no longer sometimes withheld because a patient is elderly, and it is not uncommon to undertake major surgery such as total hip replacement in a strong and healthy old person in an attempt to improve function and the quality of life.

16 Disorders of Cellular Growth, Differentiation, & Maturation

NORMAL GROWTH & MATURATION

The cells of the body continue to grow, divide, and differentiate throughout life even after all organs have developed to their full adult size and structure. The degree of growth, multiplication, and differentiation varies with different tissues; eg, in those characterized by continuous cell loss (skin, intestinal mucosa, blood), labile stem cells undergo mitosis to replace lost cells. Stem cells frequently differentiate from a primitive to a mature form during this process; eg, normoblasts in bone marrow become the erythrocytes of the peripheral blood.

Normal growth, mitotic division, and differentiation are controlled so as to maintain the normal structure of a particular tissue. In the skin, for example, as superficial keratinized cells are shed from the surface, basal cells proliferate at a suitable rate to replace them. The newly produced basal cells move upward, differentiating into squamous cells that undergo nuclear and cytoplasmic changes, and mature to become the superficial cornified layer of cells. When the epidermal turnover rate is normal, the skin appears normal on histologic examination; but if the rate is greatly increased, as occurs in psoriasis, cells do not fully mature and abnormalities are seen both on gross examination and at the histologic level.

ABNORMAL GROWTH: ATROPHY, HYPERTROPHY, & HYPERPLASIA

Definitions

Abnormal cellular growth may result in either a decrease or an increase in the mass of the involved tissue (Fig 16–1).

Atrophy is a decrease in the size of a tissue or organ, resulting from a decrease either in the size of individual cells or in the number of cells composing the tissue. Note that atrophy, which is a decrease in size of a normally formed organ, is distinct from agenesis, aplasia, and hypoplasia, which are abnormalities of organ development.

Hypertrophy is an increase in the size of a tissue due to increased size of individual cells, as exemplified by the increased thickness of the left ventricle—due to the increased size of the constituent myocardial fibers—in patients with high blood pressure. Hypertrophy occurs in tissues made up of permanent cells, in which a demand for increased metabolic activity cannot be met through cell multiplication.

Hyperplasia is an increase in the size of a tissue as a result of increased numbers of component cells. As an example, the increase in breast size that occurs during pregnancy is due to an increase in the total number of epithelial cells and lobules. Hyperplasia is the principal mechanism accounting for increased size in tissues composed of labile and stable cells.

Not uncommonly, increased size of a tissue is due to a combination of hypertrophy and hyperplasia, as occurs in the uterus during pregnancy.

Causes of Atrophy

Decrease in the size of a cell results from a reduction in the amount of cytoplasm and the number of cytoplasmic organelles and is usually associated with diminished metabolism. Degenerating organelles are taken up in lysosomal vacuoles for enzymatic degradation (autophagy). Residual organelle membranes often accumulate in the cytoplasm as brown lipofuscin pigment. A decrease in

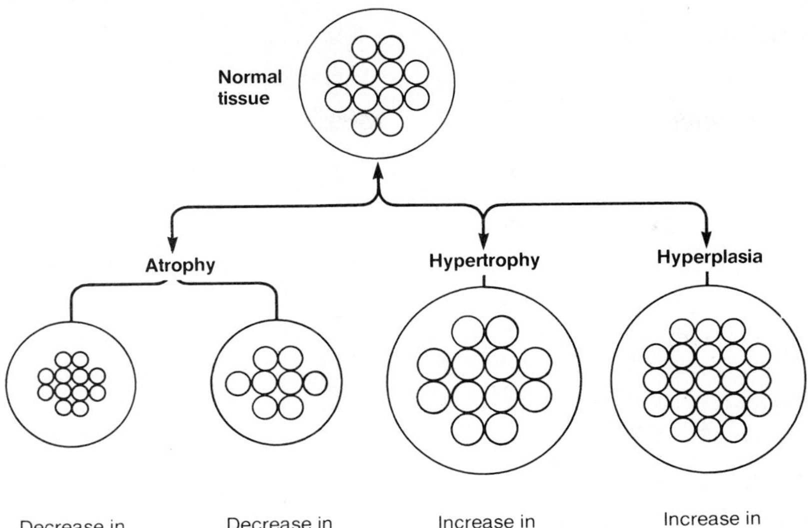

Figure 16–1. Abnormalities of growth. Definitions of the terms atrophy, hypertrophy, and hyperplasia.

cell number results from sporadic death of cells in tissue over a long period.

A. Atrophy of Disuse: Atrophy of disuse occurs in immobilized skeletal muscle and bone, as when a fractured limb is put in a cast or when a patient is restricted to complete bed rest. Skeletal muscle atrophies rapidly with disuse. Atrophy is initially the result of a rapid decrease in cell size that is readily reversible when activity is resumed. With more prolonged immobilization, muscle fibers decrease in number as well as in size. Since skeletal muscle can regenerate only to a very limited extent, restoration of muscle size after loss of muscle fibers can only occur through compensatory hypertrophy of the surviving fibers, which often requires a long rehabilitation period. Bone atrophy results when bone resorption occurs more rapidly than bone formation; it is characterized by decreased size of the trabeculae (decreased mass), leading to osteoporosis of disuse. In this type of bone atrophy, immobilization is associated with lack of functional stress on the bone, leading to failure of normal function of osteoblasts.

B. Denervation Atrophy: Skeletal muscle is dependent on its nerve supply for normal function and structure. Damage to the lower motor neuron at any point between the cell body in the spinal cord and the motor end plate leads to rapid atrophy of the muscle fibers supplied by that nerve. When denervation is temporary, physical therapy and electrical stimulation of the muscle are important to prevent muscle fiber loss and ensure that normal function can be restored when nerve function is reestablished.

C. Atrophy Due to Loss of Trophic Hormones: The endometrium, breast, and many endocrine glands are dependent on trophic hormones for normal cellular growth, and withdrawal of these hormones leads to atrophy of the target cells. When estrogen secretion by the ovary decreases at menopause, there is physiologic atrophy of the endometrium, vaginal epithelium, and breast. Pituitary disease associated with decreased secretion of pituitary trophic hormones results in atrophy of the thyroid, adrenals, and gonads. High-dose adrenal corticosteroid therapy, which is sometimes used for immunosuppression, causes atrophy of the adrenal glands because it suppresses pituitary corticotropin (ACTH) secretion. Such patients soon lose the ability to secrete cortisol and become dependent on exogenous steroids. Withdrawal of steroid therapy in such patients must be gradual enough to permit regeneration of the atrophied adrenal.

D. Atrophy Due to Lack of Nutrients: Severe protein-calorie malnutrition (marasmus) results in the utilization of body tissues such as skeletal muscle as a source of energy and protein after other sources such as adipose stores have been exhausted. Marked muscle atrophy is seen in marasmus.

A decrease in blood supply (ischemia) to a tissue as a result of arterial disease results in atrophy of the tissue due to progressive cell loss. Cerebrovascular disease, for example, is associated with cerebral atrophy, including neuronal loss.

E. Senile Atrophy: Cell loss is one of the morphologic changes of the aging process. It is most apparent in tissues populated by permanent cells, eg, the brain and heart. Atrophy due to aging is frequently compounded by atrophy resulting from coexisting factors such as ischemia.

F. Pressure Atrophy: Prolonged compression of tissue causes atrophy. A large, encapsulated benign neoplasm in the spinal canal may produce atrophy in both the spinal cord it compresses and

Table 16-1. Hypertrophy and hyperplasia of organs.

Tissue	Cause of Increased Demand
Skeletal muscle hypertrophy	Physical activity, weight lifting
Cardiac muscle hypertrophy	Increased pressure load (high blood pressure, valve stenosis) or increased volume load (valve incompetence causing regurgitation of blood)
Smooth muscle (wall of intestine, urinary bladder) hypertrophy	Obstructive lesions
Bone marrow hyperplasia Erythroid hyperplasia	Increased destruction of erythrocytes (hemolytic process); prolonged hypoxia (living at high altitudes).
Megakaryocytic hyperplasia	Increased destruction of platelets in the periphery
Myeloid hyperplasia	Increased demand for neutrophils (as in inflammation)
Lymph node hyperplasia	Antigenic stimulation (proliferative immune response)
Uterine myometrial hypertrophy	Pregnancy (hormone-induced)
Breast hyperplasia	Pregnancy and lactation (hormone-induced)
Renal hypertrophy	Unilateral disease of one kidney; removal of one kidney

the surrounding vertebrae. It is likely that such atrophy results from compression of small blood vessels, resulting in ischemia, and not from the direct effect of pressure on cells.

Causes of Hypertrophy & Hyperplasia

Hypertrophy results from increased amounts of cytoplasm and cytoplasmic organelles in cells. In secretory cells, the synthetic apparatus—including the endoplasmic reticulum, ribosomes, and the Golgi zone—becomes prominent. In contractile cells such as muscle fibers, there is an increase in size of cytoplasmic myofibrils. **Hyperplasia** results when cells of a tissue are stimulated to undergo mitotic division, thereby increasing the number of cells.

A. Physiologic Hypertrophy and Hyperplasia: Hypertrophy and hyperplasia may occur as an adaptation to increased demand (Table 16–1; Figs 16–2, 16–3, and 16–4). Hypertrophy and hyperplasia are controlled responses reflecting in-

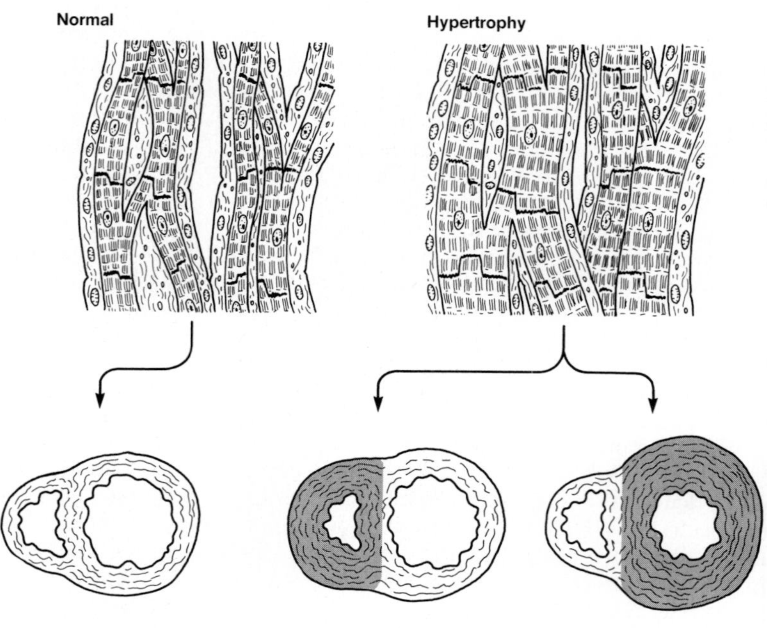

Figure 16–2. Cardiac muscle hypertrophy, showing the increase in size of cardiac muscle fibers. Hypertrophy may involve any of the cardiac chambers if they are subjected to an increased pressure or volume load (right and left ventricular hypertrophy and a few of their common causes are shown).

A

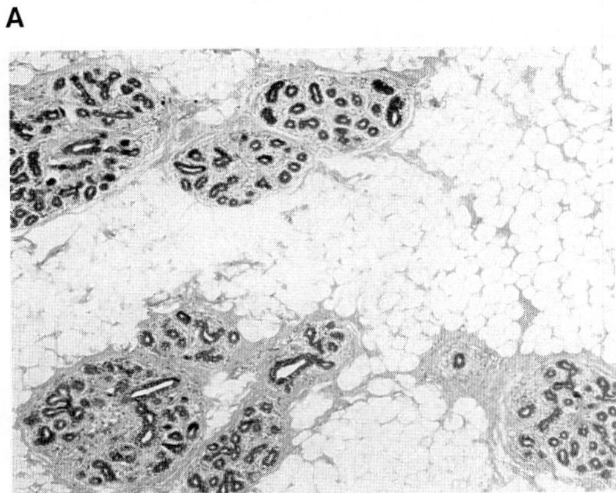

B

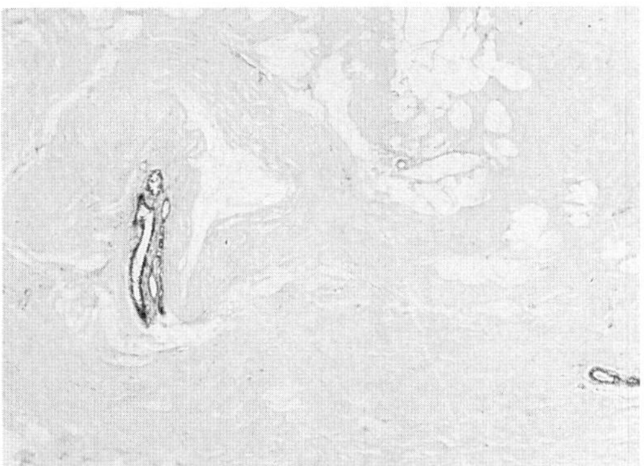

C

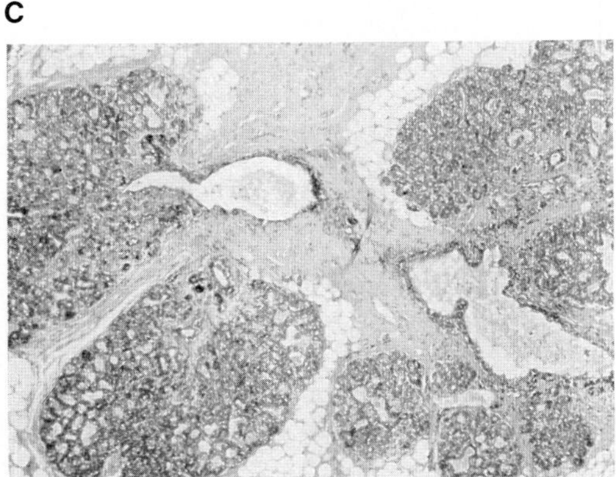

Figure 16-3. Photomicrographs of breast tissue from 3 different patients (all at the same magnification). **A:** Normal breast, showing lobules separated by adipose stroma. **B:** Atrophic breast in a postmenopausal woman, showing greatly decreased numbers of lobules. **C:** Lactating breast, showing hyperplasia of the lobules, which have increased in number at the expense of the stroma.

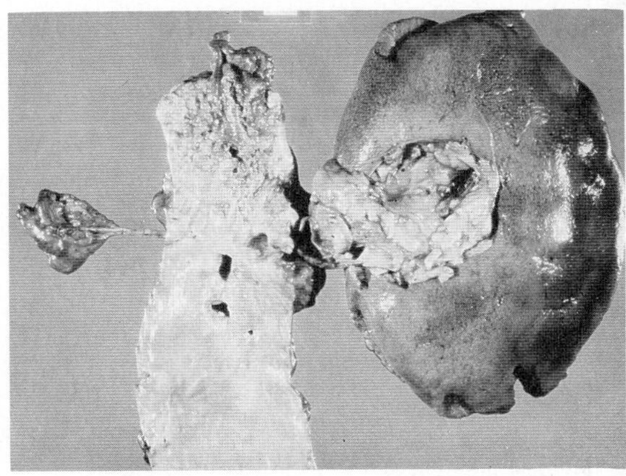

Figure 16-4. Developmental hypoplasia of one kidney associated with marked compensatory hyperplasia of the other kidney.

creased demand; if the demand is removed, the tissues revert toward normal.

B. Pathologic Hypertrophy and Hyperplasia: Abnormal hypertrophy and hyperplasia occur in the absence of an appropriate stimulus of increased functional demand. **Myocardial hypertrophy,** if it occurs without recognizable cause (eg, in the absence of hypertension or valvular or congenital heart disease), is considered an example of pathologic hypertrophy. Such hypertrophy is frequently associated with abnormal cardiac function, producing cardiomyopathy (see Chapter 23).

Endometrial hyperplasia is an important result of increased estrogen stimulation, particularly when estrogens are not opposed by progesterone secretion, as typically occurs near the menopause. It is associated with irregular, often excessive uterine bleeding and increases the risk of endometrial cancer (see Chapter 53). The presence of excessive trophic hormones causes hyperplasia of the target organs; eg, excessive secretion of ACTH causes **bilateral adrenal hyperplasia.** The hyperplastic target organs frequently show increased function. In the case of the adrenal, there is increased cortisol secretion (Cushing's syndrome; Chapter 60).

Thyroid hyperplasia (goiter; Graves' disease) results from increased TSH stimulation of the thyroid or from the action of autoantibodies that are able to bind to TSH receptors in thyroid cell membranes (Chapter 58).

Hyperplasia of the prostate gland is common in older men and is due to hyperplasia of both the glandular and the stromal elements. The cause is not known, though it is believed that waning androgen levels may be responsible (Chapter 51).

Table 16-2. Metaplasia.[1]

Type of Metaplasia	Site	Causative Factors
Epithelial metaplasia		
Squamous metaplasia	Multiple sites Bronchus Endocervix Urinary bladder	Vitamin A deficiency Cigarette smoking, chronic inflammation Chronic inflammation Chronic inflammation, schistosomiasis
Intestinal metaplasia	Esophagus Stomach	Acid reflux Alkaline reflux, chronic inflammation
Gastric metaplasia	Esophagus Intestine	Acid reflux Unknown
Mesenchymal metaplasia		
Osseous metaplasia	Fibrous scars Areas of calcification	Unknown Unknown
Myeloid metaplasia[2]	Spleen, liver	Unknown

[1]See text for details of cell types involved.
[2]Myeloid metaplasia is the appearance of myeloid (bone marrow) elements outside the bone marrow and is not metaplasia in the strict sense, since it is usually the result of extreme hyperplasia of the bone marrow with extension of hematopoiesis into extramedullary sites such as the spleen and liver. (The last-named sites are normal sites of hematopoiesis in the fetus, however.)

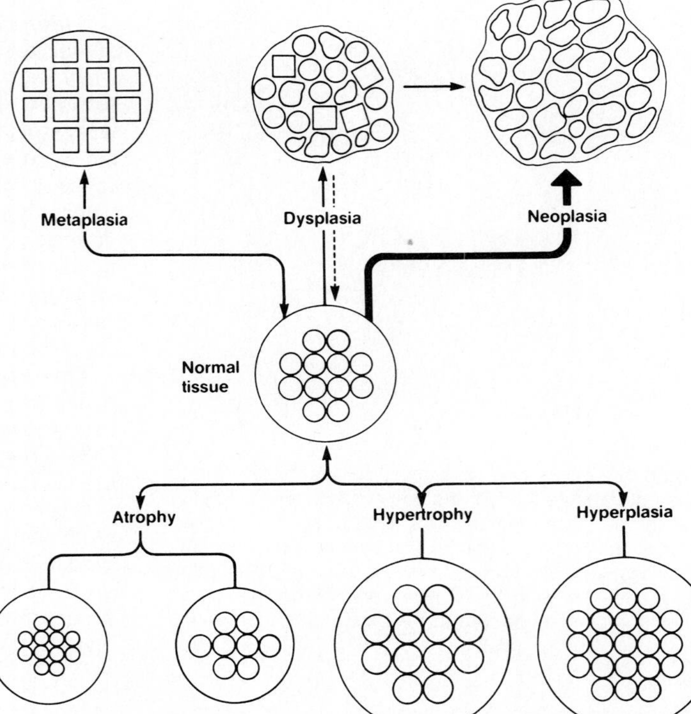

Figure 16-5. Abnormalities of cell growth and maturation. Note that more than one abnormality may be present in a given case, eg, the respiratory mucosa may show squamous metaplasia associated with dysplasia.

ABNORMAL GROWTH PRINCIPALLY INVOLVING DIFFERENTIATION: METAPLASIA (Table 16–2)

Metaplasia is an abnormality of cellular differentiation in which one type of mature cell is replaced by a different type of adult cell—and the latter is not normal for the tissue involved. Metaplasia results from abnormal differentiation of stem cells (Figs 16–5, 16–6, and 16–7). The "new" metaplastic tissue is structurally normal, however, so that the regular cellular organization is maintained. Metaplasia is reversible.

Metaplasia most commonly involves epithelium. As the germinative stem cells multiply to replace cells shed at the surface, they differentiate in a manner that is abnormal for that location, resulting in epithelium of a type different from that usually present. Epithelial metaplasia is thus a manifestation of the varied potential for differentiation in stem cells and typically occurs following chronic physical or chemical irritation.

In **squamous metaplasia**—the most common type of epithelial metaplasia—nonsquamous pseudostratified columnar or cuboidal epithelium is replaced by a normal-appearing stratified squamous epithelium. Squamous metaplasia is common in the endocervix and the bronchial mucosa (Fig 16–6); it occurs less frequently in the endometrium and urinary bladder.

Glandular metaplasia occurs in the esophagus, where the normal squamous epithelium is replaced by a glandular, mucus-secreting epithelium (either gastric or intestinal in type), usually as a result of acid reflux into the esophagus (see Barrett's esophagus, Chapter 37). Metaplasia may also occur in the stomach and intestine, where the mucosa of one part is replaced by that of another, eg, replacement of gastric mucosa with intestinal mucosa (intestinal metaplasia) or vice versa (gastric metaplasia).

Metaplasia rarely occurs in mesenchymal tissue and is best exemplified by osseous metaplasia in scars and other fibroblastic proliferations. Met-

Normal endocervical epithelium

Columnar epithelial cells

Basement membrane

Reserve cells (stem cells of endocervical epithelium) normally divide and differentiate into glandular epithelial cells that replace exfoliated surface cells.

Hyperplasia

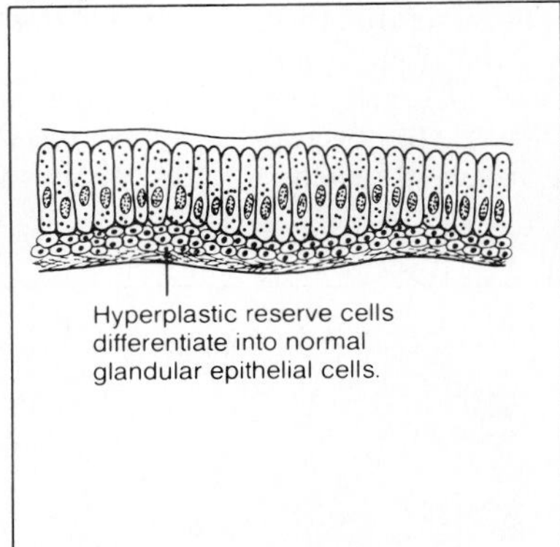

Squamous metaplasia

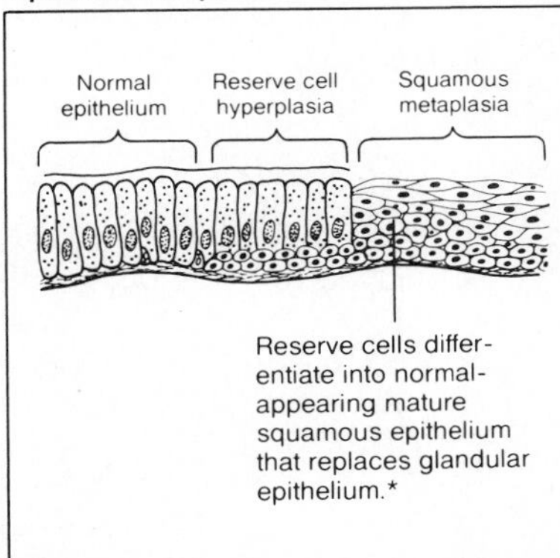

*Similar changes occur in squamous metaplasia of the bronchus.

Dysplasia

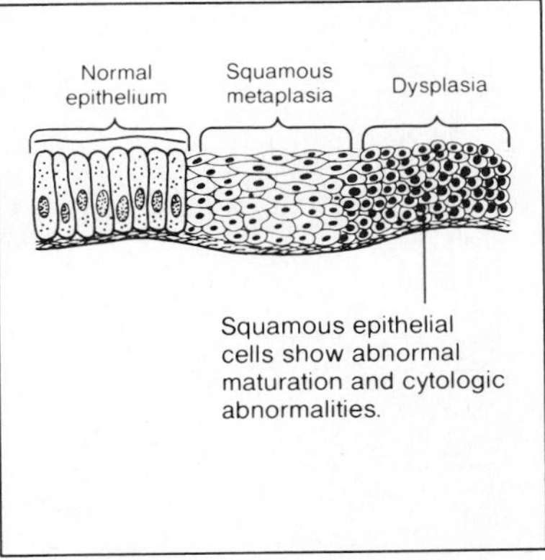

Figure 16–6. Hyperplasia, squamous metaplasia, and dysplasia occurring in the uterine endocervical epithelium. Similar changes may occur in the bronchial epithelium.

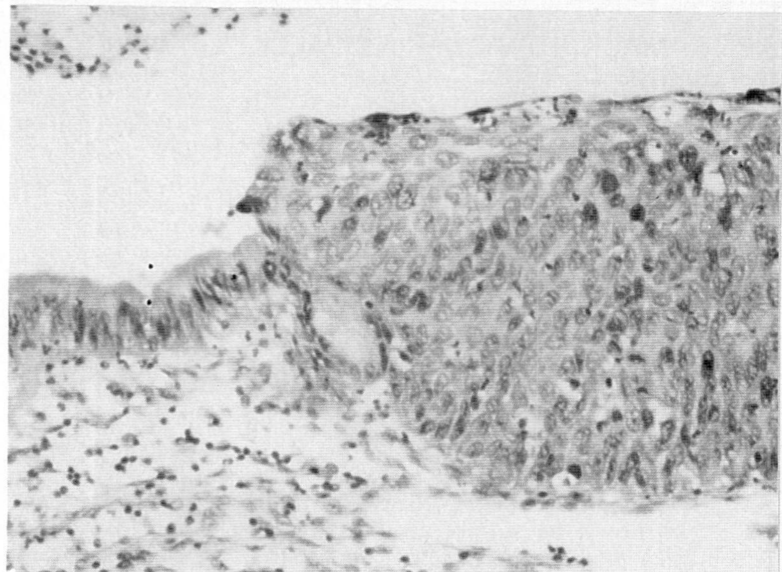

Figure 16-7. Endocervix, showing squamous metaplasia with severe dysplasia. The normal columnar epithelium (at left) has been replaced by a squamous epithelium, which in turn shows cytologic features of dysplasia and loss of maturation.

aplasia in mesenchymal tissue is the same as epithelial metaplasia in representing the potential for diverse differentiation of mesenchymal stem cells.

Most metaplasia is of little clinical significance, although important functional deficits may result in some areas; eg, loss of cilia and of mucus production in the bronchi may predispose to development of infection. Metaplastic tissue is structurally normal and itself carries no increased risk of development of cancer. However, dysplastic changes are often present as well (Fig 16-7), and cancer does occur in metaplastic epithelia under such circumstances; eg, squamous carcinoma develops in metaplastic squamous epithelium in the bronchus, and adenocarcinoma may arise in the esophagus from metaplastic glandular epithelium.

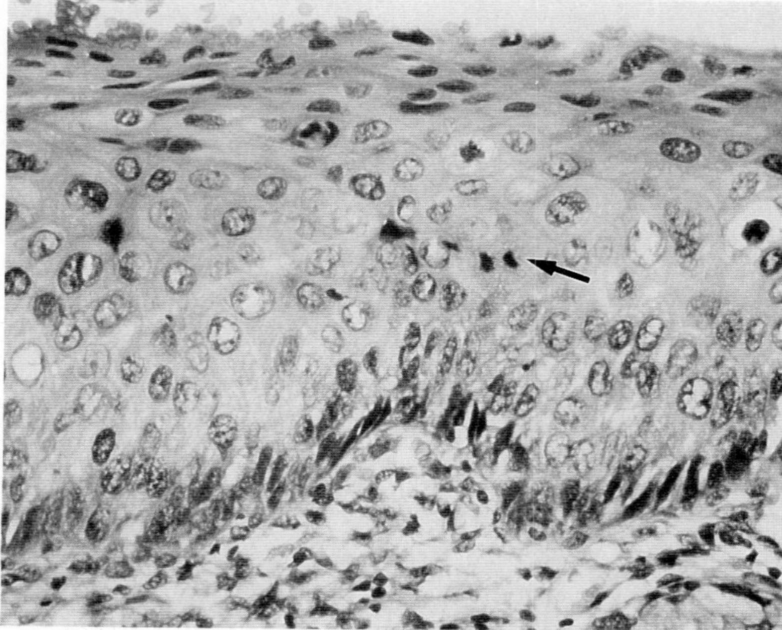

Figure 16-8. Squamous epithelium of uterine cervix, showing moderate dysplasia. The epithelium shows abnormal maturation and cytologic abnormalities, including the presence of cells with large hyperchromatic nuclei in the upper half of the epithelium. Mitotic figures (arrow) are also present above the basal layer.

ABNORMAL GROWTH INVOLVING BOTH DIFFERENTIATION & MATURATION: DYSPLASIA

Characteristics of Dysplasia

Dysplasia is an abnormality of both differentiation and maturation. Use of the term "dysplasia" should be restricted to abnormalities of cell growth with the characteristics described below and illustrated by (Figs 16–5 to 16–10). Loose application of the term dysplasia to denote any cell or tissue that does not appear quite normal is to be discouraged.

A. Nuclear Abnormalities: Dysplasia is characterized by increased size of the nucleus, both absolute and relative to the amount of cytoplasm (increased nuclear:cytoplasmic ratio); increased chromatin content (hyperchromatism); abnormal chromatin distribution (coarse clumping); and nuclear membrane irregularities such as thickening and wrinkling.

B. Cytoplasmic Abnormalities: Cytoplasmic abnormalities in dysplasia result from failure of normal differentiation, eg, lack of keratinization in squamous cells and lack of mucin in glandular epithelium.

C. Increased Rate of Cell Multiplication: In squamous epithelium, an increased rate of cellular multiplication is characterized by the presence of mitotic figures in many layers of the epithelium—in contrast to the normal state, in which mitosis is limited to the basal layer. Individual mitoses are morphologically normal in dysplasia.

D. Disordered Maturation: Dysplastic epithelial cells retain a resemblance to basal stem

A

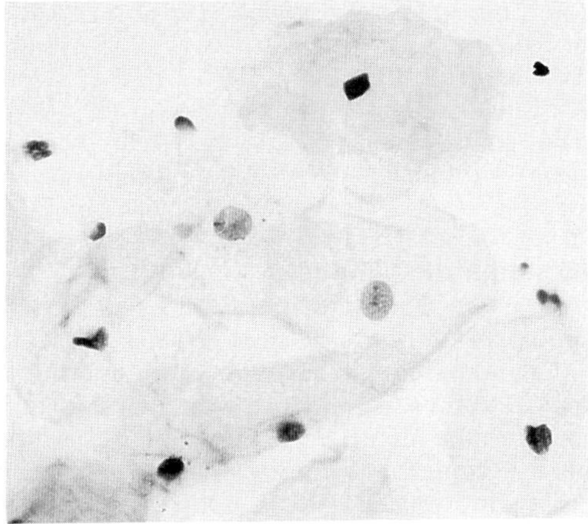

B

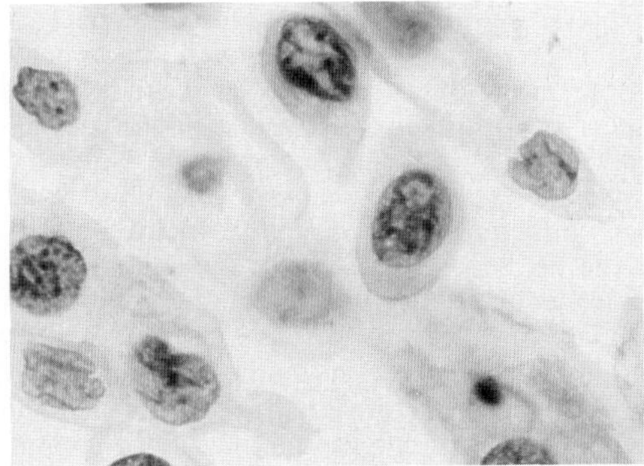

C

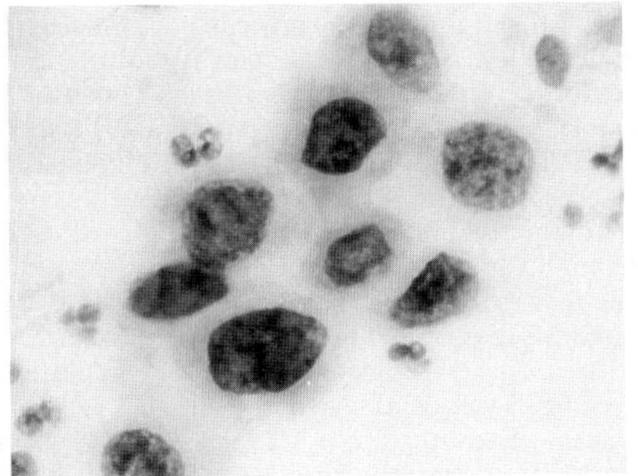

Figure 16–9. Cytologic preparations from the uterine cervix, stained by the Papanicalaou stain ("Pap smears"). **A:** Smear from normal cervix, showing flattened surface squamous cells with abundant keratinized cytoplasm and small nuclei. **B:** Severe dysplasia, showing cells with an increased nuclear:cytoplasmic ratio and enlarged hyperchromatic nuclei. **C:** Squamous carcinoma, showing marked pleomorphism, with extreme nuclear hyperchromatism and irregular distribution of chromatin.

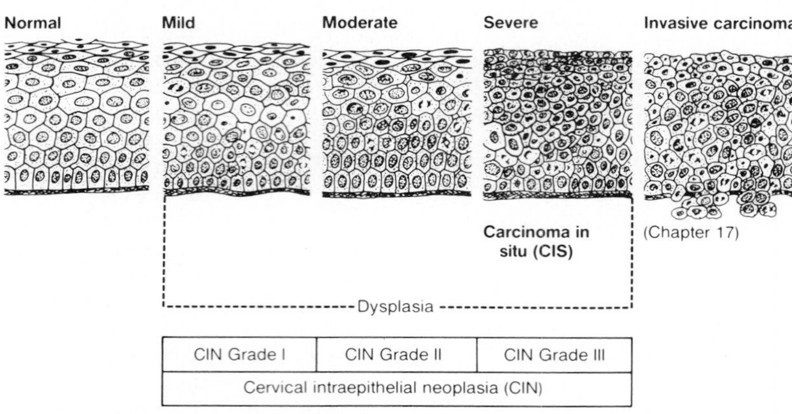

Figure 16-10. Squamous epithelium of the uterine cervix, showing criteria used for grading dysplasia (cervical intraepithelial neoplasia). The maturation defect, the nuclear:cytoplasmic ratio, and the nuclear chromatin abnormalities progressively increase as the grade of dysplasia increases. Note that infiltration of the neoplastic cells through the basement membrane distinguishes invasive carcinoma from dysplasia and carcinoma in situ.

cells as they move upward in the epithelium; ie, normal differentiation (keratin production) fails to occur. Dysplasia is usually graded as mild, moderate, or severe.

Significance of Dysplasia

When it is defined in this manner, epithelial dysplasia is a **premalignant lesion,** associated with an increased risk of development of cancer. In simple terms, dysplasia is a step short of cancer—cancer being a general term for invasive, aggressive growths that are more properly called malignant neoplasms. The process of neoplasia and the many different kinds of neoplasms are the subject of the next 3 chapters. In the uterine cervix, the relationship of dysplasia to cervical cancer is so intimate that the term cervical intraepithelial neoplasia (CIN) is used synonymously with the term dysplasia (Fig 16–10). For this reason, we include the discussion of carcinoma in situ at this point—recognizing, however, that carcinoma in situ is a true neoplasm with all of the features of malignant neoplasms except invasiveness, which will be described in the next chapter. Severe dysplasia of the cervix and carcinoma in situ of the cervix have the same clinical significance and are treated similarly.

The risk of developing invasive cancer varies with (1) the grade of dysplasia—the more severe, the greater the risk; (2) the duration of dysplasia—the longer the duration, the greater the risk; and (3) the site of dysplasia. Dysplasia in the urinary bladder is associated with a more imminent risk of cancer than is cervical dysplasia, in which several years may elapse before invasive carcinoma develops.

Differences Between Dysplasia & Cancer

Dysplasia and carcinoma in situ differ from true cancer in 2 important respects: invasiveness and reversibility.

A. Lack of Invasiveness: The abnormal cellular proliferation in dysplasia and carcinoma in situ does not invade the basement membrane. Since the epithelium contains neither lymphatics nor blood vessels, the proliferating cells do not spread from the epithelium. Complete removal of the dysplastic area is therefore curative. Cancer, in contrast, invades the basement membrane and spreads from the local (primary) site via lymphatics and blood vessels, so that excision of the primary site may not be curative.

B. Reversibility: Dysplastic tissue, particularly that affected by the milder grades of dysplasia, may sometimes spontaneously return to normal—unlike cancer, which is an irreversible process.

Diagnosis of Dysplasia

A. Gross Examination: Epithelial dysplasia, including carcinoma in situ, is usually asymptomatic, and in many cases gross examination of the mucosa shows no abnormality. Dysplasia can sometimes be identified through special examination techniques (eg, colposcopy for cervical dysplasia, fluorescent bronchoscopy for bronchial dysplasia). The **Schiller test** for cervical dysplasia exploits the lack of cellular differentiation of the dysplastic epithelium; when the cervix is painted with iodine solution, normal squamous epithelium turns brown owing to its glycogen content; dysplastic epithelium remains unstained.

B. Microscopic Examination: The diagnosis of dysplasia is usually confirmed by microscopic examination of samples from asymptomatic patients. Cytologic findings must be confirmed by biopsy. Smears are made from material scraped from the epithelium for cytologic diagnosis (Fig 16–9); tissue obtained by biopsy is necessary for histologic diagnosis (Figs 16–7 and 16–8). Microscopic examination of the nuclear and cytoplasmic features of dysplastic tissue provides evidence for both diagnosis and grading of dysplasia. The criteria for cytologic diagnosis of dysplasia are presently well established for the cervix, urinary bladder, and lung. In other sites, such as the gastrointestinal tract and breast, it may be difficult to differentiate dysplasia from other epithelial changes associated with inflammation and regeneration (repair and regeneration involve cell proliferation, so that variable degrees of cellular disorganization may occur; this so-called atypia reverts to normal and carries no increased risk of cancer).

Routine cytologic screening of Papanicolaou cervical smears has permitted early detection and treatment of cervical dysplasia. Widespread use of Pap smears has contributed to the striking decline in incidence of cancer of the uterine cervix in the past 20 years. The results of cytologic screening in other sites have not been as encouraging. Although dysplasia can be recognized in lung (sputum smears), bladder (urine smears), stomach (gastric brushings), and colon (colonic lavage), complete removal of all dysplastic epithelium from these tissues is much more difficult. As a result, routine screening for dysplasia in these tissues is not recommended, and early recognition of dysplasia has had little impact on the statistics for incidence of cancer in these sites.

17 Neoplasia: I. Classification, Nomenclature, & Epidemiology of Neoplasms

Neoplasia (L "new growth") is an abnormality of cellular differentiation, maturation, and control of growth. Neoplasms are commonly recognized by the formation of masses of abnormal tissue (tumors). The term "tumor" can be applied to any swelling—and in that context is one of the cardinal signs of inflammation—but most commonly it is used to denote suspected neoplasm. Neoplasms are **benign** or **malignant** depending on several features, chiefly the ability of malignant neoplasms to spread from the site of origin. Benign neoplasms grow but remain localized. **Cancer** denotes a malignant neoplasm (the term is thought to derive from the way in which the tumor grips the surrounding tissues with clawlike extensions, much like a crab).

Although a neoplasm may not be difficult to recognize, the process of neoplasia is hard to define. The definition of neoplasm proposed in the early 1950s by Rupert Willis, a British pathologist, is probably the best: "A neoplasm is an abnormal mass of tissue, the growth of which exceeds and is uncoordinated with that of the surrounding normal tissues and persists in the same excessive manner after cessation of the stimuli that evoked the change." This definition is analyzed in greater detail in Chapter 18.

CLASSIFICATION OF NEOPLASMS

Although all neoplasms possess certain characteristics in common—particularly the capacity for uncontrolled continuous growth (Chapter 19)—they vary enormously in their gross and microscopic features. The clinical presentation, behavior, effects, response to therapy (Chapter 19), and etiology (Chapter 18) are likewise diverse.

For these reasons, the classification of neoplasms has major implications for prognosis and therapy. Approaches to the classification of neoplasms are summarized in Table 17–1.

BIOLOGIC BEHAVIOR OF NEOPLASMS

Types of Biologic Behavior

The biologic behavior of neoplasms constitutes a spectrum (Fig 17–1) with 2 extremes:

A. Benign: At one extreme, a benign neoplasm grows slowly and is encapsulated. There is no infiltration or active destruction of surrounding tissue and no spread to distant sites (ie, no metastasis). Such neoplasms are rarely life-threatening but may become so because of hormone secretion or critical location; eg, a benign neoplasm arising in a spinal nerve root can compress the spinal cord and cause paraplegia; a benign neoplasm can cause death if it arises in a cranial nerve and compresses the medulla.

B. Malignant: At the other extreme are malignant neoplasms, which grow rapidly, infiltrate and destroy surrounding tissues, and metastasize throughout the body, often with lethal results.

Table 17-1. Approaches to classification of neoplasms.

Basis for Classification	Historical Aspect	Current Clinical Usefulness
Site	First recognized by Egyptian embalmers, who realized that tumors of the breast, uterus, soft parts, and so forth were different from one another.	The basis for all clinical classifications; neoplasms of any given site may include many different pathologic types.
Biologic behavior	Hippocrates (460–375 BC) recognized 2 broad groups: (1) "carcinos": innocuous, which included some inflammatory lesions and benign neoplasms; and (2) "carcinomas": dangerous, often causing death. Galen (130–200 AD) classified "tumors" as (1) according to nature (eg, pregnant uterus), (2) exceeding nature (inflammatory masses), or (3) contrary to nature (the true neoplasms).	The distinction between benign and malignant is the most important form of clinical classification and the one on which treatment is based (see text).
Cell (tissue) of origin (histogenetic classification)	Histologic features of neoplasms have been used since the introduction of diagnostic microscopy in 1850. Mallory (1862–1941): "Tumors are classified on a histologic basis . . . the cell type is the one important element from which a tumor should be named."	Forms the basis of modern nomenclature of most neoplasms; however, the cell type is not known for some neoplasms, and eponyms and descriptive names are used instead (see text).
Embryologic derivation	Adami (1861–1926) classified neoplasms according to their derivation from ectoderm, endoderm, or mesoderm.	The broad classification of neoplasms as epithelial or mesenchymal uses embryologic derivation to a slight extent; this classification is of little use.
Differentiation potential of cell of origin	. . .	Recognition of neoplasms arising from cells that are totipotent (germ cell neoplasms), pluripotent, or unipotent is useful theoretically but of little practical value.
Etiology	. . .	Unsatisfactory because the cause of neoplasms is largely unknown. May be of use in the future.
Gross or microscopic features	Used throughout history to classify neoplasms; ulcerating, fungating, polypoid, gelatinous, scirrhous, medullary, etc.	Of little value. Descriptive terms are used to qualify neoplasms and to describe neoplasms whose histogenesis is uncertain, eg, alveolar soft part sarcoma, granular cell tumor.

C. Intermediate: Between these 2 extremes is a smaller third group of neoplasms that are locally invasive but have low metastatic potential. Such neoplasms are called locally aggressive neoplasms or low-grade malignant neoplasms. An example is basal cell carcinoma of the skin.

Identification of Biologic Behavior by Pathologic Examination

Treatment of neoplasms is guided by their biologic behavior. Benign neoplasms are cured by excision of the tumor. Locally aggressive neoplasms must be treated by excising the tumor along with

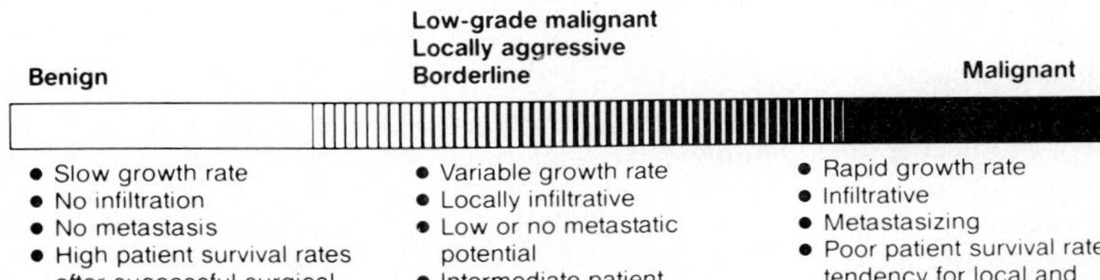

Figure 17-1. Biologic behavior of neoplasms. The behavior of neoplasms is shown as a spectrum from benign to highly malignant. There is also an intermediate group of low-grade malignant neoplasms composed of those that have the potential for local recurrence but limited or no metastatic potential.

a wide margin of surrounding tissue to ensure that infiltrating cells are removed. Malignant neoplasms require local wide removal, frequently including regional lymph nodes as well as systemic treatment for neoplastic cells that may have metastasized.

The pathologist usually classifies a neoplasm as benign or malignant on the basis of histologic and cytologic features in association with the cumulative clinicopathologic experience gained with various types of neoplasms. There are no absolute criteria for distinguishing benign from malignant neoplasms, and the characteristics listed in Table 17-2 serve as general guidelines only.

A. Rate of Growth: Malignant neoplasms generally grow more rapidly than benign ones, but there is no critical rate that distinguishes malignant from benign. Assessment of the growth rate is based upon clinical information (eg, change in size of the mass in serial examinations). On microscopic examination, the number of mitotic figures and the metabolically active appearance of nuclei (enlarged, dispersed chromatin, large nucleoli) correlate positively with the growth rate of the neoplasm.

B. Size: The size of a neoplasm generally has no bearing on its biologic behavior. Many benign neoplasms become very large; conversely, highly malignant neoplasms may be lethal by virtue of extensive dissemination even though the original primary tumor is still small. In a few neoplasms, however, size is the deciding factor in distinguishing benign from malignant growths. A carcinoid tumor of the appendix is considered benign unless it is larger than 2 cm, in which case it is regarded as malignant; this distinction is based on the observation that the risk of metastasis increases with increasing size of the primary neoplasm and that appendiceal carcinoid tumors less than 2 cm in diameter do not metastasize. Benign and malignant carcinoid tumors are histologically identical.

C. Degree of Differentiation: When the term differentiation is used to describe neoplasms, it denotes the degree to which a neoplastic cell resembles the normal adult cells of the tissue in question; this meaning is distinct from the more general use of the word to describe passage of a cell down a particular maturation pathway. Benign neoplasms are usually fully differentiated; ie, they resemble normal adult tissue (Fig 17-2). Malignant neoplasms, on the other hand, show variable degrees of differentiation and frequently demonstrate little resemblance to normal tissue (ie, they are poorly differentiated). In **anaplasia,** the neoplastic cells have no morphologic resemblance whatsoever to normal tissue. Malignant neoplasms are also usually more cellular, have a higher mitotic rate, and display the cytologic features of malignancy (Table 17-2). The importance of these individual criteria varies with different neoplasms. For example, the mitotic rate is the

Table 17-2. Summary of features differentiating benign and malignant neoplasms.[1]

Benign	Malignant
Gross features	
Smooth surface with a fibrotic capsule; compressed surrounding tissues.	Irregular surface without encapsulation; destruction of surrounding tissues.
Small to large, sometimes very large.	Small to large.
Slow rate of growth.	Rapid rate of growth.
Rarely fatal (except in central nervous system) even if untreated.	Usually fatal if untreated.
Microscopic features	
Growth by compression of surrounding tissue.	Growth by invasion of surrounding tissue.
Highly differentiated, resembling normal tissue of origin microscopically.	Well or poorly differentiated. Most malignant neoplasms do not resemble the normal tissue of origin (anaplasia).
Cells similar to normal and resembling one another, presenting a uniform appearance.	Cytologic abnormalities,[2] including enlarged, hyperchromatic, irregular nuclei with large nucleoli; marked variation in size and shape of cells (pleomorphism).
Few mitoses;[3] those present are normal.	Increased miotic activity; abnormal, bizarre mitotic figures often present.
Well-formed blood vessels.	Blood vessels numerous and poorly formed; some lack endothelial lining.
Necrosis unusual; other degenerative changes may be present.	Necrosis and hemorrhage common.
Distant spread (metastasis) does not occur.	Metastasis to distant sites.
Investigative techniques	
DNA content usually normal.	DNA content of cells increased, additional chromsomes commonly present.
Karyotype usually normal.	Karyotypic abnormalities, including aneuploidy and polyploidy, are common.[4]

[1]None of these features are absolute; metastasis, invasion, and anaplasia are the most helpful.
[2]Note that the cytologic abnormalities of malignant neoplasms resemble those of dysplasia but are more extreme.
[3]Note that some nonneoplastic states have numerous mitotic figures (eg, normal bone marrow, lymph nodes undergoing an immune response).
[4]Subtle gene deletions or translocations are being recognized with increased frequency.

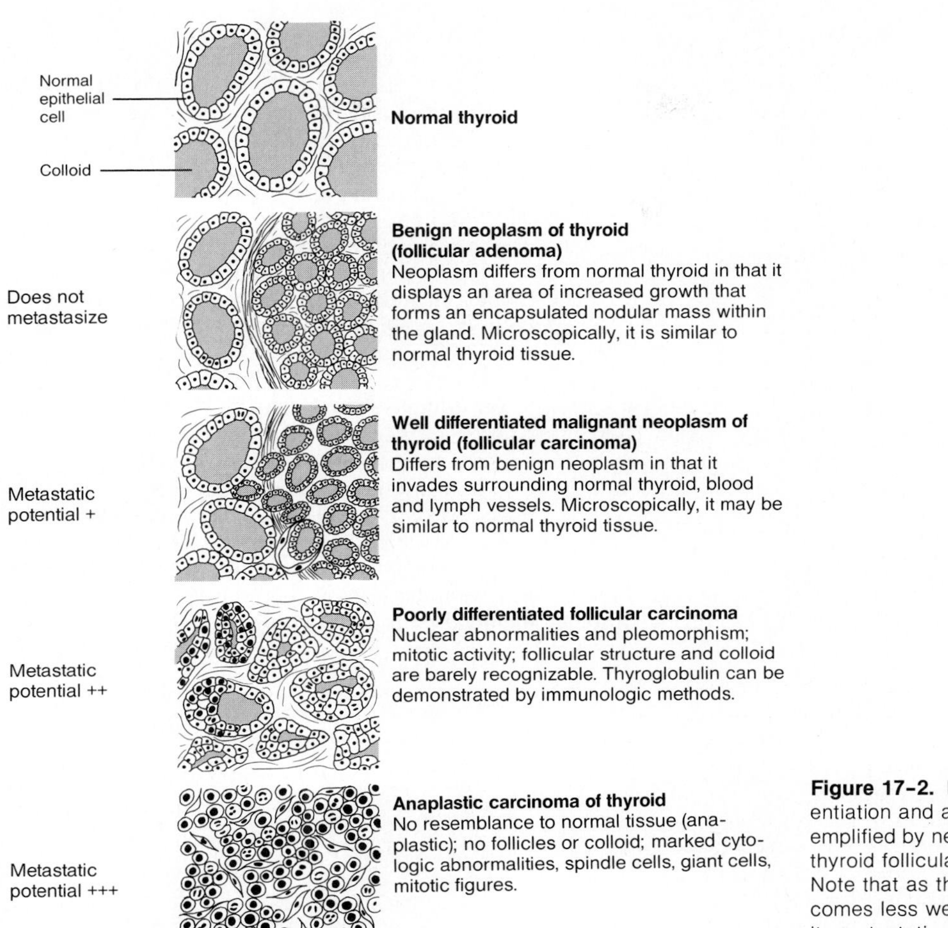

Figure 17-2. Degree of differentiation and anaplasia as exemplified by neoplasms arising in thyroid follicular epithelium. Note that as the neoplasm becomes less well differentiated, its metastatic potential increases.

major factor distinguishing benign from malignant smooth muscle neoplasms in the uterus; in many other neoplasms, the mitotic rate is of little relevance. Similarly, pheochromocytoma, a neoplasm of the adrenal medulla, may show extreme cytologic abnormalities without demonstrating malignant behavior.

D. Changes in DNA: Neoplasms are associated with abnormalities in their DNA content; this abnormality increases with the degree of malignancy. The degree of **hyperchromatism** (increased staining of the nucleus) provides a crude assessment of DNA content on microscopic examination; malignant cells are hyperchromatic. Cytogenetic studies demonstrating **aneuploidy and polyploidy** also are indicative of malignancy and are becoming more widely available. When measured precisely by flow cytometry, the DNA content of malignant cells correlates well with the degree of malignancy in malignant lymphoma, bladder neoplasms, and astrocytic neoplasms. This is a promising technique, but its use is still largely experimental.

E. Infiltration and Invasion: Benign neoplasms are generally noninfiltrative and are surrounded by a capsule of compressed and fibrotic normal tissue. Malignant neoplasms, on the other hand, have infiltrating margins. Many exceptions to this rule exist, and some benign neoplasms—eg, granular cell tumor, dermatofibroma, and carcinoid tumors—lack a capsule and have an infiltrative margin.

F. Metastasis: The occurrence of metastasis (noncontiguous or distant growth of tumor; Chapter 18) is absolute evidence of malignancy. The major reason for distinguishing benign from malignant neoplasms is to be able to predict their ability to metastasize before they do so.

Gross and microscopic examination of a neoplasm usually enables a trained pathologist to classify most neoplasms as benign or malignant. In some instances, however, this identification is difficult, and the only reliable evidence of a neoplasm's biologic behavior is the occurrence of metastasis; eg, 90% of pheochromocytomas are benign, but there are no reliable criteria for identifying the 10% that will metastasize.

CELL OR TISSUE OF ORIGIN (Histogenesis)

Neoplasms are classified and named chiefly on the basis of their presumed cell of origin. These cells have different potentials for further development into various cell types (Tables 17—3 and 17—4).

Neoplasms of Totipotent Cells

The prototype of the totipotent cell—ie, a cell that is capable of differentiating (maturing) into any cell type in the body—is the zygote, which gives rise to the fetus. In postnatal life, the only totipotent cells in the body are the **germ cells.** These are most commonly found in the gonads but also occur in the retroperitoneum, mediastinum, and pineal region.

Germ cell neoplasms (Fig 17-3) may remain with minimal differentiation as a mass of malignant primitive germ cells (seminoma and embryonal carcinoma) or may develop into a variety of tissues, including trophoblast (choriocarcinoma), yolk sac (yolk sac carcinoma), or somatic structures (teratoma) (Table 17-4). Mixtures of different tissues frequently coexist in a single neoplasm.

Teratomas show somatic differentiation and contain elements of all 3 germ layers: entoderm, ectoderm, and mesoderm. Thus, brain, respiratory and intestinal mucosa, cartilage, bone, skin, teeth, or hair may be seen in the neoplasm. The constituent tissues are not limited to those normally present in the area of origin. One theory held that teratomas represented a maldeveloped included twin (twin within a twin), but teratomas

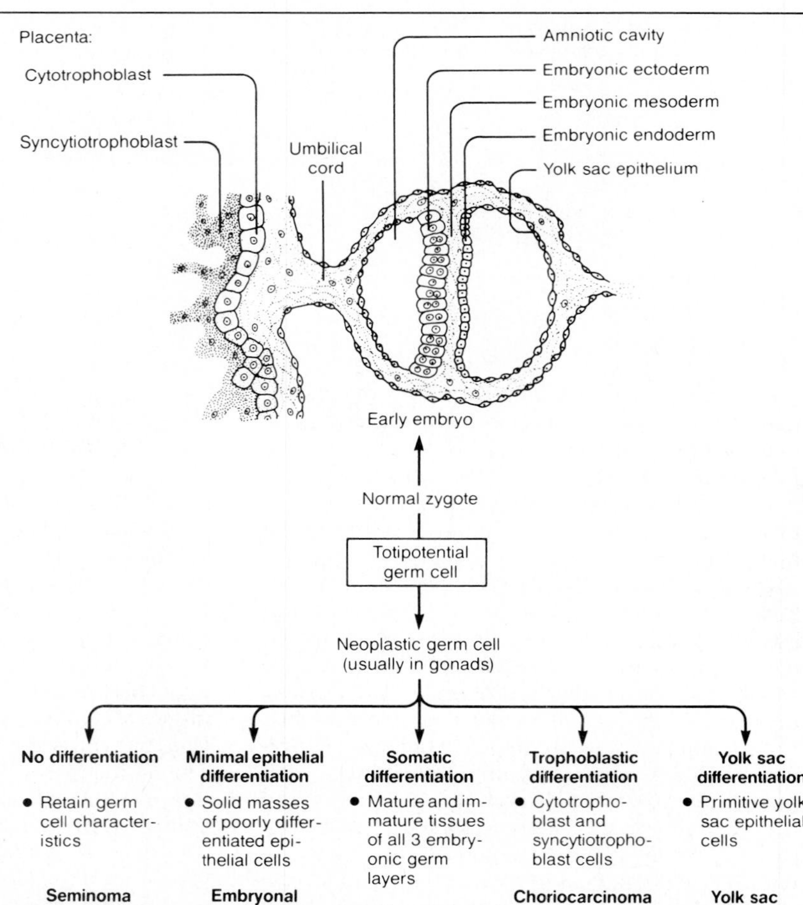

Figure 17-3. Neoplasms of totipotential cells (germ cell neoplasms, bottom), compared with the development of the normal zygote (top). Neoplastic germ cells retain the same potential for differentiation as the zygote and are classified according to the types of differentiation present.

Table 17-3. Classification of the cells on the basis of their ability to differentiate into different tissues.

Cell Type	Occurrence in Normal Development	Differentiation Capabilities Displayed in Derived Neoplasms
Totipotent cell	Zygote (fetal) Germ cells (gonads usually, extragonadal rarely)	Able to develop into any cell type (capability similar to that of zygote).
Pluripotent cell	Found in primitive cells that constitute organ anlagen (fetal). Persists in some organs (eg, cerebellum, kidney, adrenal, retina, pineal) in the first few years of postnatal life.	Able to develop into multiple cell types having a maximum of 2 germ layers. These neoplasms occur in the first few years of life.
Differentiated cell	Adult labile and stable cell: usually differentiates into one cell type only but retains limited ability to differentiate into related cells (as in metaplasia).	Most human neoplasms arise from these cells. Common in older patients. Neoplasm composed of one cell type (may have metaplastic elements).
Permanent cell	End-stage functioning cells of epithelia and permanent cells in muscle and brain. Unable to divide (postmitotic).	Does not produce neoplasms (few if any exceptions).

differ from fetuses in that the various tissues are largely disorganized.

Teratomas are further classified as mature (well-differentiated and composed of adult-type tissues) or immature (made up of fetal-type tissues). Immature teratomas are malignant, whereas mature teratomas vary in their biologic potential. Most mature teratomas are benign, eg, mature teratoma of the ovary (dermoid cyst) (Chapter 52). Mature testicular teratomas are benign when they occur in childhood but are usually malignant in adult testes. In teratomas, the distinction between benign and malignant incorporates unusual criteria such as maturity of constituent tissues, site of occurrence, and age of the patient.

Neoplasms of Embryonic Pluripotent Cells

Pluripotent cells can mature into several different cell types, and the corresponding neoplasms have the potential for formation of diverse structural elements; eg, neoplasms of the renal anlage cells (nephroblastoma) commonly differentiate into structures resembling renal tubules and less often into rudiments of muscle, cartilage, and bone. These neoplasms are generally called **embryomas** or **blastomas** (Fig 17-4).

Embryonic pluripotent cells are found only in the fetal period and during the first few years of postnatal life. The corresponding neoplasms usually occur in early childhood and only rarely in adults.

Blastomas may be completely undifferentiated—ie, are composed of small, malignant, primitive-appearing, hyperchromatic cells—or may show evidence of differentiation, eg, the presence of primitive renal tubules in nephroblastoma or of ganglion cells in neuroblastoma. Evidence of differentiation generally signifies less malignant biologic behavior.

Neoplasms of Differential Cells

Differentiated, adult-type cells make up most of the cells in the body in postnatal life. They show a restricted potential for differentiation, as seen when they undergo metaplasia. Most human neoplasms are derived from differentiated cells.

The classification and nomenclature of these neoplasms (Table 17-4) combine several of the approaches set out in Table 17-1: the distinction between benign and malignant and epithelial and mesenchymal; the cell or tissue of origin; the site; and other descriptive features.

A. Nomenclature of Neoplasms of Differentiated Cells: (Fig 17-5.)

1. Epithelial neoplasms-A benign epithelial neoplasm is called an **adenoma** if it arises from glandular epithelium (eg, thyroid adenoma, colonic adenoma) and a **papilloma** if it has a papillary architecture. Papillomas may arise from squamous, glandular, or transitional epithelium (eg, squamous papilloma, intraductal papilloma of the breast, and transitional cell papilloma, respectively). Not uncommonly, descriptive adjectives are incorporated in the nomenclature; eg, colonic adenomas may be villous or tubular.

Malignant epithelial neoplasms are called **carcinomas** (adenocarcinomas if derived from glandular epithelia; squamous carcinoma and transitional cell carcinoma if originating in those kinds of epithelia). Names may also include the organ of origin and often an adjective as well, eg, clear cell adenocarcinoma of the kidney, papillary adenocarcinoma of the thyroid, verrucous squamous carcinoma of the larynx.

2. Mesenchymal neoplasms-Benign mesenchymal neoplasms are named after the cell of origin (a Greek or Latin word is used) followed by the suffix *-oma* (Table 17-4). The names of these tumors may contain the organ of origin and an adjective, eg, cavernous hemangioma of the liver.

Malignant mesenchymal neoplasms are named

Table 17-4. Classification of common neoplasms.

Differentiation Potential and Cell Type	Cell or Site	Benign Neoplasm	Malignant Neoplasm
Totipotent cells	Germ cell	Teratoma (mature)	Teratoma (immature), seminoma (dysgerminoma), embryonal carcinoma, yolk sac carcinoma, choriocarcinoma
Pluripotent cells (embryonic blast cells of organ anlage)	Retinal anlage Renal anlage Primitive (peripheral) nerve cells Primitive neuroectodermal cells		Retinoblastoma Nephroblastoma (Wilms's tumor) Neuroblastoma Medulloblastoma
Differentiated cells Epithelial cells Squamous	Skin, esophagus, vagina, mouth, metaplastic epithelium	Squamous papilloma	Squamous carcinoma Basal cell carcinoma
Glandular	Gut, respiratory tract, secretory glands, bile ducts, ovary, endometrium of uterus	Adenoma Cystadenoma	Adenocarcinoma Cystadenocarcinoma
Transitional	Urothelium	Papilloma	Transitional cell carcinoma
Hepatic	Liver cell	Adenoma	Hepatocellular carcinoma (hepatoma)
Renal	Tubular epithelial cell	Adenoma	Adenocarcinoma
Endocrine	Thyroid, parathyroid, pancreatic islets	Adenoma	Adenocarcinoma
Mesothelium	Mesothelial cells	Benign mesothelioma	Malignant mesothelioma
Placenta	Trophoblast cells	Hydatidiform mole	Choriocarcinoma
Mesenchymal cells Fibrous tissue	Fibroblast	Fibroma	Fibrosarcoma
Cartilage	Chondrocyte	Chondroma	Chondrosarcoma
Nerve	Schwann cell	Schwannoma	Malignant peripheral nerve sheath tumor
	Neural fibroblast	Neurofibroma	Malignant peripheral nerve sheath tumor
Bone	Osteoblast	Osteoma	Osteosarcoma
Fat	Lipocyte	Lipoma	Liposarcoma
Notochord	Primitive mesenchyme		Chordoma
Vessels	Endothelial cells	Hemangioma Lymphangioma	Hemangiosarcoma, Kaposi's sarcoma Lymphangiosarcoma
Pia and arachnoid	Meningeal cells	Meningioma	Malignant meningioma
Muscle	Smooth muscle cells Striated muscle cells	Leiomyoma Rhabdomyoma	Leiomyosarcoma Rhabdomyosarcoma
Melanocytes	Melanocytes[1]	Nevi (various types)	Melanoma (malignant)
Glial cells	Astrocytes		Astroyctomas Glioblastoma multiforme
	Ependymal cells Oligodendroglial cells		Ependymoma Oligodendroglioma
Hematopoietic tissue (marrow)	Erythroblasts[2] Myeloblasts[2] Monoblasts[2]		Erythroblastic leukemia[2] (Di Guglielmo) Myeloid leukemia[2] Monocytic leukemias[2]
Lymphoid tissue	Lymphoblasts Lymphocytes[2]		Malignant lymphomas, lymphocytic leukemias, myeloma
	Histiocytes[2]		Malignant histiocytosis

[1]The origin of melanocytes is still controversial; we have placed them with mesenchymal tissues on the basis of their content of vimentin intermediate filaments (like other mesenchymal cells) as opposed to keratin (as in epithelial cells).
[2]The cells of origin, nomenclature, and relationships of these neoplasms are complex and are discussed fully in Chapters 26 and 29.

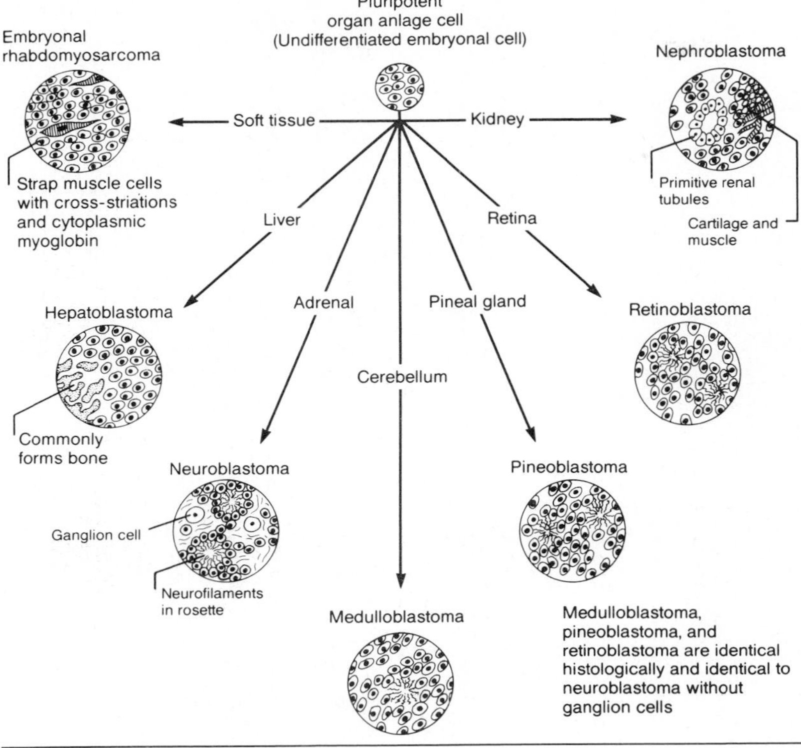

Figure 17-4. Neoplasms of pluripotent embryonic-type cells ("blastomas"). These neoplasms commonly occur in children and may be diagnosed by clinical features (eg, site, catecholamine secretion in neuroblastoma), evidence of differentiation (eg, tubules in nephroblastoma, ganglion cells in neuroblastoma), or immunohistologic methods (eg, actin in embryonal rhabdomyosarcoma). These tumors may also differentiate into mesenchymal elements (eg, bone in hepatoblastoma and cartilage and muscle in nephroblastoma.)

after the cell of origin, to which is added the suffix *-sarcoma*. Again, adjectives are commonly used; eg, liposarcomas are classified as sclerosing, myxoid, round cell, or pleomorphic.

B. Exceptions to These Rules: The simple scheme described above is complicated by several groups of neoplasms that do not conform to the pattern.

1. Neoplasms that "sound benign" but are really malignant-The names of some malignant neoplasms are formed by adding the suffix *-oma* to the cell of origin, eg, lymphoma (lymphocyte), plasmacytoma (plasma cell), melanoma (melanocyte), glioma (glial cell), and astrocytoma (astrocyte). The adjective "malignant" should be used—malignant lymphoma, malignant melanoma—but if it is not, these neoplasms are assumed to be malignant because there is no benign lymphoma, melanoma, glioma, etc.

2. Neoplasms that "sound malignant" but are really benign-Two rare bone neoplasms, osteoblastoma and chondroblastoma, may sound malignant because of the suffix *-blastoma* but are in fact benign neoplasms derived from osteoblasts and chondroblasts present in adult bone.

3. Leukemias-Neoplasms of blood-forming organs are called leukemias. These disorders are all considered malignant, though some exhibit a

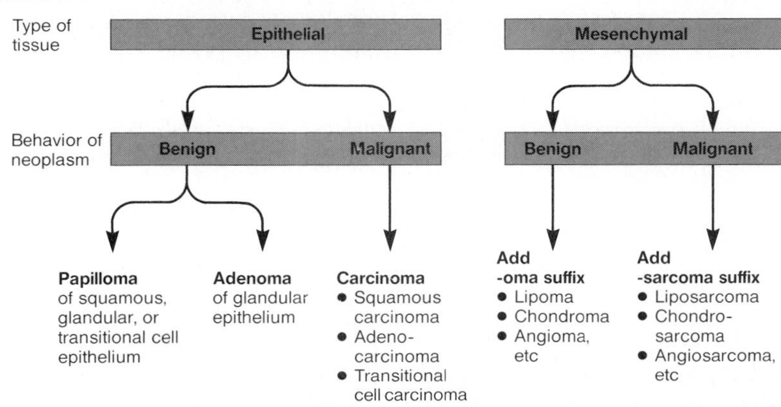

Figure 17-5. Nomenclature of neoplasms arising from differentiated (adult-type) cells.

slower clinical course than others (Chapter 26). Leukemias are classified on the basis of their clinical course (acute or chronic) and cell of origin (lymphocytic, granulocytic, myelocytic, promyelocytic, monocytic, etc). Leukemias are characterized by the presence of neoplastic cells in bone marrow and peripheral blood; they rarely produce localized tumors.

4. Mixed tumors–Neoplasms composed of more than one neoplastic cell type are called mixed tumors. Malignant mixed tumors may have 2 epithelial components, as in adenosquamous carcinoma; 2 mesenchymal components, as in malignant fibrous histiocytoma; or an epithelial and a mesenchymal component, as in carcinosarcoma of the lung and malignant mixed müllerian tumor of the uterus.

The existence of mixed tumors poses certain conceptual problems: Are they neoplasms derived from 2 separate cell lines that coincidentally became neoplastic at the same time, or are they neoplasms of a single multipotent cell type that then differentiates along more than one pathway? The latter is considered more likely.

In the case of benign mixed tumors such as fibroadenoma of the breast, most investigators believe that only the epithelial (adenoma) component is neoplastic and that fibrous tissue represents some form of reaction to the adenoma cells.

5. Neoplasms whose cell of origin is unknown–When the cell of origin is unknown, the name of the person who first described the neoplasm is commonly used to name the tumor (Table 17–5). As the histogenesis of these neoplasms is clarified, the name is often changed: Wilms's tumor is now called nephroblastoma, and Grawitz's tumor is better known as renal adenocarcinoma. Some neoplasms of uncertain histogenesis are named descriptively, eg, granular cell tumor, alveolar soft part sarcoma.

Hamartomas & Choristomas

Hamartomas and choristomas are tumorlike growths thought to be the result of developmental anomalies. They are not true neoplasms (ie, they do not show continuous excessive growth). The tumors are abnormal, disorganized, proliferating masses of several different adult cell types.

A **hamartoma** is composed of tissues that are normally present in the organ in which the tumor arises; eg, a hamartoma of the lung consists of a disorganized mass of bronchial epithelium and cartilage that may become so large that it presents as a lung mass. Its growth is coordinated with that of the lung itself.

A **choristoma** resembles a hamartoma but contains tissues that are not normally present in its site of origin. A disorderly mass of smooth muscle and pancreatic acini and ducts in the wall of the stomach is properly called a choristoma. A gastric choristoma such as this may present as an intramural mass that is clinically indistinguishable from a benign neoplasm.

Table 17–5. Common eponymous neoplasms.

Eponym	Cell of Origin
Neoplasms of uncertain histogenesis	
Ewing's sarcoma	?Primitive mesenchymal cell
Hodgkin's lymphoma	?Unidentified mesenchymal cell
Brenner tumor	Probably celomic epithelium covering ovary
Neoplasms of known histogenesis	
Burkitt's lymphoma[1]	B lymphocyte
Kaposi's sarcoma[1]	Vascular endothelial cell
Krukenberg tumor[1]	Metastatic adenocarcinoma cell involving ovary
Wilms's tumor	Pluripotent embryonic renal cell (nephroblastoma)
Grawitz's tumor	Renal tubular cell (renal adenocarcinoma)
Hürthle cell tumor	Thyroid follicular cell

[1]Though the histogenesis is known, the eponyms are retained because they denote a specific type of neoplasm that differs from others with a similar histogenesis.

INCIDENCE & DISTRIBUTION OF CANCER IN HUMANS

Incidence & Mortality Rates

Cancer is the second overall leading cause of death (after ischemic heart disease) in the USA. It caused 460,000 deaths (accounting for 22% of all deaths) in 1985, and the incidence is rising, with an estimated 490,000 deaths anticipated in 1989—probably reflecting the increasing average age of the population.

There are many reasons why the incidence of cancer varies tremendously in different populations and different areas. Epidemiologic study of cancer distribution often sheds light on the etiologic factors. Thorough knowledge of the incidence and pattern of cancer in the local population is important for the clinician evaluating the possibility of cancer in a given patient.

Both the incidence (Fig 17–6) and the death rate (Fig 17–7) of cancer must be considered. The latter reflects both the incidence and the success of diagnosis and therapy. For instance, skin cancer is

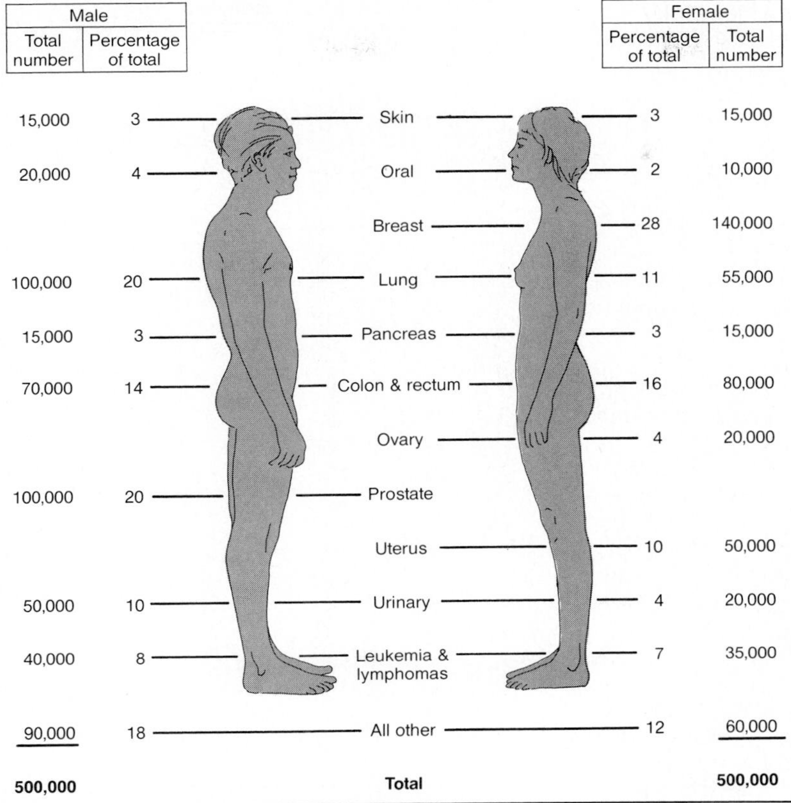

Figure 17-6. Estimated cancer incidence by site and sex (USA, 1989). Nonmelanoma skin cancer and carcinoma in situ have been excluded. There are approximately 500,000 cases of nonmelanoma skin cancer per year in the USA. (Modified and reproduced, with permission, from CA 1988;38:5.)

by far the commonest cancer in the USA (> 500,000 cases per year) but is usually diagnosed early and cured by excision; the death rate from skin cancer is thus low and does not figure prominently in the overall cancer death rate statistics. (Note that in Figs 17–6 and 17–7, nonmelanoma skin cancer has been specifically excluded and does not appear in the overall cancer incidence statistics.)

Major Factors Affecting Incidence

The presence or absence of any of the many factors influencing the incidence of cancer must be established during history taking and physical examination of a patient thought to have cancer.

A. Sex: Prostate cancer in men and uterine cancer and breast cancer in women are obviously sex-specific. In other types of cancer, the reasons for the difference in incidence between the sexes are less evident. For example, esophageal and stomach cancer are more common in men and thyroid cancer is more common in women. Both bladder and lung cancer are more common in men, partly because of greater occupational exposure (dye and rubber industries for bladder cancer; mining and asbestos for lung cancer) and smoking habits. Recent figures show that the rate of lung cancer in women is fast approaching that in men as smoking habits of women match those of men.

B. Age: The frequency of occurrence of most types of cancer varies greatly at different ages.

Carcinoma is rare in children, but leukemias, primitive neoplasms (blastomas) (Fig 17–4) of the brain, kidney, and adrenal, malignant lymphomas, and some types of connective tissue tumors are relatively common (Table 17–6). Most of these childhood neoplasms grow rapidly and are composed of small, very primitive cells with large, hyperchromatic nuclei, scant cytoplasm, and a high mitotic rate.

In adults, carcinomas make up the largest group of malignant tumors; they result from neoplastic change occurring in mature adult-type epithelial tissues. Sarcomas occur in adults but are less common than carcinomas.

Neoplasms of the hematopoietic and lymphoid cells (leukemias and lymphomas) occur at all ages. The incidence of different types of these neoplasms varies with age; eg, acute lymphoblastic leukemia is common in children, whereas chronic lymphocytic leukemia occurs more often in the elderly (Chapter 26).

C. Occupational, Social, and Geographic Factors: Occupational factors have been mentioned with reference to an increased risk of blad-

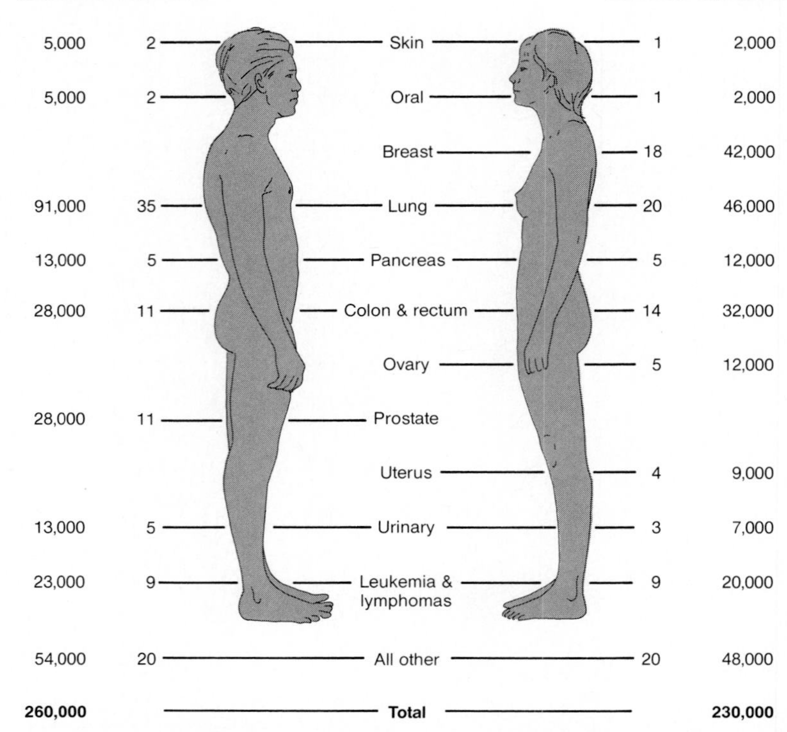

Figure 17-7. Estimated cancer deaths by site and sex (USA, 1989). Nonmelanoma skin cancer has been excluded. The incidence of lung cancer in women is increasing rapidly; in 1986, lung cancer replaced breast cancer as the leading cause of cancer deaths in women.

der cancer in workers in the dye industry and lung cancer in certain miners. These aspects are discussed more fully in Chapter 18 and usually correlate with increased exposure to carcinogens. Because the risk is so high in certain industries, an occupational history is an essential part of a full medical examination.

Similarly, such social habits as cigarette smoking—and to a lesser extent pipe and cigar smoking, snuff taking, and tobacco chewing—represent risk factors for development of several types of cancer, and the physician must evaluate the amount of exposure to these factors during history taking.

Epidemiologic studies also show that a patient's sexual and childbearing histories are important. Women who have borne several children and have breast-fed them have a significantly lower inci-

Table 17-6. Common childhood neoplasms.

Neoplasm	Site	Proposed Progenitor Cell	Chapter
Acute lymphocytic leukemia	Blood or marrow	Embryonic lymphoblasts (nonmarking, B or T)	26
Lymphoblastic lymphoma	Lymph nodes or lymphoid tissue	Embryonic T lymphoblasts	29
Burkitt's lymphoma (B cell)	Lymph nodes or lymphoid tissue	Embryonic B lymphoblasts	29
Medulloblastoma	Cerebellum	Embryonic cerebellar neuroectodermal cells	65
Retinoblastoma	Retina	Embryonic retinal blast cells	33
Neuroblastoma	Adrenal medulla; sympathetic ganglia	Embryonic neuroblasts	60
Nephroblastoma (Wilms's tumor)	Kidney	Embryonic metanephric cells	49
Hepatoblastoma	Liver	Embryonic liver cells	43
Osteosarcoma	Bone	Osteoblasts	67

dence of breast cancer than women who elect not to breast-feed or who are nulliparous. (Nuns have a high incidence of breast cancer.) This variation has been attributed to differences in levels of sex hormones in these 2 groups. Conversely, nuns have a lower incidence of cervical cancer, which appears to be most common among women who begin sexual activity early—particularly those with multiple partners. Circumcised men have a much lower incidence of carcinoma of the penis than their uncircumcised counterparts, and some studies have suggested that carcinoma of the uterine cervix is more common in women whose sexual partners have not been circumcised. Various explanations include the finding that smegma is carcinogenic in mice; associations of cervical carcinoma with standards of sexual hygiene and herpesvirus and papovavirus infections (Chapter 53) have also been reported.

Geographic variations in the overall incidence of cancer and in the incidence of specific types of cancer also occur from one country to another (Table 17–7), from one city to another, and from urban to rural areas (Figs 17–8 and 17–9). Detailed epidemiologic case control studies have sometimes uncovered associations with high-risk occupations, diet, environmental carcinogens, or endemic viruses; other occurrences remain unexplained. For example, the high incidence of stomach cancer in Japan (Fig 17–8) has been related to diet (smoked raw fish). This type of cancer does not appear to be genetically determined, since Japanese emigrating to the USA show within a single generation the lower incidence of stomach cancer demonstrated by native-born Americans. However, marked differences in the mortality rate of stomach cancer exist even within different parts of the USA for reasons that are unknown. (Areas

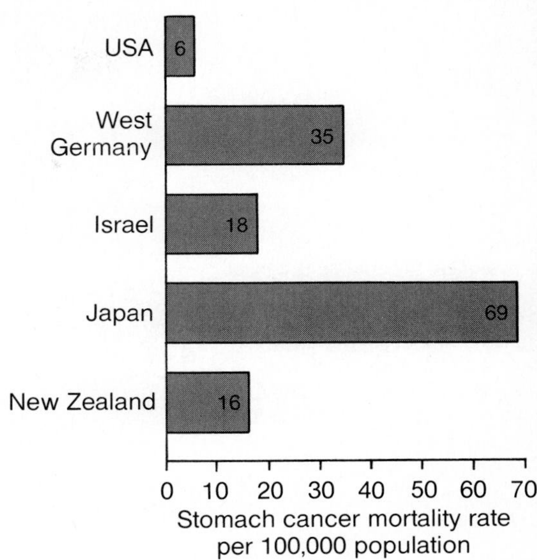

Figure 17–8. Stomach cancer mortality rate per 100,000 population in selected countries, showing marked geographic variations.

with high gastric cancer mortality death rates in the north central USA are associated with populations of northern European descent.) The factors involved clearly differ from those playing a role in lung cancer, since the distribution of deaths due to this disease is very different, although there is some association with asbestos exposure in mining or shipyards.

Marked variation in cancer incidence in different countries has in some cases provided important clues to the possible causative role of viruses

Table 17–7. The geography of cancer.

	Incidence per 100,000 Males per Site[1]									
	Total	Naso-pharynx	Tongue	Esophagus	Stomach	Colon	Liver	Lung	Prostate	Leukemia
Africa (Natal)	200	0	2	[40][2]	12	2	[28]	[40]	25	4
South America (Colombia)	200	0	3	5	[60]	4	4	20	25	5
Singapore (Chinese)	[250]	[20]	2	[20]	[45]	10	[32]	[54]	4	4
India and Sri Lanka	130	1	[14]	13	10	4	1	13	7	3
USA	[260]	1	3	6	15	[27]	4	[44]	23	10
UK	[240]	1	1	3	25	15	1	[73]	18	10
Japan	190	1	3	5	[60]	15	2	[36]	5	5

[1]These statistics are the 1979 figures for men. In women, the mortality rate from breast cancer varies between high rates of 33.8:100,000 in the United Kingdom and 27.1 in the USA to low rates of 6.0 in Japan, 2.7 in Hong Kong, and 1.2 in Thailand.

[2]Particulary high incidence figures are bracketed [ ].

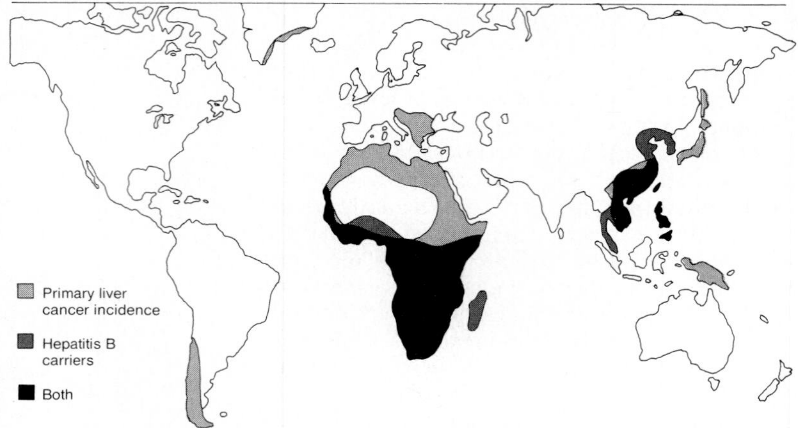

Figure 17-9. Areas of high prevalence of hepatitis B carrier state, compared with areas of high prevalence of primary liver cancer. The large area in which both of these conditions coexist suggests an etiologic relationship between hepatitis B infection and liver cancer.

Table 17-8. Diseases associated with increased risk of neoplasia.

Nonneoplastic or Preneoplastic Condition	Neoplasm
Mongolism (trisomy 21)	Acute myeloid leukemia
Xeroderma pigmentosum (plus sun exposure)	Squamous cancer of skin
Gastric atrophy (pernicious anemia)	Gastric cancer
Tuberous sclerosis	Cerebral gliomas
Café au lait skin patches	Neurofibromatosis (dominant inheritance); acoustic neuroma, pheochromocytoma
Actinic dermatitis	Squamous carcinoma of skin; malignant melanoma
Glandular metaplasia of esophagus (Barrett's esophagus)	Adenocarcinoma of esophagus
Dysphagia plus anemia (Plummer-Vinson syndrome)	Esophageal cancer
Cirrhosis (alcoholic, hepatitis B)	Hepatocellular carcinoma
Ulcerative colitis	Colon cancer
Paget's disease of bone	Osteosarcoma
Immunodeficiency states	Lymphomas
AIDS	Lymphoma, Kaposi's sarcoma
Autoimmune diseases (eg, Hashimoto's thyroiditis)	Lymphoma (eg, thyroid lymphoma)
Dysplasias (eg, cervical dysplasia)	Cancer (see Chapter 16)

and immune stimulation. The distribution of Burkitt's lymphoma, infection with Epstein-Barr virus, and malaria in Africa provides the best-known example of an association between a neoplasm and infection. A close association also exists between liver cell carcinoma and the incidence of hepatitis B virus carriers in a population (Fig 17-9).

D. Family History: A few cancers have a simple pattern of genetic inheritance (Chapter 18)—and those that do are so striking that they warrant careful study of relatives of known cases (eg, retinoblastoma, polyposis coli and carcinoma of the colon, medullary carcinoma of the thyroid).

For other cancers, the genetic link is not as strong (eg, breast cancer) or is almost nonexistent

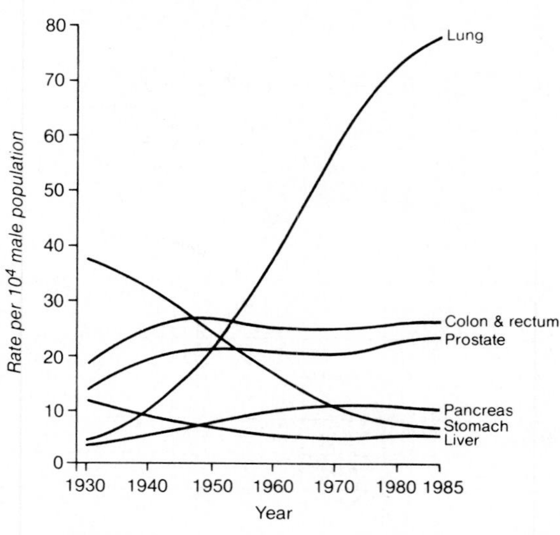

Figure 17-10. Age-adjusted cancer death rates for selected sites in males (USA, 1930–1985). (Modified and reproduced, with permission, from CA 1988;38:13.)

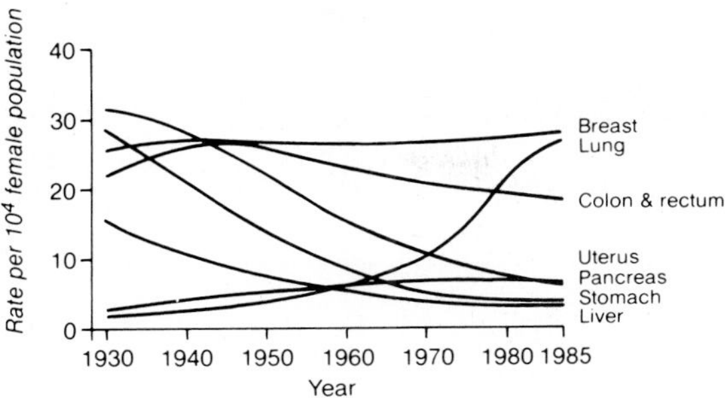

Figure 17-11. Age-adjusted cancer death rates for selected sites in females (USA, 1930–1985). (Modified and reproduced, with permission, from CA 1988;38:12.)

(eg, lung cancer). It must also be understood that familial occurrence of neoplasms may represent the action of similar environmental factors rather than a genetic predisposition.

"Cancer families" with a high incidence of cancer have also been described. In such cases the cancer is usually of a particular type but may be of different types; eg, colon, endometrial, and breast cancer occur in some families. Cancer in such families may skip generations, suggesting the possible interplay both of recessive genetic mechanisms and of environmental factors.

E. History of Associated Diseases: Perhaps the most important finding in the history of a patient with suspected cancer is a record of diagnosis or treatment of previous cancer. A positive history of cancer greatly increases the chances that the current illness represents either a metastasis (which may be delayed many years) or a second primary tumor. Statistics show that patients who have had cancer—even if the lesion was totally excised—have a much higher incidence of a second cancer, particularly in the same tissue. For example, cancer in one breast increases the chances of cancer in the opposite breast, and one occurrence of colon cancer necessitates repeated routine examinations to detect the development of another colon cancer. Second cancers of a different type—particularly leukemia and sarcomas—also occur as a complication of chemotherapy and radiation used to treat the first cancer.

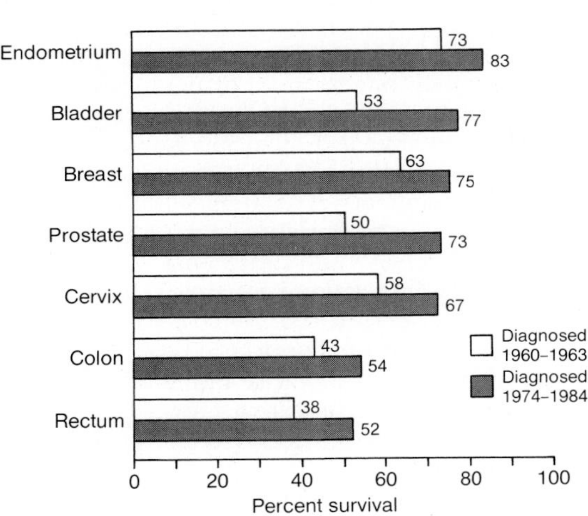

Figure 17-12. Five-year survival rates (expressed as percentages) for cancers in selected sites. Note the improvement in survival rates for cases diagnosed between 1974 and 1984 as compared with those diagnosed between 1960 and 1963.

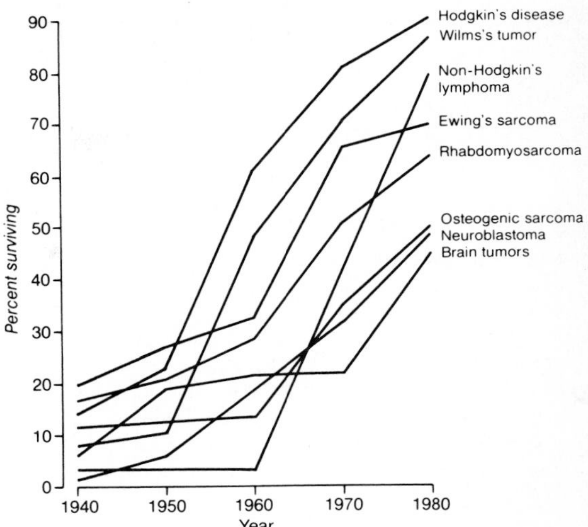

Figure 17-13. Survival in selected childhood cancers expressed as the percentage of children surviving 2 years after diagnosis. Note the marked improvement in survival statistics in the last 2 decades for all types of cancer.

In addition, certain disorders that in themselves are nonneoplastic carry an associated higher risk of development of cancer and are considered preneoplastic diseases. These diseases are uncommon, but together they constitute a significant group of risk factors (Table 17–8).

Trends in Cancer Incidence

The relative incidence of different types of cancer and their mortality rates vary over time and reflect both changes in incidence of various cancers and improvement in diagnosis and therapy (Figs 17–10 through 17–13).

18 Neoplasia: II. Mechanisms & Causes of Neoplasia

Neoplasia is an abnormality of cell growth and multiplication characterized (1) by excessive cellular proliferation that typically but not invariably produces an abnormal mass, or tumor; (2) by uncoordinated growth occurring without any apparent purpose; and (3) by persistence of excessive cell proliferation and growth even after the inciting stimulus that evoked the change has been removed—ie, neoplasia is an irreversible process.

Neoplasia is poorly understood. It cannot be defined by etiology, since the causes are largely unknown, nor can it be defined in terms of a fundamental genetic or metabolic change in the cell, since these too are unknown.

THEORIES OF ORIGIN OF NEOPLASIA

Several theories have been advanced to explain neoplasia, many of them reflecting or in response to advances in the basic sciences current at the time. For example, theories of the viral cause of neoplasia coincided with the demonstration of transmission of certain animal neoplasms by ultrafiltrable agents (Rous sarcoma, 1908; Shope papilloma, 1933; Bittner milk factor, 1935). Immunologic theories came to the fore after experiments involving tumor transplantation in animals (Ehrlich, 1908; immune surveillance, Burnet, 1950s). DNA mutations as a cause of neoplasia were proposed after the discovery of DNA structure and function (Watson and Crick, 1950s). Several of these theories have enjoyed a phase of respectability, followed by a period of discreditation and then reemergence in modified guise.

Multifactorial Origin of Neoplasia

Development of a detectable neoplasm most probably requires more than one step, expressed most simply as the action of an **initiator,** which produces the first in a series of changes leading to neoplasia (initiation), followed by prolonged action of one or more **promoters** to cause neoplastic growth (promotion). The requirement of successive insults (multiple hit theory) accounts for the long latent period that usually exists between the action of a cancer-causing agent and the clinical expression of neoplastic disease (see Fig 18–2). This concept of multiple hits is generally accepted and combines one or more of the hypotheses described below to provide a unifying explanation of the development of clinically apparent cancer. The role of the Bittner milk factor (an RNA virus) in mouse mammary carcinoma (Fig 18–1) and the genesis of African Burkitt's lymphoma in humans (Fig 18–2) clearly illustrate that cancer arises through the interaction of many factors.

Genetic Mutation Theory

Changes in the genome resulting from (1) spontaneous mutation or (2) the action of external agents may cause neoplasia if the alteration involves growth-regulating genes. Such genes have been identified in normal cells and are believed to produce growth factors. Knowledge of these genes and their products is still rudimentary.

A genetic change may be either a modification of a gene or a change in expression of a gene. In either case, abnormalities in the production of regulator proteins occur that alter the pattern of cell growth or differentiation. Many different oncogenic agents, including chemical carcinogens and viruses, may exert their effects through this mechanism.

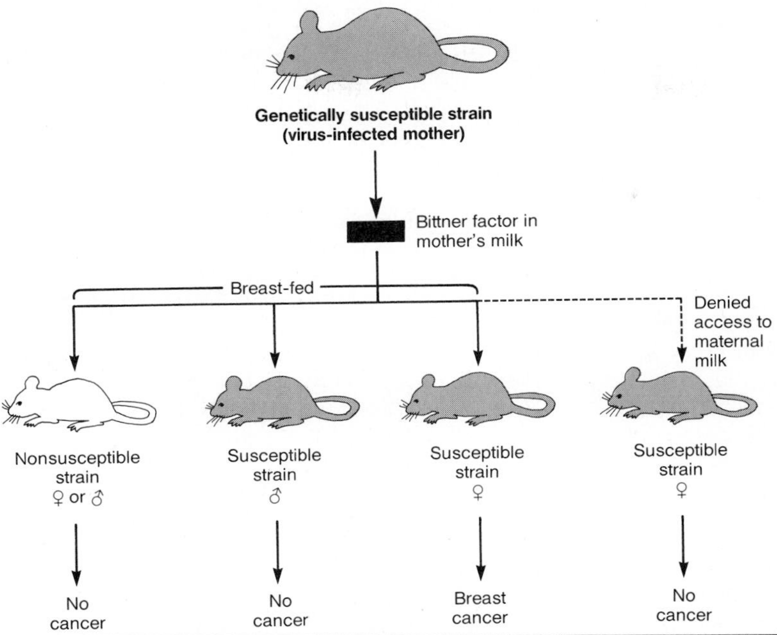

Figure 18–1. Multifactorial causation of breast cancer in experimental mice. Development of breast cancer requires genetic susceptibility, ingestion of the Bittner milk factor (a type B RNA retrovirus) in maternal milk, and an appropriate hormonal environment (female mouse or male mouse injected with estrogens). Absence of any of these factors results in failure to develop cancer.

A. Neoplasia Associated With Constant Genetic Abnormalities: The presence of constant genetic abnormalities in some neoplasms (see Chapter 19) suggests that such abnormalities may produce neoplasia.

The pedigree of families with a high incidence of retinoblastoma shows inheritance of an abnormal chromosome 13 with a partially deleted long arm; it is postulated that the missing genetic material may be involved in the normal control of growth of retinal cells. It is thought that retinoblastoma develops in these patients when the residual normal chromosome 13 undergoes a similar deletion due to an abnormal mitosis or mutation.

Over 90% of patients with chronic granulocytic leukemia show a reciprocal translocation of genetic material between chromosome 22 and chromosome 9 (Philadelphia chromosome, Ph[1] [see Fig 19–4]). It is suggested that this translocation is associated either with loss of genetic material or

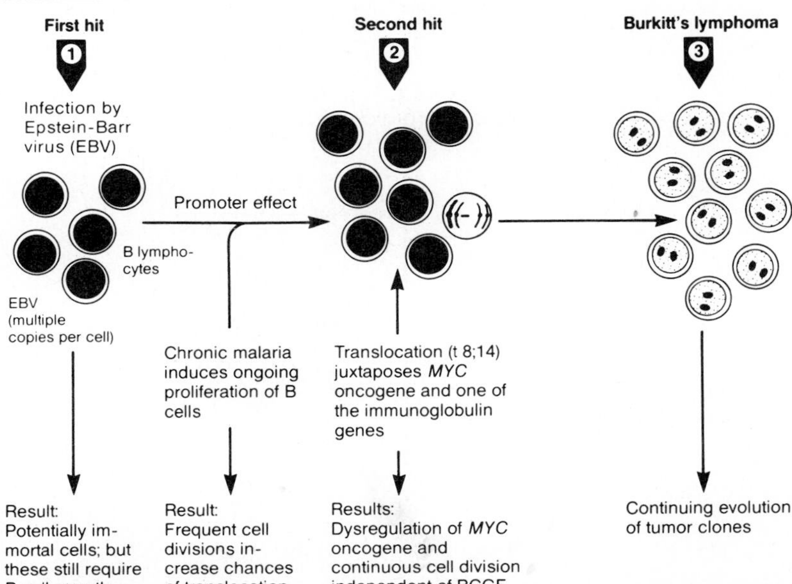

Figure 18–2. Oncogenesis in Burkitt's lymphoma. The first "hit" is infection of B lymphocytes with Epstein-Barr virus. Chronic malaria induces proliferation of B lymphocytes, increasing the likelihood of the second event, which is a chromosomal translocation that activates a cellular oncogene and leads to malignant lymphoma.

with defective gene action (dysregulation) caused by removal from the influence of normal moderator genes. The translocation of the *C-ABL* oncogene from chromosome 9 to 22 is of particular interest in this regard. In the Ph[1] chromosome, the genetic change leads to production of a novel growth-regulating protein (a tyrosine protein kinase with a molecular weight of 210) and neoplastic proliferation of granulocytes. As techniques for chromosomal analysis become more refined, genetic abnormalities will probably come to be identified in many tumors.

B. Neoplasia Associated With Chromosomal Instability: Some rare syndromes associated with chromosomal instability, frequent chromosomal breakage, and abnormal DNA repair mechanisms are also associated with cancer. These conditions include Bloom's syndrome, Fanconi's syndrome, ataxia telangiectasia, and xeroderma pigmentosum.

In xeroderma pigmentosum, there is an inherited (autosomal recessive) deficiency of enzymes that effect repair of damaged DNA in cells. When epidermal cells in the skin are exposed to ultraviolet radiation, abnormal linkages between pyrimidine bases are produced. In normal individuals, DNA-repairing enzymes remove these abnormal linkages, and the DNA molecule returns to normal. In xeroderma pigmentosum, repair does not occur. Patients with this disease have a high incidence of multiple skin cancers (ultraviolet light may be regarded as the promoter).

C. Neoplasia Associated With Aging: The incidence of most common neoplasms rises with age, leading to the hypothesis that the increase results from gene abnormalities that accumulate in aging cells because of faulty DNA repair.

Virogene Oncogene Theory

It has been suggested that neoplastic transformation occurs as a result of activation (or derepression) of specific DNA sequences (**cellular oncogenes** [C-*ONC*]) in cells. Activation may be effected by various carcinogens, including viruses, radiation, and chemicals (Fig 18–3). Cellular oncogenes are believed to control production of growth factors and may be important in normal growth regulation.

Certain RNA oncogenic viruses contain nucleic acid sequences—called **viral oncogenes** (V-*ONC*)—that are essentially identical to cellular oncogenes. Such sequences have been found in certain experimental animal neoplasms (Table 18–1).

There is debate about whether cellular oncogenes result from permanent incorporation of the viral oncogene into the host cell genome at some time during evolution or whether the RNA oncogenic virus acquired its V-*ONC* sequence by incorporation of the cellular oncogene from an animal cell (Fig 18–4)—the familiar argument about

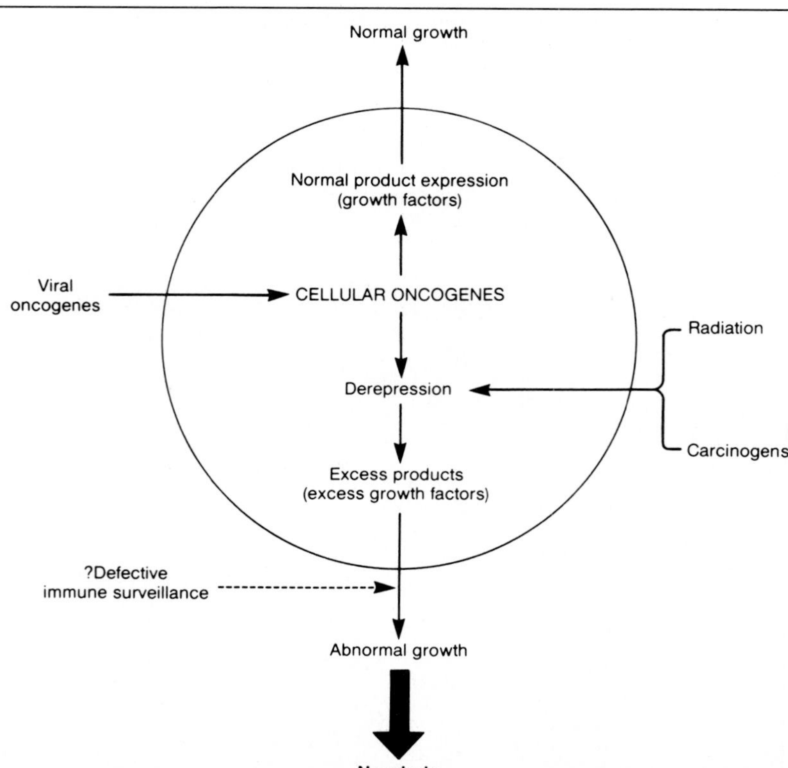

Figure 18–3. Relationship of cellular oncogenes to normal growth and neoplasia and the possible modes of oncogene activation.

Table 18-1. Representative oncogenes.

Viral Oncogene	Species Origin	Tumor Type	Virally Determined DNA in Host Cell	Tyrosine Phosphorylase Product
V-*SRC*	Chicken	Sarcoma	Yes	Yes
V-*YES*	Chicken	Sarcoma	Yes	Yes
V-*MYC*	Chicken	Carcinoma, sarcoma, leukemia	Yes	?
V-*MYB*	Chicken	Leukemia	Yes	?
V-*ABL*	Mouse	Leukemia	Yes	Yes
V-*MOS*	Mouse	Sarcoma	Yes	?
V-*RAS*	Rat	Sarcoma, leukemia	Yes	?
V-*FES*	Cat	Sarcoma	Yes	Yes
V-*SIS*	Monkey	Sarcoma	Yes	?

A
?In the course of evolution viral oncogene is permanently incorporated into host genome as a cellular oncogene (c-*ONC*)

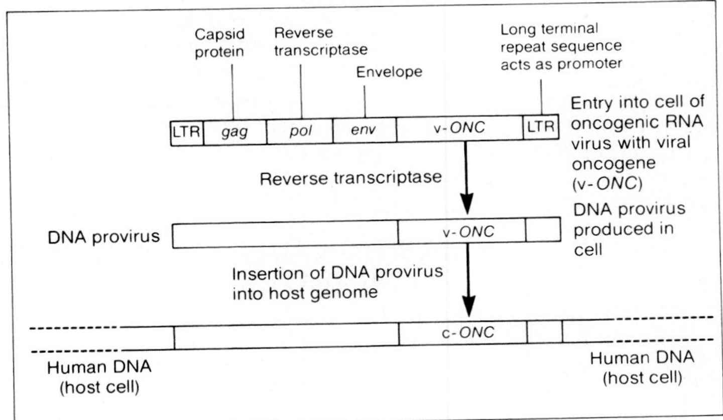

B
?In the course of evolution RNA viruses acquired the cellular oncogene from animal cells by recombination

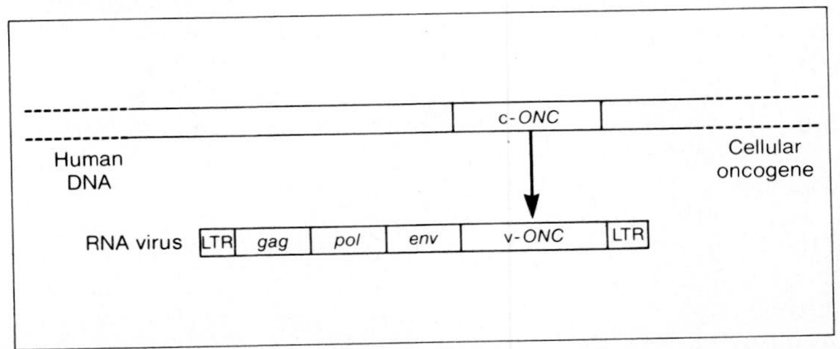

Figure 18-4. Oncogenic RNA viruses, viral oncogenes, and cellular oncogenes. Two opposing theories seek to explain the presence of essentially identical nucleic acid sequences (oncogenes) in oncogenic viruses and animal cells. **A:** In the course of evolution, a viral gene segment becomes permanently incorporated in the host genome to form a cellular oncogene. **B:** In the course of evolution, the RNA virus acquires the cellular oncogene from an animal cell through recombination. The second theory is currently favored. The cellular oncogenes are considered growth-regulating genes. Neoplasia thus represents the production of multiple copies or abnormal "switching on" of these oncogenes.

which came first, the chicken or the egg. Whatever their origin, cellular oncogenes are inherited as part of the cell genome. Cellular oncogenes are identified in cells by the use of complementary DNA (or RNA) probes (manufactured nucleotide sequences that show a reciprocal fit with segments of the oncogene).

Although many oncogenes have been recognized in human cancer cells, their role in the genesis of neoplasia is unclear, particularly since similar oncogenes **(proto-oncogenes)** have also been found in normal cells. There may be several reasons why normal cells containing oncogenes fail to show neoplastic characteristics: (1) the dosage effect, which suggests that a certain critical number of oncogenes is required before neoplastic growth can occur; (2) the necessity for a second insult—such as the action of another carcinogen—before the oncogene can be activated; (3) the possibility that the oncogene is somehow incomplete and requires some sort of modification before it can become active; and (4) the necessity of a translocation that removes an oncogene from a site where it is suppressed to another chromosomal site where it is inappropriately activated.

For many oncogenes tested to date, the gene product is a protein kinase tyrosine phosphorylase with growth-regulating properties. In other instances, the oncogene product serves as a cellular receptor for known growth factors (eg, erb B and epidermal growth factor).

DNA oncogenic viruses also appear to contain oncogene segments, which are inserted directly into the host cell genome. However, normal noninfected host cells do not appear to contain intrinsic DNA sequences (cellular oncogenes) analogous to viral oncogenes of DNA viruses.

Epigenetic Theory

According to the epigenetic theory, the fundamental cellular alteration occurs not mainly in the genetic apparatus of the cell but rather in the gene products, specifically the protein products of growth-regulating genes.

The main evidence for the role of epigenetic mechanisms in neoplasia comes from cancers produced by certain chemicals that have no known effect on the genetic apparatus of the cell. The main action of some of these chemicals is binding of cytoplasmic proteins, and it is changes in these proteins that are thought to cause the abnormal growth giving rise to neoplasms.

Theory of Failure of Immune Surveillance

The theory of immune surveillance encompasses several concepts: (1) Neoplastic changes frequently occur in the cells of the body. (2) As a result of alteration in their DNA, neoplastic cells produce new molecules (neoantigens, tumor-associated antigens). (3) The immune system of the body recognizes these neoantigens as foreign and mounts a cytotoxic immune response that destroys the neoplastic cells expressing the neoantigen. (4) Neoplastic cells produce clinically detectable neoplasms only if they escape recognition and destruction by the immune system.

This theory of immune surveillance was popular in the 1950s largely because it provided a raison d'être for the then recently discovered phenomenon of cell-mediated immunity. Evidence supporting the existence of immune surveillance is based on observations of a higher incidence of neoplasia in many immunodeficiency states and in transplant recipients receiving immunosuppressive drugs. The observation that cancer is a disease of the elderly may then be attributed to progressive failure of immune surveillance in the face of an increased frequency of neoplastic events resulting from the defective DNA repair that accompanies aging.

Challenges to the theory are based on several findings: (1) T cell-deficient strains of mice do not show higher rates of neoplasia; (2) immunodeficient humans or those who have undergone transplant operations develop mainly lymphomas and not a full spectrum of different cancers, as would be expected; (3) thymectomized humans do not show an increased incidence of neoplasia; and (4) although many tumors do possess tumor-associated antigens and an immune response can often be demonstrated, the response is clearly ineffective at the time of clinical expression of the cancer.

The complexity of interactions between the immune system and tumors is depicted in Fig 18–5.

AGENTS CAUSING NEOPLASMS (Oncogenic Agents; Carcinogens)*

Carcinogens are substances that are known to cause cancer or at least produce an increased incidence of cancer in an animal or human population. Many carcinogens have been identified in experimental animals, but because of dose-related effects and the metabolic differences between species, the relevance of these studies to humans is not always clear. The following discussion will consider mainly those carcinogens of known importance to humans. It is important to stress that (1) the cause of most common human cancers is unknown; (2) most cases of cancer are probably multifactorial in origin; and (3) except for ciga-

*An agent that causes neoplasms is an oncogenic agent; an agent causing a malignant neoplasm (cancer) is a carcinogenic agent.

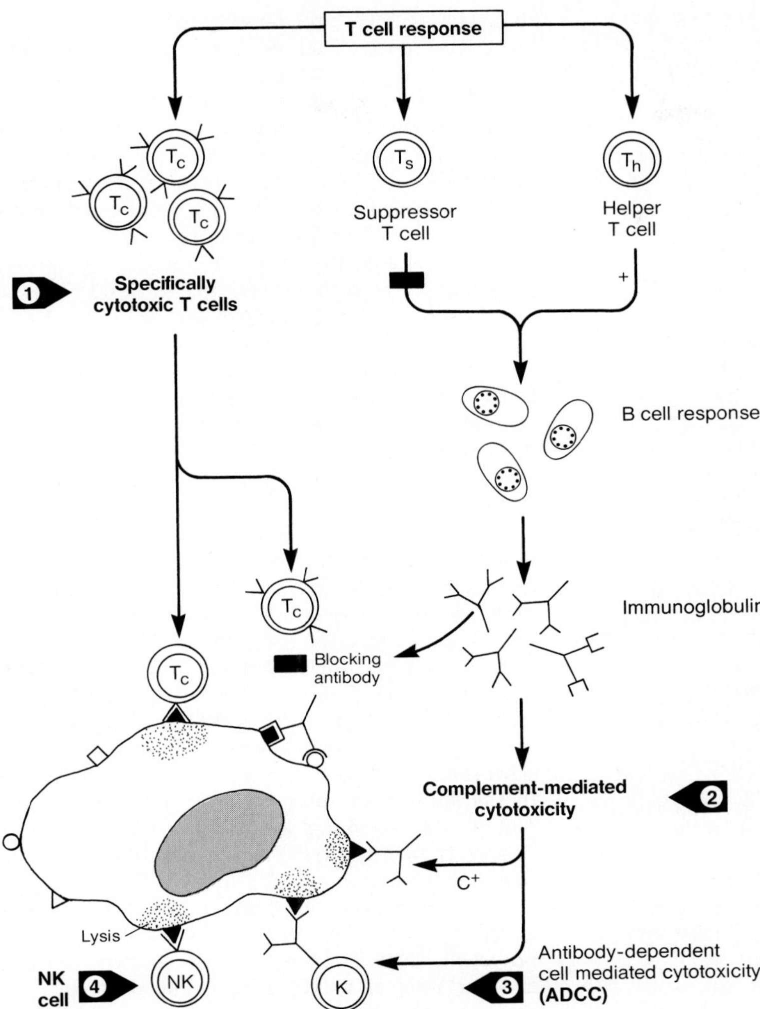

Figure 18–5. The immune response and cancer. The net effect of the immune response on neoplastic cells varies. Neoplastic cells may be killed by **(1)** cytotoxic T cells (T_c), **(2)** antibody and complement (C^+), **(3)** antibody-dependent cell-mediated cytotoxicity (ADCC), or **(4)** activity of natural killer (NK) cells. On the other hand, blocking antibodies or inappropriate suppressor T cell activity may interfere with these effects and thus enhance growth of the neoplastic cells.

rette smoking, the agents discussed below have been implicated in only a small percentage of cases.

The importance of environmental carcinogens must not be minimized simply because they may not yet have been identified. The marked geographic variation in the incidence of different cancers (Chapter 17) is thought to result more from the action of different carcinogens than from variations in genetic makeup. If this belief is valid, then still unidentified environmental agents probably play a major role in causing 95% of human cancers.

Chemical Oncogenesis (Table 18–2)

It is difficult to assess the possible carcinogenic effects of the many industrial, agricultural, and household chemicals present in low levels throughout the environment. A significant hazard is also posed by disposal of industrial waste, which may contaminate drinking water and offshore coastal waters (and marine life).

One of the major problems associated with the identification of chemical carcinogens is the long lag phase, sometimes 20 or more years between exposure and the development of cancer (Chapter 19). Unless the effects produced are dramatic, it is difficult to establish the carcinogenicity of any particular chemical in view of the huge number of substances to which people are exposed during their lives. Table 18–3 summarizes the clinical approach and experimental assays used to detect potential carcinogens.

Most chemical carcinogens act by producing changes in DNA. A small number act by epigenetic mechanisms, ie, they cause changes in growth-regulating proteins without producing genetic

Table 18-2. Major chemical carcinogens in humans.[1]

Chemical	Types of Cancer
Polycyclic hydrocarbons Soot (benzo[α]pyrene, dibenzanthracene)	Skin; scrotal cancer in chimney sweeps
Inhalation or chewing of tobacco products (mainly cigarettes)[2]	Lung, bladder, oral cavity, larynx, esophagus
Aromatic amines Benzidine, 2-naphthylamine	Bladder
Aflatoxins	Liver
Nitrosamines	?Esophagus, ?stomach
Cancer chemotherapeutic agents Cyclophosphamide, chlorambucil, thiotepa, busulfan	Leukemias
Asbestos	Lung cancer, mesothelioma
Heavy metals Nickel, chromium, cadmium	Lung
Arsenic	Skin
Vinyl chloride	Liver (angiosarcoma)

[1]Most of the chemicals listed here are those for which strong evidence exists for human carcinogenesis; several other compounds exist that are thought to be carcinogenic.
[2]Cigarette smoking is responsible for more human cancer than all of the other listed chemicals combined.

changes. Still others may act synergistically with viruses (derepressing oncogenes) or may serve as promoters for other carcinogens.

Chemical carcinogens that act locally at the site of application without having to undergo metabolic change in the body are called **proximate or direct-acting carcinogens**. Other chemicals produce cancer only after they are converted into metabolically active compounds within the body; these are termed procarcinogens, and the active carcinogenic compounds that are produced are called **ultimate carcinogens**.

A. Polycyclic Hydrocarbons: The first recognized carcinogen in humans was soot, the tarry residue of coal combustion. Sir Percivall Pott established in 1775 that soot was the agent responsible for scrotal cancer in boys who cleaned chimneys as part of their jobs as apprentices to London chimney sweeps. Because of inadequate washing, soot from the chimneys tended to collect in the rugose scrotal skin and cause cancer. Much later, it was shown that the active carcinogens in soot and coal tar were a group of polycyclic hydrocarbons, the most active of which were benzo(α)pyrene and dibenzanthracene. Application of small amounts of these polycyclic hydrocarbons to the skin of experimental animals regularly cause skin cancer.

B. Cigarette Smoking: Cigarette smoking—and to a lesser extent cigar and pipe smoking—is associated with an increased risk of cancer of the lung, bladder, oropharynx, and esophagus. Smoking filtered cigarettes and newer low-nicotine and low-tar cigarettes decreases the risk only slightly. There is also evidence that the risk of cancer associated with smoking is not limited to the smoker but may extend to nonsmoking family members, coworkers, and others in close physical proximity to the smoke for long periods. It has been estimated that smoking accounts for more cancer deaths than all other known carcinogens combined.

Cigarette smoke contains numerous carcinogens, the most important of which are probably polycyclic hydrocarbons (tars). Although these are direct-acting carcinogens in the skin, they act as procarcinogens in producing lung and bladder cancer. Inhaled polycyclic hydrocarbons are converted in the liver to an epoxide by a microsomal enzyme, aryl hydrocarbon hydroxylase. This epoxide (the ultimate carcinogen) is an active compound that combines with guanine in DNA, leading to neoplastic transformation. Smokers who develop lung cancer have been shown to have significantly higher levels of aryl hydrocarbon hydroxylase than nonsmokers or smokers who fail to develop cancer. The reported risk of developing cancer has varied in different studies, but it is about 10 times higher in someone who smokes a pack of cigarettes a day for 10 years (10 "pack years") than in a nonsmoker. If a smoker stops smoking, the risk drops almost to that of a nonsmoker after about 10 years of abstinence.

C. Aromatic Amines: Exposure to aromatic amines such as benzidene and naphthylamine is associated with an increased incidence of bladder cancer (first recognized in workers in the leather and dye industries). Similar compounds have been used in many pathology and research laboratories; their use is closely controlled by the FDA

Table 18-3. Chemical carcinogenesis: Methods for detecting potential carcinogens.[1]

- Clinical observation (physicians and patients)
- Epidemiologic studies (environment and industry)
- Experimental animal bioassays
  - By chemical and drug industries
  - By FDA (or equivalent bodies elsewhere)
  - By university and research groups
- Mutagenesis assays
  - Bacterial mutagenesis (Ames test)
  - Mammalian cell culture (Syrian hamster embryo; rodent fibroblasts; human cell lines)
  - In *Drosophila,* mice, and so forth
- Cell culture transformation assays
- Assays of chromosomal or DNA binding or damage

[1]Modified and reproduced, with pemission, from Weinstein IB: The scientific basis for carcinogen detection and primary cancer prevention. *CA* 1982:**32**:348.

(Food and Drug Administration), but as with radiation, there is no safe threshold of exposure.

Aromatic amines are procarcinogens that enter the body through the skin, lungs, or intestine and exert their carcinogenic effects predominantly in the urinary bladder. In the body they are converted to carcinogenic metabolites that are excreted in the urine. Retention of urine in the bladder maximizes the carcinogenic effect on the bladder mucosa.

Different species vary in their susceptibility to the effects of aromatic amines: Humans and dogs are quite susceptible; rats and rabbits, much less so. This variation reinforces the point that procarcinogens (which must be converted in the body to ultimate carcinogens) may have different effects in different species because of different metabolic processes. This is a serious flaw in all animal studies that attempt to establish lack of carcinogenicity of new drugs to be used in humans.

D. Cyclamates and Saccharin: These compounds are artificial sweeteners widely used by patients with diabetes mellitus. Administration of large amounts of these compounds has caused bladder cancer in experimental animals. No carcinogenic effect has been demonstrated in humans, and it is not even known whether humans metabolize these compounds to produce ultimate carcinogens.

E. Azo Dyes: These dyes were extensively used as food coloring agents ("scarlet red" and "butter yellow") until they were shown to cause liver tumors in rats. They have since been withdrawn from commercial use.

F. Aflatoxin: Aflatoxin, a toxic metabolite produced by the fungus *Aspergillus flavus,* is thought to be an important cause of liver cancer in humans. The fungus grows on improperly stored food, particularly grain, groundnuts, and peanuts, producing aflatoxin. In Africa, dietary intake of large amounts of aflatoxin has been shown to correlate with a high incidence of hepatocellular carcinoma. Ingested aflatoxin is oxidized in the liver to an ultimate carcinogen that binds with guanine in the DNA of hepatic cells. In large amounts, the toxin causes acute liver cell necrosis followed by regenerative hyperplasia and possibly cancer. When lesser amounts are ingested over a long period, the carcinogenic effect predominates.

G. Nitrosamines: Small amounts of these compounds have been shown to be carcinogenic in experimental animals. Their ability to react with both nucleic acids and cytoplasmic macromolecules provides a theoretic basis for their carcinogenic action, but their role in human carcinogenesis is uncertain.

Nitrosamines are derived mainly from conversion of nitrites in the stomach. Nitrites are ubiquitous in food because of their common use as preservatives, mainly in processed meats, ham, bacon, sausage, and so forth. The direct local action of nitrosamines is thought to be an important cause of esophageal and gastric cancer. The markedly decreased incidence of gastric cancer in the last 2 decades in the USA is believed to be due mainly to better refrigeration of food, which has decreased the need for preservatives. The high incidence of gastric cancer in Japan is thought to be related more to high intake of smoked fish (containing polycyclic hydrocarbons) than to high nitrosamine levels.

H. Betel Leaf: Chewing of betel leaf in Sri Lanka and parts of India is responsible for an extremely high incidence of cancers of the oral cavity. The carcinogenic agent has not been identified but is believed to be present either in the areca (betel) nut or in the crushed limestone or tobacco that is commonly chewed along with the betel leaf.

I. Anticancer Drugs: Certain drugs used in the treatment of cancer (alkylating agents, such as cyclophosphamide, chlorambucil, busulfan, and thiotepa) interfere with nucleic acid synthesis in cancer cells. They also interfere with DNA synthesis in normally dividing cells, particularly those in the bone marrow, and may cause oncogenic mutations. Leukemia is the most common neoplastic complication of cancer chemotherapy and is a significant problem in patients in whom cure of the primary tumor has been achieved.

J. Asbestos: Asbestos has been widely used as an insulating material and fire retardant and is found in almost all buildings constructed in the USA between 1940 and 1970. The greatest individual exposure to asbestos occurred in shipyard workers during World War II.

Asbestos is inhaled into the lung, where it produces fibrosis and chronic lung disease. Asbestosis also leads to fibrous proliferation in the pleura, where it results in fibrous plaques that are a reliable radiologic indicator of previous asbestos exposure. Asbestos is associated with 2 types of cancer.

1. Malignant mesothelioma-This uncommon neoplasm is derived from mesothelial cells, mainly in the pleura but also in the peritoneum and pericardium. Nearly all patients who develop malignant mesothelioma give a history of asbestos exposure, making malignant mesothelioma the most specific cancer associated with asbestos exposure.

2. Bronchogenic carcinoma-The most common form of lung cancer is bronchogenic carcinoma. Patients with asbestos exposure have a risk of lung cancer about twice that of the general population; this risk is greatly magnified by smoking (Fig 18–6). Although it is not as specifically associated with asbestosis as is mesothelioma, lung cancer is the commonest malignant neoplasm in patients with a history of asbestos exposure.

It has been established that the risk of malignant mesothelioma and lung cancer is not limited

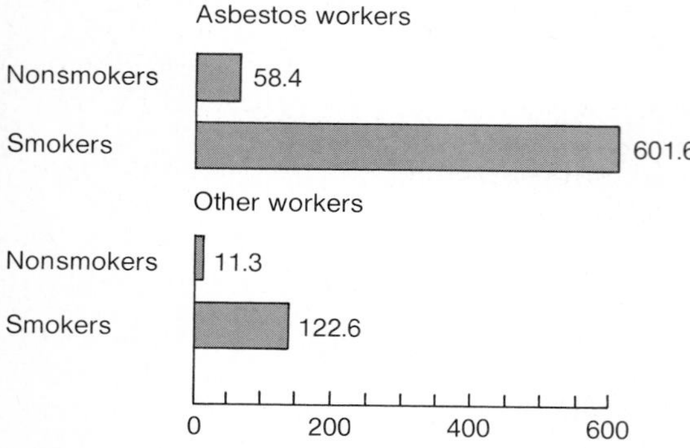

Figure 18-6. Lung cancer death rates per 100,000 man-years standardized for age, showing the additive effect of cigarette smoking and asbestos exposure.

solely to individuals with high levels of exposure to asbestos. Family members of shipyard workers and even individuals living in communities where asbestos industries exist carry an increased risk of developing cancer. Recognition of this fact has resulted in massive claims for compensation by many individuals with low levels of exposure and has created severe financial difficulties for companies involved in the manufacture of asbestos and asbestos-containing products.

K. Other Industrial Carcinogens: Many other cancer-causing agents have been identified. Miners exposed to heavy metals such as nickel, chromium, and cadmium show an increased incidence of lung cancer. Arsenic exposure, which may occur in agricultural workers exposed to arsenic-containing pesticides, is associated with a high incidence of skin cancer and a lesser risk of lung cancer. Vinyl chloride, a gas used in the manufacture of polyvinyl chloride (PVC), has been shown to be associated with a malignant vascular neoplasm (angiosarcoma) of the liver, mainly in experimental animals.

Radiation Oncogenesis

Several different types of radiation cause cancer, most probably by direct effects on DNA or possibly by activation of cellular oncogenes.

A. Ultraviolet Radiation: Solar ultraviolet radiation is associated with different kinds of skin cancer, including squamous carcinoma, basal cell carcinoma, and malignant melanoma. Neoplasms of the skin caused by exposure to ultraviolet light are especially common in fair-skinned individuals whose occupations expose them to sunlight; eg, farmers in Queensland, Australia, have an extremely high incidence of melanoma. Skin cancer is overall the most common type of cancer in the USA. The incidence of ultraviolet radiation-induced skin cancer, including melanoma, is low in dark-skinned races because of the protective effect of melanin pigment.

Ultraviolet light is believed to induce formation of linkages between pyrimidine bases on the DNA molecule. In normal individuals, this altered DNA molecule is rapidly repaired. Carcinoma occurs when DNA repair mechanisms do not operate efficiently, as occurs in older individuals and in people with xeroderma pigmentosum (see p 282). Skin cancer due to exposure to sunlight is thus a disorder seen most often in the elderly.

B. X-Ray Radiation: Early radiologists who were exposed to x-rays of low penetration developed radiation dermatitis with a high incidence of skin cancer. As x-rays capable of greater penetration were developed, the second generation of radiologists suffered an increased incidence of leukemia. Present-day radiologists are at minimal risk for cancer because of highly effective protective measures against x-rays.

In the 1950s it was believed that thymic enlargement caused respiratory obstruction in infants (this was later proved to be untrue; a large thymus is normal in infants). Infants experiencing respiratory distress therefore underwent radiation therapy of the neck to decrease thymic size; many developed papillary thyroid cancer 15–25 years later.

One complication of radiotherapy for cancer is the occurrence of additional radiation-induced malignant neoplasms, commonly sarcomas, that appear 10–30 years after radiation therapy.

Diagnostic x-rays use such small doses of radiation that no increased risk of cancer is believed to be associated with their use. A possible exception is that abdominal x-rays during pregnancy may slightly increase the incidence of leukemia in the fetus. As radiation doses increase with newer forms of radiology such as mammography and CT scans, the question of carcinogenic risk again arises.

C. Radioisotopes: The carcinogenic effect of radioactive materials was first recognized when many cases of osteosarcoma occurred among factory workers who used radium-containing paints to produce luminous watch faces. It was found that these workers shaped their brushes to a point with their tongues and lips, thereby ingesting dangerous amounts of radium. Radioactive radium is metabolized in the body in much the same way as calcium and is therefore deposited in bone, where it induces osteosarcoma.

Occupational exposure to radioactive minerals in the mines of central Europe and the western USA is associated with an increased incidence of lung cancer.

Thorotrast, a radiologic dye containing radioactive thorium, was used in diagnostic radiology between 1930 and 1955. Seventy percent of administered Thorotrast is deposited in the liver, where it appears in tissue sections as amorphous, brown, refractile granules in Kupffer cells that persist for years. Thorium has a half-life of 400 years; as it decays, it emits mostly alpha particles, which penetrate only short distances but cause multiple areas of focal damage. Thorotrast increases the risk for several types of liver cancer, including angiosarcoma, liver cell carcinoma, and cholangiocarcinoma (cancer of the bile ducts).

Radioactive iodine, which is used to treat nonneoplastic thyroid disease, is associated with an increased risk of cancer developing 15–25 years after treatment; the risk is weighed against the nature of the primary disease, the therapeutic benefits, and the patient's age.

D. Nuclear Fallout: Three groups of people have been exposed to nuclear fallout. The Japanese in Hiroshima and Nagasaki who survived the atomic bomb blasts have shown a greatly increased incidence of cancer, including leukemia and carcinoma of the breast, lung, and thyroid. Inhabitants of the Marshall Islands were accidentally exposed to fallout during atmospheric testing of a nuclear device in the southern Pacific Ocean. The fallout was rich in radioactive iodine and resulted in a high incidence of thyroid neoplasms in those exposed. The accident at the Chernobyl nuclear power plant in the USSR in 1986 also released radioactive iodine into the atmosphere and resulted in the exposure of several thousand people to radioactive contamination.

The radiation levels that would result from the destruction and detonation of current nuclear power plants and nuclear weapons are several thousand times those associated with the Hiroshima bomb. The devastation resulting from fallout produced by a nuclear accident or nuclear warfare would be compounded by the increased incidence of cancer for years afterward. Although the accident at the Three Mile Island nuclear power plant in Pennsylvania did not lead to radiation exposure, it emphasized the constant risk of nuclear fallout associated with such facilities.

To put all of this in perspective, it has been estimated that all radiation derived from x-rays, therapeutic isotopes, nuclear power plants, and the like currently accounts for less than 1% of the total radiation exposure of the population; the remainder comes from radioactive rocks, the earth itself, and cosmic rays.

Viral Oncogenesis (Table 18–4)

Both DNA viruses and RNA viruses can cause neoplasia. DNA viruses insert their nucleic acid directly into the genome of the host cell. RNA viruses require RNA-directed DNA polymerase (reverse transcriptase), an enzyme that causes the production of a DNA copy of the RNA viral genome; this DNA copy (provirus) can then be inserted in the host genome. Some RNA viruses contain a "built-in" oncogene that directly activates the cell; others insert adjacent to an endogenous cellular oncogene, which is thereby activated (Fig 18–7). Insertion of the viral DNA sequence into the host genome is a highly complex process requiring several viral enzymes that cleave the host DNA, insert the viral DNA, and then repair the break.

The insertion of viral DNA into the host genome may have a variety of effects (Chapter 13). In the case of oncogenic viruses, neoplastic transformation occurs in susceptible cells.

The presence of a viral genome in a cell can be demonstrated in various ways: (1) reciprocal hybridization studies using DNA probes, (2) recognition of virus-specific antigens on infected cells, and (3) detection of virus-specific mRNA.

A. Oncogenic RNA Viruses: Oncogenic RNA viruses (retroviruses, formerly called oncornaviruses) cause many neoplasms in experimental animals, including leukemia and lymphoma in mice, cats, and birds; various sarcomas in birds (Rous sarcoma virus) and primates; and breast carcinoma in mice (Bittner milk factor, or mouse mammary tumor virus). Retroviruses have been implicated in only a few human neoplasms.

1. Japanese T cell leukemia-This form of leukemia was first described in Japan. A retrovirus (human T lymphocyte virus type I [HTLV-I]) has been cultured from tumor cells in this disease, and the virus is believed to play a direct etiologic role.

2. Infection with HIV-Human immunodeficiency virus (HIV) is a retrovirus that infects human lymphocytes and causes acquired immune deficiency syndrome (AIDS). The malignant B cell lymphomas associated with AIDS may result from HIV oncogenesis.

3. Other disorders-There is weak evidence to suggest that other hematologic cancers may have a viral origin. Tissue samples taken from many patients with leukemias and lymphomas contain viral reverse transcriptase, and there have been reports of isolation of virus in cultures or identification of viral nucleic acid by DNA probes in human leukemia cells. Epidemiologic case clustering in some patients with Hodgkin's disease suggests that the cause is a transmissible virus. The exact significance of these findings is as yet unknown.

4. Breast carcinoma-In mice, breast carcinoma is caused by the mouse mammary tumor virus (MMTV), an RNA virus transmitted in breast milk (Fig 18–1). Serum antibodies that are able to neutralize MMTV have been identified in some women with breast cancer, and MMTV or a similar antigen can be demonstrated in human breast cancer cells, suggesting that an RNA virus identical or similar to MMTV may cause human breast cancer. In addition, viruslike particles and RNA resembling that of MMTV have been identified in human breast cancer cells and breast milk. Despite these findings, the theory that an RNA virus is the cause of human breast cancer is still considered unproved.

Table 18–4. Oncogenic viruses.

Group	Virus	Host	Tumor
RNA viruses (retroviruses) Type C	Avian leukemia-sarcoma complex	Chicken	Leukosis, Rous sarcoma
	Murine leukemia-sarcoma complex	Mouse, rat, hamster	Leukemia, sarcoma
	Feline leukemia-sarcoma complex	Cat/dog	Leukemia, sarcoma
Type B	Murine mammary tumor virus (Bittner milk factor)	Mouse	Breast cancer
Type C-like	HTLV-I	Human	T cell leukemia
	Human immunodeficiency virus (AIDS virus)	Human	AIDS-related lymphomas
DNA viruses Papovavirus	Papilloma virus	Human, rabbit, cow, dog	Papilloma (laryngeal), condylomata acuminata, verruca vulgaris, ?carcinoma of cervix
	Polyoma virus	Mouse	Many tumors in newborn hamsters
	SV40	Monkey	Tumors in hamsters only
Herpesvirus	Herpes simplex type 2	Human	?Carcinoma of cervix
	Epstein-Barr virus	Human	Carcinoma of nasopharynx, Burkitt's lymphoma
	Avian	Chicken	Marek's disease
	Rabbit	Rabbit	Lymphoma
Poxvirus	Fibroma-myxoma	Rabbit	Fibromyxoma
	Molluscum contagiosum	Human	Molluscum contagiosum[1]
Parapoxvirus	Hepatitis B	Human, rodent, duck	Hepatocellular carcinoma

[1]A self-limited proliferative disease of the epidermis: not a true neoplasm.

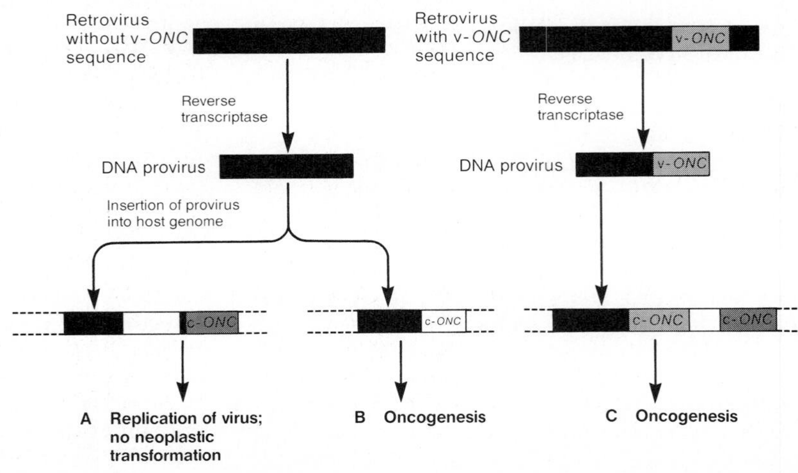

Figure 18–7. RNA virus (retrovirus) oncogenesis. Provirus (from retroviral RNA) can insert at many sites in the host genome. **A:** When a provirus lacking a V-*ONC* gene inserts at some distance from a cellular oncogene, viral replication occurs without neoplastic transformation. **B:** If the provirus inserts adjacent to a cellular oncogene, it may activate that oncogene and cause neoplasm. **C:** Retrovirus containing a V-*ONC* gene may lead to neoplasia directly on insertion. This effect is maximal if insertion occurs next to a cellular oncogene.

B. Oncogenic DNA Viruses: Several groups of DNA viruses have been implicated as the cause of human neoplasms.

1. Papilloma viruses–These viruses cause benign squamous epithelial cell neoplasms in skin and mucous membranes, including the common wart (verruca vulgaris), the venereal wart (condyloma acuminatum), and recurrent laryngeal papillomas in children (laryngeal papillomatosis).

DNA hybridization studies have revealed papilloma virus types 6 and 11 in most cases of condyloma acuminata, whereas severe dysplasia and invasive carcinoma of the uterine cervix are associated with types 16, 18, 31, and 33. Furthermore, papilloma viral DNA appears to be present in extrachromosomal episomes in the condylomas but is in an integrated form in severe dysplasia and carcinoma.

2. Molluscum contagiosum–Molluscum contagiosum is a poxvirus that causes wartlike squamous epithelial cell tumors in the skin. These are self-limited and probably not true neoplasms.

3. Epstein-Barr virus (EBV)–This herpesvirus causes infectious mononucleosis, an acute infectious disease that occurs worldwide. Epstein-Barr virus is also thought to cause Burkitt's lymphoma in Africa and nasopharyngeal carcinoma in the Far East.

Epstein-Barr virus selectively infects B lymphocytes, binding to membrane receptors on the B lymphocyte that appear to be specific for the virus. Studies using DNA probes show that the Epstein-Barr virus genome is present in over 90% of African Burkitt lymphoma cells. It is thought that infected B lymphocytes undergo neoplastic transformation when a second causative factor operates. The similarity of geographic distribution of Burkitt's lymphoma and malaria has led to speculation that the chronic immune proliferation induced by malaria may be this second inciting factor.

4. Herpes simplex virus (HSV) type 2–Epidemiologic evidence has long pointed toward herpes simplex virus type 2 as the cause of cancer of the uterine cervix. DNA probe studies have identified the herpes simplex virus type 2 genome in cervical cancer cells. It is not known whether herpes simplex virus actively causes cervical cancer or whether it is merely an opportunistic pathogen.

5. Cytomegalovirus (CMV)–The nucleic acid of this herpesvirus is present in most cells of the lesions associated with Kaposi's sarcoma, a disorder most commonly found in immunodeficient patients. It is not known whether cytomegalovirus causes Kaposi's sarcoma or whether it is an opportunistic organism.

6. Hepatitis B virus–This virus is believed to be an important cause of hepatocellular carcinoma, which is common in Africa and the Far East—areas with a high incidence of hepatitis B infection and high carrier rates. The virus can be demonstrated in liver cancer cells in some patients. Sustained liver cell proliferation (regeneration) that occurs in response to virus-induced injury may be the critical factor predisposing to neoplastic change.

7. Adenoviruses–Some adenoviruses cause cancer in certain animals, but although they commonly infect humans, they have not been shown to be carcinogenic in humans.

Nutritional Oncogenesis

Despite extensive research, there is little hard evidence linking cancer to diet, with the exception of the possible presence in the diet of known chemical carcinogens (see above).

The best evidence for the role of diet in oncogenesis is in the incidence of colon cancer. Burkitt, recognizing that Africans had a low incidence of colon cancer compared with people in Western countries, suggested that this was due to the high fiber content of the African diet, which produces bulky stools that pass rapidly through the intestine. Low-fiber "Western" diets produce a small, hard stool with a long transit time. Slow passage through the bowel is associated with longer exposure to increased numbers of anaerobic bacteria that are thought to cause bile acid dehydrogenation, producing carcinogens. Slow transit also prolongs exposure to any food-associated carcinogens.

A diet high in animal fat has been associated statistically with an increased incidence of cancer of the colon and with breast cancer; this observation remains unexplained.

Hormonal Oncogenesis

A. Induction of Neoplasms by Hormones:

1. Estrogens–Patients with estrogen-producing tumors of the ovary (granulosa cell tumor) or with persistent failure of ovulation (resulting in high levels of estrogen) have a high risk of endometrial cancer (Chapter 53). Estrogen causes endometrial hyperplasia, which is followed first by cytologic dysplasia and then by neoplasia.

2. Hormones and breast cancer–**Prolactin** may play a minor role in causing human breast cancer. Extensive studies of patients taking **oral contraceptives** have shown that the risk of breast cancer is minimally increased in patients taking preparations with a high estrogen content. The current low-estrogen contraceptives are thought not to increase the risk of breast cancer. Since only female mice develop breast carcinoma after exposure to the Bittner milk factor (Fig 18–1), it has been postulated that **estrogens** are somehow instrumental in causing the disease; it has been shown that male mice given estrogen become equally susceptible to development of cancer.

3. Diethylstilbestrol (DES)–This synthetic estrogen was used in high doses between 1950 and 1960 to treat threatened abortion. Female children who were exposed to diethylstilbestrol in utero have a greatly increased incidence of clear-cell adenocarcinoma, a rare vaginal cancer that develops in young women between 15 and 30 years of age.

4. Steroid hormones-Use of oral contraceptives and anabolic steroids is rarely associated with development of benign **liver cell adenomas.** A few cases of liver cell carcinoma have been reported.

B. Hormonal Dependence of Neoplasms: Many neoplasms that are not caused by hormones are nonetheless dependent on hormones for optimal growth. The cells of such neoplasms are thought to have receptors on their cell membranes for binding hormones; when the neoplasm is deprived of the hormone, its growth is often slowed but not halted. Treatment of some common human neoplasms takes advantage of this property.

1. Prostatic cancer-This cancer is almost always dependent on androgens. Removal of both testes or the administration of estrogens frequently results in a dramatic—though temporary—regression of prostatic cancers.

2. Breast cancer-This cancer is frequently but not consistently dependent on estrogens and less frequently on progesterone. Hormone dependence correlates strongly with the presence of estrogen and progesterone receptors on the cell membrane. Verifying the presence or absence of these receptors through biochemical and immunologic techniques (Fig 18-8) constitutes part of the diagnosis of breast cancer. Oophorectomy or treatment with the estrogen-blocking drug tamoxifen eliminates estrogen and causes regression of most receptor-positive breast cancers, but this regression is temporary.

3. Thyroid cancer-Well-differentiated thyroid cancers are consistently dependent on thyroid-stimulating hormone (TSH). Administration of thyroid hormone to suppress TSH secretion is an important aspect of treatment.

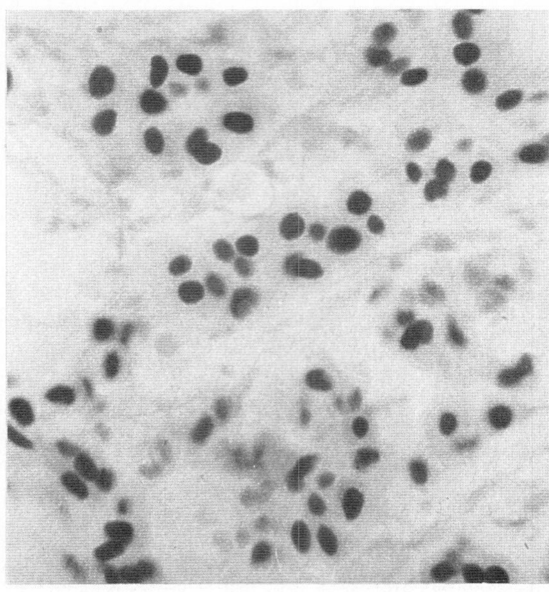

Figure 18-8. Frozen section of cells of a breast cancer that expresses a high level of estrogen receptors. The tissue has been stained by the immunoperoxidase technique using a monoclonal antibody directed against estrogen receptors. Dark nuclear staining indicates positivity for estrogen receptors and provides evidence that estrogen receptors are located mainly in the nucleus.

Genetic Oncogenesis (The Role of Inheritance in Oncogenesis)

In experimental settings, many animal strains show a genetic susceptibility for development of neoplasms. In many instances, this predisposition appears to result from the presence of one or more cellular oncogenes inherited as part of the genome. No hereditary human neoplasms have been shown to be due to oncogenes, although the possibility cannot be ignored.

A. Neoplasms With Mendelian (Single-Gene) Inheritance: Cancer-causing genes may act in a dominant or recessive manner. If dominant, they may produce a molecule that directly causes neoplasia. If recessive, lack of both normal genes may lead to failure of production of a factor necessary for maintaining control of normal growth.

1. Retinoblastoma-This uncommon malignant neoplasm of the retina occurs in children, and 40% of cases are inherited. The morphologic appearance of familial retinoblastoma is the same as that of the noninherited form. However, the familial form displays other distinguishing features: (1) it is commonly bilateral; (2) chromosomal analysis consistently shows deletion of part of the long arm of chromosome 13; and (3) spontaneous regression is common. Regression enables affected individuals to live into adult life to reproduce and transmit the gene. Examination of parents of children with familial retinoblastoma reveals signs of the regressed neoplasm in one parent.

As noted on p 281, there is inheritance of an abnormal partially deleted chromosome 13, producing a heterozygous state in which there is a greatly increased risk of developing retinoblastoma (95% of such patients develop the disease, often with multiple tumors). However, actual oncogenesis requires a second event, namely, deletion of the corresponding part of the long arm of the remaining chromosome 13, producing a homozygous state and development of retinoblastoma. In sporadic cases of retinoblastoma, it appears that 2 mutational deletions involving both chromosomes 13 must occur coincidentally in cells of the retina.

The inheritance of retinoblastoma shows an apparent dominant pattern as a result of the high rate of conversion of the heterozygous state to the homozygote (deletions involving both chromosomes 13) in which the recessive change is expressed.

Recent studies reveal the presence of a similar abnormality of chromosome 13 in cells of small cell undifferentiated carcinoma of the lung (Chapter 36). Furthermore, survivors of familial retinoblastoma have been shown to have a high risk of developing small cell undifferentiated carcinoma of the lung, especially if they smoke cigarettes.

2. Wilms's tumor (nephroblastoma)-Nephroblastoma is a malignant neoplasm of the kidney that occurs mainly in children. Many cases are associated with deletion of part of chromosome 11 (Fig 18–9). Both sporadic and familial cases occur, by mechanisms thought to resemble those described for retinoblastoma.

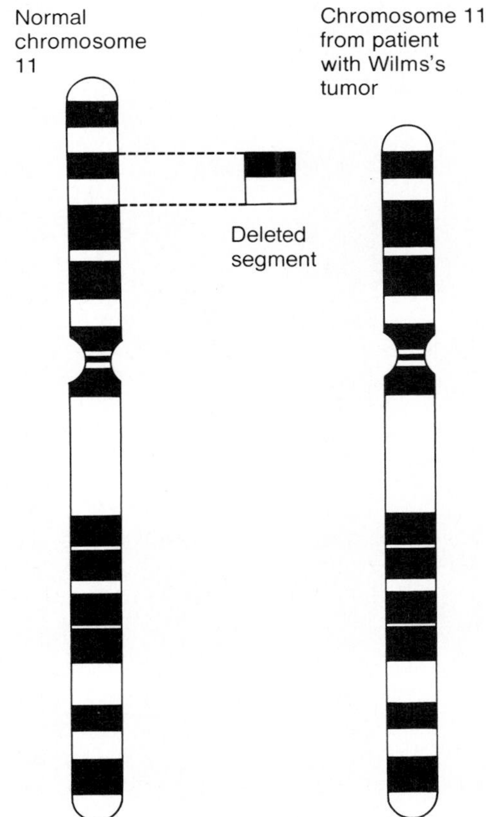

Figure 18–9. Diagrammatic representation of normal chromosome 11 and an abnormal 11 chromosome, showing a deleted segment that is commonly found in patients with nephroblastoma (Wilms's tumor).

3. Other inherited neoplasms-Other neoplasms with an autosomal dominant inheritance pattern are as follows: (1) Neurofibromatosis (von Recklinghausen's disease) is characterized by multiple neurofibromas and pigmented skin patches known as café au lait spots (expressivity and penetrance are variable—ie, the clinical severity varies) (Chapter 15). (2) Multiple endocrine adenomatosis is manifested by benign neoplasms in the thyroid, parathyroid, pituitary, and adrenal medulla. (3) Familial polyposis coli is characterized by innumerable adenomatous polyps in the colon. Cancer eventually develops in all patients unless they undergo colectomy (Chapter 41). Gardner's syndrome is a variant in which colonic polyps are associated with benign neoplasms and cysts in bone, soft tissue, and skin. (4) Nevoid basal cell carcinoma syndrome is characterized by dysplastic melanocytic nevi and basal cell carcinomas in the skin (Chapter 61).

Inheritance patterns other than autosomal dominant are uncommon in familial neoplasia. Turcot's syndrome, a very rare disease in which multiple adenomatous polyps of the colon are associated with malignant tumors (gliomas) of the nervous system, is thought to have an autosomal recessive inheritance pattern.

B. Neoplasms With Polygenic Inheritance: Many common human neoplasms are familial, ie, they occur in a group of related individuals more often than would be expected on the basis of chance alone.

1. Breast cancer-First-degree female relatives (mother, sisters, daughters) of a premenopausal woman with breast cancer have a risk of developing breast cancer that is 5 times higher than that of the general population. The risk is even greater if the patient has bilateral breast cancer.

2. Colon cancer-Cancer of the colon tends to occur in families both as a complication of inherited familial polyposis coli and independently of familial polyposis coli. A few families exist with a reported predisposition for development of colon cancer. Some of the "cancer families" also have other cancers, notably of the endometrium and breast.

It has been suggested that this familial tendency may be the result of inheritance of multiple genes that combine to influence the development of neoplasia. Some of these inherited genes may be oncogenes. It is also possible that the observed familial tendency for development of a disease simply reflects the action of some common environmental carcinogen in closely related individuals.

C. Neoplasms Occurring More Frequently in Inherited Diseases: Many inherited diseases are associated with a high risk of neoplasia. These include (1) syndromes characterized by increased chromosomal fragility (eg, xeroderma pigmentosum, Bloom's syndrome, Fanconi's syndrome, and ataxia telangiectasia), in which neoplasia is due to frequent DNA abnormalities; and (2) syndromes of immunodeficiency (Chapter 7), in which failure of immune surveillance or inappropriate immune stimulation of any remaining lymphoid cells predisposes to neoplasia. In these disorders, it is not the neoplasm itself that is inherited but rather some susceptibility to neoplasia.

Neoplasia: III. Biologic & Clinical Effects of Neoplasia

19

ORIGINS OF NEOPLASIA

Two types of origins have been proposed for neoplasms.

Monoclonal Origin

According to the theory of monoclonal origin, a carcinogen produces neoplastic change in a single cell, which then multiplies and gives rise to the neoplasm. The monoclonal origin of neoplasms has been clearly shown in neoplasms of B lymphocytes (B cell lymphomas and plasma cell myelomas) that produce immunoglobulin and in some other tumor types by isoenzyme studies (Fig 19–1).

Field Origin

A carcinogenic agent acting on a large number of similar cells may produce a field of potentially neoplastic cells. Neoplasms may then arise from one or more cells within this field. In many cases the result is several discrete neoplasms, each of which derives from a separate clonal precursor. The field change may be regarded as the first of 2 or more sequential steps that lead to overt cancer (Chapter 18).

Multifocal (neoplastic field) neoplasms occur in skin, urothelium, liver, breast, and colon. Recognizing that a neoplasm is of field origin has practical implications, since one neoplasm in any of these sites should alert the clinician to the possibility of a second similar neoplasm. In the breast, for example, cancer in one breast carries a risk of cancer in the opposite breast that is about 10 times higher than that of the general population.

CHARACTERISTICS OF NEOPLASIA

The Lag period

A constant feature of all known agents that cause neoplasms is the interval (lag period) between exposure and development of the neoplasm. In survivors of the atomic bomb blasts of Hiroshima and Nagasaki, the largest number of cases of leukemia occurred about 10 years after the event, and some cancers developed as late as 20 years afterward. In shipyard workers exposed to asbestos in World War II, neoplasms are still appearing after 40 years even though exposure stopped more than 30 years ago. In utero exposure to diethylstilbestrol may give rise to vaginal cancer 15 or more years after birth. This long lag period may account for the difficulty in identifying carcinogenic agents for common neoplasms.

The reason for the lag period is unknown. If it is assumed that a carcinogen causes fundamental neoplastic alteration in a cell, then the altered cell must be subjected to a second insult before it shows neoplastic growth **(2-hit theory).** In this

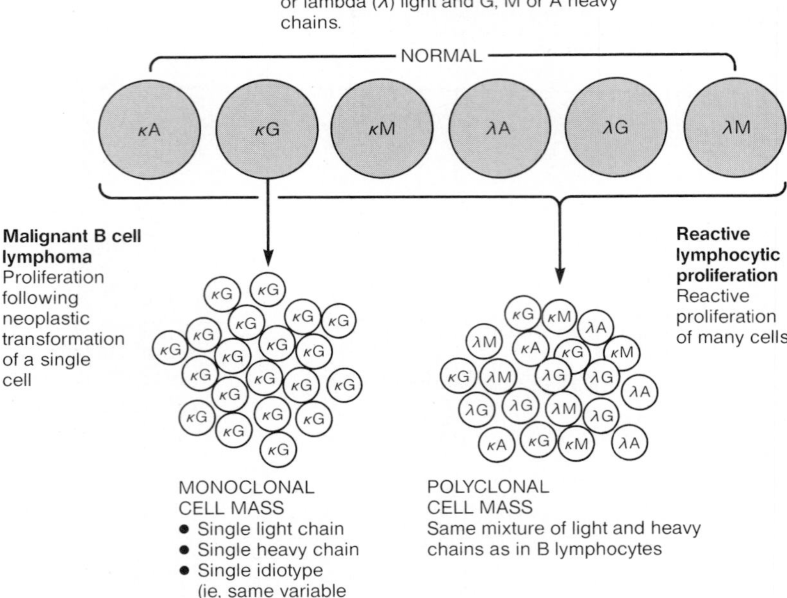

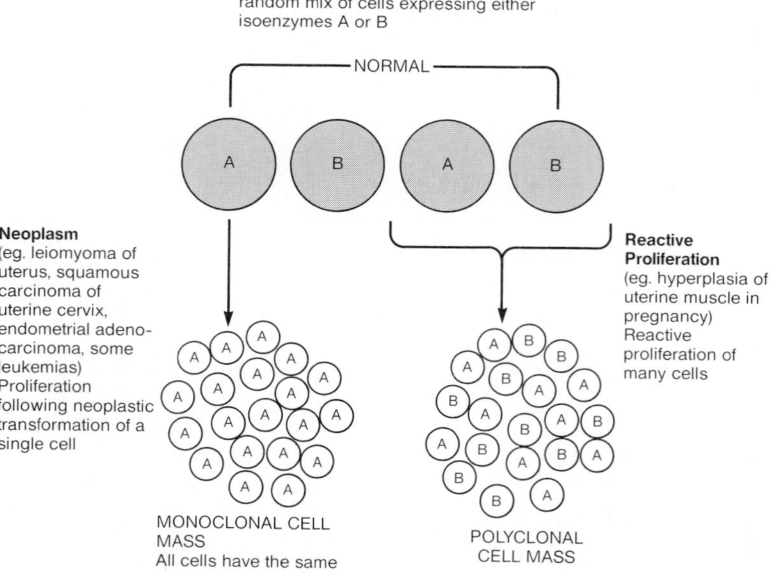

Figure 19–1. Methods of characterization of cell populations as monoclonal or polyclonal. **A:** Immunoglobulin light and heavy chain distribution in a B lymphocyte population. **B:** Glucose-6-phosphate dehydrogenase isoenzyme studies may be used in some female patients. G6PD isoenzyme inheritance is X-linked. In heterozygous females, one X chromosome codes for the A isoenzyme and the other for the B isoenzyme. Since one X chromosome is randomly inactivated in the adult cell, an adult cell will contain only one of the isoenzymes. A polyclonal population will be composed of cells containing both isoenzymes in approximately equal amounts, whereas a monoclonal population will be composed of cells that express only one isoenzyme.

theory, the first event—the neoplastic change—is **initiation** (Fig 19–2), and the carcinogen causing it is the **initiator**. The second event—which induces neoplastic growth—is **promotion,** and the agent is the **promoter**.

During the lag period, the altered cell may not show any structural or functional abnormality; eg, an epidermal cell that has been exposed to a carcinogen looks and functions the same as surrounding cells. Subtle changes are probably present in such cells, particularly in the genome, but these cannot be detected at present.

Precancerous (Premalignant) Changes (Table 19–1)

In most instances, after a lag period, a cell that has been altered by a carcinogen develops into a neoplasm through neoplastic cellular proliferation. In a few cases, an intermediate abnormal, nonneoplastic growth pattern develops in altered cells and can be recognized clinically or microscopically. Such an abnormality is a precancerous (or preneoplastic) lesion; the former term is more accurate, since this concept applies only to malignant neoplasms.

It is important to recognize precancerous lesions, because surgical excision is curative (the potentially malignant tissue having been removed). Benign neoplasms that often become malignant are also considered precancerous lesions (Table 19–1).

Occult Cancer

Invasive cancer is usually lethal, but progression of disease varies. Small prostatic cancers are

Table 19–1. Precancerous (premalignant) lesions.

Precancerous Lesion	Cancer
Hyperplasia	
Endometrial hyperplasia	Endometrial carcinoma
Breast—lobular and ductal hyperplasia	Breast carcinoma
Liver—cirrhosis of the liver	Hepatocellular carcinoma
Dysplasia[1]	
Cervix	Squamous carcinoma of cervix
Skin	Squamous carcinoma
Bladder	Transitional cell carcinoma
Bronchial epithelium	Lung carcinoma
Metaplasia[2]	
Glandular metaplasia of esophagus	Adenocarcinoma of esophagus
Inflammatory lesions	
Ulcerative colitis	Carcinoma of colon
Atrophic gastritis	Carcinoma of stomach
Autoimmune (Hashimoto's) thyroiditis	Malignant lymphoma, thyroid carcinoma
Benign neoplasms	
Colonic adenoma	Carcinoma of colon
Neurofibroma	Malignant peripheral nerve sheath tumor (malignant schwannoma)

[1]These are de novo dysplasias; dysplasia also usually precedes malignancy in the other conditions listed.
[2]Note that metaplasia of itself is usually not preneoplastic—in the lung, squamous cell metaplasia is followed by dysplasia and then neoplasia.

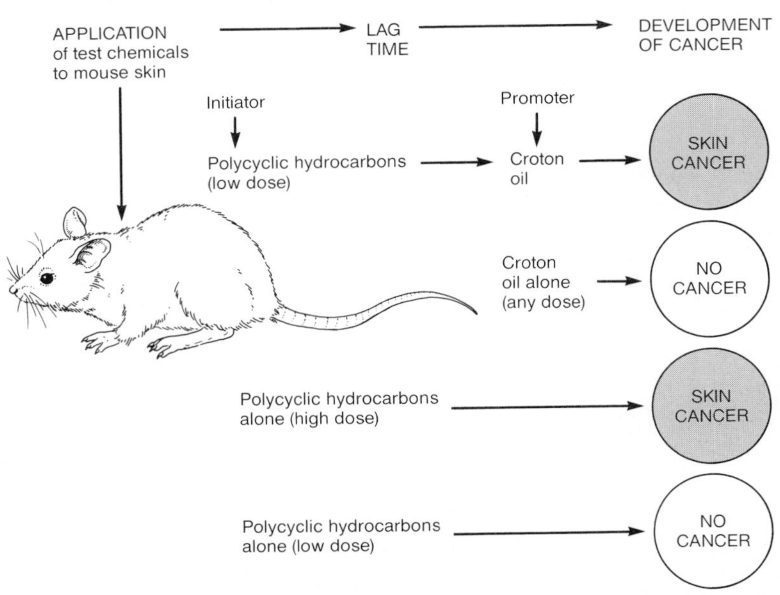

Figure 19–2. Initiation and promotion of a neoplasm. Polycyclic hydrocarbons, which are carcinogens at high doses, cause skin cancer. The action of polycyclic hydrocarcons is enhanced by croton oil, which acts as a promoter. This is best seen by the effect of croton oil in producing cancer when a subcarcinogenic (low) dose of polycyclic hydrocarbon is used. Note that croton oil in any dose does not cause cancer. Many carcinogens act as both initiators and promoters.

found incidentally—ie, in patients who died of other causes without any clinical evidence of prostate cancer—at autopsy in about 30% of men over age 60 years. This figure rises to 90% of men over age 90 years. These cancers are called occult because they remained small and did not become manifest clinically during life.

Another example of long-standing hidden cancer is delayed metastatic disease (occult metastases). Patients who have been treated for melanoma and breast cancer sometimes develop evidence of metastatic disease 15–20 years later. It has been proposed that occult cancers and delayed metastases may represent examples of partial immunologic control.

Changes in Structure & Function of Neoplastic Cells (Fig 19–3)

A. Surface Membrane Alterations: Surface membrane changes include alteration in level of activity of membrane enzymes, decrease in glycoprotein and fibronectin content, abnormalities in electrical charge, and alterations in the subjacent microtubular and microfilamentous cytoskeleton.

Normal cells in culture grow in orderly, tightly cohesive monolayers. Cell division is arrested as cells establish contact with other cells **(contact inhibition)**. In contrast, cancer cells in culture grow as disorganized, multilayered masses that pile up on one another. This loss of contact inhibition is characteristic of neoplastic cells.

It is thought that failure of contact inhibition—coupled with lack of adhesiveness among individual tumor cells—may partially explain the ability of malignant neoplastic cells to invade and metastasize.

B. Immunologic Alterations:

1. Appearance of tumor-associated antigens–Most neoplastic cells express new antigens (neoantigens, tumor-associated antigens) on their surfaces. These antigens probably represent expression of the altered genome. The term "tumor-specific antigen" is deliberately avoided, since detailed studies have shown that most (if not all) of these neoantigens are not entirely limited to cancer cells.

a. Common viral antigens–In viral-induced neoplasms, new antigens are frequently coded by the virus, and all neoplasms caused by a particular virus will show the same new antigen, regardless of the tissue, individual, or species in which the neoplasm arises. The new antigen is the same because the genomic alteration is constant (heritable) and is based on introduction of viral nucleic acid.

b. Unique antigens–Neoplasms induced by chemicals or radiation manifest new antigens that are distinctive for each different neoplasm induced. Even separate neoplasms occurring in the same tissue in the same individual will produce different antigens. This pattern reflects the random genomic alterations produced by radiation and most chemicals.

c. Oncofetal antigens–A third category of tumor-associated antigens includes the so-called oncofetal antigens: **carcinoembryonic antigen (CEA)** and **α-fetoprotein (AFP)**. These result from derepression of genes that normally are active only in fetal life. Detection of CEA or AFP has some diagnostic value (see below).

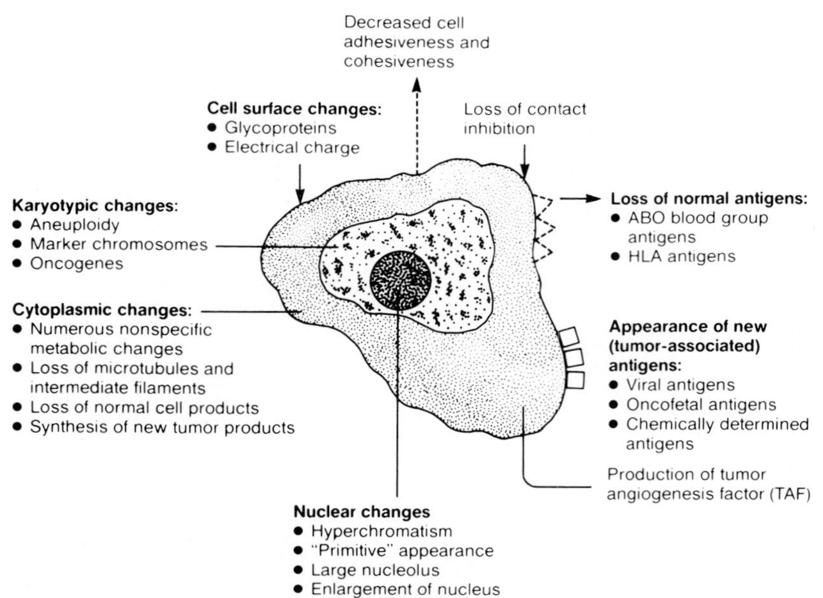

Figure 19–3. Changes in neoplastic cells.

Tumor-associated antigens are often only weakly immunogenic but may evoke humoral and cellular immune responses, as evidenced by antibody production and a lymphocytic infiltrate surrounding the neoplastic cells. Although lymphocytes are commonly present in neoplasms, evidence that they may play a role in controlling tumor growth is limited to a small number of neoplasms. **Hodgkin's disease,** for example, is classified on the basis of the number of lymphocytes present, and lymphocyte predominance implies a better prognosis than lymphocyte depletion. In another example, **medullary carcinoma of the breast** is characterized by the presence of a prominent lymphocytic infiltrate and has a more favorable prognosis than other breast cancers. And finally, the magnitude of the lymphocytic response at the margin of a **malignant melanoma** correlates somewhat with prognosis.

Very rarely, neoplasms regress spontaneously. Such regression has been reported most frequently in retinoblastoma, choriocarcinoma, neuroblastoma, malignant melanoma, and renal adenocarcinoma. The reason for tumor regression is not known, but in some instances it may represent an immunologic destructive phenomenon.

2. Loss of antigens normally present-Neoplastic cells also frequently lack antigens that are present in normal cells. Some evidence suggests that loss of antigens may correlate with the biologic behavior of the neoplasm—ie, the greater the loss of antigens, the more malignant the neoplasm. In bladder neoplasms, for example, those cancers that have lost ABO blood group antigens tend to invade and metastasize more extensively than comparable cancers that have retained these antigens.

C. Karyotypic Abnormalities: As analytic techniques improve, increasing numbers of chromosomal abnormalities are being identified in neoplastic cells (Table 19–2). Many malignant cells show major nonspecific chromosomal abnormalities such as aneuploidy and polyploidy.

Of greater importance are chromosomal abnor-

Table 19–2. Chromosomal abnormalities in neoplasms.

Abnormality	Neoplasm
Aneuploidy, tetraploidy, polyploidy	Many malignant neoplasms, especially poorly differentiated and anaplastic types
Translocations[1]	
9 ⇄ 22 t(9;22) (Philadelphia chromosome)	Chronic myeloid leukemia (90%) Acute myeloid leukemia Acute lymphocytic leukemia (FAB types L_1 and L_2 [Chapter 26])
8 ⇄ 14 t(8;14)	Burkitt's lymphoma[3] Acute lymphocytic leukemia (FAB type L_3 [Chapter 26])[3] Immunoblastic B cell lymphoma
15 ⇆ 17 t(15;17)	Promyelocytic leukemia (Chapter 26)
4 ⇄ 11 t(4;11)	Acute lymphocytic leukemia (FAB type L_2)[3] Immunoblastic B cell lymphoma
11 ⇆ 14 t(11;14)	Chronic lymphocytic leukemia
14 ⇄ 18 t(14;18)	Some B cell lymphomas
6 ⇄ 14 t(6;14)	Cystadenocarcinoma of ovary
3 ⇄ 8 t(3;8)	Renal adenocarcinoma Mixed parotid tumor (benign)
Deletions[1,2]	
Deletion of 8 and 17	Blast crisis of chronic myeloid leukemia
5q− and 7q−	Acute myeloid leukemia Acute monocytic leukemia
3p−	Small cell carcinoma of lung
1p−	Neuroblastoma[3]
13q−	Retinoblastoma[3]
11p−	Nephroblastoma[3]
−22	Meningioma
Trisomy	
Trisomy 12	Chronic lymphocytic leukemia

[1]Many of these translocations and deletions occur at the point of insertion of an oncogene.
[2]Note p = short arm and q = long arm of designated chromosome.
[3]Mainly tumors of childhood.

malities that have fairly specific associations with certain neoplasms (Table 19–2). The most important of these (and first to be identified) is the **Philadelphia chromosome** (Ph^1), an abnormally small chromosome 22 found in over 90% of patients with chronic granulocytic leukemia (CGL). Ph^1 results from reciprocal translocation of genetic material between chromosome 22 and chromosome 9 (Fig 19–4). Patients with chronic granulocytic leukemia who lack Ph^1 have a worse prognosis than those who are Ph^1-positive. Ph^1 is not entirely specific for chronic granulocytic leukemia; a few patients with acute lymphocytic and acute granulocytic leukemias have been positive for Ph^1.

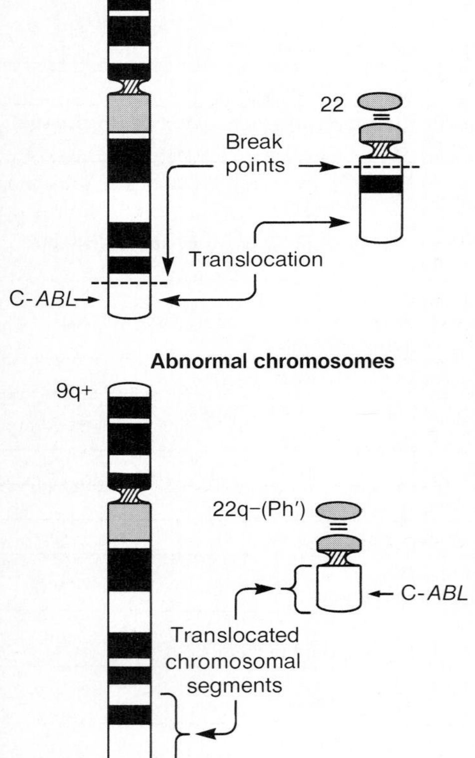

Figure 19–4. Formation of the Philadelphia (Ph^1) chromosome, which is commonly seen in chronic myeloid leukemia. Part of chromosome 9, including the Abelson oncogene (C-*ABL*) is translocated to chromosome 22, with exchange of chromosomal segments between 9 and 22. Interaction of C-*ABL* with genes on chromosome 22 produces a new chimeric (gene fusion) protein—tyrosine kinase—that appears to induce neoplastic proliferation of myeloid precursor cells.

Additional chromosomal abnormalities in chromosomes 8 and 17 in patients with chronic granulocytic leukemia usually indicate development of the accelerated phase (blast crisis) of the disease.

D. Tumor Cell Products: (Table 19–3.) The synthesis and secretion of various tumor cell products are important for 2 reasons: (1) their presence may indicate the existence of a neoplasm in the

Table 19–3. Tumor cell products.

Product	Commonly Associated Neoplasms
Oncofetal antigens	
Carcinoembryonic antigen (CEA)	Carcinoma of colon, pancreas, stomach, lung, breast
α-Fetoprotein (AFP)	Hepatocellular carcinoma, some germ cell neoplasms
Enzymes	
Prostatic acid phosphatase	Prostatic carcinoma
Alkaline phosphatase (Regan isoenzyme)	Carcinoma of pancreas
Lactate dehydrogenase	Many malignant neoplasms
Immunoglobulin (monoclonal)	B cell lymphomas, plasma cell myeloma
Hormones (from endocrine neoplasms)	
Growth hormone, prolactin, ACTH	Pituitary adenoma
Insulin, glucagon, gastrin	Pancreatic islet cell neoplasms
Parathyroid hormone	Parathyroid neoplasms
Cortisol, aldosterone	Adrenocortical neoplasms
Catecholamines	Pheochromocytoma, neuroblastoma
Calcitonin	Medullary (C cell) carcinoma of thyroid
Serotonin (5-HT)	Carcinoid (neuroendocrine) neoplasms of gut, lung
Histamine	Mast cell neoplasms
Chorionic gonadotropin (hCG)	Choriocarcinoma, some germ cell neoplasms
Androgens, estrogens	Testicular and ovarian neoplasms
Ectopic hormones (from nonendocrine neoplasms)	See Table 19–4.
Tumor angiogenesis factor (TAF)	Many malignant neoplasms
Osteoclast activating factor	Plasma cell myeloma

body—ie, they act as **tumor markers;** and (2) they may produce clinical effects **(paraneoplastic syndromes)** unrelated to direct involvement of tissue by the tumor.

1. Oncofetal antigens-Oncofetal antigens are antigens that are normally expressed only in fetal life but may be reproduced by neoplastic cells. Detection of these oncofetal antigens in adults is of some clinical value, since they are usually (not always) associated with malignant neoplasms.

Carcinoembryonic antigen (normally present in embryonic and fetal entodermal tissues) is found in most malignant neoplasms arising from tissues that develop from the embryonic entoderm, eg, colon and pancreatic cancer and some cases of gastric and lung cancer. About 30% of breast cancers also produce the antigen, which may be directly detected in tumor tissues by immunohistologic methods or may be measured in serum. Carcinoembryonic antigen is not specific for cancer, however, since slight increases in serum levels also occur in several nonneoplastic diseases, eg, ulcerative colitis and cirrhosis of the liver. The value of carcinoembryonic antigen as a tumor marker lies not so much in confirming a diagnosis as in monitoring the response to therapy and in the early diagnosis of recurrence after treatment in patients with colon cancer.

Alpha-fetoprotein is synthesized by normal yolk sac and fetal liver cells as well as by the neoplastic cells of primitive gonadal germ cell neoplasms (embryonal or yolk sac carcinomas) and liver cell carcinoma. Elevated serum levels of α-fetoprotein are of diagnostic value in patients with gonadal or hepatic masses; the protein can also be demonstrated immunohistochemically in tissue. As with carcinoembryonic antigen, elevated levels of α-fetoprotein may occur in other diseases besides cancer: mildly elevated levels may be seen in hepatic diseases such as cirrhosis in which nonneoplastic liver cell proliferation occurs.

2. Enzymes-Elevated serum levels of **prostate-specific acid phosphatase** occur in prostate cancer, usually when invasion has occurred beyond the capsule of the gland. High levels of Regan isoenzyme (an isoenzyme of alkaline phosphatase) are noted in some cases of pancreatic cancer. Levels of common cytoplasmic enzymes such as lactate dehydrogenase are elevated in many neoplasms and merely indicate increased turnover and necrosis of cells.

3. Immunoglobulins-Neoplasms of B lymphocytes (some B cell lymphomas, myeloma) frequently synthesize immunoglobulins. Since these neoplasms are monoclonal, only one type of immunoglobulin is produced. Immunoglobulin production is of great diagnostic value if the number of tumor cells and secretion of immunoglobulin are sufficient to produce a monoclonal band on serum protein electrophoresis (see Chapter 30).

4. Excessive hormone secretion-Well-differentiated neoplasms of endocrine cells are frequently associated with excessive production of hormones (Table 19–3). The hormone produced by the neoplasm is identical to that produced by the corresponding normal cell. Overproduction is due not only to the increased number of cells caused by the tumor but also to a failure of normal control mechanisms. The clinical symptoms resulting from these endocrine neoplasms are readily predictable because they represent the manifestations of excess hormone levels.

Endocrine neoplasms may be benign or malignant. The clinical course and prognosis depend more on the biologic behavior of the neoplasm than on the hormone it produces.

5. Ectopic hormone production-(Table 19–4.) Abnormal synthesis of hormones (so-called ectopic hormone production) may occur in malignant neoplasms derived from cells that normally do not secrete hormones. This phenomenon represents derepression of genes associated with the neoplastic process. Clinical effects resulting from the excessive hormone levels are as predictable as those associated with endocrine tumors.

Changes in Growth Pattern of Neoplastic Cells

The cellular growth abnormality associated with neoplasia is one of its chief attributes and serves to distinguish benign from malignant neoplasms.

Table 19-4. Ectopic hormone production by neoplasms.

Hormone	Commonly Associated Neoplasms
Chorionic gonadotropin (hCG)	Carcinoma of lung (30%), breast
Parathyroid hormone[1]	Squamous carcinoma of lung, renal adenocarcinoma, other squamous carcinomas
Adrenocorticotropic hormone (ACTH)	Small-cell carcinoma of lung, pancreatic islet cell neoplasms
Antidiuretic hormone (ADH)	Small-cell carcinoma of lung
Insulin[1]	Hepatocellular carcinoma, retroperitoneal sarcomas
Erythropoietin[1]	Renal adenocarcinoma, cerebellar hemangioblastoma, hepatocellular carcinoma

[1]The abnormal molecules of the ectopic hormone may not always be identical to those of the normal hormone but are similar enough to exert the same physiologic effect.

A. Excessive Cell Proliferation: Neoplastic cells generally multiply more rapidly than their normal counterparts. The resulting accumulation of increased numbers of cells in tissue commonly takes the form of a tumor, although in leukemia (cancer of white blood cells), the accumulated cells are spread throughout the bone marrow and blood and do not form a localized tumor mass. It is important to realize that the overall number of neoplastic cells can increase even if the rate of proliferation is slow; eg, in chronic lymphocytic leukemia, the accumulation of neoplastic cells is due to an arrest in maturation of neoplastic lymphocytes. Such cells fail to complete the cell cycle and therefore do not mature and die as normal cells do.

1. Rate of growth and malignancy-The rate of proliferation of neoplastic cells varies greatly. Some neoplasms grow so slowly that growth is measured in years; others proliferate so rapidly that an increase in size can be observed in days. As a general rule, the degree of malignancy of a neoplasm correlates with its rate of growth: the more rapid the growth, the more malignant the neoplasm. Important exceptions exist; eg, keratoacanthoma, a benign neoplasm of epidermal cells in the skin, initially grows more rapidly than does squamous carcinoma of the skin.

2. Assessment of growth rate-Clinically, the rate of growth of a neoplasm can be measured by the time needed for it to double in size. This **doubling time** varies from a few days in Burkitt's lymphoma to many months in most malignant epithelial neoplasms to many years in some benign neoplasms.

A crude histologic assessment of the growth rate is the **mitotic count,** which is usually expressed as the number of mitotic figures (Fig 19–5) counted in 10 consecutive high-power fields in the most active area of the neoplasm. In general, the higher the mitotic count, the more rapid the growth rate of the neoplasm. There are many exceptions to this general statement.

Although the growth rate is important, there is no reliable way of assessing it (Table 19–5).

B. Abnormal Differentiation and Anaplasia: When benign or slow-growing malignant neoplastic cells proliferate, they tend to differentiate normally and resemble their normal counterparts (ie, they are well-differentiated) (see Fig 17–2). For example, the cells constituting a lipoma (a benign neoplasm of adipocytes) resemble mature adipocytes on microscopic examination.

As the degree of malignancy increases, the degree of differentiation decreases, and neoplastic cells do not resemble the cell of origin so closely (see Fig 17–2). When the cell of origin cannot be recognized on microscopic examination (ie, the neoplasm does not resemble any normal cell), a neoplasm is said to be undifferentiated or anaplastic (Fig 19–6).

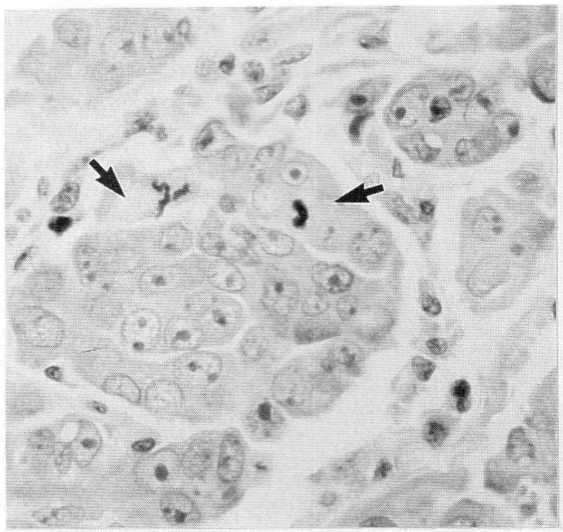

Figure 19–5. Mitotic figures in a malignant neoplasm. Two mitotic figures are present (arrows), one normal (at right) and the other tripolar (at left). Note also the large nuclei, high nuclear:cytoplasmic ratio, and large nucleoli that characterize these malignant cells.

When failure of differentiation occurs in malignant neoplasms, structural abnormalities appear both in the cytoplasm and in the nuclei of neoplastic cells (Figs 19–5 and 19–6). These changes are similar to those seen in dysplasia but are more severe. They include pleomorphism (variation in appearance of cells), increased nuclear size, increased nuclear:cytoplasmic ratio, hyperchromatism, prominent macronucleoli, abnormal chromatin distribution in the nucleus, nuclear membrane abnormalities, and failure of cytoplasmic differentiation. The severity of these cytologic abnormalities increases as the degree of malignancy increases. Most benign neoplasms have few if any of these abnormalities.

Neoplastic cells may occasionally differentiate in a manner that is abnormal for the cell of origin.

Table 19–5. Assessment of growth rate of neoplasms.

Clinical approach: serial palpation of the mass
Radiologic approach: serial x-rays or CT scans of the mass
Microscopic approach:
Cellularity (rapidly growing neoplasms are highly cellular)
Number of mitoses (mitotic count per unit area) (see Fig 19–5)[1]
Flow cytometry: percentage of cells in the S and G_2M phases of the cell cycle (high with rapid growth)
Culture approach (short-term tissue culture is unreliable because growth conditions in vitro are different from those in vivo)

[1]The number of high-power fields used for assessment varies in different neoplasms.

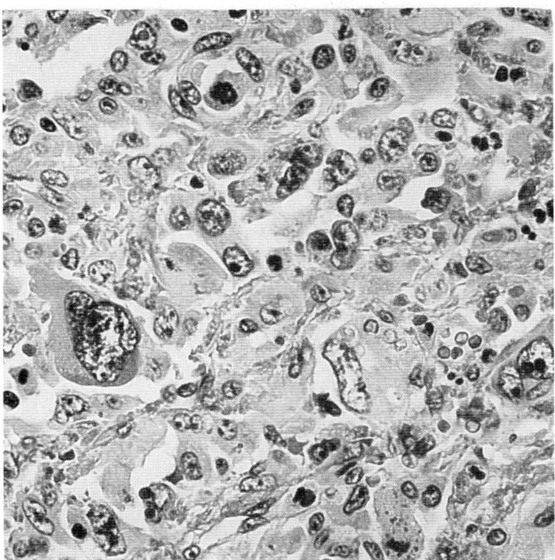

Figure 19-6. Anaplastic malignant neoplasm, showing marked pleomorphism (variation in cell size and shape). Several multinucleated tumor giant cells are present, together with other features of cancer such as a high nuclear:cytoplasmic ratio, hyperchromatism, and prominent nucleoli. This tumor, which is an anaplastic carcinoma of the pancreas, bears no resemblance to the cell of origin.

For example, neoplastic endometrial glandular epithelium sometimes differentiates to form both glandular and squamous epithelial cells (adenosquamous carcinoma), and malignant Schwann cells may give rise to bone-producing cells. The term tumor metaplasia is sometimes used for this phenomenon, though abnormal neoplastic differentiation is preferred.

C. Invasion (Infiltration): Benign neoplasms do not invade adjacent tissue but tend to expand centrifugally, forming a capsule of compressed normal tissue and collagen. Malignant neoplasms encroach on normal tissue planes and form tongues of neoplastic cells extending on all sides. Malignant neoplasms usually do not form a capsule.

Carcinomas and sarcomas demonstrate similar patterns of invasion and metastasis despite their different tissues of origin. Invasion of the basement membrane (Figs 19–7 and 19–8) by carcinoma distinguishes invasive cancer from intraepithelial (or in situ) cancer. Having penetrated the basement membrane, malignant cells gain access to the lymphatics and blood vessels, the first step toward general dissemination (Fig 19–9). Infiltrating neoplastic cells tend to follow fascial planes along the pathway of least resistance; eventually destruction of tissue occurs. The mechanisms whereby neoplastic cells invade and destroy tissues are poorly understood, but surface membrane abnormalities, loss of contact inhibition of cells, and decreased cell adhesiveness are believed to play a part.

Assessment of the extent of invasion by gross examination at the time of surgery is often difficult, because neoplastic cells can frequently remain undetected away from the apparent borders of the neoplasm. Appropriate surgical treatment of malignant neoplasms therefore involves a wide margin of excision of apparently normal tissue surrounding the tumor. The size of the margin varies; eg, a much wider surgical resection is required for gastric carcinoma than for gastric leiomyosarcoma, because malignant gastric epithelial cells tend to infiltrate more widely than malignant smooth muscle cells. Microscopic examination of rapidly frozen tissue sections must be performed to verify that the margins of resection are clear of

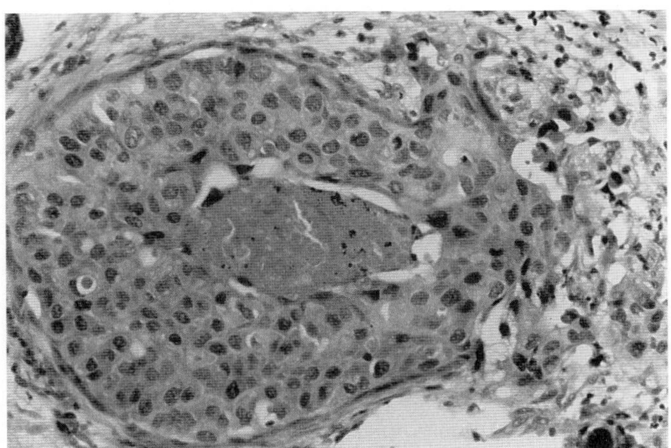

Figure 19-7. Carcinoma of the breast that is predominantly confined within the duct except at the right side, where it has infiltrated through the ductal basement membrane into the surrounding stroma.

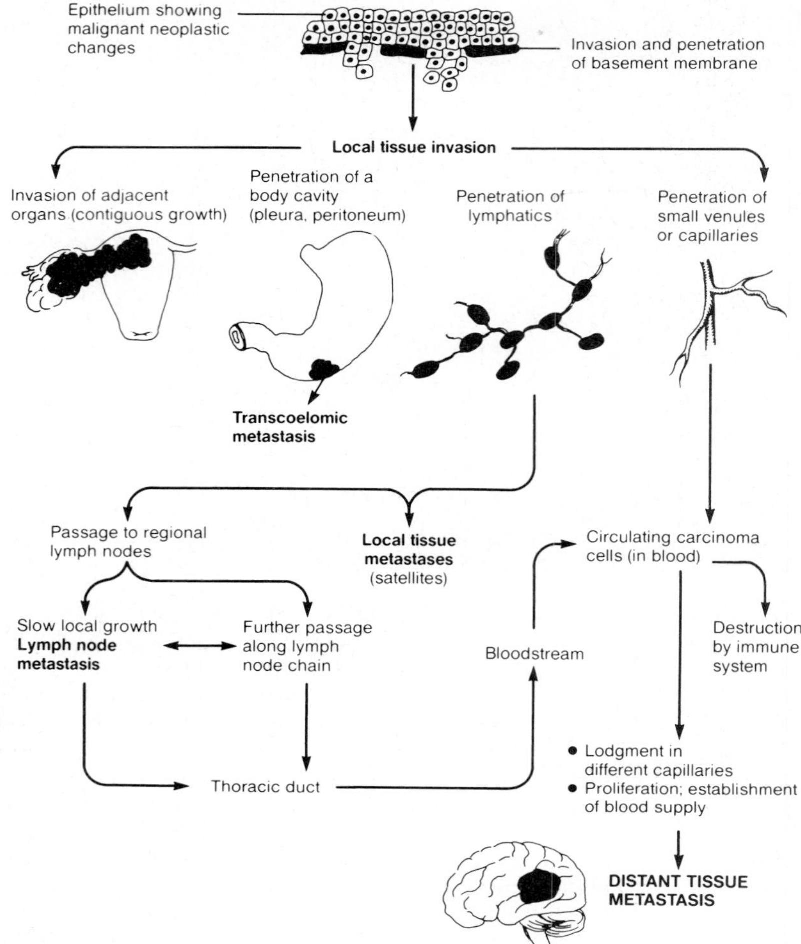

Figure 19-8. Invasion and methods of metastasis as exemplified by a carcinoma. Sarcomas arise in connective tissue and are not limited by a basement membrane. Their properties of invasion and metastasis resemble those of carcinomas, except that sarcomas generally favor hematogenous over lymphatic metastasis.

neoplastic cells. Such examination can be performed while the patient is still in surgery, so that further resection can be undertaken if necessary.

D. Metastasis: Metastasis is the establishment of a second neoplastic mass through transfer of neoplastic cells from the first neoplasm to a secondary location separate from the original tumor. Metastasis occurs only in malignant neoplasms and explains why they are life-threatening and difficult to eradicate.

1. Lymphatogenous metastasis-Metastasis via the lymphatics occurs early in carcinomas and melanomas but is an unusual occurrence in most sarcomas, which tend to spread mainly via the bloodstream.

Malignant cells are carried by the lymphatics to the regional lymph nodes (Fig 19-10). The belief that cancerous cells spread first to the regional lymph nodes—where their advance may be temporarily arrested by the immune response—is the rationale for radical surgery, which removes both the primary neoplasm and the regional lymph nodes to thereby eliminate the most likely sites of early metastases. Removal of lymph nodes is per-

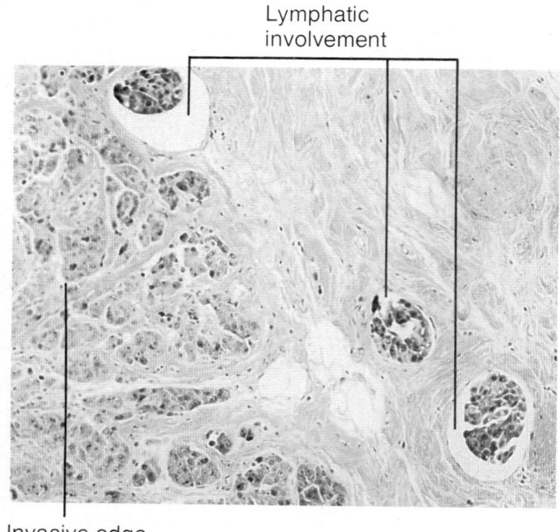

Figure 19-9. Infiltrating carcinoma, showing invasion of lymphatics by the tumor cells.

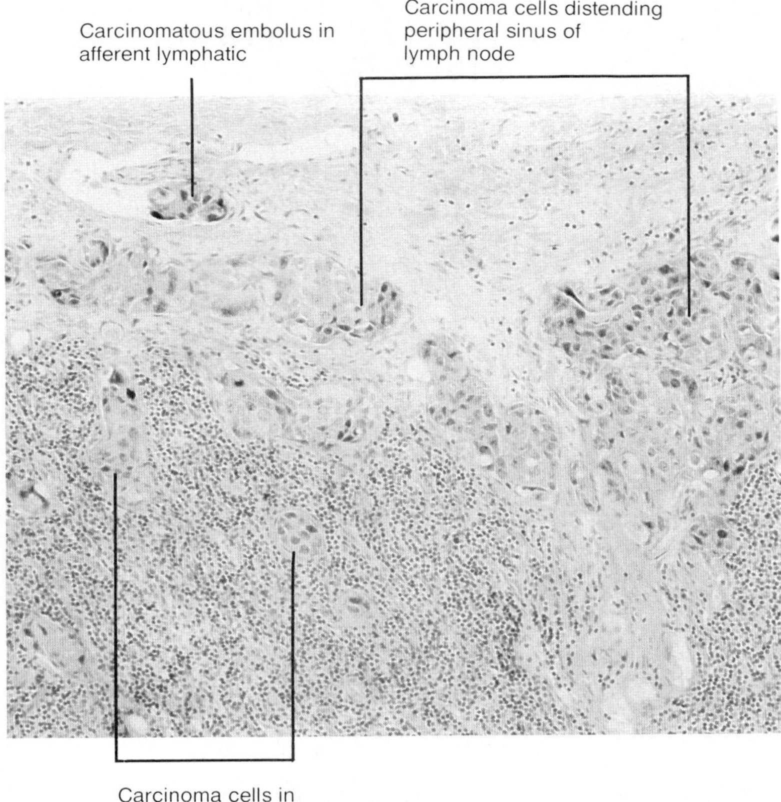

Figure 19–10. Metastatic carcinoma in a lymph node.

formed only for those neoplasms in which lymphatic metastasis is common, eg, carcinoma and melanoma. Knowledge of the lymphatic drainage of various tissues enables the clinician to predict the sites of lymph node involvement.

2. Hematogenous metastasis–Entry of cancerous cells into the bloodstream is believed to occur during the early clinical course of many malignant neoplasms. Most of these malignant cells are thought to be destroyed by the immune system, but some become coated with fibrin and entrapped in capillaries. (Anticoagulants such as heparin that keep the cells from being coated with fibrin decrease the development of metastases in experimental animals.) Metastasis can occur only if enough cancerous cells survive in the tissues to become established and proliferate at a second site (Figs 19–10, 19–11, and 19–12). The production of **tumor angiogenesis factor** (TAF) by the cancerous cells stimulates growth of new capillaries in the vicinity of tumor cells and encourages vascularization of the growing metastasis.

The site of metastasis is most commonly the first capillary bed encountered by blood draining the primary site (Fig 19–12). Some types of cancer apparently favor particular metastatic sites, though the mechanisms responsible are unknown. Skeletal metastases are common in cancer of the prostate, thyroid, lung, breast, and kidney. Adrenal metastases are common in lung cancer. Experiments using repeated animal passage have enabled researchers to select clones of human cancer cells that selectively metastasize to specific sites.

3. Metastasis in body cavities (seeding)–Entry of malignant cells into body cavities (eg, pleura, peritoneum, or pericardium) or the subarachnoid space may be followed by dissemination of the cells anywhere within these cavities (transcoelomic metastasis); eg, the rectovesical pouch and ovary are common locations for peritoneal metastasis in patients with gastric cancer.

Cytologic examination of the fluid from these body cavities for the presence of malignant cells is an excellent method of confirming the diagnosis of metastasis.

4. Dormancy of metastases–Cancerous cells that spread to distant sites may remain dormant there (or at least remain slowly growing and undetectable), sometimes for many years. The presence of such dormant cancerous cells (or slowly growing subclinical metastases) has led to attempts to eradicate them by means of systemic chemother-

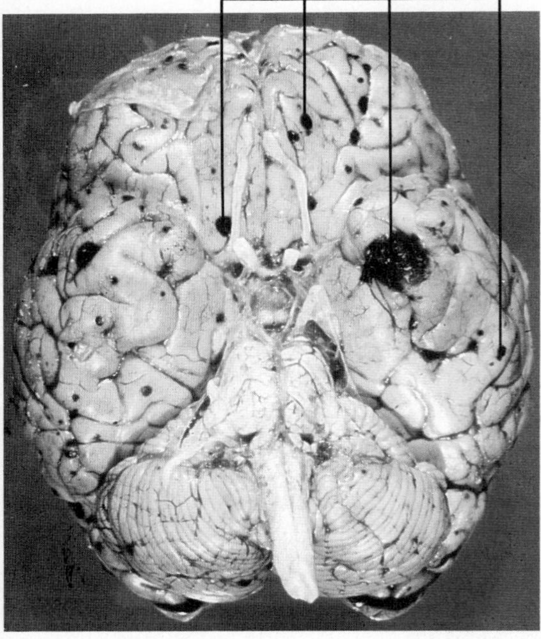

Figure 19–11. Hematogenous metastasis to the brain by a malignant melanoma, showing multiple pigmented tumor deposits.

apy after treatment of the primary tumor. Such adjuvant chemotherapy has not improved cure rates for most types of cancer.

Development of delayed metastases makes it difficult to pronounce a patient cured with any confidence. Survival for 5 years after treatment is considered a sign of cure for most cancers. However, 10- and 20-year survival rates are almost always lower than the 5-year survival rates, which suggests that many patients experience late metastases.

Disseminated metastases are incurable for the most part. However, recent advances in anticancer therapy have raised hopes of cure in a few types of disseminated cancer, including some leukemias, malignant lymphoma, choriocarcinoma, and testicular germ cell neoplasms.

Table 19–6 summarizes the properties of neoplasms.

EFFECTS OF NEOPLASIA ON THE HOST

Neoplasia may be the underlying cause of almost any sign or symptom anywhere in the body. Recognizing the ways in which neoplasms produce symptoms and signs is an important part of diagnosis.

Direct Effects of Local Growth of Primary Tumors

The signs and symptoms arising from local growth of a benign neoplasm or a primary malignant neoplasm vary with the site of the lesion, the nature of the surrounding anatomic structures, and the overall rate of growth of the neoplasm. The growing tumor may compress or destroy adjacent structures, cause inflammation, pain, vascular changes, and varying degrees of functional deficits (Table 19–7).

If the tumor is growing near a vital structure (eg, the brain stem), such local effects may be lethal, and it does not matter whether the neoplasm is benign or malignant.

Neoplasms growing in a confined area, eg, the cranial cavity, form space-occupying lesions that are associated not only with local compressive effects but also with a general—and potentially lethal—increase in intracranial pressure.

Table 19–6. Summary of properties of neoplasms.

Usually produce mass lesions (leukemia is an exception).
Grow steadily, though rate varies with different neoplasms.
Display variable degree of autonomy (some still partially hormone-dependent, eg, breast cancer and estrogen).
Mimic structure of cell or tissue of origin.[1]
Mimic function of cell or tissue of origin.[2]
Mimic antigenic properties of progenitor cell (but may lose antigens or gain new ones).
May induce immune response, but this does not prevent continued neoplastic growth.
Induce growth of supporting stroma and blood vessels.
Invade and metastasize (malignant neoplasms only).
Cause disease through compression, destruction, and distant effects (see Tables 19–7 and 19–8).

[1]Degree of mimicry of structure is termed differentiation.
[2]Mimicry of function includes production of immunoglobulin by myeloma cells (plasma cell neoplasm) and production of hormones by endocrine neoplasms. Malignant neoplasms often lose function (eg, ability to produce hormone) or gain function (eg, ability to produce inappropriate or ectopic hormone [see Tables 19–3 and 19–4]).

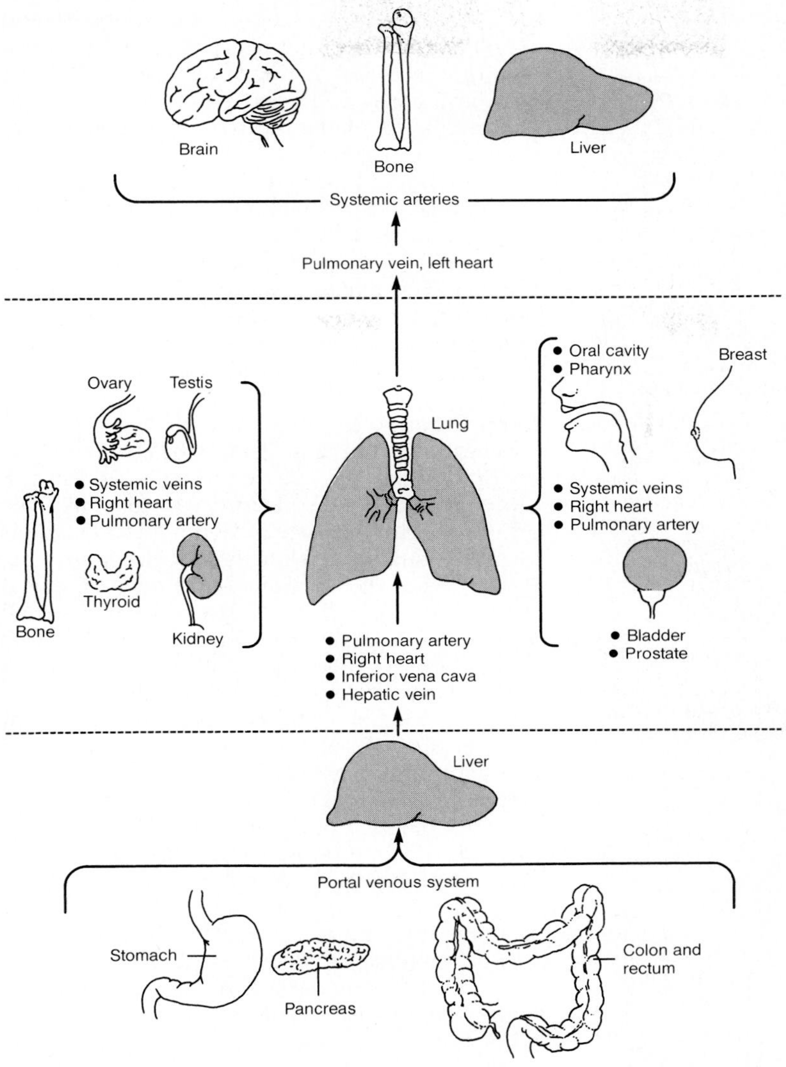

Figure 19–12. Principal anatomic routes of hematogenous metastasis. Primary neoplasms in the gastrointestinal tract and pancreas metastasize via the portal venous system to the liver. Other neoplasms tend to involve the lungs via the systemic circulation. Malignant cells may bypass the liver and lungs and enter the systemic circulation and produce metastases in any organ in the body. The systemic organs such as brain, bone, and liver are the common sites of metastasis of lung cancer.

Direct Effects of Growth of Metastases

Metastatic deposits form growing tumors that may compress and destroy adjacent tissues in the same way that a primary lesion does. The effects associated with a primary lesion are the direct result of the actions of the tumor on a single site in the body, however, whereas in metastatic disease, more than one metastasis may be present and a multiplicity of effects may occur.

Paraneoplastic (Nonmetastatic) Syndromes

Cancer may also cause various signs and symptoms distant from the primary lesion that are unassociated with metastases; these effects are termed paraneoplastic (or nonmetastatic) syndromes. Some syndromes are attributable to the production of biologically active substances by the tumor cells, including hormones by endocrine tumors, ectopic hormones by tumors of other tissues, and immunoglobulins by certain neoplasms derived from B lymphocytes (see Chapter 30). Other syndromes are less readily explained (Table 19–8). Suggested mechanisms include autoimmune phenomena, the formation of soluble immune complexes, and secretion of substances not yet characterized.

Certain paraneoplastic syndromes are so characteristic of a specific cancer that their presence should prompt a thorough investigation for the existence of the underlying cancer (eg, myasthenia gravis—thymoma; acanthosis nigricans—gastric cancer).

Table 19-7. Local effects of tumor.

Local Effect	Result
Mass	Presentation as tissue lump or tumor
Ulcer (nonhealing)	Destruction of epithelial surfaces (eg, stomach, colon, mouth, bronchus)
Hemorrhage	From ulcerated area or eroded vessel
Pain	Any site with sensory nerve endings; tumors in brain and many viscera are initially painless
Seizures	Tumor mass in brain; seizure pattern often localizes the tumor
Cerebral dysfunction	Wide variety of deficits depending on site of tumor
Obstruction	Of hollow viscera by tumor in the wall; bronchial obstruction leads to pneumonia; obstruction of bile ducts causes jaundice
Perforation	Of ulcer in viscera; in bowel may produce peritonitis
Bone destruction	Pathologic fracture, collapse of bone
Inflammation	Of serosal surface, pleural effusion, pericardial effusion, ascites
Space-occupying lesion	Raised intracranial pressure in brain neoplasms; anemia due to displacement of hematopoietic cells by metastases to the bone marrow
Localized loss of sensory or motor function	Compression or destruction of nerve or nerve trunk; classic example is involvement of recurrent laryngeal nerve by lung or thyroid cancer, with resulting hoarseness
Edema	Due to venous or lymphatic obstruction

APPROACH TO CANCER DIAGNOSIS

Clinical Suspicion

The diagnosis of cancer is particularly difficult because of its protean manifestations. Clinicians must therefore entertain the possibility that a neoplasm is the cause of symptoms in any patient in whom the diagnosis is not obvious.

A thorough clinical history is the essential first step in diagnosis. This includes a family history (for genetic predisposition or disorders associated with a high cancer rate), social history (eg, smoking), occupational history (eg, shipyard worker, miner), diet and geographic origin (eg, smoked fish, aflatoxin, high incidence of hepatitis B), and sexual and childbearing history (eg, nuns have a high rate of breast cancer, in contrast to women who have borne and breast-fed several children; and carcinoma of the cervix is more common in women who begin sexual activity at an early age and have many different partners). A complete history takes into account all of the possible causative factors as well as all of the possible effects of neoplasia for a particular patient.

Physical examination is directed toward finding localizing symptoms or signs and thereby discovering a mass lesion that may be sampled by biopsy or aspiration for a histologic diagnosis.

Early Diagnosis

When symptoms and signs associated with cancer first appear, the disease is usually already at a fairly advanced stage. In order to maximize the chances of cure, routine (screening) examinations of asymptomatic individuals may be performed. Routine cytologic screening in the form of annual cervical smears (Papanicolaou smears) in all women age 35 years and over constitutes the best example of this screening technique. These smears of exfoliated cells are a way to rapidly detect dysplastic epithelium, which can be treated to prevent development of cervical cancer. Routine use of cervical smears has resulted in a dramatically decreased incidence of cervical cancer in the screened population. Unfortunately, screening methods do not exist for most other types of cancer. In an attempt to detect cancer at an earlier stage, public education campaigns have been mounted that encourage women to examine their breasts monthly to detect small lumps and to undergo mammography to detect preclinical breast cancer. Furthermore, all people age 50 years and older are being encouraged to undergo sigmoidoscopy every 3–5 years after 2 negative examinations 1 year apart to detect early cancer or precancerous adenomas of the colon and rectum.

Apart from these screening approaches, any hemorrhage (rectal bleeding, hematuria), lump (breast lump, a mole that changes in size or color), a wound that fails to heal, or any unexplained feeling of ill health must be investigated with the possibility of cancer in mind. Cancer is still often not diagnosed until the disease is far advanced. The prognosis is worse for almost all cancers when widespread dissemination has occurred (see Fig 19–14).

Cytologic Diagnosis

Cytologic examination of cells is a useful and accurate method of diagnosing cancer. Samples for cytologic examination may be obtained by a variety of techniques.

(1) Exfoliated cells from a contiguous malignant neoplasm—eg, lung and bladder cancer and leukemic involvement of the meninges—can be

Table 19-8. Distant effects of tumors and paraneoplastic syndromes.

Clinical Effect	Causative Factors
Various hormonal effects, eg, hypoglycemia, Cushing's syndrome, gynecomastia, hypertension	Hormone produced by endocrine tumors; so-called "ectopic" hormones produced by nonendocrine neoplasms (see Tables 19-3 and 19-4).
Anemia	Chronic blood loss or unknown toxic effects cause iron deficiency type. Replacement of marrow by tumor causes leukoerythroblastic type (see Chapter 24). Thymoma may be associated with spontaneous aplastic (hypoplastic) type; such anemia may also be iatrogenic. Autoantibodies (especially from lymphoma) cause hemolytic type. Fragmentation of erythrocytes in abnormal vessels of neoplasms.
Immunodeficiency	Lymphoma especially.
Hyperviscosity syndrome, Waldenström's macroglobulinemia, Raynaud's phenomenon	Monoclonal immunoglobulin (usually IgM) from lymphoma or myeloma (see Chapter 30).
Purpura	Various causes, usually decreased platelets due to marrow involvement or effects of therapy; decreased levels of coagulation factors, especially if liver is extensively involved.
Acanthosis nigricans	Thirty percent of cases are associated with visceral carcinoma (especially of the stomach); cause is unknown.
Dermatomyositis	In adults, 50% of cases are associated with underlying cancer; mechanism is unknown.
Pruritus	Hodgkin's disease (mechanism unknown); any tumor with obstructive jaundice.
Disseminated intravascular coagulation	Widespread cancer (probably due to release of thromboplastic substances by dying tumor cells; (see Chapter 27).
Polycythemia	Renal cancer, hepatoma, uterine myoma, and cerebellar hemangioblastoma; in some instances due to erythropoietin-like substance produced by tumor.
Gout	Hyperuricemia due to excess nucleic acid turnover; may be precipitated by cytotoxic therapy.
Myasthenia gravis, myasthenic (Eaton-Lambert) syndrome	Thymoma especially; autoantibodies (see Chapter 66); other tumors; mechanism unknown.
Clubbing of fingers and hypertrophic pulmonary osteoarthropathy	Lung cancer and other intrathoracic neoplasms especially; mechanism unknown.
Peripheral neuropathy (sensory and motor)	Various cancers.
Myopathy (especially of proximal muscles)	Mechanism unknown.
Cerebral and cerebellar degeneration	Lung and breast cancer; mechanism unknown.
Migratory thrombophlebitis (especially in leg veins)	Carcinoma of stomach, pancreas, lung, and other organs; release of thromboplastins by necrotic tumor.
"Marantic" (nonbacterial thrombotic) endocarditis	Various cancers (see Chapter 22); mechanism unknown.
Hypercalcemia	Parathryoid hormone (including ectopic production), release of calcium from lysed bone (metastases), or lytic factors (as in myeloma).
Cachexia, hypoalbuminemia, fever	Advanced cancer; possible autoimmune, toxic, and nutritional mechanisms.

identified in samples of sputum, urine, cerebrospinal fluid, and body fluids. Recognition of malignant cells in blood (as in the leukemias) or bone marrow smears (leukemias, myeloma, metastatic carcinoma) is based upon similar cytologic principles.

(2) Brushing or scraping of epithelium or of a lesion that has been visualized by endoscopy (bronchoscopy, gastroscopy, colposcopy) may be performed to obtain cells for examination. Papanicolaou smears of the cervix are included in this group (see Fig 16–9).

(3) A fine (22-gauge) needle can be passed into virtually any location to aspirate material directly from a mass lesion (fine-needle aspiration). Cells obtained are smeared on slides for cytologic examination. Radiologic techniques such as CT scan and ultrasonography may help guide the needle into the mass.

Cytologic diagnosis is remarkably accurate

when performed by a trained pathologist. However, considerable experience is required to distinguish between malignant cells and cells showing cytologic abnormalities associated with regeneration, repair, metaplasia, inflammation, or some vitamin deficiencies (particularly folate). The increasing use of immunoperoxidase techniques (see below) has improved the reliability of cell and tumor identification. The general rule that cytologic diagnosis must be confirmed by histologic diagnosis before radical treatment is undertaken has been modified as confidence in cytologic and immunohistochemical techniques has grown. In many centers, radical surgery is undertaken on the basis of positive results on fine-needle aspiration for carcinomas such as those of the breast, pancreas, and thyroid.

Histologic Diagnosis

Histologic diagnosis is considered the definitive method of establishing the diagnosis of a neoplasm. A trained pathologist with an adequate specimen can provide an accurate diagnosis in most cases; in some instances, the histologic features alone do not permit conclusive diagnosis, and ancillary techniques such as immunohistology, special stains, and electron microscopy are necessary (Table 19–9). The diagnosis may be based on examination of the entire neoplasm removed at surgery (excisional biopsy) or examina-

Table 19–9. Common special stains.

Stain	Material Demonstrated	Clinical Usefulness
Histochemical		
Reticulin stain	Reticulin framework	Pattern in carcinoma differs from that of lymphoma or sarcoma.
Fontana stain	Melanin	Most melanomas are positive.
Trichrome, phosphotungstic acid-hematoxylin (PTAH)	Myofibers, glial fibers	Tumors of muscle origin, glial neoplasms.
Periodic acid-Schiff (PAS) after diastase digestion; mucicarmine	Epithelial mucin	Adenocarcinomas are positive.
Grimelius' silver stain	Argentaffin granules	Carcinoid tumors are positive.
Immunoperoxidase		
Antibodies to keratins	Keratin intermediate filaments	Present in epithelial cells only, including carcinomas.
Antibody to vimentin	Vimentin intermediate filaments	Present in mesenchymal cells, including sarcomas.
Antibody to carcinoembryonic antigen	Carcinoembryonic antigen	Present in many carcinomas, especially of colon and gastrointestinal tract.
Antibody to α-fetoprotein	α-Fetoprotein	Most hepatomas and some germ cell tumors are positive.
Antibody to prostatic acid phosphatase	Acid phosphatase specific to the prostate	Stains only prostatic epithelium, including metastatic prostatic cancer.
Antibodies to immunoglobulins	Light or heavy chain depending on the antibody	Stains certain B cell lymphomas and multiple myeloma; monoclonal pattern identifies neoplastic process.
Antibody to glial fibrillary acidic protein	Glial fibrillary acidic protein (intermediate filament)	Stains only astrocytes, ependymal cells, and their tumors.
Antibody to common leukocyte antigen	Antigen common to all lymphoid cells	Present in most lymphomas.
Antibody to human chorionic gonadotropins (hCG)	Intracellular chorionic gonadotropin	Trophoblastic neoplasms, germ cell neoplasms, some lung cancers.
Antibody to thyroglobulin	Thyroglobulin in cells	Well-differentiated thyroid carcinoma is positive.
Antibodies to chromogranin and neuron-specific enolase	Granules containing these substances	Marker for neuroendocrine neoplasms, some lung cancers.
Antibody to desmin, myoglobin	Desmin intermediate filament, myoglobin	Cells of muscle origin are positive.
Antibody to S100 protein	S100 protein	Present in melanoma, cells of neural origin, and chondrocytes.

tion of a sample of the neoplasm obtained either by incisional biopsy or with a large-bore cutting needle.

A. Techniques:

1. Frozen section method-Tissue sections are prepared from tissue quickly frozen at the time of surgery. This technique has the advantage of providing information while the patient is still on the operating table (often within 15 minutes). Speed is invaluable when information such as the histologic diagnosis of the tumor, its extent of lymph node involvement, or neoplastic infiltration of the margins of resection of the tumor is needed for surgical decision making. The major disadvantage of this method is that the cytologic details in the preparation are poor, and the diagnosis is less accurate than when processed tissue (paraffin sections) is used.

2. Paraffin section method-Small blocks of formalin-fixed tissue are dehydrated and embedded in paraffin to provide a rigid matrix for cutting sections; this process takes about 24 hours. Such permanent sections provide the best material for microscopic diagnosis. Hematoxylin and eosin (H&E) stain is the standard stain for these sections; the hematoxylin stains the nuclei blue, and the eosin stains cytoplasm and extracellular material pink. If the diagnosis is not immediately apparent, special stains may be needed (Table 19–9). Histochemical stains rely upon chemical differences in various tissues. They include silver stains to display the reticulin framework of the tissue or to stain melanin (in a melanoma) and the PAS (periodic acid-Schiff) stain to test for mucin, such as might be found in an adenocarcinoma.

3. Immunoperoxidase techniques-Immunohistochemical stains are a more recent innovation. They use specific labeled antibodies—usually horseradish peroxidase—to identify marker antigens in cells and tissues (Table 19–9). When the peroxidase reacts with a substrate, it produces a colored product that identifies the location of the antigen in the tissues. This method is analogous to the use of fluorescent labeled antibody method but gives better results on paraffin sections (Fig 19–13).

4. Electron microscopy-Electron microscopy can be performed on paraffin sections, but results are poor. Special fixation (in glutaraldehyde) and processing are required for optimal results. Ultrastructural features visible on electron microscopy are useful in recognizing many types of neoplasms, eg, anaplastic squamous carcinoma, melanoma, endocrine tumors, and muscle cell tumors.

B. Information Provided by Pathologic Diagnosis:

1. Type of neoplasm-The name of the neoplasm will be given in the pathology report.

2. Biologic behavior-The pathology report will state whether the neoplasm is benign or malignant if that information is not implicit in the name of the neoplasm. When histologic examination cannot predict the biologic behavior of the neoplasm, such a statement will be provided.

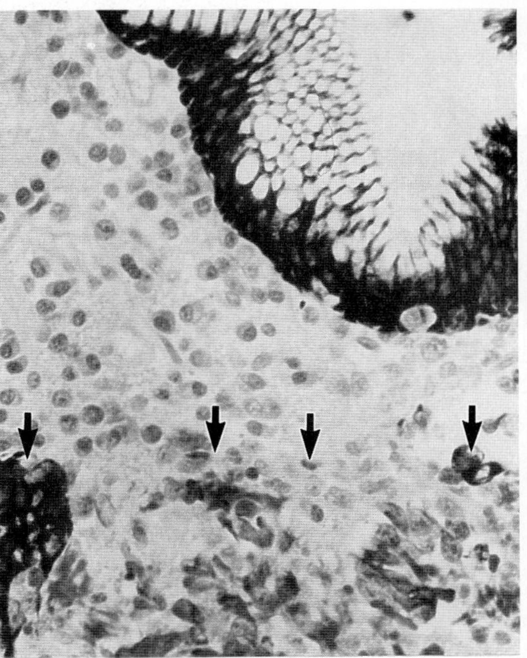

Figure 19–13. Immunohistochemical stain for keratin intermediate filaments used to diagnose a neoplasm of the stomach as a carcinoma. The surface epithelium stains positively for keratin as do malignant cells in the mucosa (arrows). These malignant cells could not be classified as lymphoid or epithelial by routine microscopy but were identified as carcinoma by positive keratin staining. Note that all cells of epithelial origin stain positively for keratin intermediate filaments.

3. Histologic grade-The histologic grade of a malignant neoplasm describes the degree of differentiation of the neoplasm, expressed either in words (eg, well, moderately, or poorly differentiated adenocarcinoma) or in numbers (eg, grade I, II, or III transitional cell carcinoma of the bladder—grade I being the least and III the most malignant). Highly specific criteria exist for histologic grading of many tumors. The histologic grade has significant implications for prognosis, metastasis, and survival.

4. Degree of invasion and spread-This information is vital in planning treatment of some neoplasms; eg, in malignant melanoma of the skin, the treatment is based on the depth of infiltration (see Chapter 61). In bladder neoplasms, it is imperative to state whether or not muscle invasion has occurred in the biopsy specimen.

5. Pathologic stage-The pathologic stage describes the extent of spread of a neoplasm. In a specimen obtained during resection, the pathologic stage is determined by the extent of infiltration and metastasis (eg, depth of invasion of the wall of a viscus, lymph node involvement). Pathologic staging is important because it determines what further treatment a patient may be given, and it is a valuable guide to prognosis. Criteria for pathologic staging vary with different neoplasms and different organs. An attempt to standardize pathologic staging is the so-called TNM classification, which classifies neoplasms on the basis of size of the primary tumor (T), lymph node involvement (N), and distant metastases (M).

Serologic Diagnosis

Theoretically, it may be possible to diagnose cancer by detecting cancer cell products in the serum, whether these be molecules secreted by malignant cells or antigens released by periodic death of such cells. No general serologic screening methods exist for cancer, but several tests are of value for certain tumors (Table 19–10).

Radiologic Diagnosis

Radiologic techniques, including CT and MRI scans, are invaluable for localizing masses as part of the primary diagnosis or for staging tumors. Occasionally, radiologic findings are so characteristic that they suggest a particular type of tumor; eg, multiple lytic lesions in the skull are typical of plasma cell myeloma, and a bone tumor with lytic areas with radial new bone formation strongly suggest osteosarcoma. As a general rule, radiologic findings suggestive of cancer must be confirmed by either cytologic or histologic examination of biopsy material before treatment can be started.

Table 19–10. Serologic assays for cancer diagnosis or follow-up.

Substance in Serum	Cancer Type
Carcinoembryonic antigen (CEA)	Gastrointestinal tract cancer (especially colon), breast and lung cancer; elevated levels in some noncancerous states.
α-Fetoprotein (AFP)	Hepatoma, yolk sac tumors.
Human chorionic gonadotropin (hCG)	Greatly elevated in choriocarcinoma; rarely elevated in other neoplasms.
Prostatic acid phosphatase; prostate-specific epithelial antigen	Two separate molecules; levels of both are elevated in metastatic prostatic cancer.
Monoclonal immunoglobulin	Myeloma, some B cell lymphomas.
Specific hormones	Endocrine neoplasms and "ectopic" hormone-producing tumors.
CA 125	Ovarian carcinoma; other neoplasms.

TREATMENT OF NEOPLASMS

The purpose of accurate diagnosis of the specific tumor type is to enable the clinician to select an appropriate mode of therapy. Even with the best treatment, survival rates vary greatly for different types of neoplasms (Fig 19–14).

Surgery

A. Benign Neoplasms: Surgical removal is curative. In a few cases, surgical removal may be difficult because of the location, eg, choroid plexus papillomas in the third ventricle.

B. Malignant Neoplasms:

1. Wide local excision–Surgical treatment of malignant neoplasms is more difficult, since they tend to infiltrate tissues. Local excision requires careful pathologic examination (including frozen sections as required) of the margins of resection to ensure complete removal. For low-grade malignant neoplasms, wide local excision is frequently sufficient for cure. Incomplete removal leads to local recurrence.

2. Lymph node removal–Malignant neoplasms with a high risk of early lymphatic metastasis are often treated by removal not only of the affected tissue but also of the lymph node group of primary drainage (radical surgery); eg, in radical mastectomy, the axillary lymph nodes are dissected and removed with the breast. Often a large mass of tissue around the lymph nodes must be removed. Radical mastectomy is curative in over 70% of cases of breast carcinoma if the primary tumor is small and if axillary lymph nodes are free of tumor at surgery. With large neoplasms or those that involve axillary lymph nodes, the cure rate achieved by radical mastectomy falls sharply.

3. Surgery for metastatic disease–Surgery was long held to be of little or no value in the treatment of metastatic disease. The rationale for this belief was that if one metastasis was present, others were probably present as well and would become clinically apparent later. In this situation, surgical removal of metastases would not improve survival. However, it is now apparent that removal of solitary or limited numbers of metastases in lung and liver from many neoplasms (sarcomas; colon, renal, and testicular cancers) can improve survival rates if combined with effective chemotherapy. In such cases, removal of metastases reduces tumor bulk, thereby enhancing the effect of chemotherapy and amplifying any residual immune response.

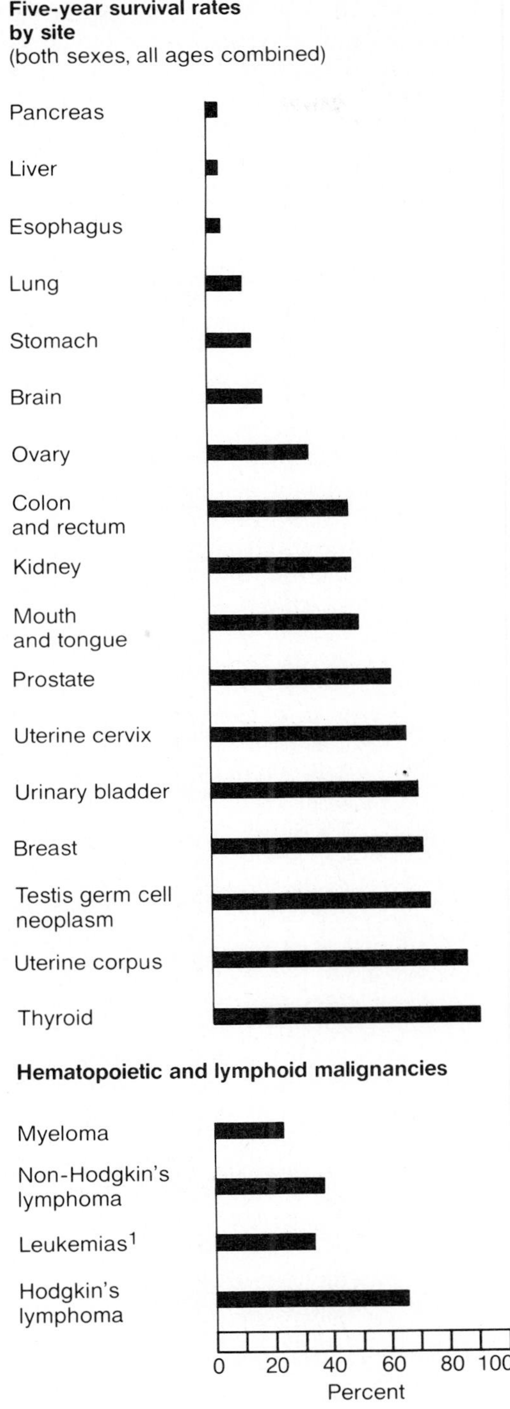

Figure 19–14. Five-year survival rates by site (both sexes, all ages combined). The rates given are the overall rates for the site and have been adjusted to include only deaths caused by the cancer. Within each site, there are different types of cancer that have greatly different survival rates. **Note:** Survival rates differ greatly for different types of leukemia (see Chapter 26).

4. **Palliative surgery**–Surgery also plays an important role in palliation of symptoms by relieving pain and restoring function in patients with incurable cancer. For example, surgical decompression of the spinal cord is performed when vertebral metastases threaten to cause paraplegia, and surgery may be used to bypass an obstructed esophagus and permit swallowing.

Radiation Therapy

Many malignant neoplasms are sensitive to radiation. In general, the more primitive and the more rapidly growing the neoplasm, the more likely it is to be radiosensitive; however, sensitivity is not synonymous with cure. The effect of radiation in a given neoplasm can be predicted on the basis of past experience with radiation therapy in similar neoplasms (see Chapter 11).

Radiation is rarely used as the sole method of treatment with cure as the objective. Its use as a main treatment is limited to therapy of radiosensitive malignant neoplasms that cannot be surgically removed, eg, those located deep in the brain such as pineal germinoma.

Radiotherapy is often used as an adjunct to surgery and is sometimes used postoperatively to remove any residual tumor cells and decrease the risk of local recurrence. Radiotherapy is also used as a palliative treatment for neoplasms that are too extensive for surgical removal.

Chemotherapy

Advances in cancer chemotherapy have greatly improved the outlook for many patients with cancer. Choriocarcinoma and testicular germ cell neoplasms—which were formerly associated with high mortality rates—are now successfully treated with drugs. Chemotherapy is the treatment of choice for many other neoplasms such as malignant lymphoma and leukemia. Chemotherapy improves survival rates when used in conjunction with surgery in breast and lung carcinoma.

Anticancer drugs act in one of several ways: (1) by interfering with cell metabolism and RNA or protein synthesis (antimetabolites); (2) by blocking DNA replication and mitotic division (antimitotic agents); or (3) by exerting hormonal effects, eg, estrogens in prostate carcinoma and antiestrogenic agents such as tamoxifen in breast carcinoma.

Immunotherapy

Immunotherapy as cancer treatment has been disappointing. Attempts to stimulate the immune system with adjuvants such as BCG have met with limited success. (Enhanced survival has been described in some melanoma patients.) Interferon and interleukin-2 (see Chapter 4) are still under investigation as treatments for such cancers as Kaposi's sarcoma, malignant melanoma, and lymphoma but clearly do not have the spectacular effects many researchers hoped for.

More specific immunotherapy using monoclonal antibodies developed against tumor-associated antigens has been used in the treatment of malignant melanoma, lymphoma, and some carcinomas but is still largely experimental. One promising approach uses the antibody to carry cytotoxic drugs, toxins, or radioisotopes to the tumor site.

Section V. The Cardiovascular System

Atherosclerotic arterial disease (Chapter 20), which is responsible for ischemic disease of the myocardium (Chapter 23), brain, and other organs, is the major cause of death in developed countries, and accounts for over 40% of all deaths in the USA. The consequences of arterial narrowing and thrombosis have been considered in Chapter 9, a brief review of which may be beneficial at this stage. Hypertension (Chapter 20) affects an estimated 25 million adult Americans.

Congenital heart diseases are considered in Chapter 21. Although the incidence has declined with decreased prevalence of rubella as a result of immunization (Chapter 15), other teratogenic factors are continually being identified as placing the fetus at risk. Current incidence of significant congenital heart disease is about 25,000 per year in the USA. The incidence of rheumatic heart disease (Chapter 22) is also decreasing, in this case due to a general decline in streptococcal infections in developed countries. However, over 1 million Americans suffer from chronic rheumatic valvular disease. This population of patients with chronic valvular disease, the use of prosthetic valve replacements, and intravenous drug abuse are associated with infective endocarditis (Chapter 22), which is the most significant infectious disease of the heart. Primary neoplasms of the heart are rare, the only common neoplasm being the cardiac myxoma (Chapter 22).

Cardiac transplantation is still considered experimental though there is an increasing tendency to use transplants for irreparable congenital diseases and primary myocardial diseases (cardiomyopathies - Chapter 23). Transplantation is not discussed in this section, and the reader should refer to Chapter 8.

20 The Blood Vessels

- Structure and Function
- Diseases of Blood Vessels
  - Congenital Disorders
    - Coarctation of the Aorta
    - Marfan's Syndrome
    - Other Inherited Disorders of Connective Tissue
    - Congenital (Berry) Aneurysms
  - Degenerative Vascular Disorders
    - Atherosclerosis
    - Systemic hypertension
    - Medial Calcification (Monckeberg's Sclerosis)
    - Aortic Dissection (Dissecting Aneurysm of the Aorta)
    - Varicose veins
  - Inflammatory Diseases of Blood Vessels
    - Syphilitic Aortitis
    - Takayasu's Disease
    - Giant Cell Arteritis (Temporal Arteritis)
    - Polyarteritis Nodosa
    - Wegener's Granulomatosis
    - Small Vessel Vasculitis
    - Thrombophlebitis
    - Lymphangitis
  - Neoplasms of Vessels

STRUCTURE & FUNCTION

The Systemic Circulation

The systemic circulation supplies arterial blood to the tissues; it begins at the aortic valve and ends with the openings of the venae cavae into the right atrium. Its component vessels and their function may be described as follows:

Elastic arteries—the aorta and its major branches—convert the spasmodic left ventricular output to a more continuous flow distally.

Muscular arteries—the internal carotid, coronary, brachial, femoral, renal and mesenteric arteries—distribute blood to the tissues.

Arterioles—by definition, arteries less than 2 mm in diameter—have muscular walls and a rich sympathetic nerve supply that permits adjustment of luminal size. Arterioles regulate the pressure decrease from aortic to capillary levels (Fig 20–1). Adjustment of resistance within the arterioles is a major factor determining systemic blood pressure and distribution of flow.

The **microcirculation** consists of capillaries, precapillary sphincters and postcapillary venules and is the site of exchange with the tissue fluids.

Veins are low pressure capacitance vessels that return blood to the heart. Forward flow in the veins is facilitated by endothelial valves.

The Pulmonary Circulation

The main function of the pulmonary circulation is to effect respiratory gas exchange in the pulmonary capillary bed; it begins at the pulmonary valve and ends in the left atrial openings.

The pulmonary circulation is at low pressure (25/10 mm Hg). Since this is lower than the plasma osmotic pressure, there is normally no fluid movement out of the alveolar capillaries, permitting the alveoli to remain dry for effective gas exchange.

The Portal Circulations

Portal circulations within the systemic circulation interpose a second capillary bed to subserve a specific function. The **hepatic portal circulation** delivers intestinal and splenic blood to the liver, giving that organ first access to substances absorbed from the intestine. A minor portal circulation in the **pituitary stalk** transports releasing hormones from the hypothalamus to the anterior pituitary gland.

The Lymphatic Circulation

Lymphatic vessels originate in the interstitial compartment of tissues and end in the opening of the thoracic duct into the jugular vein. Their main function is to transport large molecules and excess fluid from the interstitium back into the blood. Lymphatic vessels have thin walls with endothelial valves spaced at intervals that promote central flow; the lymphatic system operates under very low pressure.

Interspersed in the lymphatic system are the lymph nodes, which represent the immune system of the body (Chapter 4).

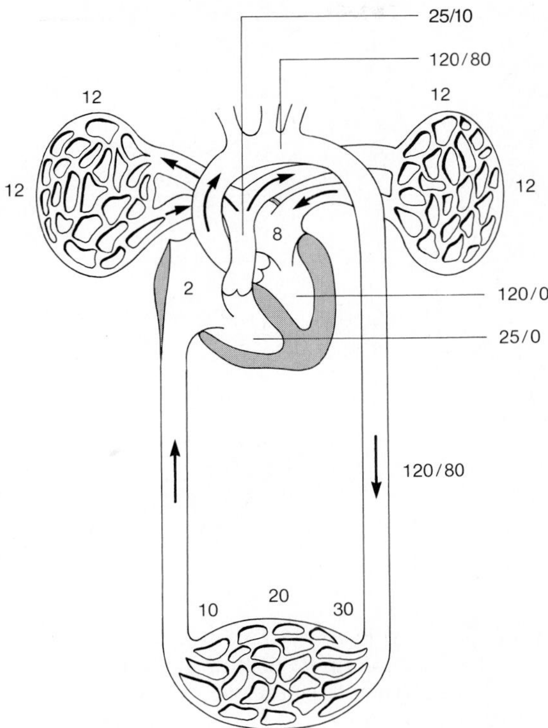

Figure 20-1. Blood pressures (mm Hg) in the pulmonary and systemic circulation.

Vascular Endothelium

The endothelium is a simple, flat layer of cells that lines the internal surface of the entire vascular system. Intercellular junctions represent "pores" through which water and small molecules can pass in and out under hydrostatic and osmotic pressure (Chapter 2). Contraction of the endothelial cells can adjust the size of these pores, permitting active control of capillary permeability, in the allergic and inflammatory responses. Luminal blood is also the source of nutrition for the walls of small vessels and the inner walls of large arteries. The outer layers of the walls of larger arteries are supplied by small arterioles in the adventitia (vasa vasorum).

The vascular endothelium synthesizes a large number of different substances, the most important of which are prostaglandins and coagulation factor VIII. Factor VIII is a useful marker for endothelial cells and can be demonstrated in tissue sections by immunohistologic techniques.

DISEASES OF BLOOD VESSELS (Table 20-1)

CONGENITAL DISORDERS

COARCTATION OF THE AORTA

Coarctation of the aorta is a congenital malformation characterized by narrowing of the vessel's lumen. Two distinct types are recognized.

Infantile (Preductal) Coarctation

Infantile coarctation of the aorta is a rare defect characterized by extreme narrowing of a segment of aorta proximal to the ductus arteriosus. The upper half of the body is supplied by the aorta proximal to the coarctation; the lower half is supplied from the pulmonary artery through a patent ductus arteriosus, producing cyanosis restricted to the lower part of the body. (Blood from the pulmonary artery is deoxygenated venous blood.) The defect is often fatal early in life unless corrected.

Adult Coarctation (Fig 20-2)

Adult coarctation of the aorta is a more common defect, seen oftener in males than in females. It is characterized by localized narrowing of the aorta immediately distal to the closed ductus arteriosus. It may be asymptomatic, the lower half of the body receiving an adequate blood supply

Table 20-1. Diseases of blood vessels.

Congenital diseases
Coarctation of the aorta
Marfan's syndrome
Congenital (berry) aneurysm
Degenerative diseases
Atherosclerosis
Hypertension
Medial calcification
Aortic dissection
Varicose veins
Inflammatory diseases
Syphilitic aortitis
Takayasu's aortitis
Giant cell arteritis
Polyarteritis nodosa
Wegener's granulomatosis
Thromboangiitis obliterans
Small vessel vasculitis
Neoplasms
Hemangioma, pyogenic granuloma, glomus tumor, lymphangioma
Angiosarcoma
Kaposi's sarcoma
Lymphangiosarcoma

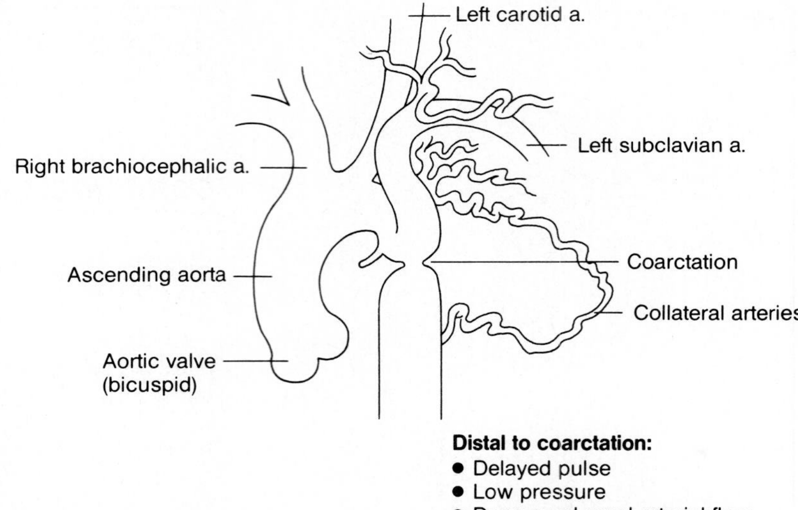

Figure 20–2. Adult type coarctation of the aorta. Decreased renal blood flow stimulates increased renin secretion, which is the main cause of hypertension.

through well developed collaterals. Coarctation of the aorta is common in patients with Turner's syndrome.

With severe adult coarctation, **ischemia** in the lower half of the body results in pain in the leg muscles during exercise (intermittent claudication) and **hypertension,** due mainly to decrease in renal blood flow, which stimulates the renin-angiotensin-aldosterone mechanism. Mechanical obstruction to aortic flow plays only a minor role in causing hypertension. Development of **collateral arteries,** mainly around the shoulder girdle, may be seen clinically or on x-rays. The circuitous passage of blood to the lower aorta through these collaterals causes the femoral pulse to be delayed and the blood pressure in the legs to be lower than that in the arms.

Coarctation of the aorta is frequently associated with **bicuspid aortic valve.** An important complication in patients with coarctation is **infective endocarditis** (Chapter 22) involving the abnormal aortic valve.

MARFAN'S SYNDROME

This rare single-gene autosomal dominant abnormality has a variable degree of expression. The exact biochemical defect is not known, but increased urinary excretion of hydroxyproline indicates high collagen turnover. Connective tissues all over the body are defective, but the most significant changes occur in the media of the aorta, which shows patchy replacement of muscle by myxomatous material. This medial degeneration causes weakness, with dilatation of the aortic root, leading to aortic valvular incompetence; and a tendency to aortic dissection (see below) and spontaneous rupture. Similar accumulation of myxomatous material in the mitral valve produces mitral valve prolapse syndrome, which may cause mitral incompetence.

Skeletal abnormalities such as increased height, arachnodactyly (thin, long, "spiderlike" fingers), and a high-arched palate are characteristic. Ligamentous abnormalities cause dislocation of the lens and hypermobile joints. Abraham Lincoln is believed to have had Marfan's syndrome. Clinically, most patients with Marfan's syndrome are asymptomatic. Athletes with Marfan's syndrome who undergo severe physical stress are prone to develop aortic dissection and rupture, which may cause sudden death.

OTHER INHERITED DISORDERS OF CONNECTIVE TISSUE

Other rare inherited diseases in which there is defective connective tissue formation include **Ehlers-Danlos syndrome, pseudoxanthoma elasticum, osteogenesis imperfecta,** and the **mucopolysaccharidoses**—all associated with aortic medial degeneration and weakening, predisposing to aortic root dilatation and aortic rupture.

CONGENITAL (BERRY) ANEURYSMS

"Congenital" aneurysms occur in small muscular arteries, such as the cerebral, renal, and splenic arteries, particularly at points of bifurcation. They are most commonly found in the circle of Willis (Fig 20–3), where their rupture causes sub-

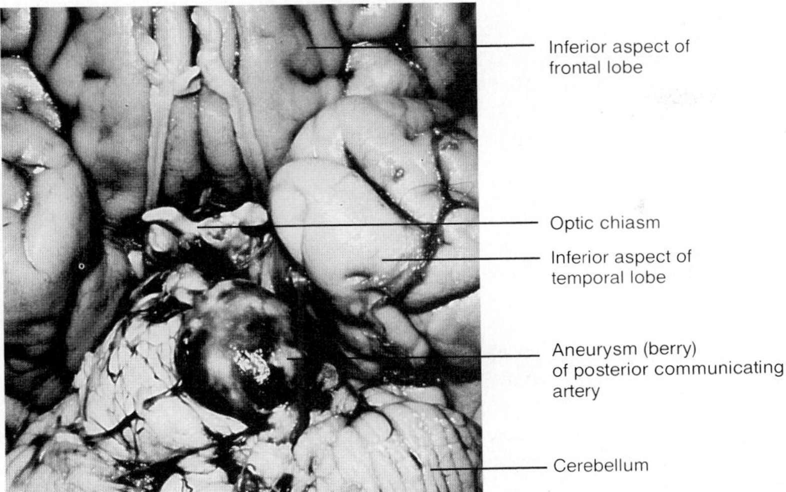

Figure 20-3. Berry aneurysm of the circle of Willis at the base of the brain.

arachnoid hemorrhage (Chapter 64). Berry aneurysms are not truly congenital since they are not present at birth, but there is a congenital defect in the arterial media that permits development of the aneurysm in adult life. Rupture of such aneurysms is particularly apt to occur in hypertensive patients.

DEGENERATIVE VASCULAR DISORDERS

ATHEROSCLEROSIS*

Incidence

Atherosclerosis is the main cause of ischemic heart disease and cerebrovascular disease and the major primary cause of death in most developed countries. The incidence of deaths due to atherosclerotic arterial disease increased in the United States until about 1970, when it leveled off; and since 1975 it has declined. The cause of this highly desirable trend is uncertain, though it is probably related to changes in diet and exercise habits.

In most developed countries, some degree of atherosclerosis is almost invariably present in the aorta and muscular arteries after middle age. The incidence and severity are generally less in underdeveloped countries.

*Atherosclerosis is thickening of the artery resulting from deposition of specific atheromatous lesions. "Arteriosclerosis" is a nonspecific term that denotes thickening and loss of elasticity ("hardening") of the arteries from any cause. Changes associated with aging and hypertension often lead to arteriosclerosis.

Etiology

Atherosclerosis is best regarded as a degenerative arterial disease characterized by deposition of complex lipids in the intima. Its cause is uncertain, though numerous risk factors have been identified, most importantly age, sex, hyperlipidemia, hypertension, and cigarette smoking (Table 20–2).

A. Hypertension: Hypertension is the strongest risk factor for atherosclerosis in older people. Ischemic heart disease is 5 times more common in a hypertensive individual (blood pressure > 160/95 mm Hg) than in one who is normotensive (blood pressure < 140/90 mm Hg). Diastolic hypertension imposes a greater risk than systolic hypertension.

B. Hyperlipidemia: Hyperlipidemia is the strongest risk factor for atherosclerotic arterial disease in patients under 45 years old. The risk exists with both hypercholesterolemia and hypertriglyceridemia (Table 20–3). In a patient under 45 years of age, a serum cholesterol level over 265 mg/dL is associated with a 5-fold increased risk compared with a level under 220 mg/dL. A serum cholesterol of less than 200 mg/dL is now considered desirable.

Low density lipoproteins (LDLs) and cholesterol levels correlate directly with the severity of atherosclerosis. Serum levels of cholesterol associated with high density lipoprotein (HDLs) correlate inversely; ie, a high serum HDL cholesterol level has a protective effect, while low HDL cholesterol levels increase the risk. Low HDL cholesterol levels are seen more commonly (1) in males than in females at all ages, (2) in cigarette smokers, (3) in patients with diabetes mellitus, and (4) in inactive individuals.

Intimal arterial deposition of lipid in the hyperlipidemias occurs mainly in type II, III, and IV

Table 20-2. Risk factors for atherosclerosis.

Age: Significant disease is rare under 30 years.

Sex: Males are affected more than females; female incidence increases after menopause; sex incidence is equal after age 75 years. Estrogens probably have a protective effect.

Hypertension: The major risk factor in patients over 45 years of age. Hypertensives have a 5-fold risk compared to normotensives.

Hyperlipidemia: The major risk factor in patients under 45 years. Both primary and secondary hyperlipidemias carry a 5-fold risk.

Low levels of HDL cholesterol: HDL cholesterol levels are low in males, people who do not exercise, smokers, and diabetics.

Cigarette smoking: One pack per day produces a 3-fold increased risk.

Diabetes mellitus: A risk factor independent of all others.

Lack of exercise: Incidence greater in persons in sedentary occupations; regular exercise (15 minutes at least twice weekly) decreases risk. Effect probably due to increase in serum HDL with exercise.

Obesity: An independent risk factor when the weight is more than 20% above normal for height and frame.

Type A personality (controversial): Aggressive, ambitious persons have an increased risk.

Inheritance: Probably a minor factor; familial tendency reflects common life-style and diet and inheritance of hypertension, hyperlipidemia, and diabetes mellitus.

hyperlipoproteinemias and produces a high risk of ischemic heart disease due to narrowing of the coronary arteries. Deposition of lipid in **macrophages in the skin** produces yellow plaques and nodules (xanthoma, xanthelasma). Deposition in **tendons** causes thickening and yellow discoloration (xanthoma tendinosum).

C. Cigarette Smoking: In individuals who smoke, ischemia resulting from arterial narrowing is aggravated by increased blood levels of carboxyhemoglobin, which reduces the total oxygen-carrying capacity of the blood.

D. Diabetes Mellitus: Diabetics have an increased risk of atherosclerotic vascular disease that is independent of other commonly associated factors such as hypertension and obesity. There is some evidence that rigid control of diabetes may reduce the risk.

Pathology

A. Atheromatous Plaque: (Figs 20–4 and 20–5.) The intimal plaque is the pathologic lesion that characterizes atherosclerosis.

1. Early lesion–The earliest recognizable change is the accumulation of complex lipids within smooth muscle cells in the intima of large vessels. These cells soon become disrupted, and the lipid is released to accumulate in the connective tissue of the intima. The lipid is composed mainly of cholesterol, with smaller amounts of triglyceride and phospholipid. Fibroblasts enter the

Table 20-3. Hyperlipidemic disorders.

Type	Elevated Lipoprotein	Serum		Plasma on Standing[1]	Familial Disease (Inherited)	Secondary
		Cholesterol	Triglyceride			
I	Chylomicrons	N	↑	Creamy	Lipoprotein lipase deficiency (autosomal recessive)	. . .
IIa	LDL	↑	N	Clear	Familial hypercholesterolemia (autosomal dominant; varies)	Hypothyroidism, nephrotic syndrome, dietary, diabetes mellitus
IIb	LDL plus VLDL	↑	↑	Usually clear	Familial mixed lipoproteinemia (autosomal dominant; varies)	
III	Beta-VLDL	↑	↑	Turbid	Familial dysbetalipoproteinemia (autosomal recessive)	Obstructive jaundice
IV	VLDL	N	↑	Clear or turbid	Familial triglyceridemia (variable)	Diabetes mellitus, alcoholism, dietary
V	Chylomicrons plus VLDL	N	↑	Creamy	Very rare	. . .

[1]On standing, the plasma normally clears. Chylomicrons are large particles and tend to stay on the surface without precipitating, producing a creamy supernatant. This is a simple test to detect lipoprotein abnormalities.
VLDL = very low density lipoproteins (high content of triglyceride).
LDL = low-density lipoproteins (high content of cholesterol).
N = normal serum level; normal levels are defined statistically for men and women, separately for different age groups.

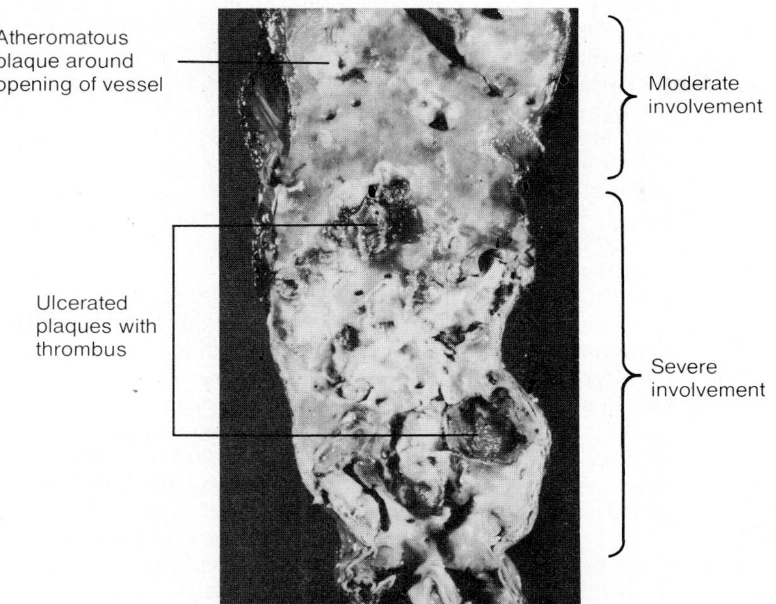

Figure 20-4. Severe atherosclerosis of the lower abdominal aorta. Note multiple areas of ulceration with adherent mural thrombus.

plaque at an early stage and lay down collagen, which becomes intimately admixed with the lipid.

The atheromatous plaque appears grossly as a flat yellow-white elevation on the intimal surface (Fig 20-4). It is covered by endothelium. When cut across, the center of the plaque consists of semisolid yellow lipid material. (The word "atheroma" is from the Greek word for porridge.) Microscopically, the well-formed plaque appears as a mass of palely eosinophilic debris in the intima in which needle-shaped cholesterol crystals are commonly seen (Fig 20-5). Collagen and smooth muscle cells may be present in varying amounts.

2. Distribution–The aorta is affected in most cases, with maximal change in the abdominal aorta (Fig 20-4). Involvement of muscular arteries such as the coronary, carotid, vertebrobasilar, mesenteric, renal, and iliofemoral arteries is com-

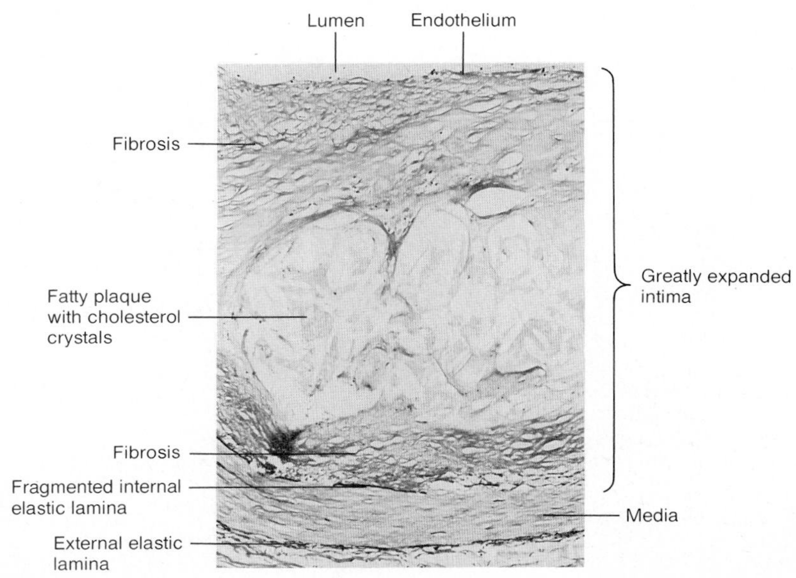

Figure 20-5. Atherosclerotic plaque. Low magnification.

mon and is responsible for many of the clinical manifestations. Plaques tend to be most prominent at points of branching of the major arteries.

3. Complications-(Fig 20–6.) **Thrombosis** is the most important complication of atherosclerosis, since it may cause complete occlusion of the artery. Thrombosis is caused by (1) slowing and turbulence of blood in the artery in the region of the plaque and (2) ulceration of the plaque.

Dystrophic calcification of the plaque is very common. Severely affected vessels (including the aorta) become converted to calcified tubes. Ulceration of the overlying endothelium may precipitate thrombosis overlying the plaque. **Ulceration** may also cause the lipid contents of the plaque to be discharged as **emboli** into the bloodstream (Chapter 9). **Vascularization** of the plaque may lead to hemorrhage into the plaque, which expands the plaque and may occlude the lumen of the artery. Hemorrhage may also precipitate ulceration and thrombosis.

Aneurysms may develop in vessels weakened by extensive plaque formation; the abdominal aorta is a favored site.

B. Fatty Streaks: Fatty streaks are thin, flat yellow streaks in the intima produced by lipid deposition in the cytoplasm of intimal mesenchymal cells. They occur maximally around the aortic valve ring and thoracic aorta. Fatty streaks occur very early in life, often in the first year, and are seen all over the world irrespective of sex, race or environment. They increase in number until about age 20 years and then decrease. It is most likely that fatty streaks are harmless and not related to atherosclerosis; the earlier view that they progress to atheromatous plaques is probably incorrect.

Pathogenesis

The mechanism of formation of atheromatous plaques is unknown. Theories advanced to explain their pathogenesis are not mutually exclusive.

A. Lipid Imbibition Theory: According to this theory, the primary cause of atherosclerosis is an abnormality in the endothelium that permits entry (1) of lipoproteins, which become deposited in the intima; and (2) of factors that stimulate smooth muscle proliferation (certain lipoproteins and platelet growth factors). This would explain why certain types of lipoproteins and not others are associated with a high risk of atherosclerosis.

Endothelial abnormalities may be due to injury from turbulence, which is maximal at points of arterial branching (the sites most commonly involved by atherosclerosis). High arterial blood

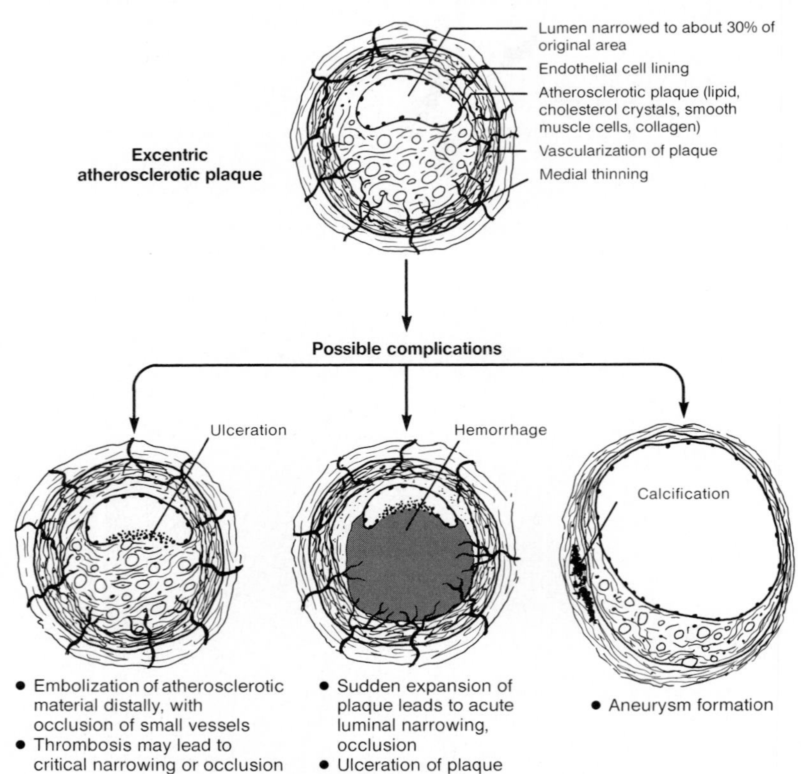

Figure 20–6. Complications of atherosclerosis.

pressure (hypertension) would aggravate this tendency to injury. Nicotine, carbon monoxide, and other factors that cause endothelial abnormalities have been identified in the serum of cigarette smokers.

B. Thrombus Encrustation Theory: An early theory held that endothelial injury resulted in formation of small thrombi that became incorporated into the intima by reendothelialization and organized, with subsequent lipid degeneration initiating plaque formation. It is unlikely that this is the primary mechanism, but it may contribute to enlargement of established lesions.

C. Monoclonal Hypothesis: The smooth muscle proliferation that occurs in the atheromatous plaque has been shown, by glucose-6-phosphate dehydrogenase isoenzyme studies, to be monoclonal, which means that all the cells of the lesion are derived from a single parent cell, somewhat in the manner of a neoplasm—though plaques do not behave as neoplasms in other ways. According to this theory, monoclonal smooth muscle proliferation is the critical event in the pathogenesis of atherosclerosis, and subsequent fatty degeneration is an inevitable change that may be aggravated by hyperlipidemia and physical forces causing endothelial injury. Various substances in the serum known to cause smooth muscle proliferation include endogenous lipoproteins and platelet factors and exogenous substances associated with cigarette smoking. While many different chemicals in cigarette smoke cause smooth muscle proliferation in vitro, the actual substance responsible in vivo has not been identified.

Clinical Features (Fig 20–7)

A. Narrowing of Affected Arteries: Ischemia from arterial narrowing is responsible for most of the clinical effects of atherosclerosis (Fig 20–8). A decrease in blood flow usually occurs only with

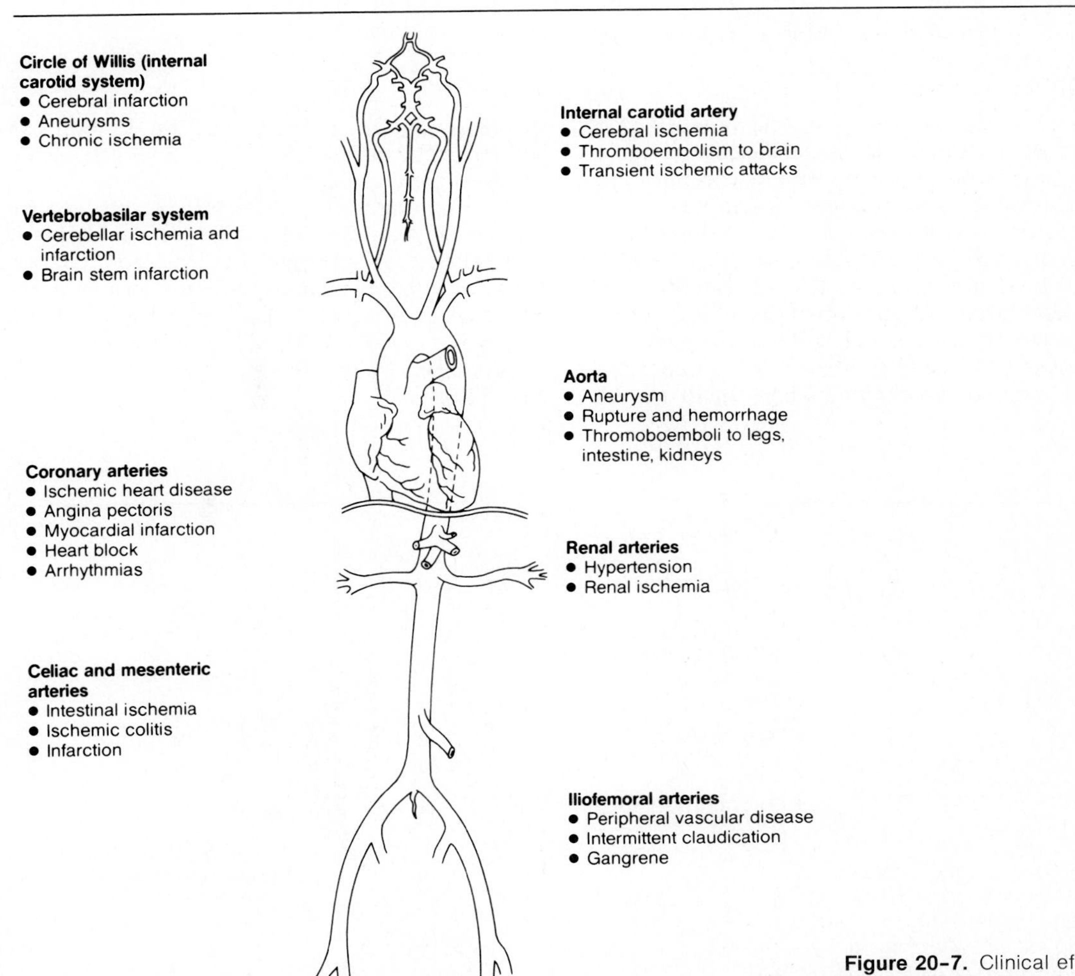

Figure 20–7. Clinical effects of atherosclerosis related to the major arteries involved.

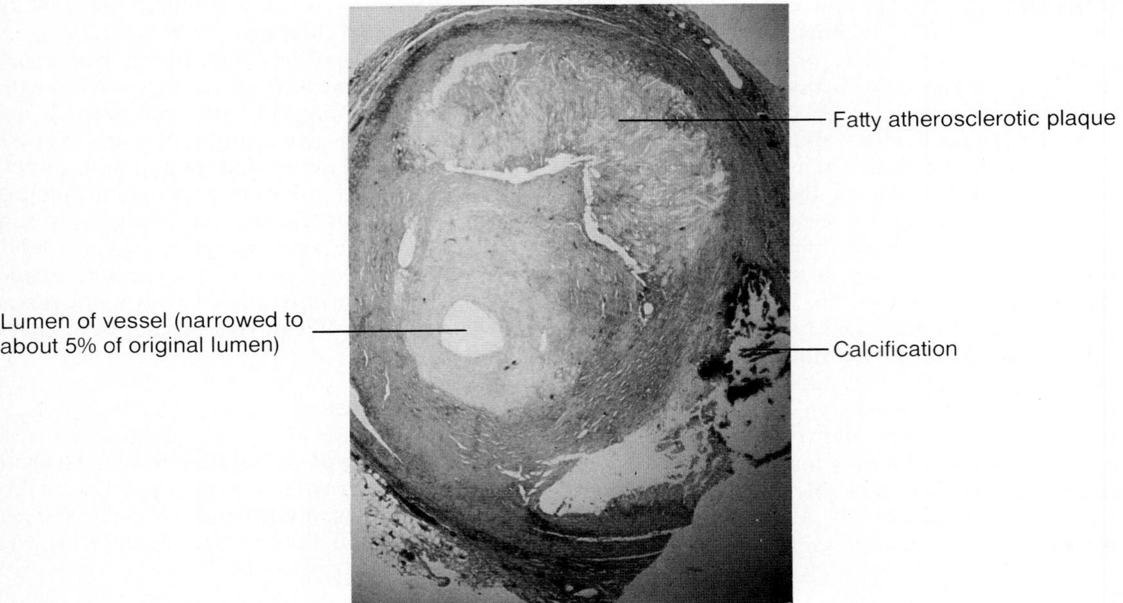

Figure 20-8. Coronary artery narrowing caused by atherosclerosis. Low magnification.

severe (> 70%) narrowing of the vessel. Aortic narrowing is almost never sufficient to cause symptoms. However, narrowing of coronary, cerebral, renal, mesenteric, and iliofemoral vessels often causes ischemic changes in the organs and tissues supplied. Superimposed thrombotic occlusion of these arteries may cause **infarction.**

B. Embolism: Ulceration of the atheromatous plaque may result in embolization of the lipid contents of the plaque (Fig 20-6). This is important in the cerebral circulation, where small emboli produce transient ischemic attacks. Emboli can sometimes be visualized in the retinal arteries on funduscopic examination.

C. Aneurysm: (Fig 20-9.) In severe atherosclerotic involvement of the aorta, the wall may be weakened to an extent that leads to dilatation or aneurysm formation. Atherosclerotic aneurysms occur mainly in the lower abdominal aorta and may appear as a fusiform dilatation of the whole vessel circumference or a saccular bulge on one side of it.

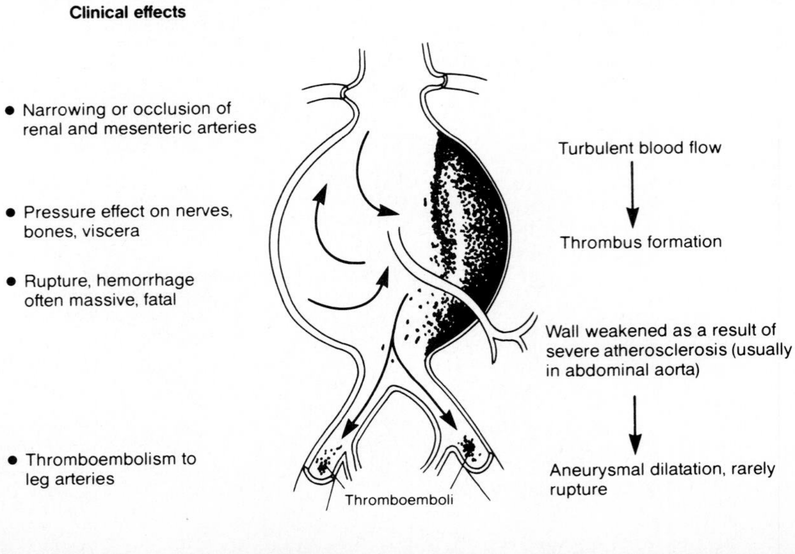

Figure 20-9. Clinical effects of an atherosclerotic aneurysm of the abdominal aorta. This is now the commonest type of aortic aneurysm and has superseded syphilitic aneurysms which involved the thoracic aorta.

SYSTEMIC HYPERTENSION

Hypertension is defined as sustained elevation of systemic arterial blood pressure. While the concept is clear, the exact pressure that constitutes hypertension is an arbitrary determination. Normal blood pressure is defined statistically and varies with age and sex (Fig 20–10). A pressure under 140/90 mm Hg is considered normal, and 160/95 mm Hg is generally accepted as hypertensive. Pressures between 140 and 160 mm Hg systolic and 90–95 mm Hg diastolic are regarded as borderline. Diastolic pressure is a more reliable indicator of significant hypertension than systolic.

Incidence

About 15–20% of adults in the United States have blood pressures over 160/95 mm Hg. These individuals have increased mortality rates, related mainly to the associated atherosclerotic arterial disease.

Etiology & Pathogenesis (Fig 20–11)

A. Essential Hypertension: Essential hypertension occurs as a primary phenomenon without known cause. It is the commonest type of hypertension, usually occurring after age 40 years, with a familial incidence suggestive of polygenic inheritance upon which environmental factors are superimposed.

The pathogenesis is uncertain. No constant changes have been identified in plasma levels of renin, aldosterone, or catecholamines—or in the activity of the sympathetic nervous system or baroreceptors—that could account for the elevated blood pressure.

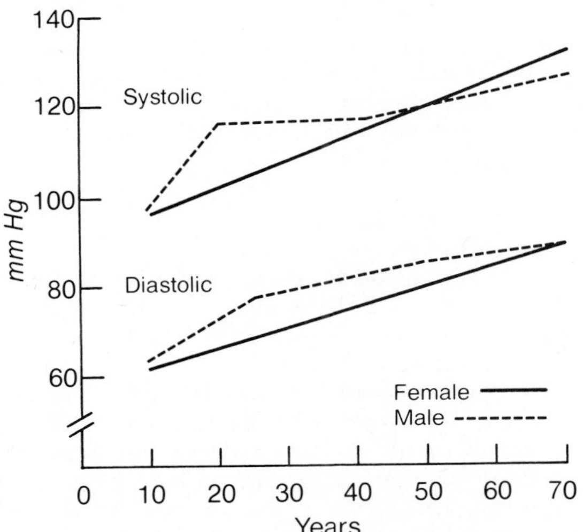

Figure 20–10. Variation in mean normal blood pressure with age in males and females.

The currently favored theory is that essential hypertension is due to high dietary intake of sodium in a genetically predisposed individual. There may be associated failure of excretion by the kidney in the face of a prolonged high sodium load. Sodium and water retention results in an increase in plasma volume, cardiac output and peripheral resistance. Associated risk factors include stress, obesity, cigarette smoking, alcohol consumption and environmental factors such as hardness of water; all of these appear to be minor factors. Age, race, and sex differences produce significant statistical variation in the prevalence of hypertension (Table 20–4).

B. Secondary Hypertension: Secondary hypertension is that due to a preceding defined disease process (Table 20–5). Even though an underlying cause can be identified in less than 10% of cases of hypertension, this group is important because many of the diseases can be treated. Secondary hypertension must be strongly suspected in a patient under 40 years of age who develops hypertension. Sodium retention is the usual mechanism of secondary hypertension and may occur in any of the following circumstances (Fig 20–11).

1. Decreased glomerular filtration–As in acute glomerulonephritis, chronic renal failure, and coarctation of the aorta.

2. Increased secretion of renin–As in renal artery stenosis, coarctation of the aorta, accelerated hypertension, and rarely with renal neoplasms that secrete renin, such as benign neoplasms of the juxtaglomerular apparatus and rare cases of renal adenocarcinoma. Renin stimulates aldosterone secretion by the adrenal cortex (secondary aldosteronism).

3. Increased secretion of mineralocorticoids–This occurs independently of renin secretion with aldosterone-secreting adrenal neoplasms **(Conn's syndrome)** or with excess cortisol production in **Cushing's syndrome**. High plasma levels of cortisol result in sodium retention. In 11-hydroxylase deficiency (congenital adrenal hyper-

Table 20–4. Percentage prevalence of hypertension in USA.[1]

	Black		White	
	Male	Female	Male	Female
< 25 years	5	5	5	1
25–44 years	35	25	15	10
45–64 years	45	50	25	25
> 65 years	50	60	35	40

[1]Hypertension is defined here as sustained systolic blood pressure > 160 mm Hg or diastolic pressure > 95 mm Hg.

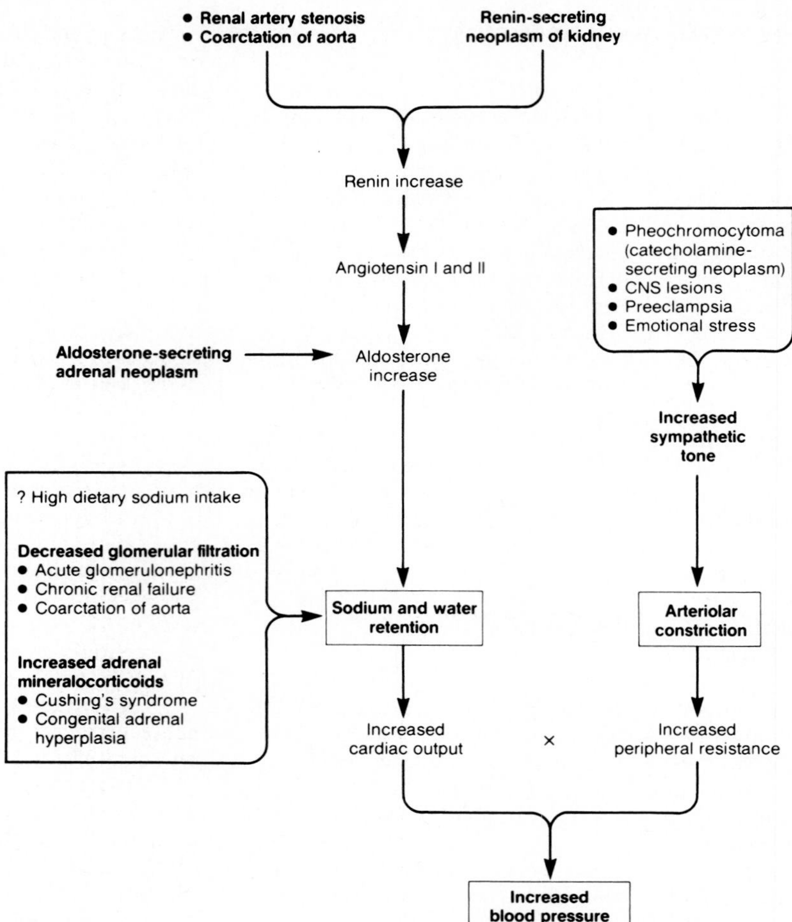

Figure 20–11. Factors involved in the pathogenesis of hypertension. Note that more than one of the factors listed may operate in a given patient.

plasia), abnormal mineralocorticoids accumulate leading to sodium retention.

4. Increased sodium intake with reduced sodium excretion–Hypertension in chronic renal failure is the result of failure of renal control of sodium balance and is directly related to sodium intake in these patients.

Pathology

A. Benign Hypertension: In the earliest phase of hypertension, vasoconstriction is produced by smooth muscle contraction and there are no microscopic changes in blood vessels. Following sustained vasoconstriction, there is thickening of the media due to muscle hypertrophy, progressing to hyaline degeneration and intimal fibrosis. These changes are known as hyaline arteriolosclerosis and are found with long standing hypertension of mild to moderate degree **(“benign” hypertension)**. The tissues supplied by affected vessels may show changes of chronic ischemia.

B. Malignant Hypertension: The accelerated (“malignant”) phase of hypertension is characterized by very severe hypertension (diastolic pressure > 110 mm Hg) and **fibrinoid necrosis** of the media with marked intimal fibrosis and extreme narrowing of the arteriole (Fig. 20–12). The tissues supplied by affected vessels show acute ischemia with microinfarcts and hemorrhages. Accelerated hypertension is frequently associated with elevated serum renin levels, establishing a vicious cycle that tends toward further elevation of the blood pressure.

Clinical Features (Table 20–6)

A. Early Hypertension: The early phase of hypertension is asymptomatic and the diagnosis can be made only by detecting the elevation of blood pressure.

B. Hypertensive Heart Disease: Systemic hypertension results in increased work for the left ventricular muscle, which undergoes hypertrophy, thereby maintaining cardiac output. With severe hypertension, particularly in the accelerated phase, left ventricular failure occurs.

Hypertension is a major risk factor for coronary atherosclerosis and ischemic heart disease.

Table 20-5. Etiology and classification of hypertension.

Essential (primary) hypertension

Secondary hypertension
- Renal diseases
  - Renal vascular diseases
    - Renal artery stenosis (atherosclerosis, fibromuscular hyperplasia, posttransplantation)
    - Arteritis, polyarteritis nodosa
    - Renal artery embolism
  - Renal parenchymal diseases
    - Acute glomerulonephritis
    - Chronic glomerulonephritis
    - Chronic pyelonephritis
    - Polycystic disease of the kidney
  - Renal neoplasms
    - Juxtaglomerular apparatus neoplasm
    - Renal carcinoma
    - Wilms' tumor
- Endocrine diseases
  - Pheochromocytoma
  - Primary aldosteronism (Conn's syndrome)
  - Cushing's syndrome
  - Congential adrenal hyperplasia due to 11-hydroxylase deficiency
- Coarctation of the aorta
- Drug-induced hypertension
  - Corticosteroids
  - Amphetamine use
  - Chronic licorice ingestion[1]
  - Oral contraceptives
- Neurologic diseases
  - Raised intracranial pressure
  - ?Psychogenic
- Hypercalcemia

[1]Licorice has an aldosteronelike effect ("pseudoaldosteronism").

Table 20-6. Clinical features and diagnosis of hypertension.

Clinical features
- Asymptomatic
- Headache: occipital, throbbing, early morning
- Heart disease
  - Left ventricular hypertrophy
  - Left ventricular failure[1]
  - Atherosclerotic ischemic heart disease: angina, myocardial infarction[1]
- Renal disease
  - Chronic renal failure
  - Rapidly progressive renal failure (malignant nephrosclerosis)[1]
- Cerebral disease
  - Atherosclerotic cerebral thrombosis and infarction[1]
  - Cerebral hemorrhage[1]
  - Hypertensive encephalopathy
- Visual disturbances (hypertensive retinopathy)

Diagnosis
- Blood pressure measurement
- Funduscopic examination (see Fig 20-13)
- Electrocardiography (evidence of left ventricular hypertrophy)
- Laboratory tests
  - Serum urea and creatinine (elevated in renal disease)
  - Serum electrolytes (low serum K^+ in aldosteronism)
  - Urinalysis (red cells and protein in renal disease)
  - Serum catecholamines and urinary metanephrine (pheochromocytoma)
  - Plasma cortisol and urinary 17-hydroxycorticosteroids (Cushing's disease)
  - Serum aldosterone and renin levels
- Angiography, urography (evidence of renal disease, neoplasms)
- Renal biopsy

[1]Common causes of death in hypertensives.

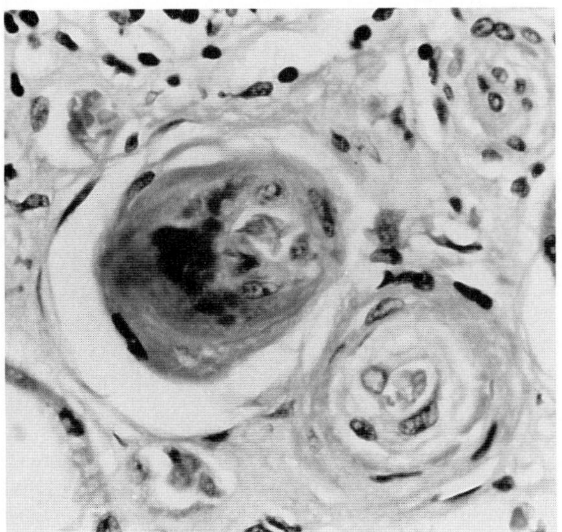

Figure 20-12. Vascular changes in malignant hypertension. The arteriole in the center shows fibrinoid necrosis, which appears as a dark area in the media, with marked luminal narrowing. The adjacent arteriole shows concentric intimal fibrosis. High magnification.

Ischemia is aggravated by the increased oxygen demand of the hypertrophied myocardium.

C. Hypertensive Renal Disease: Changes in renal arterioles occur in most cases of hypertension, resulting in decreased glomerular filtration, progressive fibrosis, and loss of nephrons in the kidneys. Renal ischemia resulting from these changes sets up a vicious cycle (falling glomerular filtration rate, renin release, angiotensin production, salt retention) that aggravates the hypertension.

Renal failure with elevation of serum creatinine usually occurs only in patients with accelerated hypertension. Fibrinoid necrosis is present in renal arterioles (Fig 20–12). Hematuria occurs, and marked reduction in glomerular filtration rate may progress to acute renal failure.

D. Hypertensive Cerebral Disease: Hypertensive patients have a greatly increased incidence of cerebrovascular disease, both thrombosis and hemorrhage ("strokes"). Cerebral thrombosis is the result of atherosclerosis; cerebral hemorrhages result from rupture of microaneurysms in small intracerebral perforating arteries.

Hypertensive encephalopathy is due to spasm of small arteries in the brain induced by very high blood pressures. The temporary spasm, though insufficient to cause infarction, leads to cerebral edema, which produces headache and transient cerebral dysfunction.

E. Hypertensive Retinal Disease: The retinal arterioles show all the changes of hypertension on funduscopic examination (hypertensive retinopathy). Narrow, irregular arteries with thickened walls characterize mild to moderate hypertension. Accelerated hypertension leads to retinal hemorrhages; fluffy exudates ("cotton wool spots")—ill-defined areas of edema, hemorrhage, and repair resulting from ischemia (Fig 20–13); and edema of the optic disk (papilledema).

Diagnosis (Table 20-6), Treatment, & Prognosis

The blood pressure should be measured several times over a period of several weeks to make certain that hypertension is sustained. It is important to look for clinical effects due to hypertension and for treatable causes, especially in patients under 40, since essential hypertension is uncommon in this age group.

When a treatable cause of hypertension such as renal artery stenosis or an adrenal neoplasm is present, surgery is curative. Patients with essential hypertension must receive lifelong antihypertensive drugs, which act by causing increased excretion of sodium and water by the kidneys (diuretics) and by decreasing peripheral resistance (sympathetic blocking agents). The prognosis for patients with essential hypertension depends on how well the blood pressure is controlled with these drugs. With modern effective drugs, the prognosis is good.

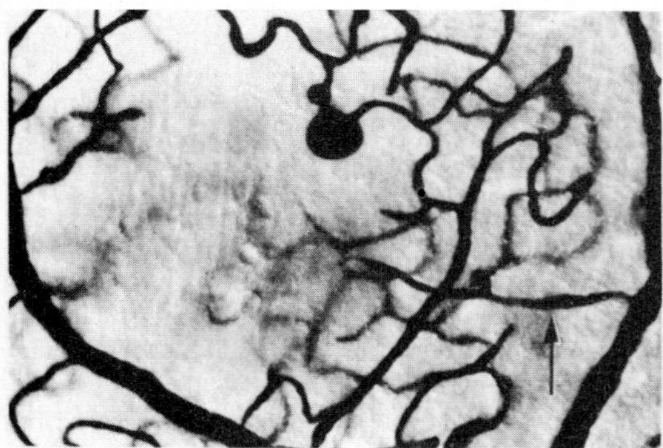

Figure 20–13. Retina of a patient with hypertensive retinopathy showing an exudate and failure of capillary filling in affected area. A microaneurysm is also present. (Injected with India ink; stained with oil red O; magnification × 90.) (Reproduced, with permission, from Ashton N: Pathophysiology of retinal cotton wool spots. Br Med Bull 1970;26:143.)

MEDIAL CALCIFICATION (Monckeberg's Sclerosis)

Medial calcification is a clinically unimportant but very common degenerative change affecting muscular arteries such as the femoral, radial, and uterine arteries. The tunica media shows extensive calcification. There is no luminal narrowing or endothelial damage. Medial calcification does not produce any clinical abnormality—it is seen in elderly people and is regarded as an aging change.

AORTIC DISSECTION (Dissecting Aneurysm of the Aorta)

Incidence & Etiology (Fig 20–14)

In aortic dissection, there is disruption of the media of the aorta by entry of blood under high pressure through an intimal tear. Dissection is usually preceded by a form of myxomatous degeneration of the media known as **Erdheim's cystic medial degeneration**. While this degenerative change is not uncommon, only a small proportion of patients develop dissection. **Hypertension** is an important factor, leading to rupture of the endothelium and intima and permitting entry of blood at high pressure into the weakened media.

Pathology

Aortic dissection is commonly associated with an intimal tear, usually just above the aortic valve or immediately distal to the ligamentum arteriosum. Blood enters the media at this intimal tear and dissects between the layers of smooth muscle in the media, particularly where weakened by cystic medial degeneration (Figs 20–14 and 20–15).

Cystic medial degeneration appears microscopically as ill defined mucoid lakes with associated patchy loss of elastin fibers and smooth muscle. Cystic medial degeneration and aortic dissection are much more common in patients with **Marfan's syndrome,** in whom there is primary deficiency of collagen synthesis.

Lathyrism is a similar condition induced experimentally in animals by feeding a diet of sweet peas. The high content of ß-aminopropionitriles in sweet peas interferes with collagen synthesis, causing myxomatous degeneration of the media.

Clinical Features

The clinical effects of aortic dissection depend upon its site and extent. Actual dissection of the media produces sudden severe pain, which is usually retrosternal and mimics the pain of myocardial infarction. Arteries taking origin from the aorta may become occluded, or rupture may occur leading to massive hemorrhage (Fig 20–14).

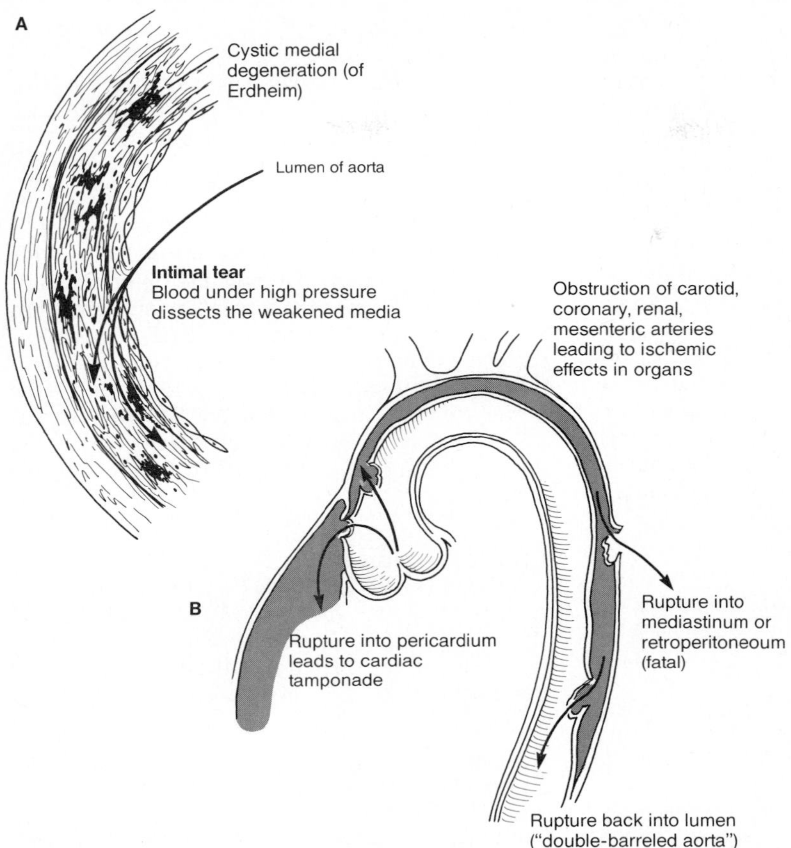

Figure 20-14. Aortic dissection. **A:** Mechanism of dissection, showing an intimal tear and blood under high pressure dissecting the media, which shows Erdheim's degeneration. **B:** Possible outcomes of aortic dissection. Shown here is a type I dissection that involves both ascending and descending aorta. Type II dissection, involves only the ascending aorta, and type III involves only the descending aorta.

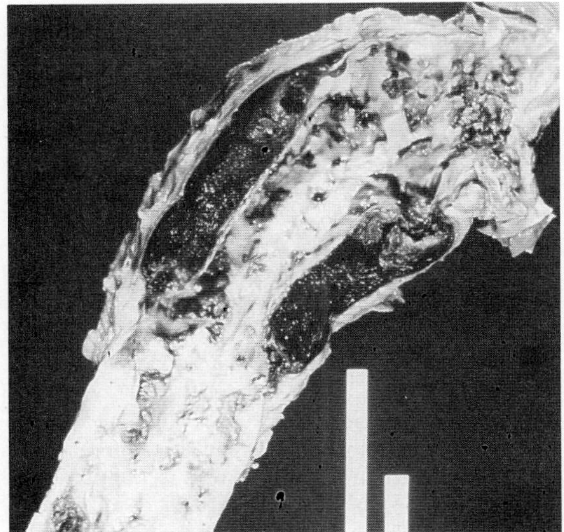

Figure 20-15. Aortic dissection, showing blood clot in the media.

VARICOSE VEINS

Abnormally dilated and tortuous veins occur in several sites—in the legs, rectum (hemorrhoids), esophagus (varices in portal hypertension), or spermatic cord (varicocele). They are associated with increased pressure in the affected vessels, obstruction to adequate venous drainage, or increased blood flow in the affected vessels.

Etiology

In the legs, varicose veins involve the superficial saphenous venous system and result (1) from obstruction to the deep veins of the leg, the superficial varicose veins representing the collateral venous drainage to the leg; and (2) from incompetence of the valves in the saphenous veins and in the perforating veins that normally prevent flow of blood from the deep to the superficial veins. The latter mechanism relating to valve incompetence is responsible for most cases of varicose veins. The cause of valve incompetence is unknown but is probably a degenerative phenomenon.

Clinical Features

Varicose veins are visible in the leg as markedly dilated tortuous veins (Fig 20–16) whose distribution depends upon which valves are competent. They are associated with obesity and pregnancy, and there may be a familial predisposition.

Varicose veins produce adverse cosmetic effects and chronic aching and swelling, and they serve as sites for recurrent thrombophlebitis, stasis dermatitis, and skin ulceration. Stasis ulcers typically occur in the region of the ankle.

Treatment

Treatment consists of surgical removal of the varicose superficial leg veins or, for small varices, local injection of sclerosing agents. Before such treatment is undertaken, deep venous occlusion must be excluded; otherwise, the venous drainage of the entire leg may be compromised.

INFLAMMATORY DISEASES OF BLOOD VESSELS

Inflammation of blood vessels (vasculitis) is a feature of many diseases (Table 20–7).

SYPHILITIC AORTITIS

Syphilitic aortitis occurs in the tertiary stage of syphilis, often many decades after the primary infection. The spirochete cannot be demonstrated in the lesions, and it has been suggested that immunologic hypersensitivity plays a part in pathogenesis.

Though syphilis remains a common disease, syphilitic aortitis has become rare today because of successful treatment of early syphilis.

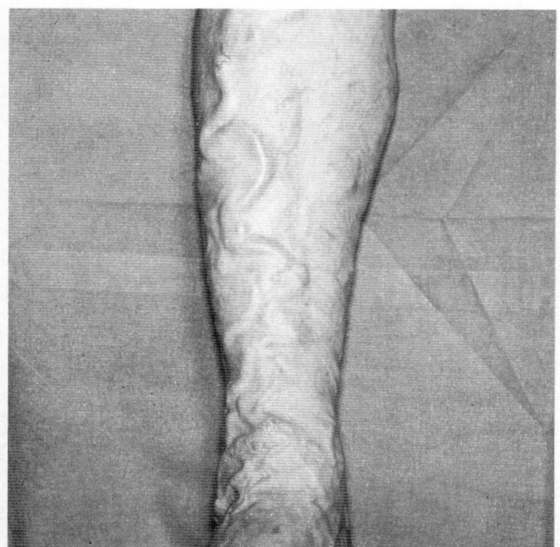

Figure 20–16. Varicose veins of the saphenous system.

Pathology (Fig 20–17)

The vasa vasorum, which normally provide blood supply to the adventitia and outer media of the aorta, are primarily involved by inflammation and luminal narrowing due to intimal fibrosis (endarteritis obliterans). Ischemia leads to degeneration and fibrosis of the outer two-thirds of the aortic media, which is supplied by the vasa vasorum. There is compensatory irregular fibrous thickening of the intima ("tree bark appearance").

Clinical Features

Weakening of the aortic wall causes (1) dilatation of the aortic root and aortic incompetence, (2) aneurysmal dilatation of the aorta, and (3) narrowing of the openings of the coronary arteries ("ostial stenosis"), causing myocardial ischemia.

TAKAYASU'S DISEASE

Takayasu's disease (also called occlusive thromboaortopathy, aortic arch syndrome, and pulseless disease) is a disease of unknown cause that is uncommon in the United States but has a relatively high incidence in Japan. Females are affected more often than males in a 9:1 ratio. About 90% of cases occur in people under 30 years of age.

Pathology

The disease process usually is restricted to the aortic arch, though in 30% of cases the whole aorta is involved and in 10% only the descending aorta.

Marked fibrosis involves all layers of the wall, causing narrowing and occlusion of arteries taking origin from the aorta. Microscopic examination shows infiltration of the media and adventitia by neutrophils and chronic inflammatory cells, particularly around the vasa vasorum. In a few cases, granulomas with giant cells are seen.

Clinical Features

Occlusion of the origin of the aortic arch vessels leads to loss of radial pulses and ischemic neurologic lesions. Ocular ischemia with visual impairment is typical. In cases that involve the descending aorta, involvement of renal arteries may lead to hypertension.

The course is variable and may end in death

Table 20-7. Classification of inflammatory vascular diseases.

Disease	Etiology	Vessels Involved	Usual Age Range
Syphilitic aortitis	*Treponema pallidum*	Vasa vasorum of aortic wall, small arteries of brain.	>40
Takayasu's aortitis	Unknown	Aorta	< 30
Giant cell arteritis	?Autoimmune	Scalp, shoulder, eye	> 50
Polyarteritis nodosa	?Immune complex	Muscular arteries	< 50
Wegener's granulomatosis	Immunologic	Nose, lung, kidney	> 50
Small vessel vasculitis	Immune complex	Arteriole (systemic)	Any
Thromboangiitis obliterans	Uncertain; associated with smoking	Lower extremity (arteries and veins)	< 50
Thrombophlebitis	Several factors	Veins	Any
Lymphangitis	Several factors	Lymphatics	Any

either in the acute phase or after several years of slowly progressive disease.

GIANT CELL ARTERITIS (Temporal Arteritis)

Giant cell arteritis is an uncommon disease, virtually confined to individuals over 50 years of age. The cause is uncertain. Type IV hypersensitivity against arterial wall antigens has been demonstrated in a few cases.

Pathology

Giant cell arteritis is so named because its microscopic features are dominated by granulomatous inflammation and the presence of numerous giant cells. Fragmentation of the internal elastic lamina is followed by fibrosis. Thrombosis may occur in the acute phase.

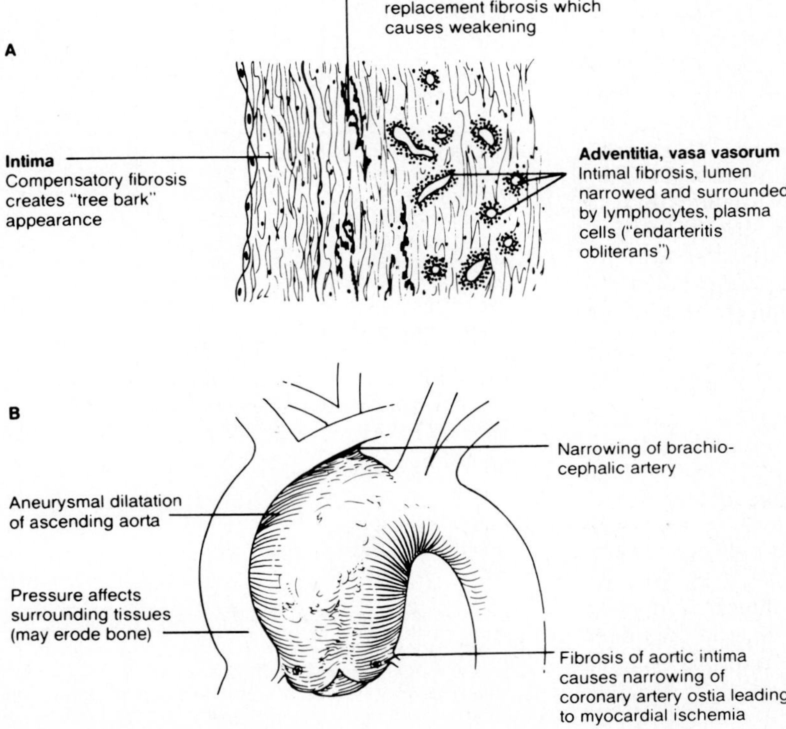

Figure 20-17. Pathologic changes of syphilitic aortitis. **A:** The inflammation in the vasa vasorum causes endarteritis obliterans, resulting in ischemic loss of smooth muscle in the media. **B:** The weakening of the media causes aneurysmal dilatation of the aorta, most commonly in the ascending thoracic aorta.

The inflammation affects medium-sized muscular arteries, with a predilection for the superficial temporal artery and intracranial arteries, including those supplying the retina.

Clinical Features

The most common clinical presentation is with "temporal arteritis," which causes severe headache associated with thickening and tenderness of the superficial temporal artery. Diagnosis is by biopsy of the artery; because involvement may be focal, it is important to attempt biopsy of tender inflamed segments. Elevation of the erythrocyte sedimentation rate, though not specific, is a useful diagnostic test.

Diagnosis followed by treatment with corticosteroids is important, because involvement of the retinal artery may cause permanent blindness. Cranial nerve paralyses may also occur.

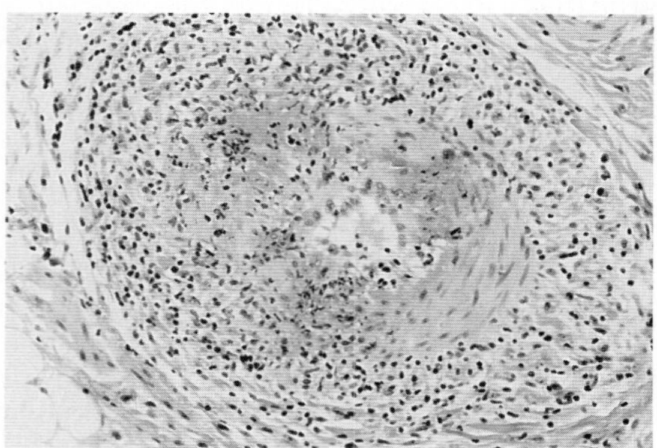

Figure 20-18. Polyarteritis nodosa, showing marked acute inflammation involving the entire thickness of a medium-sized artery. The media shows focal fibrinoid necrosis. Low magnification.

POLYARTERITIS NODOSA

Polyarteritis nodosa is an uncommon disease that occurs most frequently in young adults. Males are more frequently affected than females. The disorder is believed to be a type III immunologic hypersensitivity (immune complex) reaction. Hepatitis B surface antigen is present in the complexes in 30–40% of patients; the antigen involved in other cases is unknown.

Pathology

Medium-sized and small arteries throughout the body show characteristic segmental lesions consisting of nodular reddish swellings and multiple microaneurysms. Arterial rupture with tissue hemorrhages and thrombosis with tissue ischemia may occur in the acute phase. In the chronic phase, the involved artery is thickened by fibrosis.

Microscopic examination shows fibrinoid necrosis of the media and acute inflammation involving all layers (Fig 20–18). In the chronic phase, the artery shows less specific concentric fibrosis of the wall. A typical feature of polyarteritis is the coexistence of acute and chronic lesions at different sites.

Clinical Features

The usual course is progressive, with exacerbations and remissions. Without treatment, the 5-year survival rate is less than 20%; with steroid therapy, 50% of patients are alive after 5 years.

In the acute phase, patients develop fever, with variable signs and symptoms according to the pattern of organ involvement (Table 20–8).

Diagnosis of polyarteritis is clinical. Biopsy of acutely affected tissue such as muscle or kidney may provide histologic confirmation.

Table 20-8. Clinical and laboratory findings in polyarteritis nodosa.

	Percentage of Cases

Fever
Renal changes
  Microscopic hematuria
  Glomerulonephritis
Hypertension
	> 50

Skin rashes (nonspecific)
Arthritis and arthralgia
Neuropathy and mononeuritis, such as isolated cranial nerve palsy
Myalgia and myositis
Pulmonary changes[1]
  Hemoptysis
  Asthma
	30–50

CNS changes (nonspecific)
Cardiac changes
  Pericarditis
  Myocardial ischemia
Intestinal (ischemia)
  Abdominal pain
  Diarrhea
  Perforation
Hepatomegaly (painful)
	< 30

Hematologic abnormalities
  Anemia
  Leukocytosis and eosinophilia
  Thrombocytosis and thrombocytopenia
  Elevated erythrocyte sedimentation rate
	> 50

Serum abnormalities
  Hepatic B surface antigen
  Rheumatoid factor
  Cryoglobulins
  Decreased complement factor
	20–50

[1]Pulmonary changes do not occur in classic polyarteritis; they are seen in a variant form of the disease known as allergic granulomatosis and angiitis of Churg and Strauss.

WEGENER'S GRANULOMATOSIS

Wegener's granulomatosis is characterized by **necrotizing vasculitis,** similar to that seen in polyarteritis nodosa but with extensive extravascular necrosis and granulomatous reaction; and, in most cases, involvement of the lungs, nasopharynx, and kidney (glomerulonephritis). The course is rapidly progressive. The disease responds partially to immunosuppressive therapy, but the overall prognosis is poor. Wegener's granulomatosis is discussed in greater detail in Chapter 35.

THROMBOANGIITIS OBLITERANS (Buerger's Disease)

Thromboangiitis obliterans is rare in the United States and Europe but is a common cause of peripheral vascular disease in Israel, Japan, and India. The disease occurs most often in young men in the age group from 20 to 30 years and is largely restricted to heavy cigarette smokers. Exacerbations and remissions of the disease are closely related to changes in smoking habits. The mechanism by which smoking provokes the disease is unknown.

Pathology

Thromboangiitis obliterans is characterized by segmental involvement of small and medium-sized arteries, mainly in the lower extremities. The lesion frequently involves adjacent veins and nerves.

In the acute phase, there is marked swelling and neutrophilic infiltration of the entire neurovascular bundle. Thrombosis is common. Healing by fibrosis and organization of thrombi produces thick cordlike vessels with occluded lumens.

Clinical Features

Progressive ischemia of the lower limbs produces intermittent claudication, with pain in the calf muscles precipitated by exercise and relieved by rest. As the disease progresses, the amount of exercise necessary to produce pain (called the claudication distance) decreases, leading to progressively greater disability.

With severe disease, pain is present at rest along with trophic changes in the skin, culminating in dry gangrene.

The disease is progressive. Abstinence from smoking frequently results in remissions, but it is not uncommon for these patients to continue smoking cigarettes even as disease progresses to extreme disability and amputation of their limbs.

SMALL VESSEL VASCULITIS

Necrotizing vasculitis affecting small vessels occurs in a large number of different diseases, most of which are mediated by type III immune complex hypersensitivity (Table 20–9). Noninflammatory small vessel disease occurs in diabetes mellitus. (See Diabetic Microangiopathy, Chapter 46.)

Raynaud's disease is a distinct process of unknown cause characterized by small vessel spasm without anatomic abnormalities. **Raynaud's phenomenon,** which has similar clinical consequences, occurs as a secondary manifestation of many diseases in which small vessel vasculitis occurs. Both disorders are characterized by numbness and pallor or cyanosis of hands and feet in response to cold.

Pathology

The changes are similar to those seen in polyarteritis nodosa except that smaller arterioles are in-

Table 20–9. Diseases in which small vessel immune vasculitis is commonly present.

	Sites Involved	Antigen (Probable) in Immune Complex
Connective tissue diseases (Chapter 68)		
Systemic lupus erythematosus	Systemic	Nuclear antigens
Progressive systemic sclerosis	Skin, gut, lung, kidney	
Mixed connective tissue diseases	Systemic	
Mixed cryoglobulinemia	Systemic	Patient's IgG (the anti-IgG antibody is commonly IgM)
Henoch-Schönlein purpura	Skin, kidney, gut	Patient's IgA(?)
Drug hypersensitivity	Skin, other	Penicillin, sulfonamides, gold salts, antithyroid drugs, etc
Focal infective vasculitis, infective endocarditis	Skin, kidney, retina	Bacterial antigens
Erythema nodosum	Skin	Various (tuberculosis, sarcoidosis, acute rheumatic fever, fungal infections, leprosy, drugs)

volved. Fibrinoid necrosis of the arteriolar walls is accompanied by intense neutrophil infiltration of the vessels. Degeneration of neutrophils in the lesions causes lysis and fragmentation of nuclei (leukocytoclasia) and deposition of nuclear fragments ("nuclear dust") in and around the affected vessel. Thrombosis and hemorrhage are common. Immunoglobulin and complement can be demonstrated by immunologic techniques in these lesions.

Clinical Features

These diseases are characterized by involvement of multiple organs. Skin involvement leads to raised purpuric patches ("palpable purpura"). Renal involvement is associated with glomerulonephritis. Individual diseases are considered elsewhere.

THROMBOPHLEBITIS

Thrombophlebitis and phlebothrombosis have been discussed in Chapter 9. Two specific types of thrombophlebitis will be discussed briefly here.

Phlegmasia Alba Dolens (Painful White Leg)

This is a rare but specific type of deep leg vein thrombophlebitis that occurs during the later months of pregnancy. There is extreme swelling of the leg associated with severe pain, tenderness, and increased temperature. The cause is not known.

Migratory Thrombophlebitis

Episodic inflammation of superficial veins at multiple sites occurs in association with thromboangiitis obliterans or with carcinomas of internal organs such as the pancreas, stomach, lung, or colon. (This is called Trousseau's syndrome after the French physician who described it in himself. He died of pancreatic cancer.) The mechanism by which the neoplasm produces thrombophlebitis is unknown.

LYMPHANGITIS

Bacterial Lymphangitis

Lymphangitis commonly complicates bacterial infections of the skin, *Streptococcus pyogenes* being the commonest cause. The inflamed lymphatics appear as painful, red streaks, frequently associated with acute lymphadenitis.

Filarial Lymphangitis

Filarial lymphangitis is extremely common in the tropics and is caused by *Wuchereria bancrofti* and *Brugia malayi* transmitted by mosquitoes of the *Aedes* and *Culex* species. Microfilariae reaching the lymphatics mature into adult worms, and death of the worms causes acute lymphangitis. This is followed by fibrotic occlusion of the lymph channels, resulting in obstruction and chronic lymphedema (elephantiasis).

NEOPLASMS OF VESSELS

BENIGN NEOPLASMS

Hemangioma

Hemangiomas are common. About 70% are present at birth, which suggests that they may be hamartomas rather than true neoplasms. The skin, liver, and brain are common sites, but any organ may be involved. Hemangiomas are composed of well-formed vascular spaces lined by endothelial cells that show no cytologic atypia. They are classified as capillary hemangiomas, composed of vessels of capillary size; or cavernous hemangiomas, composed of large thin-walled vascular spaces.

Capillary hemangiomas are usually found in the skin and mucous membranes as small (< 1 cm), red to blue plaques or nodules. Most grow slowly with the growth of the individual. One specific type ("strawberry" hemangioma) grows rapidly during the first few months of life and then regresses (80% regress completely by 5 years).

Cavernous hemangiomas occur in skin as well as in the viscera, forming a soft spongy mass that may reach 2–3 cm in size. They grow slowly.

Hemangiomas in deep subcutaneous tissues and skeletal muscle (intramuscular hemangiomas) tend to be ill-defined and require wide excision to prevent local recurrence. They do not metastasize.

Pyogenic Granuloma

There is debate over whether this lesion is an inflamed angioma or simply a nodule of reactive granulation tissue. It occurs in the skin and oral cavity, particularly during pregnancy or after trauma. Pyogenic granulomas are histologically similar to capillary hemangiomas but often have ulcerated surfaces and are acutely inflamed. They appear as polyps that grow rapidly to reach 1–2 cm in a few weeks, whereupon they may regress spontaneously. They do not recur after surgical removal.

Glomus Tumor (Glomangioma)

A glomus is a small temperature receptor "organ" situated in small arterioles. Benign neoplasms of glomi may occur anywhere in the skin but are most common under the fingernails and toenails. They occur in adults, forming small, firm, red-blue lesions that are extremely painful. They vary in size from 1 mm to 1 cm.

Microscopically, glomangiomas are composed of vascular spaces separated by nests of small, regular round cells with scant cytoplasm.

Lymphangioma

Cavernous lymphangioma (also called cystic hygroma) is a benign tumor that occurs mainly in the neck in infancy, causing considerable enlargement of the neck. It is common in Turner's syndrome. The larger tumors may obstruct delivery through the birth canal. Lymphangiomas also occur in the mediastinum and retroperitoneum in adults. They probably should be considered hamartomas rather than neoplasms. Lymphangiomas can grow to large size, making complete surgical removal difficult. They do not metastasize.

MALIGNANT NEOPLASMS

Angiosarcoma (Hemangiosarcoma)

Angiosarcoma is a rare neoplasm of adults. It may occur anywhere in the body, but the skin, soft tissue, bone, liver, and breast are the common sites. Hepatic angiosarcomas have been etiologically associated with thorium dioxide (Thorotrast), a radiologic dye that was used in 1930–1950, and vinyl chloride, used in the plastics industry.

Angiosarcoma is a malignant neoplasm of endoethelial cells. It typically forms interdigitating vascular spaces but may be anaplastic. Angiosarcomas are destructive, infiltrative neoplasms that metastasize early via the bloodstream. The endothelial nature of the cells can be established by positivity for factor VIII in immunohistochemical staining.

Angiosarcoma usually presents as a large, hemorrhagic, rapidly growing mass. The prognosis is poor, mainly because of early and widespread metastasis.

Kaposi's Sarcoma

Kaposi's sarcoma was a rare neoplasm in the United States until 1979. It occurred mainly in elderly patients and involved the lower extremities as a slowly growing, ulcerative skin lesion with a protracted course.

In 1979, Kaposi's sarcoma occurred in epidemic proportions in patients with AIDS. These patients had a much more aggressive variant of Kaposi's sarcoma that involved viscera such as intestine, lung, lymph nodes, and liver as well as the skin. Cases of disseminated Kaposi's sarcoma occur also in other immunocompromised patients, particularly after renal transplantation.

The cause of Kaposi's sarcoma and how it is related to immune deficiency are unknown. The genome of cytomegalovirus is found in many neoplastic cells, but whether this is incidental or has an etiologic relationship is uncertain.

Kaposi's sarcoma is an infiltrative lesion composed of spindle shaped endothelial cells that form poorly developed vascular slits. Erythrocyte extravasation and hemosiderin deposition occur commonly. The neoplastic cells are poorly differentiated and have an increased mitotic rate. Factor VIII stain is positive, providing evidence that the neoplastic cells are endothelial. Disseminated Kaposi's sarcoma is believed to be due to the occurrence of multiple neoplasms all over the body rather than to metastasis.

Lesions of Kaposi's sarcoma appear as purple patches, plaques, or nodules in the skin which may ulcerate (Chapter 7). In the viscera, they appear as hemorrhagic masses. In the immunodeficient individual, Kaposi's sarcoma is rapidly progressive; death occurs within 3 years in most patients with AIDS.

Lymphangiosarcoma

Lymphangiosarcoma is a malignant neoplasm of lymphatic endothelium. It is rare, occurring with greatest frequency in patients who develop lymphedema in the upper extremity after radical mastectomy followed by radiation therapy for breast carcinoma. Removal of axillary lymphatics causes lymphedema, and the use of radiation may contribute to malignant transformation. The neoplasm grows rapidly and metastasizes early. The prognosis is poor.

21 The Heart: I. Structure & Function; Congenital Diseases

STRUCTURE & FUNCTION

Layers of the Heart

The heart is composed of (1) the endocardium, which lines the internal surfaces of the cardiac chambers and valves; (2) the myocardium; (3) the pericardium, composed of an inner visceral layer covering the heart and an outer parietal layer completing the pericardial sac; and (4) a specialized conducting system consisting of the sinoatrial (SA) and atrioventricular (AV) nodes, the bundle of His, and the arborizing Purkinje fibers.

Sides of the Heart (Fig 21–1)

The muscular interatrial and interventricular septa divide the heart longitudinally into a **right side,** which accepts the deoxygenated systemic venous return and pumps it into the low pressure pulmonary circulation; and a **left side,** which accepts the oxygenated pulmonary venous blood and pumps it into the aorta. The left side and the systemic arterial circulation are at much higher hydrostatic pressures than the right side and the pulmonary arterial circulation.

Chambers of the Heart

Each side of the heart is further divided by the atrioventricular valves into an atrium and a ventricle.

A. Atria: The 2 atria are low-pressure chambers that accommodate venous return and are protected from high ventricular systolic pressure by closure of the atrioventricular valves. The muscular atrial walls normally have a thickness not exceeding 2 mm.

B. Ventricles: The ventricles represent the muscular pump of the heart. The **right ventricle** pumps blood into the relatively low-pressure pulmonary circulation (systolic pressure 15–30 mm Hg) and has a wall thickness of less than 0.5 cm. The **left ventricle** develops a systolic pressure of 100–150 mm Hg to maintain the high pressure systemic circulation (Fig 21–2). The left ventricle normally has a wall thickness of up to 1.5 cm.

Cardiac Valves

The pump mechanism of the heart is made possible by the presence of valves that isolate one part of the heart from another when they close (Fig 21–2). The cardiac valves are thin, translucent fibrous membranes that are attached circumferentially to the valve ring. Blood flow through normal open valves is nonturbulent and laminar and therefore not perceived by auscultation. When a valve closes, the free edges come firmly into apposition, effectively closing the orifice.

A. Atrioventricular Valves: The atrioventricular valves lie between the atrium and ventricle on each side. They are composed of 2 (mitral

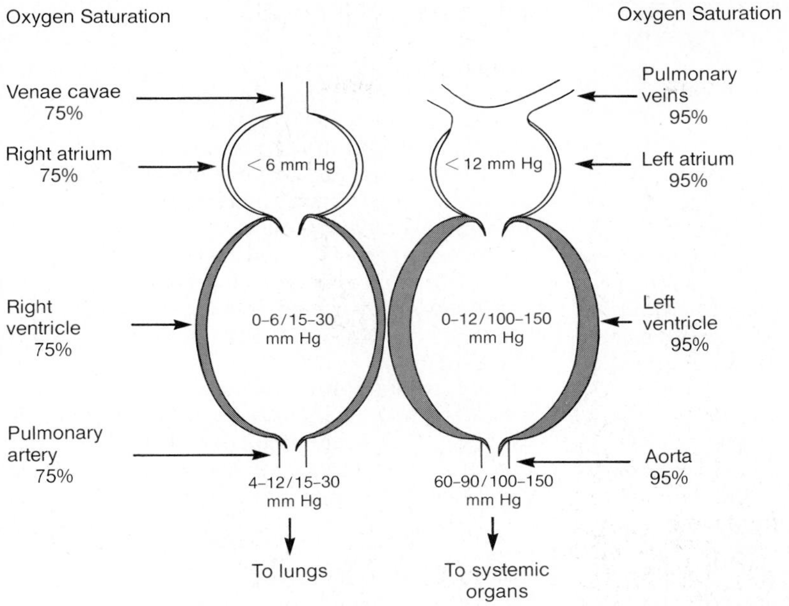

Oxygen Saturation

Venae cavae 75%

Right atrium 75%

Right ventricle 75%

Pulmonary artery 75%

< 6 mm Hg

0–6/15–30 mm Hg

4–12/15–30 mm Hg

To lungs

< 12 mm Hg

0–12/100–150 mm Hg

60–90/100–150 mm Hg

To systemic organs

Oxygen Saturation

Pulmonary veins 95%

Left atrium 95%

Left ventricle 95%

Aorta 95%

Figure 21–1. Normal pressures and oxygen saturation in the different chambers of the heart and great vessels.

valve) or 3 (tricuspid valve) cusps. The free edges of the atrioventricular valves are attached to the papillary muscles of the ventricle by fibrous cords (chordae tendineae). Atrioventricular valve closure produces the first heart sound, which signals the onset of ventricular contraction. Closure of the valves in systole prevents regurgitation of blood into the atrium.

B. Semilunar Valves: The semilunar (aortic and pulmmonary) valves lie between the ventricles and the great vessels. Closure at the end of systole produces the second heart sound, which signals the end of ventricular ejection. The valves remain closed during diastole, preventing regurgitation of blood from the great vessels into the ventricles.

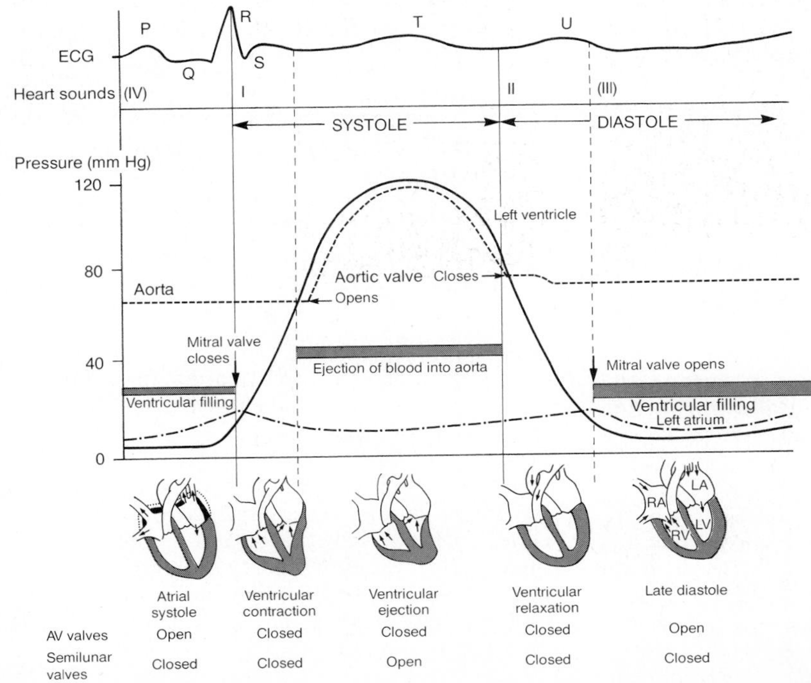

Figure 21–2. Cycle of contraction and valve action for the left side of the heart. The right side of the heart acts in parallel except that pressures are lower and valve motions are not quite synchronous.

METHODS OF EVALUATING CARDIAC STRUCTURE & FUNCTION

Physical Examination

A. Arterial Pulse: Palpation of the carotid and radial artery pulses permits recognition of the rate and rhythm of ventricular contraction as well as subtle changes in the pressure wave associated with certain cardiac diseases—exemplified by the sustained low-volume pulse in aortic valve stenosis or the bounding pulse in aortic valve incompetence.

B. Jugular Venous Pulse: The height of the jugular vein pulse wave is an accurate estimation of central venous pressure. It is increased in right heart failure, volume overload, and pericardial tamponade or constriction. Alteration of the wave form of the jugular venous pulse also provides important information. For example, accentuation of the first or a wave indicates that the pressure in the right side of the heart is increased; absence of the a wave is a sign of atrial fibrillation.

C. Cardiac Apex Beat: Localization of the cardiac apex beat by palpation permits rough evaluation of cardiac enlargement. A sustained heave at the apex is characteristic of left ventricular hypertrophy; a heave at the left parasternal border occurs with right ventricular hypertrophy.

D. Auscultation of the Heart: The normal heart usually has 2 sounds, the first due to closure of the atrioventricular valves and the second due to closure of the semilunar valves (usually slightly "split" because of asynchronous closure of pulmonary and aortic valves) (Fig 21–2). Various additional sounds usually signify disease (Fig 21–2). A third heart sound (triple, or gallop, rhythm) may occur as a result of rapid ventricular filling in diastole and is seen in heart failure and mitral incompetence. An opening snap suggests mitral stenosis; a fourth heart sound, pulmonary or systemic hypertension; and a friction rub, pericarditis.

Cardiac murmurs result from turbulence of blood flow through the heart, usually across damaged valves and abnormal pressure gradients. Soft "innocent" ejection systolic murmurs occur in high-output states such as fever or anemia and during vigorous exercise. Murmurs signifying congenital and valvular heart disease will be discussed later.

Electrocardiography

The electrocardiogram (ECG) is a graphic display of the electrical activity of the heart as recorded on the body surface by appropriately placed electrodes. The normal electrocardiographic tracing can be divided into (1) the **P wave,** due to atrial depolarization; (2) the **PR interval,** which is a rough measure of conduction time through the atrioventricular node; (3) the **QRS complex,** due to ventricular depolarization; and (4) the **T wave,** due to ventricular repolarization (Fig 21–2). The ST segment is isoelectric (ie, level with the baseline) in the normal person.

The ECG provides valuable information for assessment of (1) cardiac hypertrophy, (2) arrhythmias and conduction delays, (3) myocardial ischemia and infarction, (4) pericardial disease, and (5) electrolyte abnormalities (especially K^+, Mg^{2+}, Ca^{2+}) and some drug effects (eg, digitalis).

Imaging

Echocardiography is a means of evaluation of cardiac structure with sound waves reflected from the heart. **Chest radiography** evaluates gross cardiac structure and size. **Magnetic resonance imaging (MRI)** is beginning to have clinical application.

Cardiac Catheterization

Cardiac catheterization requires insertion of a catheter through a vein (to the right heart) or artery (to the left heart). This permits evaluation of pressures and oxygen saturation in the various chambers. Injection of radiopaque dye (angiography) permits visualization and photography of the contracting heart and the coronary arteries.

Endomyocardial Biopsy

Tissue can be taken from the inner surface of the heart with a biopsy forceps passed in a manner similar to a cardiac catheter. The main indications for endomyocardial biopsy are for verification of diagnosis of suspected myocarditis, cardiomyopathy, and rejection after heart transplantation.

MANIFESTATIONS OF CARDIAC DISEASE

PAIN

Ischemic Pain

The commonest cause of cardiac pain is myocardial ischemia. Pain is believed to be caused by stimulation of nerve endings by the lactic acid produced during anaerobic glycolysis. Ischemic pain is retrosternal and usually described as constricting in nature. It may radiate to the back, to either arm (especially the left), or up the neck into the jaw. Pain varies in severity from mild to excruciating. **Angina pectoris** is ischemic pain usually induced by exercise (sometimes by stress or cold) and relieved by rest.

Pericardial Pain

Inflammation of the parietal pericardium produces a sharp lower retrosternal pain that tends to vary with posture and respiration. It is often accompanied by signs of pericardial inflammation such as pericardial rub and effusion.

CARDIAC ENLARGEMENT

Enlargement of the heart may result from dilatation of the cardiac chambers (eg, in heart failure, myocarditis) or hypertrophy of the walls (eg, in hypertension, many valvular defects). Cardiac enlargement itself does not cause clinical symptoms, but it is a useful indication of the presence of cardiac disease. It may be recognized by clinical examination (the apex), radiography, or electrocardiography.

Documentation of cardiac hypertrophy at autopsy is usually done by measuring the thickness of the walls. Right ventricle thickness exceeding 0.5 cm and left ventricular thickness exceeding 1.5 cm constitutes hypertrophy. A more accurate assessment of ventricular muscle hypertrophy is obtained by weighing the muscle. This requires dissection of the muscle away from other structures and is rarely done in routine autopsies.

ABNORMAL CARDIAC RHYTHM (Arrhythmia; Dysrhythmia)

Normal cardiac contraction is initiated in the sinoatrial (SA) node and conducted across the atrium to the atrioventricular (AV) node (His-Purkinje system). Ventricular contractions are coordinated by the branches of the AV node. Arrhythmias reflect (1) altered activity of the SA node, (2) the development of "new" ectopic foci that drive the heart at an accelerated or irregular rate, and (3) conduction defects (Table 21–1).

Table 21–1. Classification of cardiac arrhythmias.

Altered activity of the SA node
Sinus tachycardia
Sinus bradycardia
Sinus arrhythmia
Ectopic rhythms
Supraventricular (atrial or AV nodal)
Supraventricular extrasystoles
Paroxysmal supraventricular tachycardia
Atrial flutter
Atrial fibrillation
Ventricular
Ventricular extrasystoles
Ventricular tachycardia
Ventricular filbrillation
Heart block
Sinoatrial block (partial or complete)
Atrioventricular block (partial or complete)
Bundle branch block

Patients are sometimes aware of arrhythmias, complaining of "missed beats" or palpitations. Some forms of arrhythmia produce characteristic alterations in the pulse. Electrocardiography is valuable in identifying cardiac arrhythmias.

Etiology

The principal cause of significant cardiac arrhythmia is ischemia. Other causes include infection (myocarditis), various inflammatory conditions (systemic lupus erythematosus, rheumatic fever, sarcoidosis), drugs (digitalis, quinine derivatives, antidepressants, catecholamines, beta-blockers, calcium channel blockers), electrolyte abnormalities (hyperkalemia), endocrine disease (thyrotoxicosis), and congenital abnormalities of the conduction system. Various tachycardias, usually benign, may be precipitated by anxiety or caffeine ingestion.

Effects

Cardiac output during arrhythmias depends on the stroke volume and heart rate. In bradyarrhythmias (slow heart rate), cardiac output falls when the reduction in heart rate cannot be compensated for by an increased stroke volume. In tachyarrhythmias (rapid rate), cardiac output may also fall because of decreased ventricular filling resulting from shortened diastole. In addition, ventricular oxygen consumption is increased and myocardial blood supply decreased because of inadequate coronary perfusion. Acute heart failure is therefore common in patients with ventricular tachycardia. The severity of cardiac arrhythmia is directly related to the decrease in cardiac output. Supraventricular tachycardias and incomplete heart block do not cause serious effects. Ventricular fibrillation results in cessation of effective ventricular ejection and causes rapid death. Ventricular tachycardia and complete heart block are serious arrhythmias associated with a variable decrease in cardiac output.

CARDIAC FAILURE

Cardiac failure is inability to maintain an adequate cardiac output despite normal venous return. Cardiac output also falls below normal if venous return is reduced, as in the noncardiogenic types of shock (Chapter 9).

Etiology

Causes of cardiac failure are classified according to whether they produce predominantly left-sided or right-sided failure (Table 21–2) or low-output or high-output failure (Table 21–3).

Pathology & Clinical Effects

The effects of cardiac failure are classified as **(1) "forward" failure,** resulting from decreased

Table 21-2. Common causes of heart failure.

Primarily left-sided
Ischemic heart disease
Hypertensive heart disease
Aortic valve disease (stenosis, incompetence)
Mitral valve disease (stenosis,[1] incompetence)
Myocarditis
Cardiomyopathy
Cardiac amyloidosis
High-output states (thyrotoxicosis, anemia, arteriovenous fistula)
Primarily right-sided
Left-sided heart failure[2]
Chronic pulmonary disease ("cor pulmonale")
Pulmonary valve stenosis
Tricuspid valve disease (stenosis, incompetence)
Congenital heart disease (ventricular septal defect, patent ductus arteriosus)
Pulmonary hypertension (primary and secondary)
Massive pulmonary embolism

[1]Mitral stenosis produces functional failure of the left side of the heart; although the left ventricle itself is not in failure, the left atrium is.
[2]Left heart failure is the most common cause of right heart failure because of back pressure effects via the pulmonary circulation.

cardiac output; or **(2) "backward" failure,** due to accumulation of venous return within the heart (cardiac dilatation) or in the tissues draining to the heart (Fig 21-3). Although both occur together, one may dominate the clinical picture.

In addition, clinical changes associated with cardiac failure depend on (1) whether the left or right side is predominantly affected, (2) the magnitude of the decrease in cardiac output, and (3) whether failure is acute or chronic.

Table 21-3. Low- and high-output cardiac failure: Definition and causes

Definition	Causes
Low-output failure Inability to maintain a normal systemic cardiac output, eg, normal = 5 L/min; failure = 3—4 L/min.	Disorders of the myocardium Ischemic heart disease Myocarditis Cardiomyopathy Amyloidosis Arrhythmias Increased pressure load Systemic hypertension Valve stenosis All causes of right ventricular failure secondary to lung disease (cor pulmonale)
High-output failure Inability to maintain an abnormally high cardiac output because of demand for increased blood flow, eg, normal = 5 L/min; increased demand = 7 L/min; failure = 5-6 L/min.	Valve incompetence Anemia Thyrotoxicosis (hyperthyroidism) Fever Arteriovenous malformation Paget's disease of bone Plasma volume overload Beriberi

A. Left-Sided Heart Failure:

1. Acute cardiac arrest–Cessation of effective left ventricular contraction (cardiac arrest) leads to **sudden death**. The causes include ventricular asystole (no contractions) or ventricular fibrillation (ineffective, uncoordinated contractions). Cerebral anoxia leads to loss of consciousness and death within a few minutes. Emergency cardiac resuscitation by external cardiac massage, if started immediately, can maintain an adequate circulation, allowing time for treatment of the cause.

2. Acute severe decrease in output–An acute severe decrease in cardiac output may lead to **cardiogenic shock**. The decreased cardiac output evokes reflex sympathetic stimulation, which results in increased heart rate (tachycardia) and vasoconstriction in skin, muscle, intestine and kidney, diverting blood to the brain and heart (Chapter 9). The decreased glomerular filtration pressure resulting from vasoconstriction causes decreased urine output and an increased serum level of urea (prerenal uremia). Prolonged vasoconstriction diminishes tissue perfusion and renders shock irreversible. Death then follows rapidly.

In severe cardiogenic shock, the phase of compensation by reflex sympathetic activity may be very short.

3. Acute "backward" failure–The backward failure component of acute left heart failure is **pulmonary edema**. Failure of the left heart to pump the pulmonary venous return causes increased hydrostatic pressure in the pulmonary capillaries with transudation of fluid into the alveolar space (pulmonary edema).

Clinically, pulmonary edema is manifested as severe difficulty in breathing (dyspnea) accompanied by cough productive of pink, frothy sputum (the alveolar fluid transudate). The edema fluid produces "wet sounds" (rales or crepitations) on auscultation.

4. Chronic "backward" failure–Chronic left heart failure is dominated by the changes of **chronic pulmonary venous congestion,** which if prolonged induces fibrous thickening of the alveolar septa. The thickened alveolar septa represent increased resistance to lung expansion, causing dyspnea. The dyspnea is maximal when congestion of the lung is greatest, as in exercise (exertional dyspnea), and during sleep (recumbency), when peripheral edema fluid is mobilized, increasing venous return to the heart. Orthopnea (dyspnea in the recumbent position) and paroxysmal nocturnal dyspnea (dyspnea during sleep) are typical symptoms of chronic left heart failure.

Entry of small amounts of blood into the alveoli leads to the accumulation of hemosiderin-laden macrophages in the alveoli (Chapter 9), imparting a brown color to the fibrotic lung ("brown induration of the lung").

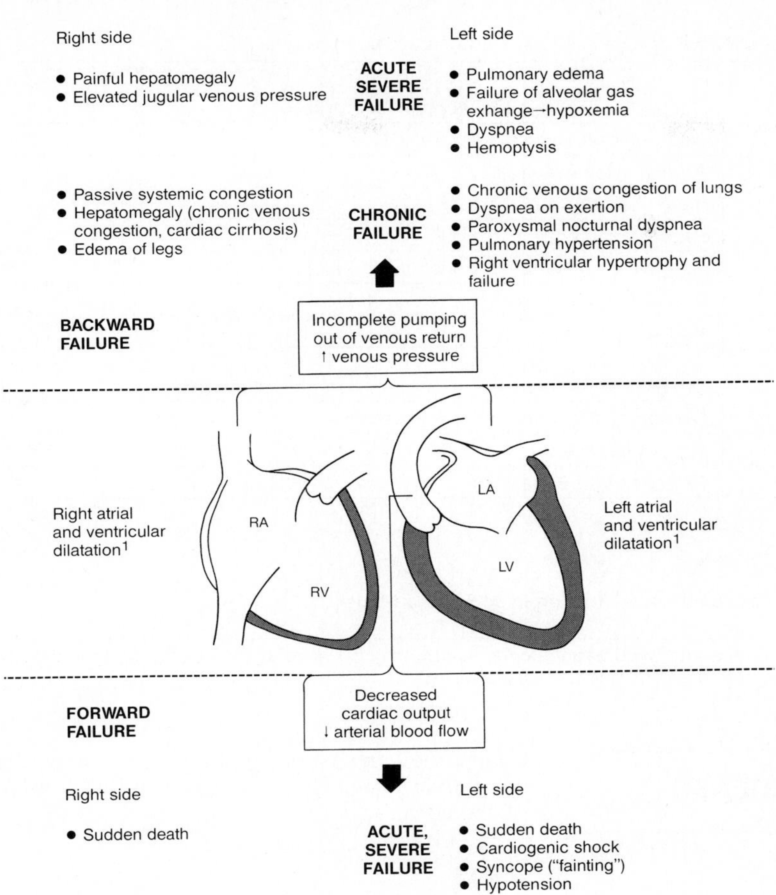

Figure 21-3. Effects of cardiac failure. **Note 1:** Dilatation partly represents a compensatory mechanism for increasing cardiac output. The stretching of myocardial fibers results in increased force of myocardial contraction.

Progressive fibrosis of the alveolar septa causes pulmonary hypertension which leads to right ventricular hypertrophy and ultimately, right ventricular failure. The commonest cause of right ventricular failure is left heart failure.

B. Right-Sided Heart Failure:

1. Acute severe decrease in output–Acute right heart failure occurs most commonly when a massive pulmonary embolus becomes impacted in and obstructs the outflow tract of the right ventricle and main pulmonary artery. This results in arrest of the circulation and **sudden death.**

Cardiac tamponade is another form of acute right heart failure. A sudden increase in pericardial cavity pressure due to fluid accumulation interferes with right ventricular diastolic filling, resulting in decreased right ventricular output.

2. Chronic "backward" failure–Chronic right heart failure is manifested clinically by **systemic venous congestion**. The jugular venous pulse is elevated. The liver is enlarged as a result of congestion and tender as a result of stretching of the liver capsule. Within the hepatic lobule, congestion occurs first around the central vein, which becomes darker than the periphery of the lobule, producing an appearance that resembles a cut nutmeg (''nutmeg liver''). Associated fatty change (due to anoxia) enhances this appearance. Cardiac ''cirrhosis'' may follow.

Peripheral edema is the most obvious feature of right heart failure, occurring in dependent areas—the ankles in ambulatory patients and the sacrum in recumbent ones.

C. Cardiac Edema:

Edema occurs in both left and right heart failure. In left heart failure, edema fluid accumulates in the lungs, whereas in right heart failure the fluid gravitates to the dependent systemic veins. Chronic cardiac edema is primarily the result of sodium and water retention in the kidneys, which increases total body water as well as total plasma volume. Stimulation of the renin-angiotensin-aldosterone mechanism by the lowered cardiac output is the main factor (Chapter 2).

Treatment

See Table 21–4.

Table 21-4. Pathologic rationale of treatment of heart failure.

Treat primary cause of failure	
Coronary artery disease	Coronary artery bypass, angioplasty, drugs
Arrhythmia	Defibrillation, pacemaker, drugs
Hypertension	Antihypertensive drugs
Valve defects	Valve repair or replacement
Cardiomyopathy	Heart transplant
Pulmonary embolism	Surgical embolectomy, fibrinolysins, anticoagulants
Cardiac tamponade	Aspiration of pericardial effusion fluid
Constrictive pericarditis	Pericardiectomy
Treat consequences of failure	
Increase cardiac output	Drugs that stimulate myocardial contraction (digitalis)
Reverse sodium and water retention	Diuretics,[1] salt restriction, venesection
Treat shock	Dopamine, electrolytes, fluid
Relieve pulmonary congestion	Diuretics,[1] sit patient up
General measures	
Correct anemia.	
Withdraw any drugs that may be myocardial depressants.	
Provide physical and emotional rest.	
Administer oxygen (compensates for abnormal ventilation in congested lungs).	
Maintain electrolyte balance.[1]	

[1]Certain diuretics may cause hypokalemia and hypomagnesemia, which not only have direct effects on the myocardium but also potentiate the toxic effects of drugs such as digitalis.

CONGENITAL HEART DISEASE

ETIOLOGY

In most cases of congenital heart disease, there is no identifiable cause. Many cases probably result from the action of unknown teratogens in the first trimester of pregnancy, which is when fetal cardiac development takes place. Most congenital cardiac defects are not inherited.

In a few patients, a specific cause can be identified.

Rubella

Transplacental infection of the fetus by rubella virus in the first trimester of pregnancy is a cause of many cardiac anomalies, such as patent ductus arteriosus and pulmonary stenosis. Congenital rubella has decreased in frequency as a consequence of rubella immunization. Other viral infections, notably mumps and influenza, have been suggested as causing congenital cardiac defects, but the evidence is not convincing.

Chromosomal Abnormalities

Down's syndrome (trisomy 21) is associated with a 20% incidence of defects of the atrioventricular valves or the atrial and ventricular septa. **Turner's syndrome** (45,XO) is associated with cardiac anomalies in about 20% of cases. Coarctation of the aorta is the commonest anomaly. **Trisomy 18** is associated with right ventricular origin of the aorta.

Drugs

Thalidomide caused severe structural abnormalities in the fetus, including cardiac anomalies. More recently, consumption of alcohol during early pregnancy has been shown to cause congenital cardiac defects (fetal alcohol syndrome).

CLASSIFICATION

Congenital heart defects (Table 21–5) can occur in either side of the heart at the atrial, ventricular. or aortopulmonary level. The common defects are classified according to (1) which side of the heart is involved; (2) whether there is a communication or shunt between the 2 sides; and (3) in those defects where there is a shunt, the presence or absence of cyanosis.

Cyanosis is bluish discoloration of the skin and mucous membranes caused by increased amounts of reduced hemoglobin in arterial blood. In congenital cyanotic heart disease, cyanosis is caused by right-to-left shunt, which allows unoxygenated venous blood to bypass the lungs and enter the systemic circulation (central cyanosis).

Table 21-5. Classification and frequency[1] of congenital heart disease.

Without shunt (20%)	
Right-sided	
Pulmonary stenosis	10%
Ebstein's anomaly	Rare
Left-sided	
Coarctation of the aorta	10%
Aortic stenosis	Rare
Dextrocardia	Rare
With shunt (80%)	
Acyanotic	
Atrial septal defect	15%
Ventricular septal defect	25%
Patent ductus arteriosus	15%
Cyanotic	
Tetralogy of Fallot	10%
Transposition of great vesels	10%
Truncus arteriosus	Rare
Tricuspid atresia	Rare
Total anomalous pulmonary venous return	Rare
Hypoplastic left heart syndromes	Rare
Eisenmenger's syndrome[2]	Rare

[1]Relative frequencies of individual anomalies in children.
[2]The term "Eisenmenger's syndrome" is applied to the development of pulmonary hypertension and reversal of shunt direction in patients with atrial septal defect, ventricular septal defect, and patent ductus arteriosus. Surgery to close the defect in the presence of this degree of pulmonary hypertension has a high mortality rate.

ATRIAL SEPTAL DEFECT (ASD)

Ostium Secundum ASD (Fig 21-4)

The most common type of ASD is a defect in the development of the septum secundum, which produces mild disease that is frequently not detected until adult life.

In most cases of ostium secundum ASD, the defect is large enough (> 2 cm) to cause near equalization of left and right atrial pressure, with flow of blood from left to right through the ASD. In the usual case, pulmonary flow is increased to about twice that of systemic output, and the right ventricle is dilated and hypertrophied owing to the volume overload. This is usually well tolerated, and right ventricular failure is uncommon.

Clinically, there is right ventricular hypertrophy and delayed pulmonary valve closure, causing a widely split second heart sound that does not vary with respiration ("fixed" split). Increased flow through the pulmonary valve produces an ejection systolic murmur and loud pulmonary valve closure. The diagnosis is confirmed by cardiac catheterization, echocardiography, or isotope studies.

The main complication of ostium secundum ASD is the development of **pulmonary hypertension,** increased right side pressure, and either right heart failure or reversal of the shunt and cyanosis. Paradoxic embolization to the systemic circulation and infective endocarditis may occur.

Ostium Primum ASD

Ostium primum defects are rare, constituting about 5% of all cases of ASD. They occur as large defects in the lower part of the atrial septum and are often associated with mitral valve lesions. Ostium primum defect is common in Down's syndrome. Ostium primum ASD produces severe disease in early childhood, with features of mitral incompetence superimposed on the ASD.

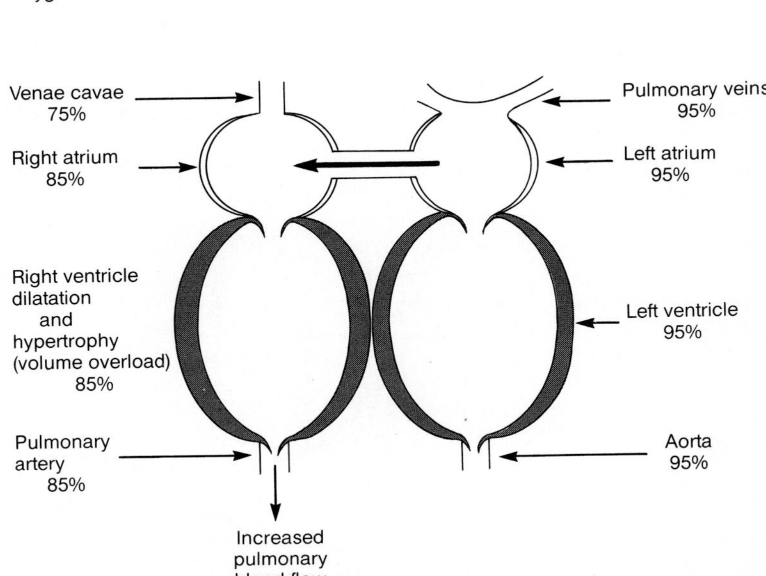

Figure 21-4. Pathophysiology of atrial septal defect. The net left-to-right shunt through the atrial septal defect results in volume overload of the right atrium, right ventricle, and pulmonary circulation. The volume of the shunt can be calculated from cardiac output and the amount of increase in oxygen saturation occurring at right atrial level. In the early stages, the pressures in the right side of the heart are not increased. With time, pulmonary vascular changes may occur, leading to increasing pulmonary arterial pressure. Reversal of the direction of flow through the shunt may occur with severe pulmonary hypertension.

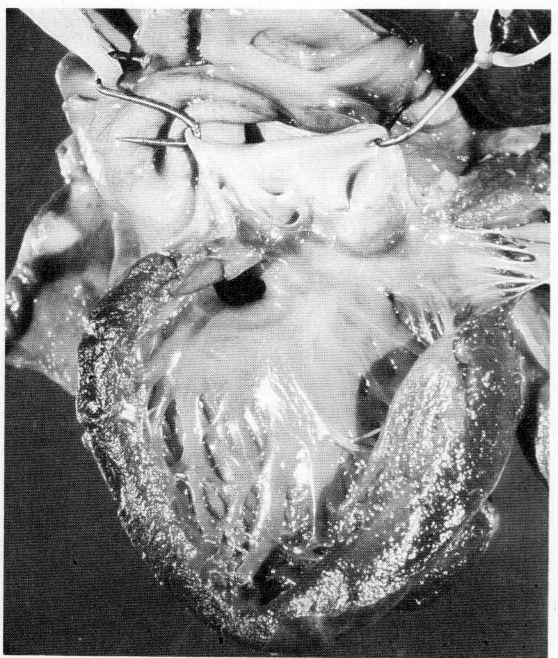

Figure 21-5. Ventricular septal defect seen from the left ventricular side. Note the hypertrophied left ventricle.

VENTRICULAR SEPTAL DEFECT (VSD)

VSD is the most commonly encountered cardiac anomaly in children. Most defects occur in the membranous part of the interventricular septum just below the orifices of the semilunar valves (Fig 21-5). VSD is classified according to its size.

Small VSD (Maladie de Roger)

Small VSDs (< 0.5 cm in diameter) are common. They produce a low-volume shunt from the left to the right ventricle during systole. This shunt across a high pressure gradient produces a loud pansystolic murmur heard best at the left sternal edge. With a small defect, right ventricular pressure is increased only slightly. Cardiac catheterization shows entry of oxygenated blood into the right ventricle (Fig 21-6).

Patients with small VSDs have few symptoms. The defect tends to decrease in relative size as the heart grows and may even close spontaneously.

Large VSD

A large VSD is much more serious, with clinical manifestations appearing in early childhood. Initially, a large volume of blood is shunted from the left to the right ventricle during systole, producing volume overload of both ventricles, hypertrophy of both ventricles, and a pansystolic murmur.

Increased blood flow through the pulmonary circulation induces pulmonary hypertension and a loud pulmonary valve closure sound. Progressive increase in right ventricular pressure leads to thickening and narrowing of the small pulmonary arteries, reduction in shunt volume, and, finally, shunt reversal. This produces cyanosis (Eisenmenger's syndrome). Shunt reversal in VSD occurs some time after birth (tardive cyanosis) and is associated with decrease or disappearance of the pansystolic murmur. Patients with VSD are at risk for infective endocarditis (Chapter 22).

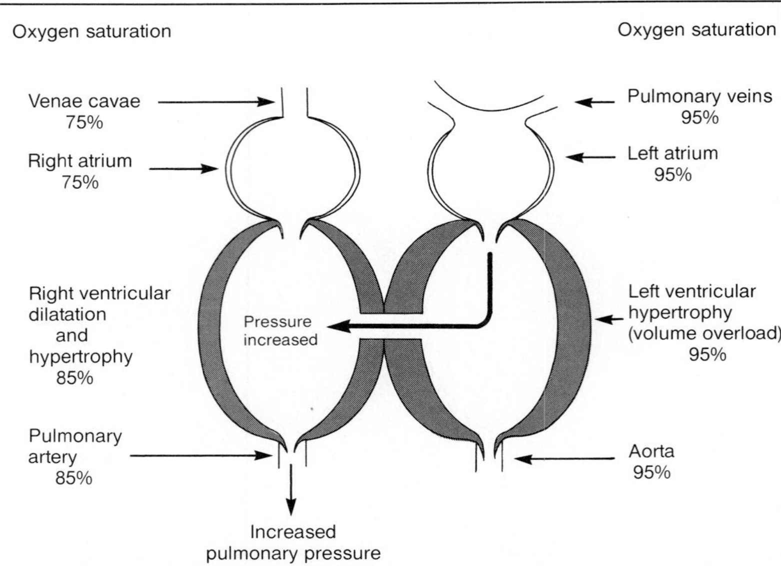

Figure 21-6. Pathophysiology of ventricular septal defect. The defect results in a left-to-right shunt at the ventricular level, resulting in increased volume and pressure in the right ventricle, the magnitude of which depends on the size of the defect. The right ventricle undergoes hypertrophy because of volume and pressure overload. The left ventricle, which must handle the shunted blood in addition to the normal output into the aorta, also undergoes hypertrophy and dilatation. Pulmonary arterial pressure may increase with time as a result of changes occurring in the pulmonary vasculature. This causes a progressive decrease in shunt volume and, if severe enough, may result in shunt reversal.

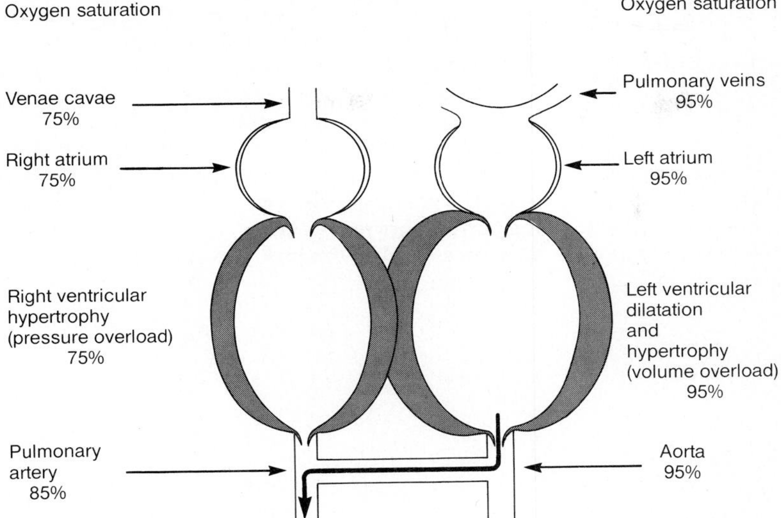

Figure 21-7. Pathophysiology of patent ductus arteriosus. Blood is shunted from the aorta to the main pulmonary artery via the patent ductus. This results in increased pressure and volume in the pulmonary artery, the magnitude of which depends on the size of the shunt. Pulmonary hypertension causes right ventricular hypertrophy. The left ventricle, which pumps a volume equal to the shunt plus the systemic output, also undergoes hypertrophy. Increasing pulmonary hypertension due to secondary pulmonary vascular changes may result in shunt reversal.

PATENT DUCTUS ARTERIOSUS (PDA)

The ductus arteriosus is a normal fetal vascular channel that connects the pulmonary artery and the aorta, permitting right ventricular output to bypass the inactive fetal lungs. At birth, when the lungs expand, pulmonary vascular resistance falls; flow across the ductus decreases, and it closes by muscle spasm. Permanent fibrotic occlusion is usually complete by 8 weeks. In premature infants, anatomic closure may be delayed several months. Indomethacin promotes the closure of a PDA.

A **small PDA** leads to a small left-to-right shunt, continuous throughout the cardiac cycle, because there is a pressure gradient from the aorta to the pulmonary artery throughout the cycle. This causes the typical continuous (''machinery'') murmur of PDA. A small PDA causes only mild elevation of pulmonary artery pressure and minimal symptoms. Cardiac catheterization shows an increase in oxygen saturation of blood at the pulmonary artery level, the degree of this increase providing a measure of the shunted volume (Fig 21-7). The patent ductus may also be involved by a process analogous to infective endocarditis.

With a **large PDA**, the high aortic pressure is transmitted to the pulmonary artery, causing marked pulmonary hypertension and ultimately

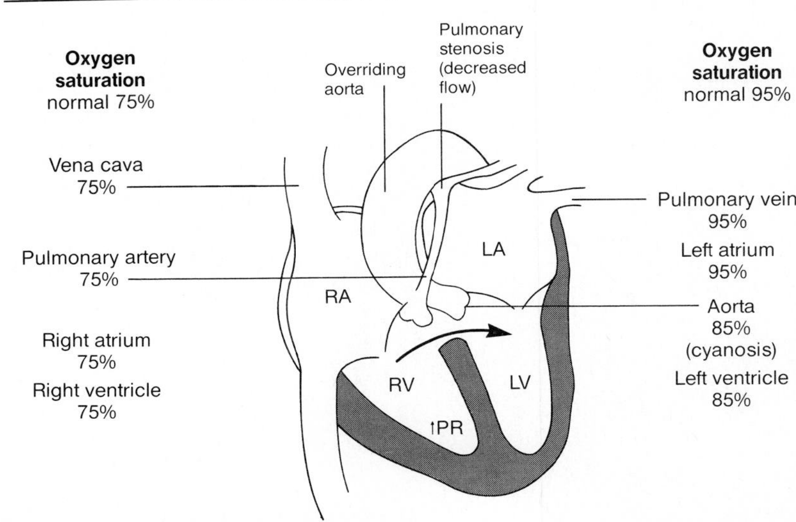

Figure 21-8. Fallot's tetralogy. The marked narrowing of the pulmonary outflow tract results in a right-to-left shunt through the ventricular septal defect, resulting in central cyanosis. The right ventricle is hypertrophied.

resulting in shunt reversal (Eisenmenger's syndrome).

TETRALOGY OF FALLOT

Tetralogy of Fallot (Fig 21–8) is the commonest cyanotic congenital cardiac anomaly. It is characterized by (1) a large ventricular septal defect; (2) stenosis of the pulmonary outflow tract; (3) dextroposition of the aorta, which overrides the right ventricle; and (4) hypertrophy of the right ventricle. The pulmonary stenosis raises right ventricular pressure so that the shunt across the VSD is right-to-left, with venous admixture of systemic arterial blood causing cyanosis.

Tetralogy of Fallot is a severe defect that presents at birth with central cyanosis ("blue babies"). The prognosis is very poor without treatment. With corrective surgery, which has become very successful in the past 2 decades, normal survival is the rule.

The Heart: II. Endocardium & Cardiac Valves

22

- Acute Rheumatic Fever
- Systemic Lupus Erythematosus (SLE)
- Infective Endocarditis
- Disorders of Cardiac Valves
  - Mitral Stenosis
  - Mitral Incompetence
  - Aortic Stenosis
  - Aortic Incompetence
  - Pulmonary Valve Lesions
  - Tricuspid Valve Lesions
- Neoplasms of the Endocardium
  - Cardiac Myxoma

ACUTE RHEUMATIC FEVER

Incidence

Acute rheumatic fever occurs in children, commonly between 5 and 15 years of age—the same age group in which streptococcal pharyngitis occurs frequently. The disease is more common among children of lower socioeconomic backgrounds and is still prevalent in underdeveloped countries. In the United States and Western Europe, there has been a marked decline in streptococcal infections and acute rheumatic fever in the past 2 decades.

Etiology

Acute rheumatic fever is an immunologic hypersensitivity reaction affecting the endocardium, myocardium, and pericardium **(pancarditis)**. The endocardium is the site of maximal involvement.

Rheumatic fever occurs 2–6 weeks after streptococcal sore throat (Fig 22–1) and is caused by an immune response to streptococcal antigens. Most of the serologic types of group A *Streptococcus* that cause pharyngitis have been associated with acute rheumatic fever, but only a few patients with streptococcal pharyngitis develop rheumatic fever (the attack rate is generally less than 5%). The factors that make an individual susceptible to this complication of streptococcal infection are unknown, but there is an association with the histocompatibility antigen **HLA-B5**. More rarely, the disease follows streptococcal infections at sites other than the pharynx.

Pathogenesis

The exact relationship between streptococcal infection and cardiac injury is unknown. Injury is not the result of direct infection, as shown by negative streptococcal cultures in affected heart tissue. That rheumatic fever occurs 2–3 weeks after streptococcal infection strongly suggests an immunologic hypersensitivity mechanism. High levels of antistreptococcal antibodies (antistreptolysin O, anti-DNAse, antihyaluronidase) commonly occur in patients who develop rheumatic fever and are indicative of the preceding streptococcal infection.

Many theories have been advanced to explain the cardiac damage that occurs in rheumatic fever (Table 22–1). The immunologic reaction is probably a form of type II hypersensitivity. Immunoglobulin and complement can be demonstrated in myocardial fiber membrane by immunologic techniques in patients with acute rheumatic fever. Cross-reacting antibodies with activity against both streptococcal protein and myocardial sarcolemma have been demonstrated in the sera of patients with acute rheumatic fever. It must be emphasized that the presence of such antibodies does not by itself constitute evidence of an etiologic relationship, since similar antibodies have been detected in a small percentage of patients following myocardial infarction.

The frequent presence of immune complexes, especially in HLA-B5 patients with rheumatic fever is persuasive evidence for a causative role for type III hypersensitivity. Finally, it has been postulated that type IV cell-mediated hypersensitivity may play a role, though there is little direct evidence for that view.

Clinical Features (Table 22–2)

Acute rheumatic fever affects multiple organs. It has a sudden onset characterized by high fever and one or more of the following major features:

A. Carditis: Carditis is the most serious manifestation and occurs in about 35% of patients with a first attack of rheumatic fever.

B. Polyarthritis: Acute Inflammation affecting multiple large joints is the presenting feature in 75% of patients. The joints are involved asym-

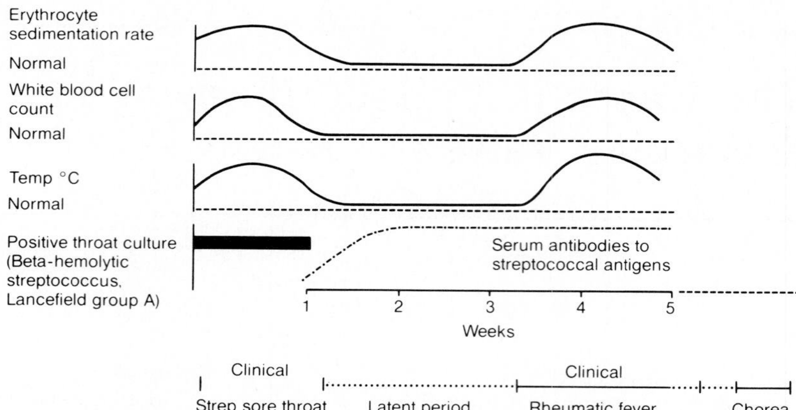

Figure 22-1. The temporal relationship between streptococcal infection and acute rheumatic fever.

metrically, and the inflammation tends to move from joint to joint (migratory polyarthritis). Affected joints are swollen, red, warm, and painful.

C. Chorea: Random involuntary movements (chorea) are caused by involvement of the basal ganglia of the brain. Chorea may develop up to 6 months after the streptococcal pharyngitis. It may persist for weeks but has an excellent prognosis.

D. Skin Lesions: Erythema marginatum (a circular ring of erythema surrounding central normal skin) is specific for rheumatic fever but occurs only in about 10% of cases. It is of short duration. **Erythema nodosum** (a nodular, red, tender rash typically seen over the anterior tibia) is less specific but occurs more commonly.

E. Subcutaneous Rheumatic Nodules: These occur mainly over bony prominences in the extremities. They are pea-sized, nontender, and last 6–10 weeks. Their presence usually indicates concurrent cardiac involvement. Pathologically, rheumatic nodules consist of foci of fibrinoid necrosis with a surrounding granulomatous reaction.

Pathology of Carditis

Cardiac involvement involves all layers of the heart (pancarditis). Endocarditis occurs in all patients with rheumatic carditis, whereas myocarditis and pericarditis are present only in severe cases.

The **Aschoff body** is the microscopic lesion that is diagnostic of rheumatic fever (Fig 22–2). Aschoff bodies occur in the connective tissue of the heart, most commonly in the subendocardial region and the myocardial interstitium.

A. Endocarditis (Valvulitis): The valvular endocardium shows maximum involvement. The valves of the left side are affected more often and more severely than the right and the mitral valve more than the aortic. Involved valves show edema and denudation of the lining endocardium, particularly in areas of maximum trauma at the line of apposition of the free edge of the valve. Platelet-fibrin thrombi (**rheumatic vegetations**) form in areas of endocardial damage (Fig 22–3). Rheumatic vegetations do not become detached as emboli. Valve edema and vegetations may cause turbulence of blood and produce various transient murmurs (eg, Carey-Coombs diastolic murmur);

Table 22-1. Postulated mechanisms of immunologic "autohypersensitivity" in rheumatic fever.

- Induced chemical change in cardiac antigens (eg, by hyaluronidase)
- *Streptococcus* or streptococcal products acting as hapten with cardiac components
- Release of sequestered cardiac antigens by *Streptococcus*-induced inflammation
- Streptococcal products act as adjuvant, abnormally stimulating immune response
- Production of immune complexes containing streptococcal antigens
- Cross-reacting antibodies: streptococcal protein and myocardial protein; streptococcal carbohydrate and valve glycoproteins

Table 22-2. Clinical features for diagnosis of rheumatic fever (Jones criteria).[1]

Major Criteria	Minor Criteria
Polyarthritis (75%)	Arthralgia
Carditis (35%)	Fever
Chorea (10%)	Preceding group A streptococcal infection
Subcutaneous nodules (10%)	Preceding bout of rheumatic fever
Erythema marginatum (10%)	Elevated ESR Elongated PR interval on ECG

[1]Diagnosis requires 2 major criteria or one major and 2 minor; thus, individual features are not present in all cases. Figures in parenthesis show approximate frequency of feature and vary widely in different series. The incidence of carditis is falling; 50 years ago, 80% of patients with acute rheumatic fever had clinical carditis. Fever occurs in 70–80% of cases.

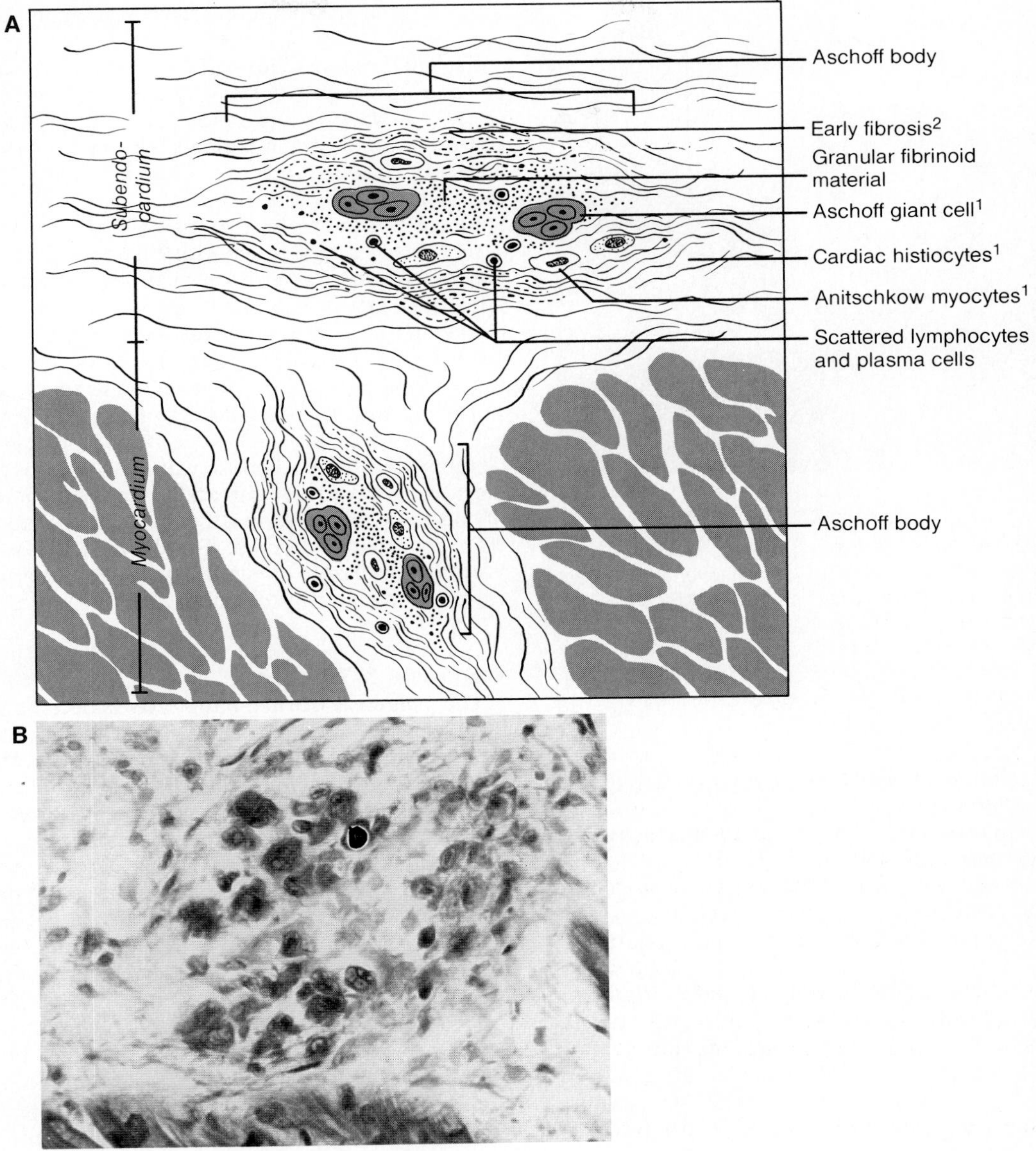

Figure 22-2. A: Diagrammatic representation of Aschoff bodies in the subendocardium and myocardial interstitial tissue in acute rheumatic fever. **Note 1:** Note that many authorities regard Aschoff giant cells, Anitschkow myocytes, and cardiac histiocytes as variants of macrophages. **Note 2:** Fibrosis becomes more prominent as healing occurs. The end result of an Aschoff body is a fibrous scar. **B:** Aschoff body in myocardial interstitium. Note the typical multinucleated giant cells. High magnification.

murmurs occur in most patients with cardiac involvement.

B. Myocarditis: Acute myocardial involvement, characterized by the presence of numerous Aschoff bodies in the myocardium, causes tachycardia and dilatation of the heart. Cardiac failure occurs in a small number of cases.

C. Pericarditis: Acute inflammation of the pericardium (fibrinous pericarditis) occurs only in severe cases, causing chest pain and a pericardial rub. Pericardial effusion is rarely of sufficient magnitude to cause problems.

Sequelae

A. Immediate: The great majority of patients with acute rheumatic fever recover completely from the acute attack, usually within 6 weeks. A very small number of patients (less than 5%) die

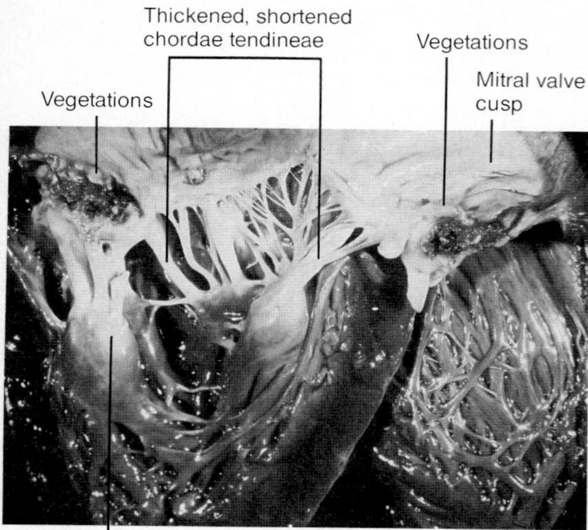

Figure 22-3. Rheumatic heart disease, showing small vegetations typical of acute rheumatic fever at line of apposition of the mitral valve cusps. Note that the chordae tendineae are thickened and shortened, suggesting chronic rheumatic heart disease. This patient gave a history of recurrent attacks of acute rheumatic fever over several years.

in the acute phase of severe myocarditis (heart failure and arrhythmia).

B. Recurrences: A patient who has recovered from an attack of rheumatic fever is apt to develop recurrences. Recurrent attacks produce additional scarring and greatly increase the risk of later development of chronic rheumatic heart disease.

C. Chronic Rheumatic Heart Disease: Rheumatic endocarditis heals by fibrosis. Fibrosis may occur in the free endocardium, most commonly in the posterior wall of the left atrium (McCallum's patch) but is of greatest significance when it involves the valves, causing valve dysfunction (chronic rheumatic heart disease) (Figs 22-3 and 22-4).

Chronic disease tends to follow recurrent acute episodes of rheumatic fever by a variable interval (2-20 years). In some cases, chronic rheumatic heart disease occurs in patients with no history of an acute episode. In these cases, it is likely that the acute attack was subclinical.

Fibrosis of the valve with fusion of the commissures leads to a rigid valve with a narrowed orifice **(valve stenosis)**. Severe destruction of the valve apparatus may cause valve ring dilatation, with thickening and shortening of chordae tendineae, resulting in regurgitation of blood through the valve when it is closed **(valve incompetence)**.

The mitral valve is the most commonly affected and is the only affected valve in 50% of cases. Combined mitral and aortic valve lesions are next most frequent (40%), with additional involvement of the tricuspid valve in a few cases. Pulmonary valve involvement is rare. The different valve lesions are discussed fully in the section on acquired valve lesions later in this chapter.

Prognosis & Treatment

The prognosis of rheumatic fever is determined by (1) the severity of the acute illness; (2) whether or not there is cardiac involvement, since all other manifestations, including chorea, resolve completely; and (3) whether or not there are recurrences. The greater the number of recurrences, the higher the incidence of subsequent chronic rheumatic heart disease. This is the rationale for prolonged prophylactic penicillin therapy in patients who have had an attack of acute rheumatic fever (to prevent streptococcal infection and hence recurrence of rheumatic fever).

Treatment of the acute attack of rheumatic fever with penicillin has no effect on the course of the disease. Salicylates and corticosteroids are useful for symptomatic treatment of rheumatic fever, but, again, have no effect on its course.

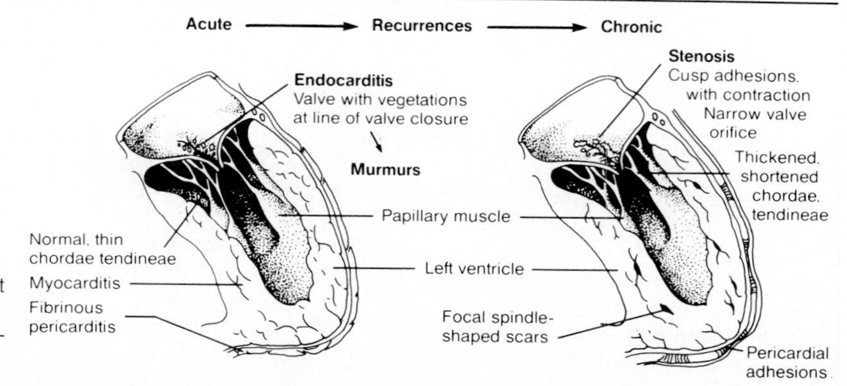

Figure 22-4. Rheumatic heart disease, contrasting the features of acute and chronic disease.

SYSTEMIC LUPUS ERYTHEMATOSUS (SLE)

The heart is involved in 10–20% of cases of SLE. The immune complex-mediated injury may involve any layer of the heart. SLE is one of the most common causes of **acute pericarditis** in the United States. Pericarditis is fibrinous, with little effusion.

Libman-Sacks endocarditis is the most characteristic cardiac lesion of SLE. Multiple, small, flat vegetations occur on the mitral and tricuspid valves. Both the atrial and ventricular surfaces of the valve, the chordae tendineae, and the mural endocardium are involved. SLE valvulitis is rarely severe enough to cause valve dysfunction.

INFECTIVE ENDOCARDITIS

The incidence of infective endocarditis has decreased with the availability of antibiotics. Death from infective endocarditis is now largely restricted to those cases caused by virulent organisms.

Classification

It has been customary to classify infective endocarditis as acute or subacute. There is, however, considerable overlap, and it is probably best to consider this condition as a spectrum of clinical features ranging between the 2 extremes. It is much more important to identify the causative infectious agent than to classify the disease as acute or subacute. A large number of bacteria and fungi have been isolated from cases of infective endocarditis (Table 22–3).

A. Acute Infective Endocarditis: This is the most severe form of infective endocarditis and is less common than the subacute variety. It is caused by virulent organisms, most commonly *Staphylococcus aureus, Streptococcus pyogenes,* and *Neisseria gonorrhoeae*. Gram-negative enteric bacilli are less common causes. These organisms can infect healthy valves, which means that a previous valvular defect need not be present. Destruction of the affected valves may be associated with severe bacteremia and abscesses in many other organs.

B. Subacute Infective Endocarditis: Subacute involvement is more common. It is caused by organisms of low virulence such as *Streptococcus viridans, Streptococcus faecalis, Staphylococcus epidermidis,* and *Candida albicans*. The infection usually occurs in a previously damaged valve. Subacute infective endocarditis is a less severe illness characterized by low grade bacteremia, often developing over weeks to months and commonly presenting as fever of unknown origin. Valvular destruction is less severe and abscesses in other organs are rarely seen. With treatment, the mortality rate is low.

Table 22-3. Organisms most commonly causing infective endocarditis.[1]

	Usual Clinical Picture	
	Acute	**Subacute**
Staphylococcus aureus, Streptococcus pyogenes, Neisseria gonorrhoeae, Proteus, Pseudomonas	■■■■	
Bacteroides, Escherichia coli, Klebsiella	■■	■■
Staphylococcus epidermidis, Streptococcus viridans, Streptococcus pneumoniae, Streptococcus faecalis, Haemophilus, Listeria, Candida albicans, Histoplasma, Aspergillus, Rickettsia		■■■■

[1]*S aureus* causes more than 50% of acute cases, *S viridans* more than 50% of subacute cases. Many other organisms are occasionally causative.

Pathogenesis

Two factors are usually operative in the causation of infective endocarditis:

A. Bacteremia (or Fungemia): Entry of infectious agents into the blood is a prerequisite for infective endocarditis. Bacteremia is apt to occur in the following clinical circumstances:

1. Following oral surgical procedures, including dentistry–*S viridans,* which is a low-virulence α-hemolytic streptococcus normally found in the oral cavity, is the cause of over half of cases of subacute infective endocarditis.

2. Following urologic procedures such as bladder catheterization–*S faecalis* and gram-negative enteric bacilli, which are normally found in the perineal region, are the common organisms.

3. Intravenous drug abuse–Virulent organisms, commonly *S aureus,* frequently contaminate unsterilized needles used by drug addicts.

4. Severe infection–Severe infection anywhere in the body may be associated with bacteremia.

B. Endocardial Injury: While the more virulent organisms can cause infection in normal valves, less virulent ones can only infect previously abnormal endocardium. Most cases of endocarditis occur in patients with endocardial abnormalities. Certain factors important in the pathogenesis of infective endocarditis are common to all the clinical settings listed below, ie, high pressure gradients and jet effects, which together increase the likelihood of endocardial injury and local thrombosis, providing a nidus for infection if there are microorganisms in the blood at the time the thrombosis occurs.

1. Chronic rheumatic heart disease-Mitral incompetence and aortic valve disease impose a high risk. Pure mitral stenosis is rarely complicated by infective endocarditis. Chronic rheumatic valvular disease is the most common antecedent endocardial abnormality associated with infective endocarditis.

2. Congenital heart disease-Congenital heart disease, most commonly a small ventricular septal defect or bicuspid aortic valve, is the antecedent endocardial abnormality in a small number of cases. Its relative frequency may, however, increase as the incidence of chronic rheumatic heart disease decreases.

3. Degenerative valvular disease-Calcification of valves and mitral valve prolapse syndrome are rarely complicated by infective endocarditis.

4. Prosthetic cardiac valves-Prosthetic valves are widely used for valve replacement and frequently become infected. *C albicans* and staphylococci are common causes of prosthetic valve endocarditis.

Pathology

Infected thrombi (vegetations) are the characteristic pathologic finding in infective endocarditis (Figs 22–5 to 22–7; see also Chapter 9). The colonies of organisms within the vegetations are relatively protected from host defenses because the valves are avascular and cannot mount an adequate acute inflammatory response and because the surface of the vegetation is covered by dense fibrin and platelets, which limits access of leukocytes or antimicrobial substances in the blood, including antibiotics, to the interior of the vegetation where the organisms are found.

The vegetations of infective endocarditis are multiple, large, and friable and commonly become detached from the valve as emboli. Vegetations tend to be larger and more friable in acute than in subacute endocarditis.

Vegetations occur principally on the valves of the left side of the heart, following the distribution of chronic rheumatic heart disease (mitral > aortic > tricuspid > pulmonary). Right-sided endocarditis is uncommon but may occur in (1) intravenous drug abusers, in whom the tricuspid valve is commonly affected; (2) patients with indwelling venous catheters extending into the right atrium; (3) patients with gonococcal endocarditis;

VEGETATION

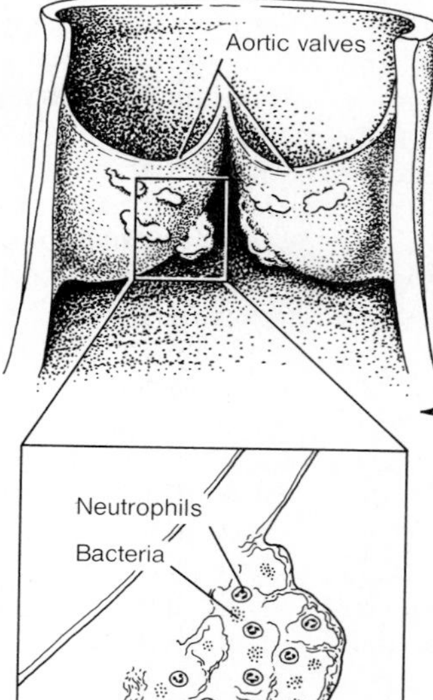

EFFECTS

Valve distortion
- Changing murmurs

Valve perforation
- Acute valvular incompetence

Bacteremia
- Splenomegaly
- Fever, malaise, weight loss
- Microabscesses (with virulent organisms)
- Involvement of viscera
- Pustular skin rashes

Immune complexes
- Osler's nodes (tender red nodules)
- Janeway lesions (red papules in palms and soles)
- Proliferative glomerulonephritis
- Vasculitis, arthritis

Emboli
- Focal embolic glomerulonephritis
- Petechial hemorrhages
  - In nail bed (splinter hemorrhages)
  - In retina (Roth's spots)
  - Cutaneous
- Mycotic aneurysms
- Microinfarcts
  - CNS dysfunction
  - Intestinal pain
  - Myocardial ischemia
  - Lung: hemoptysis

Laboratory tests
- Positive blood culture (95%)
- Leukocytosis, chronic anemia
- ↑ ESR
- Hyperglobulinemia
- ↓ Complement levels

Figure 22–5. Clinical effects of infective endocarditis resulting from infection and formation of vegetations on the valve.

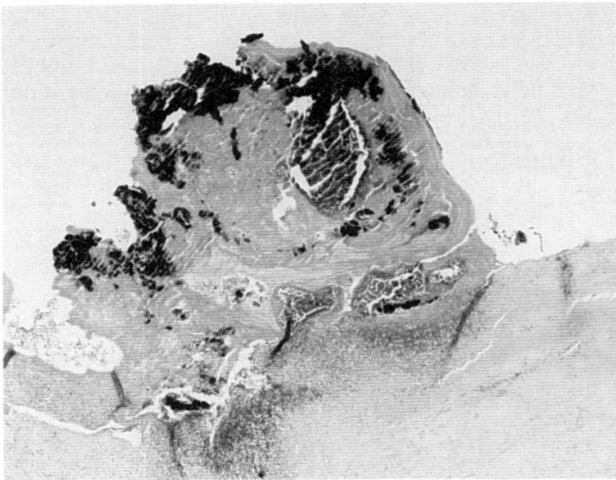

Figure 22-6. Vegetation of infective endocarditis. Dark areas represent collections of neutrophils and bacterial colonies. Low magnification.

and (4) patients with ventricular septal defect, because the jet of shunted blood causes endocardial injury in the right ventricle.

Clinical Features (Fig 22-5)

A. Bacteremia (or Fungemia): Blood culture is positive in over 95% of cases and is the most important diagnostic test. Most patients have constant bacteremia; a few have intermittent bacteremia. For this reason, it is recommended that multiple blood cultures be drawn at intervals before the patient is given antibiotics.

Fever is the most common symptom. It is low-grade and persistent in subacute endocarditis and high with rigors in acute disease. Chronic bacteremia causes phagocytic and endothelial cell hyperplasia in the spleen, leading to **splenomegaly**. Bacteremia also causes **petechial hemorrhages** in the skin, retina (Roth spots), and nails ("splinter hemorrhages"). Weight loss and chronic anemia also occur in subacute disease. Finger clubbing is a common but late sign; its pathogenesis is unknown.

When infection is caused by virulent pyogenic organisms, **miliary abscesses** are produced in all organs of the body.

B. Immune Complexes: Antibodies and bacterial antigens combine to form circulating immune complexes. Deposition of immune complexes in the glomerular capillaries causes focal or diffuse proliferative glomerulonephritis (Chapter 48). Microscopic hematuria and proteinuria occur in over 50% of patients with infective endocarditis.

Cutaneous immune complex-mediated vasculitis is responsible for erythematous papules in the palms and soles (Janeway lesions) and characteristic tender red nodules in the fingers or toes (Osler's nodes). These occur in 25% of patients.

C. Valvular Dysfunction: Large vegetations on the valves impinge on the flow of blood causing turbulence and **cardiac murmurs**. With changes in size of vegetations, the character of the murmurs changes, a feature that is typical of infective endocarditis.

Progressive destruction of the valve may produce **valve perforation** (Fig 22-7), currently the commonest cause of acute mitral and aortic incompetence.

D. Embolism: Emboli from the friable vegetations are common. With left-sided endocarditis, systemic embolism causes multifocal areas of infarction in the brain, kidney, heart, intestine, spleen, and extremities. With right sided vegetations, embolism involves the pulmonary vessels.

In about 10% of cases of infective endocarditis, the organisms in the embolus produce a local infection in the artery at the site of lodgment, causing weakening of the arterial wall and formation of an aneurysm. These infective **mycotic aneurysms** may rupture and cause massive hemorrhage. (*Note:* The term "mycotic aneurysm" denotes an aneurysm resulting from any infection—not necessarily a fungal infection, as suggested by the adjective.)

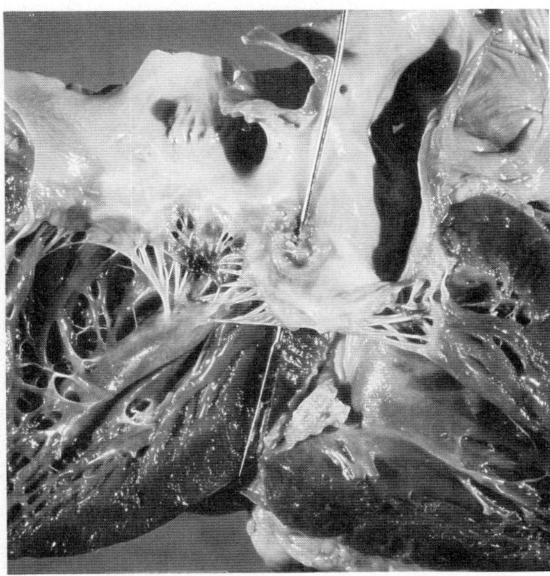

Figure 22-7. Perforation of the mitral valve in infective endocarditis. (**Note:** A metal probe has been passed through the perforation in the valve.) The perforation has occurred in the area of a vegetation.

Differential Diagnosis (Table 22-4)

Infective endocarditis must be distinguished from other diseases causing fever of unknown origin and noninfective causes of endocarditis in

Table 22-4. Differential features of diseases in which valve vegetations and plaques occur.

	Infective Endocarditis	Rheumatic Fever	Systemic Lupus Erythematosus	Noninfective Endocarditis	Carcinoid Syndrome[1]
Vegetation size	Large	Small	Small	Medium	Plaques
Valves affected	Mitral, aortic	Mitral, aortic	Mitral	Mitral, aortic	Pulmonary, tricuspid
Site	Leaflet	Free edge	Atrial and ventricular surfaces	Leaflet	Both surfaces
Embolism	+ + +	−	−	+	−
Acute inflammatory cells	+	−	−	+	−
Organisms	+ + +	−	−	−	−
Valve destruction	+ +	−	−	−	−
Valve fibrosis	−	+ + +	−	−	+

[1] see page 358.

which vegetations occur. These include acute rheumatic fever, collagen diseases such as systemic lupus erythematosus, and noninfective thrombotic endocarditis.

Noninfective endocarditis was at one time thought to be a clinically insignificant cause of valvular vegetations occurring in terminally ill patients—it was also called marantic (wasting) endocarditis for that reason. Recently it has been recognized that these vegetations may occur early in the course of many diseases, notably cancer. The vegetations occur mainly on the mitral and aortic valves and may be large and friable. Their detachment as systemic emboli is common and may result in significant abnormalities in these patients.

Prevention & Treatment

When dental, oral, or urologic procedures are planned in patients with known cardiac valvular disease, antibiotic cover during and immediately after the procedure is necessary to kill any organisms that enter the bloodstream before they reach the cardiac valves. Such antibiotic prophylaxis is effective in preventing infective endocarditis in these patients.

Antibiotic therapy, based on the antibiotic sensitivity of the organism cultured from the blood, is the mainstay of treatment of infective endocarditis. Even with appropriate antibiotic therapy, 10–20% of "subacute" cases and up to 50% of acute cases end in death. Therapy should be continued for 4–6 weeks to eradicate all organisms from the vegetations. Where there is severe valve damage and in prosthetic valve endocarditis, valve replacement is required.

DISORDERS OF CARDIAC VALVES

MITRAL STENOSIS

Etiology

Mitral stenosis (Fig 22–8) is almost always the result of chronic rheumatic heart disease. Females are affected more than males in a ratio of 9:1.

Pathophysiology (Figs 22-9 and 22-10)

Mitral stenosis causes resistance to blood flow through the open mitral valve during diastole. The resulting turbulence produces a murmur. In mild

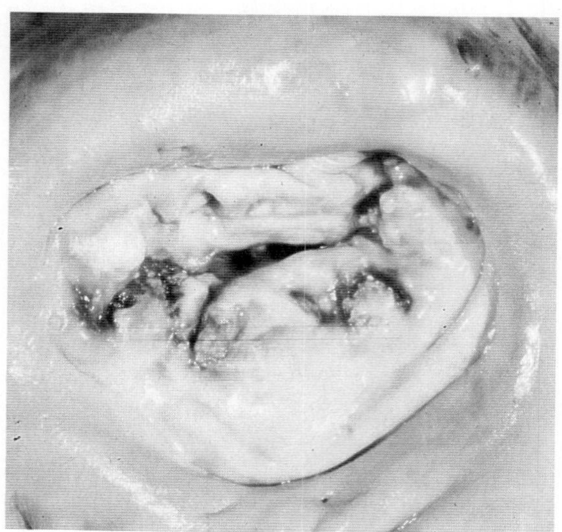

Figure 22-8. Mitral stenosis. The mitral valve orifice is visualized from the left atrium and shows the typical "fish-mouth" appearance.

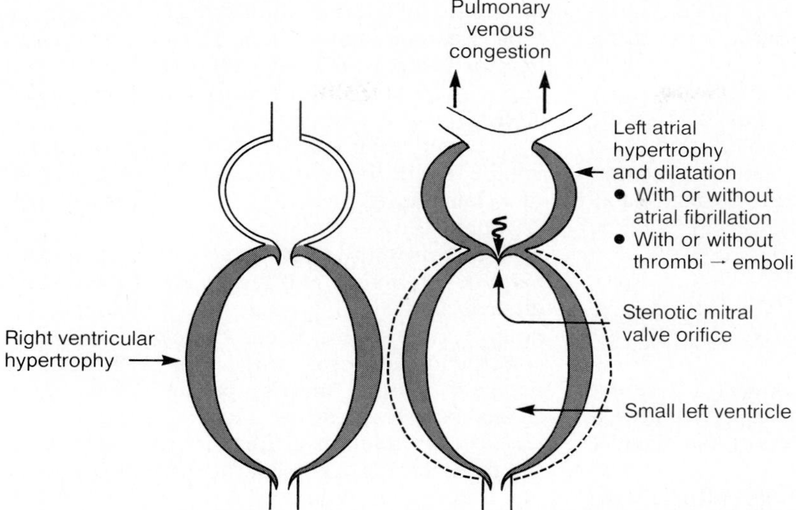

Figure 22-9. Pathophysiology of mitral stenosis. Resistance to flow at the mitral orifice leads to dilatation and increased pressure in the left atrium, which is transmitted to the pulmonary veins. Pulmonary venous hypertension causes changes in the pulmonary vessels that result in pulmonary arterial hypertension, which in turn leads to right ventricular hypertrophy.

mitral stenosis, the pressure across the valve rapidly equalizes, and the murmur is restricted to the mid-diastolic part of the cycle. With increasing stenosis, the length of the diastolic murmur increases. The murmur is accentuated by atrial systole which precedes ventricular systole (presystolic accentuation). Closure of the abnormal mitral valve is often loud (loud first heart sound).

Normally, the mitral valve opens silently soon after aortic valve closure (S_2) (Chapter 21). However, an abnormal stenotic mitral valve opens with a clicking sound (opening snap, OS); the shorter the interval between S_2 and OS, the higher the left atrial pressure and the more severe the stenosis. If the valve becomes rigid as a result of calcification, the opening snap disappears.

Obstruction to flow through the mitral orifice leads to left atrial dilatation and hypertrophy (Fig 22–9). Blood tends to stagnate in the left atrium, predisposing to thrombus formation, especially if atrial fibrillation develops (a common complication of mitral stenosis). Left atrial thrombi may then cause systemic embolism. Or it may obstruct the narrowed mitral orifice, causing sudden death ("ball valve thrombus").

Mitral stenosis leads to increased pulmonary venous pressure and features of left heart failure. If acute, pulmonary edema and pulmonary hemor-

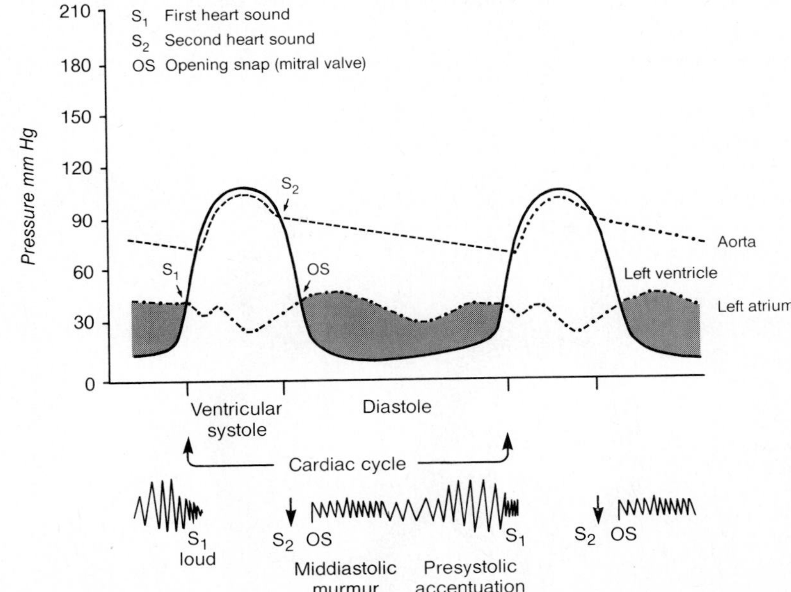

Figure 22-10. Mitral stenosis, showing pressure changes in the left side of the heart and aorta and abnormal heart sounds in a typical case. Compare with normal (Fig 21–2). Note the pressure gradient between the left atrium and left ventricle during mid diastole owing to the stenotic mitral opening. This corresponds to the murmur.

rhage may occur; if chronic, the results are interstitial fibrosis, pulmonary arterial hypertension and right ventricular hypertrophy.

In mild mitral stenosis, left ventricular filling is normal and cardiac output is normal. With severe stenosis, left ventricular end-diastolic volume and cardiac output are decreased. The left ventricle, which pumps less blood than normal, may undergo mild atrophy.

MITRAL INCOMPETENCE

Etiology

Rheumatic heart disease accounts for about 50% of cases of mitral incompetence, usually associated with mitral stenosis. Males and females are equally affected.

Mitral valve prolapse ("floppy valve") syndrome is a degenerative change that is present in about 1% of the population (especially young women), the result of accumulation of mucopolysaccharides in the valve leaflet. Clinical mitral incompetence occurs in only a small percentage of cases. A similar abnormality of the mitral valve is present in patients with Marfan's syndrome.

Chronic left ventricular failure with dilatation of the mitral valve ring may cause functional mitral incompetence. Acute mitral incompetence may occur with rupture of chordae tendineae due to **infective endocarditis** or **trauma** or to rupture of papillary muscles due to **myocardial infarction**.

Rarely, **calcification of the valve ring** in the elderly may lead to mitral incompetence.

Pathophysiology (Figs 22-11 and 22-12)

When the mitral valve is incompetent, regurgitation of blood from the left ventricle to the atrium occurs throughout systole, producing a typical **pansystolic murmur**. During diastole, regurgitant blood flows back across the mitral valve, producing a third heart sound and a diastolic flow murmur.

Left ventricular volume is greatly increased, being the sum of the cardiac output plus the regurgitant flow; the left ventricle is thus dilated and hypertrophied.

The left atrium, which accepts both the pulmonary venous return and regurgitant flow, is also dilated. Left atrial pressure and pulmonary venous pressure are increased. Acute mitral valve incompetence, as occurs with valve perforation or papillary muscle rupture, produces pulmonary edema and acute left heart failure. In chronic disease, there is pulmonary fibrosis, pulmonary arterial hypertension, and right ventricular hypertrophy followed by failure.

AORTIC STENOSIS

Etiology

Rheumatic aortic stenosis is commonly accompanied by mitral valve defects. Isolated aortic stenosis is uncommon in chronic rheumatic heart disease.

Congenital bicuspid aortic valves may undergo progressive fibrosis and calcification; this is now believed to be the cause of more than 50% of cases of aortic stenosis.

Calcification of the valve in the elderly may cause mild aortic stenosis.

Congenital narrowing of the left ventricular outflow tract above or below the aortic valve produces the same functional defect as aortic stenosis. **Hypertrophic cardiomyopathy** may also pro-

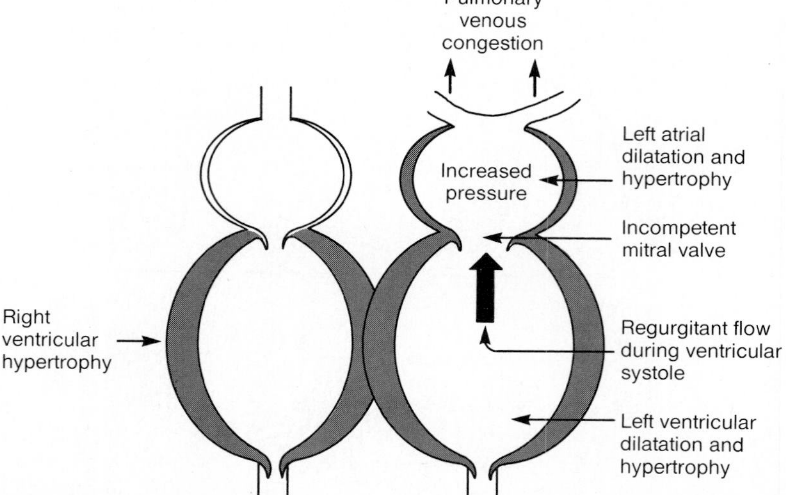

Figure 22-11. Pathophysiology of mitral incompetence. Regurgitation of blood from left ventricle to left atrium during systole causes dilatation and increased pressure in the left atrium. This results in pulmonary venous congestion, pulmonary vascular changes, and pulmonary arterial hypertension, leading to right ventricular hypertrophy. The left ventricle, which must pump out the cardiac output plus the regurgitant flow, undergoes dilatation and muscular hypertrophy.

amine), which promotes fibrosis in the endocardium, leading to plaquelike fibrotic lesions in the valves with fusion of commissures. The right-sided valves are chiefly affected in carcinoid syndrome because serotonin is rapidly metabolized in the lung and is present only in low concentration in pulmonary venous blood.

Pulmonary incompetence is rare and most often "functional" owing to valve ring dilatation in right heart failure.

Pathophysiology

Pulmonary stenosis causes a rough **ejection systolic murmur** over the pulmonary valve, delayed closure of the pulmonary valve, and very soft valve closure owing to the low pressure in the pulmonary artery. Typically, the pulmonary component of the second heart sound is not heard. Right ventricular hypertrophy and failure occur.

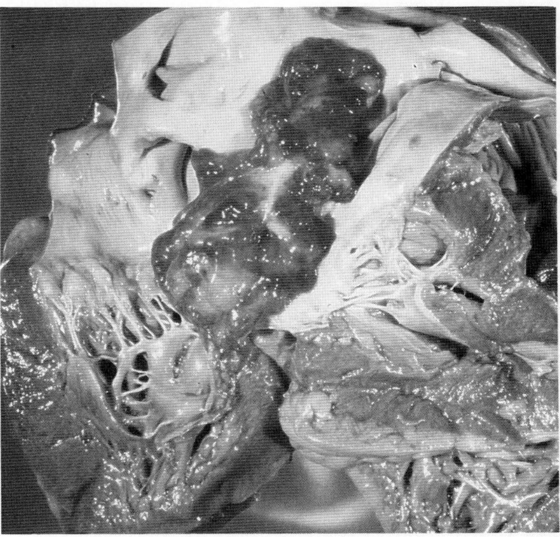

Figure 22–15. Left atrial myxoma projecting into the lumen of the opened left atrium. Note protrusion of tumor into the mitral valve orifice. This patient died suddenly from circulatory arrest caused by prolapse of the tumor into the mitral orifice.

TRICUSPID VALVE LESIONS

Tricuspid incompetence is usually due to right ventricular dilatation in right heart failure. This causes a pulsatile jugular venous pulse and pulsatile enlargement of the liver owing to transmission of right ventricular systole to the venae cavae through the incompetent tricuspid valve.

Tricuspid stenosis rarely occurs in chronic rheumatic heart disease, and it is then almost always associated with mitral and aortic valve lesions. Tricuspid stenosis and incompetence may also occur in carcinoid syndrome and as congenital defects.

NEOPLASMS OF THE ENDOCARDIUM

CARDIAC MYXOMA

Myxoma is a benign neoplasm of the endocardium. Although it occurs rarely, it is by far the commonest primary neoplasm of the heart. The neoplasm is derived from endocardial mesenchymal cells and usually forms a firm gelatinous polypoid mass that protrudes into the lumen of the heart (Fig 22–15). Myxomas occur almost exclusively in the atria, particularly the left atrium. Histologically, it is composed of small stellate cells embedded in an abundant mucopolysaccharide stroma.

Clinical features of cardiac myxoma include systemic effects such as irregular, prolonged fever, weight loss, anemia, and increased plasma globulin levels. The reason for these systemic symptoms is unknown.

Additional features in left atrial myxoma include systemic embolism, resulting from detachment of fragments of the neoplasm; and mitral orifice obstruction. Turbulence of blood around the tumor produces a middiastolic murmur that resembles the murmur of mitral stenosis. Prolapse of the polypoid neoplasm into the mitral orifice may obstruct circulation and is a rare cause of sudden death.

23 The Heart: III. Myocardium & Pericardium

ISCHEMIC HEART DISEASE

Incidence

Ischemic heart disease is responsible for 500,000 deaths a year in the Unites States—or 25–30% of all deaths—and is the leading cause of death in most developed countries.

Etiology

Ischemic heart disease is caused by narrowing of one or more of the 3 major coronary artery branches (Fig 23–1). These are functional end-arteries, and sudden occlusion of any one leads to infarction in the area of supply. However, gradual narrowing may permit development of collaterals that are sufficient to prevent infarction.

Atherosclerosis accounts for 98% of cases of ischemic heart disease. The risk factors for ischemic heart disease are those for atherosclerosis (Chapter 20).

Other rare causes of coronary artery narrowing include coronary artery spasm (Prinzmetal angina); coronary artery embolism, most commonly in infective endocarditis; coronary ostial narrowing in syphilis and Takayasu's aortitis; coronary ostial occlusion in dissecting aneurysm of the aorta; and various types of arteritis involving the coronary arteries, including polyarteritis nodosa, thromboangiitis obliterans, and giant cell arteritis.

Clinical Features

Ischemic heart disease may be manifested clinically in many ways (Fig 23–2). The more important ones—myocardial infarction, angina pectoris, sudden death, cardiac arrhythmias, and cardiac failure—are discussed below. An individual patient with ischemic heart disease may manifest more than one of these conditions.

MYOCARDIAL INFARCTION

Incidence

Approximately 1.25 million people in the United States suffer a myocardial infarction (heart attack) every year; of these 35–40% die. Most patients are over 45 years of age, and men are affected 3 times more frequently than women, paralleling the incidence of atherosclerosis.

Etiology

Except in those rare causes of nonatherosclerotic coronary artery narrowing listed above, most patients who suffer myocardial infarction have **severe atherosclerotic narrowing** of one or more coronary arteries (Fig 23–3; see also Chapter 20). A fresh thrombus overlying an atherosclerotic plaque is found in 40–90% of cases (Fig 23–4), the frequency varying greatly in different studies. Thrombosis may be precipitated by slowing and turbulence of blood flow in the region of a plaque or by ulceration of a plaque.

In cases where no thrombus is found, infarction may be precipitated by increased myocardial demand for oxygen, as occurs during exercise and excitement; reduction of coronary blood flow through a greatly narrowed artery due to cardiac slowing during sleep; or segmental muscular spasm of coronary arteries. In some cases, the thrombus may undergo lysis by the fibrinolytic system after infarction has occurred.

Distribution of Infarction (Fig 23–1)

Myocardial infarction involves principally the left ventricle, interventricular septum, and conducting system. The atria and right ventricle are rarely involved, probably because their thin mus-

A
Normal blood supply

Left coronary artery
Anterior descending branch
Right coronary artery
Right marginal branch
Left circumflex branch
Right coronary artery
Posterior descending branch
Anterior
Posterior

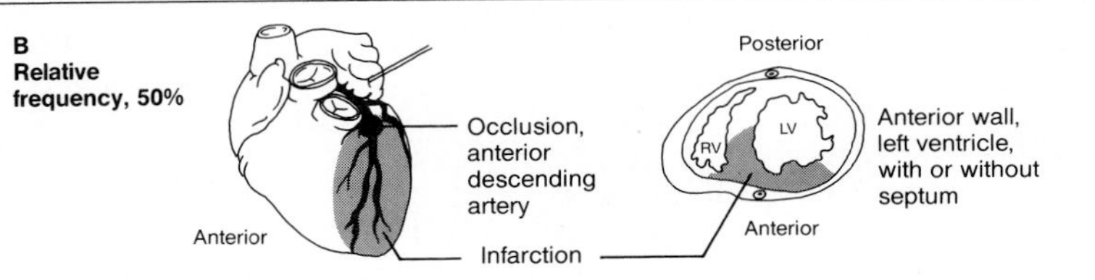

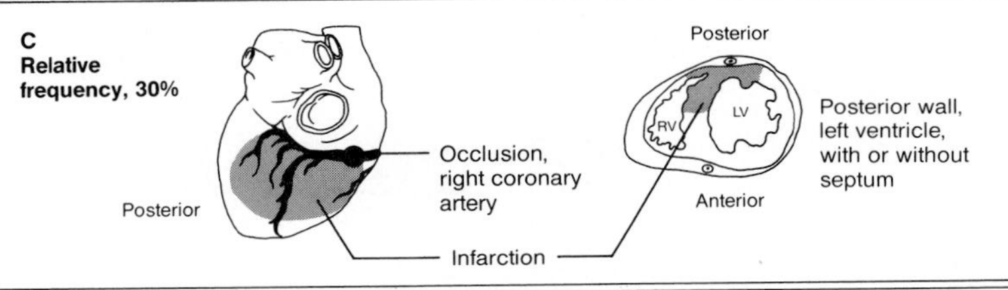

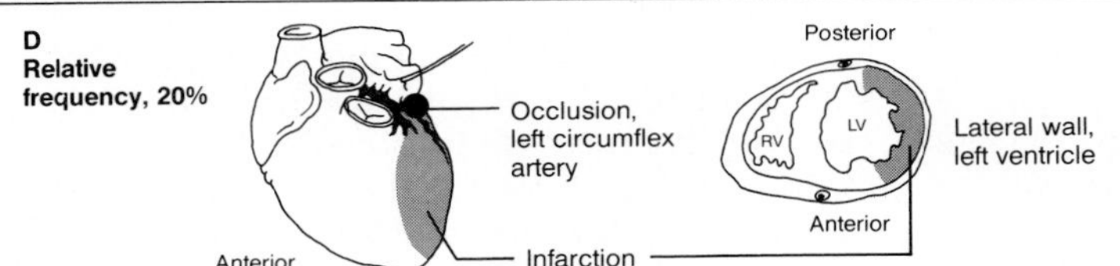

Figure 23–1. Blood supply to the myocardium **(A)** and areas of infarction resulting from the most frequent sites of coronary artery occlusion (relative frequency expressed as a percentage). The exact area of myocardium affected will vary depending on normal anatomic variation in blood supply and the extent of collateral circulation that exists at the time of coronary occlusion.

cle walls derive a considerable part of their nutritional supply directly from the blood in the cardiac lumen. The distribution of infarction depends on which vessel is occluded. However, because collaterals develop in a chronically narrowed coronary circulation, the blood supply may traverse circuitous routes, leading to infarcts in unusual sites (paradoxic infarction).

Infarction may be **transmural,** involving the full thickness of the wall (Fig 23–5), or **subendocardial**. The subendocardial region has the most critical blood supply.

Pathology

For 2 hours after the onset of myocardial infarction (as indicated by onset of pain or arrhythmias and shock), there are no morphologic changes in the necrotic myocardial fibers. At about 2 hours, electron microscopic changes appear (swelling of mitochondrial endoplasmic reticulum, fragmentation of myofibrils). Light microscopic changes may appear in 4–6 hours but are rarely detectable with certainty before 12–24 hours. **Coagulative necrosis** of the myocardial fibers is recognized by nuclear pyknosis and dark pink staining of the cytoplasm and loss of striations in the cytoplasm (Fig 23–6; Table 23–1; see also Chapter 9).

The tetrazolium test. Incubation of a slice of normal myocardium in tetrazolium produces a red-brown color resulting from reaction of tetrazolium with a dehydrogenase enzyme; infarcted myocardium remains pale because the enzyme is lost from the cells within hours after infarction. The value of this technique is limited.

Clinical Features

Ischemic pain is the dominant symptom of myocardial infarction—a tightening retrosternal pain that varies in severity from mild to excruciating. It resembles angina but is not relieved by rest or vasodilators. Rarely, myocardial infarction may occur without pain ("silent infarction"). The onset of ischemic pain is sudden and may occur

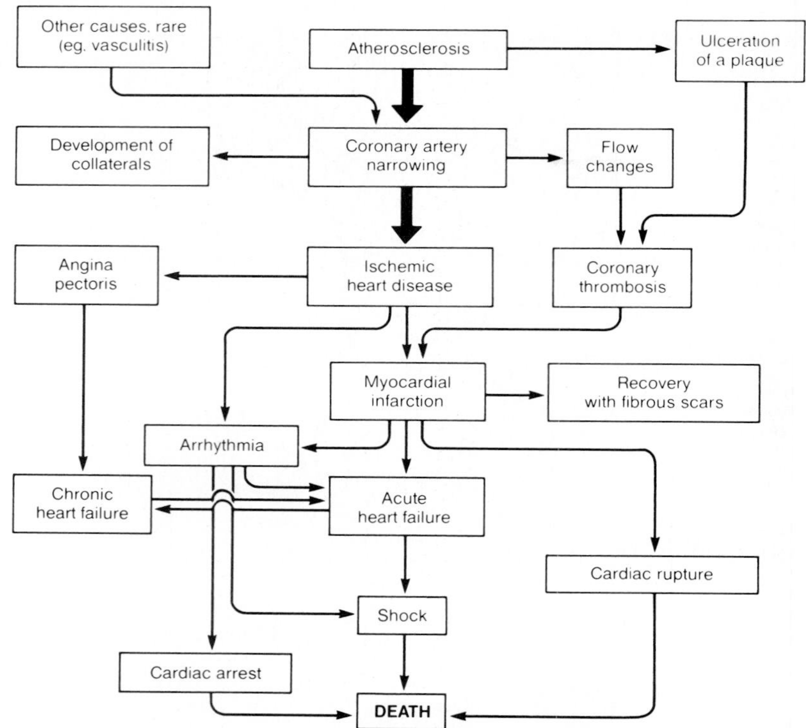

Figure 23-2. Causes and clinical consequences of ischemic heart disease.

during exercise, excitement, rest or even sleep. Cardiac pain is often accompanied by signs of autonomic stimulation such as sweating, changes in heart rate, a lowered blood pressure (with or without shock), and faint or additional heart sounds.

The diagnosis of myocardial infarction, when suspected clinically, is based on electrocardiographic and serum enzyme changes. Electrocardiography shows elevation of the ST segment above the isoelectric line within a few hours, representing an abnormal electrical potential associated with acute injury. The T wave becomes inverted, and in transmural infarction the dead muscle acts as an electrical window, producing an abnormal Q wave. As healing takes place, the ST segment returns to the isoelectric line, but T wave inversion and the Q wave persist.

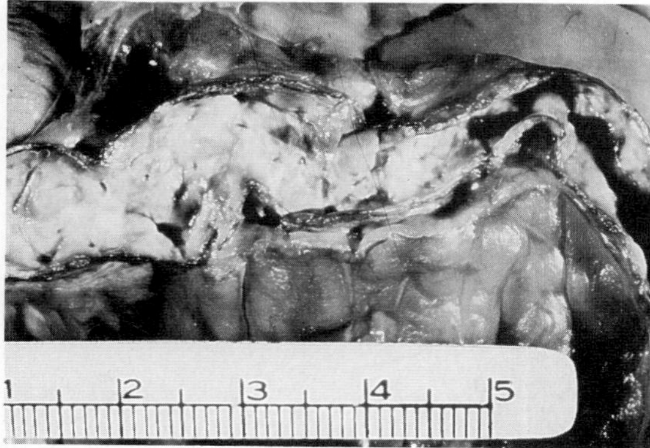

Figure 23-3. Coronary atherosclerosis. The left coronary artery has been opened longitudinally to show extensive plaque formation that has produced marked surface irregularity. Marked narrowing of the vessel was present, but this is better seen in transverse sections (see Fig 20-8).

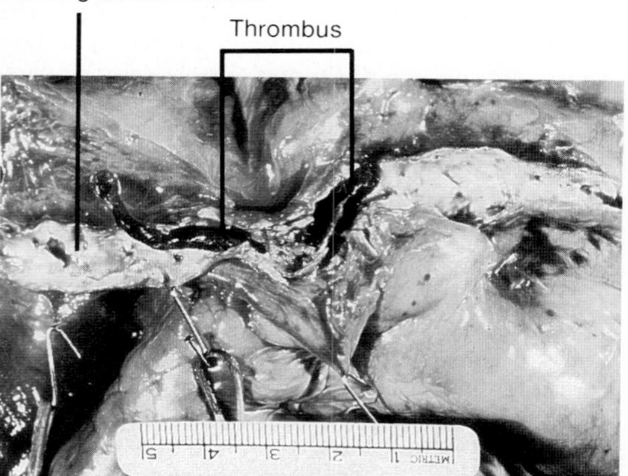

Figure 23-4. Thrombosis in an atherosclerotic coronary artery, resulting in occlusion of the vessel.

Right ventricle

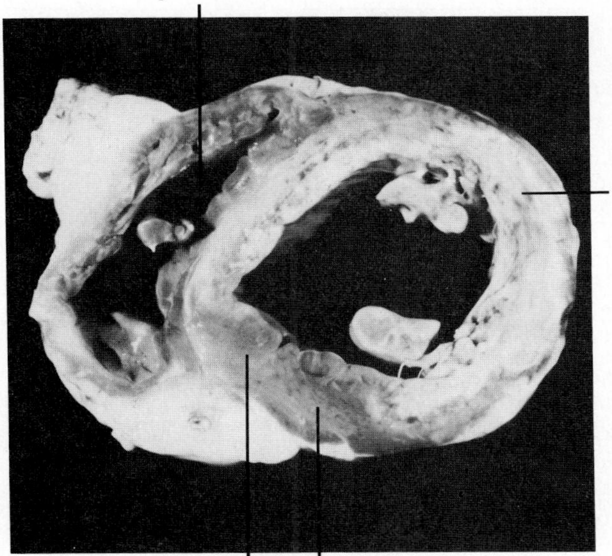

Infarcted myocardium, lateral left ventricle

Normal myocardium of the posterior left ventricle and septum. This area is supplied by the right coronary artery.

Figure 23-5. Myocardial infarction. The infarcted zone, which is pale, includes the anterior and lateral wall of the left ventricle and the anterior two-thirds of the interventricular septum. This infarct was associated with thrombotic occlusion of the main left coronary artery.

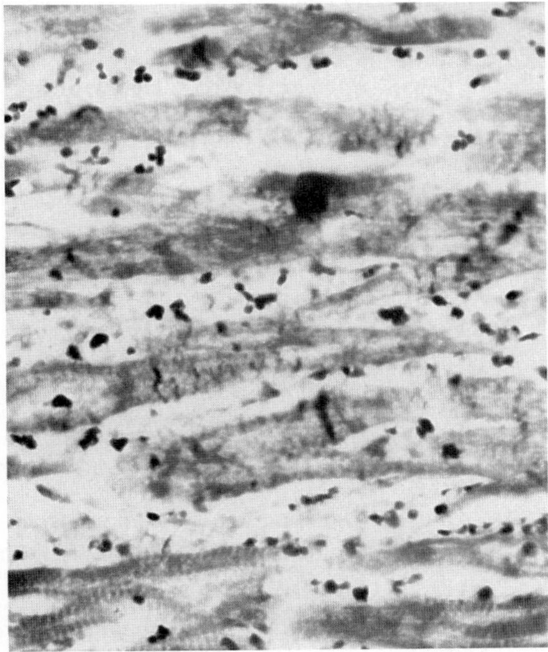

Figure 23-6. Acute myocardial infarction 1–3 days after onset. Note loss of striations and lysis of myofibers, with acute inflammation. Striations are still visible in a few myofibers at the bottom of the figure. High magnification.

Necrotic myocardial fibers release a variety of enzymes into the bloodstream (Fig 23–7). When both creatine kinase (CK)-MB isoenzyme and lactic acid dehydrogenase-isoenzyme 1 (LDH–1) serum levels are elevated, a specific diagnosis of acute myocardial infarction can be made. When a patient with chest pain shows no elevation of either of these enzymes on serial samples, myocardial infarction can be ruled out. Sequential CK-MB levels are helpful in following the evolution of an infarct—eg, a secondary increase indicates new infarction or extension of the area of infarction.

Myocardial infarction is followed by elevation of temperature, increased neutrophil count in the peripheral blood, and changes in plasma proteins. Increases in acute phase reactants such as fibrinogen and haptoglobin cause elevation of the erythrocyte sedimentation rate. These changes are due to the release of chemical mediators in the area of infarction.

Complications

A. Arrhythmias: Abnormalities in cardiac rhythm occur in about 70% of cases of myocardial infarction, mainly during the first few hours. They represent a serious and preventable cause of death.

1. Ectopic electrical foci develop in the injured myocardium. Ventricular extrasystoles are common; ventricular tachycardia is less common but can lead to impaired ventricular filling and acute

Table 23-1. Dating of an infarct.[1]

Elapsed Time	Gross or Naked Eye Features (at Autopsy)	Light Microscopic Features
0-12 hours	None	Usually None
12-24 hours	Softening, irregular pallor	Loss of striations Cytoplasmic eosinophilia Nuclear pyknosis Mild edema Occasional neutrophils
1-3 days	Pale infarct surrounded by a red (hyperemic) zone	As above, plus: Nuclear lysis More neutrophils Inflammatory capillary dilatation
4-7 days	Pale or yellow (caused by liquefaction by neutrophils), definite red margin	As above, plus: Liquefaction of muscle fibers Neutrophils Macrophages remove debris Ingrowth of granulation tissue from margins
7-14 days	Progressive replacement of yellow infarct by red-purple (granulation) tissue	As above, plus: Disappearance of necrotic muscle cells Reduced numbers of neutrophils Macrophages, lymphocytes Beginnings of fibrosis and organization of granulation tissue
2-6 weeks	Becomes gray-white	As above, plus: Development of fibrous scar Decreasing vascularity Contraction of scar

[1]The time course is influenced by the size of the infarct.

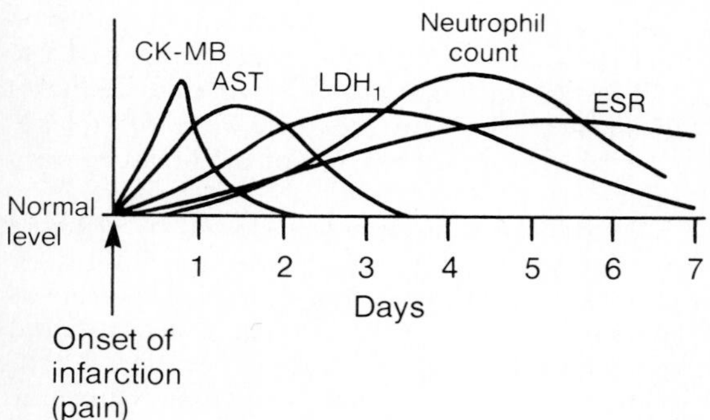

Figure 23-7. Changes in serum enzymes, neutrophil count, and erythrocyte sedimentation rate (ESR) following acute myocardial infarction. The serum level of MB isoenzyme of creatine kinase (CK-MB) rises rapidly, and CK-MB elevation is the test of choice in the first 24 hours. Since CK-MB levels return to baseline rapidly, isoenzyme 1 of lactate dehydrogenase (LDH_1) is the test of choice from 2 to 7 days. A test combination that includes CK-MB and LDH_1 is extremely effective in the diagnosis of acute myocardial infarction. Aspartate aminotransferase (AST) is of limited usefulness because of its lack of specificity, AST being present also in high concentration in liver and skeletal muscle.

left ventricular failure. The most dangerous arrhythmia is ventricular fibrillation, which causes cardiac arrest.

The occurrence of tachyarrhythmias bears no relationship to the size of the infarct. Successful management may therefore be followed by full recovery. Since most arrhythmias occur within the first 2 hours—often before the patient reaches a hospital—training of the lay community in cardiopulmonary resuscitation (CPR) is an important part of overall management. Community CPR training is recommended by the American Heart Association.

2. Heart block resulting from involvement of the conducting system occurs more commonly with posterior myocardial infarcts. It is usually due to involvement of the conducting fibers by edema around an infarct, in which case the heart block is temporary. Permanent heart block due to necrosis of the conducting fibers is less common. Complete heart block is characterized by severe bradycardia and reduced cardiac output. Death may occur.

3. Autonomic stimulation is a common occurrence in acute myocardial infarction, producing either tachycardia (sympathetic stimulation) or bradycardia (vagal stimulation).

B. Left Ventricular Failure: Acute left ventricular failure results from arrhythmia or massive necrosis of myocardium. The clinical effects are sudden death, cardiogenic shock, and acute pulmonary edema. The last 2 syndromes have a high mortality rate, even with treatment.

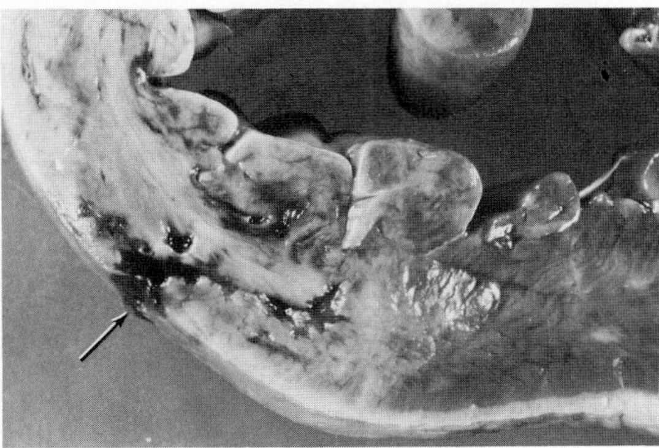

Figure 23–8. Myocardial infarction with rupture of the left ventricular wall. (Courtesy of O Rambo. Reproduced, with permission, from Sokolow M, McIlroy MB: *Clinical Cardiology,* 5th ed. Appleton & Lange, 1990.

C. Progressive Infarction: Extension of the initial infarcted area to adjacent muscle is uncommon, but it must be recognized because it can be prevented. The muscle around the infarcted area has a marginal blood supply that may become inadequate if there is an increased myocardial oxygen demand, eg, during exercise or under conditions of emotional stress. This is one reason why patients are kept at bed rest in the first week after myocardial infarction. Vascular supply to the muscle is at risk also if there is a decrease in coronary perfusion, due either to extension of a thrombus or to decreased cardiac output. Progression of an infarct can be diagnosed by following the serum CK-MB levels.

D. Pericarditis: Fibrinous or hemorrhagic pericarditis complicates myocardial infarction in about 30% of cases. It usually occurs within the first few days and may cause pericardial pain, pericardial rub, or pericardial effusion. Effusion sufficient to impair cardiac function is uncommon.

E. Systemic Embolism From Mural Thrombi: Involvement of the endocardium by the infarct leads to the formation of mural thrombi over the area of infarction. Such thrombi may become detached as emboli that enter the systemic arteries.

F. Myocardial Rupture: The infarcted muscle represents an area of weakness that is maximal at 5–7 days as the neutrophil enzymes cause liquefaction of the necrotic muscle fibers (Fig 23–8). Rupture may occur into the pericardial sac, producing hemopericardium and rapid death from cardiac tamponade; through the interventricular septum, producing an acute ventricular septal defect, with a left-to-right shunt and acute right ventricular failure; or within the papillary muscles, producing acute mitral incompetence.

G. Ventricular Aneurysm: (Fig 23–9.) High intraventricular pressure may cause progressive outward bulging of the area of infarction during systole. This paradoxic motion of part of the ventricular wall during systole is called a ventricular aneurysm. Aneurysms may develop either in the first 2 weeks or after several months in the healed infarct and may cause left ventricular failure. Mural thrombi forming in an aneurysm may become detached as systemic emboli.

ANGINA PECTORIS

Angina pectoris is characterized by episodic ischemic cardiac pain not associated with myocardial infarction. Two types of angina are recognized: angina of effort and variant (Prinzmetal's) angina.

Angina of Effort

Angina of effort is a common disorder usually caused by severe atherosclerotic narrowing of the coronary arterial system. The coronary arteries can provide the myocardium with adequate blood during rest but not during periods of exercise,

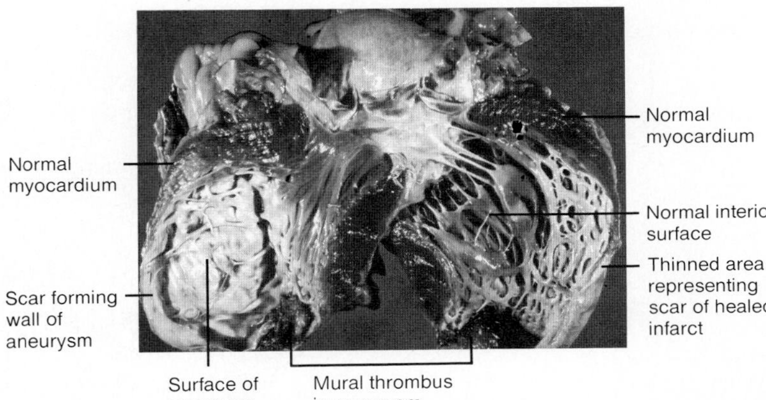

Figure 23–9. Aneurysm of the left ventricle in a patient who died from intractable heart failure 2 months after an acute myocardial infarction. The left ventricle has been cut and the 2 halves splayed out.

stress, or excitement, which precipitate ischemic pain; the pain is relieved by resting or by administration of amyl nitrite or nitroglycerin (glyceryl trinitrate).

Pathologic changes associated with angina are variable (Fig 23–10). Infarction is not present; serum enzyme levels are not elevated; and the ECG does not show changes of acute injury. Nonspecific changes in the ST segment such as ST depression and T wave inversion may reflect chronic ischemic damage. Electrocardiography during carefully graded exercise (treadmill test) is a sensitive method for detecting ischemic heart disease.

Patients with angina of effort have an increased risk of myocardial infarction, which may be preceded by an increase in the severity of anginal attacks ("crescendo or unstable angina").

Variant Angina

Variant (Prinzmetal's) angina is uncommon and occurs independently of atherosclerosis—which may, however, be present as an incidental finding. Variant angina occurs at rest and is not related to myocardial work. It is believed to be caused by coronary artery muscle spasm of insufficient duration or degree to cause myocardial infarction.

SUDDEN DEATH

Sudden death is a well-recognized occurrence in patients whose only abnormality at autopsy is severe coronary atherosclerosis. This has been attributed to **ventricular fibrillation,** leading to cardiac arrest. Studies of patients surviving such episodes (ie, in hospitalized patients) have shown that ventricular fibrillation often leads to death before myocardial infarction can develop. Many patients who die suddenly in this manner are heavy smokers.

CARDIAC ARRHYTHMIAS

Ventricular arrhythmias (Chapter 20) commonly occur in ischemic heart disease. Ventricular fibrillation, ventricular tachycardia, and complete

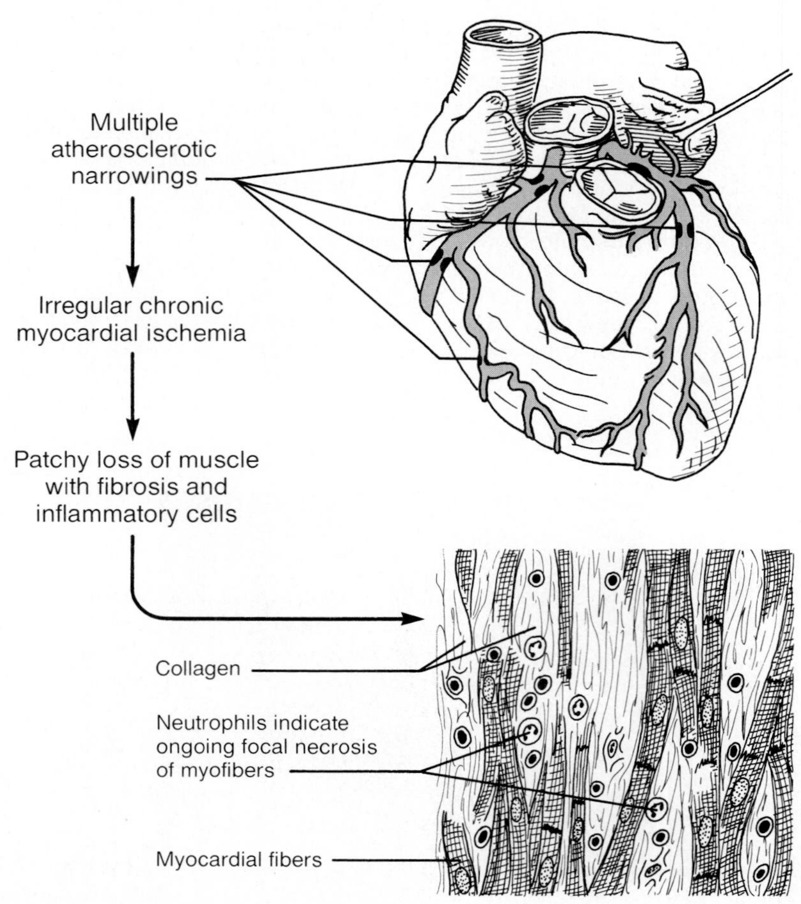

Figure 23–10. Pathologic changes commonly seen in chronic ischemic heart disease. Patients with these changes may be asymptomatic or suffer from angina pectoris.

heart block may lead to cardiac failure or sudden death.

CARDIAC FAILURE

Ischemic heart disease may be manifested by chronic left ventricular failure with or without a history of infarction or angina. Clinical and electrocardiographic features are not specific for ischemic heart disease. T wave inversion on the ECG is a common finding.

Pathologic examination shows atherosclerotic narrowing of the coronary arteries and diffuse myocardial fibrosis (Fig 23–10). The total number of myocardial fibers is often diminished, and residual fibers may show compensatory hypertrophy. Cardiac failure occurs when hypertrophy of surviving muscle can no longer compensate for progressive loss of myocardial cells.

Causes

- Idiopathic (Fiedler's)
- Autoimmune diseases: rheumatic fever, SLE, polyarteritis, others
- Toxic: doxorubicin, alcohol, other drugs
- Sarcoidosis
- Irradiation
- Toxoplasmosis
- Trichinosis
- Trypanosomiasis (Chagas' disease)
- Diphtheria toxin
- Rickettsiae: Q fever, typhus
- Viruses: coxsackie B viruses

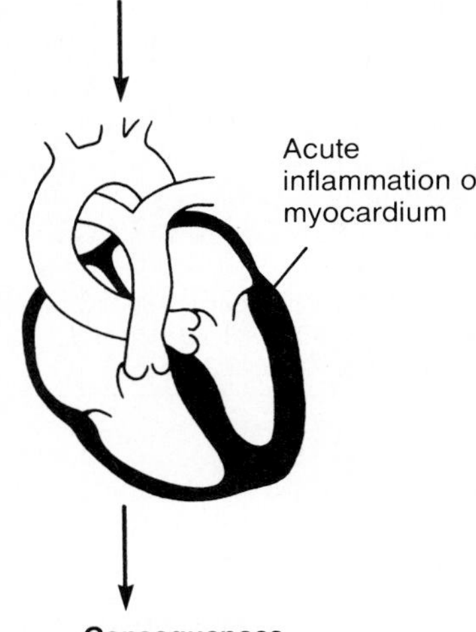

Consequences

- Fever, chest pain, leukocytosis, $\uparrow$ESR
- Left ventricular failure
- Arrhythmias
- Heart block
- ECG changes

Figure 23–11. Causes and clinical consequences of acute myocarditis.

MYOCARDITIS & CARDIOMYOPATHY

Myocarditis and cardiomyopathy are a group of diseases that chiefly involve the myocardium in the absence of hypertensive, congenital, ischemic, or valvular heart disease. The distinction between myocarditis and cardiomyopathy is somewhat arbitrary and not always made. Indeed, many authorities list myocarditis as a subset of cardiomyopathy. The term "**myocarditis**" is generally used to denote an acute myocardial disease characterized by inflammation. The cause may or may not be known. The term "**cardiomyopathy**" is then reserved for more chronic conditions in which inflammatory features are not conspicuous, including degenerative diseases and various diseases of unknown origin.

MYOCARDITIS

Incidence

The incidence of myocarditis is difficult to establish, in part because of the rarity with which cardiac muscle biopsy is performed as a means of precise diagnosis. Even when the diagnosis of myocarditis is established, a definite cause is not usually recognized during life. Myocarditis is rarely (< 1% of cases) the cause of death in autopsy studies.

Etiology (Fig 23–11)

A. Infectious Myocarditis: Viruses are believed to be the most common cause of myocarditis in developed countries (Fig 23–12). Coxsackie B virus is most frequently implicated; others include mumps, influenza, echo, polio, varicella, and measles viruses.

Clinical myocarditis may be seen in certain **rickettsial diseases** such as Q fever, typhus, and Rocky Mountain spotted fever.

Myocardial inflammation in **diphtheria** is the result of an exotoxin. The diphtheria bacillus does not enter the bloodstream, but as it multiplies in the upper respiratory tract it produces exotoxin that does enter the bloodstream. Diphtheria exotoxin inhibits protein synthesis, leading to myocardial cell degeneration and necrosis. Diphtheria is now rare in countries with immunization programs.

American trypanosomiasis (Chagas' disease) is endemic in South America, where it is a common

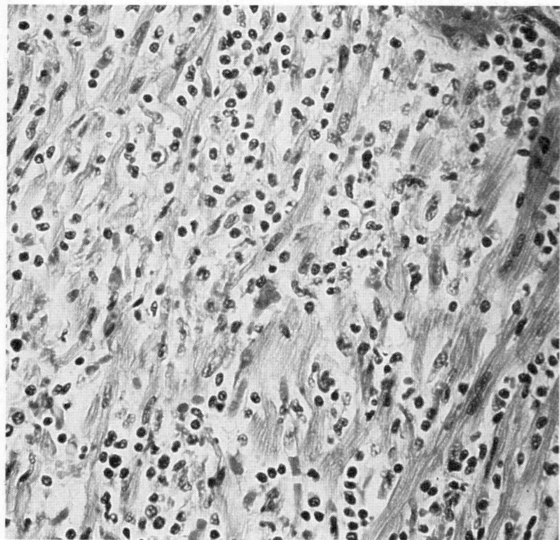

Figure 23-12. Viral myocarditis, showing extensive myofibril destruction and marked lymphocytic infiltration. High magnification.

cause of myocarditis. In the acute phase, parasitization of myofibrils leads to focal necrosis and inflammation characterized by the presence of many eosinophils. The parasites are seen as pseudocysts in myocardial fibers (Fig 23-13). The chronic phase is characterized by interstitial fibrosis and lymphocytic infiltration. The conducting system is frequently involved. Parasites are scarce in the chronic phase.

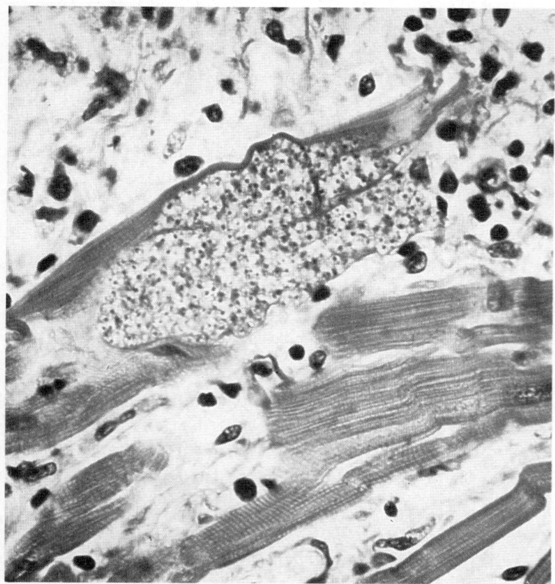

Figure 23-13. Chagas' disease of the myocardium, showing *Trypanosoma cruzi* in a distended myocardial fiber and the associated inflammation.

The acute phase of **trichinosis**, in which numerous larvae of *Trichinella spiralis* enter the bloodstream, is characterized by myocarditis. The larvae enter myocardial fibers, causing necrosis and acute inflammation with numerous eosinophils.

The myocardium is involved rarely in the acute disseminated form of **toxoplasmosis** that occurs in immunocompromised patients. *Toxoplasma gondii* pseudocysts are present in myocardial fibers.

B. Autoimmune (Hypersensitivity) Myocarditis: Myocarditis occurs in various diseases believed to have an autoimmune pathogenesis. These disorders include rheumatic fever, rheumatoid arthritis, systemic lupus erythematosus, progressive systemic sclerosis, and polyarteritis nodosa. All are characterized by focal myocardial fiber necrosis, lymphocytic infiltration, and fibrosis; vasculitis may be present. Rheumatic fever may show Aschoff bodies.

C. Toxic Myocarditis: Many drugs may injure the myocardium. The more common ones are ethyl alcohol, doxorubicin, rubidomycin, cyclophosphamide, hydralazine, phenytoin, procainamide, and the tricyclic antidepressants. Inflammatory change is often minimal, and these myocardial diseases are sometimes regarded as cardiomyopathies (eg, alcoholic cardiomyopathy; see below).

Doxorubicin (Adriamycin), one of the most effective anticancer drugs in current use, has a dose-related toxic effect on the myocardium, producing cytoplasmic vacuolation followed by necrosis. The occurrence of cardiotoxicity limits the clinical use of the drug.

D. Sarcoid Myocarditis: Sarcoidosis may produce significant cardiac involvement with noncaseating granulomatous lesions identical to those found elsewhere. Myocardial cell necrosis and inflammation are rarely severe enough to cause heart failure.

E. Radiation Myocarditis: The myocardium is relatively resistant to the effects of radiation, but clinical myocarditis may develop from large doses of radiation to the mediastinum.

F. Idiopathic Myocarditis: Myocarditis may occur without known cause, characterized by diffuse inflammation, sometimes with giant cells **(Fiedler's myocarditis)** and eosinophils. Progressive acute heart failure or sudden death may occur.

Pathology

In acute myocarditis, the heart is dilated, flabby, and pale. There may be small scattered petechial hemorrhages. Microscopically, there is edema, which separates myocardial fibers; hyperemia; and infiltration by lymphocytes, plasma cells, and eosinophils (Fig 23-12). Neutrophils may also be present if there is necrosis of individual muscle fibers. Recovery from acute myocarditis is associated with resolution. If myofibrillary necrosis has occurred, there may be irregular fibrosis.

Chronic myocarditis is a controversial entity characterized by cardiac failure, ventricular hypertrophy, and the presence of lymphocytes and plasma cells in the interstitium. This pathologic appearance may follow many of the causes listed above. Clinically, it appears as cardiomyopathy (see below).

Clinical Features

Many cases of myocarditis are asymptomatic, and its true incidence is difficult to establish. The onset is acute, with fever, chest pain, leukocytosis, and elevation of the erythrocyte sedimentation rate. Left ventricular failure may occur, manifested by a third heart sound (gallop rhythm) and mitral regurgitation caused by dilatation of the mitral valve ring. Arrhythmias include extrasystoles, atrial and ventricular tachycardia, and atrial and ventricular fibrillation and may cause sudden death. Complete heart block is manifested by bradycardia and cardiac failure. Necrosis of myocardial fibers produces injury potentials in the ST segment and elevations of serum concentration of creatine kinase, lactate dehydrogenase, and aspartate transaminase.

CARDIOMYOPATHIES

As defined above, cardiomyopathies are primary myocardial diseases characterized by a chronic course and minimal features of inflammation. Cardiomyopathy should be suspected in a young normotensive patient who develops cardiac failure in the absence of congenital, valvular, or ischemic heart disease. The term "cardiomyopathy" is also sometimes used to denote myocardial diseases associated with certain toxic, metabolic, and degenerative diseases, including alcoholism, amyloidosis, hemochromatosis, myxedema, thyrotoxicosis, beriberi (thiamine deficiency), certain glycogen storage diseases and mucopolysaccharidoses, Friedreich's ataxia, and the muscular dystrophies.

Incidence & Etiology

Cardiomyopathy is rare. It may be familial or sporadic. In most cases, no cause can be found (idiopathic), and the disorders listed above account for a relatively small proportion of cases.

Classification

Cardiomyopathies, both idiopathic and those secondary to known diseases, are classified according to type of functional abnormality. The following 4 types are recognized.

A. Congestive Cardiomyopathy: Congestive cardiomyopathy is characterized by failure of the ventricle to empty in systole. The ventricular end-systolic and diastolic volumes are increased, causing bilateral ventricular dilatation and failure. Arrhythmias are common and sometimes cause sudden death.

Histologic features are nonspecific. There is irregular atrophy and hypertrophy of myocardial fibers with progressive fibrosis.

Most cases are sporadic (10% are familial) and most have no detectable cause (idiopathic congestive cardiomyopathy). A few cases are associated with (1) metabolic diseases such as hypothyroidism, hyperthyroidism, hemochromatosis, and thiamine deficiency; (2) toxic diseases such as alcoholism and cobalt poisoning; (3) neuromuscular diseases such as Friedreich's ataxia; or (4) late pregnancy (peripartal cardiomyopathy).

Chronic alcoholism causes cardiac disease by several different mechanisms: **(1) Direct toxicity** of ethyl alcohol to myocardial cells produces congestive cardiomyopathy. **(2) Beer drinker's cardiomyopathy** is a specific variant believed to be due to the combined toxic effects of alcohol and cobalt. Specific brands of beer that had cobalt compounds added as antifrothing agents were implicated. **(3) Thiamine deficiency** associated with alcoholism causes myocardial damage (wet beriberi) and cardiac failure.

B. Hypertrophic Cardiomyopathy: Hypertrophic cardiomyopathy is characterized by marked hypertrophy of the ventricular muscle with resistance to diastolic filling. Both ventricles are diffusely involved in most cases.

Asymmetric septal hypertrophy (also called **hypertrophic obstructive cardiomyopathy**, or HOCM; also called idiopathic hypertrophic subaortic stenosis, or IHSS) is a variant characterized by selective hypertrophy of the septum immediately below the aortic valve, obstructing the left ventricular outflow tract. Clinically, this condition mimics aortic stenosis.

About 20–30% of cases of hypertrophic cardiomyopathy are familial, and in some of these there is a suggestion of an autosomal dominant inheritance pattern.

C. Restrictive Cardiomyopathy: Restrictive cardiomyopathy is characterized by decreased compliance of the ventricular muscle, increased resistance to filling, and cardiac failure. Many cases are now recognized as being due to amyloidosis.

Cardiac amyloidosis occurs in several different situations (see also Chapter 2): (1) senile amyloidosis, where the heart is frequently the only organ involved; (2) primary amyloidosis, where cardiac involvement is accompanied by deposition of amyloid in the tongue, intestine etc; and (3) secondary amyloidosis, in which the heart is affected infrequently. Amyloid deposition occurs in the myocardial interstitium and around small blood vessels. When involvement is diffuse, the myocardium is thickened and leathery-firm and has a waxy, pale gray color.

D. Obliterative Cardiomyopathy: Obliterative cardiomyopathy is characterized by marked subendocardial fibrosis resulting in encroachment of the lumen, decreased ventricular filling, and cardiac failure. Both left and right ventricles may be involved.

Two different diseases exist within this category. **(1)** In **endocardial fibroelastosis,** collagen and elastic tissue are laid down beneath the endocardium, with clinical features appearing during infancy. Some cases appear to be familial; others may be secondary to anoxia or fetal viral infection. **(2) Endomyocardial fibrosis** is an acquired disease in which there is fibrosis of the endocardium and inner myocardium. It is common in Africa and has been attributed to a diet rich in serotonin (eg, bananas), perhaps mimicking the carcinoid syndrome, in which elevated serotonin levels produce endocardial fibrosis.

DISEASES OF THE PERICARDIUM

ACUTE PERICARDITIS

Incidence

Acute pericarditis is relatively common in hospital practice.

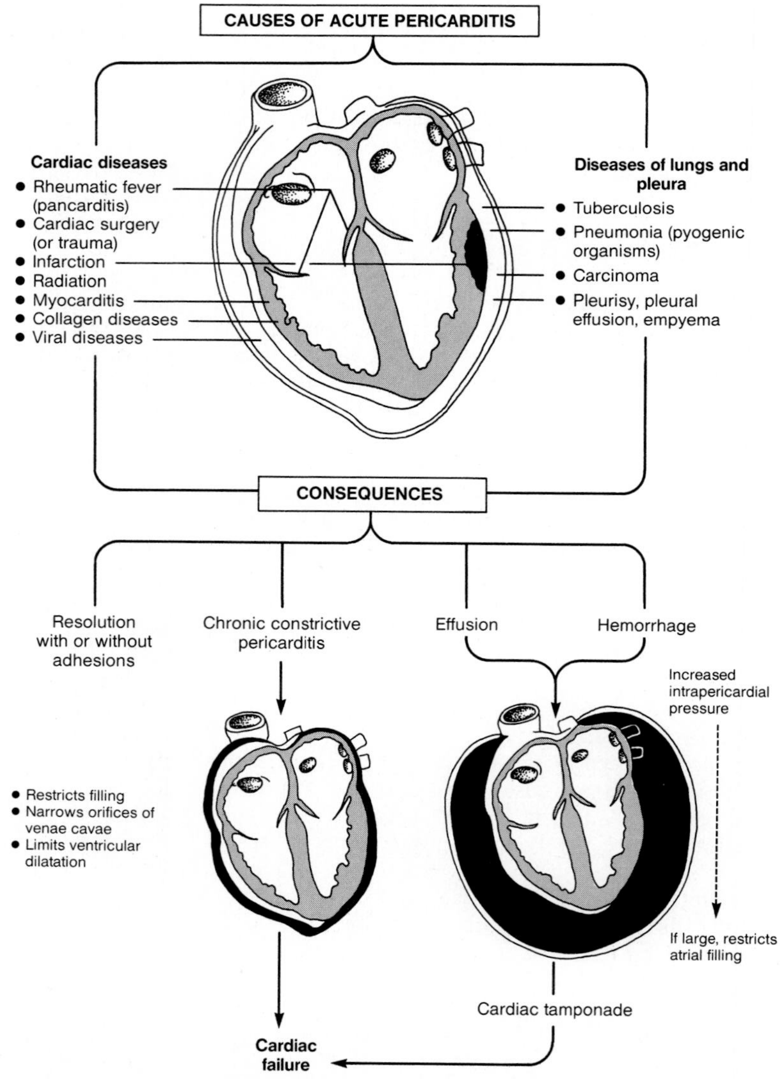

Figure 23–14. Causes and clinical consequences of acute pericarditis.

Etiology (Fig 23–14)

The common causes are infection, ischemic heart disease, uremia, and the connective tissue diseases.

A. Infectious Acute Pericarditis:

1. Viral pericarditis-Viruses known to cause pericarditis include coxsackievirus B, echovirus, and the agents of mumps, infectious mononucleosis (Epstein-Barr virus), and influenza. Viruses can be cultured from pericardial fluid.

2. Acute idiopathic pericarditis-This disorder is very similar clinically to viral pericarditis. It occurs in young adults and commonly follows a respiratory viral infection by 2–3 weeks, suggesting the possibility of hypersensitivity reaction. The disease is self-limited, with recovery in 1–2 weeks.

3. Tuberculous pericarditis-Tuberculous pericarditis is due to direct spread of infection from a caseous mediastinal lymph node leading to acute followed by chronic pericarditis. It is now rare in developed countries.

4. Pyogenic pericarditis-Infection of the pericardium by pyogenic organisms is caused by direct spread from a suppurative focus in the lung or pleura. *Streptococcus pneumoniae,* staphylococci, and gram-negative bacilli are the common causes. Effective antibiotic therapy of lung infections has reduced the frequency of this condition.

B. Noninfectious Acute Pericarditis: Acute pericarditis frequently complicates acute rheumatic fever, myocardial infarction, chronic renal failure (uremia), and connective tissue diseases such as systemic lupus erythematosus and rheumatoid arthritis. Malignant neoplasms may directly involve the pericardium and cause inflammation. Pericarditis may also occur after cardiac trauma and cardiac surgery. There is typically a delay of weeks after the trauma, suggesting that immunologic hypersensitivity may play a role. Delayed pericarditis occurring 2–3 weeks after myocardial infarction (Dressler's syndrome) probably has a similar hypersensitivity basis. Acute pericarditis may follow radiation therapy to the mediastinum in the treatment of cancer.

Pathology

The smooth pericardial surface is transformed into a reddened membrane roughened by adherent clumps of fibrin (see Fig 3-5). Infiltration by neutrophils causes yellow discoloration. The visceral and parietal layers of pericardium are thus thickened and loosely adherent—said to peel apart like 2 slices of buttered bread ("bread and butter appearance"). Fluid exudation into the pericardial sac varies from minimal ("dry," or fibrinous, pericarditis) to significant (pericarditis with effusion). The fluid is usually serous. Hemorrhagic effusions commonly occur in renal failure, malignant neoplasms, and tuberculosis.

Clinical Features

Pericarditis causes pericardial pain and a pericardial rub. When there is significant effusion, the inflamed pericardial layers separate, and both the rub and the pain diminish. Pericardial effusion causes cardiac enlargement, dullness to percussion, and muffled heart sounds. With large effusions, raised intrapericardial pressure impairs diastolic filling of the right atrium, leading to acute right heart failure (cardiac tamponade). With rapidly developing effusions, cardiac tamponade may cause death very rapidly.

Systemic features of acute inflammation include acute onset of fever and leukocytosis.

Diagnosis

Pericarditis can be diagnosed clinically by the presence of a pericardial rub or effusion, confirmed by chest x-ray, echocardiography, and examination of aspirated pericardial fluid (culture and cytologic examination).

CHRONIC ADHESIVE PERICARDITIS

Recovery from acute pericarditis frequently produces fibrous plaques ("milk spots") in the visceral pericardium or adhesions between the 2 pericardial layers (chronic adhesive pericarditis). These are of no clinical significance.

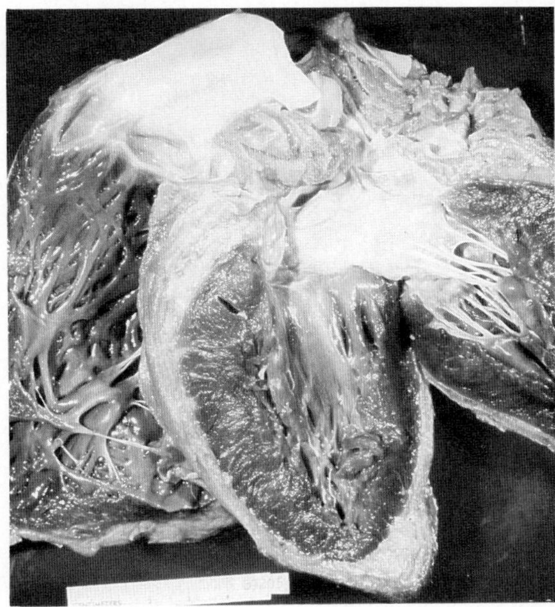

Figure 23–15. Chronic constrictive pericarditis caused by tuberculous pericarditis. The heart is encased by a thickened fibrous pericardium, and the ventricular luminal size is decreased as a result of restriction of filling.

CHRONIC CONSTRICTIVE PERICARDITIS

Chronic constrictive pericarditis is uncommon, and in most cases the cause is not known. Tuberculosis and pyogenic infections were common causes in the past. Immunologic mechanisms may account for most noninfectious cases.

Chronic constrictive pericarditis is characterized by encasement of the heart in a greatly thickened fibrotic pericardium (Fig 23–15). Chronic inflammatory cells are frequently present, along with dystrophic calcification. The pericardial sac is obliterated.

The fibrous pericardium constricts the cardiac chambers, particularly reducing right atrial filling. Elevation of jugular venous pressure and decreased cardiac output result. Ascites and hepatic enlargement are common clinical features. Chest x-ray frequently shows calcification. Surgical removal of the thickened pericardial sac (pericardiectomy) is effective treatment.

NEOPLASMS OF THE MYOCARDIUM & PERICARDIUM

The myocardium and pericardium are occasionally involved by metastatic tumor or by direct local invasion by lung carcinoma or malignant lymphoma.

Rhabdomyoma, which is composed of a disorganized mass of cardiac muscle, is a hamartoma that occurs in patients with tuberous sclerosis (see Chapter 62). It is very rare.

Primary cardiac malignant neoplasms include pericardial malignant mesothelioma and angiosarcoma. They are very rare.

Section VI.
The Blood & Lymphoid System

Changes in different types of blood cells occur in many diseases (Chapters 24, 26), eg, changes in leukocyte count provides useful information in infectious diseases (Chapter 13). Anemia is an extremely common clinical problem that has many causes (Chapters 24, 25). Neoplasms of the hemopoietic system include myeloproliferative disorders (Chapter 25 and 26), leukemias (Chapter 26), malignant lymphomas (Chapter 29), and plasma cell myeloma (Chapter 30). Leukemias and lymphomas represent the commonest malignant neoplasms under age 30 years. Successful treatment of these hematopoietic neoplasms has made their early and accurate diagnosis very important. Students may find it worthwhile to review the discussion of normal hemostasis in Chapter 9 before undertaking a study of bleeding disorders (Chapter 27).

Chapters 28–30 deal with diseases of the lymph nodes, spleen, and thymus. These include infections, reactive proliferations, and malignant lymphomas. The student may find it helpful to review earlier chapters relating to the immune system (Chapter 4) and immunodeficiency (Chapter 7) prior to embarking on these chapters.

24 Blood: I. Structure & Function; Anemias Due to Decreased Erythropoiesis

STRUCTURE & FUNCTION OF BLOOD ELEMENTS

PERIPHERAL BLOOD

The peripheral blood is composed of formed elements or cells suspended in plasma (Table 24–1).

Erythrocytes (Red Blood Cells)

Erythrocytes are nonnucleated biconcave disks with a uniform diameter of 7.5–8 μm. Erythrocytes are extremely pliable cells, able to change shape as they squeeze through the microcirculation. The erythrocyte cytoplasm contains hemoglobin, a protein complexed to an iron containing porphyrin that gives the cell its characteristic red color. Hemoglobin is vital to oxygen transport in the blood—the main function of the erythrocyte.

Erythrocytes have a life span in the peripheral blood of approximately 120 days. They are derived from normoblasts in the bone marrow, which lose their nucleus in the final stage of development prior to release into the peripheral blood (Figs 24–1 and 24–3).

Newly released erythrocytes are slightly larger than mature cells and slightly basophilic because of the presence of residual ribosomes and mitochondria. (They demonstrate a finely reticular pattern with supravital stains such as cresyl violet—hence the term **"reticulocytes."**) At any given time, approximately 1% of erythrocytes in the peripheral blood are newly released (reticulocytes). Nucleated normoblasts are not normally found in the peripheral blood.

Granulocytes

There are approximately 1000 red cells for every white cell in the blood.

Granulocytes are nucleated white blood cells that have been classified according to the nature of their cytoplasmic granules as neutrophils, eosinophils, or basophils. They are derived from the myeloid precursor series in the bone marrow (Fig 24–1) and have a life span of a few hours in peripheral blood. Myelopoiesis is described more fully in Chapter 26.

Neutrophils have a multilobate nucleus (for this reason they are also called polymorphonuclear leukocytes) and fine cytoplasmic granules. Nuclear lobation increases with maturity; when cells are released from the marrow, they have a band-like nucleus **("band forms")**. Fully mature neutrophils have 4 or 5 nuclear lobes connected by fine lines of chromatin (Fig 24–2).

Neutrophils participate in the nonspecific acute inflammatory response to injury. They are particularly active against extracellularly multiplying infectious agents, notably bacteria, but are also involved in repair and immune responses.

Eosinophils have large eosinophilic cytoplasmic

Table 24-1. Normal values for peripheral blood elements.[1]

	Male	Female
Hemoglobin (g/dL)	14–18	12–16
Erythrocytes (per μL)	4.6–6. $\times 10^6$	4.2–5.4 $\times 10^6$
Hematocrit (packed cell volume; PCV)	42–50%	37–47%
Mean corpuscular volume (MCV)[2]	76–96 fL	
Mean corpuscular hemoglobin concentration (MCHC)[3]	32–35%	
Total white blood cells (per μL)	4000–11,000	
Neutrophils	2500–7500[4]	
Lymphocytes	1500–3500	
Monocytes	200–800	
Eosinophils	60–600	
Basophils	0–100	
Platelets (per μL)	150,000–400,000	

[1]Normal values vary with age; adult values are given here.

[2]$\text{MCV} = \frac{\text{PCV}}{\text{Red cell count}}$. It is a measure of the size of individual red cells.

[3]$\text{MCHC} = \frac{\text{PCV}}{\text{Hemoglobin}}$. It is a measure of the hemoglobinization of individual red cells in relation to size.

[4]Recognize that absolute counts of the different types of leukocytes are more valuable than percentages.

granules. Nuclear lobation rarely progresses beyond 2 lobes. Eosinophils are prominent in parasitic infections and allergic reactions.

Basophils have large basophilic granules that obscure the nucleus. Like their counterparts the tissue mast cells, they are involved in type I hypersensitivity reactions.

Monocytes & Lymphocytes

Monocytes are part of the macrophage or mononuclear phagocyte system. Lymphocytes belong to the immune system. These 2 cell types are more fully discussed with the lymphoid system in Chapters 4 and 28.

Platelets

Platelets are very small, nonnucleated cytoplasmic fragments of megakaryocytes. Platelets have a vital function in control of hemorrhage (Chapter 27).

Plasma

Plasma is the fluid in which the formed elements of the blood are suspended. The normal ratio of erythrocytes to plasma is approximately 40:60 (also expressed as the hematocrit: normal is 42–50%). The hematocrit is an important determinant of blood viscosity. Disorders in which the proportion of erythrocytes is greatly increased (polycythemia) are associated with increased blood viscosity.

Plasma is composed of water, electrolytes, proteins, and a large number of other constituents such as glucose, products of protein and nucleic acid metabolism, and enzymes. Plasma proteins include albumin and a variety of globulins. **Al-**

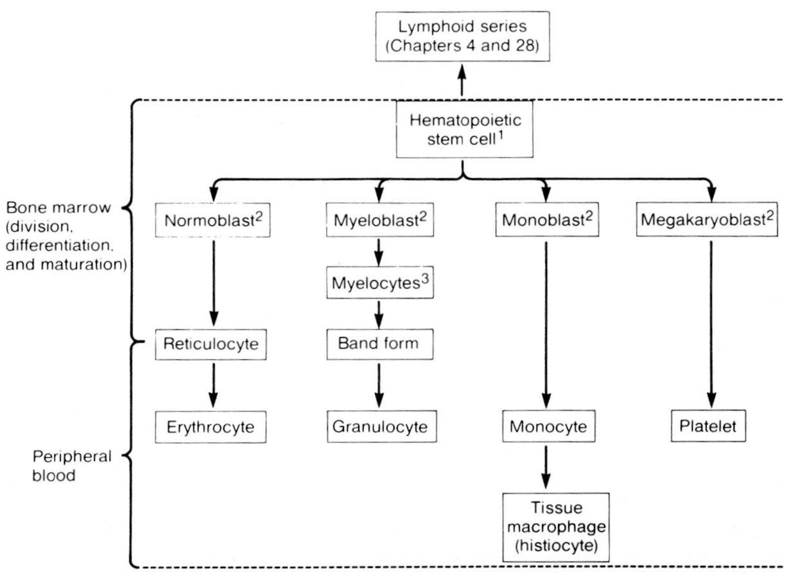

Figure 24-1. Normal hematopoiesis. **(1)** The resting hematopoietic stem cell cannot be positively identified in bone marrow but is probably a small round cell resembling a "nonmarking" or "null" lymphocyte. Once stimulated to divide, it assumes the appearance of a "blast" cell with a primitive nucleus and basophilic cytoplasm. **(2)** These are the stem cells of the various series, which proliferate and replenish the blast cell pool as well as differentiating into the mature cells of the series. **(3)** Neutrophils, basophils, and eosinophils diverge at the myelocyte stage, developing their characteristic secondary cytoplasmic granules.

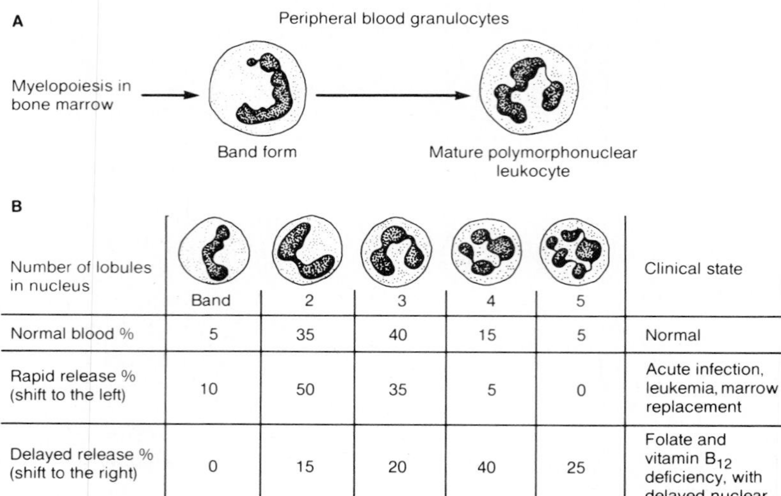

Number of lobules in nucleus	Band	2	3	4	5	Clinical state
Normal blood %	5	35	40	15	5	Normal
Rapid release % (shift to the left)	10	50	35	5	0	Acute infection, leukemia, marrow replacement
Delayed release % (shift to the right)	0	15	20	40	25	Folate and vitamin B_{12} deficiency, with delayed nuclear maturation

Figure 24–2. Maturation of polymorphonuclear leukocytes **(A)** and changes observed in nuclear lobation (Arneth count) in disease states **(B).**

bumin, which is synthesized by the liver, is the major determinant of plasma oncotic pressure, which governs fluid exchange in systemic capillaries. **Globulins** include immunoglobulins, complement, enzymes, factors involved in blood coagulation, fibrinolysis, and several transport proteins for hormones, minerals, lipids, and nutrients. Measurements of various plasma constituents may provide evidence of disease.

Serum

Serum is the fluid that remains after blood has been allowed to clot in a tube. It resembles plasma except that fibrinogen and other coagulation factors will have been depleted by the process of clot formation.

"Blood tests" may be performed on whole blood (eg, hemoglobin, blood cell counts), plasma (eg, plasma protein), or serum (eg, serum amy-

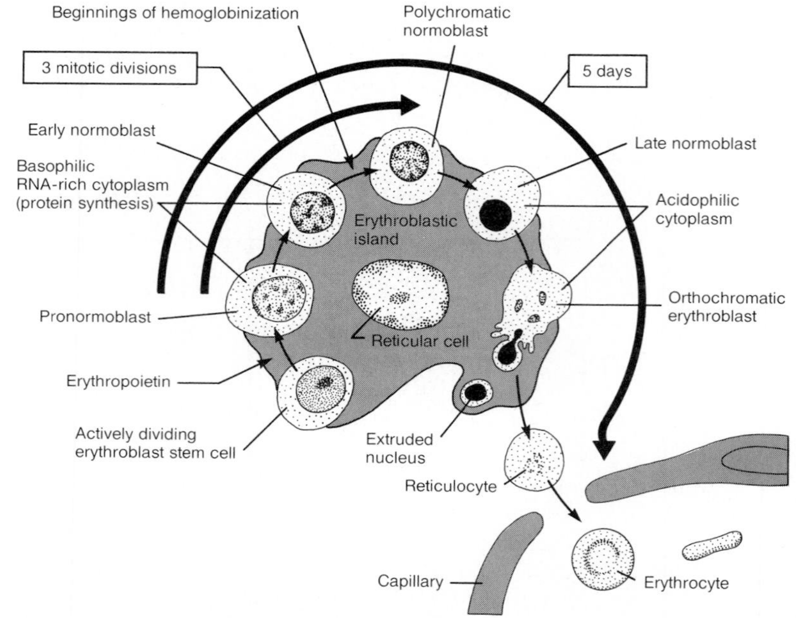

Figure 24–3. Erythrocyte maturation sequence. Nuclear division and maturation requires vitamin B_{12} and folic acid; deficiency of these vitamins results in retarded nuclear maturation (megaloblastic anemia). Hemoglobin, which is synthesized from protoporphyrin and iron, stains with eosin, producing a progressive change in the cytoplasmic staining reaction from basophilic (pronormoblast) through polychromatic (intermediate normoblast) to eosinophilic (late normoblast and erythrocyte).

lase, iron). Tests performed on whole blood and plasma require collection in tubes containing anticoagulant to prevent clotting. Tests performed on serum require clotted blood.

BONE MARROW

Normal Bone Marrow

The bone marrow is the sole site of production of erythrocytes, granulocytes, and platelets after birth. It also produces blood monocytes which are part of the macrophage system. At birth, hematopoietic marrow is present in the medullary cavity of all the bones of the body. With increasing age, the hematopoietic marrow is replaced by adipose tissue in the bones of the extremities, and hematopoietic marrow is found only in the axial skeleton.

Bone Marrow Examination

Specimens of bone marrow in adults must be obtained from an axial bone, most commonly the iliac crest or sternum. In children, bone marrow for biopsy may also be recovered at the tibial tuberosity. **Aspiration biopsy** utilizes a thin needle and provides material for smears and for histologic sections of centrifuged particles. **Trephine biopsy** utilizes a larger needle that provides a core of tissue (including bone spicules) from the marrow for histologic sections. **Open marrow biopsy** is sometimes performed in difficult cases.

The following criteria are evaluated in a bone marrow examination:

(1) Cellularity: the proportion of hematopoietic cells to fat cells; this varies with site and age, from near 100% in a child, to 50% in adult axial marrow, to 0% in peripheral marrow from the elderly (ie, marrow is all fat).

(2) Amount and maturation of erythropoiesis.

(3) Amount and maturation of myelopoiesis.

(4) Myeloid:erythroid ratio (normally 3:1 or 4:1).

(5) Numbers and morphology of megakaryocytes.

(6) Numbers and morphology of plasma cells.

(7) Tumor cells: leukemia, lymphoma, carcinoma.

(8) Microbial parasites (bacteria, fungi, protozoa).

(9) Iron content (by iron stain).

(10) Presence of fibrosis.

All stages of maturation of erythroid, myeloid, and megakaryocytic series should be present, with more mature cells outnumbering the blasts. The earliest precursors of the various cell lines (stem cells, or hemocytoblasts) cannot be distinguished by light microscopy.

If systemic infection is suspected (eg, tuberculosis, brucellosis), part of the bone marrow specimen should be cultured using appropriate techniques.

PRODUCTION OF BLOOD CELLS

Red Cell Production (Erythropoiesis)

Erythrocyte production in the bone marrow is under the influence of **erythropoietin,** which is produced by the kidneys in response to arterial blood oxygen content. Erythrocyte maturation (Fig 24–3) involves **nuclear maturation,** characterized by decreasing size of the nucleus and pyknosis by the late normoblast stage, and **cytoplasmic hemoglobinization,** which imparts an increasing eosinophilia to the basophilic cytoplasm of the early normoblast.

White Cell Production (Myelopoiesis) & Platelet Production

Production of white blood cells is described in Chapter 26 and production of platelets in Chapter 27.

ANEMIAS

Anemia is by far the commonest disorder affecting erythrocytes. It is defined as a reduction in the hemoglobin concentration of the blood (with reference to an established normal range for age, sex, and geography), usually associated with a reduction of total circulating red cell mass. Whatever its cause, anemia decreases the oxygen-carrying capacity of the blood and, when severe enough, causes clinical symptoms and signs.

Clinical Features (Fig 24–4)

Anemia is characterized by pallor of the skin and mucous membranes and by manifestations of hypoxia (decreased oxygen content of the blood), most commonly weakness, fatigue, lethargy, dizziness, or syncope (fainting). Myocardial hypoxia may result in anginal pain. A hyperdynamic circulation, with an increase in heart rate and stroke volume, occurs in response to hypoxia. Ejection type flow murmurs may develop, and if the anemia is severe, cardiac failure may ensue (Fig 24–4).

Classification

Anemias are classified in one of 2 ways.

A. Etiologic Classification: (Table 24–2.) In this book, we will consider anemias from the

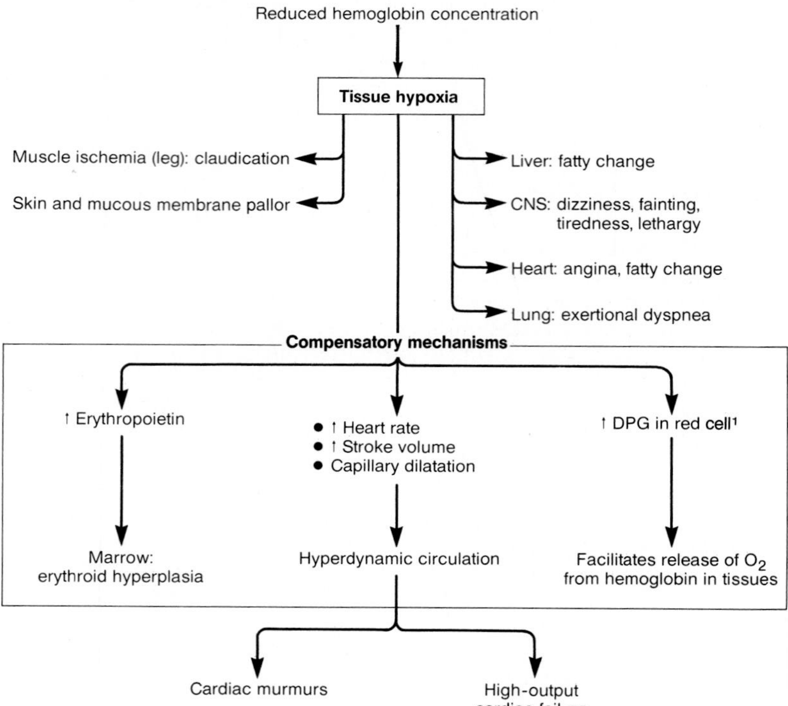

Figure 24-4. Clinicopathologic effects and physiologic compensatory mechanisms in anemia.
[1]See page 392.

Table 24-2. Etiologic classification of anemia.

- **I. Decreased erythropoiesis**
  - A. Erythroid stem cell failure.
    1. Aplastic anemia
    2. Pure red cell aplasia
  - B. Replacement of the bone marrow
    1. Malignant neoplasms: leukemias, plasma cell myeloma, malignant lymphoma, metastatic carcinoma
    2. Myelofibrosis
  - C. Inadequate erythropoietin stimulation: chronic renal disease
  - D. Defective DNA synthesis (megaloblastic anemias)
    1. Vitamin B_{12} deficiency
    2. Folic acid deficiency
  - E. Defective hemoglobin synthesis
    1. Iron deficiency
    2. Anemia of chronic disease
    3. Sideroblastic anemias
  - F. Other nutritional and toxic factors
    1. Scurvy
    2. Protein malnutrition
    3. Chronic liver disease
    4. Hypothyroidism
    5. "Chronic" disease, including infection and cancer
- **II. Blood loss**
  - A. Acute
  - B. Chronic
- **III. Hemolytic anemias (see Chapter 25)**
  - A. Due to intrinsic red cell defects
  - B. Due to extrinsic factors

standpoint of their causes: (1) decreased production of erythrocytes by the marrow, (2) blood loss too extensive for replacement by the marrow, and (3) increased rate of destruction of erythrocytes (hemolytic anemias). Anemias due to decreased erythropoiesis or blood loss will be discussed in this chapter; hemolytic anemias are the subject of the next chapter.

B. Morphologic Classification: (Table 24-3.) Classification of anemias according to changes in size and hemoglobin content of erythrocytes in the peripheral blood is shown in Table 24-3 and in Fig 24-5.

Incidence

The incidence of anemia varies from 2% to 15% in different studies in Britain and the USA. Anemia is about twice as common in females. Mild anemia without symptoms is quite common, but anemia may be the presenting sign of serious disease. If "normal range" USA values are used, anemia is much more common in underdeveloped countries; this observation raises questions about what the normal range really is and whether it should be defined differently for different populations.

Diagnosis

When a patient presents with symptoms of anemia—eg, pallor of mucous membranes, fatigue,

Table 24–3. Morphologic classification of anemia. (See also Fig 29–5.)

Type	MCV	MCHC	Common Causes
Macrocytic anemia[1]	Increased	Normal	Folic acid deficiency Vitamin B_{12} deficiency Liver disease Hypothyroidism Posthemorrhagic[2]
Microcytic anemia Hypochromic	Decreased	Decreased	Iron deficiency Thalassemia Sideroblastic anemias
Normochromic	Decreased or normal[3]	Normal	Spherocytosis
Normocytic anemia Normochromic	Normal	Normal	Aplastic anemia Anemia of chronic disease Chronic renal failure Posthemorrhagic[2] Some hemolytic anemias
Leukoerythroblastic anemia[4]	Normal	Normal	Replacement or infiltration of bone marrow

[1]A subset of macrocytic anemias shows abnormal maturation in the marrow; these are the "megaloblastic" anemias. Macrocytic anemias are normochromic.
[2]Becomes macrocytic as a result of increased numbers of reticulocytes as erythropoiesis increases.
[3]Spherocytes are erythrocytes that have lost their disk shape and are usually smaller than normal (microspherocytes). They are commonly associated with hemolysis and, therefore, the presence of increased numbers of reticulocytes, which may cause the MCV to be increased from low to normal levels.
[4]Leukoerythroblastic anemias are characterized by the presence of early forms of both white and red cells (including normoblasts) in the peripheral blood.

and breathlessness—the initial diagnosis may be confirmed by demonstration of a decreased hemoglobin level. Morphologic classification of the anemia into macrocytic, normocytic-normochromic, microcytic-hypochromic, and dimorphic is done by examination of blood values (MCV, MCHC) and a peripheral blood smear. Identification of the cause of anemia may require bone marrow examination, hemoglobin electrophoresis, and determination of serum iron, vitamin B_{12}, and folate levels. The tests required will vary with different patients; eg, bone marrow examination is critical in macrocytic anemia and of limited value in microcytic-hypochromic anemia.

ANEMIAS DUE TO DECREASED RED CELL PRODUCTION

There are many mechanisms by which production of erythrocytes by the marrow is decreased. Since there is no mechanism to decrease the rate of peripheral destruction of erythrocytes, anemia results. The more important of these conditions will be discussed below.

APLASTIC ANEMIA

Aplastic anemia is the result of failure of production or suppression, or destruction of stem cells in the bone marrow, which leads to decreased generation of erythrocytes, leukocytes, and platelets (pancytopenia). The bone marrow shows marked decrease in cellularity.

Etiology

Drugs are the commonest cause of aplastic anemia in clinical practice (Table 24–4).

Pathology & Clinical Features

Aplastic anemia shows a markedly hypocellular bone marrow with a reduction of all cell lines. The peripheral blood smear shows the following characteristic features:

A. Anemia: Erythrocytes are decreased in number, but those that remain are normocytic and normochromic. There is an absence of reticulocytes in the peripheral blood.

B. Granulocytopenia: Granulocytopenia (neutropenia) occurs rapidly, because these cells have a very short life span; infections and oral ulcers result.

C. Thrombocytopenia: Thrombocytopenia results in a bleeding tendency.

Treatment & Prognosis

Treatment is symptomatic, plus corticosteroids. The prognosis is poor. In severe, irreversible cases, death results from the effects of infections (eg, pneumonia, septicemia), bleeding (eg, intracranial hemorrhage), or anemia (eg, cardiac failure).

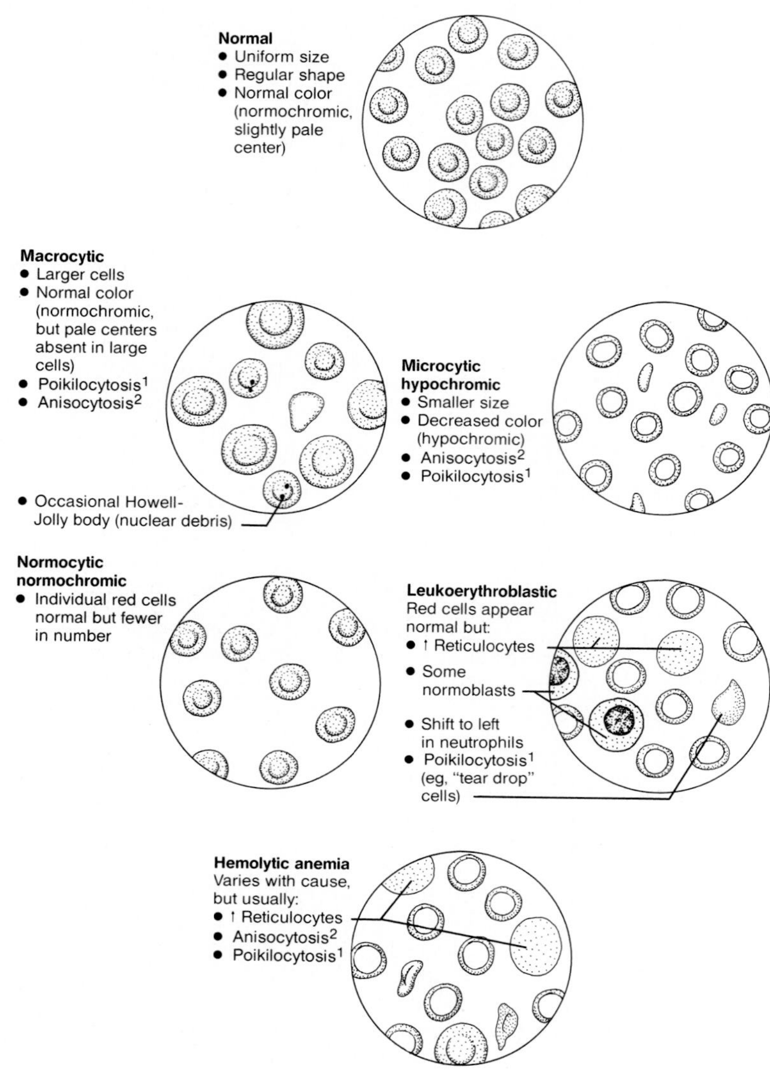

Figure 24-5. Peripheral blood appearance of different morphologic types of anemias. **(1)** Poikilocytosis: variation in shape. **(2)** Anisocytosis: variation in size.

RED CELL APLASIA

Pure red cell aplasia occurs rarely. It may be a **congenital** disorder (Blackfan-Diamond disease), manifested in early life by anemia and erythroid hypoplasia. This disorder frequently remits spontaneously or in response to corticosteroid therapy. **Acquired** red cell aplasia is usually a transient complication that occurs in congenital hemolytic anemias such as sickle cell anemia. Adult red cell aplasia may also occur as a complication of thymoma by an unknown mechanism.

MARROW REPLACEMENT (LEUKOERYTHROBLASTIC) ANEMIAS

Involvement of the bone marrow cavity by metastatic neoplasms, lymphoma, or leukemia, disseminated granulomatous diseases (such as tuberculosis), fibrosis, or multiple abscesses displaces and replaces the normal marrow elements. Replacement of proliferating marrow cells of sufficient degree may result in anemia, leukopenia, or thrombocytopenia.

Compensatory phenomena include (1) the development of active marrow in sites outside the marrow cavity (extramedullary hematopoiesis or myeloid metaplasia, especially in spleen and liver)

Table 24–4. Causes of aplastic anemia.[1]

Primary (idiopathic): no known cause
Secondary (toxic) Drugs (a) Predictable, dose-related—primarily cytotoxic anticancer drugs: amethopterin, mechlorethamine, vincristine, daunorubicin, etc (b) Unpredictable idiosyncratic reactions: rare, do not require prior exposure, nonimmune Antiepileptic drugs (hydantoins) Oral antidiabetic agents (tolbutamide, chlorpropamide) Tranquilizers (chlorpromazine, chlordiazepoxide, etc) Antirheumatic drugs (phenylbutazone, indomethacin, colchicine, gold salts) Antibacterial agents (sulfonamides, streptomycin, isoniazid, tetracyclines, chloramphenicol[2]) Many others (hydralazine, mepacrine, thiazide diuretics) (c) Unpredictable hypersensitivity: immune reaction, requires prior exposure; many drugs (antibodies to drugs often detectable)
Industrial and household chemicals Benzene, trinitrotoluene (TNT), some organic solvents, "glue sniffing," certain insecticides (DDT, chlordane, lindane)
Associated diseases (a) Familial hypoplastic anemia (Fanconi; chromosomal abnormalities and a high incidence of leukemia) (b) With infective hepatitis (c) With pancreatitis (d) With paroxysmal nocturnal hemoglobinuria (e) Preleukemia

[1]***Note:*** May present with total marrow failure, failure of red cell production alone, or failure of white cell production alone (neutropenia).
[2]Chloramphenicol may produce both a direct toxic effect (dose-related) and an idiosyncratic reaction.

and (2) release of cells from the marrow before maturation is complete. The latter results in a "shift to the left" (immature white cells, including myeloblasts and myelocytes) and the presence of nucleated red cells (normoblasts) in the peripheral blood—hence the designation leukoerythroblastic anemia. The blood picture is characteristic (Fig 24–5).

MEGALOBLASTIC ANEMIAS

Megaloblastic anemias are a subset of macrocytic anemias in which the maturation phase of erythropoiesis in the bone marrow is abnormal, resulting in erythroid precursors that are enlarged and show failure of nuclear maturation ("megaloblasts").

Etiology

Megaloblastic anemias result from conditions in which nucleic acid synthesis is abnormal, as in vitamin B_{12} and folic acid deficiency (Table 24–5). Vitamin B_{12} and folic acid play roles as cofactors in the conversion of deoxyuridine to deoxythymidine, an essential step in the synthesis of DNA (Fig 24–6). Note that vitamin B_{12} stores in the liver are normally sufficient for several years; following gastrectomy (which removes the source of intrinsic factor, thereby reducing vitamin B_{12} absorption), a decade may pass before megaloblastic anemia becomes apparent.

Vitamin B_{12} is present in high concentration in animal liver and to some degree in most meats but is absent in plants. Folate is widely distributed, especially in leafy green vegetables. Dietary deficiency of vitamin B_{12} is rare except in strict vegetarians. Dietary deficiency of folic acid is

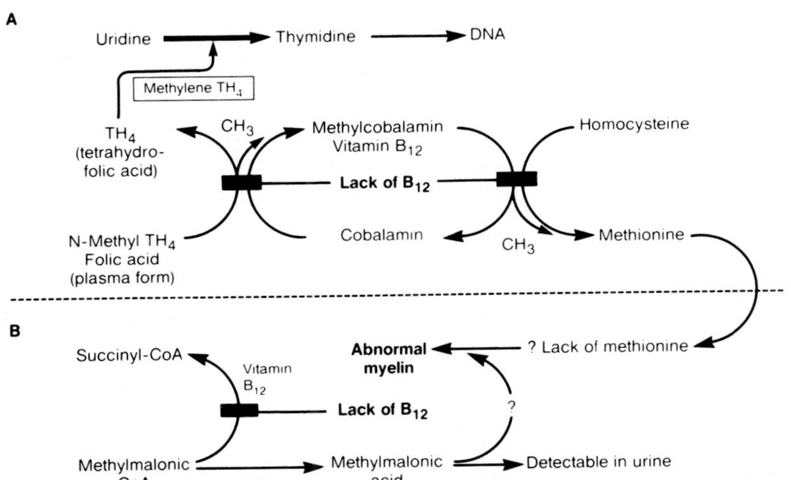

Figure 24–6. Role of vitamin B_{12} and folic acid in nucleic acid and myelin metabolism. Lack of either vitamin B_{12} or folic acid retards DNA synthesis **(A)**. Lack of vitamin B_{12} leads to abnormal myelin synthesis, possibly via a deficiency of methionine **(B)**.

Table 24–5. Causes of megaloblastic anemia.

Vitamin B_{12} deficiency
- Inadequate dietary intake: very rare; only in strict vegetarians
- Failure of absorption due to intrinsic factor deficiency[1]
  - Pernicious anemia
  - Total and subtotal gastrectomy
- Terminal ileal disease[1]
  - Crohn's disease
  - Strictures and fistulas that bypass the terminal ileum
  - Surgical removal of the terminal ileum
- Competition for vitamin B_{12} by intestinal microorganisms
  - Bacterial overgrowth (blind loop syndromes)
  - *Diphyllobothrium latum* (fish tapeworm) infection
- Drugs: para-aminosalicylic acid (antituberculous agent)
- Congenital deficiency of transcobalamin II (the vitamin B_{12} transport protein in blood)

Folic acid deficiency
- Inadequate intake
  - Chronic alcoholism
  - Malnutrition
- Failure of absorption[2]
  - Tropical sprue
  - Other malabsorptive states
- Increased demand
  - Pregnancy and infancy
  - States of increased DNA synthesis (malignant neoplasms with high rate of cell turnover, erythroid hyperplasia in congenital hemolytic anemias)
- Drugs with folic acid antagonistic activity
  - Anticancer drugs such as methotrexate
  - Anticonvulsants such as hydantoins

Other causes
- Arsenic poisoning
- Nitrous oxide inhalation
- Some forms of chemotherapy (in addition to folic acid antagonists)
- Orotic aciduria (a rare condition with abnormal synthesis of purines and pyrimidines)

[1]Vitamin B_{12} absorption depends on formation of a complex with intrinsic factor and absorption of this complex in the terminal ileum.
[2]Folate is absorbed throughout the small intestine; it does not require an "intrinsic factor."

common and occurs in many states of malnutrition.

Pathology

A. Red Cell Changes: When DNA synthesis is abnormal, erythropoiesis changes from normoblastic to megaloblastic.

Megaloblasts differ from normoblasts in that they are larger and show delayed nuclear maturation but normal cytoplasmic hemoglobinization (nuclear-cytoplasmic asynchrony) (Fig 24–7). The late megaloblast, for example, shows a primitive nucleus and fully hemoglobinized cytoplasm—in contrast with the late normoblast, which has a pyknotic nucleus.

Delayed maturation leads to accumulation of erythrocyte precursor cells. The bone marrow is hypercellular and contains large numbers of early megaloblasts; prior to the discovery of the beneficial effect of liver extract (contains vitamin B_{12}) on pernicious anemia, this picture was mistaken for that of acute leukemia.

Intramedullary hemolysis or ineffective erythropoiesis–Many megaloblasts undergo destruction in the bone marrow before maturation, aggravating the anemia and producing mild elevation of serum bilirubin and lactate dehydrogenase (LDH isoenzymes 1 and 2).

The **peripheral blood smear** shows **macrocytosis** (large red cells with elevated MCV) and marked variation in size **(anisocytosis)** and shape **(poikilocytosis)** (Fig 24–5). Oval forms (macro-ovalocytes) are prominent, and Howell-Jolly bodies, consisting of nuclear debris, are occasionally seen. Megaloblastic anemias are therefore macrocytic anemias if the morphologic classification of anemia is used. Note that not all macrocytic anemias are megaloblastic.

B. Neutrophil Changes: The neutrophils are also affected. Neutrophil precursors in the bone marrow show marked enlargement; giant metamyelocytes are characteristic. In the peripheral blood, neutrophils show **hypersegmented nuclei,** with many cells showing more than 5 nuclear lobes (Figs 24–2 and 24–7).

C. Changes in Other Cells in the Body: The abnormality in DNA synthesis affects many other cells in the body, notably those that have a high rate of cell turnover. These include the intestinal mucosa and other epithelia that show cell enlargement and nuclear abnormalities. Recognition of these changes is important if cytologic studies are undertaken—eg, in uterine cervical smears, the nuclear changes of folate deficiency may resemble those of dysplasia.

Clinical Features & Diagnosis

Patients with megaloblastic anemia present with symptoms of severe anemia. Megaloblastic anemia should be suspected upon finding macrocytic anemia with hypersegmented neutrophils in the peripheral blood. Bone marrow examination is necessary for confirmation and shows megaloblastic erythropoiesis.

Establishment of the precise cause of megaloblastic anemia requires further clinical examination and laboratory testing (Table 24–6).

There are 2 principal forms of megaloblastic anemia: folate deficiency, which has several underlying causes (Table 24–5); and vitamin B_{12} deficiency, again with several causes, including pernicious anemia, which will be discussed below at some length.

Note that the megaloblastic anemia of folate deficiency is identical to that of vitamin B_{12} deficiency; administration of folic acid may thus mask (partially correct) the anemia of vitamin B_{12} deficiency, and vice versa; however, folic acid ad-

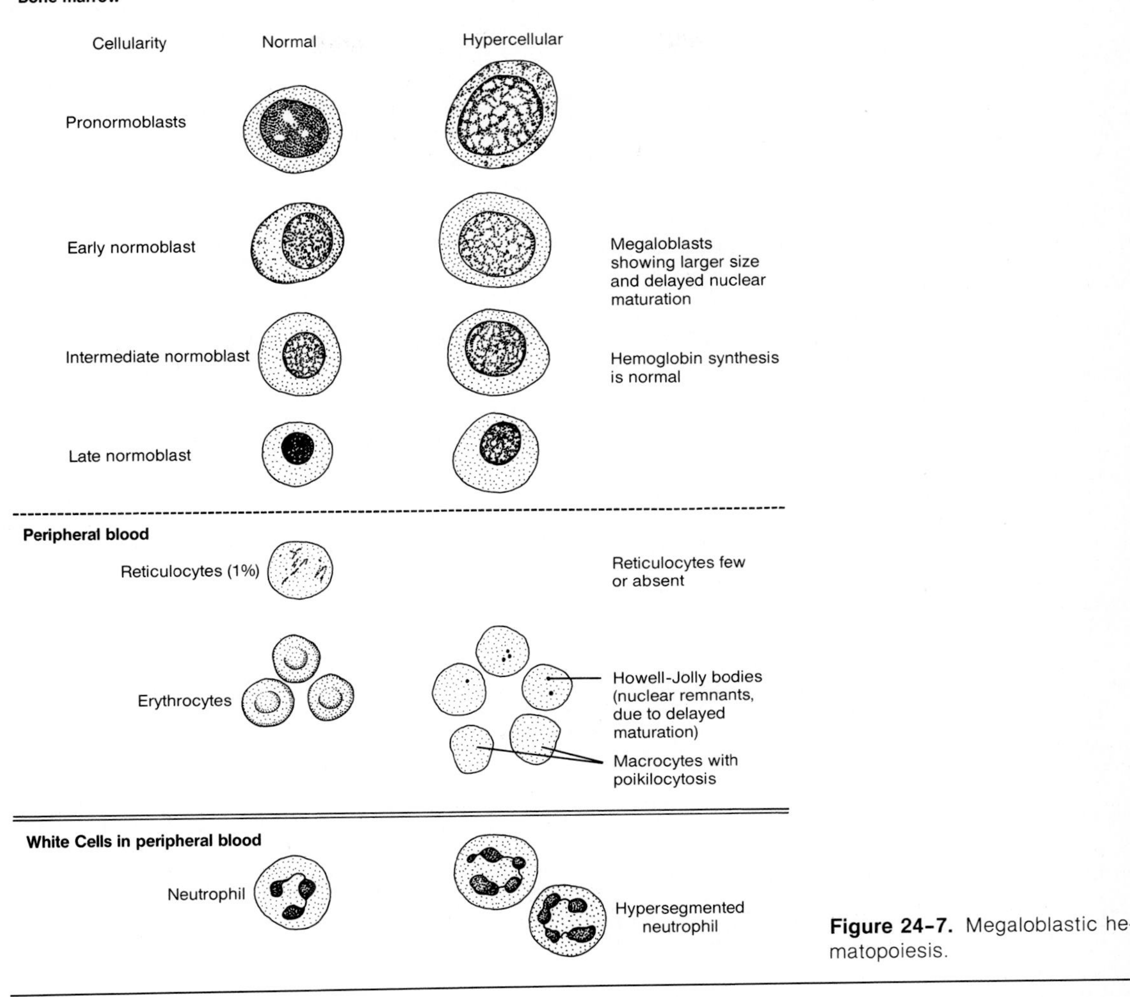

Figure 24–7. Megaloblastic hematopoiesis.

ministration does not correct the neurologic effects of B_{12} deficiency. For this reason, it is important to exclude vitamin B_{12} deficiency before treating megaloblastic anemia with folate.

1. PERNICIOUS (ADDISONIAN) ANEMIA

Pernicious anemia is a form of megaloblastic anemia due to vitamin B_{12} deficiency. It is common in western Europe and among Caucasians (particularly of Northern European descent) in the United States but rare in Asia and Africa. Pernicious anemia occurs predominantly after the age of 50 years, slightly more often in males than females. Family members show an increased incidence of achlorhydria, decreased vitamin B_{12} absorption, or overt pernicious anemia. A rare form of the disease called juvenile pernicious anemia occurs in childhood.

Pathogenesis

Adult pernicious anemia is an **autoimmune disease,** caused by immunologic destruction of the gastric mucosa. The mucosa of the body and fundus of the stomach is characterized by lymphocytic infiltration and progressive loss of parietal cells (chronic atrophic gastritis). This process is associated with failure of secretion of acid and **intrinsic factor**. Achlorhydria is invariably present in these patients and can be demonstrated by sampling gastric fluid after appropriate stimulation tests. In the absence of intrinsic factor, vitamin B_{12} absorption is drastically reduced.

The exact mechanism of immune destruction is not fully known (Fig 24–8). Three types of autoantibodies may be demonstrated in both serum

Table 24-6. Differential diagnosis of folic acid and vitamin B_{12} deficiency anemias.

	Vitamin B_{12} Deficiency	Folate Deficiency
Megaloblastic anemia	+	+
Peripheral blood features	Identical	
Subacute combined degeneration of the spinal cord	+	–
Serum vitamin B_{12}[1]	Low	Normal
Serum folate[1]	Normal	Low
Red cell folate	Normal	Low
Response to vitamin B_{12} by injection[2]	+	–
Vitamin B_{12} absorption test (Schilling)	Abnormal[3]	Normal
Antiparietal or intrinsic factor antibodies in serum	±[4]	–

[1]Serum levels measured by radioimmunoassay.
[2]Response consists of an almost immediate increase in reticulocytes.
[3]Test uses radiolabeled dose of vitamin B_{12}. It is normal in dietary deficiency and abnormal in bacterial overgrowth, general malabsorption, and pernicious anemia; in pernicious anemia it corrects to normal if intrinsic factor is added.
[4]Positive in pernicious anemia (see text); negative in general malabsorption states.

and gastric juice: (1) About 75% of patients have an antibody that blocks vitamin B_{12} binding to intrinsic factor (blocking antibody); (2) about 50% have an antibody that binds with the intrinsic factor-vitamin B_{12} complex, interfering with the binding of the complex to ileal mucosal receptors, a prerequisite for vitamin B_{12} absorption; and (3) about 90% of patients have antibodies against gastric parietal cells. This antibody is also present in the serum of a minority of patients with other autoimmune diseases (Addison's disease, Hashimoto's thyroiditis) and rarely in "normal" elderly individuals.

The serum antibodies are frequently IgG, and gastric juice antibodies are IgA.

While useful for the diagnosis of pernicious anemia, the role played by these autoantibodies in producing the disease is uncertain. A few patients with pernicious anemia have none of the 3 antibodies. It has been suggested without proof that the gastric mucosal destruction may be mediated by autoreactive T lymphocytes (cell-mediated hypersensitivity).

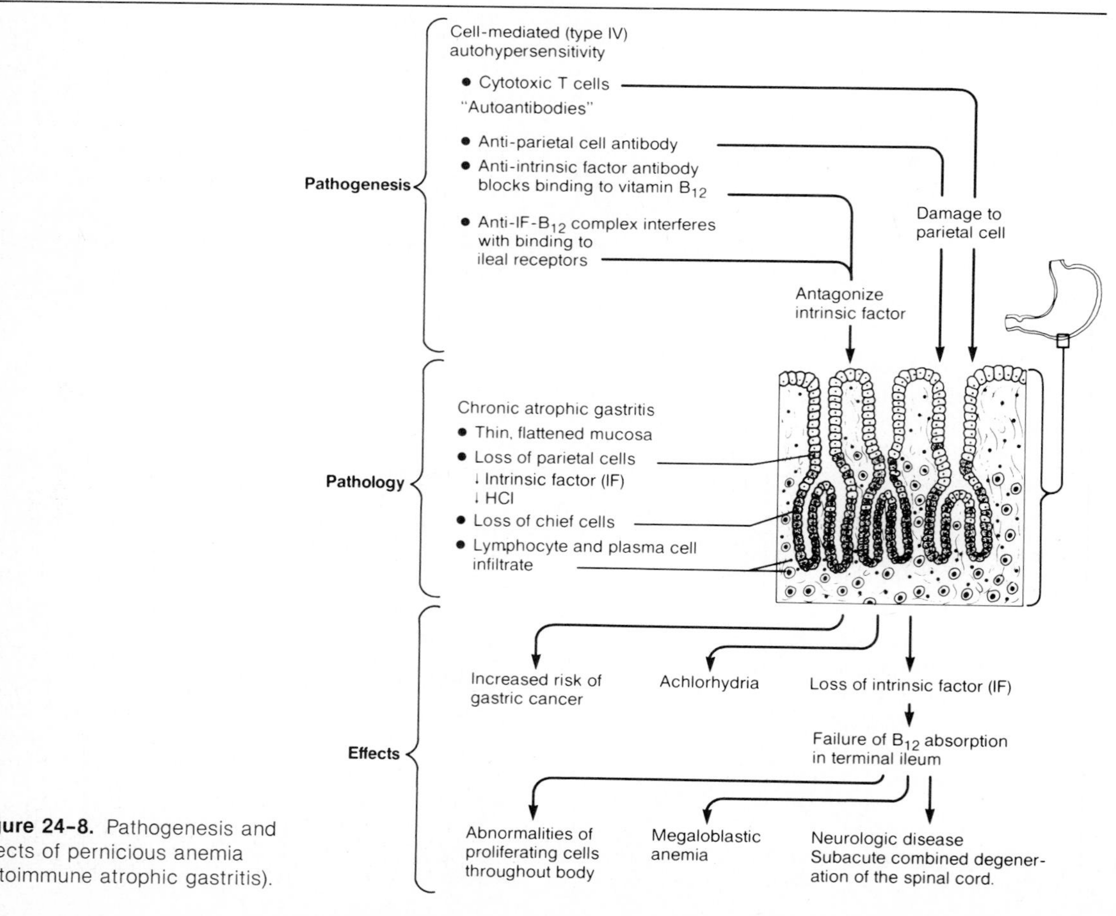

Figure 24-8. Pathogenesis and effects of pernicious anemia (autoimmune atrophic gastritis).

Pathology & Clinical Features (Fig 24-8)

Chronic atrophic gastritis with achlorhydria is constantly associated with the failure of intrinsic factor secretion that leads to vitamin B_{12} deficiency. Megaloblastic anemia and other changes resulting from failure of nucleic acid synthesis have been described above. Neurologic changes are due to demyelination by uncertain mechanisms (Fig 24–7).

The most characteristic neurologic abnormality in pernicious anemia is **subacute combined degeneration of the spinal cord,** which is characterized by demyelination of the posterior and lateral columns of the cord (Chapter 64). This leads to loss of position and vibration sense, loss of deep tendon reflexes, and, in the later stages of the disease, pyramidal dysfunction.

Peripheral neuropathy is due to segmental demyelination of nerves. These neurologic changes do not occur in patients with folic acid deficiency (Table 24–6).

Treatment & Prognosis

Patients with pernicious anemia die without treatment (the adjective indicates the high mortality rate in the past). With adequate replacement therapy with injected vitamin B_{12} (cyanocobalamin), these patients live a normal life. The anemia reverses rapidly, the bone marrow reverting to normal. Neurologic changes improve slowly and often incompletely.

Patients with pernicious anemia remain at increased risk for development of **gastric carcinoma** in the atrophic gastric mucosa and must be followed carefully for this complication. Precancerous epithelial dysplasia usually occurs before invasive carcinoma develops and can be detected in gastric biopsies.

IRON DEFICIENCY ANEMIA

Iron deficiency anemia is by far the commonest cause of anemia worldwide. It is common in underdeveloped as well as developed countries, but the causes differ in the 2 settings. In countries of the third world, hookworm infections account for most cases. In the United States, pregnancy and chronic blood loss due to gastrointestinal ulcers or neoplasms are the commonest causes. It has been estimated that in the USA, 50% of pregnant women, 20% of all women, 20% of preschool children, and 3% of men suffer from iron deficiency.

Normal iron balance is regulated mainly by changes in the intestinal absorption of iron to match the normal loss of iron from the body in secretions, exfoliated cells, and menstrual blood (Fig 24–9).

Plasma iron is complexed with the iron-binding protein transferrin. Normal plasma has enough transferrin (iron binding capacity) to bind 250–400 μg of iron per deciliter of blood. In a normal adult, approximately 30% of the transferrin is saturated, the normal plasma iron being 50-150 μg/dL (Fig 24–10).

Note that the massive iron turnover associated with normal erythropoiesis and red cell breakdown is internalized, with the iron from erythro-

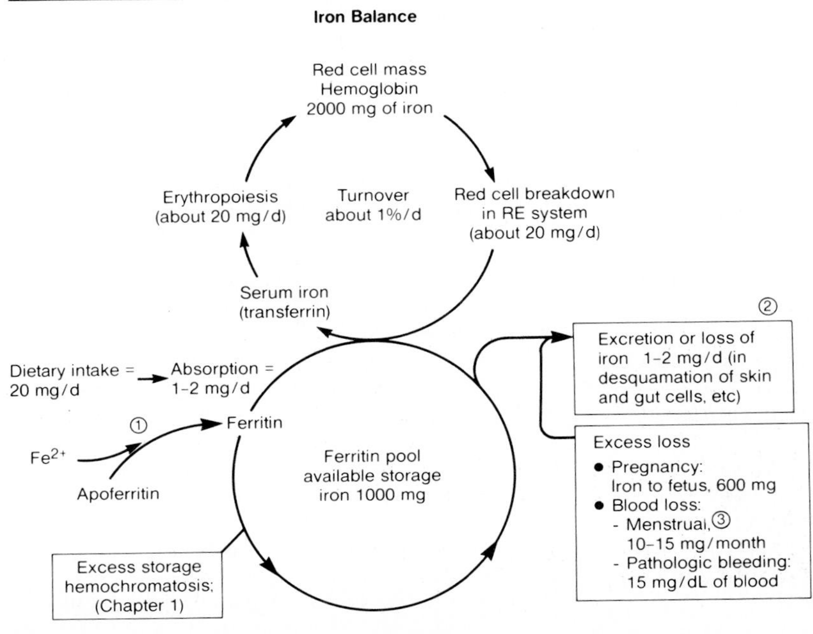

Figure 24-9. Iron balance. **(1)** Absorption of ferrous iron (Fe^{2+}) occurs in the upper small intestine and is facilitated by the presence of gastric acid. Upon demand, absorption of iron can increase only to a limited degree (to about 20% of dietary iron). **(2)** There is no mechanism for excretion of excess iron. **(3)** Increased absorption of iron in women usually compensates for normal menstrual loss.

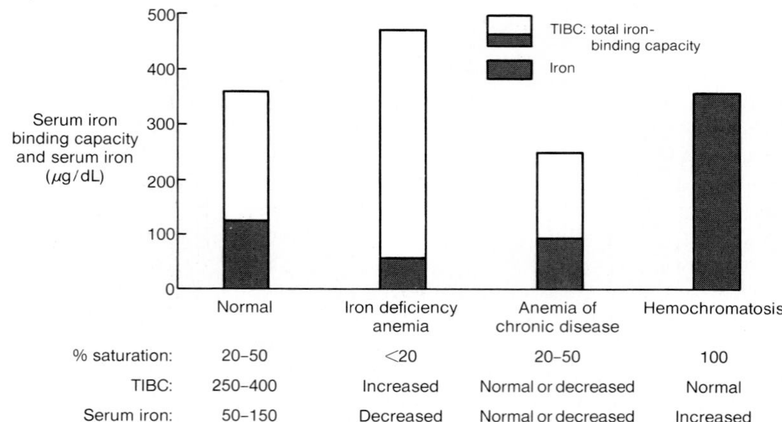

Figure 24–10. Serum iron and iron binding capacity in health and disease.

cyte destruction in the reticuloendothelial cells passing to the ferritin storage pool and thence to the plasma and bone marrow for reutilization in erythropoiesis. The plasma iron turnover for erythropoiesis is about 20 mg/d.

Causes of Iron Deficiency (Table 24–7)

A. Dietary Deficiency: The daily dietary iron requirement is 5–10 mg/d (equivalent to 0.5–1 mg of absorbed iron) for men and 7–20 mg/d for women. The normal diet in the United States contains about 15 mg of iron, marginally adequate for women. Iron deficiency due to dietary deficiency occurs commonly in underdeveloped countries, where the dietary iron intake is chronically less than required.

B. Increased Demand for Iron: In developed countries, iron deficiency occurs in individuals on marginal diets or when there is an increased demand for iron, ie, in the growth phase of early childhood and during pregnancy and lactation. Premature infants are especially at risk. Dietary iron supplements are essential during these times.

C. Malabsorption of Iron: Iron deficiency may occur in severe generalized malabsorptive states such as celiac disease and tropical sprue. It also occurs after total gastrectomy because (1) gastric acid is necessary for optimal iron absorption and (2) the transit time of food in the small intestine is decreased after gastrectomy.

D. Chronic Blood Loss: Loss of blood is a major cause of iron deficiency throughout the world. One hundred milliliters of whole blood with a hemoglobin of 15 g contains about 50 mg of iron (1 g hemoglobin contains 3.5 mg iron). Excessive menstrual blood loss from any cause and occult gastrointestinal blood loss (due to hookworm infection, peptic ulcer disease, chronic aspirin ingestion, esophageal varices, hemorrhoids, and neoplasms) are the commonest causes of iron deficiency anemia; chronic loss of as little as one teaspoonful (5 mL) of blood per day will tip most people into negative iron balance. Note that the normal marrow is able to compensate for this degree of blood loss. However, with chronic loss the onset of iron deficiency interferes with erythropoiesis, and this leads to anemia.

Pathology

Iron deficiency is first reflected in a decrease in iron stores, demonstrated by a decreased serum ferritin level and an absence of iron in a specimen of bone marrow. Serum ferritin reflects the amount of storage iron in the body. Bone marrow biopsies are routinely examined by the Prussian blue stain for their iron content.

When iron stores are exhausted, the serum iron level falls. This is usually associated with an increase in the plasma transferrin level (also called total iron binding capacity, or TIBC). The net result is a decrease in saturation of the TIBC, which is a sensitive indicator of iron deficiency (Fig 24–10).

The main effect of iron deficiency is to reduce erythropoiesis, with several consequences.

A. Anemia: Anemia is due both to a decreased amount of hemoglobin in individual red cells and to a decrease in the total red cell mass. The poorly hemoglobinized erythrocytes appear as pale hypochromic cells with an expanded central clear zone and a thin ring of pink cytoplasm (Fig 24–5). The MHC is decreased.

B. Microcytosis: The erythrocytes are abnormally small (Fig 24–5) and have a decreased MCV. **Hypochromic microcytic anemia** is the typical result of iron deficiency; however, it is not specific for iron deficiency anemia.

C. Increased Free Erythrocytic Porphyrin: Reduced availability of iron for chelation with protoporphyrin results in accumulation of increased amounts of free protoporphyrin in the erythrocyte.

D. Bone Marrow Changes: The bone marrow

Table 24–7. Iron deficiency anemia: Possible causes and investigations.

Possible Causes	
Infancy and childhood	Dietary
	Chronic blood loss
	Chronic infection
	Prematurity
Adult female (reproductive years)	Dietary
	Excessive menstrual loss
	Pregnancies and miscarriages
	Gastrointestinal blood loss
	Hematuria, other blood loss
Adult male (and postmenopausal female)	Gastrointestinal blood loss
	Drugs (eg, aspirin)
	Dietary (rare)
	Epistaxis, hematuria, other blood loss
	Hereditary hemorrhagic telangiectasia[1]
Investigations	
History	Diet
	Drugs (aspirin)
	Gastrointestinal symptoms (pain, indigestion, black or bloody stools, dysphagia)
	Menstrual history
Examination	Rectal, sigmoidoscopy (cancer, hemorrhoids)
	Pelvic, in female
	Evidence of telangiectases
X-rays	Barium swallow: esophageal varices
	Barium meal: peptic ulcer, gastric cancer, hiatus hernia
	Barium enema: carcinoma, colitis
	Chest: lung cancer, other causes of hemoptysis
Fecal occult blood[2]	Tests for blood in feces
Urinalysis[3]	Tests for blood in urine

[1]Osler-Weber-Rendu disease: Hereditary hemorrhagic telangiectasia produces multiple pinpoint bleeding foci in the gastrointestinal tract, mouth, lips, and skin.
[2]The fecal occult blood test (performed with commercially available strips or pellets) is a sensitive test for bleeding in the gastrointestinal tract; it will also be positive after eating red meat, especially if cooked rare.
[3]Simple screening test using a commercial reagent strip; more formal analysis by microscopic examination of fresh urine sediment.

shows variable normoblastic hyperplasia. The normoblasts are small, have decreased hemoglobin, and show an irregular frayed cell membrane. **Storage iron is absent,** and the number of sideroblasts (normoblasts containing cytoplasmic iron) is decreased.

E. Epithelial Changes: Iron deficiency also results in atrophy of many epithelial surfaces, eg, the mucous membrane of the mouth, tongue, pharynx, esophagus, and stomach. In the esophagus, atrophy may be associated with mucosal webs and dysphagia. Gastric changes may result in hypochlorhydria (decreased acid secretion). Koilonychia (concave fingernails with abnormal ridging and splitting) is a specific result of iron deficiency. The association of iron deficiency anemia, koilonychia, atrophic glossitis, and dysphagia is known as Plummer-Vinson syndrome (Chapter 37).

Treatment

It is vital to establish the underlying cause prior to treatment (Table 24–7). Iron replacement, either orally or parenterally, is effective in treating iron deficiency anemia and replenishing body stores. It is important in the management of patients with iron deficiency anemia to find and correct the reason for anemia.

ANEMIA OF CHRONIC DISEASE

Anemia occurs as a complication of many chronic diseases such as chronic infections, collagen diseases and malignant neoplasms. The anemia in these cases is caused by **failure of transport of storage iron** into the plasma and therefore into developing erythrocytes. This leads to failure of hemoglobinization and anemia. In most cases, the red cells are normocytic and normochromic (Fig 24–5), but they may be hypochromic.

The diagnosis is made by finding increased iron stores in the bone marrow and elevated plasma ferritin levels, decreased serum iron and TIBC, decreased numbers of sideroblasts in the bone marrow, and increased free erythrocytic protoporphyrin. The percentage saturation of plasma transferrin (TIBC) is usually within normal limits (Fig 24–10).

Anemia is usually mild to moderate, but it is difficult to treat. Iron therapy does not help and may actually cause harm by increasing the tissue iron stores.

ANEMIA OF CHRONIC RENAL FAILURE

Patients with chronic renal failure develop a normochromic, normocytic anemia due to failure of normal erythropoietin secretion by the kidney. The bone marrow may show mild hypoplasia of the erythroid series.

SIDEROBLASTIC ANEMIA

Sideroblastic anemia is an uncommon type of anemia characterized by the presence in the bone marrow of increased numbers of sideroblasts (erythroid precursors with demonstrable cytoplasmic iron). It has a variety of causes (Table 24–8).

Sideroblastic anemias are characterized by either a **hypochromic, microcytic,** or **dimorphic** peripheral blood erythrocyte appearance. A di-

Table 24-8. Causes of sideroblastic anemia.

Hereditary (X-linked)
Primary acquired; no other associated disease
Secondary acquired
Chronic alcoholism
Pyridoxine deficiency
Drugs: antituberculous drugs, chloramphenicol
Lead poisoning

morphic peripheral blood picture is one in which there is an admixture of hypochromic, microcytic erythrocytes and macrocytic erythrocytes.

Serum iron, TIBC, and saturation are increased. The marrow shows erythroid hyperplasia, markedly increased amounts of storage iron, increased number of sideroblasts and defective hemoglobinization. A characteristic feature is the presence of ring sideroblasts—normoblasts in which the amount of iron is so greatly increased that it appears as cytoplasmic granules arranged in a complete ring around the nucleus. It appears that there is a defect in incorporating iron into the hemoglobin molecule within the erythrocyte. In general, the number of sideroblasts is greater in primary acquired sideroblastic anemia than in the secondary type of disease. Secondary sideroblastic anemia frequently responds to treatment with pyridoxine.

In some patients with refractory sideroblastic anemia, increased numbers of immature white cells (mainly myeloblasts) are present. This is believed to be a premalignant change (dysmyelopoiesis), with many (10%) of these patients going on to develop acute leukemia.

ANEMIA DUE TO BLOOD LOSS

ACUTE BLOOD LOSS

Acute hemorrhage results in loss of whole blood from the vascular compartment, leading to hypovolemia and compensatory mechanisms to maintain perfusion to vital organs (see Shock, Chapter 9). In the acute bleeding phase, blood values—including red cell count, hemoglobin, and hematocrit—are normal because equivalent amounts of red cells, hemoglobin, and plasma are lost. An important compensation for hypovolemia is retention of water and electrolytes by the kidneys to restore blood volume. This begins immediately and causes dilution of the blood. Within hours, the effect of this dilution is seen as a progressive decrease in red cell count, hemoglobin, and hematocrit in the peripheral blood. The amount of decrease of these values depends on the amount and rate of blood loss and the effectiveness of renal compensation. Regeneration of erythrocytes lost during the hemorrhage occurs over the next several weeks and slowly restores the red cell count, hemoglobin, and hematocrit levels. During this regenerative phase, the bone marrow shows erythroid hyperplasia and depletion of iron stores, and the peripheral blood shows a reticulocytosis proportionate to the increased rate of erythrocyte production. The anemia is therefore temporary. The body's iron stores are replenished over the next few months. In patients who have depleted iron stores and a marginal dietary intake of iron, an episode of acute hemorrhage may precipitate iron deficiency anemia.

CHRONIC BLOOD LOSS

Chronic bleeding is compensated for initially by erythroid hyperplasia of the bone marrow and increased production of erythrocytes. This persists until iron stores have been depleted, at which time iron deficiency prevents adequate compensation. Anemia due to chronic blood loss is therefore an iron deficiency anemia and is discussed under that heading.

Blood: II. Hemolytic Anemias; Polycythemia

25

HEMOLYTIC ANEMIAS *(Table 25–1)*

Hemolytic anemias are a group of diseases characterized by shortened survival of red blood cells in the circulation. Red cell destruction may occur chiefly in the reticuloendothelial system (extravascular hemolysis—the usual situation in most types of hemolytic anemia) or in the blood (intravascular hemolysis—uncommon, largely restricted to physical lysis of red cells, as in microangiopathy, or to complement mediated lysis), or in some combination of the two (Fig 25–1).

Extravascular Hemolysis

Extravascular hemolysis is characterized by the following features.

A. Hemolytic Jaundice: Increased production of unconjugated bilurubin occurs because of increased breakdown of hemoglobin. Unconjugated bilirubin is complexed with plasma albumin and transported to the liver, where it is taken up by the liver cells for conjugation (Fig 25–1; see also Chapter 1). Jaundice appears only when the amount of unconjugated bilirubin delivered to the liver exceeds the capacity of that organ to conjugate and excrete it. Even when present, the degree of jaundice in hemolytic processes is usually mild.

Unconjugated bilirubin is not excreted in the urine (acholuric jaundice).

B. Increased Bilirubin Excretion in Bile: The liver excretes increased amounts of conjugated bilirubin in the bile, which is why patients with chronic hemolytic processes tend to develop bilirubin pigment stones in the gallbladder. The bile enters the duodenum, where it is converted to urobilinogen by bacterial action. Increased excretion of fecal urobilinogen is present in hemolytic anemias. The urobilinogen is also absorbed in the portal vein and excreted in increased amounts in the urine (Fig 25–1; see also Chapter 1).

C. Erythroid Hyperplasia: The anemia stimulates erythroid hyperplasia in the bone marrow, sometimes to a remarkable degree, with expansion of the marrow cavity that can be recognized on x-rays. Anemia occurs only when the erythroid hyperplasia cannot compensate for the hemolysis. The increased rate of erythropoiesis also results in an increase in the number of reticulocytes in the peripheral blood. In severe cases, normoblasts may enter the peripheral blood. The maximum marrow response is an 8- to 10-fold increase in red cell production.

D. Hemosiderosis: Iron produced by degradation of hemoglobin is retained in the reticuloendothelial cells to cause hemosiderosis. The tendency to hemosiderosis in chronic hemolytic anemias is aggravated by increased intestinal absorption of iron and use of blood transfusions.

Intravascular Hemolysis

Intravascular hemolysis is characterized by the following features.

A. Hemolytic Jaundice: The hemoglobin re-

Table 25-1. Classification of hemolytic anemias.

Intrinsic defect of erythrocytes
Congenital hemolytic anemias
Membrane defects
Hereditary spherocytosis
Hereditary elliptocytosis
Enzyme deficiency
Glucose-6-phosphatase deficiency
Pyruvate kinase deficiency
Abnormal hemoglobin synthesis (hemoglobinopathies)
Sickle cell disease
Thalassemia
Unstable hemoglobins
Acquired hemolytic anemias
Paroxysmal nocturnal hemoglobinuria
Hemolysis due to extrinsic factors
Immune hemolytic anemias
Autoimmune hemolytic anemias
Associated with warm antibodies
Associated with cold antibodies
Isoimmune hemolytic anemias
Hemolytic blood transfusion reactions
Hemolytic disease of the newborn
Drug-induced immune hemolytic anemias
Direct-acting external agents
Infections: malaria
Snake venom
Physical trauma: microangiopathy, hypersplenism

leased into the circulation is taken up and degraded by the reticuloendothelial system, causing unconjugated hyperbilirubinemia.

B. Erythroid Hyperplasia: Marked only if hemolysis becomes chronic.

C. Decreased Plasma Haptoglobin: Haptoglobin is an α_2 globulin that rapidly binds free hemoglobin in the plasma. Normal blood has sufficient haptoglobin to bind about 100–200 mg of hemoglobin.

D. Hemoglobinemia: Free hemoglobin in the plasma appears when hemolysis has exhausted the capacity of plasma haptoglobin to bind hemoglobin. Hemoglobin imparts a pink color to the plasma and can be identified definitively by its typical spectrophotometric bands.

E. Hemoglobinuria: The hemoglobin molecule is filtered by the glomerulus and appears unchanged in urine, imparting a pink color. The hemoglobin may be taken up by renal tubular cells and degraded therein with deposition of hemosiderin in the cytoplasm. Desquamated tubular epithelial cells containing hemosiderin may appear in the urine (**hemosiderinuria**).

F. Methemalbuminemia: Part of the released hemoglobin is oxidized to methemoglobin. This substance may be bound to albumin to form methemalbumin or complexed with hemopexin, a beta globulin, and cleared by the liver. The presence of methemalbumin in the plasma (detected by Schumm's test) is good evidence for intravascular hemolysis.

G. Increased serum levels of lactate dehydrogenase are commonly present in intravascular hemolysis due to release of this enzyme from red cells.

INTRINSIC ERYTHROCYTE DEFECTS

ERYTHROCYTE MEMBRANE DEFECTS

The Erythrocyte Membrane

The cell membrane of the erythrocyte is a trilaminar bipolar phospholipid structure in which are situated many kinds of integral structural proteins such as glycophorin. It is flexible and is often referred to as a "fluid mosaic structure."

Rhesus (Rh) blood group antigens represent integral structural molecules of the membrane. Very rare patients who lack Rh antigens (Rh null) have severe membrane abnormalities that result in deformed erythrocytes known as stomatocytes which have greatly shortened survival times. **ABO glycoprotein blood group antigens,** on the other hand, are not integral structural proteins of the membrane. They are located on the outer part of the membrane.

The inner surface of the cell membrane is supported by a latticelike fibrillar network of contractile proteins that include actin and spectrin. Spectrin is believed to control red cell shape and deformability. The membrane also has many **enzyme systems** (cAMP, ATP, and GTP-dependent protein kinases) that appear to regulate membrane functions.

1. HEREDITARY SPHEROCYTOSIS

Etiology & Pathogenesis

Hereditary spherocytosis is a congenital autosomal dominant disease with variable penetrance. Patients may present with severe hemolysis in childhood or with mild hemolysis manifested first during adult life. The exact expression of the abnormal gene has not been elucidated. Abnormal polymerization of spectrin and defective membrane autophosphorylation have been demonstrated.

The obvious abnormality in hereditary spherocytosis is a change in the shape of the red cell from its normal biconcave shape to a spherical shape. These spherocytes are less pliable than normal erythrocytes and tend to lose membrane substance as they traverse the splenic sinusoids, becoming progressively smaller (microspherocytes); spherocyte life span is shortened, with destruction occurring in the spleen.

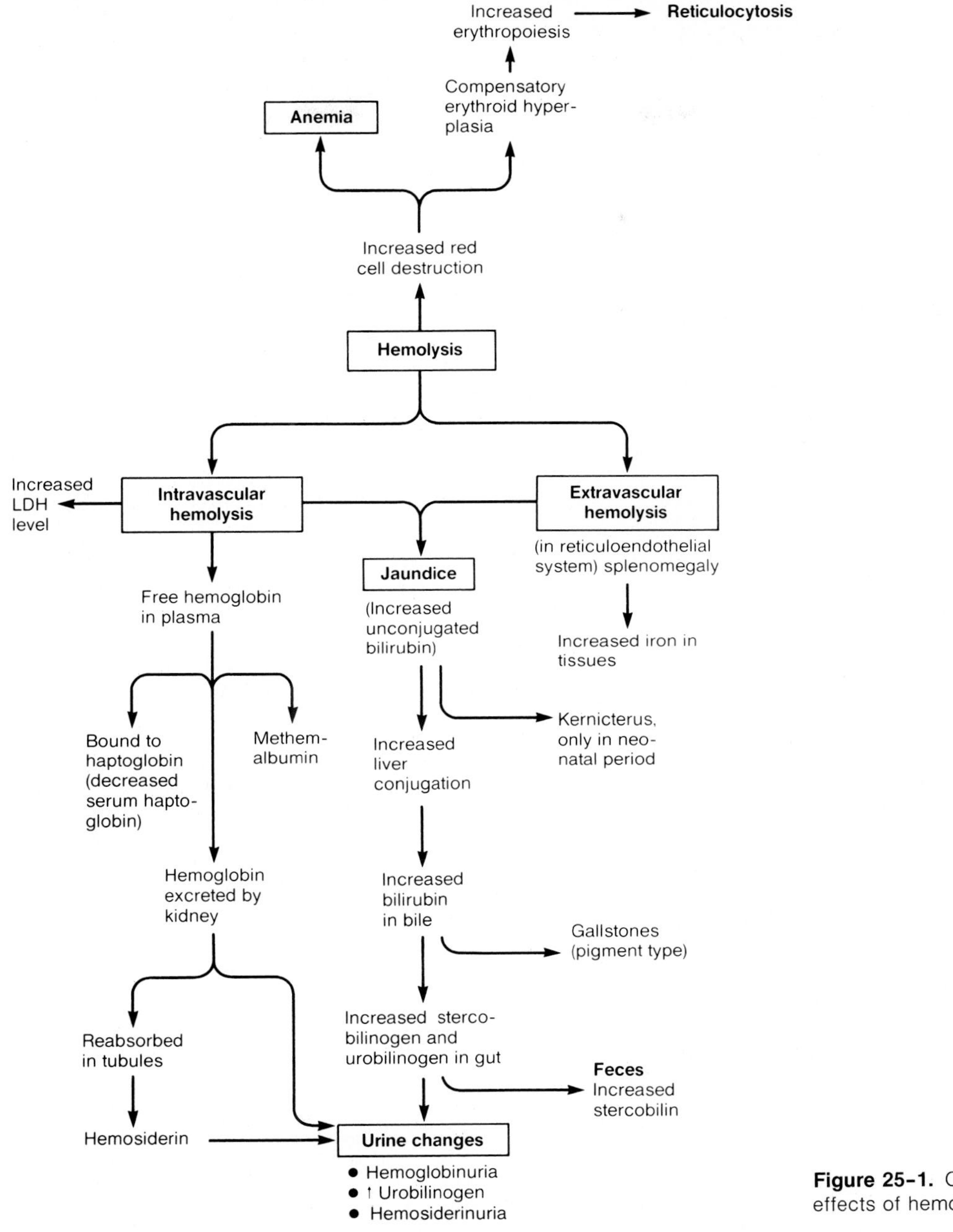

Figure 25-1. Clinicopathologic effects of hemolysis.

Clinical Features

Patients present with hemolytic anemia and jaundice. Splenic enlargement is usually present as a result of reticuloendothelial hyperplasia. Life-threatening aplastic crises may occur in association with infection. The diagnosis of hereditary spherocytosis is established by demonstration of hemolysis, the family history, peripheral blood examination showing microspherocytes plus reticulocytosis, and increased fragility in the osmotic fragility test (spherocytes are more susceptible to lysis by saline solution). Spherocytes also show autohemolysis when incubated at 37 °C for 24–48 hours; autohemolysis is reduced by the addition of glucose.

Treatment

The erythrocyte membrane defect cannot be reversed by any known therapy. The only treatment available is splenectomy, which acts by removing the site of maximum erythrocyte destruction. The peripheral blood still shows the typical changes of spherocytosis after splenectomy; however, hemolysis is much reduced.

2. HEREDITARY ELLIPTOCYTOSIS

Hereditary elliptocytosis (ovalocytosis) resembles spherocytosis except that the red cells are oval and the disease is usually less severe, associated with mild splenomegaly. Inheritance is by autosomal dominant transmission.

3. PAROXYSMAL NOCTURNAL HEMOGLOBINURIA

Paroxysmal nocturnal hemoglobinuria is a rare acquired disease of red cells characterized by increased sensitivity of the membrane to complement. Erythrocyte lysis in the circulation results in hemoglobinemia, hemoglobinuria and hemosiderinuria.

Complement activation occurs mainly through the alternative pathway and is precipitated (1) by decreased pH (acidification) in vivo during sleep, as a result of slower respiration and accumulation of carbon dioxide—hence "paroxysmal nocturnal"; (2) by acidification of serum in vitro (Ham's test); and (3) by addition of sucrose to serum in vitro (sucrose lysis test). The sucrose lysis test is a useful screening test for this disorder.

Patients with paroxysmal nocturnal hemoglobinuria are usually young adults, and the anemia may be severe. The disease has a close association with aplastic anemia, either preceding it or following an episode of aplasia. It is believed that paroxysmal nocturnal hemoglobinuria represents a clone of abnormal erythrocytes developing in a hypoplastic bone marrow.

ERYTHROCYTE ENZYME DEFICIENCY

Normal Erythrocyte Metabolism

The erythrocyte has no mitochondria and lacks enzymes of the citric acid cycle and oxidative phosphorylation. ATP synthesis therefore occurs via glycolysis (Fig 25–2). Pyruvate kinase is essential for this reaction. ATP is required mainly for the transport functions and structural integrity of the cell membrane. An important constituent in the glycolytic pathway is 2,3 diphosphoglycerate (2,3-DPG), increased levels of which favor oxygen release from hemoglobin to the tissues; 2,3-DPG production is stimulated by hypoxia, and high erythrocyte 2,3-DPG levels are present in chronic anemia.

The **pentose phosphate pathway** is important in

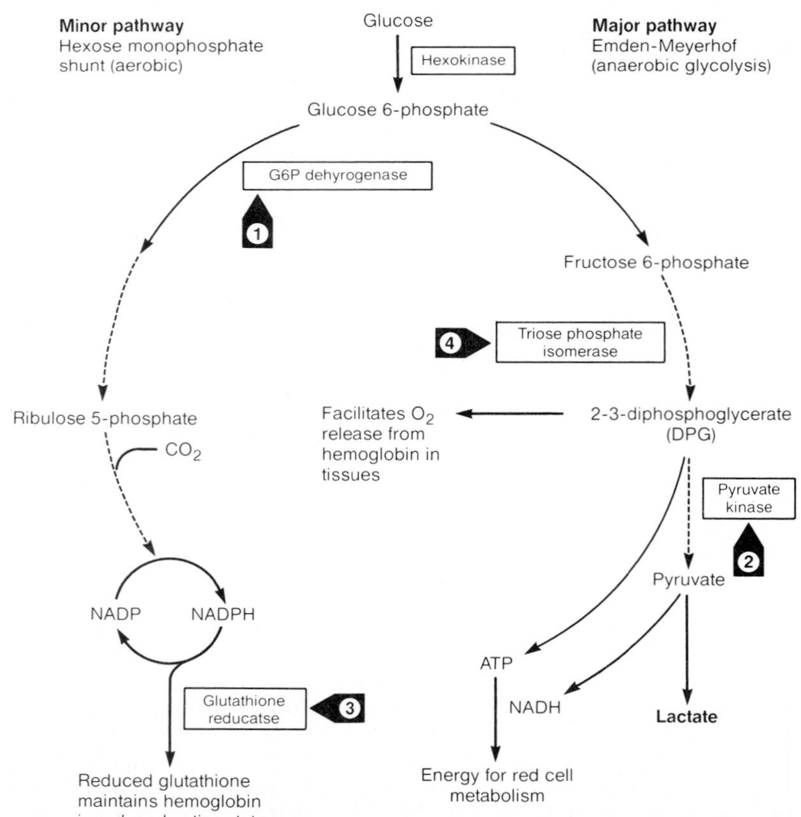

Figure 25–2. Glucose metabolism in the erythrocyte. The 4 enzymes that are most commonly deficient to a degree that results in clinical disease are indicated by numbers.

preventing hemoglobin oxidation (Fig 25–2). Failure of this mechanism results in oxidation, denaturation, and precipitation of hemoglobin as **Heinz bodies.** Heinz bodies adhere to the erythrocyte membrane, interfering with membrane deformability and making them more susceptible to phagocytosis in the splenic sinusoids. In addition, splenic macrophages remove those parts of the membrane with adherent Heinz bodies ("pitting"), causing membrane loss and formation of microspherocytes. **Glucose-6-phosphate dehydrogenase** is an important enzyme in this pathway.

1. GLUCOSE-6-PHOSPHATE DEHYDROGENASE (G6PD) DEFICIENCY

G6PD deficiency is the most common erythrocyte enzyme abnormality. Several variants are recognized; most do not cause disease. The G6PD-A (−) variant, inherited as an X-linked trait, is present in about 10% of blacks in the United States and has a worldwide distribution. It is the result of 2 point mutations and is probably the most common mutation-induced disease of humans. Full expression of the enzyme deficiency occurs in males. Heterozygous female carriers may have mild enzyme deficiency (resulting from random expression of the normal or affected X chromosome).

Deficiency of G6PD increases as the cell ages, and hemolytic episodes therefore tend to affect the older cells. G6PD-deficient red cells are more vulnerable to oxidants, which cause oxidative denaturation of hemoglobin and lead to formation of Heinz bodies and hemolysis. The main oxidant agents concerned are drugs such as primaquine, sulfonamides and nitrofurantoin.

Most patients with G6PD deficiency are asymptomatic, though the diagnosis may be confirmed by quantitative spectrophotometric assays. **Acute intravascular hemolysis** may occur after exposure to an oxidant drug; however, because all of the older G6PD-deficient cells have lysed, G6PD levels may appear normal, and the diagnosis is difficult to make in the acute stage. Rarely, patients develop a mild chronic hemolytic anemia.

The Mediterranean variant of G6PD deficiency occurs in Middle Eastern populations and produces G6PD deficiency in red cells of all ages; the disease is therefore more severe.

2. OTHER ERYTHROCYTE ENZYME DEFICIENCIES

Pyruvate kinase deficiency is less common than G6PD deficiency but more often produces clinical effects. It is inherited as an autosomal recessive trait and occurs with equal frequency in both sexes. Patients present with acute or chronic hemolytic anemia. The diagnosis is made by enzyme assay.

Deficiencies of other enzymes such as **glutathione reductase and triosephosphate isomerase** are rare.

HEMOGLOBINOPATHIES

Several different types of hemoglobin occur in humans. All have 4 polypeptide chains per molecule of hemoglobin, each chain linked with one heme group composed of an iron-chelated protoporphyrin molecule (Figs 25–3 and 25–4). Diseases manifesting abnormalities of hemoglobin synthesis are termed hemoglobinopathies. Three broad types are recognized: (1) **qualitative** hemoglobinopathies characterized by synthesis of an abnormal hemoglobin molecule, commonly due to a single gene abnormality (eg, sickle cell disease, hemoglobin C disease); (2) **quantitative** hemoglobinopathies (thalassemias), characterized by failure of secretion of one chain type, leading to lack of certain types of hemoglobin and a compensatory increase of other hemoglobins; and (3) **combined** qualitative and quantitative hemoglobinopathies.

The most common hemoglobinopathies are in-

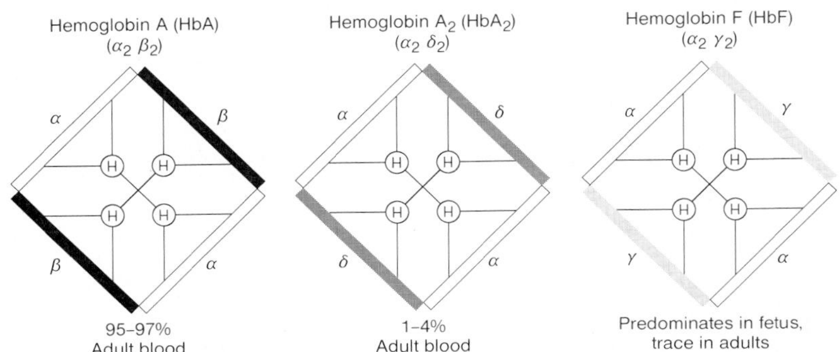

Figure 25–3. Types of hemoglobins normally found in the adult and fetus. Hemoglobin F levels rapidly decrease in the blood after birth. Ⓗ = heme group.

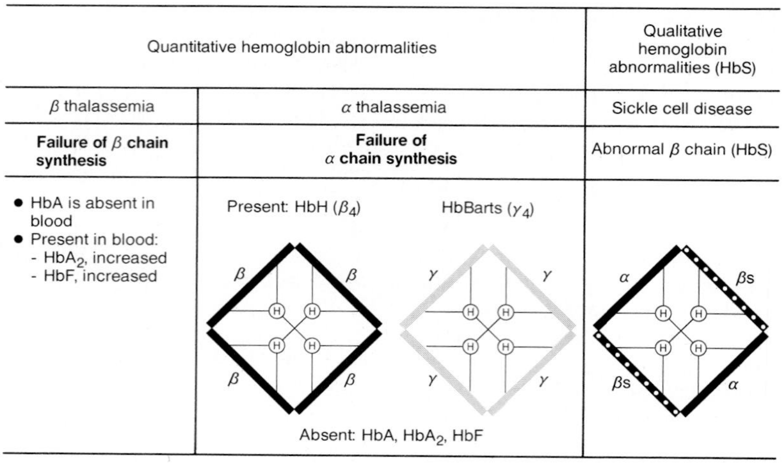

Quantitative hemoglobin abnormalities			Qualitative hemoglobin abnormalities (HbS)
β thalassemia	α thalassemia		Sickle cell disease
Failure of β chain synthesis	**Failure of α chain synthesis**		Abnormal β chain (HbS)
• HbA is absent in blood • Present in blood: - HbA_2, increased - HbF, increased	Present: HbH (β_4)	HbBarts (γ_4)	
	Absent: HbA, HbA_2, HbF		

Figure 25–4. Hemoglobinopathies. In beta thalassemia, complete failure of beta chain synthesis results in absence of HbA. HbA_2 and HbF levels are increased to a varying degree. In alpha thalassemia, complete failure of alpha chain synthesis results in an absence of HbA, HbA_2, and HbF and the presence in the blood of beta and gamma chain tetramers. Numerous qualitative abnormalities of hemoglobin exist; sickle cell disease is illustrated here because it is the most common.

herited as single gene abnormalities that dictate insertion of a single abnormal amino acid into the beta polypeptide chain. Several different abnormal genes are recognized, each producing a different abnormal hemoglobin. The most common abnormal hemoglobin is HbS (which results in sickle cell disease); less common abnormal hemoglobins are HbC, HbD, and HbE. Individuals who are homozygous for the abnormal gene have high levels of the abnormal hemoglobin, whereas heterozygotes have lower levels (Fig 25–5). HbS-C disease is double-heterozygous for the S and C genes.

1. SICKLE CELL DISEASE

The abnormal HbS gene is common in Africa, India and among blacks in the United States. It is rare in Caucasian and Oriental races.

A. Sickle Cell Trait: One abnormal gene is present in 9% of American blacks. These heterozygous (A/S) individuals suffer from the sickle cell trait, which usually causes no symptoms. Sickle cell trait confers some protection on the erythrocyte against infection with *Plasmodium falciparum;* this selective advantage is believed to have favored the persistence of the HbS gene in malaria-endemic areas.

B. Sickle Cell Disease: Sickle cell disease represents the homozygous (S/S) state and occurs in 0.1–0.2% of blacks born in the United States; about 50,000 black Americans suffer from sickle cell disease.

Pathology

A single point mutation (codon beta-6 GAG → GTG) dictates replacement of the normal glutamic acid at position 6 in the beta chain with valine. The result is HbS. This amino acid substitution is on the surface of the molecule and results

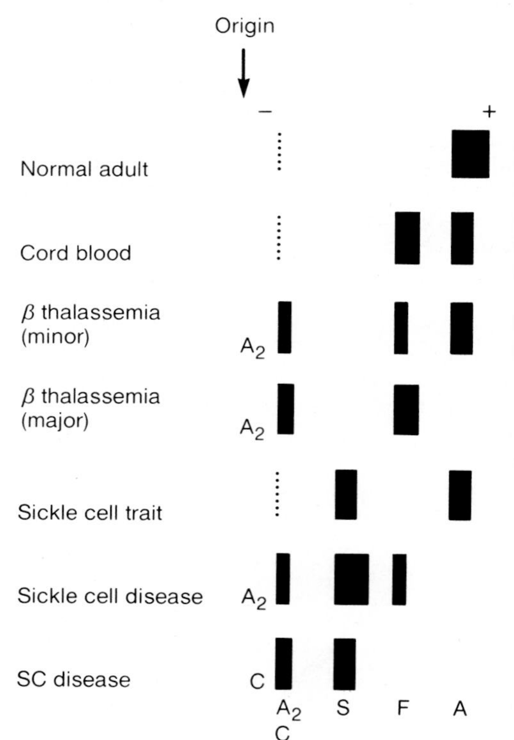

Figure 25–5. Hemoglobin electrophoretic patterns in normal adult blood, cord blood (fetus), and different hemoglobinopathies. Note that HbA_2 and HbC migrate identically in this electrophoresis medium.

in a tendency to polymerization, yielding semisolid crystalline structures called **tactoids,** under conditions of decreased oxygen tension. The degree of anoxia required to induce tactoids is very small in homozygous (S/S) patients (sickle cell disease), in whom the red cells contain up to 80% HbS, and much greater in heterozygous (A/S) patients (sickle cell trait), in whom the red cells contain about 30% HbS and 70% HbA.

Tactoid formation causes (1) decreased solubility of hemoglobin, (2) change in shape of the erythrocyte to a sickle cell, and (3) decreased deformability of the erythrocyte. Change in shape is due to interaction between the tactoids and the spectrin-actin cytoskeleton. Initially, sickling reverses when oxygenation improves, but with repeated or sustained anoxia, the erythrocyte assumes a permanently sickled shape. Decreased deformability leads to phagocytosis and destruction in the splenic and liver sinusoids.

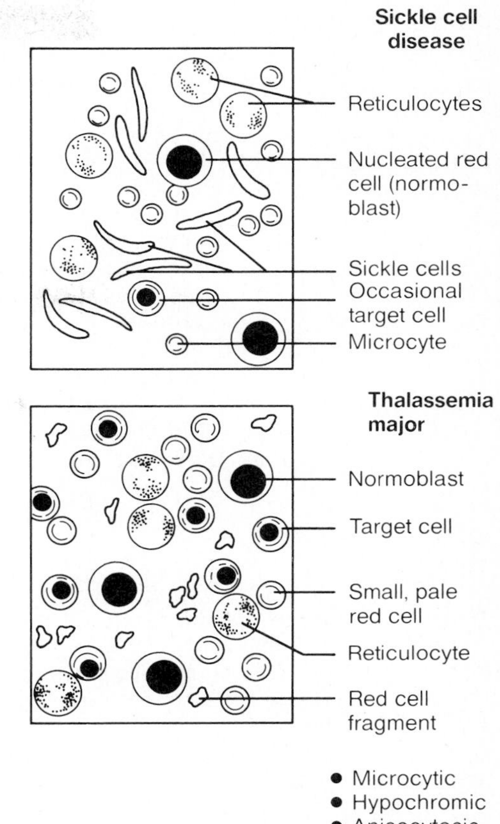

Figure 25–6. Peripheral blood smear features in sickle cell disease and beta thalassemia major. The presence of nucleated red cells and increased numbers of reticulocytes reflects the rapid rate of erythropoiesis. The peripheral blood findings are not specific for these diseases, and other tests such as hemoglobin electrophoresis are required for diagnosis.

Clinical Features

The onset of sickle cell disease is in childhood, and death often occurs during early adult life. With improvements in management, many patients now survive longer.

Patients present with evidence of chronic extravascular hemolysis and severe anemia. Growth retardation is common, as is heart failure (high-output type). Mild hemolytic jaundice with absent urinary bilirubin and increased fecal and urinary urobilinogen are usual. The bone marrow shows marked compensatory normoblastic hyperplasia, often leading to expansion of the marrow cavity in bones and causing bony deformities ("tower skull" and "hair-on-end" appearance on skull x-rays). Chronic leg ulcers that fail to heal are a typical feature of sickle cell disease but are of unknown pathogenesis.

Diagnosis

Sickle cells in peripheral blood smears are diagnostic (Fig 25–6) but not always present. Addition of metabisulfite to the blood smears induces sickling (metabisulfite sickle preparation). The dithionine solubility test detects decreased solubility of hemoglobin, and hemoglobin electrophoresis permits identification and quantitation of HbS in the blood (Fig 25–5). Patients with sickle cell disease have over 80% HbS in the blood with absent HbA; HbF and HbA_2 may be variably increased. Patients with sickle cell trait (heterozygous) have HbA (50–70%) and smaller amounts of HbS (30–35%), with normal HbF and HbA_2 levels. Sickle cell disease is not manifested in neonates because of their naturally high levels of HbF.

Complications

Aplastic crisis is sudden failure of hematopoiesis in the bone marrow, which may be precipitated by infections, drugs, or other causes. It is usually transient. **Hemolytic crisis** of unknown cause is characterized by a sudden increase in the level of hemolysis of erythrocytes.

Hemosiderosis and **secondary hemochromatosis** are common in long-term survivors. A positive iron balance results from stimulation of iron absorption in the intestine due to chronic erythroid hyperplasia and to multiple blood transfusions, which these patients commonly receive as treatment for anemia.

Vaso-occlusive crisis is probably due to plugging of the microcirculation by aggregates of sickle cells. Multiple microinfarcts are characterized by fever and ischemic pain, which may affect the heart, muscles, bone (aseptic necrosis of the femoral head is common), kidneys (papillary necrosis and renal failure may occur), lungs, central nervous system, and intestine.

Splenic changes are characteristic. The spleen

may be slightly enlarged in early childhood as a result of reticuloendothelial hyperplasia. Subsequently, repeated ischemic episodes cause infarction, fibrosis, and progressive decrease in splenic substance ("autosplenectomy"). In adults with sickle cell disease, the spleen is usually quite shrunken and composed of multiple brown scars containing hemosiderin (Gamna-Gandy bodies).

The functionally asplenic state predisposes patients with sickle cell disease to systemic infections with encapsulated bacteria. Pneumococcal bacteremia and *Salmonella* osteomyelitis are uncommon infections that occur with greater frequency in these patients. The presence of hyposplenism may be deduced by the presence of nuclear debris (Howell-Jolly bodies) in red cells. Howell-Jolly bodies are normally removed by the spleen.

2. OTHER ABNORMAL HEMOGLOBINS

Many other amino acid substitution hemoglobinopathies occur (Table 25-2) and may alter hemoglobin function. Hemoglobin electrophoresis is of value in recognizing the different variants (Fig 25-5). The double-heterozygous states, HbS-C and HbS-D, produce lower levels of HbS than homozygous S/S and have a disease of lesser clinical severity than sickle cell disease.

Abnormal hemoglobins may have the following consequences: (1) an increased rate of erythrocyte destruction, ie, hemolytic anemia. In most cases, the severity of hemolysis is less than that seen in sickle cell disease. (2) Instability of the hemoglobin molecule, causing precipitation of Heinz bodies and decreased red cell survival. (3) Altered affinity of the hemoglobin molecule for oxygen. When the affinity for oxygen is increased, oxygen release to the tissues is decreased, leading to hypoxia and compensatory polycythemia. When the affinity for oxygen is decreased, oxygen release to the tissues is increased, leading to decreased erythropoietin secretion and anemia and increased amounts of reduced hemoglobin in the blood (cyanosis). In these patients, tissue oxygenation is normal despite the anemia.

Table 25-2. Selected[1] amino acid substitution hemoglobin variants.[2]

Anemias in Homozygous state	
HbS-beta 6 val	Severe hemolytic anemia (sickle cell)
HbC-beta 6 lys	Mild hemolytic anemia
HbD (Punjab)-beta 121 Gln	Minimal anemia
HbE-beta 26 Lys	Mild anemia
Disease in heterozygous state	
Methemoglobinemia with cyanosis HbM (Boston)-alpha 58 Tyr HbM (Hyde Park)-beta 92 Tyr	Forms stable oxidized heme group (methemoglobin); reversible O_2 binding is prevented, and patients appear cyanosed.
Increased O_2 affinity Hb Chesapeake-alpha 92 Leu Hb Malmö-beta 97 Gln	The oxygen dissociation curve is shifted to the left; release of O_2 in tissues is reduced, leading to compensatory polycythemia.
Decreased O_2 affinity Hb Kansas-alpha 102 Thr Hb Beth Israel-beta 102 Ser	The oxygen dissociation curve is shifted to the right; increased amounts of reduced hemoglobin are present (cyanosis), but erythropoietin levels are low (anemia).
Unstable hemoglobins Hb Torino-alpha 42 Val Hb-Köln-beta 98 Met Hb Bristol-beta 67 Asp Hb Hammersmith-beta 42 Ser	Unstable hemoglobin precipitates as Heinz bodies, decreasing erythrocyte survival with varying degrees of hemolysis that is improved by splenectomy in some cases (eg, Köln, Torino).

[1]In all these conditions, substitution of a single amino acid results in a configurational change in the hemoglobin molecule.
[2]Many additional variants are known. See Winston RM, Anderson WF: the hemoglobinopathies. Chap 76, pp 1666-1710, in: *The Metabolic Basis of Inherited Disease,* 5th ed. Stanbury JB et al (editors). McGraw-Hill, 1983.

3. THALASSEMIAS (Table 25-3)

The thalassemias are characterized by a decreased rate of synthesis of hemoglobin chains that are structurally normal. **Beta thalassemia** is due to a decreased rate of synthesis of beta chains and is the most common form. **Alpha thalassemia,** in which there is a decreased synthesis of alpha chains, and **delta-beta thalassemia,** in which both delta and beta chain synthesis are affected, are rare.

Thalassemia syndromes are common in persons of Mediterranean, African, and Asian ancestry. Approximately 3% of the world's population carry the beta-thalassemia gene, which is inherited as an autosomal recessive. In beta thalassemias, the beta gene is usually present but contains one of more than 50 different known point mutations, resulting in either deficient production of messenger RNA or production of nonfunctional RNA. In most cases of alpha thalassemia, one or more of the alpha genes are deleted.

Table 25-3. Thalassemias.

	Genotype[1]	Severity of Disease	Hemoglobins Present
Beta[2]			
Beta thalassemia major	Homozygous β^0/β^0	Severe anemia	HbA absent or reduced ↑ HbA_2 ↑ HbF
Beta thalassemia minor	Heterozygous β^0/β	Mild to moderate anemia	HbA present; slight ↑ HbA_2, HbF
Alpha			
Hydrops fetalis (deletion of all 4 α genes)	$--/--$	Stillborn	Hb Barts (γ^4) HbH (β^4) Hb Portland (zeta[2], gamma[2]-embryonic)
HbH disease (deletion of 3 α genes)	$--/-\alpha$	Hemolytic anemia	HbA HbH Hb Barts
Alpha thalassemia minor (deletion of 2 genes)	$-\alpha/-\alpha$ $--/\alpha\alpha$	Mild hemolysis	HbA; trace Hb Barts
Carrier (deletion of 1 gene)	$\alpha\alpha/-\alpha$	No abnormality	Normal

[1]Only the β gene status is shown in beta thalassemias. β^0 = abnormal gene. Only the α gene status is shown in alpha thalassemias. Note that there are 2 alpha genes per haplotype.
[2]Other variants exist depending upon the exact effect of the defective beta gene.

Homozygous Beta Thalassemia (Cooley's Anemia)

Homozygous beta thalassemia is characterized by total or near total absence of synthesis of beta chains, with a marked decrease in the amount of HbA. Gamma chain production then persists into adult life, resulting in persistently elevated HbF levels (to about 40–60%, but sometimes as high as 90%). Delta chain synthesis is also increased to compensate for the absent beta chains, causing an increase in HbA_2 levels. In addition, excess free alpha chains precipitate in the cytoplasm of affected erythrocytes and are visible as inclusions. Alpha chain precipitates damage the red cells, resulting in their destruction.

Clinically, homozygous beta thalassemia begins in early childhood, with severe anemia, hemolytic jaundice, and splenomegaly. Growth retardation and delayed puberty are common features. Extreme erythroid hyperplasia causes expansion of the bone marrow and thinning of cortical bone. Involvement of the facial bones produces a characteristic facial appearance.

The peripheral blood picture is commonly that of hypochromic microcytic anemia with marked anisocytosis and numerous target forms (Fig 25–6). Reticulocytosis and the occasional presence of normoblasts attest to the increased rate of erythropoiesis. Hemoglobin electrophoresis shows elevation of HbF and HbA_2 with greatly decreased or absent HbA (Fig 25–6).

The main complication of thalassemia is the occurrence of a positive iron balance due to increased iron absorption in the gut and multiple blood transfusions. This **secondary hemochromatosis** affects many organs and is the most common cause of death, usually from myocardial or liver failure.

Heterozygous Beta Thalassemia (Cooley's Trait)

The heterozygous state of beta thalassemia may be asymptomatic or may present clinically with a mild hemolytic process characterized by mild anemia, jaundice, splenomegaly, and a hypochromic microcytic blood picture. Hemoglobin electrophoresis shows slight elevation of HbA_2 (4–7%) and HbF (2–6%). Most of the hemoglobin is HbA.

Sickle Cell-Beta Thalassemia

Sickle cell-beta thalassemia is caused by heterozygosity for both the sickle cell gene and the thalassemia gene. Clinically, it produces a hemolytic process that is intermediate in severity between sickle cell disease and sickle cell trait. The diagnosis is made by positive dithionine solubility or metabisulfite sickle tests, which demonstrate the ability to produce tactoids; and hemoglobin electrophoresis, which shows the presence of both HbS and HbA, with the former being present in greater concentration. HbF and HbA_2 are variably increased.

Alpha Thalassemia

Whereas there is only one beta gene per haplotype, there are 2 alpha genes, for a total of 4 in the normal situation. Deletion of all 4 leads to complete absence of alpha chain, severe fetal anemia with edema, erythroblastosis, and stillbirth. Absence of 3 or 2 alpha genes leads to progressively less severe disease, with varying levels of tetramer hemoglobins (β_4 and γ_4) compensating for reduced levels of HbA (Fig 25–4). Deletion of a single alpha gene has no clinical effect.

IMMUNE-MEDIATED HEMOLYTIC ANEMIAS

AUTOIMMUNE HEMOLYTIC ANEMIAS

Autoimmune hemolytic anemias are a group of diseases (Table 25–4) in which hemolysis occurs as a result of the presence of autoantibodies, with specificity against a variety of blood group antigens, including anti-I (in mycoplasmal pneumonia), anti-i (in infectious mononucleosis), and anti-P (in paroxysmal cold hemoglobinuria). Binding of the autoantibody to the erythrocyte membrane may occur maximally at body temperature (37 °C, warm antibodies) or at 4 °C (cold antibodies). The antibodies may be IgG (usually "warm"), IgM (usually "cold"), or rarely IgA. Antibody acts as a lysin, opsonin, or agglutinin (Fig 25–7; see also Chapter 4). Paroxysmal cold hemoglobinuria is an exception, being caused by an IgG antibody (Donath-Landsteiner antibody) that binds to the erythrocyte membrane in the cold, with complement fixation and intravascular hemolysis occurring as the temperature rises.

1. IDIOPATHIC WARM AUTOIMMUNE HEMOLYTIC ANEMIA

Idiopathic warm autoimmune hemolytic anemia (AIHA) occurs mainly in patients over 40 years of age and in women more frequently than in men. It is caused by an IgG autoantibody (Fig 25–7), occurring in isolation (idiopathic) or as a complication of systemic disease (Table 25–4).

Table 25–4. Classification of autoimmune hemolytic anemias.[1]

Associated with warm antibodies	70%	
Idiopathic autoimmune hemolytic anemia		40%
Complicating malignant lymphoma, chronic lymphocytic leukemia (CLL), myeloma		13%
Complicating systemic lupus erythematosus		5%
Other autoimmune diseases: polyarteritis nodosa, rheumatoid arthritis, Felty's syndrome		7%
Complicating drugs, eg, methyldopa		5%
Associated with cold antibodies	30%	
Idiopathic cold hemagglutinin disease		13%
Complicating mycoplasmal pneumonia		8%
Complicating malignant lymphoma		2%
Complicating infectious mononucleosis		2%
Paroxysmal cold hemoglobinuria		5%

[1]Warm antibodies are those that have maximum binding to the erythrocyte membrane at 37 °C (body temperature). Cold antibodies bind maximally at 4 °C.

Pathology & Clinical Features

AIHA has an insidious onset and a chronic course. Patients may present with symptoms of anemia or jaundice. Destruction of red cells or partial removal of damaged red cell membranes by splenic macrophages leads to mild splenomegaly and microcytosis.

The peripheral blood shows a normochromic normocytic anemia with microspherocytes, fragmented forms, and poikilocytes. The reticulocyte count is increased. Indirect hyperbilirubinemia, often mild, is common. Fecal and urinary urobilinogen levels are increased. The bone marrow shows normoblastic hyperplasia.

Osmotic fragility is usually increased. As in hereditary spherocytosis, autohemolysis is increased. The diagnosis of AIHA is established by demonstrating the autoantibody in serum by the antiglobulin (Coombs) test (Fig 25–8). It is necessary to exclude diseases that can cause warm antibody hemolytic anemia (Table 25–4) before making the diagnosis of **idiopathic AIHA**.

Treatment & Course

Corticosteroids represent the mainstay of treatment and are very effective. Splenectomy and immunosuppressive agents such as azathioprine may be used if steroids are not effective. Most patients have a chronic course, with relapses and remissions occurring at variable intervals.

2. IDIOPATHIC COLD HEMAGGLUTININ DISEASE

Idiopathic cold hemagglutinin disease is a rare cause of hemolysis that occurs mainly in older patients, more commonly in women. It is caused by an IgM autoantibody that binds to erythrocytes at low temperatures, fixes complement, and results in hemolysis (Fig 25–7).

Patients present with cold-induced hemolysis or **Raynaud's phenomenon,** in which ischemia causes blanching and numbness of the hands on exposure to cold, followed successively by cyanosis, redness (reactive hyperemia), throbbing pain and tingling. Ischemia is caused by sludging of red cells in capillaries, which is due either to agglutination or to hyperviscosity produced by high levels of IgM antibody.

The diagnosis is made by a positive Coombs test, with anti-IgM antibodies showing maximum reactivity at 4 °C. The Coombs test with anti-IgG at 37 °C is negative.

Cold hemagglutinin disease also occurs in association with malignant lymphoma and as a com-

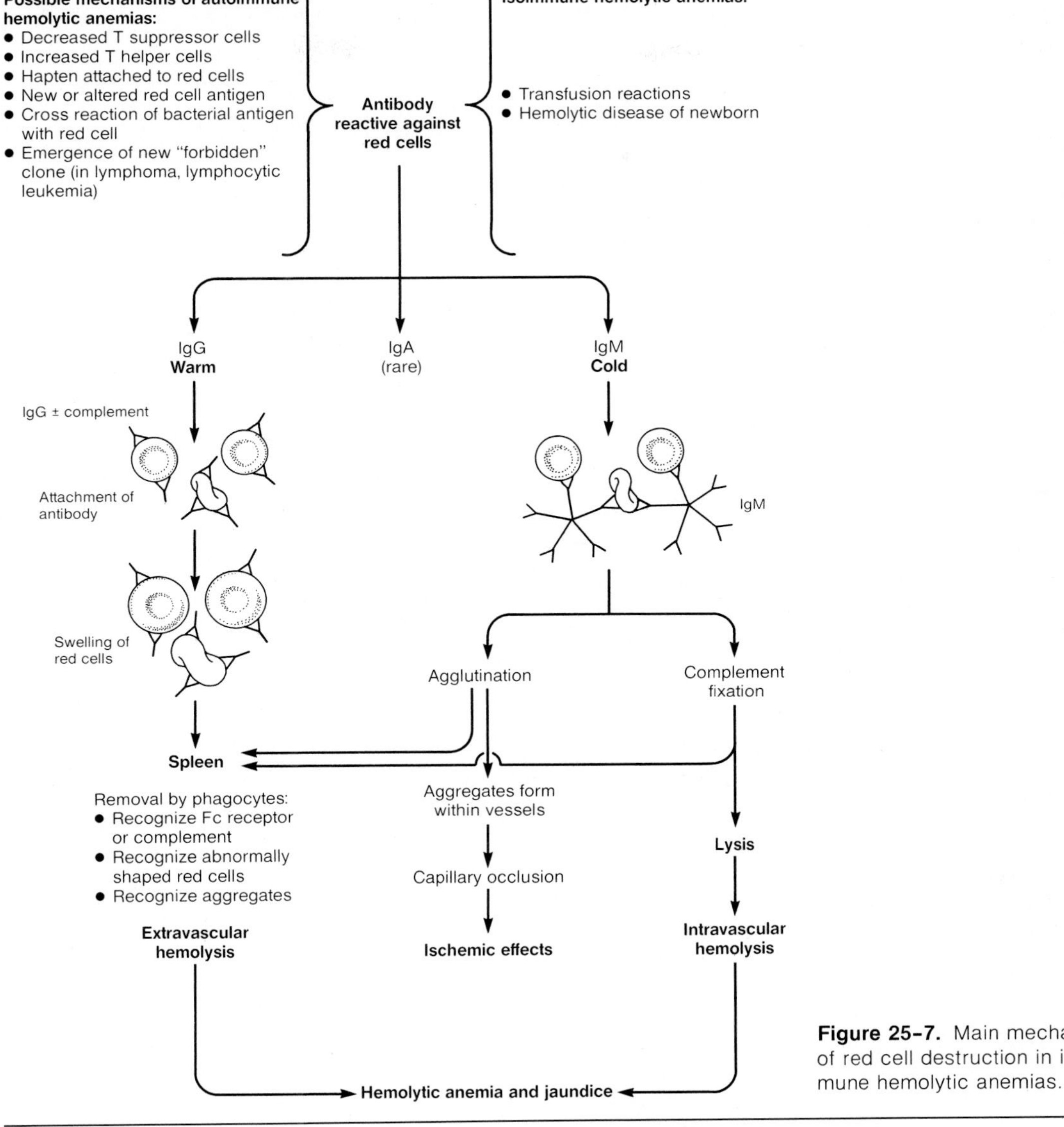

Figure 25-7. Main mechanisms of red cell destruction in immune hemolytic anemias.

plication of certain infections (eg, *Mycoplasma pneumoniae*).

3. PAROXYSMAL COLD HEMOGLOBINURIA

This rare disorder is due to the presence of a cold antibody, but in this instance the antibody is of the IgG class (directed against the P antigen on the erythrocyte membrane). Complement fixation is initiated by cold but does not proceed to lysis until the blood temperature rises to 37 °C. Patients suffer chills, fever, muscle pain, and hemoglobinuria following exposure to cold.

An acute variant of the disease follows certain viral infections. A more chronic form occurs in syphilis.

The Donath–Landsteiner test, demonstrating hemolysis of a blood sample following cooling to 4 °C and warming to 37 °C, is a useful pointer to the diagnosis.

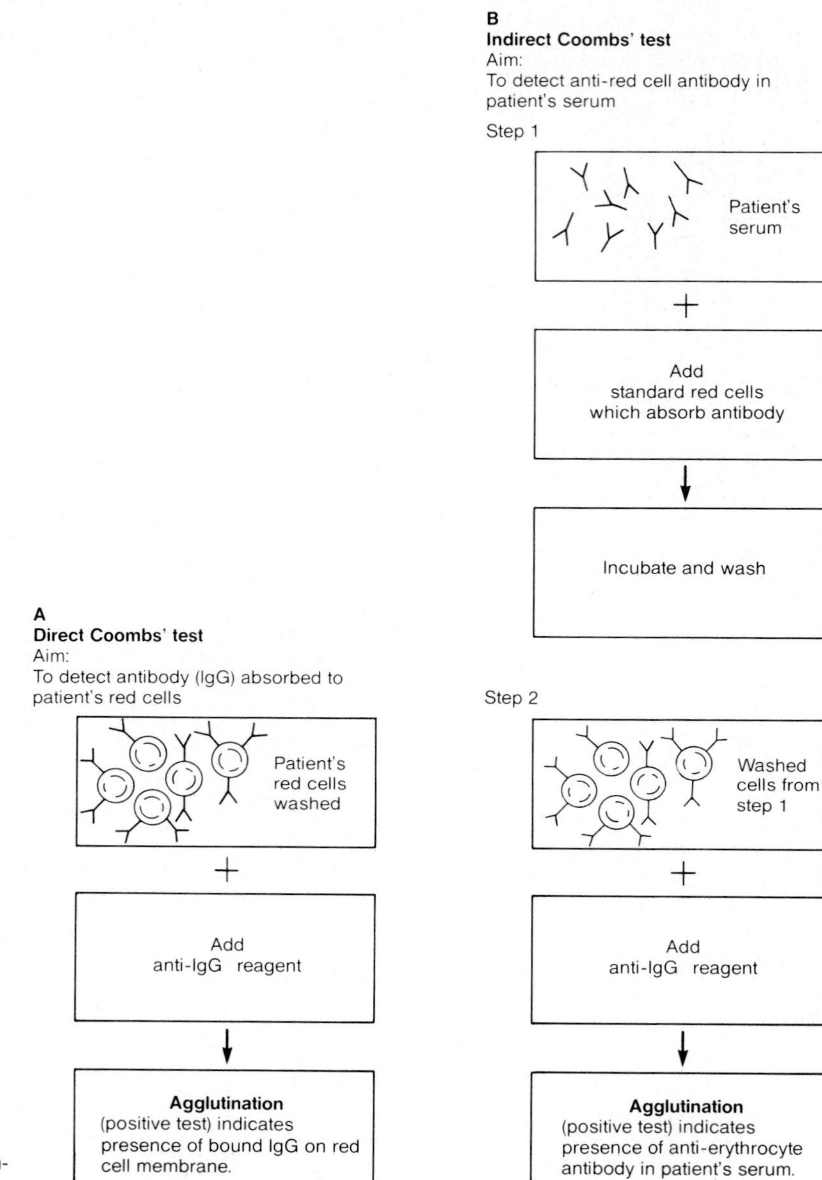

Figure 25-8. The antiglobulin (Coombs) test. Anti-IgG and standardized red cells are commercially available reagents.

ISOIMMUNE HEMOLYTIC ANEMIA

Isoimmune hemolytic anemias are those in which the red cells of one individual are lysed as a result of the action of antibodies of another individual—either in blood transfusion, where incompatible donor red cells are lysed by antibody in recipient plasma; or in hemolytic disease of the newborn, where fetal red blood cells are lysed by maternal antibodies that have traversed the placenta.

1. HEMOLYTIC BLOOD TRANSFUSION REACTIONS

Hemolytic transfusion reactions follow transfusion of incompatible blood. The more severe forms produce intravascular hemolysis and occur within minutes to hours. The transfused (donor) red cells are destroyed by antibody present in the recipient's plasma (Table 25–5). ABO incompatibility is the commonest cause of serious hemolytic reactions. Note that the presence of antibodies in the donor blood usually does not damage recipient red cells because of the dilution effect of donor

Table 25–5. Hemolytic blood transfusion reactions due to ABO system.[1]

Recipient's Blood Group	Serum Antibodies	Donor's Blood Group	Hemolytic Reaction
A	Anti-B	A or O B or AB	No Yes (destruction of donor red cells)
B	Anti-A	B or O A or AB	No Yes (destruction of donor red cells)
AB	None	A, B, or O	No
O	Anti-A and -B	O A, B, or AB	No Yes (destruction of donor red cells)

[1]The ABO system is characterized by the presence in the serum of "natural" antibody when the corresponding antigen is absent from the erythrocyte. Individuals of blood group AB have no anti-A or anti-B antibody and can receive blood of any group (universal recipients). Individuals of group O have no antigens on the red cells, and their blood can be transfused into a recipient of any group (universal donors). The only limiting factor here is the possibility that the anti-A and anti-B antibodies in the O donor's serum will react with recipient red cells (A, B, or AB); this usually presents a problem only in large transfusions and may be minimized by use of packed red cells. "Natural" antibodies are in fact induced by cross-reactive antigens present in the intestinal flora or in plant foods in individuals who lack the corresponding red cell antigen and are therefore not "tolerant."

plasma in the recipient blood pool; this risk may be further reduced by administration of packed red cells from which almost all of the donor plasma (and hence donor antibody) has been removed.

Prevention of Incompatible Transfusions

ABO hemolytic transfusion reactions are theoretically avoided by **ABO grouping** (Table 25–6). In practice, those reactions that do occur are almost all due to human (clerical) error. More rarely, serious transfusion reactions result from incompatibility in another blood group system (Table 25–7). The possibility that these rarer reactions may occur is usually revealed by the crossmatch (which reacts the donor's red cells with the recipient's serum in vitro prior to transfusion) (Table 25–6).

Hemolytic transfusion reactions are typically acute. If severe (as in most cases of ABO incompatibility), they cause severe intravascular hemolysis with hemoglobinemia (Fig 25–7). Such patients may rapidly proceed to shock and are at considerable risk of death. Less severe reactions due to non-complement-fixing antibodies produce predominantly extravascular hemolysis and may be manifested several days after the transfusion (delayed hemolytic reactions).

Table 25–6. Blood grouping and crossmatching.

1. ABO grouping of patients by agglutination reaction uses standardized anti-A and anti-B sera.

Forward Grouping			Reverse Grouping				Interpretation (Patient's Blood Group)
	Known Antisera			Cells of Known Group			
	Anti-A	Anti-B		A	B	O	
Patient's erythrocytes	+	–	Patient's serum	–	+	–	A
	–	+		+	–	–	B
	–	–		+	+	–	O
	+	+		–	–	–	AB

Note: Subgroups of A (A_1, A_2) exist and may give weaker reactions.

2. The rhesus (Rh) antigens form a complex group of which only the strongest antigen (RhD) is routinely tested. Rh(D) typing is performed using special enhanced agglutination methods or the Coombs test, because anti-Rh antibodies will not directly agglutinate red cells under the usual conditions.
3. Screening the recipient for unexpected antibodies (of other blood groups) is usually performed using standard group cells and direct agglutination or the Coombs test.
4. Crossmatching of donor cells versus patient's serum serves as a final check for possible unusual antibodies.
5. Give blood only as needed; 1 unit of whole blood contains approximately 450 mL of blood, with 60–70 g of hemoglobin; shelf life (refrigerated) is 3–5 weeks, depending on the storage method, which varies in different countries.

Table 25-7. Major blood group antigens producing transfusion reactions and hemolytic disease of the newborn.

System	Antibodies[1]	Frequency	Cause of Transfusion Reactions	Possible Cause of Hemolytic Disease of the Newborn
ABO	Anti-A[2] Anti-B[2]	"Natural" always present in appropriate group	+	+[2]
Rhesus (Rh)	Anti-D Anti-E Anti-C	Common Rare Rare	+ + +	+ + +
MNS_s	Anti-M Anti-S Anti-s	Rare Rare Rare	– + +	– + +
Kell	Anti-Kell	Rare	+	+
Duffy	Anti-Fy[a]	Rare	+	+

[1]Antibodies of the Lewis, P, and other blood group systems rarely cause hemolysis, mostly because these antibodies are active only at 20 °C.
[2]The "natural" anti-A or anti-B is IgM; however, immune anti-A or anti-B also occurs on exposure to A or B antigen producing IgG antibody. This may occur in fetal maternal bleeds across the placenta; hemolytic diease of the newborn may then result, since IgG crosses the placenta.

2. HEMOLYTIC DISEASE OF THE NEWBORN

Clinically significant hemolytic disease of the newborn is usually caused by Rh incompatibility. More rarely, ABO or other group incompatibility is responsible (Table 25–7).

The Rh system is complex, consisting of 3 pairs of alleles (D,d, C,c, E,e), which produce a variety of phenotypes. D is the strongest antigen and the one routinely tested; thus, usage of the terms "Rh-positive" and "Rh-negative" is intended to denote the presence or absence of D antigen. Note that the allele d is hypothetical and that the corresponding antigen and antibody (d and anti-d) have not been identified, while additional variants of the other 5 basic antigens have been recognized, adding to the complexity of this system.

Anti-Rh Antibodies

Contrary to the situation in the ABO system, an Rh-negative individual does not have natural anti-Rh antibodies. However, an Rh-negative individual may develop "immune" anti-Rh antibodies (IgG) if Rh-positive erythrocytes enter the circulation, either (1) when Rh-positive blood is transfused into an Rh-negative individual; or (2) during pregnancy, when fetal Rh-positive erythrocytes may enter the maternal circulation from an Rh-positive fetus. Fetomaternal passage of cells occurs across the placenta late in pregnancy, particularly during delivery. Note that the first Rh-positive pregnancy usually serves only to sensitize the Rh-negative mother; the fetus is unlikely to be affected. Subsequent Rh-positive fetuses are, however, at risk.

Effect on Fetus

If a sensitized Rh-negative woman becomes pregnant, the anti-Rh IgG crosses the placenta into the fetus, producing hemolysis of the fetal erythrocytes in utero if the fetus is Rh-positive. This may cause (1) intrauterine death of the fetus or (2) hemolytic disease of the newborn, characterized by anemia, severe jaundice, edema, and the presence of numerous normoblasts in the peripheral blood ("erythroblastosis fetalis"). Kernicterus may occur (Chapter 1).

Prevention

Hemolytic disease of the newborn is prevented by avoiding sensitization of Rh-negative women. This can be achieved (1) by accurate Rh typing when blood transfusions are given and (2) by administration of high doses of Rh antibody (Rhogam) to an Rh-negative woman during childbirth or abortion. The passively administered antibody destroys any fetal Rh-positive cells that enter the mother's blood, thereby preventing sensitization.

Hemolytic disease of the newborn occurs less often with ABO incompatibility, because anti-A and anti-B natural antibodies in the mother's plasma are usually IgM and do not cross the placenta. However, ABO incompatibility causes hemolytic disease of the newborn in those rare mothers who have immune IgG antibodies against A and B antigens in the plasma.

DRUG- & CHEMICAL-INDUCED HEMOLYSIS

A large number of drugs are known to cause immune hemolysis with a positive antiglobulin (Coombs) test. Hemolysis in these cases comes about by several different immune mechanisms, described below. Nonimmune types of drug-induced hemolysis exist also (see below).

IMMUNE HEMOLYSIS

Induction of autoantibody occurs with the antihypertensive agent methyldopa, which leads to a clinical syndrome resembling idiopathic autoimmune hemolytic anemia. The exact mechanism by which autoantibody is produced is not known; it has been postulated that a reduction in suppressor T cells may be involved.

A **hapten effect** occurs in which the drug combines with an erythrocyte membrane protein to form an antigenic complex that stimulates production of antibody. This occurs with penicillin and cephalosporins.

Hemolysis due to **immune complex** formation results when a drug induces antibody formation and then combines with the antibody to form a circulating soluble immune complex that adsorbs to the erythrocyte membrane, activating complement. Quinidine, phenacetin, and the antituberculous drug aminosalicylic acid are examples.

Direct alterations in the erythrocyte membrane (cephalosporins) lead to the adsorption of immunoglobulins and macrophage-mediated hemolysis.

NONIMMUNE DRUG-INDUCED HEMOLYSIS

Certain chemicals and toxins directly affect red cell membranes (amphotericin B, mushroom toxin, snake venoms, lipid solvents) or red cell enzymes (lead, saponin), leading to hemolysis.

Drug-induced hemolysis in G6PD deficiency is discussed earlier in this chapter.

HEMOLYSIS CAUSED BY INFECTIOUS AGENTS

Several possible mechanisms are involved, eg, (1) development of autoimmune hemolysis (infectious mononucleosis, mycoplasma pneumonia); (2) production of lytic toxins, especially in clostridial infections or in severe streptococcal septicemia (streptolysin release); and (3) direct infection of red cells, as in bartonellosis or malaria.

In **malaria,** red cell lysis occurs episodically upon release of proliferating merozoites from infected red cells (Fig 25–9). Intermittent fever coincides with hemolysis every 48 hours (tertian fever—*Plasmodium vivax, Plasmodium falciparum*) or every 72 hours (quartan fever—*Plasmodium malariae*). Red cell debris is cleared by the reticuloendothelial system and splenomegaly is common. Complications include "blackwater fever," glomerulonephritis, and cerebral malaria (Fig 25–9).

In most cases of malaria, the malarial parasite can be identified within red cells in peripheral blood smears, and the different species of plasmodia can be identified by their morphologic features.

Antimalarial drugs such as chloroquine are extremely effective in killing the malarial parasite in erythrocytes. A different drug (primaquine) is required to kill the liver stage in *P vivax* infections. Chloroquine-resistant species of *P falciparum* have appeared and complicate treatment.

MICROANGIOPATHIC HEMOLYTIC ANEMIA

Microangiopathic hemolytic anemia is caused by fragmentation of erythrocytes as they traverse an abnormal microcirculation.

Etiology

A. Disseminated Intravascular Coagulation (DIC): The fibrin strands in the microcirculation cause fragmentation of erythrocytes, slicing through the red cell membrane, which reseals over the defect (leaving a smaller red cell [microspherocyte] or deformed red cell [schistocyte]). Any of the many diseases that cause DIC (Chapter 9) may be associated with hemolytic anemia.

DIC and fragmentation hemolysis are especially important in **(1) hemolytic uremic syndrome,** a disorder of unknown cause affecting many young children characterized by renal failure and microangiopathic hemolytic anemia; and **(2) thrombotic thrombocytopenic purpura,** a serious disease of unknown cause in young adults characterized by fever, microangiopathic hemolytic anemia, marked central nervous system changes, and renal failure.

B. Abnormal Blood Vessels: Disorders associated with blood vessel abnormalities include (1) vasculitides of all types, (2) malignant hypertension, (3) vascular anomalies such as giant capillary hemangioma (Kassabach-Merritt syndrome) and arteriovenous malformations, and (4) malignant neoplasms when abnormal new vessels form in and around the neoplasm.

C. Prosthetic Cardiac Valves or Aortic Prostheses: Red cells are traumatized during passage through the prosthesis.

Pathology & Diagnosis

Microangiopathic hemolytic anemia can be diagnosed by the finding of abnormal fragmented erythrocytes (called schistocytes) in the peripheral blood smear (Fig 25–10). These cells have variable shapes with pointed ends ("helmet cells"). Microspherocytes are also present, caused by loss of

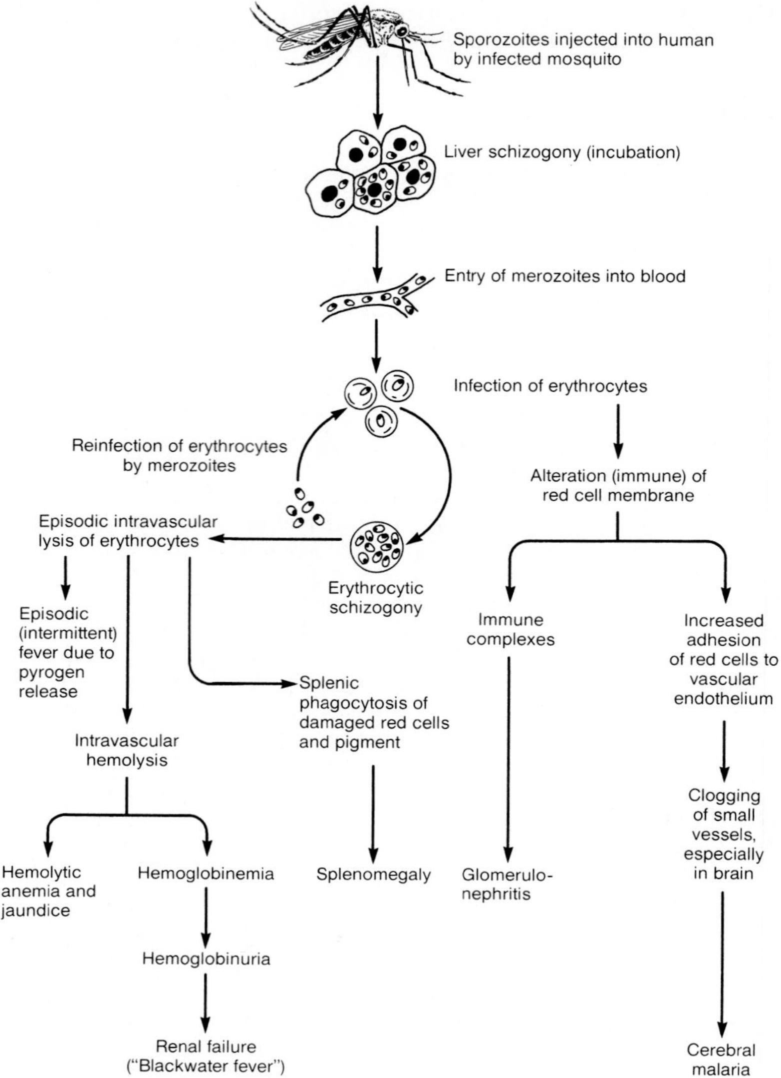

Figure 25-9. Clinicopathologic effects of malaria. All the changes shown may occur in a severe infecton with *Plasmodium falciparum.* Other *Plasmodium* species usually cause an illness characterized only by episodic hemolysis.

red cell membrane during fragmentation. Reticulocytosis and evidence of intravascular hemolysis, including hemoglobinemia, are commonly present.

POLYCYTHEMIA

Polycythemia is defined as an increased number of red cells in the peripheral blood. It is uncommon and may result from (1) An increase in the total red cell mass (absolute polycythemia) or (2) decreased plasma volume without an increase in total red cell mass (relative polycythemia), as in dehydration. Relative polycythemia is a temporary condition not discussed further.

SECONDARY ABSOLUTE POLYCYTHEMIA

Secondary polycythemia is a normal compensatory increase in the red cell volume resulting from **chronic hypoxemia,** mediated by increased production of erythropoietin. It occurs in patients with chronic lung disease or congenital cyanotic heart disease; in individuals acclimatized to living at high altitudes; in cigarette smokers, who have

Table 25-8. Anemias: Approach to diagnosis.

1. All patients: Check severity of anemia: Pallor, breathlessness, cardiac failure.
   Identify possible cause: History of blood loss; dietary, drug, family history; menstrual history; pregnancies, etc.
2. Confirm presence and severity of anemia: hemoglobin level in blood
3. Determine morphologic category of anemia - red cell morphology in peripheral blood

	Macrocytic Normochromic		Microcytic Hypochromic			Normocytic Normochromic			Dimorphic (2 red cell populations)
Reticulocytes	N/↓		N	↑		N/↓		↑	↓
Other features	Hypersegmented neutrophils	. . .	. . .	Target cells, sickle cells	Spherocytes, red cell fragments	. . .	↓ Platelets ↓ White cells	White cell left shift, nucleated red cells	Stippling; iron stain shows granules
Serum iron	N	N	↓	N/↑	N/↑	N/↓	N	N	↑
Hemoglobin electrophoresis	N	N	N	Abnormal	N	N	N	N	N
Bone marrow	↑ Erythropoiesis, megaloblasts	Variable normoblasts	↑ Erythropoiesis ↓ Iron stores	↑ ↑ Erythropoiesis ↑ Iron stores	↑ Erythropoiesis	Variable ↑ Iron stores	Degrees of aplasia	↓ Erytrhopoiesis; fibrosis, tumor cells	↑ Erythropoiesis ↑ Sideroblasts Abnormal myelopiesis in some
Vitamin B_{12}/folate levels	↓ B_{12} or ↓ folate or both	N	N	N	N	N	N	N	N
Probable diagnosis	Megaloblastic anemia	Simple macrocytic anemia	Iron deficiency anemia	Hemolytic anemia: hemoglobinopathy	Hemolytic anemia: Red cell defect Immune Other	Anemia of chronic disease	Aplastic anemia	Leukoerythroblastic anemia	Sideroblastic anemia

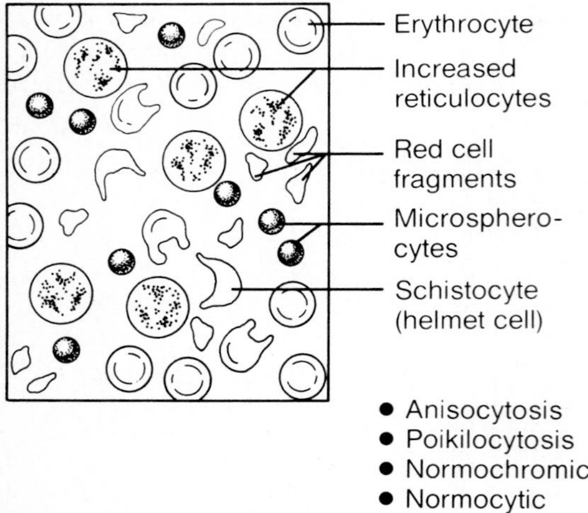

Figure 25-10. Peripheral blood erythrocyte abnormalities in microangiopathic hemolytic anemia.

increased carbon monoxide levels in the blood that bind hemoglobin and lead to hypoxia; and in patients with abnormal hemoglobins that have an increased affinity for oxygen.

Inappropriate Erythropoietin Secretion

Abnormal and uncontrolled erythropoietin secretion occurs in rare patients with neoplastic diseases, most commonly renal adenocarcinoma, cerebellar hemangioblastoma, and hepatocellular carcinoma; and nonneoplastic renal conditions such as renal cysts or hydronephrosis.

POLYCYTHEMIA RUBRA VERA ("Primary" Polycythemia)

Polycythemia rubra vera is a neoplastic myeloproliferative disorder (Chapter 26) that affects chiefly the erythroid series. Granulocytes and platelet numbers are also commonly increased. The bone marrow is hypercellular, with proliferation of all 3 cell lines. Megakaryocyte clustering is characteristic.

Patients who develop polycythemia rubra vera are usually over 40 years of age. They commonly present with ruddy cyanosis of the face and plethora due to the polycythemia. The increased viscosity of the blood caused by the increased hematocrit often results in vascular thrombosis. Many patients present with venous thrombosis, often affecting the portal circulation.

The diagnosis is made by demonstrating an increased total red cell mass in the absence of hypoxemia. Neutrophils have markedly elevated levels of the enzyme alkaline phosphatase, a feature that permits differentiation from granulocytic leukemia, in which neutrophil alkaline phosphatase is greatly reduced.

Treatment is aimed at reducing red cell mass by repeated venesection. Survival for 10–15 years is usual. As with other myeloproliferative diseases, there is an increased incidence of progressive myelofibrosis and acute leukemia in patients with polycythemia rubra vera.

Table 25-8 summarizes the approach to the diagnosis of the anemias.

Blood: III. The White Blood Cells 26

The peripheral blood contains white blood cells of several types in numbers and proportions that vary between quite narrow limits in health but more widely in disease.

NORMAL WHITE BLOOD COUNT & DIFFERENTIAL

As with many biologic parameters, there is no strict definition of "normal"; however, normal ranges are established by laboratories for their population group. Table 26–1 shows a typical set of "normal" values for the United States.

Variations in these parameters, along with changes in leukocyte morphology as seen in blood smears, are important indicators of disease (Table 26–2).

ABNORMALITIES IN LYMPHOCYTE COUNT

Lymphocyte and monocyte origin and function have been considered with the immune system (Chapter 4).

Lymphocytosis—increased lymphocyte count in peripheral blood—is best considered in relationship to causes of lymphoproliferation (Chapter 28). It may occur as (1) an acute immune response, with many "activated" or transformed lymphocytes circulating in the blood; (2) a chronic immune response, in which most of the circulating lymphocytes resemble resting small lymphocytes; or (3) neoplastic proliferation (Table 26–3).

Likewise with **lymphopenia**—decreased peripheral blood lymphocyte count—immunologic analysis by techniques such as flow cytometry is often vital to determine the cause (discussed fully in Chapter 7).

ABNORMALITIES IN MONOCYTE COUNT

Monocytosis is less commonly encountered (Table 26–4) than lymphocytosis and is of less importance diagnostically (bearing in mind that the "mononuclear" cells of "infectious mononucleosis" are activated lymphocytes and not monocytes). If the distinction of monocytes from par-

Table 26-1. White blood count (WBC), differential: "Normal values."

Total White Blood Cell Count	Adult	4000–11,000/μL
	Child (3–11 years)	6000–15,000/μL
	Infant	8000–20,000/μL
Differential White Cell Count (Adult)[1]	**Total Number**[2]	**Percentage**[2]
Neutrophils	2500–7500/μL	40–75%
Lymphoctyes	1500–3500/μL	20–50%
Monocytes	200–800/μL	2–10%
Eosinophils	60–600/μL	1–5%
Basophils	0–100/μL	< 1%

[1]In infancy and childhood, the proportion of lymphocytes is higher; in the first hours after birth, a lymphoycte count of 8000/μL is considered normal.

[2]In general, changes in absolute numbers are of more significance than changes in percentages.

Table 26-2. Broad categories of variation in leukocyte number and morphology[1]

	Increased Count	Decreased Count	Important Morphologic Changes
Neutrophils	Neutrophil leukocytosis (Table 26-5)	Neutropenia (Table 26-8)	Changes in maturity, staining, or granules (Fig 26-3; Table 26-5)
Eosinophils	Eosinophilia	—	—
Basophils	Basophilia (rare)	—	—
Lymphocytes	Lymphocytosis (Table 26-3)	Lymphopenia (Table 26-3)	Changes in maturity or changes of lymphocyte transformation (Table 26-3)
Monocytes	Monocytosis (Table 26-4)	—	Changes in maturity

[1]Individual categories are discussed in the text and expanded in further tables as indicated.

tially transformed lymphocytes is in doubt, the following may be of help: (1) monoclonal antibody markers (Leu-M1, OKM1 for monocytes; B and T cell monoclonal antibodies or the presence of surface or cytoplasmic immunoglobulin for lymphocytes; see Chapter 4); or (2) enzyme reactions such as naphthylacetate (nonspecific) esterase, which is positive in monocytes.

ABNORMALITIES IN GRANULOCYTE COUNT

NEUTROPHILS

Neutrophils develop from the precursor stem cell in the bone marrow (Fig 26-1). Early forms, which include the myeloblast, promyelocyte, and myelocyte, are actively dividing cells normally re-

Table 26-3. Variation in lymphocyte parameters in peripheral blood.

	Major Conditions	Immunology
Lymphocytosis		
With features of lymphocyte transformation, ie, medium and large lymphocytes and plasmacytoid cells[1]	Active immune responses, especially in children. Immunizations; bacterial infections (pertussis); viral infections (infectious mononucleosis, mumps, measles, viral hepatitis, rubella, influenza); toxoplasmosis.	Mixed T and B cell (polyclonal)
	Primary neoplasms—some variants of chronic lymphocytic leukemia (CLL), lymphoma	T or B cell (monoclonal)[2]
Majority resemble resting small lymphocytes	Chronic infections (tuberculosis, syphilis, brucellosis); autoimmune diseases (myasthenia gravis); metabolic diseases (thyrotoxicosis, Addison's disease).	Mixed T and B cell (polyclonal)
	Primary neoplasms—CLL, some small cell lymphomas	T or B cell (monoclonal)[2]
Lymphocytes resemble fetal lymphoblasts	**Primary neoplasms**—acute lymphoblastic leukemia, lymphoblastic lymphoma	Nonmarking or T cell or B cell (monoclonal)[2]
Admixture of abnormal lymphoid cells (rare)	**Primary neoplasms**—involvement of blood by lymphoma or myeloma	Abnormal cells are T or B cells (monoclonal)[2] often admixed with residual normal cells
Lymphopenia		
Deficiency of T cells or B cells (or subsets thereof) or of both T and B cells (see Chapter 7)	Toxic drugs and chemicals; steroid therapy, Cushing's disease; early phase of marrow involvement by leukemia; immunodeficiency states	See Chapter 7 for approach to diagnosis

[1]These medium-sized and large lymphocytes represent circulating partly transformed lymphocytes involved in disseminating the immune response (see Chapter 4). Previously they were often termed "atypical" lymphocytes, and on morphology alone they may be difficult to distinguish from neoplastic lymphocytes.
[2]Clonality as defined in Chapter 29.

Table 26-4. Causes of monocytosis.

Infections Bacteria: Tuberculosis, brucellosis, typhoid fever, subacute infective endocarditis Rickettsiae: Rocky Mountain spotted fever, typhus fever Protozoa: Malaria, trypanosomiasis, leishmaniasis
Chronic diseases Ulcerative colitis, Crohn's disease, rheumatoid arthritis, systemic lupus erythematosus
Sarcoidosis
Lipid storage disease
Primary histiocytic (monocytic) neoplasms Monocytic leukemia, myeloproliferative diseases, malignant histiocytosis
Other neoplasms Hodgkin's disease, carcinomatosis

stricted to the marrow. Maturing cells, which include the metamyelocyte, the band form, and the segmented neutrophil, are nondividing cells. Normally, the segmented neutrophil and band form are released into the peripheral blood. The maturing pool in the marrow also serves as a storage pool, amounting to 20 times the number of neutrophils present in the peripheral blood. This pool provides a mechanism for very rapid (within hours) increase in the peripheral blood neutrophil count.

Neutrophils in the peripheral blood commonly adhere to the vascular endothelium (margination) and do not figure in the neutrophil count. Neutrophils have a very short half-life in the blood, passing out into the tissues within a few hours after being released from the bone marrow.

During development, primary granules (containing myeloperoxidase, hydroxylases, etc) make their appearance at the promyelocyte stage (Fig 26–1). Specific secondary granules (containing lysozyme, lactoferrin, leukocyte alkaline phosphatase, etc) appear at the myelocyte stage, when the neutrophil, eosinophil, and basophil series diverge. The presence of these granules (and the enzymes therein) is of value in recognizing different

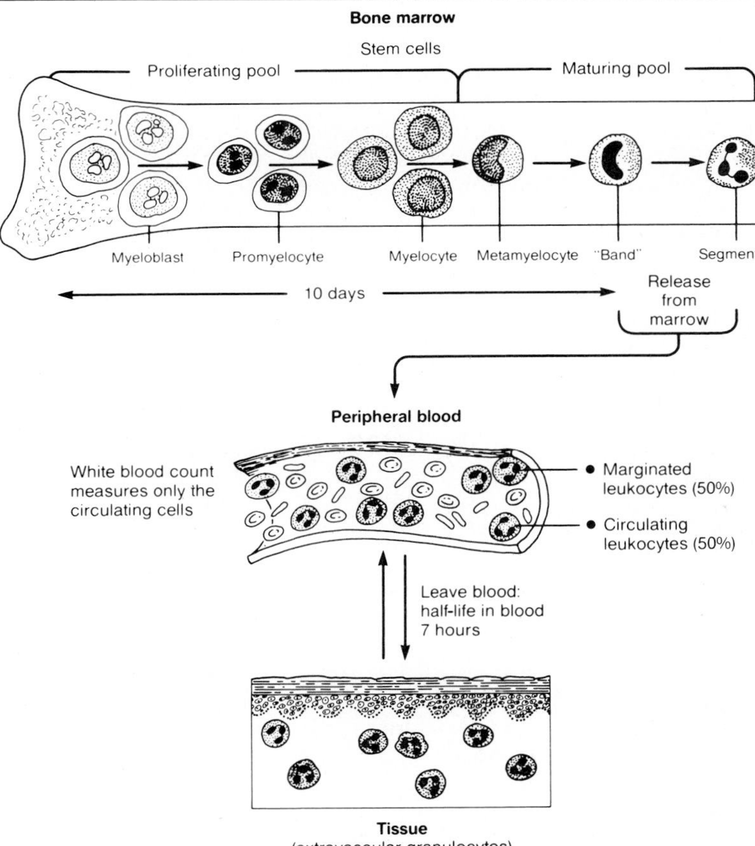

Figure 26–1. Granulocyte production and storage in the bone marrow. The proliferating pool of cells (myeloblast, promyelocyte, and myelocyte) undergo mitotic divisions and produce the mature cells that are stored in the marrow until they are mobilized, usually at the band stage. The granulocytes outside the marrow may be freely circulating in the blood, marginated in the small vessels, or in extravascular tissues. Only the free circulating granulocytes are measured by the white blood cell count.

types of normal and leukemic cells and evaluating the stage of maturation.

Abnormalities in peripheral blood neutrophil parameters (Table 26–5) may relate to alterations in the neutrophil count (neutrophil leukocytosis and neutropenia) or morphology.

Neutrophil Leukocytosis (Neutrophilia; Granulocytosis)

Neutrophil leukocytosis is present when the absolute neutrophil count exceeds 7500/μL. The term "leukemoid reaction" is used for a very severe reactive neutrophil leukocytosis, sometimes in excess of 50,000/μL, with a leftward shift owing to early release of storage pool granulocytes. The peripheral blood picture of leukemoid reaction resembles that of chronic myelocytic leukemia but may be distinguished from it by the neutrophil alkaline phosphatase level (Table 26–6), which is elevated in the leukemoid reaction and decreased in chronic myelocytic leukemia.

Neutrophil leukocytosis does not usually produce clinical symptoms and is detected by the white blood cell count. When counts are extremely high (over 100,000/μL—usually only in chronic myelocytic leukemia), the blood viscosity may increase to such an extent as to produce thrombosis and occlusion of vessels.

Neutrophil leukocytosis may result from a variety of mechanisms (Table 26–7). Redistribution of the bone marrow storage pool or tissue neutrophils into the peripheral blood results in rapid increases in the neutrophil count, often within hours after a stimulus. Increased proliferative activity of early neutrophil precursors leads to a slower (several days) increase in peripheral neutrophil count.

Examination of the peripheral blood smear provides valuable clues to etiology (Table 26–5). Reactive neutrophilias are characterized by the presence of predominantly mature forms. In neoplastic proliferations of granulocytic cells, less mature forms are present in the peripheral blood.

EOSINOPHILIA

Eosinophilia is an absolute eosinophil count in the peripheral blood that exceeds 600/μL.

Etiology

Eosinophilia is a common manifestation of parasitic infections, especially with metazoan parasites; type I hypersensitivity, eg, allergic rhinitis (hay fever), bronchial asthma, urticaria, and eczema; immunologic diseases, eg, pemphigus vulgaris, polyarteritis nodosa, and eosinophilic gastroenteritis; and neoplasms, most commonly Hodgkin's disease and mycosis fungoides. Hypereosinophilic syndromes include eosinophilic leukemia and Löffler's syndrome (Chapter 34).

NEUTROPENIA (Granulocytopenia)

Neutropenia is a decrease in the absolute neutrophil count below 1500/μL. There are numerous causes (Table 26–8). The most severe form of neutropenia is agranulocytosis, which is an absence of neutrophils in the peripheral blood.

Neutropenia is clinically significant when the neutrophil count drops below 1000/μL. Infections, usually with pyogenic bacteria, occur frequently in such patients. When the level falls below 500/μL, such infections are inevitable. Oral infections with ulceration of the throat, skin infections, opportunistic infections, and fever are the commonest manifestations. This is a common terminal event in acute leukemia and aplastic anemia. Management in cases not associated with malignant neoplasms is aimed at preventing infection (antibiotics, leukocyte infusions, patient isolation) until the marrow recovers. High doses of steroids produce improvement in some cases. Granulocyte-rich transfusions may provide temporary improvement.

NEUTROPHIL DYSFUNCTION SYNDROMES

This is a rare group of diseases in which patients manifest clinical complications similar to those seen in severe neutropenia but without a decrease in the neutrophil count in the peripheral blood. A variety of different diseases in which different functions of the neutrophil are affected have been described (Table 26–9). The net result is increased susceptibility to infection, and the differential diagnosis is from other immunodeficiency diseases (Chapter 7). Some of these conditions produce characteristic morphologic changes in the peripheral blood (Table 26–10).

NEOPLASMS OF HEMATOPOIETIC CELLS

LEUKEMIAS

The leukemias are malignant neoplastic proliferations of hematopoietic cells in the bone marrow. In most cases, the neoplastic cells are also present in increased numbers in the peripheral blood.

Table 26-5. Variations in neutrophil parameters.

	Peripheral Blood Morphology	Conditions	Comments
Normal numbers of neutrophils With shift to the left	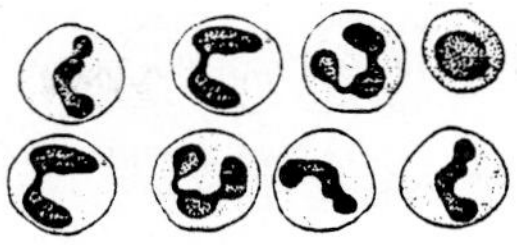	Leukoerythroblastic anemia	Physical replacement of normal marrow by fibrosis, neoplasms
		Primary neoplasms: early "preleukemic" myeloid leukemia	Leukemic marrow
With shift to the right	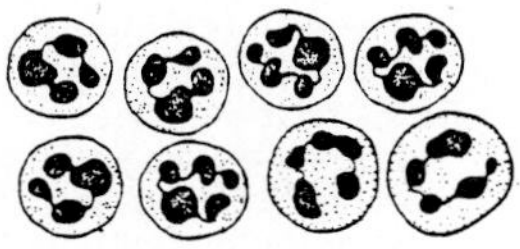	Megaloblastic anemias; folate antagonists.	Vitamin B_{12} or folate levels decreased in blood; may also produce neutropenia
With abnormal giant granulocytes or inclusions	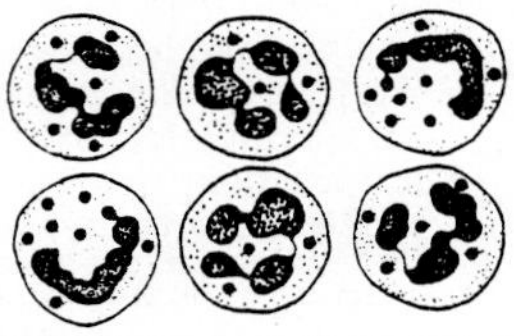	Mucopolysaccharidosis (Alder-Reilly; rare)	See Chapter 15
		Chédiak-Higashi syndrome (rare)	See Chapter 7
		Toxic granules in severe infection (more common)	
Neutrophil leukocytosis Mainly mature segmented forms; mild left shift	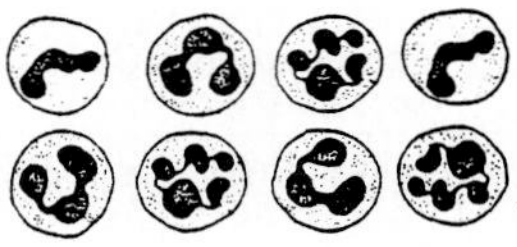	Metabolic diseases (uremia, gout); drugs (phenacetin, digitalis); postnecrosis (myocardial infarction, burns); postsurgery; acute infections (pyogenic cocci, *Escherichia coli, Proteus, Pseudomonas,* less often typhus, cholera, diphtheria)	Toxic granulation Giant toxic granules (Döhle bodies)
With high proportion of less mature cells (bands and metamyelocytes); marked left shift	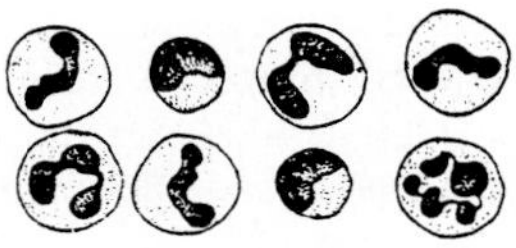	Leukemoid reaction (very severe acute infections, especially in child)	High leukocyte alkaline phosphatase level.
		Primary neoplasms: chronic myelocytic leukemia; less often, polycythemia rubra vera or myelosclerosis	Low leukocyte alkaline phosphatase level
With high proportion of "blasts"; extreme left shift	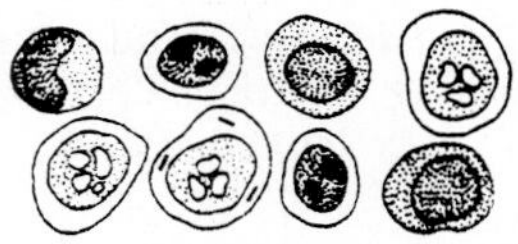	Primary neoplasms; acute myelocytic leukemia and variants	Auer rods in blast cells
Neutropenia May occur alone or may accompany lymphopenia, thrombocytopenia, anemia	Variable	Infections: Many viral infections (hepatitis, measles); some rickettsial infections; rare bacterial infections (typhoid fever, brucellosis); malaria; any very severe infection (septicemia, miliary tuberculosis)	
		Acute leukemia in early phase of marrow involvement	
		Marrow aplasia	
		Vitamin B_{12}, folate deficiency	
		Autoimmune diseases: Felty's syndrome	Antileukocyte antibodies
		Familial cyclic neutropenia	Cyclic stem cell failure (?)

Table 26-6. Leukocyte (neutrophil) alkaline phosphatase.[1]

Low	High
Chronic myelocytic leukemia[2]	Leukemoid reactions[2]
Paroxysmal nocturnal hemoglobinuria (see Chapter 25)	Infections
Aplastic anemia	Pregnancy
Metabolic diseases: diabetes, cirrhosis, gout	Hodgkin's disease, myelofibrosis, polycythemia rubra vera, Down's syndrome

[1]Scored by counting degree of positivity in 100 neutrophils.
[2]Of greatest value in distinguishing leukemoid reactions from chronic myelocytic leukemia (CML).

Abbreviations in This Section

ALL = **Acute lymphoblastic leukemia**
Acute lymphocytic leukemia
AML = **Acute myeloblastic leukemia**
Acute myelocytic leukemia
Acute myeloid leukemia
Acute granulocytic leukemia (AGL)
CLL = **Chronic lymphocytic leukemia**
CML = **Chronic myelocytic leukemia**
Chronic myeloid leukemia
Chronic granulocytic leukemia (CGL)

Preferred terminology in this book (bold type) reflects morphologic appearance of leukemic cells (eg, lymphocyte in CLL versus lymphoblast in ALL).

Table 26-7. Etiologic mechanisms that lead to neutrophil leukocytosis.

Increased bone marrow proliferation Pyogenic bacterial infections (chemical mediators) Other causes of acute inflammation (chemical mediators) Chronic myelocytic leukemia Other myeloproliferative diseases
Release from marrow storage pool into peripheral blood Acute response to endotoxin Corticosteroids Stress
Shift from marginal and extravascular pool to blood Acute pyogenic bacterial infections Hypoxia Exercise, stress
Decreased egress from circulating pool Corticosteroid therapy
Increased granulocyte survival Chronic myelocytic leukemia

Table 26-8. Etiologic mechanisms and causes of neutropenia.

Decreased marrow proliferation Infantile neutropenia (Kostmann): a rare autosomal recessive disease manifesting with severe neutropenia at birth. Cyclic neutropenia: usually familial, autosomal dominant, with onset in childhood. Profound neutropenia lasts 3–4 days and occurs in cycles of about 3 weeks, returning to normal between episodes. Possibly due to cyclic stem cell failure. Drugs that suppress granulopoiesis: anticancer drugs, certain antihistamines, antithyroid drugs, tranquilizers, gold salts, diuretics, penicillins, chloramphenicol, and antituberculous drugs. Radiation. Megaloblastic anemia (decreased DNA synthesis). Aplastic anemias, certain "refractory" anemias such as sideroblastic anemia. Marrow replacement by leukemia, lymphoma, fibrosis: leukoerythroblastic anemia.
Reduced peripheral granulocyte survival Viral and rickettsial infection Severe bacterial sepsis Drugs that cause immune destruction of granulocytes: phenylbutazone, cephalothin, aminopyrine Systemic lupus erythematosus and Felty's syndrome (immune destruction) Hypersplenism
Increased egress from circulation (pseudoneutropenia) Viral and rickettsial infections Histamine

Incidence

The number of new cases of leukemia in the United States is about 25,000 per year, with 15,000–20,000 deaths. Death rates have fallen in the past decade because of increasing effectiveness of treatment.

Acute leukemias account for 50–60% of all leukemias, with acute myeloblastic leukemia (AML) being slightly more common than acute lymphoblastic leukemia (ALL).

ALL occurs predominantly in young children (peak age incidence 3–4 years) (Fig 26–2). **AML** occurs at any age but is most common in young adults (peak 15–20 years).

Chronic leukemias account for 40–50% of leukemias, with chronic lymphocytic leukemia (CLL) being slightly more common than chronic myelocytic leukemia (CML).

CLL occurs mainly in patients over the age of 60 years.

CML occurs at all ages, with a peak incidence in the age group from 40 to 50 years (Fig 26–2).

Etiology

The cause of most kinds of leukemia is unknown.

A. Viruses: Viruses are known to cause animal leukemias and are highly suspect in humans. A retrovirus (human T lymphotropic virus type I; HTLV-I) has been identified as the causative agent

Table 26–9. Neutrophil dysfunction syndromes.

Disease	Inheritance	Age at Onset	Defect
Chédiak-Higashi syndrome	Autosomal recessive	Variable	Increased fusion of cytoplasmic granules in many cell types: a. Melanosomes → albinism b. Defective neutrophil degranulation → infections c. Abnormal giant granules in cytoplasm of monocytes, neutrophils, lymphocytes
Lazy leukocyte syndrome	Very rare; uncertain	Birth	Defective movement of neutrophils to chemotaxis
Chronic granulomatous disease of childhood	X-linked recessive	Childhood	Failure to produce peroxide by neutrophils, monocytes, leading to recurrent infections with catalase-producing organisms (*Staphylococcus aureus, Candida* spp, gram-negative enteric bacilli, *Aspergillus* spp)
Myeloperoxidase deficiency	Autosomal recessive	Asymptomatic	Myeloperoxidase deficiency in neutrophils, monocytes: usually no clinical effect
Corticosteroid therapy	—	—	Inhibits neutrophil movement and phagocytosis

Table 26–10. Morphologic leukocyte abnormalities and disease.

Abnormality	Appearance	Disease
Toxic granulation	Cytoplasmic granules become coarse and more darkly staining	Infections and inflammatory disease
Döhle bodies	1- to 2-μm blue granules in cytoplasm	As toxic granulation, plus myeloid leukemias (also seen in cyclophosphamide therapy)
Auer rods	1- to 4-μm red rods in "blast cells"	Acute myeloblastic leukemia
Pelger-Huët anomaly	Bilobed or nonsegmented neutrophils	Hereditary; also myeloid leukemias
May-Hegglin anomaly	Basophil inclusions that resemble Döhle bodies	May-Hegglin syndrome (giant platelets and thrombocytopenia)
Chédiak-Higashi anomaly	Large gray inclusions; resemble Döhle bodies	Chédiak-Higashi syndrome
Tart cell	Neutrophil containing a recognizable phagocytised granulocyte nucleus	Drug reactions
Lupus erythematosus cell	Neutrophil containing unrecognizable phagocytized nuclear material	Systemic lupus erythematosus

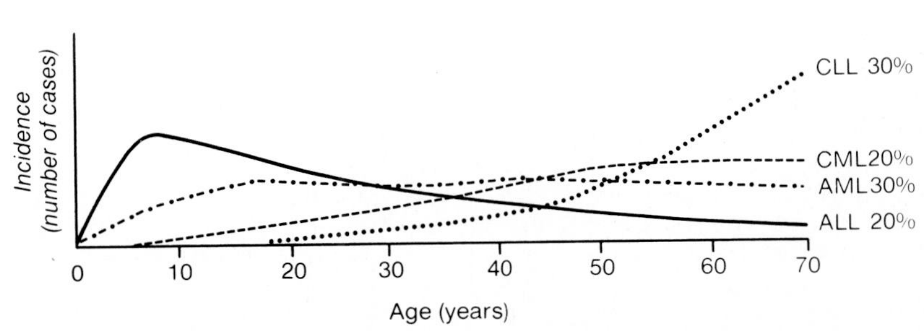

Figure 26–2. Incidence of different types of leukemias according to age. Note that ALL is predominantly a childhood disease and CLL occurs mainly in the elderly. AML and CML have a wider age distribution. The percentages given reflect the frequency of the different types of leukemias within the group. CLL = chronic lymphocytic leukemia; AML = acute myeloid (myeloblastic: granulocytic, AGL) leukemia; CML = chronic myeloid (myelocytic: granulocytic, CGL) leukemia; ALL = acute lymphoblastic (lymphocytic) leukemia.

in one type of acute T lymphocytic leukemia first described in Japan, while a related virus, HTLV-II, causes more chronic types of T cell leukemia. However, no causal agent has been identified for most cases of human leukemia.

B. Radiation: Exposure to radiation resulted in an increased incidence of leukemia in the first generation of radiologists, and leukemia occurred with increased frequency among survivors of the Hiroshima and Nagasaki bombs. Fetuses who have been exposed to radiation in utero and patients who have received radiation in the treatment of ankylosing spondylitis and Hodgkin's disease have an increased incidence of leukemia.

C. Chemical Agents: The same cytotoxic drugs used in treatment of leukemia produce an increased incidence of leukemia when used in the treatment of lymphomas and other cancers. In addition, arsenic, benzene, phenylbutazone, and chloramphenicol have been implicated in some cases.

D. Marrow Aplasia: Marrow aplasia due to any cause appears to be associated with an increased incidence of subsequent leukemia, as do the **refractory sideroblastic anemias**.

E. Immune Deficiency: Immune deficiency states are associated with an increased incidence of leukemia, suggesting that immunologic surveillance is important in preventing the emergence of neoplastic hematopoietic cells.

F. Genetic Factors: Chromosomal abnormalities are present in a high proportion of patients with leukemia if sensitive chromosomal analytic techniques are utilized (Table 26–11). The first reported was the association of the Philadelphia chromosome (a small chromosome 22 resulting from the reciprocal translocation of genetic material from chromosome 22 to chromosome 9) with chronic myelocytic leukemia. Also interesting is the increased incidence (20 times normal) of leukemia in patients with Down's syndrome (trisomy 21). Chromosome fragility syndromes (Bloom's syndrome, Fanconi's anemia) also carry a high risk of acute leukemia.

Classification

Leukemias are classified in several ways:

A. According to Onset and Clinical Course: This was the earliest approach, since the identity of the cells involved was not known. It still has clinical merit.

1. Acute leukemias have a sudden onset with a rapidly progressive course leading to death within months if untreated. They are usually characterized by primitive cells ("blasts") that are morphologically poorly differentiated.

2. Chronic leukemias have an insidious onset and a slow clinical course, patients often surviving several years even if untreated. Chronic leukemias are usually characterized by more mature type cells.

Table 26–11. Chromosomal abnormalities associated with leukemias.

Type of Leukemia	Chromsomal Abnormality
Chronic myelocytic leukemia (CML)	Philadelphia chromosome t(9;22)[1]
CML in blast crisis	t(9;22)(X2) +8,[2] isochromosome of 17 or 4
Acute myeloblastic leukemia (AML)	t(8;21), t(15;17), t(9;22) +8, 7−, 5−, 7q−, 5q−
Erythroleukemia	7q−, 5q−
Acute monocytic leukemia	t(9;11)
Acute myelomonocytic leukemia	11q−
Polycythemia rubra vera	20q−
Acute lymphoblastic leukemia (ALL)	6q−, t(4;11), t(9;22), t(8;14)
Chronic lymphocytic leukemia (CLL)	+12

[1]Note that Phi chromosome t(9;22), while typical of CML, also is seen in CML blast crisis (multiple copies), AML, and some cases of ALL (25% of adult cases).
[2]Deletions are signified by a − suffix (eg, 7q−), trisomy by a + prefix (eg, +12).

B. According to the Peripheral Blood Picture: The disadvantage of this approach is that a minority of leukemias do not involve the peripheral blood but only the bone marrow.

1. Leukemic, characterized by elevation of the white blood cell count and numerous leukemic cells. This is the common form.

2. Subleukemic, in which the total white count is normal or low but recognizable leukemic cells are present in the peripheral blood.

3. Aleukemic, where the total white count is normal or low and no recognizable leukemic cells are present in the peripheral blood.

C. According to Cell Type: Classification by cell type becomes more complex as new criteria evolve for cell recognition (Table 26–12, Fig 26–3).

1. Lymphocytic leukemias are neoplasms of lymphocytes. Their close relationship to certain of the lymphomas is considered in Chapter 29.

a. ALL is characterized by the presence in the bone marrow and peripheral blood of uniform large cells that resemble the proliferating lymphoblast of fetal development (Chapter 4). Acute lymphoblastic leukemia is further classified by its morphologic features (French-American-British—FAB—system; Table 26–13) or by its immunologic or genetic features.

b. CLL is characterized by the proliferation of small "mature" lymphocytes with a round nucleus that has dense chromatin and no nucleoli occupying almost the entire cell. In 95% of cases, the lymphocytes are B cells; in the rest, they are T cells.

Table 26-12. Traditional classification of leukemias by cell type.

Cell	Acute	Chronic
Lymphocyte	Acute lymphoblastic (ALL)	Chronic lymphocytic (CLL)
		Sézary syndrome
Granulocyte Neutrophil	Acute myeloblastic (AML)	Chronic myelocytic (CML)
Eosinophil		Eosinophilic[1] (rare)
Basophil		Basophilic[1] (very rare)
Monocyte	Acute monocytic	Chronic monocytic (rare)
Erythroid	Acute erythroblastic (erythroleukemia)	Chronic erythroleukemia[1]
		Polycythemia rubra vera
Megakaryocyte	Megakaryocytic	Thrombocythemia[1]
Plasma cell	—	Plasma cell leukemia[2] (rare)
Unknown cell[3]	—	Hairy cell leukemia (rare)
Mixed cell types	Acute myelomonocytic (AMML)	Chronic myelomonocytic (rare)

[1]Often regarded as variants of CML (chronic myelocytic leukemia) with predominant differentiation to the various cell types.
[2]Leukemic dissemination of multiple myeloma.
[3]The progenitor cell of hairy cell leukemia is now known to be a B lymphocyte, but the relationship of this cell to other B lymphocytes is still unclear.

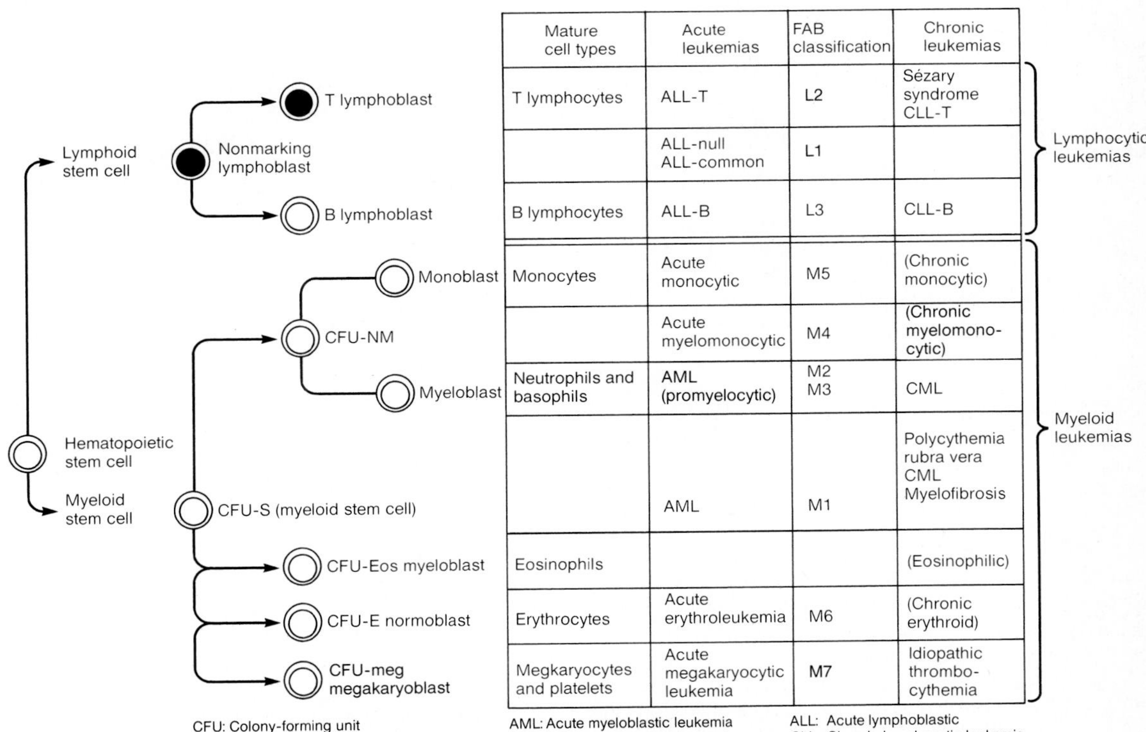

Figure 26-3. Classification of leukemias according to cell type and lineage.

Table 26-13. The French-American-British (FAB) classification of acute leukemias.

Acute lymophoblastic leukemia (ALL)	
L1	Morphology medium-sized "homogeneous" blasts; immunologically nonmarking but embraces several types, including common ALL and pre-B ALL; common in childhood; has the best prognosis.
L2	Heterogeneous blast cells; again a mixed group, some nonmarking, most T cell type; usual type seen in adults and has a bad prognosis.
L3	Homogeneous basophilic Burkitt-type blast cells, mark as B cells; bad prognosis
Acute myeloblastic leukemia	
M1	Consists of only myeloblasts without maturation.
M2	Myeloblasts with evidence of maturation.
M3	Acute promyelocytic leukemia; promelocytes have numerous darkly staining azurophilic cytoplasmic granules.
M4	Acute myelomonocytic leukemia is believed to arise from a cell that is the common precursor for monocytes and granulocytes (see Fig 26-3).
M5	Acute monocytic leukemia
M6	Erythroleukemia (Di Guglielmo's syndrome); predominance of erythroblasts along with myeloblasts.
M7	Megakaryoblastic leukemia

When lymphocytic leukemia involves lymph nodes, it has the appearance of malignant lymphoma (Chapter 29). ALL in lymph nodes is identical to lymphoblastic lymphoma (B, T or nonmarking type—formerly classified within the broader category of poorly differentiated lymphocytic lymphoma). CLL in lymph nodes is identical to small lymphocytic lymphoma (B or T type—formerly termed well-differentiated lymphocytic lymphoma).

In each case, this phenomenon represents part of the spectrum of a single disease process, **lymphoma-leukemia.** This concept is discussed further in Chapter 29.

2. Myeloid (granulocytic) leukemias are characterized by the proliferation of cells of the granulocyte series, usually neutrophils, though concomitant proliferation of eosinophils and basophils is not uncommon.

a. AML is characterized by proliferation of myeloblasts. Myeloblasts are difficult to differentiate morphologically from lymphoblasts except (1) when they contain **Auer rods,** which are purple, crystalline cytoplasmic inclusions; (2) when they show some maturation into promyelocytes, in which coarse granules are seen in the cytoplasm; and (3) when cytochemical or immunologic markers are used (Tables 26-14 and 29-5). AML is further classified (FAB system M1, M2, M3, M4) by its morphologic features. (Note that the FAB classification of AML includes monocytic leukemia [M5], erythroleukemia [M6], and megakaryoblastic leukemia [M7], which others consider separately [Table 26-13, Fig 26-3]).

b. Chronic myelocytic leukemia is characterized by proliferation of cells of the granulocyte series that have matured beyond the myeloblast stage. Less than 5% of cells in the marrow are myeloblasts. When a patient with chronic myelocytic leukemia has a bone marrow containing more than 5% myeloblasts, that patient is defined as being in the accelerated or blast phase of the disease.

3. Monocytic leukemia–Traditionally, 2 forms were distinguished: acute monocytic (Schilling type) and acute myelomonocytic (Naegeli type). Both are now included under acute myeloblastic leukemia in the FAB classification, in recognition of the known common origin with granulocytes. There is no well-defined chronic form of monocytic or myelomonocytic leukemia, though some myeloproliferative disorders do show monocytic proliferation.

a. Acute monocytic leukemia (FAB–M5) is characterized by proliferation of monoblasts. These be can reliably distinguished from other blasts only with the use of cytochemical markers (Table 26-14).

b. Acute myelomonocytic leukemia (FAB–

Table 26-14. Cytochemical identification of acute leukemias.

Type	Peroxidase	Sudan Black	Chloroacetate Esterase	Nonspecific Esterase	Periodic Acid-Schiff	Morphologic Features
Lymphoblastic (ALL)[1]	–	–	–	–	+	Single nucleolus
Myeloblastic (AML)	+	+	+	–	–	Multiple nucleoli, Auer rods
Monocytic	–	–	–	+	–	–
Myelomonocytic	+	+	+	+	–	–
Unclassified[2]	–	–	–	–	–	–

[1]Note the subtypes of ALL may be distinguished from other acute leukemias by positivity for TdT (terminal deoxynucleotide transferase), presence of CALLA (common ALL antigen or other lymphocytic antigens [see Table 29-5]), immunoglobulin or T-cell receptor gene rearrangement (see Chapter 4).

[2]Cannot be characterized cytochemically; may be identifiable by other techniques (footnote 1).

M4) is characterized by blasts that have the characteristics of myeloblasts and monoblasts, both morphologically and in cytochemical studies.

4. Other types–Erythroleukemia (Di Guglielmo's disease), plasma cell leukemia, eosinophilic leukemia, and megakaryocytic leukemia (Fig 26–3) are all rare.

Clinical Features (Fig 26–4)

A. Acute Leukemias: Acute leukemia is characterized by an acute clinical onset and rapid progression of disease. Patients usually present with evidence of a decrease in one or more of the normal hematopoietic elements because the bone marrow is overrun by the leukemic cells. Anemia, often severe and rapidly developing, causes pallor and hypoxic symptoms. Thrombocytopenia may produce abnormal bleeding or purpura. Neutropenia results in infections, fever, and ulceration of mucous membranes. Patients with acute promyelocytic leukemia (M3) frequently present with disseminated intravascular coagulation, due to the coagulant properties of the cytoplasmic granules.

Enlargement of lymph nodes is common in ALL and acute monocytic leukemia but usually absent in AML. Involvement of tissue other than lymph nodes occurs rarely in all types of acute leukemia. Rarely, a local tissue mass (chloroma or granulocytic sarcoma) may be the first manifestation of AML. Similarly, tissue masses may occur in acute monocytic leukemia.

B. Chronic Leukemias: Chronic leukemias usually have an insidious onset and a slow rate of progression. Most patients present with slowly developing anemia and enlargement of organs infiltrated by leukemia cells.

Generalized lymph node enlargement is present in CLL; histologic features of affected nodes are indistinguishable from those of small-cell (well-differentiated) lymphocytic lymphoma (Chapter 29). Splenomegaly—often massive—and hepatomegaly are usually obvious at presentation in all chronic leukemias. Patients may also manifest nodular masses in the skin, liver, heart, and kidneys.

Massive splenomegaly and hepatomegaly are common presenting complaints in patients with CML. Pain in the left lower chest is evidence of splenic infarction due to vascular occlusion by aggregates of granulocytes.

The **accelerated phase of CML,** which is characterized by the appearance of myeloblasts in the bone marrow and peripheral blood, occurs after a median period of 3–4 years. It resembles AML clinically and progresses rapidly to death if not treated (interestingly, some cases of CML blast

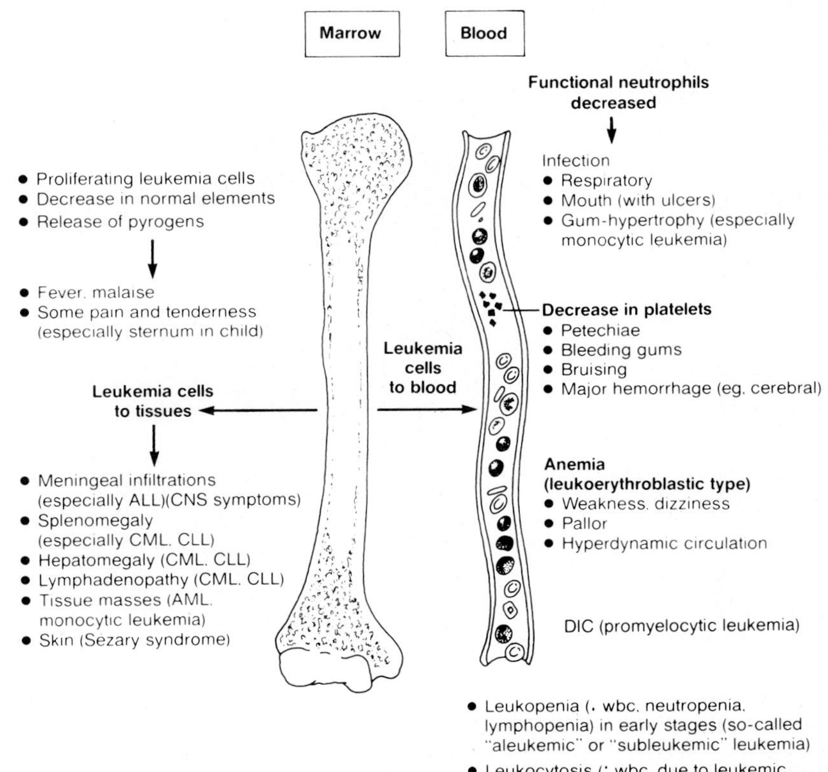

Figure 26–4. Clinicopathologic effects of leukemias.

crisis show features in common with ALL, probably representing regression to an earlier common precursor). The occurrence of the accelerated phase is associated with the appearance of new karyotypic abnormalities; cytogenetic studies may predict imminent blast crisis.

Diagnosis

A. Acute Leukemias: Acute leukemias are characterized by the proliferation of primitive cells (''blasts'') that mature little if at all. In both AML and ALL, the peripheral blood usually shows an increased total white cell count with increased numbers of blasts. Rarely, the total white count is not increased, though the diagnosis may be made by the finding of blasts in the peripheral blood smear. Extremely rarely, no blasts are seen in the peripheral blood (aleukemic leukemia).

The peripheral blood picture is diagnostic of acute leukemia in most cases (Fig 26–5). Rarely, marked lymphocytosis as seen in whooping cough or a viral infection may mimic ALL. Infectious mononucleosis, in which there are activated atypical lymphocytes in the blood, may cause considerable diagnostic difficulty (Table 26–3).

The bone marrow is abnormal in all cases of acute leukemia, being the primary site of the disease. Involvement is diffuse. The bone marrow is hypercellular, with proliferation of the cell type involved at the expense of the normal hematopoietic elements (Fig 26–6). Diagnosis of the type of acute leukemia and subclassification according to the FAB system depends on identification of the cell type.

1. In AML, the primitive myeloblasts may not show any maturation (in the M1 subtype in the FAB classification), or show minimal maturation into promyelocytes and myelocytes (M2 subtype). Acute promyelocytic leukemia (M3 subtype) is characterized by a predominance of promyelocytes. In M1 AML, the identification of the undifferentiated blasts as myeloid requires a battery of cytochemical (Table 26–14) and immunologic stains. In the future, the use of monoclonal antibodies, chromosome analysis, and genetic probes promises more accurate subclassification of AML.

2. In ALL, there is proliferation of lymphoblasts (Fig 26–5B). While these may be difficult to differentiate from myeloblasts on morphologic

A

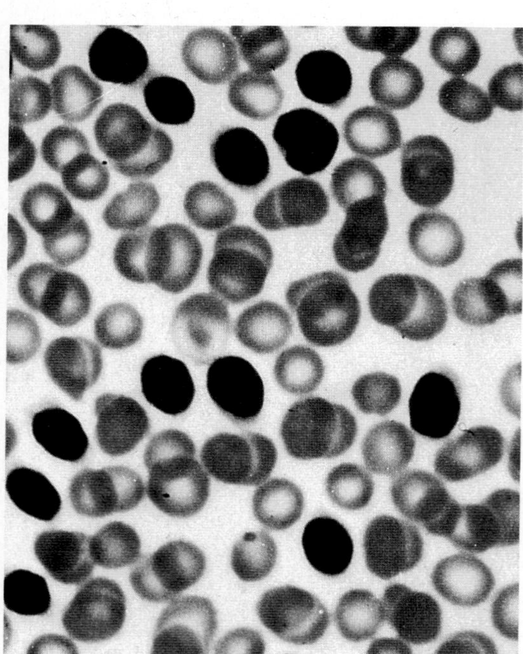

B

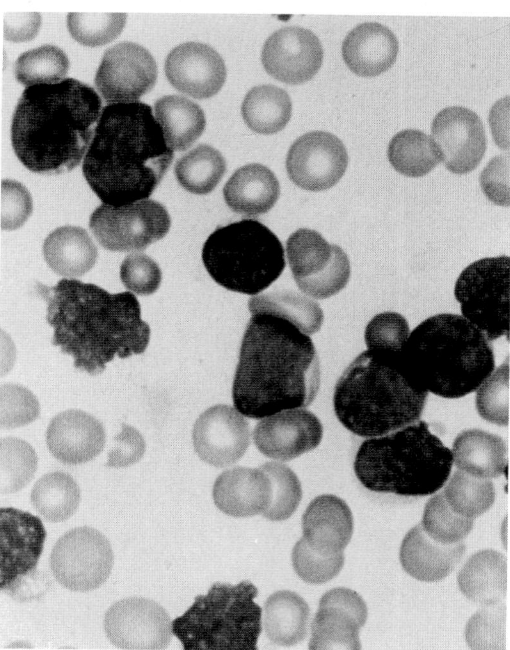

Figure 26–5. Peripheral blood changes in leukemias. In most cases of leukemia, the peripheral blood is involved. Both **A** and **B** show a marked increase in the number of leukocytes. In **A,** which represents chronic lymphocytic leukemia (CLL), the cells resemble small lymphocytes. In **B,** which is acute lymphoblastic luekemia (ALL), the cells are larger and resemble the lymphoblasts seen in early stages of lymphocytic differentiation. Note the fragmentation of the fragile leukemic cells, which is a common finding in peripheral blood smears of patients with acute leukemia.

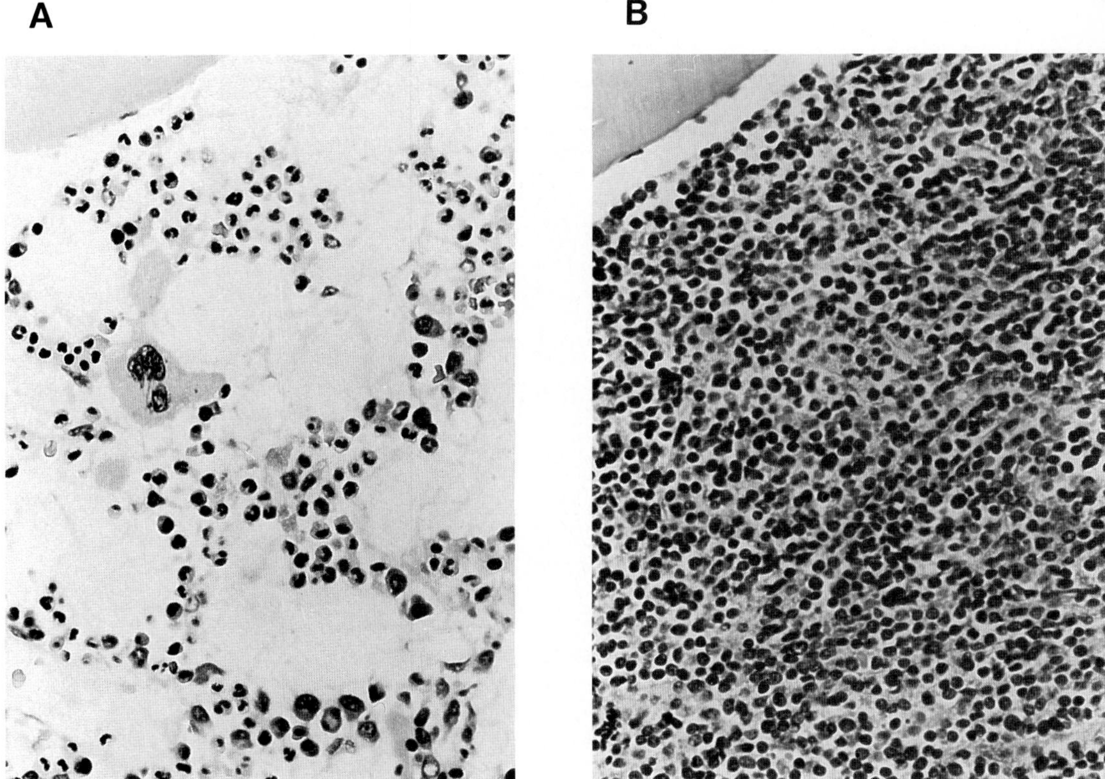

Figure 26-6. Bone marrow involvement in leukemias. The bone marrow is considered to be the site of origin of leukemias. **A** represents normal adult bone marrow, showing multinucleated megakaryocytes and myeloid and erythroid precursors distributed in a matrix containing adipocytes. In leukemia **(B),** the marrow fat and normal hematopoietic cells have been replaced by leukemic cells. In this example of CLL, the leukemic cells resemble small lymphocytes.

grounds, the use of cytochemical (Table 26–14) and immunologic stains permits accurate diagnosis. New markers for T and B lymphocytes and early lymphoid precursor cells are increasing the accuracy of subclassification of ALL.

B. Chronic Leukemias: Chronic leukemias are characterized by the presence of very high peripheral white blood cell counts. The cells are mature cells. The peripheral blood picture is diagnostic of chronic leukemia in most cases (Fig 26–5). Rarely, a leukemoid reaction (severe neutrophil leukocytosis in response to an acute inflammatory process) may be difficult to distinguish from CML (Table 26–5). The bone marrow is always abnormal, showing diffuse hypercellularity.

1. In CML, the dominant cells in the peripheral blood and bone marrow are myelocytes, metamyelocytes, and granulocytes. The granulocytes are usually neutrophils, but it is not uncommon to find increased numbers of basophils and eosinophils. Very rarely, the eosinophils are the dominant cells (eosinophilic leukemia). In the bone marrow, general myeloproliferation is present, involving not only the granulocyte series but also erythroid cells and megakaryocytes. Myelofibrosis commonly complicates CML. The Philadelphia chromosome (Chapter 19) is present in all these cell lineages and remains detectable even after remission of the CML.

2. In CLL, the neoplastic cells resemble resting small lymphocytes morphologically (Fig 26–5A) but can be shown to be monoclonal. The bone marrow is infiltrated by similar cells, but normal hematopoietic elements remain until an advanced stage of the disease.

Treatment & Prognosis

Combination chemotherapy, using several anticancer agents (Fig 26–7) simultaneously in various combinations, has improved the prognosis of patients with acute leukemias dramatically. "Common ALL" in children is now considered to be a curable disease in many cases (70% 5-year survival rate). The rate of cure in other types of ALL (T and B cell, 10% 5-year survival rates), AML, and acute monocytic leukemia (both with 5-year

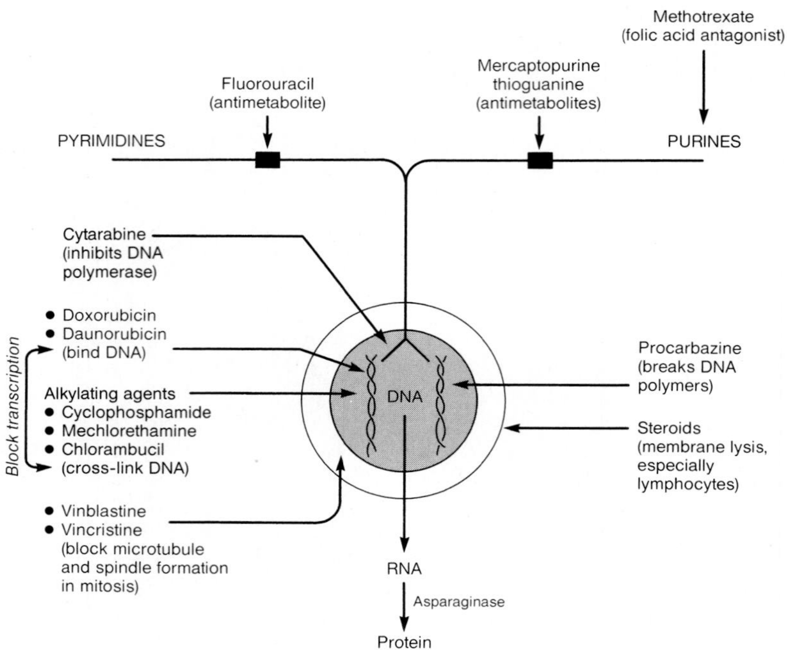

Figure 26–7. Mechanisms of action of chemotherapeutic agents used in the treatment of leukemias.

survival rates near zero) is much worse. However, chemotherapy does increase the duration of survival in comparison to nontreated cases.

Paradoxically, treatment has little effect on the survival rate of chronic leukemias. Many of these patients survive many years after diagnosis of disease without treatment, and their overall course and outcome does not seem to be altered by therapy.

Recently, acute leukemias have been treated more aggressively with the intention of destroying all the hematopoietic cells in the marrow, including leukemic cells, followed by rescue of the patient by bone marrow transplantation (see Chapter 10). The transplant consists either of matched heterologous marrow or of autologous marrow taken prior to therapy and purged of leukemic cells by in vitro treatment with monoclonal antibodies.

Hemorrhage and infection are the major causes of death of patients with leukemia, occurring as a direct effect of the leukemia or as a complication of cytotoxic therapy.

OTHER RELATED NEOPLASTIC PROCESSES

HAIRY CELL LEUKEMIA (Leukemic Reticuloendotheliosis)

Hairy cell leukemia is a rare neoplasm of the hematopoietic system that chiefly affects individuals over the age of 50 years. The neoplastic cell is medium-sized, with an ovoid nucleus, a fine chromatin pattern, and inconspicuous nucleoli. The abundant cytoplasm has a frayed cell membrane (on electron microscopy, the cell membrane shows hairy processes). Electron microscopy also reveals the presence in the cytoplasm of a specific spiral organelle (lamellar ribosomal complex). The cytoplasm contains tartrate-resistant acid phosphatase, the demonstration of which is of diagnostic value. The neoplastic cell has been demonstrated to be a B lymphocyte on the basis of the presence of immunoglobulin gene rearrangement.

Patients present commonly with anemia, neutropenia and thrombocytopenia, and splenomegaly, often massive. The disease responds poorly to chemotherapy and has a relatively poor prognosis, median survival being 2–3 years after diagnosis. Splenectomy is of value in some cases, but results are unpredictable.

MYELOPROLIFERATIVE DISEASES

The term "myeloproliferative disease" is used for a group of disorders characterized by proliferation of granulocytic, monocytic, erythroid, and megakaryocytic cell lines in the marrow. The definition includes CML, polycythemia rubra vera, idiopathic thrombocythemia, and myelofibrosis (with myeloid metaplasia; see below). The primary abnormality probably resides in the myeloid stem cell (Fig 26–3). The proliferation is considered neoplastic but low-grade; a monoclonal origin is shown by the presence of one type of G6PD isoenzyme in all the proliferating cells. Chromosomal abnormalities are present in 50% or more of cases, including translocations involving the long arm of chromosome 1, complete or partial deletions of chromosomes 5, 7, and 20, and the appearance of the Philadelphia chromosome.

Aspiration of marrow is often unsuccessful because of extensive fibrosis of the bone marrow (myelofibrosis). Residual marrow is markedly hypercellular, with proliferation of all cell lines. Eventually, one cell line may evolve to dominance, giving rise to CML (granulocyte), polycythemia rubra vera (erythrocyte), or idiopathic thrombocythemia (platelets). Clusters of dysplastic megakaryocytes are characteristic. Other organs such as spleen, liver, and lymph nodes commonly show marked extramedullary hematopoiesis, again with dysplastic features. The peripheral blood typically shows leukoerythroblastic anemia (except in polycythemic cases) with neutrophil leukocytosis and a marked shift to the left.

Myelofibrosis tends to have a slow clinical course. As marrow fibrosis progresses, extramedullary hematopoiesis may cause massive enlargement of the spleen and liver. Hemorrhage, thromboembolism, and infection are common complications.

MYELODYSPLASTIC DISORDERS (Refractory Sideroblastic Anemias)

Although uncommon, these conditions are important because they may progress to AML. Several variants exist, all characterized by dyshematopoiesis, particularly evident in erythroid cells, the precursors of which show abnormal accumulations of granular iron (sideroblasts—hence sideroblastic anemia).

Sideroblastic anemia may occur as an idiopathic or primary form with or without excess blasts and pancytopenia. Approximately 10% of patients develop AML. Secondary sideroblastic anemia occurs in vitamin B_{12} or folate deficiency or following cytotoxic therapy; it rarely progresses to AML.

Iron stains of the bone marrow are valuable in diagnosis (reveal sideroblasts). The peripheral blood typically shows a mixed (dimorphic) hypochromic and macrocytic picture.

27 Blood: IV. Bleeding Disorders

NORMAL HEMOSTASIS

The normal vascular system maintains a delicate balance between clotting mechanisms and clot lysis, with the result that internal or external bleeding is controlled and pathologic thrombosis prevented (see Chapter 9).

Several factors acting in concert maintain this equilibrium:

(1) Blood vessels maintain anatomic integrity and a smooth endothelium. Following minor injuries, the blood vessels undergo vasoconstriction, thereby preventing bleeding from the injured site and permitting repair. Vasoconstriction is an effective method of hemostasis in small vessel injuries but is not adequate when large vessels are damaged.

(2) Platelets form the initial hemostatic plug that seals a site of vascular injury. Platelets also play a major role in forming the permanent thrombus that seals the injury.

(3) Blood coagulation is the formation of fibrin from plasma precursors. Fibrin and platelets constitute the permanent hemostatic plug.

(4) Fibrinolysis is the production of factors such as plasmin from plasma precursors that lyse and remove fibrin thrombi which have formed in the circulation.

Disturbance of any one of these mechanisms may produce **abnormal bleeding** on the one hand (Table 27–1) or **abnormal thrombosis** on the other. Pathologic thrombosis is discussed in Chapter 9.

The clinical effects of abnormal bleeding disorders (Table 27–2) are similar regardless of the mechanisms. Laboratory testing is generally required to reach a precise clinical diagnosis, following which appropriate therapy may be selected.

VASCULAR DEFECTS

Along with thrombocytopenia, vascular defects represent the most common cause of bleeding diathesis. In certain vascular disorders, the underlying defect relates to production of abnormal collagen or elastin (Table 27–1); in vasculitis, inflammation is the cause.

Henoch-Schönlein purpura (anaphylactoid purpura) deserves special mention as a poststreptococcal disease of childhood. It occurs 1–3 weeks after streptococcal infection and is thought to be mediated by deposition of cross-reactive IgA or immune complexes plus complement on the endothelium. Occasional cases have been reported with apparent hypersensitivity to other bacteria, insect bites, or food (milk, eggs, crab, strawberries). Clinically, there is purpura, abdominal pain (due to mucosal involvement in the gut, often with frank bleeding), arthralgia or arthritis, and glomerulonephritis. Fever is often present. The prognosis is determined by the severity of the renal lesion (focal glomeronephritis with deposition of IgA and complement; see Chapter 48).

Hereditary hemorrhagic telangiectasia (Osler-Weber-Rendu disease) is inherited as an autosomal dominant and manifested by multiple capillary microaneurysms in the skin and mucous membranes. The lesions tend to become more conspicuous with age and are exceedingly fragile,

Table 27-1. Hemorrhagic disorders: Principal causes.

Vascular defects
- Simple and senile purpura (increased capillary fragility, especially in the elderly)
- Hypersensitivity vasculitis; many autoimmune disorders (inflammation)
- Vitamin C deficiency (scurvy, defective collagen)
- Amyloidosis (affected vessels fail to constrict)
- Excess adrenocorticosteroids (therapeutic or Cushing's disease)
- Hereditary hemorrhagic telangiectasia (Osler-Weber-Rendu syndrome)
- Ehlers-Danlos disease (defective collagen)
- Henoch-Schönlein purpura (IgA and complement damage endothelium)

Disorders of platelets
- Decrease (thrombocytopenia)
- Abnormal platelet function

Disorders of coagulation
- Deficiency of coagulation factors
- Presence of anticoagulant factors

Excessive fibrinolysis
- Disseminated intravascular coagulation
- Primary fibrinolysis

predisposing both to episodes of acute severe bleeding and to chronic blood loss from the intestinal tract with iron deficiency anemia.

PLATELETS

NORMAL STRUCTURE & FUNCTION

Platelets are anucleate cytoplasmic fragments 2–4 μm in diameter derived from megakaryocytes. The normal platelet count in peripheral blood is 150,000–400,000/μL. The platelets have a clear outer zone and an inner zone containing cytoplasmic organelles (Fig 27–1), which include contractile microfilaments and several types of granules that contain a variety of enzymes, phospholipid, ADP, ATP, serotonin, calcium, and thromboplastic substances. Platelets have a life span of 8–10 days in the peripheral blood.

Table 27-2. Common clinical manifestations of hemorrhagic disorders.

Hemorrhage into skin
- Petechiae: pinhead-sized focal hemorrhage; purpura; confluent petechiae; multiple, irregularly shaped or oval (2–5 mm or larger).
- Ecchymoses: confluent purpura; all show sequential color change—red, purple, brown—as extravasated red cells are broken down in tissues.

Excessive or prolonged bleeding
- Posttrauma, often minimal trauma; postsurgery (eg, dental extraction); "spontaneous" hemorrhage (without a history of trauma) into skeletal muscle, joints, and brain.

Bleeding from mucosal surfaces
- Epistaxis, bleeding from gums, hemoptysis, hematuria, and melena.

Bleeding from multiple sites

In peripheral blood smears, platelets appear as small granular cytoplasmic fragments about one-fourth the size of an erythrocyte. Platelets that have exited the marrow recently are larger, and a finding of many large forms is evidence that the rate of release of platelets from the marrow is increased.

The main function of platelets is in hemostasis. In the early phase of hemostasis after vascular injury, platelets plug and seal injured areas in the wall of the blood vessel (Fig 27–2). The process of formation of the platelet plug involves 2 mechanisms: adhesion and aggregation.

(1) Platelet adhesion: Platelets in the blood are attracted to collagen exposed by endothelial damage. Adherence is followed by clumping and release of cytoplasmic granules. Degranulation is an active phenomenon that involves contraction of the platelet microskeleton; it is dependent on the presence of prostaglandins and is inhibited by aspirin. Platelet adhesion is a function of the outer zone of the platelet cytoplasm.

(2) Platelet aggregation: The release of platelet granules containing ADP induces accumulation and aggregation of large numbers of platelets, to form the hemostatic plug that prevents bleeding from the injured zone. Aggregation is promoted by collagen, epinephrine, and serotonin.

ABNORMALITIES OF BLOOD PLATELETS

Abnormalities of blood platelets include (1) decreased numbers (thrombocytopenia), (2) increased numbers (thrombocytosis), and (3) abnormal platelet function. There are numerous causes for such abnormalities (Table 27–3). In general, thrombocytopenia and abnormal platelet function impair the normal hemostatic mechanism and cause increased bleeding. Thrombocytosis is associated with an increased tendency to thrombosis.

1. IDIOPATHIC THROMBOCYTOPENIC PURPURA

Incidence & Etiology

Idiopathic thrombocytopenic purpura (ITP) is a common disease in which severe reduction of platelet numbers in the blood is caused by immune destruction of platelets. It occurs in 2 clinical forms:

(1) Acute ITP is seen mainly in children. About 50% of cases are associated with a history of viral infection 2–3 weeks before onset. The exact rela-

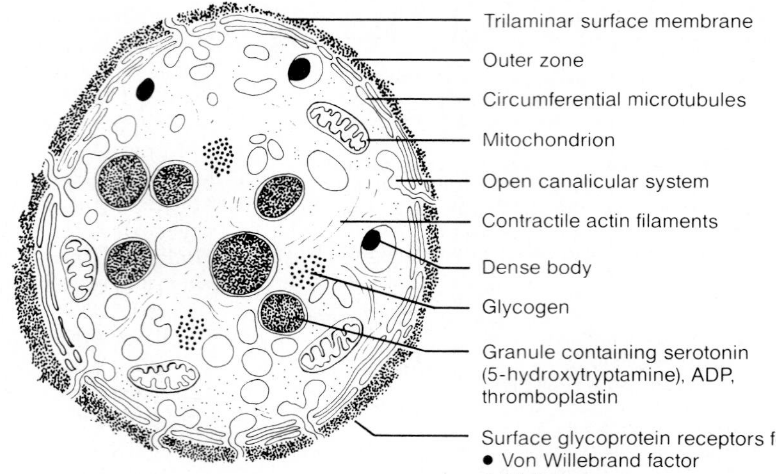

Figure 27-1. Structure of a platelet.

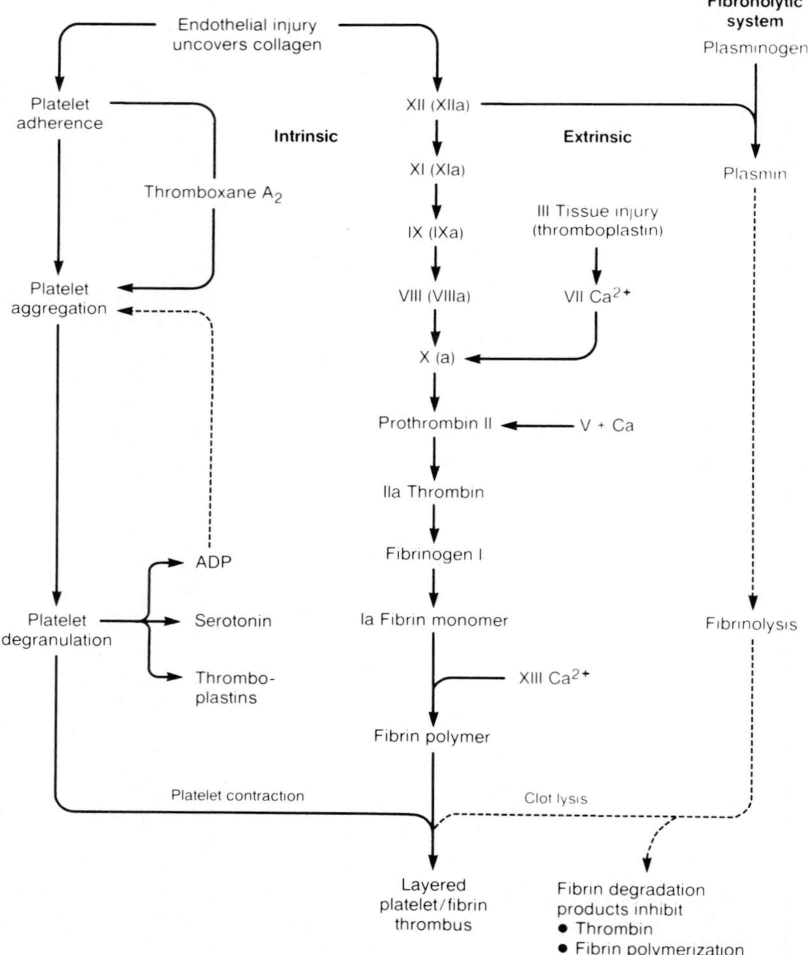

Figure 27-2. Coagulation and fibrinolytic systems. The balance between these 2 systems is very finely tuned. If this balance is disturbed, pathologic thrombosis or excessive bleeding may result.

Table 27-3. Causes of platelet abnormalities.

Thrombocytopenia
- Decreased production in the bone marrow
  - Aplastic anemia: any of numerous causes, including idiopathic
  - Radiation
  - Marrow infiltration by leukemia, metastatic neoplasms, infections
  - Vitamin B_{12} and folate deficiency
  - Hereditary, autosomal dominant form: Wiskott-Aldrich syndrome, May-Hegglin syndrome
- Pooling (sequestration) of platelets in an enlarged spleen
- Increased peripheral destruction of platelets
  - Immune mechanisms
    - Idiopathic thrombocytopenic purpura
    - Systemic lupus erythematosus
    - Drug-induced thrombocytopenia (gold salts, quinine, sulfonamides)
    - Neonatal thrombocytopenia: transfer of maternal IgG antibodies with activity against fetal platelets
    - Posttransfusion: due to alloantibodies to platelet antigen $P1^{A1}$ (rare but severe)
  - Hypersplenism
  - Increased platelet consumption
    - Disseminated intravascular coagulation
    - Thrombotic thrombocytopenic purpura
    - Hemolytic uremic syndrome
    - Valve prosthesis, artificial vascular grafts
- Dilution of platelets: massive transfusions

Thrombocytosis
- Myeloproliferative diseases, including essential thrombocythemia
- Postoperative, especially postsplenectomy
- Response to hemorrhage, exercise
- Inflammatory disorders
- Malignant neoplasms
- Sometimes in iron deficiency

Qualitative platelet disorders (abnormal function)
- Congenital
  - Defects of adhesion: Bernard-Soulier disease
  - Defects of aggregation: thrombasthenia (Glanzmann's disease)
  - Abnormal granule release: storage pool disease
  - Wiskott-Aldrich syndrome
  - Von Willebrand's disease
  - Albinism
- Acquired
  - Uremia
  - Dysproteinemias
  - Chronic liver disease, especially alcoholic
  - Drug-induced: aspirin, phenylbutazone
  - Myeloproliferative diseases
  - Vascular disorders: many diseases producing vascular damage also affect platelet function

tionship of thrombocytopenia to the infection is uncertain, but it is believed that immune complexes bind to the surface of platelets, resulting in phagocytosis by splenic macrophages. Acute ITP is characterized by spontaneous recovery in the majority of patients; 80% are normal after 6 months; and many recover within 6 weeks.

(2) Chronic ITP occurs mainly in adults, with a predilection for females (3:1) and frequent occurrence of relapse during pregnancy, suggesting a role for estrogens. Thrombocytopenia is the result of peripheral destruction of platelets that have bound an **IgG antiplatelet autoantibody** on their surface. Chronic ITP rarely resolves spontaneously but is a long-standing disorder characterized by multiple relapses and remissions.

Neonatal thrombocytopenic purpura occurs in children born to mothers with chronic ITP. It results from transfer of the IgG antibodies across the placenta.

Pathology

Platelet survival is impaired. The platelet count is markedly decreased, often to the 10,000–50,000/μL range. The bone marrow typically shows increased numbers of megakaryocytes (compensatory hyperplasia). The megakaryocytes are more basophilic, less granular, and have a smoother ("nonbudding") surface than usual, probably as a result of premature release of platelets.

The spleen is the major site of destruction of antibody-coated platelets. It is usually either normal in size or slightly enlarged and shows sinusoidal congestion and hyperplasia of macrophages.

As with any patient with severe thrombocytopenia, the bleeding time is prolonged and capillary fragility (tourniquet test) increased. Tests of coagulation (clotting time, partial thromboplastin time, and prothrombin time) are normal. Clot retraction, which depends on platelets, is defective.

Clinical Features & Treatment

Patients present with a bleeding tendency. Clinical bleeding occurs when the platelet count falls to very low levels (< 40,000/μL). The most common clinical feature is purpura. Bleeding may also occur from mucosal surfaces, leading to hematuria, melena, menorrhagia, and hemoptysis. Rarely, intracerebral hemorrhage occurs—a complication associated with a high mortality rate.

The diagnosis of ITP is one of exclusion, reached by ruling out all other causes of thrombocytopenia. The peripheral blood and bone marrow findings are suggestive but not specific, and there is no laboratory test to confirm the diagnosis.

Treatment with high dosage corticosteroids prolongs the life span of the antibody-coated platelets, probably by suppressing splenic phagocytic activity. There is evidence that autoantibody synthesis is also decreased. The response to steroids has a lag phase of several days during which platelet transfusions are frequently necessary to provide adequate hemostasis. **Splenectomy** is effective in treatment by removing the main site of platelet destruction but does nothing to correct the basic abnormality.

2. ABNORMALITIES OF PLATELET FUNCTION

Platelet function abnormalities are characterized by symptoms and signs of platelet deficiency (ie, abnormal bleeding) but with a normal platelet count. Tests of platelet function such as clot retraction, platelet adhesion, and aggregation in response to different agents are abnormal and are valuable in separating the different disease processes (Table 27–4).

BLOOD COAGULATION

NORMAL BLOOD COAGULATION

Coagulation represents the method of permanent healing of a vascular injury. It follows vasoconstriction and formation of the platelet plug and maintains hemostasis when normal blood flow is restored. Coagulation is achieved by the interaction of several plasma protein factors (Table 27–5) that ultimately results in formation of fibrin when they are activated sequentially (Fig 27–2).

DISORDERS OF BLOOD COAGULATION

Etiology

There are 3 principal groups of coagulation disorders.

(1) Deficiency of coagulation factors. Deficiencies of individual coagulation factors may occur as inherited diseases (Table 27–6). Of these, factor VIII deficiency (hemophilia A and von Willebrand's disease) and factor IX deficiency (Christmas disease) are the most common. Acquired deficiencies of coagulation factors occur in severe liver disease (all factors produced by the liver) and in vitamin K deficiency (prothrombin and factors VII, IX, and X).

(2) Presence of circulating anticoagulants. Factor deficiencies may also be induced by anticoagulant therapy with coumarin derivatives (which interfere with vitamin K, thereby inhibiting synthesis of prothrombin and of factors VII, IX, and X). Directly acting anticoagulants that antagonize some of the coagulation cascade include (a) drugs such as heparin (an antithrombin), (b) antibodies (factor VIII inhibitor and lupus anticoagulant, an antibody in systemic lupus erythematosus), and (c) natural anticoagulants (antithrombin and fibrin degradation products).

(3) Increased fibrinolytic activity in the blood resulting from increased activation of the plasmin system.

Table 27–4. Abnormalities of platelet function.

Disease	Inheritance	Platelet Adhesion[1]	Platelet Aggregation: Collagen[2]	ADP[2]	Ristocetin[2]	Other Features
Congenital						
Bernard-Soulier disease	AR	↓	N	N	↓	Giant platelets
Glanzmann's thrombasthenia	AR	N	↓	↓	N	Absent clot retraction
Storage pool disease	Variable	N	↓	↓	N	Absent dense bodies
von Willebrand's disease	AD	↓	N	N	↓	Corrected by factor VIII.vWF
Acquired						
Aspirin	–	N	↓	↓	N	Decreased cyclooxygenase
Uremia	–	↓	↓	↓	N	Pathogenesis not known
Myeloproliferative diseases	–	↓	↓	↓	N	Pathogenesis not known

AR = autosomal recessive; AD = autosomal dominant; N = normal.
[1]Tests of adhesiveness are difficult to standardize.
[2]Aggregation induced by collagen, adenosine diphosphate (ADP), or ristocetin in vitro. Other inducers of aggregation include arachidonic acid and epinephrine; the normal range is 60–100% of control.

Table 27-5. Blood coagulation factors.[1]

Factor	Name	Source
Factor I	Fibrinogen	Liver
Factor II	Prothrombin	Liver[2]
Factor III	Tissue thromboplastin	
Factor IV	Calcium	
Factor V	Proaccelerin; labile factor	Liver
Factor VI	Obsolete; activated Factor V	
Factor VII	Proconvertin; stable factor	Liver[2]
Factor VIII	Antihemophilic globulin (AHG)	Vascular endothelial cell
Factor IX	Plasma thromboplastin component (PTC); Christmas factor	Liver[2]
Factor X	Stuart-Prower factor	Liver[2]
Factor XI	Plasma thromboplastin antecedent (PTA)	?Liver
Factor XII	Hageman factor	Uncertain
Factor XIII	Fibrin-stabilizing factor	Platelets

[1]These factors occur in an inactive form in plasma. When they are activated, they are designated by an "a" after the Roman numeral.
[2]The synthesis of factors VII, IX, X, and prothrombin in the liver is dependent on the presence of vitamin K.

Clinical Features

Patients with disorders of coagulation tend to bleed excessively following minor trauma such as dentistry. In severe cases, spontaneous bleeding occurs (ie, bleeding without evident trauma)—commonly into joints (hemarthrosis) and muscles. Bleeding is usually slow but persistent and can be halted by replacement of the deficient factor.

All coagulation disorders have similar clinical manifestations. Determination of the cause of the abnormality requires bleeding and coagulation testing (Fig 27–3 and Tables 27–7 and 27–8).

FACTOR VIII DEFICIENCY

Factor VIII is a complex molecule (Fig 27–4) composed of 3 subunits: (1) Factor VIII-related antigen (VIII:RAg) is the largest part of the molecule and is detected by immunologic methods. It has no function in coagulation. (2) Factor VIII coagulant (VIII:C) is the functional part of the molecule (antihemophilic globulin). Deficiency produces hemophilia A. (3) Factor VIII-von Willebrand factor (VIII:VWF) is required in platelet aggregation. Deficiency produces von Willebrand's disease.

1. HEMOPHILIA A

Incidence & Etiology

Hemophilia A (classic hemophilia) is inherited as an **X-linked recessive trait,** occurring mainly in males. Females develop hemophilia only when they have the abnormal gene on both X chromo-

Table 27-6. Diseases resulting from an inherited coagulation factor deficiency.

Deficient Factor	Disease	Inheritance	Frequency[1]	Disease Severity
Fibrinogen	Afibrinogenemia	AR	Rare	Variable
	Congenital dysfibrinogenemia	AD	Rare	Variable
Prothrombin	. . .	. . .	Very rare	Variable
Factor V	Parahemophilia	AR	Very rare	Moderate to severe
Factor VII	. . .	AR	Very rare	Moderate to severe
Factor VIII	Hemophilia A	XR	Common	Mild to severe
	von Willebrand's disease	AD	Common	Mild to moderate
Factor IX	Hemophilia B	XR	Uncommon	Mild to severe
Factor X	. . .	AR	Rare	Variable
Factor XI	Rosenthal's syndrome	AR	Uncommon	Mild
Factor XII	Hageman trait	AR/AD	Rare	Asymptomatic
Factor XIII	. . .	AR	Rare	Severe

AR = autosomal recessive; AD = autosomal dominant; XR = X-linked recessive.
[1]Frequency: very rare = fewer than 100 reported cases; compare to hemophilia A with a frequency of 1/10,000 males.

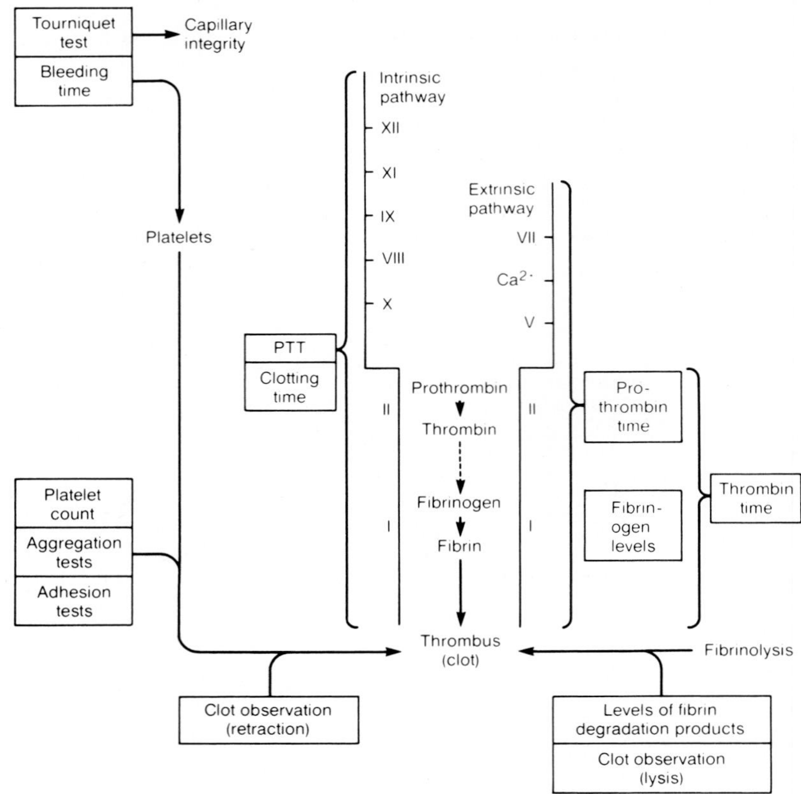

Figure 27-3. Tests used clinically to detect abnormalities in the blood coagulation and fibrinolytic systems. PTT = partial thromblastin time.

somes (homozygous)—a rare event that occurs when a hemophiliac male mates with a carrier female or when a single functional X chromosome carries the abnormal gene. The incidence in the United States is 1:10,000 males. Hemophilia occurs throughout the world.

The presence of the abnormal gene results in deficient synthesis of the coagulant subunit of the factor VIII molecule (VIII:C, Fig 27-4). Factor VIII-related antigen and factor VIII-von Willebrand factor continue to be present in normal amounts.

The heterozygous female carrier shows a mild decrease in plasma level of the coagulant subunit of factor VIII (VIII:C). Because factor VIII-related antigen level (VIII:RAg) is normal, the ratio of VIII:C to VIII:RAg is less than 0.75 (normal is 1). Observation of a reduced VIII:C to VIII:RAg ratio is a reliable means of detecting heterozygous carriers of the hemophilia A gene.

Pathology & Clinical Features

Patients with severe hemophilia have less than 1% of factor VIII coagulant activity and bleed spontaneously. Moderately affected patients (1–5% activity) bleed excessively after minor trauma, and mild cases (5–25% activity) are usually asymptomatic. The cause of the variable expression of disease in different patients is not well understood.

Spontaneous bleeding (probably caused by minimal trauma resulting from normal activity) occurs into subcutaneous tissues, skeletal muscle, joints, and mucous membranes. Intracranial hemorrhage is rare but is a major cause of death. Hemorrhage into muscle and joints occurs mainly in the extremities and is followed by organization and fibrosis leading to contractures in affected muscles and to stiffness of joints.

Bleeding after dental surgery is typical. The bleeding is not dramatic but consists of a slow and persistent ooze lasting many days. Oozing commonly begins several hours after surgery and not in the immediate postoperative period.

Diagnosis & Treatment

The partial thromboplastin time is prolonged in almost all patients, and there is a significant decrease in factor VIII coagulant activity (to less than 20% of normal). Factor VIII-related antigen is normal, and the VIII:C to VIII:RAg ratio is markedly decreased. Prothrombin time and bleeding time are normal, indicating that the defect is in the intrinsic pathway. Assays for factor VIII

Table 27-7. Tests used to evaluate hemorrhagic (bleeding) disorders. (See also Fig 27-3.)

Platelet count and morphology; peripheral blood smear.
Clotting time (whole blood coagulation time): the time taken for the patient's blood to clot in a test tube (normal, 5-10 min). This is a very insensitive test; even severe abnormalities of coagulation may be missed.
Clot observation: the formed clot is observed for 24 hours; failure of clot retraction in 1-4 hours indicates thrombocytopenia or abnormal platelet function. Clot fragmentation or lysis indicates excessive fibrinolysis.
Bleeding time (normal, 3-8 min): the time taken for a standardized skin puncture to stop bleeding. It is not a test of coagulation. Rather, it tests the ability of the vessels to vasconstrict after injury and the ability of the blood platelets to form a hemostatic plug.
Tourniquet test: inflation of blood pressure cuff above diastolic pressure for 5 minutes produces scattered petechiae in some normals, but the presence of numerous (100 or more) petechiae indicates capillary fragility, thrombocytopenia, or platelet abnormalities.
Prothrombin time[1] (PT): the time taken for clotting to occur when tissue thromboplastin (brain extract) and calcium are added to the patient's plasma (normal, approximately 12 s; 100% when expressed as a percentage of control). Tests for adequate amounts of factors V, VII, X, prothrombin and fibrinogen, ie, the extrinsic pathway of coagulation (see Fig 27-3).
Partial thromboplastin time[1] (PTT; also known as the kaolin-cephalin clotting time [KCCT]): the time taken for clotting when surface activation of factor XII is effected by Kaolin (cephalin provides platelet factors; normal, 40-50 s). Tests the adequacy of the intrinsic pathway of coagulation (factors XII, XI, IX, VIII, X, V, prothrombin, and fibrinogen; see Fig 27-3).
Thrombin time (TT): the time taken for clotting to occur when thrombin is added to the patient's plasma (normal, < 15 s). It tests the conversion of fibrinogen to fibrin and depends on adequate fibrinogen levels.
Tests for circulating anticoagulants should be performed if PT or PTT is abnormal; this involves mixing patient's plasma with known normal plasmas to determine nature of the anticoagulant factor.
Measurements of fibrinogen levels and **fibrin degradation products** is particularly useful in assessing fibrinolysis and disseminated intravascular coagulation.
Protamine sulfate test: This test is positive when fibrin monomer is present in serum and is good evidence for the presence of disseminated intravascular coagulation.

[1]The prothrombin time and the partial thromboplastin time are the 2 tests used most extensively for screening purposes.

coagulant activity and factor VIII-related antigen are diagnostic and reflect the severity of the disease.

Treatment of hemophilia consists of maintaining plasma factor VIII coagulant activity at a level that permits normal physical activity without bleeding. This may require prophylactic treatment in severe cases. Factor VIII.C is labile and must be provided as fresh plasma, or in concentrated form as cryoprecipitate, or as lyophilized factor VIII concentrate. The availability of cryoprecipitate and lyophilized factor VIII concentrate has markedly improved the outlook for patients with hemophilia. Treatment with synthetic vasopressin analogues has recently been shown to produce elevation of factor VIII levels, producing benefit in mild cases.

Cryoprecipitate is prepared in blood banks from fresh individual plasma units. Lyophilized factor VIII concentrate is made from pooled plasma obtained from a large number of blood donors. As with all such blood components prepared from multiple donors, administration of factor VIII concentrate greatly increases the risk of infections such as hepatitis B, cytomegalovirus infection, and, more recently, AIDS. Consequently, hemophiliacs represent a high-risk group for AIDS, and many have developed overt disease. Factor VIII concentrate is now heat-treated, a procedure believed to eliminate these risks.

2. VON WILLEBRAND'S DISEASE

Von Willebrand's disease is inherited as an autosomal dominant trait characterized by deficiency of the entire factor VIII molecule. Factor VIII coagulant activity and factor VIII-related antigen are decreased to the same extent, so that the ratio of these 2 components is normal.

Clinically, patients show bleeding after minor trauma. The onset of symptoms is in childhood and may decrease with age. The commonest sites of bleeding are the skin (easy bruising) and mucous membranes (epistaxis). Hemarthrosis, muscle hemorrhage, and intracranial hemorrhage are uncommon.

The diagnosis is made by demonstrating (1) prolonged partial thromboplastin time with normal prothrombin time, (2) decreased factor VIII coagulant activity and factor VIII related antigen, and (3) prolonged bleeding time due to platelet dysfunction (Table 27-8). In vitro, there is decreased platelet aggregation after addition of the antibiotic ristocetin, and the "ristocetin test" is useful for the diagnosis of von Willebrand's disease. Von Willebrand factor is present in cryoprecipitate, which can therefore be used in treating von Willebrand's disease.

FACTOR IX DEFICIENCY (Christmas Disease; Hemophilia B)

Christmas disease is uncommon, with an incidence of 1:50,000 population, and results from a deficiency of factor IX.

Christmas disease is characterized by X-linked recessive inheritance, greater prevalence in males, and a clinical picture identical to that of hemophilia A. The diagnosis is made when factor VIII coagulant activity is normal in a patient with

Table 27-8. Major bleeding disorders: Differential laboratory features.

	Tourniquet Test	Bleeding Time	Whole Blood Clotting Time	Platelet Count	Partial Thromboplastin Time (PTT)	Prothrombin Time (PT)	Comments
Vascular defects	+	↑ or N	N	N	N	N	
Platelet defects							
Thrombocytopenia	+	↑	N	↓	N	N	Abnormal clot retraction.
Platelet function defects	+	↑	N	N	N	N	See Table 27-4.
Coagulation defects							
Hemophilia A	N	N	↑	N	↑	N	VIII.C ↓ VIII.RAg and VIII.vWF normal.
von Willebrand's disease	+ or N	↑	↑ or N	N	↑	N	VIII.C ↓ VIII.RAg ↓ VIII.vWF ↓ abnormal ristocetin test.
Christmas disease (hemophilia B)	N	N	↑	N	↑	N	IX ↓
Deficiency of vitamin K-dependent factors (II, VII, IX, X)	N	N	↑ or N	N	↑	↑	Corrected by vitamin K therapy.
Liver diseases	N	N	↑ or N	N	↑	↑	Not corrected by vitamin K.
Disorders of fibrinolysis							
Disseminated intravascular coagulation	+ or N	↑	↑	↓	↑	↑	Presence of fibrin degradation products; positive protamine sulfate test.
Primary fibrinolysis	N	N	↑	N	↑	↑	

N = normal.

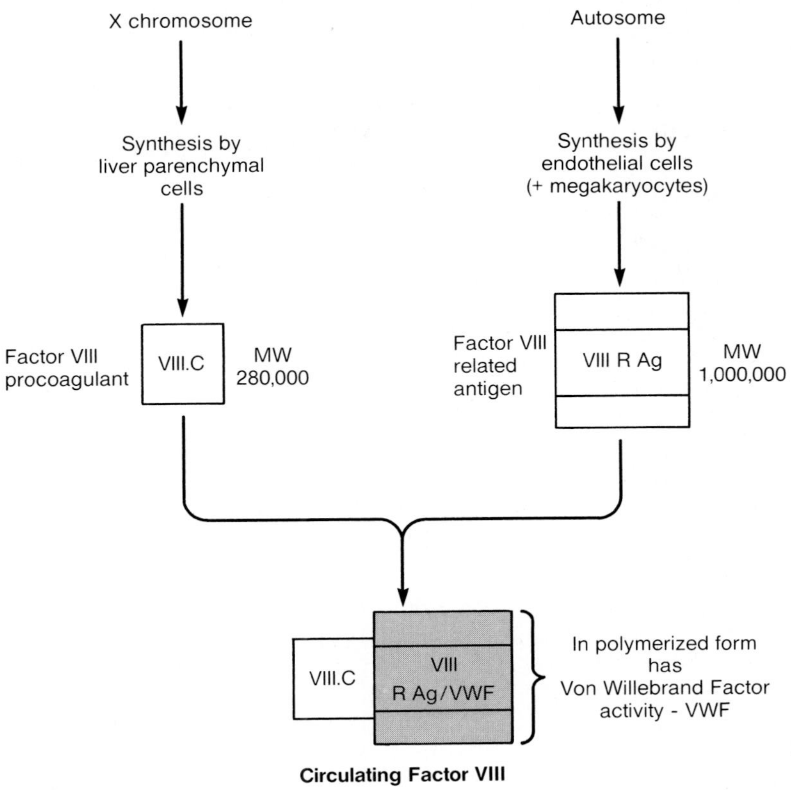

Role in intrinsic pathway of coagulation cascade (Fig. 27-3)

Deficiency
Hemophilia A

Specific laboratory tests
- Bioassay

Role in platelet agglutination/ adhesion

Deficiency
Von Willebrand's disease

Specific laboratory tests
- Bioassay (ristocetin cofactor-activity [VIII R.Co] in platelet aggregation in vitro)
- Immunoassay (F VIII R Ag)

Figure 27-4. Structure and inheritance of the factor VIII molecule. The function, the result of deficiency, and the method of testing of the various components are also shown.

symptoms of hemophilia. Plasma factor IX assay shows greatly decreased levels and is diagnostic. Treatment is with fresh plasma or factor IX concentrate; factor IX is not present in cryoprecipitate.

DISSEMINATED INTRAVASCULAR COAGULATION & FIBRINOLYSIS

Disseminated intravascular coagulation (DIC) is an important cause of bleeding that is due to consumption of platelets and several clotting factors during widespread thrombosis in the microcirculation (consumption coagulopathy). DIC and fibrinolysis are discussed in Chapter 9.

28 The Lymphoid System: I. Structure & Function; Infections & Reactive Proliferations

STRUCTURE & FUNCTION

THE LYMPHOCYTE CIRCULATION

The lymphoid system is the anatomic seat of the complex cellular and molecular interactions that make up the immune response (Chapter 4). The cells of the lymphoid system must have access to all parts of the body, both for the detection of and the response to antigen (humoral and cellular immunity). As noted in Chapter 4, lymphocytes bearing antigen receptors, both B and T cells, circulate extensively in the bloodstream. Immune cells that leave the blood in any tissue are collected in lymphatics and passed centrally, often through one or more series of lymph nodes, in which they may pause before reentering the blood. Lymphocytes also enter the lymph nodes directly from the blood through postcapillary venules (Fig 28–1).

LYMPHOID TISSUE

Within the lymphoid system there are several focal concentrations of immune cells (lymph nodes, spleen, tonsils etc) wherein lymphocytes, macrophages, and other immune cells are arranged in a manner advantageous to the various interactions that make up the immune response. It is no accident that major accumulations of lymphoid tissue occur at portals of antigen entry: the tonsils (mouth and nose), the respiratory and gastrointestinal submucosa (for inhaled and ingested antigens), the lymph nodes (for lymph drainage of skin and organs), and the spleen (as the blood filter).

The thymus and bone marrow are often termed **central lymphoid tissues** in that they are central to the development of the immune system in the embryo but do not participate in the immune response in the adult. The remaining lymphoid organs are actively involved in the immune response and constitute the **peripheral lymphoid tissue**.

The detailed microanatomic structure of the principal lymphoid organs has been described in Chapter 4. The intimate juxtaposition of macrophages—which phagocytose and process antigen—and lymphocytes provides for an optimal immune response.

It is important to recognize that this microanatomic arrangement is subject to rapid modification in the presence of an active immune response. The histologic appearances of lymphoid tissue are largely dependent upon the degree of antigenic stimulation. Reactive follicles (foci of B cell pro-

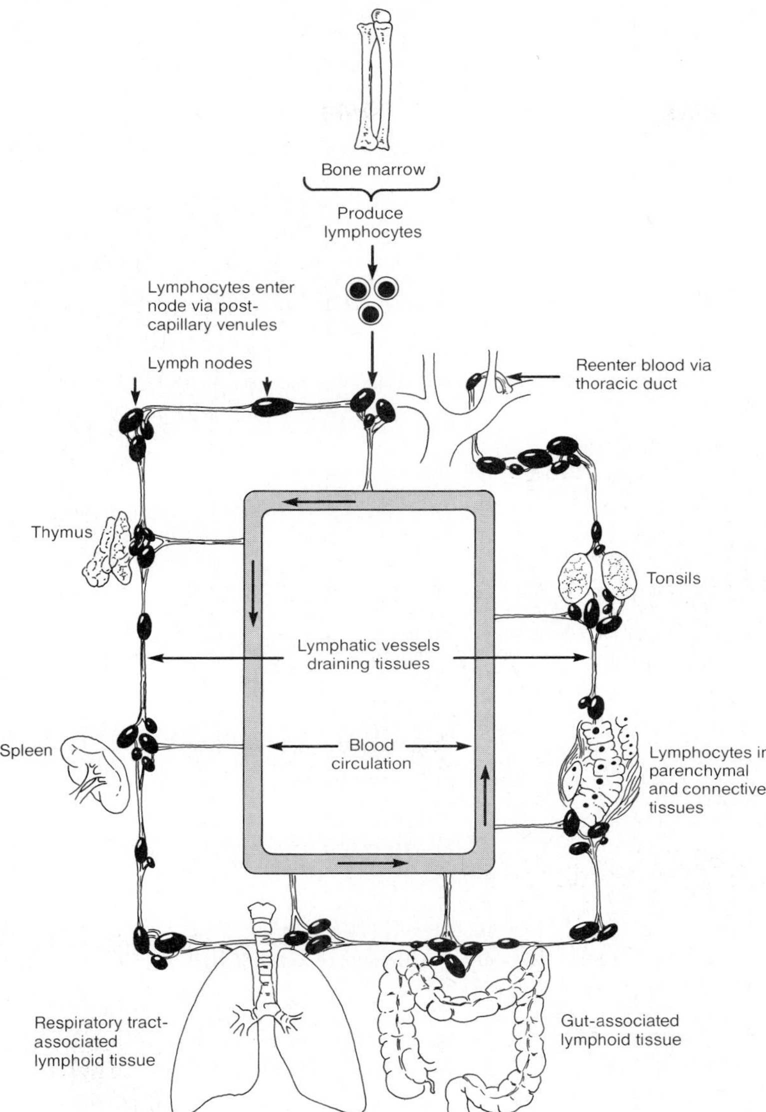

Figure 28–1. The components of the lymphoid system and the circulation of lymphocytes in blood and lymphatic vessels. Obvious lymphoid organs are the lymph nodes, spleen, and thymus. Lymphoid tissue in the tonsils, respiratory tract, gastrointestinal tract, and virtually all tissues of the body contribute heavily to the lymphoid system.

liferation) only appear following exposure to antigen. Likewise, immunoblasts are only present in the face of recent antigenic stimulation, while plasma cells indicate activity of some weeks' duration. The cellularity of the lymph node (ie, the number of immune cells present) and the overall size of the node also depend upon the extent of antigenic stimulation—likewise for the spleen and other lymphoid tissues. A normal lymph node shows some degree of baseline activity owing to the normal low-level antigen load; in the face of an additional antigen load (eg, infection), these changes are greatly exaggerated, usually with a combination of B and T cell responses.

MANIFESTATIONS OF DISEASES OF THE LYMPHOID SYSTEM

IMMUNE DEFICIENCY (Chapter 7)

Depletion of total lymphocytes in the tissues or in peripheral blood (lymphopenia) and abnormalities relating to specific subpopulations of lymphocytes may be associated with defective immunity. For example, decreased T helper cells and increased T suppressor cells, causing reversal of the normal helper:suppressor cell ratio, occurs in acquired immunodeficiency syndrome (AIDS) and in some postinfectious immunodeficiency states. Lymphocyte depletion occurring as a consequence of radiotherapy or administration of cytotoxic drugs or corticosteroids typically is associated with general immunodeficiency, which may be reversible.

Selective atrophy of lymphoid tissues occurs in the congenital immune deficiency syndromes. In the combined immune deficiency syndrome (Swiss type), both T and B zones are depleted, while in Bruton's agammaglobulinemia, the B cell areas are depleted and the T zones are normal. In DiGeorge's syndrome, the paracortical T zone is depleted in lymph nodes with preservation of follicles (B cell zones).

PERVERTED IMMUNE FUNCTION (Chapter 8)

Immunologic hypersensitivity and autoimmunity are manifestations of an abnormal immune response that leads to disease. There may be some proliferation of lymphoid tissue in these conditions, but the primary pathologic features and clinical effects occur in the organs that are the target of the abnormal immune response.

LYMPHADENOPATHY (Table 28-1)

The term "lymphadenopathy" signifies enlarged lymph nodes. Lymphadenopathy may be localized to one lymph node group in the body or may be generalized, affecting multiple groups of lymph nodes all over the body. Conditions that cause generalized lymphadenopathy may also involve lymphoid tissues elsewhere (eg, splenomegaly). In the same way, because of the extensive circulation of lymphoid cells, the peripheral blood may also show increased numbers of lymphocytes (lymphocytosis; see below).

Table 28-1. Causes of lymphadenopathy.[1]

Causes
Reactive hyperplasia (the immune response)
Nonspecific
Usually a local response to introduction of antigen, most commonly bacterial (eg, strep throat, syphilis, plague), or postvaccination, or draining a cancer site
Occasionally generalized, as a response to viremia (eg, rubella) or drug hypersensitivity
With specific features
Dermatopathic lymphadenitis
Lymphangiography reaction
Persistent generalized lymphadenopathy (AIDS-related complex)
Reactive hyperplasia (associated with specific infections)
Pyogenic lymphadenitis
Measles
Infectious mononucleosis
Toxoplasmosis
Granulomatous (eg, tuberculosis, histoplasmosis, coccidioidomycosis)
Granulomatous and suppurative (lymphogranuloma venereum, cat scratch disease)
Lymphadenopathy of uncertain cause
Sarcoidosis
With autoimmune diseases and hypersensitivity states (eg, rheumatoid arthritis, systemic lupus erythematosus, polyarteritis nodosa, serum sickness)
Sinus histiocytosis with massive lymphadenopathy
Giant lymph node hyperplasia
Abnormal immune response and immunoblastic lymphadenopathy
Primary neoplastic proliferations: the lymphomas
Non-Hodgkin's lymphomas and lymphocytic leukemias
Hodgkin's disease
Neoplasms of histiocytes
Secondary neoplasms: metastases
Carcinoma
Melanoma

[1]Most of the conditions listed may also affect lymphoid tissue elsewhere (eg, spleen, gut-associated lymphoid tissue).

LYMPHOCYTOSIS

The number of circulating lymphocytes in the peripheral blood may be increased either as a function of the immune response or as a result of neoplastic proliferation of lymphoid cells in lymphocytic leukemia and lymphoma. In leukemia, the bone marrow is always involved also, while lymphoma may or may not involve the marrow. The distinction between lymphocytic leukemias and lymphomas is somewhat arbitrary, based upon the site of clinical presentation and the extent of involvement of blood or marrow (leukemia) or lymph nodes and tissues (lymphoma).

MONOCLONAL GAMMOPATHY

Neoplasms of B cell derivation that show evidence of plasmacytoid differentiation (myeloma, plasmacytoid lymphocytic lymphoma, heavy chain disease) may secrete sufficient amounts of monoclonal immunoglobulin for this to be detectable in the serum as a discrete "spike" or M (malignant) protein—a monoclonal gammopathy (Chapter 30). The presence of such a monoclonal gammopathy provides a means of diagnosis and is of value in monitoring response to therapy of these neoplasms.

SPLENOMEGALY (Chapter 30)

Splenomegaly is enlargement of the spleen beyond the normal adult range of 120–160 g. In a lean patient, a spleen weighing 300 g or more usually is palpable.

Splenomegaly is often a result of the same factors that cause lymphadenopathy (Table 28–1), particularly acute and chronic infections that have a blood-borne phase (infectious mononucleosis, malaria). However, the spleen also is a highly vascular organ and may become enlarged owing to simple congestion or involvement by proliferating hematopoietic cells, as in the leukemias.

THYMIC ATROPHY & THYMIC ENLARGEMENT

The thymus reaches maximum size in relation to the whole body in fetal life and maximum absolute size in childhood. Thereafter, involution occurs, with gradual loss of lymphocytes and replacement by fibrofatty tissue. In the adult, the thymus weighs approximately 30 g, is essentially nonfunctional, and with rare exceptions does not participate in immunoproliferative responses.

Thymic agenesis or atrophy is characteristic of some of the immunodeficiency states described in Chapter 7; cell-mediated (T cell) immunity is affected.

Thymic hyperplasia is a rare event but is characteristic of certain "autoimmune" diseases, most commonly myasthenia gravis. The only other notable causes of thymic enlargement relate to primary or secondary neoplasms in the thymus or the occasional presence of thymic cysts (Chapter 30).

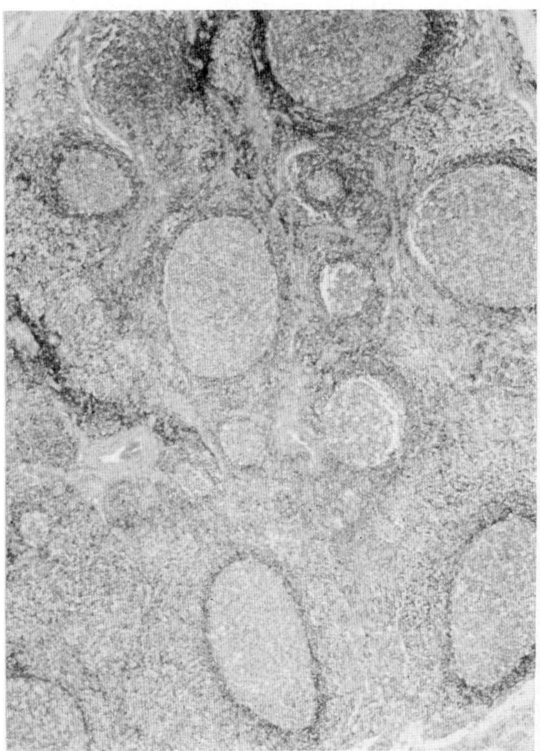

Figure 28–2. Reactive hyperplasia of a lymph node showing features of a predominantly B cell response, characterized by enlarged follicles with prominent reactive centers.

REACTIVE LYMPHOID HYPERPLASIAS

NONSPECIFIC REACTIVE HYPERPLASIA

Reactive hyperplasia within lymphoid tissue represents the tissue manifestation of the immune response and consists of 3 interrelated elements: (1) follicular hyperplasia (the B cell response), (2) paracortical hyperplasia (the T cell response), and (3) sinus histiocytosis (the histiocyte [macrophage] response). In practice, any one of these may predominate, but most responses represent an admixture of all three.

In B cell hyperplasia, the reactive follicles are usually large and conspicuous (Fig 28–2), consisting of actively proliferating B cells among which are scattered variable numbers of histiocytes and dendritic reticulum cells. The reactive follicles develop from small clusters of B cells, sometimes called **primary follicles,** in the outer part (cortex) of the lymph node. The first phase of follicular formation appears to be the trapping of antigen by dendritic reticulum cells, which then serve to stimulate local B cell proliferation, leading to development of a collection of actively transforming B lymphocytes (the secondary or reactive follicle).

A similar reaction occurs among T cells in the paracortex following trapping of antigen by interdigitating reticulum cells. In some instances, the T cell response may predominate; follicles may then be inconspicuous. This type of response particularly is seen in viral infections or postvaccination, eg, in lymph nodes draining the vaccination site.

Lymph nodes draining a malignant neoplasm frequently show reactive hyperplasia, and in many instances the most prominent component is marked expansion of the sinuses, which are filled with histiocytes **(sinus histiocytosis).**

Many cases of nonspecific reactive hyperplasia

are localized in that the antigen source also is confined to a particular region of the body. An example is enlargement of lymph nodes in the neck in conjunction with streptococcal pharyngitis. Generalized reactive hyperplasia may occur with an antigen that is distributed throughout the body, eg, in the viremic phase of viral infections, of which rubella is an excellent example.

SPECIFIC REACTIVE HYPERPLASIAS

In some instances, the general changes of reactive hyperplasia are associated with "specific" features that suggest a particular cause.

1. DERMATOPATHIC LYMPHADENITIS

Dermatopathic lymphadenitis is a form of reactive hyperplasia occurring in lymph nodes draining skin that has suffered chronic damage, such as chronic radiation dermatitis, psoriasis, and exfoliative dermatitis. The most conspicuous feature is the presence of numerous pale histiocytes containing lipid material and melanin released by the damaged epidermis.

2. LYMPHANGIOGRAPHY-ALTERED LYMPH NODES

Lymph nodes may show florid hyperplasia of histiocytes following lymphangiographic examination with lipid-containing contrast media. The histiocytes contain globules of the oily dye in the cytoplasm. This is of importance only in that it may obscure underlying pathologic processes.

3. PERSISTENT GENERALIZED LYMPHADENOPATHY

Acquired immunodeficiency syndrome (AIDS) has been described elsewhere in relation to immunodeficiency states (Chapter 7). Patients who are at risk for AIDS commonly show persistent enlargement of lymph nodes, often generalized and often associated with fever. These patients, who do not have AIDS as defined by the clinical criteria for the disease, nonetheless have antibodies for the human immunodeficiency virus (HIV), and the virus can often be isolated from involved lymph nodes. The T helper:suppressor cell ratio is reversed in blood. Persistent generalized lymphadenopathy is one of the manifestations of what is called the **AIDS-related complex (ARC).**

At present in the United States, it is estimated that there are 2 million people who have contracted the virus and give a positive serum test for HIV antibody. Of these, 10% have evidence of persistent generalized lymphadenopathy or ARC, while 1% have definitive AIDS. The percentage of HIV antibody-positive individuals without overt disease who proceed to develop persistent generalized lymphadenopathy or AIDS is not known, but it is believed that about 25% of persistent generalized lymphadenopathy patients progress to AIDS. The proportion may rise with a longer lapse of time.

Histologically, the lymph nodes in persistent generalized lymphadenopathy show follicular and paracortical hyperplasia, with very large conspicuous follicles in the early stages. Irregular loss or fragmentation of the mantle zone (the rim of small lymphocytes around the follicle) is characteristic. The helper:suppressor ratio typically is reversed in the nodes. (In other forms of reactive hyperplasia, T helper cells predominate in the lymph node.) In later stages, there is progressive depletion of lymphoid cells.

It should be emphasized that lymph nodes from patients with AIDS have identical histologic appearances, the only difference being that patients in the latter group have in addition the criteria for AIDS as defined by the Centers for Disease Control (see Chapter 7).

SPECIFIC INFECTIONS OF LYMPH NODES

Infections of the lymph nodes combine (1) features of the immune response to microbial antigens, (2) features of inflammation, and (3) specific changes that may be produced by the infectious agent. The presence of the specific agent in the lymph nodes often permits diagnosis by culture of the node, which should be requested at the time of biopsy.

ACUTE PYOGENIC (BACTERIAL) LYMPHADENITIS

Bacterial lymphadenitis is usually secondary to the spread of bacteria via lymphatics from a focus of infection in the area drained by the node. Acute inflammation with neutrophil infiltration of the node causes lymph node enlargement, pain, and tenderness. Fever is commonly present, as is a neutrophil leukocytosis in peripheral blood. Abscess formation is common. Precise diagnosis requires culture.

MEASLES

As noted above, in viral lymphadenitis, there is a marked T cell response with expansion of the paracortical zone. The follicles are usually widely separated and inconspicuous. Specific features may be present in some viral infections.

Measles is characterized by the presence of large multinucleated cells called Warthin-Finkeldey giant cells, which are thought to represent lymphocytes that have either fused or have failed to complete cytoplasmic cleavage during cell division.

INFECTIOUS MONONUCLEOSIS

Infectious mononucleosis is also characterized by a florid T cell hyperplasia, often so extensive that the follicles are totally obscured. In addition, the number of immunoblasts and T cells in intermediate stages of transformation is so high that the node may appear to be totally replaced by large cells (Figs 28–3 and 28–4), leading to possible misdiagnosis as malignant lymphoma. These large transformed lymphocytes are the same cells that appear in increased numbers in the peripheral blood (so-called Downey cells) from which the name infectious mononucleosis is derived. (The term mononucleosis was used when the disease was first described, since the nature of these large primitive-appearing mononuclear cells was unknown.)

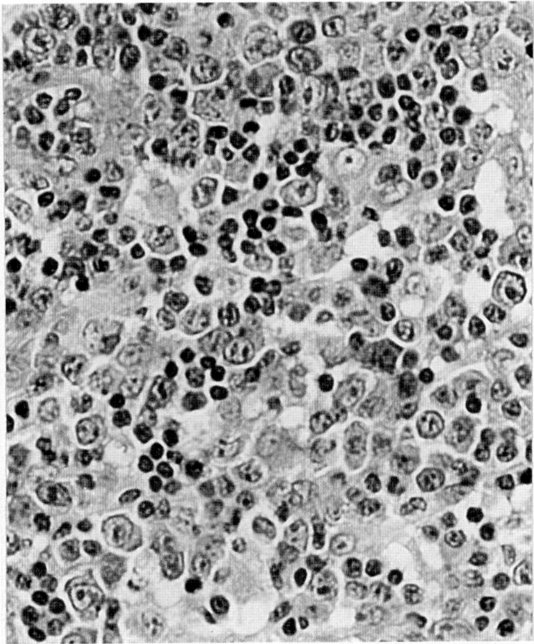

Figure 28–3. Infectious mononucleosis involving a lymph node. This is a high-magnification photograph showing the expanded paracortical region and T cells in different stages of transformation. Numerous large nuclei with prominent nucleoli scattered throughout the region represent T immunoblasts.

Infectious mononucleosis is caused by the **Epstein-Barr virus,** which specifically infects B cells (which have a receptor for the EB virus on their surface). Infected B cells then express viral antigens on their surfaces to which the T cells mount a vigorous immune response (Fig 28–4). The histologic appearance of infectious mononucleosis may be mimicked closely by other acute viral illnesses, including infection with cytomegalovirus, hepatitis virus, herpes simplex (type 2), rubella, and adenovirus; or by vaccination with attenuated live viruses.

Infectious mononucleosis is more common in children and young adults and is transmitted via the upper respiratory tract, commonly through kissing ("kissing disease"). Patients present with acute onset of fever, sore throat, lymphadenopathy, and hepatosplenomegaly. Mild liver dysfunction may be present. The disease is often milder in young children and more severe in young adults.

Infectious mononucleosis may be diagnosed by the peripheral blood appearance (lymphocytosis with Downey cells) but should be confirmed serologically as described below. Lymph node biopsy is not necessary in the face of serologic confirmation unless there is continuing enlargement of lymph nodes in the face of clinical resolution of the viral infection.

The traditional serologic test for infectious mononucleosis is the detection of heterophil antibodies by the **Paul-Bunnell test,** of which the Monospot test is a well-known example. Heterophil antibodies are cross-reactive with a variety of different tissues in different species and are not specific for infectious mononucleosis. Their detection, however, does provide a useful screening test.

Recently, tests for specific antibodies against EB virus antigens have become available, and these now represent the most specific tests for infectious mononucleosis. IgM antibody to **viral capsid antigen** (VCA) appears early in the disease, followed by IgG antibodies that persist over a long period; antibodies to Epstein-Barr membrane antigen (MA) and nuclear antigen (EBNA) appear late but persist for life.

TOXOPLASMOSIS

Toxoplasmosis is a relatively common illness caused by a protozoon, *Toxoplasma gondii,* which commonly infects cats, rodents, and livestock. Human infection is usually acquired by ingestion of oocysts from soil contaminated by cat feces. (Changing cat litter boxes daily is an effective preventive measure, since the oocysts only become in-

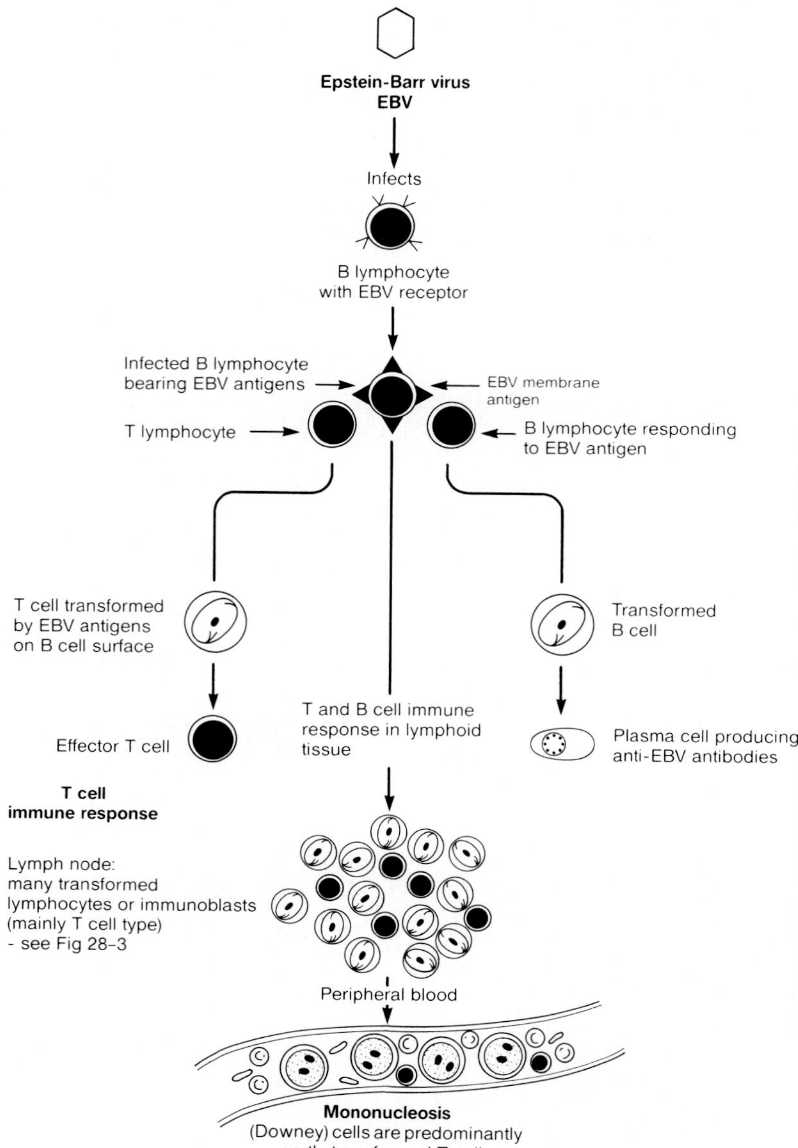

Figure 28–4. Pathogenesis and pathologic features of infectious mononucleosis.

fective for humans about a week after passage by the cat.) Less often, infection may be by ingestion of tissue cysts from undercooked pork. Because of the danger of transplacental infection of the fetus, pregnant women are advised to avoid contact with cats, kittens, and their excreta.

Acquired toxoplasmosis, which occurs in the adult, presents as an acute febrile illness with malaise and generalized lymphadenopathy resembling infectious mononucleosis. The illness may be so mild as to be asymptomatic. The presence of enlarged lymph nodes may lead to lymph node biopsy.

Histologically, the changes are quite characteristic, with extensive follicular hyperplasia and histiocytic proliferation; the histiocytes typically occur in clusters in the paracortex and within reactive centers (Fig 28–5). The pseudocysts of *Toxoplasma* may be seen occasionally; tachyzoites are almost never seen. Immunohistologic techniques using specific antibody are helpful in detecting the organisms.

Congenital toxoplasmosis is a much more serious condition in which infection is transmitted transplacentally from mother to fetus. It is characterized by necrosis in the brain, often severe, and retinal involvement. Organisms are seen in large numbers in both brain and retina in such

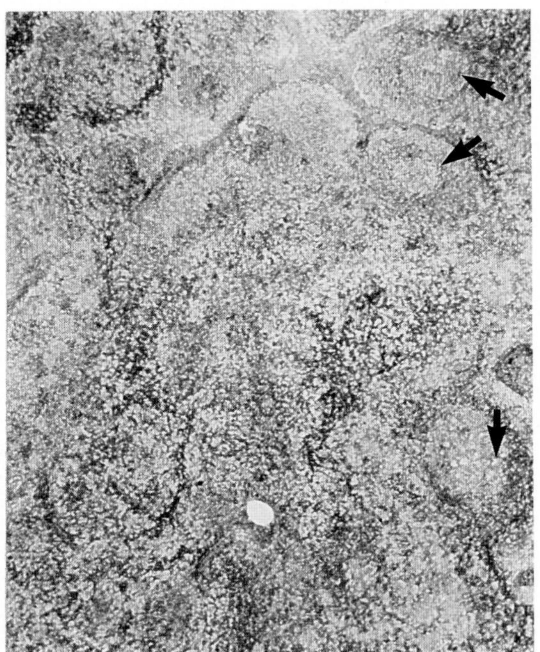

Figure 28–5. Toxoplasmosis involving a lymph node. The enlarged lymph node shows hyperplastic follicles as well as an expanded paracortical region. The follicles are poorly defined (arrows). A feature is the presence of numerous histiocytes seen in the reactive follicles as well as the paracortex.

cases. Congenital toxoplasmosis may cause stillbirth, microcephaly, hydrocephalus, and blindness in the neonatal period; or delayed neurologic and learning defects.

Diagnosis is by serologic techniques or isolation of the organism by animal inoculation (intraperitoneally into mice). The standard serologic test is the Sabin-Feldman dye test: serum containing anti-*Toxoplasma* antibody renders living *Toxoplasma* permeable to methylene blue. This test is being replaced by more sensitive fluorescence or enzyme-linked immunoassay (ELISA) tests, which do not require the use of live organisms.

GRANULOMATOUS LYMPHADENITIS

The immune response against facultative intracellular organisms is mediated by T cells, lymphokines, and macrophages and results in the formation of **epithelioid granulomas** (Chapter 5). Superimposed delayed hypersensitivity associated with the T cell response results in caseous necrosis.

The organisms most commonly responsible for caseous granulomatous lymphadenitis are *Mycobacterium tuberculosis,* atypical mycobacteria, *Histoplasma capsulatum*, and *Coccidioides immitis,* the relative frequency varying widely in different parts of the world. Lymphadenopathy usually affects only one or 2 lymph node groups, representing those nodes draining the sites of primary infection. Cervical nodes are most commonly affected. Lymphadenopathy may be the only manifestation of the disease, or lymph node involvement may be secondary to known disease elsewhere.

Histologically, the paracortical T cell response predominates. Granulomas may be small, or large and coalescent (Figs 28–6 and 28–7), with caseous necrosis replacing the entire lymph node. Marked fibrosis is commonly present.

Diagnosis is by culture. Mycobacteria may be demonstrated in histologic sections using special acid fast stains (Ziehl-Neelsen); in classic tuberculosis, organisms are few, but in atypical mycobacterial infections occurring in the elderly or immunodeficient host, numerous mycobacteria are present in the lesions. *Histoplasma* (a dimorphic soil fungus) may be seen intracellularly as 2–4 μm yeasts by silver staining. Coccidioidomycosis typically forms refractile spherules (30–80 μm in diameter) packed with endospores (Fig 28–8).

Consistent with histologic evidence of delayed hypersensitivity, these infections are associated with delayed hypersensitivity type skin tests (PPD and tuberculin for *M tuberculosis;* histoplasmin for *H capsulatum;* coccidioidin for *C immitis).* Serologic (complement fixation) tests are available for the diagnosis of histoplasmosis and coccidioidomycosis.

SUPPURATIVE GRANULOMATOUS LYMPHADENITIS

In suppurative granulomatous lymphadenitis, the histologic appearances are much the same as for granulomatous lymphadenopathy, described above, but with the addition of acute inflammation and suppuration, with neutrophils in the center of the granulomas. The fully formed suppurative granuloma tends to be stellate (star-shaped). Several different organisms may produce this form of lymphadenopathy, which usually is localized to the site of infection (eg, in cat-scratch disease, the nodes draining the site of the skin scratch are involved; in lymphogranuloma venereum, groin nodes are involved). Note that these organisms may also cause granulomatous lymphadenitis without suppurative features.

1. LYMPHOGRANULOMA VENEREUM

Lymphogranuloma venereum (LGV) is a sexually transmitted disease, most common in tropical

A

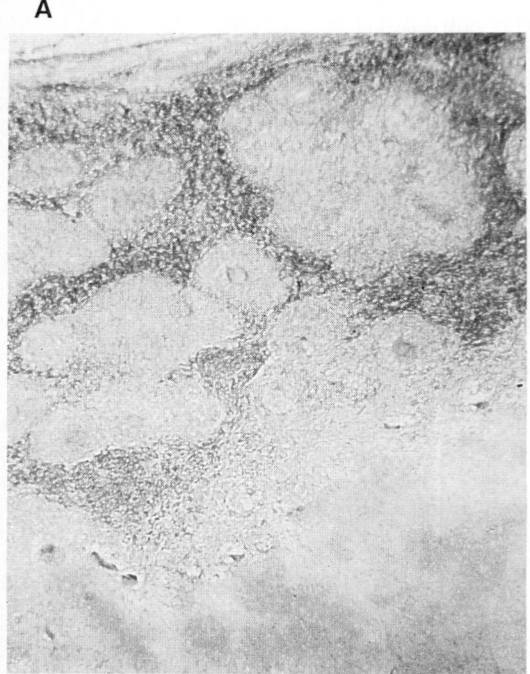

B

Figure 28-6. Granulomatous lymphadenitis. A: Low magnification showing coalescent epithelioid cell granulomas with caseous necrosis present at the bottom edge. B: High magnification showing epithelioid cells and Langhans type giant cells. Culture of node tissue was positive for *Mycobacterium tuberculosis*.

areas, caused by a strain of *Chlamydia trachomatis*. A local papule at the site of infection on the external genitalia is typically followed by marked regional lymphadenopathy, with suppuration and discharge of pus through multiple sinuses. The diagnosis may be suspected histologically (stellate granulomas) and confirmed serologically (complement fixation test) or by skin test (using heat-inactivated LGV for intradermal injection). Sulfonamides and tetracycline are effective treatment.

2. CAT-SCRATCH DISEASE

Cat-scratch disease is an uncommon cause of suppurative granulomas in lymph nodes. It is caused by a small gram-negative bacterium that stains positively with silver stains. The disease is manifested as acute onset of fever with lymphadenopathy. A history of a wound and exposure to cats is common. The diagnosis is clinical, confirmed by the pathologic features and demonstration of the organism by special stains and culture. A skin test utilizing heat-inactivated pus from known cases is positive in most individuals with the disease but also in about 10% of veterinarians with no history of the disease. The condition is self-limited.

3. OTHER CAUSES

Other infections that may produce suppurative granulomatous lymphadenitis include (1) mesenteric lymphadenitis in young children due to Yersinia enterocolitica and *Yersinia pseudotuberculosis;* (2) brucellosis, caused by various species of *Brucella;* (3) tularemia, due to *Pasteurella tularensis;* (4) plague, due to *Yersinia pestis* (the bubonic form of the disease affects lymph nodes draining the site of the flea bite); and (5) glanders and melioidosis, caused by *Pseudomonas* mallei and *Pseudomonas pseudomallei.*

All of these organisms are short gram-negative rods; in all, there may be a septicemic phase, and lymphadenopathy with suppuration (bubo formation) may occur. The severity of disease is variable, plague being the most severe.

LYMPHADENOPATHY OF UNCERTAIN CAUSE

SARCOIDOSIS

Sarcoidosis is a systemic disease characterized by the presence of noninfectious epithelioid cell

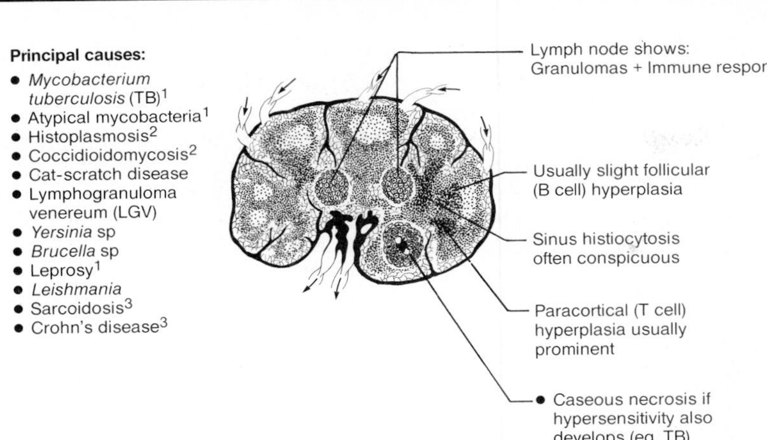

Figure 28–7. Granulomatous lymphadenitis. **Note 1:** Tuberculosis, atypical mycobacteriosis, and leprosy may be positive with acid-fast stains. **Note 2:** Histoplasmosis and coccidioidomycosis may be positive with fungal stains. **Note 3:** Sarcoidosis and Crohn's disease produce noncaseating epithelioid cell granulomas. Crohn's disease usually involves abdominal lymph nodes.

granulomas in many tissues, particularly lung, liver, lymph nodes, and skin. It ranges from asymptomatic to a severe febrile debilitating illness with cough and dyspnea, characterized by a chronic course with remissions and relapses. It is more common in men than in women, in blacks than in whites, and in the age group from 20 to 30 years. The incidence is high in Scandinavia, Western Europe, and North America.

Histologically, the granulomas resemble those occurring in tuberculosis and fungal infections except for the absence of caseous necrosis in sarcoid granulomas (Fig 28–7). Sarcoid granulomas frequently contain calcified bodies called Schaumann bodies. These are not specific for sarcoidosis. No etiologic agent has been identified.

Immunologically, patients with sarcoidosis show depressed cell-mediated immunity (eg, loss of positive skin tests to tuberculin, mumps antigen), excessive B cell activity (hyperglobulinemia), and sometimes an excess of helper T cells. The **Kveim test** (a skin test utilizing an extract of known sarcoid tissue) is usually positive.

Berylliosis produces a histologic picture identical to that of sarcoidosis, and a history of beryllium exposure should be excluded before a diagnosis of sarcoidosis is made. Similar granulomas may be found in intravenous drug users due to contaminants (especially talc) in the materials used. In these cases, the diagnosis can be made by identification of beryllium or talc in the granuloma.

LYMPHADENOPATHY OF AUTOIMMUNE DISEASE

As described in Chapter 8, the autoimmune diseases are a diverse group of disorders in which the underlying pathogenesis is believed to involve some form of immune reaction against the patient's own tissues.

Lymphadenopathy is not a conspicuous feature of most autoimmune diseases. However, significant lymph node enlargement may be seen in systemic lupus erythematosus, rheumatoid arthritis—particularly the juvenile form (Still's disease; Chapter 68)—and Sjögren's syndrome (Chapter 33).

In **systemic lupus erythematosus** and **rheumatoid arthritis,** affected lymph nodes show nonspecific follicular hyperplasia, with occasional evidence of vasculitis. In **Still's disease,** the lymphadenopathy may be the presenting clinical feature. **Sjögren's syndrome** may occur alone or in conjunction with SLE or rheumatoid arthritis. Lymphadenopathy is frequently present and typically shows a diffuse hyperplasia with inconspicuous follicles. Immunoblasts may be so numerous as to lead to a mistaken diagnosis of lymphoma. True lymphoma rarely supervenes.

Hypersensitivity states such as serum sickness and chronic drug reactions (eg, reactions to aminosalicylic acid [PAS], an antituberculous drug) may also produce lymphadenopathy, with features of mixed B and T cell response.

SINUS HISTIOCYTOSIS WITH MASSIVE LYMPHADENOPATHY

This condition is uncommon outside North Africa. In the United States, it occurs mainly in blacks. The cause is unknown. Children are mainly affected, and clinical presentation is with massive cervical lymphadenopathy, often bilateral. Affected children may have fever and mild

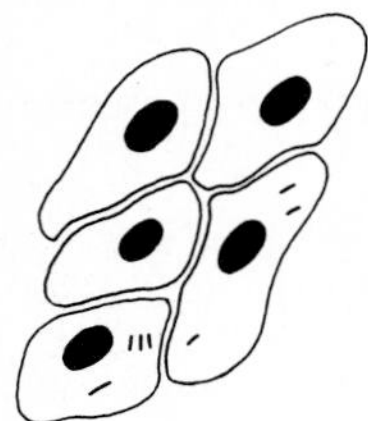

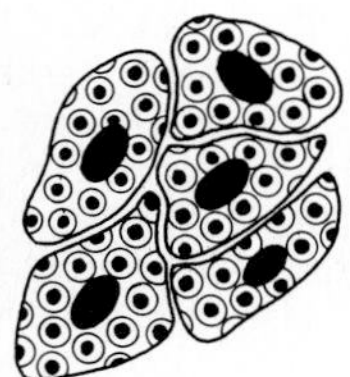

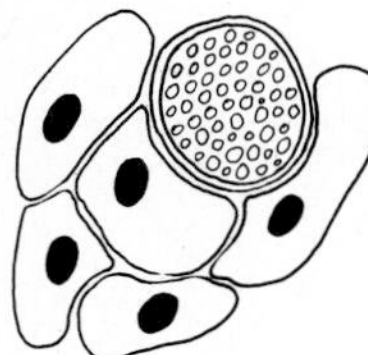

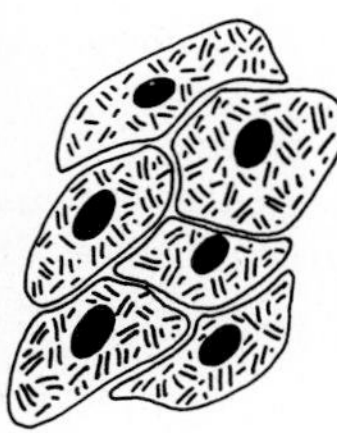

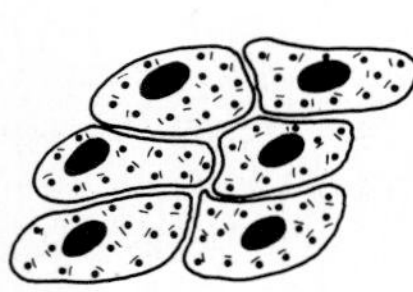

Figure 28-8. Common causative agents of granulomatous lymphadenitis, showing their morphologic characteristics and stains used for their identification in tissue sections. **Note 1:** Acid-fast stains include Ziehl-Neelsen stain for *M tuberculosis* and Fite's stain for *M leprae*. **Note 2:** Commonly used stains for fungi include methenamine silver and periodic acid Schiff (PAS) stains. Note that fungi can also be seen in routine hematoxylin and eosin-stained sections.

anemia but do not appear ill. The disease is self-limited.

The histologic picture is remarkable in that affected lymph nodes contain large numbers of cytologically benign-appearing histiocytes filling the sinuses. The histiocytes contain normal-appearing lymphocytes within their cytoplasm (this phenomenon of live cell ingestion is called "emperipolesis"); its significance is unknown.

GIANT LYMPH NODE HYPERPLASIA (Castleman-Iverson Disease)

Giant lymph node hyperplasia is an uncommon condition characterized by benign nonprogressive lymphadenopathy, usually in the mediastinum or retroperitoneum. There has been debate about whether this disease represents a hamartoma (developmental abnormality) or some form of chronic immune response to an agent or agents unknown. Two variants are recognized: plasmacellular and angiofollicular. It is unclear whether these variants represent 2 separate diseases or are 2 ends of a spectrum of changes.

In the **plasmacellular form** of giant lymph node hyperplasia, the lymph nodes show large follicles with numerous plasma cells in the remainder of the lymph node. The plasma cells are polyclonal (ie, reactive) in almost all cases. There is often an associated polyclonal hyperglobulinemia and low-grade fever; both return to normal on resection of the involved nodes. A small number of cases progress to malignant lymphoma.

In the **angiofollicular form** of giant lymph node hyperplasia, there are numerous small follicles associated with excessive numbers of peculiar hyalinized vessels. This form is not believed to be associated with an increased incidence of malignant lymphoma.

ANGIOIMMUNOBLASTIC LYMPHADENOPATHY

Angioimmunoblastic lymphadenopathy (or immunoblastic lymphadenopathy which represents a narrower definition of the same process) is a relatively uncommon condition primarily affecting older patients (over 50 years of age). Patients are debilitated, with weight loss, fever, hepatosplenomegaly, skin rashes, and generalized lymphadenopathy. In most studies, 50% of patients have died within 3 years, either of infection or because of development of an aggressive malignant lymphoma (immunoblastic sarcoma) in 15–20%. The cause is unknown.

Histologically, the lymph nodes show progressive depletion of lymphoid cells with obliteration of normal architecture and loss of follicles. Immunoblasts (both B and T) are conspicuous among the residual cells, along with a variable admixture of histiocytes, plasma cells, and eosinophils. There is amorphous cellular debris in the background.

In many instances of generalized lymphadenopathy, some but not all of these features are present. Such cases are said to show an "abnormal immune response" or "atypical hyperplasia." The outcome in such patients is unknown.

The Lymphoid System: II. Malignant Lymphomas

29

THE MALIGNANT LYMPHOMAS

Malignant lymphomas—primary neoplasms of lymphoid tissue derived from lymphocytes—occur as solid tumors, usually within lymph nodes and less often in extranodal lymphoid tissues such as the tonsil, gastrointestinal tract, and spleen.

Malignant lymphomas are classified as **non-Hodgkin's lymphomas,** which are derived from lymphocytes and histiocytes in lymphoid tissue; and **Hodgkin's lymphomas**. Hodgkin's lymphomas have retained their eponymous designation because the cell of origin remains uncertain.

NON-HODGKIN'S LYMPHOMAS

LYMPHOMA VERSUS LEUKEMIA

Neoplastic lymphocytes circulate (mimicking normal lymphocytes) and frequently are found widely distributed throughout the lymphoid tissues. If bone marrow involvement and circulating cells predominate or if they constitute the first recognized manifestation of the disease, the process is termed **leukemia**. If the proliferation dominantly affects the lymphoid tissues or if a tissue mass is the presenting feature, the process is termed **lymphoma.** This distinction is arbitrary, and in children the term lymphoma-leukemia is sometimes used because the 2 forms may coexist and because lymphoma frequently evolves toward a leukemic state (Table 29–1).

MALIGNANT LYMPHOMA VERSUS "BENIGN LYMPHOMA"

The observation that neoplastic lymphocytes circulate extensively—coupled with widespread tissue involvement in many cases—has resulted in classification of all of these conditions as malignant lymphomas. This obscures the fact that many malignant lymphomas have relatively "benign" biologic behavior (ie, are slow-growing and compatible with long survival). The widespread distribution of the disease in the body represents mimicry of normal lymphocyte circulation rather than metastatic potential. Neoplastic proliferation of lymphocytes in one area of the body without the potential for dissemination—to which the term "benign" may be applied—occurs rarely, if at all.

INCIDENCE OF NON-HODGKIN'S LYMPHOMAS

Leukemias and lymphomas, including Hodgkin's lymphoma, account for approximately 8% of all malignant neoplasms and together represent the sixth most common type of cancer. Leukemia-lymphoma is the most common lethal disease of

Table 29-1. Sites of involvement in lymphoma-leukemia.

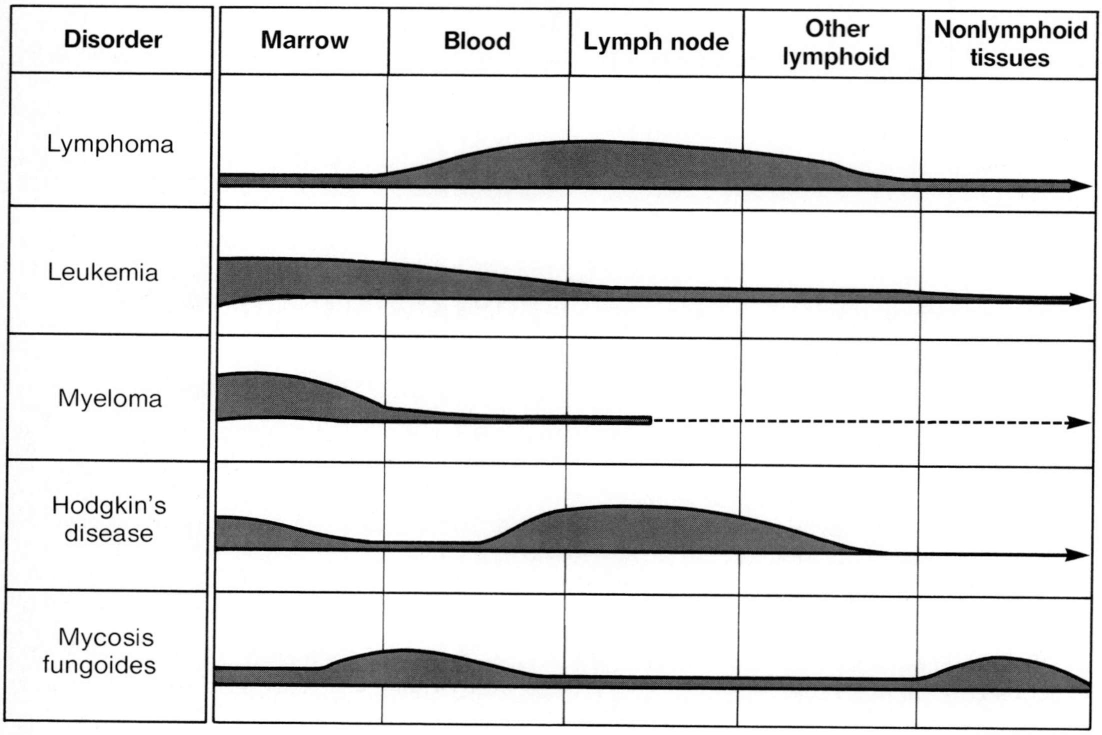

Disorder	Marrow	Blood	Lymph node	Other lymphoid	Nonlymphoid tissues
Lymphoma					
Leukemia					
Myeloma					
Hodgkin's disease					
Mycosis fungoides					

children in the United States. About 25,000 cases of non-Hodgkin's lymphoma occur annually in the United States. The relative incidence of the subtypes of lymphoma varies greatly with age (Table 29-2) and to a lesser extent with sex and geographic factors.

ETIOLOGY OF NON-HODGKIN'S LYMPHOMAS

Many animal lymphomas and leukemias have a viral etiology (eg, feline leukemia, Marek's disease—a leukemialike process—in chickens, bovine leukemia, some murine lymphomas). In humans, the viral relationship is less clear-cut.

Autoimmune & Immunodeficiency Diseases

Autoimmune and immunodeficiency diseases are associated with an increased incidence of lymphoma, presumably related to the sustained or abnormal lymphoproliferation that occurs under these circumstances. The immunodeficiency induced by drugs in transplant recipients is also associated with malignant lymphoma. There is a greatly increased incidence of non-Hodgkin's lymphomas in AIDS.

Epstein-Barr Virus Infection

EBV infection shows a close association with Burkitt's lymphoma in Africa. Burkitt's lymphoma is distributed in Africa in malaria-endemic areas. It has been postulated that EBV infection initiates B cell proliferation, which in the presence of chronic malarial infection escapes control, leading to lymphoma (see Chapter 18).

Table 29-2. Relative incidence of lymphomas in adults and children.

	Adult	Child
Hodgkin's lymphoma	15%	Rare
Follicular center cell[1]	35% (mostly small cleaved)	50% (all small noncleaved including Burkitt's)
Lymphocytic[1]	10%	Rare
Immunoblastic[1]	10%	Rare
Plasmacytoid[1]	10%	Rare
Convoluted[1] (lymphoblastic)	10%	40%
Others	Rare	Rare

[1]Subtypes of non-Hodgkin's lymphoma.

HTLV-I (Human T Lymphotropic Virus I)

HTLV-I shows a strong association with T cell lymphoma-leukemia in Japan and is considered to be causal. A viral cause of Japanese T cell lymphoma was first suspected on the basis of observed clustering of cases in southern Japan. HTLV-II, a related retrovirus, causes some forms of chronic T cell leukemia, and HTLV-V has been implicated in cutaneous T cell lymphomas.

Oncogenes & Chromosomal Markers

Oncogenes and chromosomal markers have been detected in many lymphomas. With improved methods for chromosomal identification, it has become clear that most lymphomas show distinctive chromosomal markers (eg, Burkitt's lymphoma shows an 8;14 translocation). Furthermore, in many cases the breakpoint for the translocation has been shown to be at the insertion point of an oncogene (c-myc oncogene in Burkitt's lymphoma).

DIAGNOSIS OF NON-HODGKIN'S LYMPHOMAS

Neoplastic proliferations of lymphoid cells must be distinguished from the proliferation that occurs normally as part of the immune response (reactive hyperplasia). This distinction is often difficult, and many of the criteria utilized for recognition of neoplasia in other tissue sites, such as cytologic criteria, degree of differentiation, and evidence of spread in the body (Chapter 17), do not apply. Helpful criteria for diagnosis of malignant lymphoma include loss of normal lymph node architecture and evidence of monoclonality.

Cytologic Criteria

The usual cytologic criteria for distinguishing malignant neoplasms are not reliable in identifying a lymphoid proliferation as neoplastic. The degree of cellular pleomorphism in lymphocytes involved in the immune response is often marked. Some lymphocytic neoplasms are pleomorphic; others are not. Cytologic nuclear features such as dispersed chromatin, primitive-appearing nuclei, and the presence of nucleoli are seen both in neoplastic and in reactive immunoblasts (transformed lymphocytes).

Mitotic Rate

The number of mitotic figures is very high in reactive lymph nodes. Malignant lymphomas may or may not have a high mitotic rate.

Degree of Differentiation

In most other tissues, the presence of "poorly differentiated cells" raises a suspicion of malignancy. In the lymphoid system, cells that were once termed "poorly differentiated" in that they show little resemblance to normal small lymphocytes are now known to include normal immunoblasts.

Evidence of Spread in the Body

Both normal and neoplastic lymphocytes circulate extensively. Immunologically reacting cells and neoplastic lymphocytes may be seen in the blood and in distant lymph nodes—and in lymphoid tissues generally. The extent of spread does not correlate, therefore, with the degree of malignancy.

Loss of Normal Lymph Node Architecture

Loss of the normal nodal architecture, particularly if coupled with a lack of the normal admixture of cell types seen in the immune response, is evidence that the lymphoproliferation is neoplastic.

Monoclonality

In the proliferation of lymphoid cells as part of an immune response, several clones of lymphoid cells are involved (polyclonal). The vast majority of neoplastic lymphoid proliferations arise from one clone of lymphocytes (ie, monoclonal). The monoclonal nature of lymphoid proliferation is currently the best evidence for lymphocytic neoplasia and can be established by showing any of the following:

A. The presence of monoclonal light or heavy chain immunoglobulin on the cell surface or in the cytoplasm of a B cell population. The commonest technique utilizes the fact that a polyclonal population of lymphoid cells will have nearly equal numbers of kappa- or lambda-positive cells, whereas a monoclonal population will express exclusively kappa or lambda light chain (Fig 29–1).

B. Clonal immunoglobulin gene rearrangement (B cell).

C. Clonal T receptor gene rearrangement (T cell).

D. Presence of a clonal chromosomal marker (eg, the 8;14 translocation in Burkitt's lymphoma).

NOMENCLATURE & CLASSIFICATION OF NON-HODGKIN'S LYMPHOMAS

It is still true, as Willis wrote in 1948, that "Nowhere in pathology has the chaos of names so clouded clear concepts as in the subject of lymphoid tumors."

Lymphomas show enormous variation in clinical behavior and response to therapy. The aim of classification is to identify homogeneous sub-

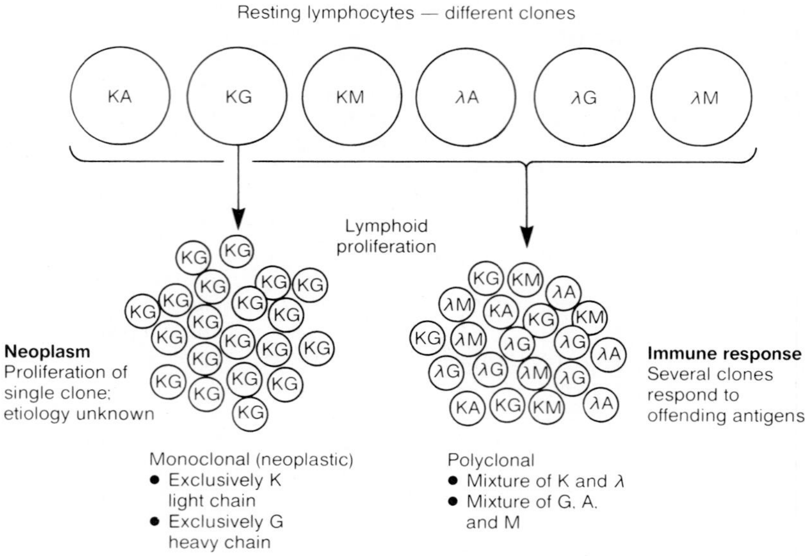

Figure 29-1. Monoclonal versus polyclonal proliferation of B lymphocytes. The monoclonal population contains one type of light and heavy chain (in the example given, kappa and G chains), whereas the polyclonal population consists of lymphocytes containing both kappa and lambda light chains and several different heavy chains.

groups that behave in a predictable way. The lymphomas, like neoplasms of other tissues, are named according to the normal cell they most closely resemble (Fig 29-2); confusion has arisen because the nomenclature of the normal cells of lymphoid tissues has changed several times during this century.

The classification of non-Hodgkin's lymphomas has changed many times in the past several years and will continue to evolve as our understanding of the lymphoid system improves. The following represents a summary of the evolution of the nomenclature, some elements of which are still in use.

Morphologic Classifications

Prior to 1950, the large, primitive-appearing cells (now called immunoblasts) in lymphoid tissues were termed reticulum cells, and it was thought that they served as stem cells for all lymphoid cells—indeed, for all hematopoietic cells. This concept is now acknowledged to be false, and the term "reticulum cell sarcoma," which was used for many large cell lymphomas, has become obsolete.

In 1956, Rappaport and colleagues published a new classification of non-Hodgkin's lymphomas (Table 29-3) based upon the belief that the reticulum cell was actually a form of histiocyte. The corresponding neoplasms were therefore called histiocytic lymphomas. The Rappaport classification was relatively simple and was of clinical value in separating some of the lymphomas into more aggressive and less aggressive types. While still used in many hospitals for its clinical relevance, the Rappaport classification is scientifically inaccurate and will eventually be replaced by one of the immune-based classifications.

Immune-Based Classifications

As modern immunologic concepts developed, several different immune-based classifications were proposed. Of these, that of Lukes and Collins (1974) is widely used in the United States, while the Kiel classification (Lennert, 1974) is prevalent in Europe. These classifications are conceptually similar, and the simpler Lukes-Collins classification is presented here (Table 29-4).

Table 29-3. The Rappaport classification (morphologic) of non-Hodgkin's lymphoma.

Type of Lymphoma[1]	Cells of Origin[2]
Well-differentiated lymphocytic lymphoma	Small T lymphocyte Small B lymphocyte Effector T lymphocyte
Poorly differentiated lymphocytic lymphoma	Stem cell (nonmarking lymphoblast) Embryonic T lymphoblast Embryonic B lymphoblast Follicular center B cells
Mixed	Follicular center B cells
Histiocytic lymphoma[3]	T immunoblast B immunoblast Follicular center B cell True histiocyte

[1]Any of these types could occur in a follicular or a diffuse pattern, the former having a more favorable prognosis.
[2]As currently understood; see Fig 29-2.
[3]Note that "histiocytic" lymphomas, as the term is used here, are mainly derived from activated lymphocytes. True histiocytic lymphomas are extremely rare.

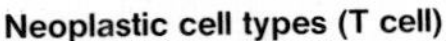

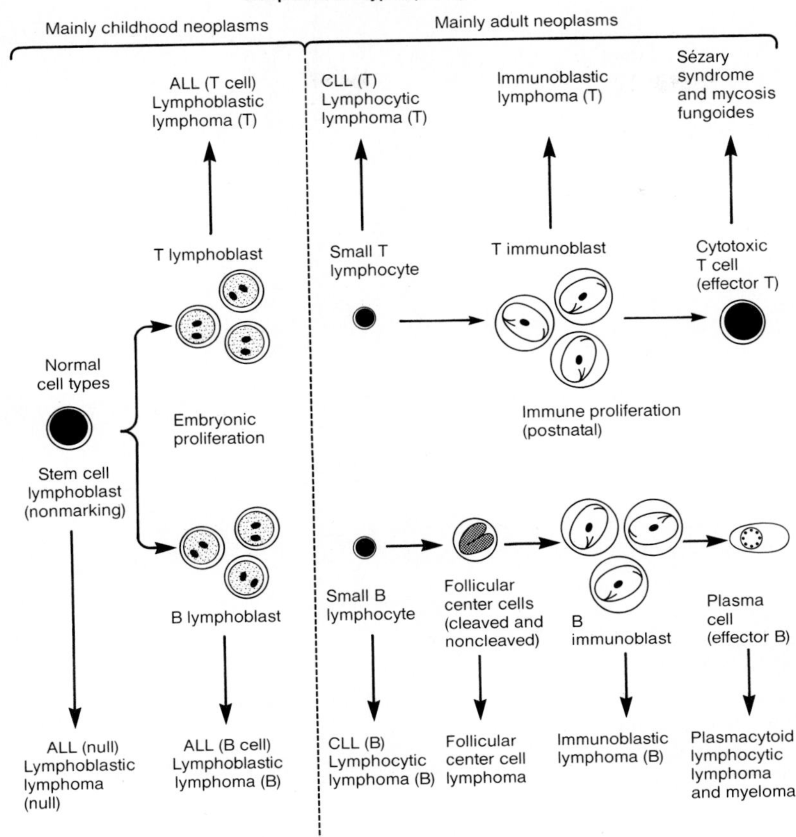

Figure 29-2. Lymphomas and leukemias derived from lymphocytes, showing relationships of the neoplastic lymphoid cells to normal lymphocyte counterparts. The cells drawn in the central area represent normal embryonic and adult lymphoid cells. Neoplasms derived from these cells are shown at top (T cell neoplasms) and bottom (B cell neoplasms). ALL = acute lymphoblastic leukemia; CLL = chronic lymphocytic leukemia.

While these immune-based classifications fit the theoretic concepts of development of lymphoid cells, they have not gained widespread acceptance because of their complexity and the need for ancillary tests to reach precise diagnoses.

At present, newly developed immunologic techniques such as surface marker phenotyping with monoclonal antibodies, gene rearrangement studies in B and T lymphocytes, and studies relating to oncogenes are being extensively used (Table 29-5) in the study of malignant lymphomas. It is expected that the information provided by these studies will lead to further evolution in the classification of these neoplasms.

The Working Formulation Classification (Table 29-6)

In 1975, in an attempt to resolve the many conflicts in classifying non-Hodgkin's lymphomas, the National Cancer Institute sponsored a multi-institutional study that resulted in a classification system called "The Working Formulation of Non-Hodgkin's Lymphoma for Clinical Usage." This classification is currently in use in the United States.

The Working Formulation sorts non-Hodgkin's lymphomas into 3 main prognostic groups: (1) low-grade lymphomas, which are clinically indolent diseases with long median survival times but rarely cured by therapy; (2) intermediate-grade lymphomas; and (3) high-grade lymphomas, which have an aggressive natural history but are responsive to chemotherapy and, as more effective treatment protocols are developed, are potentially curable.

The Working Formulation is primarily a morphologic and clinical classification. As immunologic information accumulates, there is no doubt that this classification will change. Furthermore, as newer lymphoma subtypes are recognized, they will be added to the basic classification in the appropriate prognostic group, depending on their clinical course.

Table 29-4. The Lukes-Collins (immune-based) classification of non-Hodgkin's lymphoma (modified).

Neoplasm	Corresponding Normal Cell
Nonmarking cells[1]	
Acute lymphoblastic leukemia (ALL; null cell) Lymphoblastic lymphoma (null)	Stem cell (nonmarking lymphoblast)
T cells	
Convoluted T cell lymphoma T cell ALL	T cell lymphoblast
T-cell chronic lymphocytic leukemia (CLL)/lymphocytic lymphoma	Small T cell lymphocyte
T-cell immunoblastic lymphoma[2]	T cell immunoblast
Mycosis fungoides/Sézary syndrome	Effector T cell
B cells	
B cell ALL B-cell lymphoblastic lymphoma	B lymphoblast
B cell CLL/lymphocytic lymphoma	Small B lymphocyte
Follicular center cell lymphoma	Follicular center B cell[3]
B-cell immunoblastic lymphoma[2]	B immunoblast
Plasmacytoid lymphocytic lymphoma	Effector B cell
Histiocyte	
True histiocytic lymphoma	Histiocyte

[1]Nonmarking category was designated as U (or undefined) in original classification.
[2]Immunoblastic lymphoma is sometimes called immunoblastic sarcoma.
[3]The follicular center contains several morphologic variants of the B lymphocyte, including small cleaved, large cleaved, small noncleaved, and large noncleaved cells. Follicular center cell lymphomas corresponding to these cell types have been recognized. Burkitt's lymphoma is usually included in this category; others would place it under B lymphoblastic. These are closely related categories (see Fig 29-2), and the decision is somewhat arbitrary.

SPECIFIC TYPES OF NON-HODGKIN'S LYMPHOMAS

The different types of non-Hodgkin's lymphomas have greatly differing clinical and histologic features. The more important types are set forth in Table 29-7 and illustrated in Figs 29-3 to 29-6.

1. B CELL LYMPHOMAS

B cell lymphomas are common. Most of them arise from the follicular center in lymph nodes

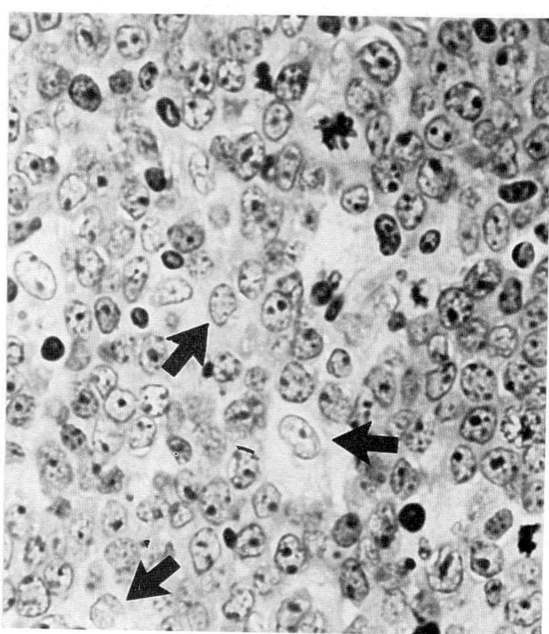

Figure 29-3. Malignant lymphoma, B cell lymphoblastic, small noncleaved, Burkitt type. The cells resemble embryonic B lymphoblasts and are characterized by small size, round nuclei with prominent nucleoli, a high mitotic rate, and the presence of scattered histiocytes that give a "starry sky" appearance. This is a high-grade lymphoma.

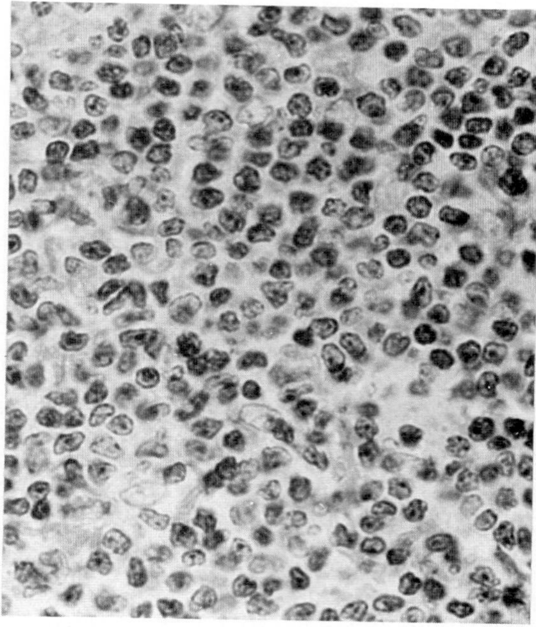

Figure 29-4. Malignant lymphoma, B cell, follicular center cell, small cleaved cell. The neoplastic lymphocytes are small and have irregular nuclei with cleavage planes and inconspicuous nucleoli, resembling cells in the follicles. The mitotic rate is low. This is a low-grade lymphoma.

Table 29-5. Immunologic findings in malignant lymphomas and leukemias (phenotyping).[1]

	T Cell Lymphoma/ Leukemia	B Cell Lymphoma/ Leukemia	Null Cell Lymphoma/ Leukemia	Histiocytic Neoplasms	Granulocytic and Monocytic Leukemias
Surface Ig (SIg)	−	+(−)	−	−	−
Cytoplasmic Ig (CIg)	−	−(+)	−	−	−
E rosette (obsolete)	+	−	−	−	−
Complement rosette (obsolete)	−	+	−	+	−
Fc rosette (obsolete)	−	+	−	+	+(−)
T cell antigens (CD1, CD2, CD5)[2]	+	−	−	−	−
B cell antigens (CD20, CD24)[2]	−	+	−	−	−
Monocyte antigens (CD11, CD15)[2]	−	−	−	+	+(−)
Ig gene rearranged[3]	−	+	+(−)	−	−
T receptor gene rearranged[3]	+	−	−(+)	−	−
Common ALL Ag (CALLA)[4]	−	−(+)	+	−	−(+)

+ or − indicates usual situation: not absolute. (+) or (−) indicates a significant minority finding.
[1]Note that the phenotypic pattern relates the different leukemias and lymphomas to phases of leukocyte development (see Fig 26-3 for leukemias, Fig 29-2 for lymphomas).
[2]Numerous monoclonal antibodies are available, and fashions change (see Chapter 4). Among the T cell lymphomas, some can be shown to be predominantly helper phenotype (CD4) and a few are predominantly suppressor (CD8), although the corresponding function is not necessarily manifest. Cases of ALL, T cell type, often show early T cell or thymocyte markers.
[3]See Chapter 4: considered the earliest markers of B or T cell differentiation.
[4]CALLA (CD10) was first described as present in the cells of "common" ALL (acute lymphoblastic leukemia); it also is present in some normal lymphoid precursor cells and granulocytes.

Table 29-6. The working formulation of non-Hodgkin's lymphomas for clinical use.[1]

Low-grade
- Small lymphocytic lymphoma; includes chronic lymphocytic leukemia and plasmacytoid lymphocytic lymphoma.
- Follicular, small, cleaved cell lymphoma.
- Follicular, mixed small cleaved and large cell lymphoma.

Intermediate-grade
- Follicular, large cell lymphoma.
- Diffuse, small cleaved cell lymphoma.
- Diffuse, mixed small and large cell lymphoma.
- Diffuse, large cell (cleaved and noncleaved) lymphoma.

High-grade
- Large cell, immunoblastic lymphoma.
- Lymphoblastic (convoluted and nonconvoluted cell) lymphoma.
- Small noncleaved cell (Burkitt's) lymphoma.

Miscellaneous
- Composite, mycosis fungoides, histiocytic lymphoma; extramedullary plasmacytoma, unclassifiable, others.

[1]Assignment to grades is based on overall pattern (follicular or diffuse) and cell type.

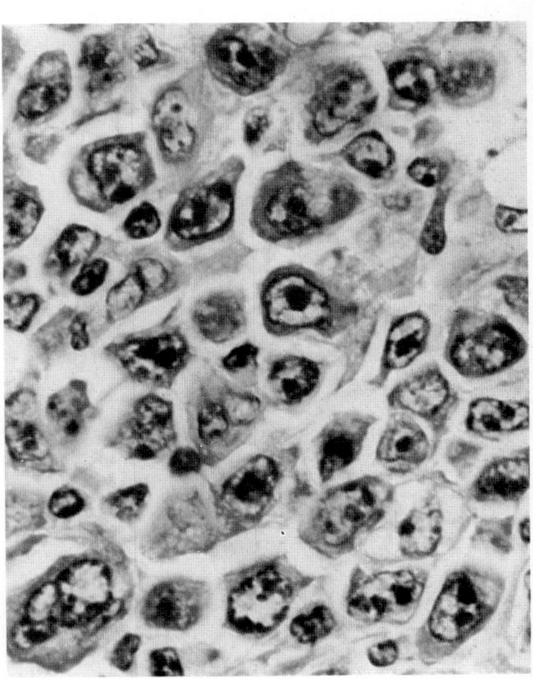

Figure 29-5. B-immunoblastic sarcoma. The neoplastic cells resemble B immunoblasts, with large nuclei, prominent nucleoli, abundant amphophilic cytoplasm, and a high mitotic rate. This is a high-grade lymphoma.

Table 29–7. Classification of non-Hodgkin's lymphomas.[1]

Morphology	Lymphoma Type[2]	Morphologic Description	Important Clinical Features	Marker Results
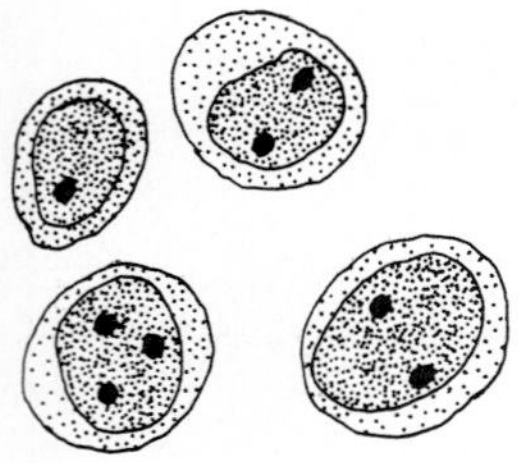	B lymphoblastic lymphoma including FCC, small noncleaved, and Burkitt's lymphoma (see Fig 29–3); ALL B-cell type is related leukemia	Cells resemble small transformed lymphocytes or lymphoblasts. Nuclei round but variable in size (by definition do not exceed size of histiocyte nucleus). Nuclear chromatin finely dispersed. 1–3 small nucleoli. Moderate amount of basophilic cytoplasm. "Starry sky" reactive histiocytes common. Generally diffuse, obliterating lymph node architecture. (See Fig 29–3.)	Abdominal presentation characteristic in US cases, often children. May become manifest as leukemia (then equals L3 subtype of ALL). Rapidly growing tumor. Includes classic Burkitt lymphoma of Africa that typically presents in the jaw and is associated with Epstein-Barr virus. If present in blood or marrow, termed B ALL. Prognosis worse than non-B, non-T ALL.	Majority monoclonal SIg:IgM.
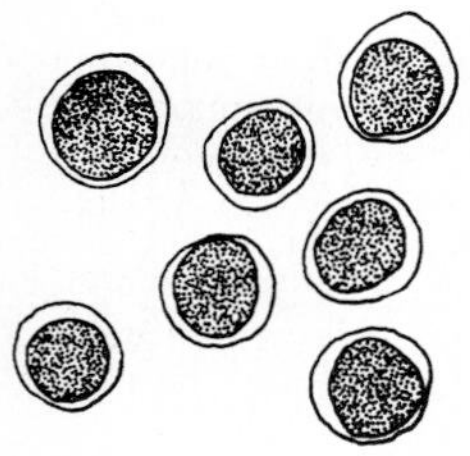	Small lymphocytic lymphoma: B cell; CLL B-cell type is related	Diffuse proliferation of small lymphocytes. Uniform, round nuclei with basophilic compact chromatin and inconspicuous nucleoli. Narrow rim of pale cytoplasm. Large transformed lymphocytes and mitoses rare.	Typically prolonged "benign" course in elderly. Merges with spectrum of CLL. Rarely transforms to large cell (IBS) with rapid turnover (Richter syndrome).	Most show monoclonal surface Ig pattern, usually IgM or IgD.
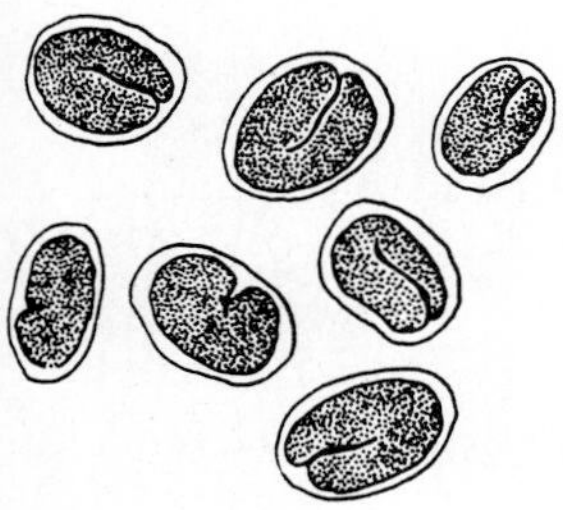	FCC: small cleaved lymphoma (see Fig 29–4)	Wide range of cell sizes, but small cells predominate. Nuclei have basophilic compact chromatin, and many show deep cleavage planes. Nucleoli are inconspicuous, and cytoplasm is indistinct or scanty. Transformed lymphocytes present in small numbers. Mitoses rare. 75% are follicular, remainder diffuse. (See Fig 29–4.)	Asymptomatic presentation typical. Low cell turnover rate. Marrow involved at presentation in > 70%. Paradox of widespread distribution but prolonged median survival. Occasionally leukemic, resembling CLL, but "cleaved" nuclear morphology.	Most show monoclonal surface Ig pattern, usually IgM or IgG.
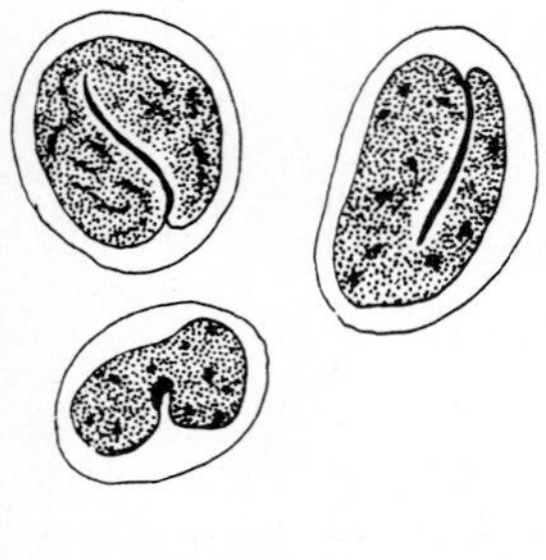	FCC; large cleaved lymphoma	Nuclei larger than nuclei of reactive histiocytes. Prominent nuclear irregularity with exaggerated cleavage planes. Cytoplasm moderate. Small cleaved and noncleaved cells generally present in small numbers. Predominance of large cleaved cells determines cell type.	Commonly present in mesenteric, retroperitoneal, or inguinal nodes. Also often extranodal.	Typically monoclonal SIg: IgM, IgG, IgA.

Table 29-7. Classification of non-Hodgkin's lymphomas.[1] (Continued)

Morphology	Lymphoma Type[2]	Morphologic Description	Important Clinical Features	Marker Results
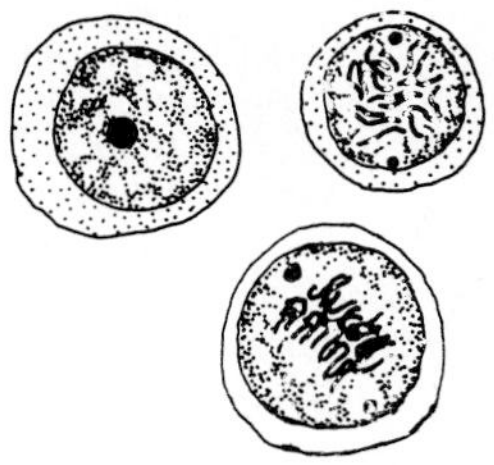	FCC; large non-cleaved lymphoma	Similar to small non-cleaved (or lymphoblastic), but cells and nuclei larger. Mitoses numerous. Follicular in approximately 10% of cases.	Aggressive neoplasm with high turnover rate. Rapid dissemination.	Typically shows monoclonal SIg: IgM or IgG.
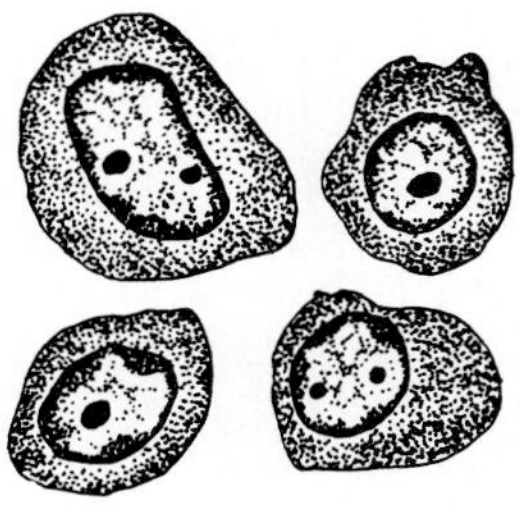	Immunoblastic sarcoma; B cell (see Fig 29–5)	Immunoblasts resemble large non-cleaved FCC, but more deeply staining basophilic cytoplasm. Often plasmacytoid features. Nucleoli often central and prominent; nucleus appears vesicular owing to margination of chromatin. (See Fig 29–5).	Abnormal immune states (immunosuppression, alpha-chain disease, SLE, drug hypersensitivity, IBL) frequently precede development of lymphoma. Rapidly progressive neoplasm.	Majority monoclonal for SIg or cytoplasmic Ig: IgG, IgA, or IgM.
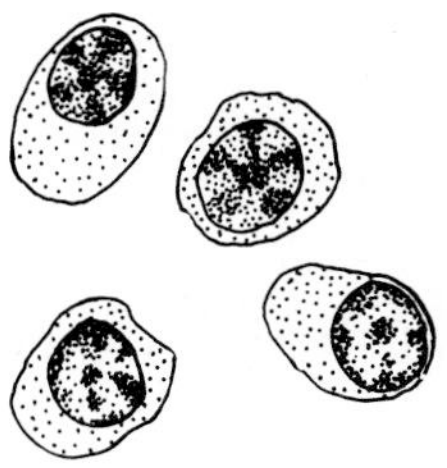	Plasmacytoid lymphocytic lymphoma	Similar to small lymphocytic lymphoma but has abnormal plasmacytoid cell component of variable prominence. These cells possess cytoplasm resembling plasma cell, but nucleus more like lymphocyte. Some cells have PAS-positive intranuclear structures (Dutcher bodies).	Waldenström's macroglobulinemia is part of this group. Monoclonal serum "spike" present.	Usually monoclonal IgM, at times IgG. SIg type same as serum spike.
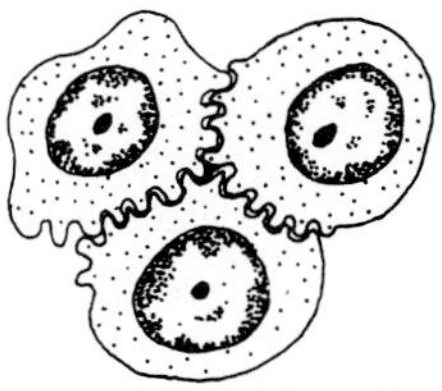	Hairy cell leukemia (leukemic reticuloendotheliosis)	In tissue sections, cells appear medium-sized with abundant pale cytoplasm and round-to-oval nuclei	Manifestations of pancytopenia and splenomegaly. Benign course, particularly following splenectomy. Cytotoxic therapy may hasten demise.	Tartrate-resistant acid phosphatase in cytoplasm. Monoclonal SIg; Ig synthesis and Ig gene rearrangement reported.
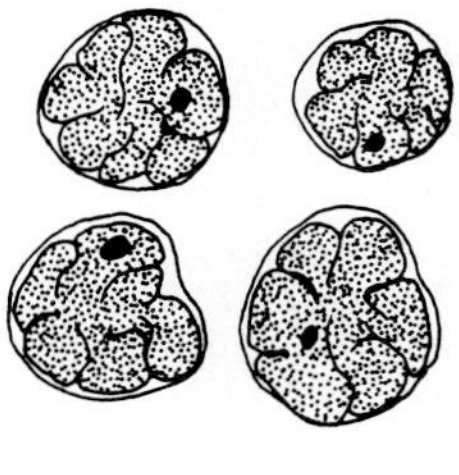	Lymphoblastic (convoluted T cell lymphoma); ALL T-cell type is related leukemia	Diffuse proliferation of "primitive" cells. Nuclear chromatin finely stippled, and nucleolus inconspicuous. Mitoses numerous. Some cells have convoluted or complexly folded nucleus.	Primarily a lymphoma-leukemia of children but may be of any age. Male predominance. Presentation usually in lymph nodes or mediastinum. Response to therapy poor. If present in blood or marrow, termed T ALL. Prognosis worse than non-B, non-T ALL.	Diagnostic cells mark with anti-T cell antibodies.

(cont.)

Table 29-7. Classification of non-Hodgkin's lymphomas.[1] (Continued)

Morphology	Lymphoma Type[2]	Morphologic Description	Important Clinical Features	Marker Results
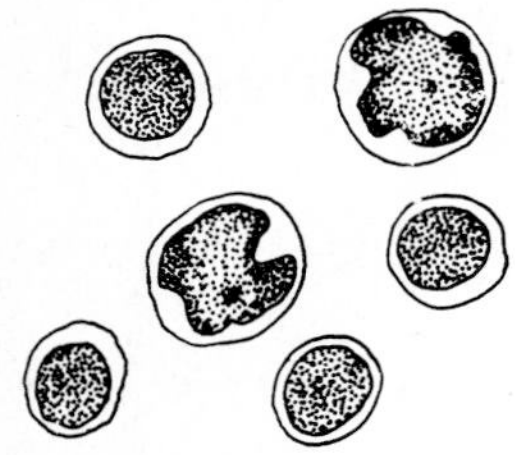	Small lymphocytic lymphoma, T cells; CLL T-cell type is related leukemia	Cells resemble small lymphocytes. Nuclei with compact chromatin. Rim of pale cytoplasm. Nuclei occasionally irregular in form.	May be leukemic resembling B cell CLL. Variant is common in Japan.	Diagnostic cells mark with anti-T cell antibodies. Often helper phenotype.
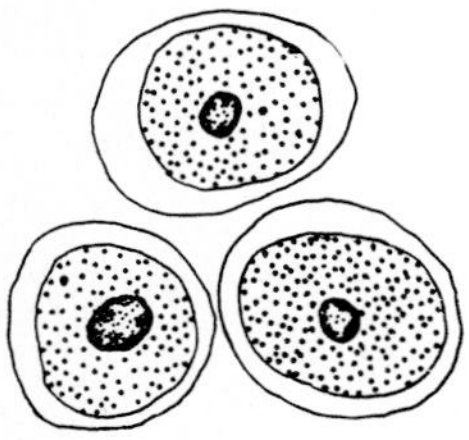	Immunoblastic sarcoma; T cell	Admixture of small and transformed lymphocytes. Latter predominate. In sections they have pale, water-clear cytoplasm.	Less common than B-IBS from which it may be distinguished immunologically. Prognosis poor.	Lymphoma cells mark with anti-T cell antibodies.
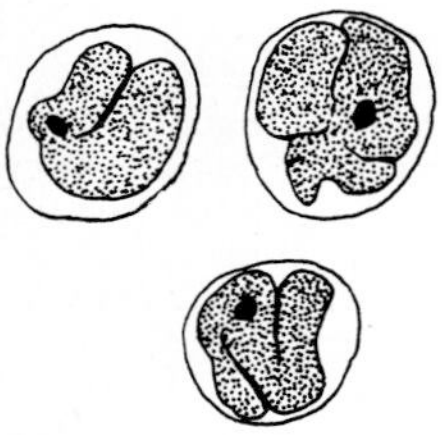	Mycosis fungoides (MF) and Sézary cell (see Fig 29–6)	MF/Sézary cells have compact chromatin and few mitoses resembling normal small lymphocytes, except that they are larger and the nuclei often show complex folding. (See Fig 29–6).	MF and Sézary syndrome closely related. Affinity of cells for skin consistent with affinity of T cell for skin. MF may progress to involvement of nodes, spleen, and blood. Sézary involves blood *ab initio.*	Cells mark with anti-T cell antibodies. Frequently helper phenotype.
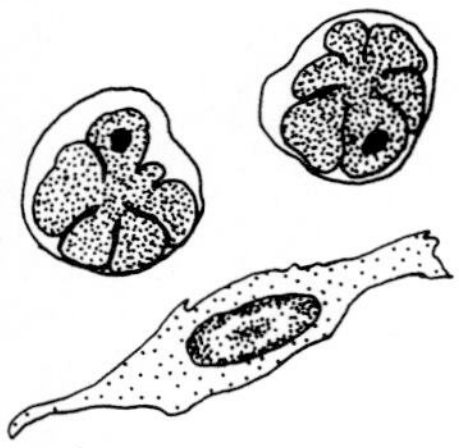	Lymphoepithelioid cell lymphoma	Neoplastic T lymphocytes are admixed with reactive histiocytes. Sometimes confused with Hodgkin's disease.	Relatively rare. Intermediate grade of malignancy.	Lymphoid component marks as T cells.
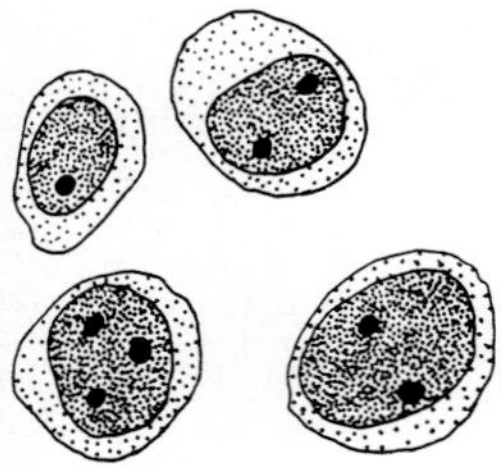	Lymphoblastic lymphoma; ALL—null; non-B, non-T—is related leukemia	Relatively monotonous population of lymphoblasts with numerous mitoses.	Most often presents as leukemia, so-called null; non-B, non-T; or common ALL; has the best prognosis among ALL. Less often presents as a lymphoblastic lymphoma.	Neoplastic cells lack the usual B or T cell markers (hence non-B, non-T or null cell). However, most cases express common ALL antigen (CALLA). Most show Ig gene rearrangement and thus are really B cell.

ALL = acute lymphoblastic leukemia; CLL = chronic lymphocytic leukemia; IBS = immunoblastic sarcoma (B-IBS = IBS of B cell type); FCC = follicular center cell lymphoma; IBL = immunoblastic lymphadenopathy; SLE = systemic lupus erythematosus; SIg = surface immune globulin; PAS = periodic acid-Schiff.

[1]Modified from Lukes RJ et al: Immunologic approach to non-Hodgkin lymphomas and related leukemias. *Semin Hematol* 1978;**15:**322.

[2]Histologic type; related tumors having monoclonal serum proteins are discussed later with "myeloma."

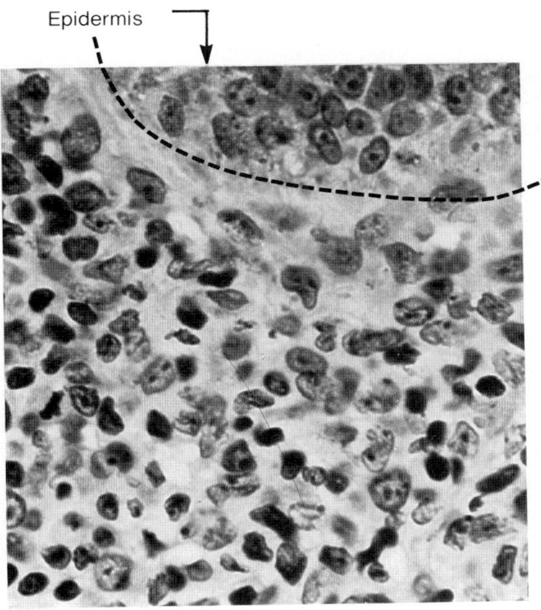

Figure 29-6. Mycosis fungoides (cutaneous T cell lymphoma), showing infiltration of dermis and epidermis by T cells characterized by irregular nuclei with lobation (cerebriform nuclei). The dotted line represents the plane of the epidermal basement membrane, which has become obliterated.

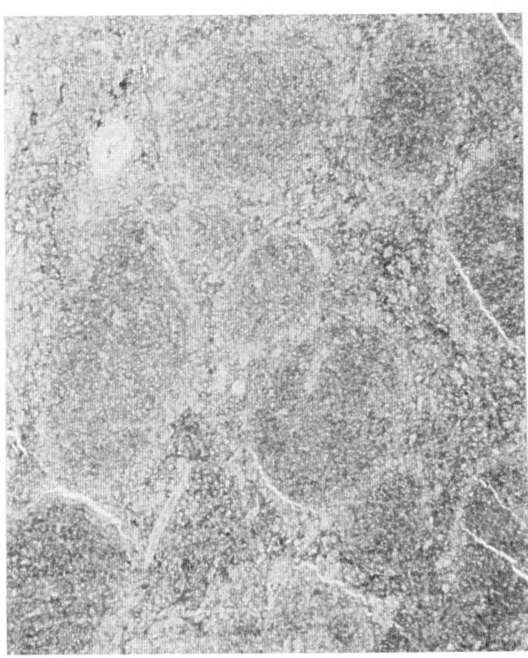

Figure 29-7. Follicular pattern in malignant lymphoma. Such a follicular pattern is seen only in B cell lymphomas and is a favorable histologic feature.

(follicular center cell lymphomas). Histologically, they replace the lymph node in which they arise and may have either a diffuse or follicular pattern. In general, follicular lymphomas have a better prognosis than diffuse lymphomas (Fig 29-7).

B cell lymphomas arise from cells that display the full range of transformation of B cells and are classified as low-grade, intermediate-grade, and high-grade according to the cell type involved. The morphologic and clinical features of these specific types of B cell lymphomas are considered in Table 29-7.

Low-grade (by Working Formulation; see Table 29-6) **B cell lymphomas** include (1) small lymphocytic lymphoma, which is the lymph node counterpart of chronic lymphocytic leukemia; (2) plasmacytoid lymphocytic lymphoma, which is commonly associated with Waldenström's macroglobulinemia (see Chapter 30); (3) small cleaved cell lymphoma, follicular; and (4) mixed small cleaved and large cell lymphoma, follicular.

Intermediate-grade B cell lymphomas include (1) large cell lymphoma, follicular and diffuse, cleaved and non-cleaved; (2) small cleaved cell lymphoma, diffuse (Fig 29-4); and (3) mixed small cleaved and large cell lymphoma, diffuse.

High-grade B cell lymphomas include (1) B immunoblastic sarcoma (Fig 29-5); and (2) small, non-cleaved cell lymphoma, which includes Burkitt's lymphoma (Fig 29-3).

2. T CELL LYMPHOMAS

T cell lymphomas are less common than B cell lymphomas. A low percentage of small lymphocytic lymphomas (chronic lymphocytic leukemia) are T cell, and this represents the only low-grade T cell lymphoma. T immunoblastic sarcoma and lymphoblastic T cell lymphoma, which includes convoluted T cell lymphoma, are the 2 common types of T cell lymphoma, and they are both high grade lymphomas. Cutaneous T cell lymphoma (mycosis fungoides) is a special extranodal type of T cell lymphoma (Fig 29-6). The morphologic and clinical features of these specific types of T cell lymphomas are considered in Table 29-7.

FACTORS DETERMINING PROGNOSIS IN NON-HODGKIN'S LYMPHOMAS

Histologic Type

The prognosis varies markedly with different histologic types of non-Hodgkin's lymphoma (Table 29-8). It is useful to classify malignant lymphomas as low-grade, intermediate-grade, and

Table 29–8. Histology and prognosis of non-Hodgkin's lymphomas.

Type of Non-Hodgkin's Lymphoma	Grade and Approximate Five-Year Survival Rate (Treated)
Lymphocytic Plasmacytoid lymphocytic Most follicular center cell lymphomas with follicular pattern	Good (60%) (low-grade)
Most follicular center cell lymphomas with diffuse pattern	Intermediate (40%)
Immunoblastic lymphoma Lymphoblastic lymphoma (includes convoluted T lymphoma and Burkitt's)	Bad (25%) (high-grade)

high-grade, since the grades correlate well with survival. In general, lymphomas with a follicular histologic pattern are of lower grade (longer survival times) than those with a diffuse pattern. A follicular pattern occurs only in follicular center cell lymphomas (Fig 29–7).

Stage of Disease

The stage of the disease is an expression of the extent of spread of the neoplasm. Specific criteria have been developed for staging Hodgkin's lymphoma and the non-Hodgkin's lymphomas. The aim is to define the extent of disease precisely as a basis for rational decisions about therapy (surgery, radiotherapy, chemotherapy, etc). The staging procedure given here (Table 29–9) was developed for Hodgkin's lymphoma and has been extended for use in management of non-Hodgkin's lymphomas.

The stage may be the **clinical stage,** which is determined by the history and physical examination, radiologic studies, isotopic scans, laboratory tests of urine, blood, and liver, and the initial biopsy results; or the **pathologic stage,** which is based on histologic findings in tissue removed by biopsy or laparotomy, with symbols indicating the tissue samples taken (N = node, H = liver, S = spleen, L = lung, M = marrow, P = pleura, O = bone, D = skin) and the results of histopathologic examination (+ indicates involved, − indicates not involved).

It must be emphasized that the clinical and pathologic staging classifications are unique to the main subtypes of lymphomas and apply only at the time of disease presentation and before definitive therapy is started.

TREATMENT OF NON-HODGKIN'S LYMPHOMA

Survival depends on rational choice of treatment. The use of combined (multiple-agent) chemotherapy (Table 29–10) has favorably influenced the prognosis of these neoplasms. Paradoxically, treatment of previously bad prognostic types of lymphoma (lymphoblastic and immunoblastic) is sometimes more successful in providing complete remission than treatment of the less aggressive histologic types. This probably reflects the fact that most chemotherapeutic agents act only on dividing cells, which are plentiful in high-grade lymphomas but sparse in low-grade lymphomas. Cyclic chemotherapeutic regimens are used so that neoplastic cells that are not in the dividing phase during one dose and therefore survive are treated by the next dose, when they may have entered the dividing phase. Radiotherapy is useful for patients with localized disease.

Table 29–9. Staging of Hodgkin's and non-Hodgkin's lymphomas.[1]

Stage I:	Involvement of a single lymph node region (I) or of a single extralymphoid site (I_E).
Stage II:	Involvement of 2 or more lymph node regions on the same side of the diaphragm.
Stage III:	Involvement on both sides of the diaphragm (III), which may also be accompanied by localized involvement of a single extralymphoid site (III_E) or the spleen (III_S).
Stage IV:	Diffuse or disseminated involvement of one or more extralymphoid organs or tissues with or without associated lymph node involvement.

[1]Each of these stages is divided into A and B categories—B for those with defined general symptoms and A for those without. The B classification is given those patients with unexplained weight loss, unexplained fever, and night sweats; it has a worse prognosis.

Table 29–10. Multiple-agent chemotherapy for Hodgkin's lymphoma and the non-Hodgkin lymphomas.[1]

MOPP	*M*echlorethamine (nitrogen mustard), *O*ncovin (vincristine), *p*rocarbazine, *p*rednisone
C-MOPP	*C*yclophosphamide, *m*echlorethamine, *O*ncovin, *p*rocarbazine, *p*rednisone
COP	*C*yclophosphamide, *O*ncovin, *p*rednisone
CHOP	*C*yclophosphamide, *h*ydroxydaunorubicin, *O*ncovin, *p*rednisone
BACOP	*B*leomycin, *A*driamycin (doxorubicin), *c*yclophosphamide, *O*ncovin, *p*rednisone
ABVD	*A*driamycin, *b*leomycin, *v*inblastine, *d*acarbazine

[1]All are given in spread doses and recycled at 4 weeks for 6 or more cycles, depending upon when (if) remission is achieved and upon patient tolerance.

HODGKIN'S LYMPHOMA

Hodgkin's lymphoma (also called Hodgkin's disease) is a malignant lymphoma characterized by the presence of Reed-Sternberg cells in the involved tissue (Figs 29–8 and 29–9). It accounts for 30–40% of all lymphomas and is usually considered separately from the other (non-Hodgkin's) lymphomas. Eight thousand cases occur annually in the United States. Hodgkin's lymphoma shows a bimodal age incidence, with a peak in early adulthood and another in old age.

ETIOLOGY OF HODGKIN'S LYMPHOMA

The cause of Hodgkin's lymphoma is not known. Early controversy over whether the disease was a peculiar infection (once thought to be a form of tuberculosis) or a form of cancer has given way to general acceptance of Hodgkin's lymphoma as a neoplastic process. That the neoplastic cells are often so sparsely distributed among reactive lymphoid cells has led to the hypothesis that the histologic features reflect some form of host response against the neoplastic Reed-Sternberg cells (Fig 29–10).

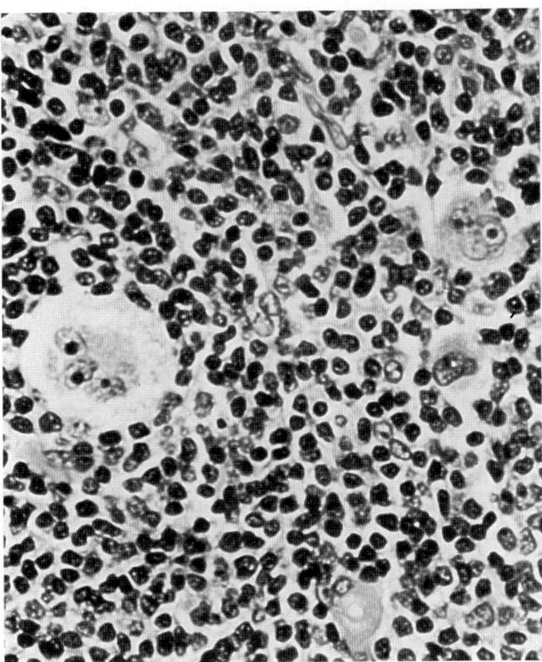

Figure 29–8. Hodgkin's lymphoma, mixed cellularity, showing multinucleated Reed-Sternberg cells in a background of cells that include lymphocytes, plasma cells, eosinophils, histiocytes, and mononuclear Reed-Sternberg cells.

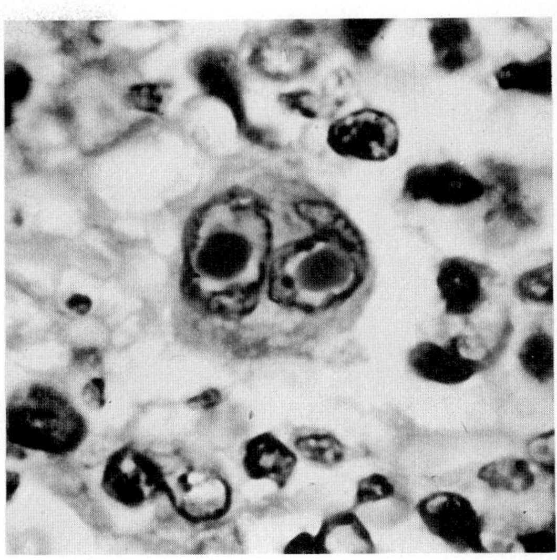

Figure 29–9. Hodgkin's lymphoma. High magnification of a classical Reed-Sternberg cell with 2 nuclei containing the typical large nucleoli.

Immunologic responses are abnormal in Hodgkin's lymphoma, and mice with chronic low-grade graft-versus-host reactions may show similar histologic features. Cell-mediated (T cell) immunity is depressed in Hodgkin's lymphoma, but it is not clear whether that is a cause or a consequence of the disease. Clusters of cases of Hodgkin's lymphoma in restricted geographic areas have been suggestive of some infective or other environmental agent, but no such agent has been identified.

Immunologic studies have not resolved the problem of the cellular origin of Hodgkin's lymphoma, and if anything have complicated the issue. There is a developing consensus that Hodgkin's lymphoma may not be a single entity but may represent several morphologically similar processes of diverse cellular origin. For example, there is immunologic evidence that lymphocyte-predominant Hodgkin's lymphoma is B lymphocyte-derived. In addition, nodular sclerosing Hodgkin's lymphoma has distinctive clinical and epidemiologic features that have led some to suggest it might be a separate process. Candidates for the cell of origin for the different types of Hodgkin's lymphoma include the lymphocyte, the histiocyte, and the interdigitating reticulum cell.

PATHOLOGIC FEATURES OF HODGKIN'S LYMPHOMA

Though the diagnosis of Hodgkin's lymphoma depends upon the finding of classic Reed-Sternberg cells, these cells show little evidence of nucleic

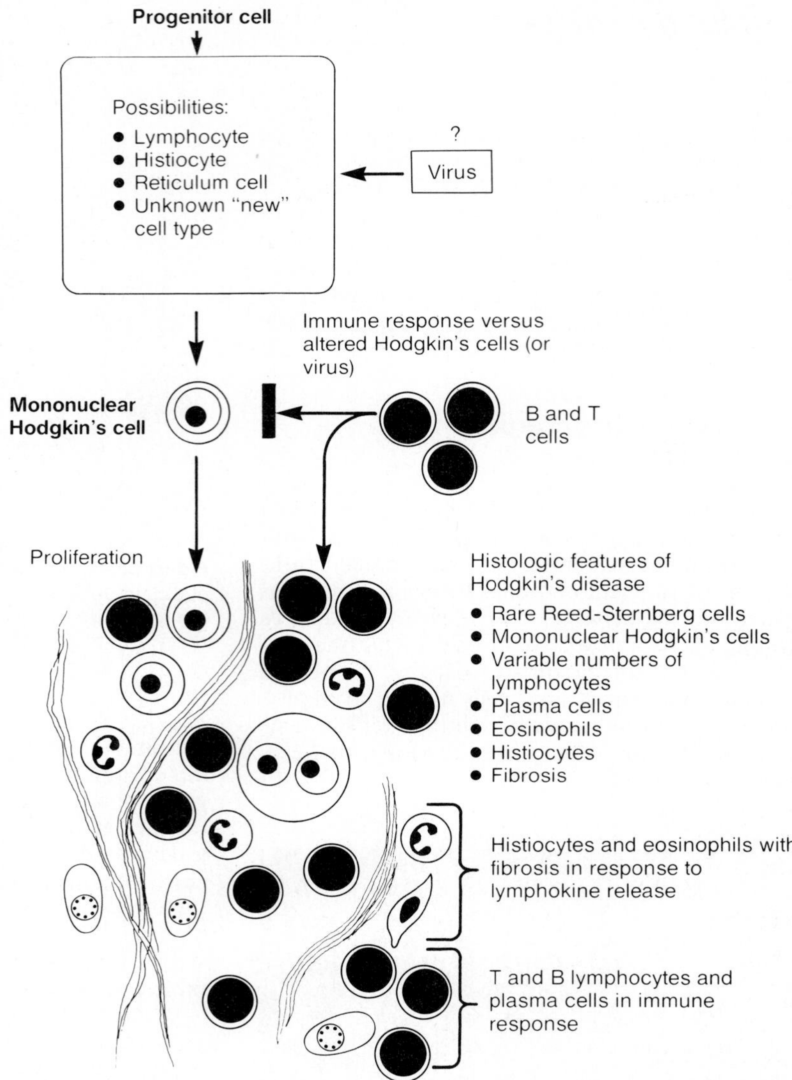

Figure 29–10. Pathogenetic mechanisms leading to the histologic features of Hodgkin's lymphoma.

acid synthesis or proliferative activity. Large mononuclear cells (called Hodgkin's cells) that resemble Reed-Sternberg cells are the proliferative cells in Hodgkin's lymphoma (Fig 29–10).

The histologic picture of Hodgkin's lymphoma is particularly distinctive in that the neoplastic Reed-Sternberg cells are few in number and are admixed with variable numbers of lymphocytes, plasma cells, histiocytes, eosinophils, neutrophils, and fibroblasts, all of which are considered to be reactive (Figs 29–8 and 29–10). Yet the lymph node may be totally destroyed, and an identical process may progress to involve many lymph nodes, spleen, liver, bone marrow, and extralymphatic tissues. This is a contrast with other malignant neoplasms, in which the malignant cells predominate in the involved tissues.

Staging, both clinical and pathologic, is similar to that for non-Hodgkin's lymphoma (Table 29–9).

CLASSIFICATION OF HODGKIN'S LYMPHOMA

The varying relative proportions of Reed-Sternberg cells (and mononuclear variant cells), lymphocytes, histiocytes, and areas of fibrosis have permitted subclassification of Hodgkin's lymphoma into 4 subtypes that have epidemiologic, prognostic, and therapeutic differences (Tables 29–11 and 29–12).

Table 29–11. Histologic subclassification of Hodgkin's lymphoma.

	Sclerosis (Fibrosis)	Number of Lymphocytes	Number of Reed-Sternberg Cells	Other Cells
LP (lymphocyte predominant)	–	++++	+	±Histiocytes
MC (mixed cellularity)	± → +	++	++	+ Plasma cells, histiocytes, eosinophils
LD (lymphocyte depleted)	+ → ++ Diffuse	+	++ → ++++	± Plasma cells, histiocytes, eosinophils
NS (nodular sclerosis)	++++ (Broad bands)	+ → +++	+ → ++++	± Plasma cells, histiocytes, eosinophils

Lymphocyte-Predominant Hodgkin's Lymphoma

This subtype, which is characterized by the presence of numerous lymphocytes and few classic Reed-Sternberg cells, has the best prognosis. It may occur in nodular or diffuse form and may include a conspicuous component of reactive histiocytes (earlier known as the L&H—lymphocytic and histiocytic—form of Hodgkin's lymphoma). The presence of large polyploid variants of the Reed-Sternberg cell with lobulated nuclei ("popcorn" cells) is characteristic. It typically presents as stage I disease and progresses slowly.

Lymphocyte-Depleted Hodgkin's Lymphoma

This form has the worst prognosis and typically presents as stage III or stage IV disease. Lymph nodes are replaced by a destructive process containing numerous pleomorphic mononuclear and classic Reed-Sternberg cells, variable amounts of diffuse fibrosis, and very few lymphocytes. Lymphocyte-depleted Hodgkin's lymphoma is often refractory to therapy.

Mixed-Cellularity Hodgkin's Lymphoma

This subtype has an intermediate histologic appearance with numerous lymphocytes, plasma cells, eosinophils, and Reed-Sternberg cells (Figs 29–8 and 29–10). The prognosis is intermediate between that of lymphocyte-predominant and lymphocyte-depleted lymphoma. The response to therapy is usually good.

Nodular Sclerosing Hodgkin's Lymphoma

This subtype has a good prognosis, usually presenting as early stage disease. Young women are particularly affected, and mediastinal involvement is common. Nodular sclerosis is histologically characterized by broad bands of collagen circumscribing nodules of involved tissue and by the presence of large Reed-Sternberg cell variants that have multilobated nuclei and abundant pale cytoplasm (lacunar cells).

DIAGNOSIS & TREATMENT OF HODGKIN'S LYMPHOMA

In spite of intensive research and a wealth of immunologic data, the diagnosis of Hodgkin's lymphoma is still based entirely upon histologic examination—the finding of the classic Reed-Sternberg cell in pathologic tissue is considered essential for diagnosis. Subclassification is then accomplished by examination of other histologic

Table 29–12. Histologic subtypes of Hodgkin's lymphoma as correlated with clinical presentation and survival.

Histologic Type	Sex	Stage of Presentation	Symptoms[1]	Approximate 5-Year Survival Rate (1974)[2]	Common Primary Site
LP	M > F	Usually I, II	None (all A)	90%	Neck
MC	M > F	I, II, III, IV	A > B	50%	Any
LD	M > F	Usually III, IV	B > A	40%	Any/multiple
NS	F > M	Usually I, II	A > B	70%	Mediastinum

[1]Symptoms: B = with any 2 of fever, weight loss, or night sweats; A = without these symptoms.
[2]Survival figures for 1974 are given because they more clearly indicate differences in the natural history of the histologic types. Current aggressive combined chemotherapy has decreased the differences in the survival rates of the different types; the 5-year survival rate in all groups is over 70% today.

parameters (Table 29–11). Note that although Reed-Sternberg cells are characteristic of Hodgkin's lymphoma, morphologically similar cells may be seen occasionally in non-Hodgkin's lymphomas and in reactive hyperplasias (such as Epstein-Barr virus infection).

Selection of therapy depends not only upon the histologic type but on the stage and other clinical parameters. Localized forms of Hodgkin's lymphoma may be treated with either radiation or chemotherapy. Chemotherapy is highly effective when multiple agents are used and may lead to cures even in patients with disseminated (late stage) disease. The evolving treatment of Hodgkin's lymphoma has provided a model of the team approach to management of neoplastic diseases, requiring close consultation among pathologists, radiologists, oncologists, surgeons, and radiotherapists (Table 29–13).

NEOPLASMS OF HISTIOCYTES

As noted above, the term histiocytic lymphoma (in the Rappaport classification) is a misnomer, and almost all of these tumors are neoplasms of large lymphocytes (large follicular center cells and immunoblasts). True histiocytic neoplasms do occur but are uncommon. They fall into 3 main categories, discussed below.

Table 29–13. Rules for biopsy of suspected lymphoma, including Hodgkin's lymphoma.

1. Clinical workup prior to biopsy.
2. Physician and surgeon *talk to each other.*
3. Notify pathologist prior to biopsy. (May wish to arrange special studies, eg, culture, immunologic markers. It is optimal to have the pathologist pick up the removed lymph node from surgery.)
4. Surgeon: Examine patient prior to anesthesia.
5. Sutton's law:[1] Take the biggest, juiciest node, even if this means a deeper dissection; remove intact.
6. Get it to pathology lab *urgently* and in fresh state. Do not fix in formalin or other fixative.
7. Histologic diagnosis includes immunotyping.
8. Staging: Clinical examination—special x-ray techniques (CT scan, lymphangiogram); surgical staging by laparotomy in some cases, looking for spleen, liver, lymph node involvement.
9. Staging conference. Pathologist, surgeon, physician *talk to one another.*
10. Selection of therapy: surgery, radiotherapy, chemotherapy.

[1]Sutton's law: Willie Sutton was an incorrigible robber of US banks. When asked by a judge why he repeatedly robbed banks, he replied, "Because that's where the money is." Sutton himself denied the truth of this story, but it persists in medical mythology.

TRUE HISTIOCYTIC "LYMPHOMA"

This tumor is rare, accounting for less than 5% of primary neoplasms of lymph nodes. The neoplastic cells are large and pleomorphic, typically with granular pink cytoplasm. Distinction from large cell lymphomas is difficult without immunologic tests. The malignant histiocytes may show phagocytosis and variable reactivity with anti-monocyte/histiocyte antibodies such as Leu M1, Mo 1 (Chapter 4). Histiocytic lymphomas are usually aggressive and refractory to treatment. Early disease is confined to lymph nodes and appears clinically like malignant lymphoma. Advanced disease is difficult to distinguish from histiocytic medullary reticulosis (see below).

MALIGNANT HISTIOCYTOSIS & HISTIOCYTIC MEDULLARY RETICULOSIS

These 2 terms are used interchangeably to denote a highly malignant systemic neoplasm of histiocytes, involving lymph nodes and soft tissue. The malignant histiocytes first involve medullary sinuses within lymph nodes but rapidly spread to destroy lymph nodes and other tissues, producing hepatosplenomegaly, lymphadenopathy, and pancytopenia. Typically there is extensive erythrophagocytosis by the neoplastic cells. The prognosis is poor.

HISTIOCYTOSIS X

The term histiocytosis X is used to denote 3 related diseases:

(1) Eosinophilic granuloma is a relatively benign unifocal disease that involves bone, particularly the skull and ribs of children and young adults, though long bones are sometimes involved. Radiologically, it presents as a well-demarcated lytic lesion. Histologically, the lesion is seen as a diffuse infiltrate composed of histiocytes, giant cells, and eosinophils.

(2) Hand-Schüller-Christian disease is morphologically similar to eosinophilic granuloma but is multifocal and has a less favorable prognosis. The base of the skull is characteristically involved, producing the triad of proptosis, lytic bone lesions in skull, and diabetes insipidus—the last due to destruction of the posterior pituitary.

(3) Letterer-Siwe disease (generalized histiocytosis) appears to represent the aggressive end of the spectrum, with widespread lesions of bone and lymphoid tissue. The condition is uncommon and occurs only in young children. Lymphadenopathy and skin lesions are due to infiltration by large pale neoplastic histiocytes.

In all of these conditions, the neoplastic histiocytes show a resemblance to the Langerhans cells of the skin (ie, react with monoclonal antibody OKT6 and contain tennis racket-shaped Birbeck granules on electron microscopy). Langerhans cells are thought to be antigen handling cells.

METASTATIC NEOPLASMS

Metastatic neoplasms—most commonly carcinomas and malignant melanoma—are a common cause of lymph node enlargement. Not infrequently, an enlarged lymph node is the method of clinical presentation of a carcinoma, the primary tumor being occult; eg, cervical lymphadenopathy is a common mode of presentation of nasopharyngeal carcinoma.

The histologic diagnosis of metastatic neoplasms is easy when the neoplasm is well differentiated. When it is poorly differentiated, the distinction between large-cell ("histiocytic") lymphoma, poorly differentiated carcinoma, and amelanotic malignant melanoma is very difficult to make on histologic examination. The demonstration of specific markers (common leukocyte antigen for lymphomas; keratin for carcinomas; and S100 protein and melanosomes for melanomas) by immunoperoxidase techniques is essential for accurate diagnosis.

30 The Lymphoid System: III. Plasma Cell Neoplasms; Spleen & Thymus

PLASMA CELL NEOPLASMS

MONOCLONAL GAMMOPATHY

As described elsewhere (Chapter 29), neoplastic proliferations of B lymphocytes are demonstrably monoclonal; if plasmacytoid differentiation occurs, the neoplastic cells may secrete immunoglobulin that will accumulate in the serum and produce a monoclonal "spike" or M protein. The terms "monoclonal gammopathy" and "plasma cell dyscrasia" are employed synonymously for disorders in which a monoclonal spike is present in serum. Most conditions associated with monoclonal gammopathy (Table 30–1) show evidence of proliferation of plasma cells or plasmacytoid cells—hence the term "plasma cell dyscrasia." It is important to distinguish those forms of monoclonal gammopathy that are malignant, since they require treatment.

Diagnosis

A. Serum Protein Electrophoresis: The serum contains numerous proteins that may be separated according to differences in size and charge by electrophoresis. Protein molecules are allowed to migrate on special paper or in a gel under the influence of an electrical field. Identical molecules migrate to an identical point within the field, and each different protein accumulates at a characteristic point under specified conditions (Fig 30–1). Protein accumulations, or bands, may be visualized by staining and quantitated by densitometry: the higher the density of the band, the more protein is present.

A monoclonal gammopathy is characterized by the appearance of a high narrow peak ("spike") in the globulin region of the protein electrophoretic strip. The nature of this spike generally permits differentiation from a polyclonal immunoglobulin increase—as occurs in chronic infections—which produces a broad elevation of the globulins (Fig 30–2).

B. Serum Immunoelectrophoresis: Serum proteins separated by electrophoresis in agarose may be identified by immunologic means using antibodies to precipitate the various proteins (Fig 30–3). The precipitation arcs so formed may be identified by their characteristic position in the electrophoretic pattern—or more precisely by using defined antibodies of known specificity (Fig 30–4). Protein electrophoresis thus provides a rapid means of evaluating the serum proteins, while immunoelectrophoresis is particularly valuable in analyzing the immunoglobulins. Analysis of precipitation patterns in immunoelectrophoresis can prove that a band in the gamma globulin region is a monoclonal immunoglobulin.

C. Urine Electrophoresis: Electrophoresis of proteins in urine is a valuable adjunct to serum electrophoresis in that if the kidneys are damaged, as they frequently are in plasma cell myeloma, the monoclonal proteins leak into the urine where they are easily detected. Furthermore, excess (free) light chains are frequently produced in myeloma; these form dimers, which, having a molecular weight of 50,000, pass into the urine and can be detected by urine electrophoresis (Bence Jones protein).

D. Bence Jones Protein: Bence Jones protein

Table 30-1. Causes of monoclonal gammopathy (ie, the presence of a monoclonal or M spike in serum).

		Monoclonal "Spike"
Neoplastic		
Multiple myeloma	Multiple plasma cell neoplasms in bone	IgG, IgA, IgM, IgD, or free light chains
Plasmacytoid lymphocytic lymphoma[1]	Lymph node or tissue mass containing neoplastic plasmacytoid lymphocytes	Usually IgM (macroglobulinemia)
Alpha heavy chain disease[2]	Plasmacytoid cell neoplasm especially involving gut wall	Alpha chain only
Amyloidosis	Usually associated with an underlying plasmacytic neoplasm	IgG or light chain
Nonneoplastic		
Benign monoclonal gammopathy	Mild reactive plasmacytosis in marrow: by definition not malignant[3]	Usually low-level stable IgG
Transient gammopathies	Probably a phase of florid immune response when one clonal product (antibody type) dominates; seen in some infections and with some cancers	Usually IgG, low-level
"Autoimmune" gammopathy	Monoclonal immunoglobulins are found as part of mixed cryoglobulinemia and cold agglutinin disease (see text); rare	Usually IgM, low-level

[1]Other B cell neoplasms (chronic lymphocytic leukemia, follicular center cell lymphomas, and immunoblastic sarcoma of B cell type) may also produce detectable "spikes" if very sensitive techniques are utilized.
[2]Gamma and mu chain diseases also occur but are very rare (see text).
[3]It is not known whether the condition represents a benign neoplasm or a reactive clone that becomes predominant and persists.

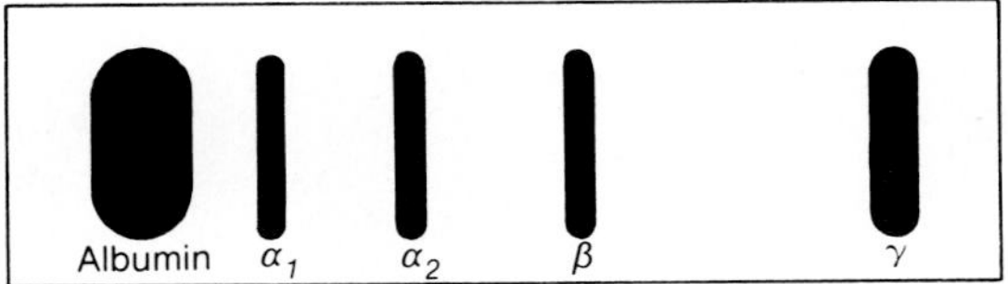

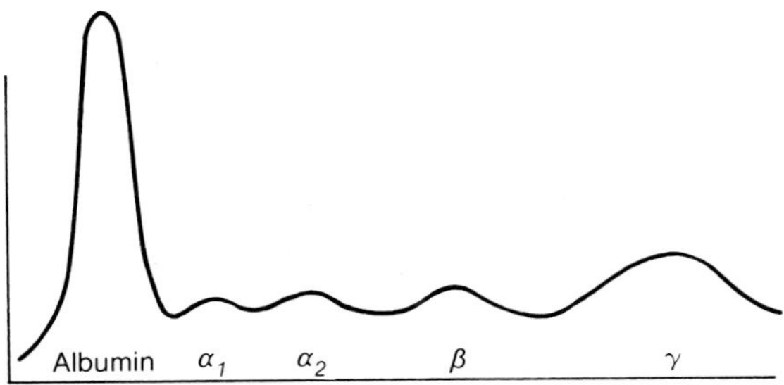

Figure 30-1. Serum protein electrophoresis. In normal individuals, all molecules of albumin are identical in charge and molecular weight and therefore accumulate in one narrow band on electrophoresis. Since the serum contains a large amount of albumin, this produces a high peak on densitometry. The globulins in serum are made up of several different proteins and produce several broad bands. The immunoglobulins fall in the gamma globulin band, which is normally low and broad since there are many different immunoglobulins in normal serum.

represents free immunoglobulin light chains that have been filtered by the glomeruli and are excreted in urine. The detection of Bence Jones protein is historically important, since for many years this was a standard diagnostic test for plasma cell neoplasms. The original test involved heating urine and observing a precipitate forming at 40–60 °C, which then redissolved as the temperature reached 80 °C (other proteins also precipitate but do not redissolve). With the more recent recognition that Bence Jones protein consists of light chain dimers, immunoelectrophoresis demonstrating the presence of monoclonal light chain has superseded the heat method.

MULTIPLE MYELOMA

Incidence & Etiology

Multiple myeloma is so named because the disease is characterized by the presence of multiple small tumors within the bone marrow. The tumors are composed of plasma cells. Alternative names include multiple plasmacytoma, plasma cell myeloma, and Kahler's disease.

Myeloma is the most common form of plasma cell dyscrasia, accounting for about one-sixth of all hematopoietic neoplasms, a frequency roughly equal to that of Hodgkin's disease. The peak incidence is in the eighth decade, and the disease is very rare in persons under 40 years of age.

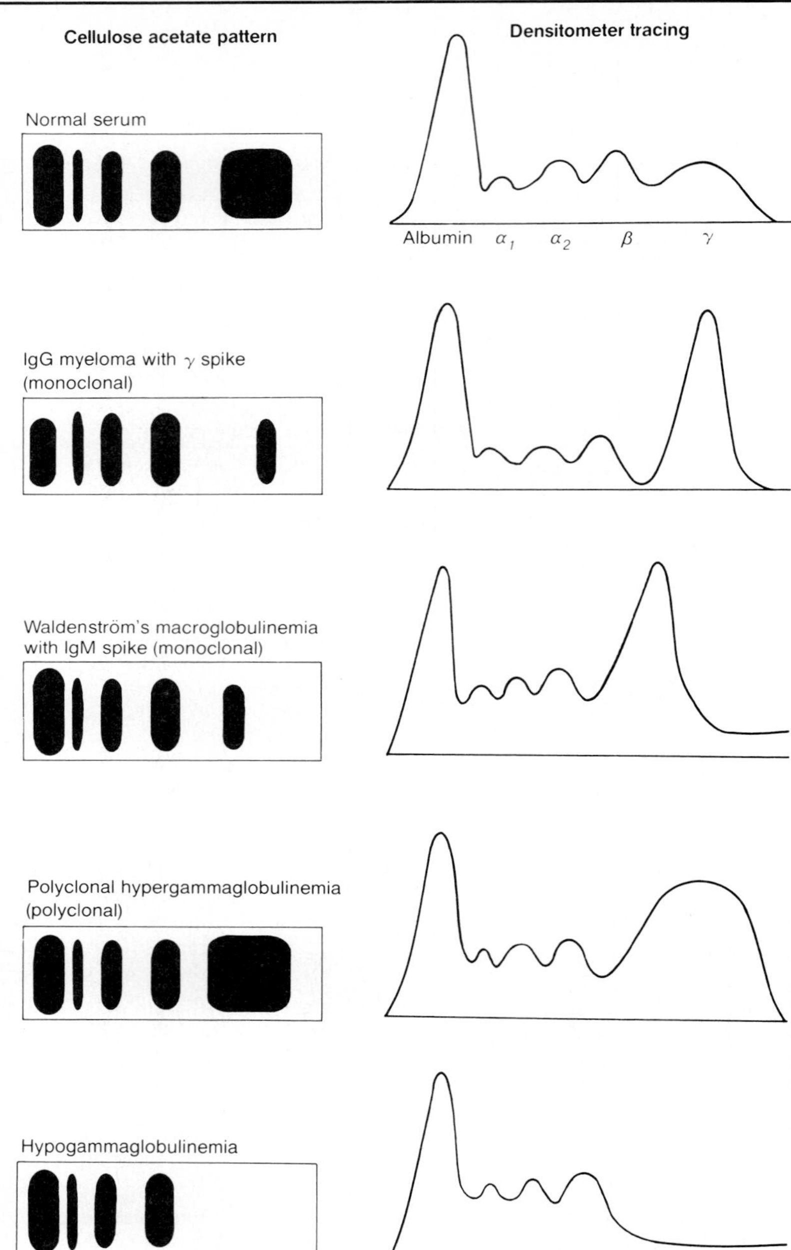

Figure 30-2. Serum protein electrophoresis, showing patterns seen in normal serum, monoclonal gammopathies, polyclonal hypergammaglobulinemia, and hypogammaglobulinemia.

The etiology of myeloma is unknown; however, in induced murine plasmacytoma—a plasma cell neoplasm of the mouse—sustained immune stimulation (by mineral oil and bacterial antigens) is causal. In murine plasmacytoma, a chromosomal translocation results in the juxtaposition of C-*MYC* oncogene with the murine immunoglobulin gene, and it is postulated that immune stimulation then serves to produce continuing activity not only of the immunoglobulin gene but of the adjacent C-*MYC* gene as well.

Clinical Features & Diagnosis

The clinical features of plasma cell myeloma relate to the underlying pathologic process (Table 30–2). Presentation is usually due to symptoms of anemia, bone pain and fractures due to bone marrow involvement, infection, renal disease, or hyperviscosity. The release of an osteoclast activating factor contributes to bone lysis in myeloma.

Diagnosis is based upon (1) radiologic findings (multiple lytic lesions, especially in ribs, long bones and skull); (2) bone marrow examination

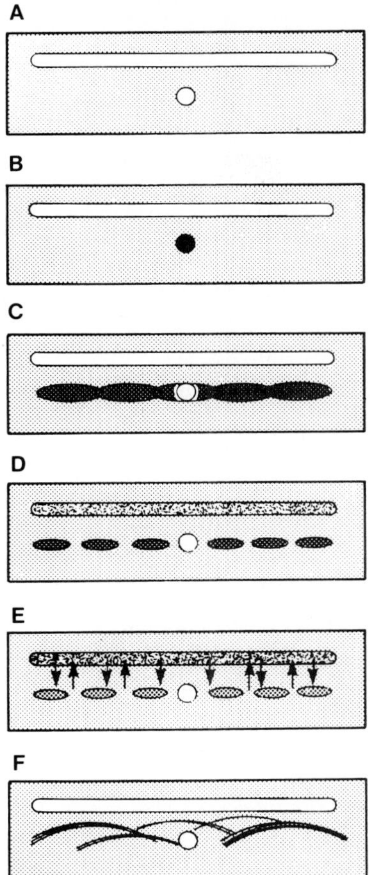

Figure 30–3. Technique of immunoelectrophoresis. **A:** Semisolid agar poured onto glass slide and antigen well and antiserum trough cut out of agar. **B:** Antigen well filled with human serum. **C:** Serum separated by electrophoresis. **D:** Antiserum trough filled with antiserum to whole human serum. **E:** Serum and antiserum diffuse into agar. **F:** Precipitin lines form for individual serum proteins.

Table 30–2. Clinicopathologic correlates in myeloma.

Clinical Features	Underlying Pathology
Anemia (usually normochromic, occasionally macrocytic or leukoerythroblastic)	Due to combination of accelerated red cell destruction, nutritional factors, and replacement of marrow by tumor.
Bone pain	Lytic lesions weaken bone, causing compression with or without collapse; may compress nerve roots in spine. Release of osteoclast-activating factor (OAF) contributes to lysis.
Renal disease	Due to combination of light chain deposition in tubules, hypercalcemia, amyloid, and renal infection.
Hypercalcemia symptoms	Due to lytic lesions and effects of OAF.
Infections	Due to decreased ability to produce specific antibody (especially bacteria such as pneumococcus).
Hyperviscosity syndrome	Due to high levels of Ig, producing microcirculatory impairment; typically seen in plasmacytoid lymphoma producing IgM (macroglobulinemia) but may occur with myeloma producing IgG or IgM.
Bleeding diathesis	Due to combination of thrombocytopenia, hyperviscosity, and amyloid.
Arthritis	Due to amyloid deposits or rarely uric acid (secondary gout, especially following treatment).
Neuropathy	Due to root compression or amyloidosis.

(smear or biopsy showing large numbers of abnormal plasma cells); and (3) the presence of a monoclonal spike (M protein) in serum or urine. The monoclonal immunoglobulin in the serum can be composed of light chain only, heavy chain only, or whole immunoglobulin of classes IgG, IgA, IgD, or IgE as well as IgM. In classic myeloma, IgG is most commonly present, followed by free light chains and then IgA. IgD and IgM are much less common, and IgE is very rare.

In advanced disease, the diagnosis is not difficult; the tumor cell burden is then estimated at 10^{11} malignant cells. It is believed that by the usual diagnostic techniques, diagnosis is made with a tumor burden of approximately 10^8 malignant cells. In theory, earlier diagnosis would enhance the success of therapy. Immunohistologic techniques such as staining for kappa and lambda light chains or for heavy chains, may be used to detect monoclonal plasma cells in bone marrow at an early stage, when the tumor burden may be less (Fig 30–5).

Plasma cell myeloma is treated by multiple-agent chemotherapy (eg, using melphalan or cyclophosphamide and adrenocorticosteroids) with local radiotherapy for painful bone lesions. The prognosis is poor, with a median survival of approximately 3 years.

PLASMACYTOID LYMPHOCYTIC LYMPHOMA & WALDENSTRÖM'S DISEASE

As noted earlier, B cell lymphomas may show plasmacytic differentiation of some of the cells within the neoplastic clone, with resultant production of monoclonal immunoglobulins. Detectable

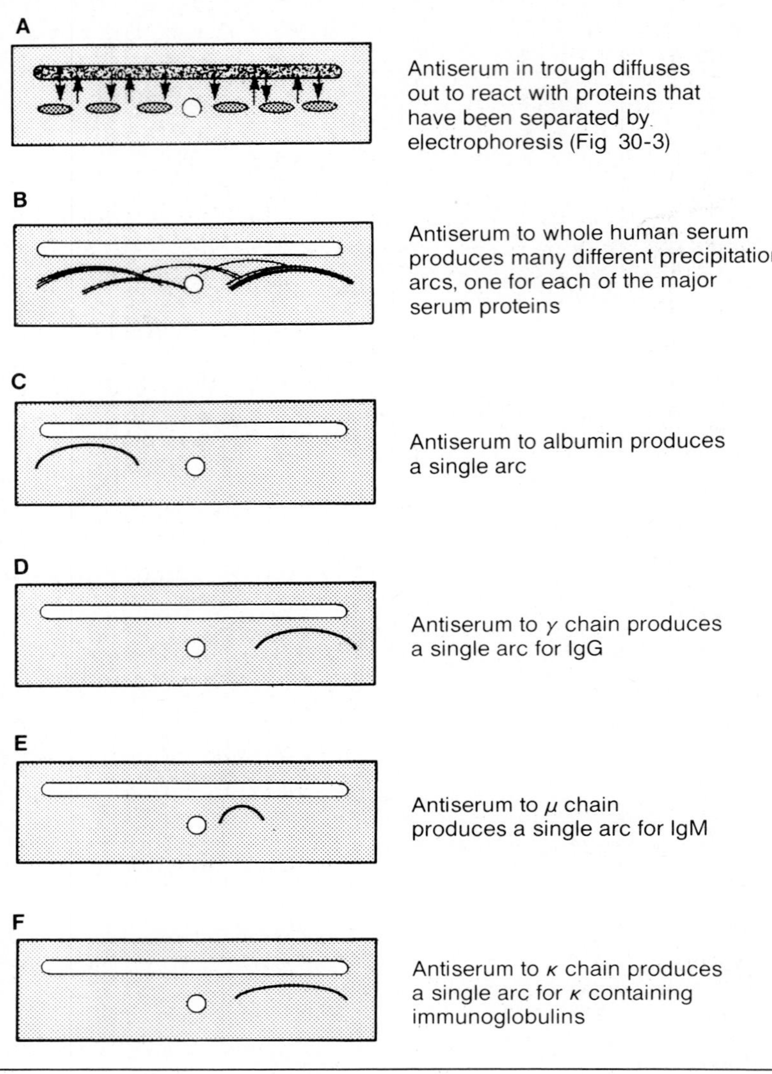

Figure 30-4. Immunoelectrophoresis, showing ability to identify major serum proteins by use of specific antisera. Several examples are shown.

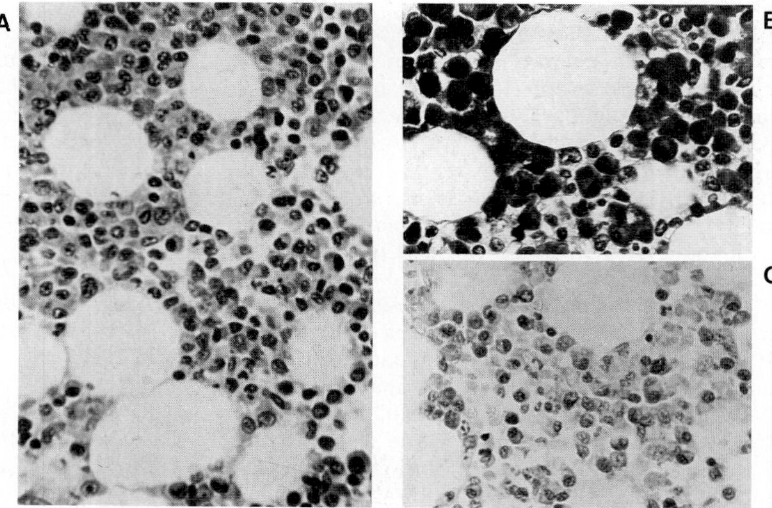

Figure 30-5. Section of a needle biopsy of bone marrow from a patient with marrow involvement by multiple myeloma. **A:** Numerous plasma cells have replaced most of the marrow; a few fat cells remain. **B and C:** Same case after staining for immunoglobulin light chains by the immunoperoxidase technique. In **B,** staining with anti-kappa reveals a positive reaction (black) in the plasma cells, whereas in **C,** staining with anti-lambda shows no reactivity. This demonstrates the monoclonal nature of this neoplasm. An IgA kappa monoclonal spike was detected in serum.

serum monoclonal immunoglobulins occur infrequently in B-immunoblastic sarcoma, follicular center cell lymphoma, and well-differentiated lymphocytic lymphoma (or CLL) but are the rule in plasmacytoid lymphocytic lymphoma. This is in keeping with the presence of numerous plasmacytoid lymphocytes in this condition, having condensed lymphocytelike nuclei (as opposed to the more open clockface nuclei of plasma cells) but plasma cell-like cytoplasm rich in endoplasmic reticulum (see Table 29–7).

Plasmacytoid lymphocytic lymphoma is almost exclusively a disease of the elderly (50 years of age or older) and usually presents with anemia and manifestations of bleeding or hyperviscosity syndrome (Waldenström's disease). These effects result from high levels of monoclonal IgM present in this condition; IgG and IgA monoclonal proteins are present much less frequently.

Diagnosis is by (1) biopsy of involved lymph nodes or tissue masses and (2) serologic studies demonstrating an IgM monoclonal protein. Bence Jones protein (urinary light chain dimers) is detectable in about 30% of cases. The bone marrow frequently is focally involved, as in other lymphomas, but shows small collections of plasmacytoid lymphocytes and not extensive infiltration by plasma cells, as in myeloma. Lytic bone lesions are rare.

Elevated IgM levels account for many of the clinical findings, in part due to increased viscosity of blood caused by the large IgM molecules. Viscosity can be measured directly (with an Ostwald viscometer); levels above 3.0 (normal is less than 2.0) are considered abnormal. **Hyperviscosity** produces sludging and slowing of blood in capillaries, which may produce transient neurologic symptoms due to multiple small ischemic foci within the central nervous system plus visual impairment if retinal vessels are involved. IgM may also act as a cryoglobulin, precipitating in small vessels in the relatively cooler peripheral tissues. **Raynaud's phenomenon,** characterized by cold sensitivity, pain, and focal gangrene, may result. **Anemia** is due to a combination of bleeding, impaired red cell production due to bone marrow involvement, and accelerated red cell destruction. **Bleeding manifestations** relate to thrombocytopenia, sludging, and complexing of IgM with clotting factors.

Treatment of this condition is in part symptomatic, to relieve the consequences of hyperviscosity, and in part aimed at the primary B cell lymphoma. Plasmapheresis, a technique for selective removal of IgM from the patient's serum, is of value in alleviating the symptoms temporarily. Chlorambucil and corticosteroids are the drugs of choice for direct treatment of the tumor.

LIGHT & HEAVY CHAIN DISEASES

As noted above, surplus light chains frequently are present in multiple myeloma along with whole immunoglobulin molecules and often are seen in the urine as Bence Jones protein. In some cases of myeloma, only light chains are produced, and this condition has been termed **light chain disease** or **Bence Jones myeloma**. The clinicopathologic findings are identical to those of other forms of plasma cell myeloma. Kappa light chain disease and lambda light chain disease are identical pathologically.

The production of heavy chains alone is a much less common phenomenon, and different types of heavy chains are associated with distinctly different pathologic conditions. These are summarized in Table 30–3. Mu chain disease is the least common and shows some resemblance to CLL; gamma chain disease is slightly more common than mu chain disease and resembles plasmacytoid lymphocytic lymphoma, while alpha chain disease is the most common form of heavy chain disease and typically presents as a lymphomatous infiltration of the gut.

These conditions may be diagnosed by demonstration of the monoclonal heavy chain in serum by immunoelectropheresis or in tissue sections using immunohistologic techniques.

Table 30–3. Heavy chain diseases.

	Alpha Chain Disease	Gamma Chain Disease	Mu Chain Disease
Approximate number of reported cases	150	50	15
Age at onset	10–30 years	10–40 years	> 50 years
Morphologic features	IPSID:[1] Plasma cell hyperplasia, Mediterranean lymphoma, immunoblastic sarcoma (B cell)	Usually resembles plasmacytoid lymphocytic lymphoma	Usually resembles chronic lymphocytic leukemia
Tissue site	Most often gut (IPSID);[1] rarely respiratory tract	Lymph node, spleen	Lymph nodes, marrow
Associated with amyloid	No	Yes	Yes

[1]IPSID = immunoproliferative small intestinal disease spectrum with 3 phases.

Alpha chain disease is of particular interest in that it includes a spectrum of disease ranging from plasma cell hyperplasia, usually involving the lamina propria of the small intestine, through progressive hyperplasia to frank neoplasia, all in association with a detectable monoclonal serum and urine immunoglobulin component that contains alpha chain fragments but no light chains. The term "immunoproliferative small intestinal disease (IPSID)" has been proposed for this spectrum of conditions. The initial nontumor phase of this disease is characterized by a diffuse plasma cell infiltrate that morphologically appears benign but shows an alpha chain-restricted pattern on immunohistologic staining. This stage is succeeded by a mixed plasmacellular and lymphocytic infiltrate that is sometimes known as Mediterranean lymphoma or Middle East lymphoma. Finally, there is the stage of frank destructive lymphoma, with marked cellular atypia and destructive invasion. Such cases show a high proportion of immunoblasts and indeed sometimes have been classified as immunoblastic sarcomas. There have been some claims that the early stages may represent sustained immunostimulation and may be reversible by the use of broad-spectrum antibiotics.

PRIMARY AMYLOIDOSIS

The tissue manifestations of amyloidosis have been described elsewhere (Chapter 2). With the recognition that in many cases the amyloid fibril appears to be composed of immunoglobulin or immunoglobulin fragments, it has become clear that primary amyloidosis and multiple myeloma are in fact closely related conditions. Indeed, in some instances it is difficult to distinguish them, the chief distinguishing criterion being the presence of multiple plasmacellular lytic lesions within bone marrow in myeloma and their absence in primary amyloidosis.

Like myeloma, primary amyloidosis has a peak incidence in the elderly. It tends to have an insidious onset, presenting with evidence of peripheral neuropathy, malabsorption syndrome, or renal or cardiac insufficiency. In the presence of a monoclonal gammopathy, primary amyloidosis is diagnosed on the basis of tissue biopsy showing typical histochemical reactions of amyloid (Congo red) in the absence of multiple myeloma or B cell lymphoma.

THE SPLEEN

Structure & Function

The spleen is located in the upper abdomen underneath the left rib cage. It weighs 120–160 g and is that part of the peripheral lymphoid system that is in the path of the blood circulation. The spleen is made up of **(1) white pulp**, composed of the lymphoid follicles (malpighian corpuscles), which contain both B cell (germinal centers) and T cell (periarteriolar lymphoid sheath) zones (see Chapter 4); and **(2) red pulp**, composed of the sinusoids, which are lined by endothelium and separated by the splenic cords.

The main function of the spleen is subserved by the phagocytic cells (littoral cells) that lie in the cords and sinusoids. These macrophages remove senescent erythrocytes from the blood. The macrophages have Fc receptors that permit them to recognize antibody-complexed particles in the blood and phagocytose them. Thus, in patients with autoimmune hemolytic anemias and thrombocytopenia, the spleen represents a major site of cell destruction.

The immunologic function of the spleen is not vital. In otherwise normal adults, splenectomy results in minimal immunodeficiency. In young children, splenectomy is followed by an increased susceptibility to infection with encapsulated bacteria such as *Streptococcus pneumoniae* and *Salmonella* species.

SPLENOMEGALY

The main clinical manifestation of splenic disease is splenic enlargement. The normal spleen is not palpable. When splenic enlargement occurs, the spleen can be palpated under the left costal margin.

The causes of splenomegaly (Table 30–4) are similar to the causes of lymphadenopathy (Chapter 28), with an additional set of features that relate to the role of the spleen as a filter for the blood and as a potential hematopoietic organ.

Splenomegaly in acute and chronic infections and in autoimmune and hypersensitivity diseases primarily results from proliferation of lymphocytes participating in the immune response to blood-borne antigens. In these situations, the malpighian nodules are generally much enlarged and may show conspicuous reactive centers that are foci of B cell proliferation. In most infections, a combined T and B cell response is seen. In the autoimmune diseases, the features of B cell reactivity may be particularly conspicuous. In leishmaniasis and in malaria, histiocytic proliferation also

Table 30-4. Causes of splenomegaly.

Nonneoplastic	
Acute infections	Various (eg, infectious mononucleosis, typhoid fever, malaria)
Chronic infections	Various (eg, brucellosis, infective endocarditis, malaria, leishmaniasis)
Autoimmune diseases	Rheumatoid arthritis (especially Still's disease),[1] systemic lupus erythematosus, idiopathic thrombocytopenic purpura
Hypersensitivity reactions	To drugs; serum sickness
Sarcoidosis	
Amyloidosis	
Storage diseases	Gaucher's disease; Niemann-Pick disease, ceroid histiocytosis
Portal venous hypertension	Cirrhosis, portal vein thrombosis
Hematologic disorders	Hemolytic anemias (thalassemia, autoimmune); extramedullary erythropoiesis, myelofibrosis
Splenic cysts and hamartomas	
Neoplastic	
Lymphocytic leukemias	Especially large in chronic lymphocytic leukemia and hairy cell leukemia
Non-Hodgkin's lymphomas	
Hodgkin's disease	
Polycythemia rubra vera	
Monocytoid leukemias	
Myeloid leukemias	Especially chronic myelocytic leukemia
Histiocytosis X	Hand-Schüller-Christian disease; Letterer-Siwe disease; histiocytic medullary reticulosis
Secondary neoplasms	Relatively rare

[1]Still's disease = juvenile rheumatoid arthritis.

contributes to the splenomegaly, and in leishmaniasis the characteristic organisms are usually readily observable within histiocytes.

Sarcoidosis produces numerous discrete granulomatous lesions resembling those seen in lymph nodes. Disseminated tuberculosis may produce an identical appearance, and the distinction may depend upon successful culture of the causative organism.

The "**storage diseases**" typically show proliferation of histiocytes. Splenomegaly is especially marked in Gaucher's disease, Niemann-Pick disease, and ceroid histiocytosis (sea-blue histiocyte syndrome). In H&E sections, these may all look similar, and special staining techniques and enzymatic analyses are required to make the distinction.

In **portal vein congestion,** the picture is of an expanded red pulp consisting of dilated sinuses packed with red blood cells. If chronic, there may be extensive fibrosis, hemorrhage, and deposition of iron pigment. The destruction of red cells in hemolytic anemias may produce a similar appearance. Multiple small infarcts are especially typical of the spleen in sickle cell anemia, in which the spleen decreases in size through childhood to become a shrivelled fibrotic structure ("autosplenectomy").

Of the **neoplasms** involving the spleen, chronic lymphocytic leukemia and hairy cell leukemia almost always produce significant splenomegaly, with extensive infiltration of the white pulp by neoplastic lymphocytes in CLL and the white pulp and sinuses in hairy cell leukemia. Similarly, non-Hodgkin's lymphomas may involve the spleen, exemplified by extensive involvement of the white pulp in many of the small-cell lymphomas or the formation of large destructive nodules in large-cell lymphomas such as immunoblastic sarcoma. **Hodgkin's disease** typically appears multifocally in the spleen, initially within the white pulp but later forming large confluent nodules throughout the spleen. **Myelocytic and monocytic leukemias** involve especially the red pulp of the spleen, and splenomegaly is marked in chronic myelocytic leukemia. In these conditions, leukemic cells may be admixed with areas showing extramedullary erythropoiesis.

Both **Hand-Schüller-Christian disease** and **Letterer-Siwe disease** (related manifestations of histiocytosis X) may involve the spleen. In the former condition, involvement may be diffuse or nodular, with numerous foamy histiocytes and eosinophils distributed throughout the spleen. In Letterer-Siwe disease, there is extensive involvement of the red pulp by proliferating histiocytes. **Histiocytic medullary reticulosis** typically produces marked splenomegaly with extensive replacement of red pulp by atypical histiocytes that show varying degrees of phagocytosis of red blood cells. Involvement is diffuse, akin to that seen in monocytic leukemias, and distinct nodules usually are not formed.

While small foci of metastatic tumor are found not uncommonly in spleens from patients dying from disseminated carcinoma, these metastatic deposits within the spleen seldom become large enough to produce clinical splenomegaly.

HYPERSPLENISM

Regardless of its cause, splenic enlargement may rarely result in anemia, leukopenia, and thrombocytopenia due to increased sequestration and destruction of these cells in the spleen. Red cells undergo membrane damage in their passage through the spleen and show anisocytosis and poikilocytosis in the peripheral blood. Splenectomy is curative.

THE THYMUS

The thymus, which is located in the superior mediastinum, reaches peak size and functional activity before birth, playing a vital role in the development and differentiation of T lymphocytes (see Chapter 4). This function is largely complete at birth, and thymectomy even in the neonatal period produces little immunologic impairment. The thymus undergoes gradual involution after childhood. In adults, the thymus is composed mainly of a pad of fat in which are scattered lymphoid nodules and Hassal's corpuscles.

Abnormalities in thymic structure associated with congenital immunodeficiency diseases have been described in Chapter 7.

Table 30-5. Pathology of the thymus.

Agenesis, dysgenesis	In congenital immunodeficiency states, the thymus may be rudimentary or absent (eg, DiGeorge syndrome, combined immunodeficiency; see Chapter 7).
Atrophy, involution	A "normal" age change in adults; a similar more acute loss of lymphocytes may occur in utero in "fetal stress" syndromes, as "accidental thymic involution."
Hyperplasia	Presence of immunoblasts plus B cell-reactive follicles in thymic medulla in myasthenia gravis and occasionally in systemic lupus erythematosus, Hashimoto's disease, Graves' disease, Addison's disease, rheumatoid arthritis, etc.[1]
Thymic epithelial cysts	Either cysts of Hassall's corpuscles or branchial cleft remnants; usually contain thymic tissue within the walls.
Thymic neoplasms	Primary thymomas are uncommon. Seminomas occur even more rarely. The thymus may be involved by leukemias, especially T-cell acute lymphoblastic leukemia.

[1]Status thymolymphaticus was once considered a cause of "sudden infant death"; the "thymic hyperplasia" described in this condition was nothing more than the normal large newborn thymus. Many of these cases were unfortunately treated by radiation, with a subsequent high incidence of thyroid cancer.

THYMIC HYPERPLASIA & MYASTHENIA GRAVIS

The thymus does not participate in the general lymphoid hyperplasia that occurs in systemic immune responses, and there is no thymic response that mirrors the normal proliferation of lymphoid cells that occurs in the lymph nodes, spleen, or gut-associated lymphoid tissues. The term "thymic hyperplasia" is thus a misnomer. However, it persists in current usage and denotes the presence of reactive follicles (foci of B cell proliferation) in the thymic medulla. This phenomenon is seen very rarely in normal individuals, but occurs in myasthenia gravis and to a lesser extent in other autoimmune diseases (Table 30–5).

Approximately 80% of patients with myasthenia gravis show germinal or reactive centers within the thymic medulla; another 10% of patients with myasthenia gravis have thymomas. A variety of abnormal immunologic findings have also been described in myasthenia gravis, including lymphocyte infiltrates in muscle, depressed mitogen responses for T cells, anti-DNA antibodies, anti-thymocyte antibodies, and, most significant in terms of the pathology of the disease, antibodies to acetylcholine receptors on the motor endplate (Chapter 66). Thymectomy leads to a gradual improvement in symptoms in many patients, particularly young women with disease of short duration. It is postulated that this change may be due to removal of a cross-reacting antigen or of a T helper cell population within the thymus that promotes production of the antireceptor antibody.

THYMIC NEOPLASMS

Any of the cells normally present in the thymus gland may give rise to primary neoplasia; thus, connective tissue cells (fibroblasts, fat cells, myoid cells, vascular cells, etc) may rarely give rise to tumors, as may scattered neuroendocrine cells (argentaffin cells—producing thymic carcinoid tumors). These types of neoplasms are mostly benign and no different from the comparable neoplasms of other tissues.

1. MALIGNANT LYMPHOMAS

Non-Hodgkin's lymphomas of T cell type may involve the thymus and occasionally appear to originate in the thymus. B cell lymphomas less often involve the thymus but may extend into the organ from involved mediastinal lymph nodes. Nodular sclerosing Hodgkin's disease typically involves the mediastinum and thymus.

Acute lymphoblastic leukemia (ALL) of T cell type particularly involves the thymus. As noted in Chapter 29, T-ALL forms a spectrum of disease with T lymphoblastic (or convoluted) lymphoma. The lymphomatous presentation of this disease typically is as a mediastinal mass, which many believe to originate in the thymus (so-called Sternberg's sarcoma). This characteristically is a disease of young men and classically terminates in acute lymphoblastic leukemia. The neoplastic T lymphoblasts show immunologic features in common with thymic lymphocytes (ie, positive for the monoclonal antibodies OKT6, OKT10, OKT4, and OKT8).

2. THYMOMA

The term "thymoma" is now reserved for neoplasms derived from the thymic epithelium, though certain types of thymic lymphoma were once included in this category.

Thymomas, even though they are epithelial neoplasms, typically contain large numbers of nonneoplastic T lymphocytes admixed with the epithelial cells; the lymphocytes may be so numerous and the epithelial cells so inconspicuous that the distinction from lymphoma is difficult.

Thymomas are rare, but several histologic subtypes have been described. Well-differentiated thymomas resemble normal thymus and are usually encapsulated and benign. In other cases, the epithelial cells are larger and more numerous. In poorly differentiated tumors, the epithelial cells may assume a spindle appearance (spindle-cell thymoma). Capsular invasion occurs in some tumors and may be followed by local invasion in a minority of cases; distant metastases are rare.

Table 30-6. Thymoma and associated "paraneoplastic" syndromes.[1]

Myasthenia gravis: 10% of myasthenia patients have thymoma.
Pure red cell aplasia: 50% of aplastic patients have thymoma.
Neutropenia with or without thrombocytopenia
Hypogammaglobulinemia
Polymyositis
Myocarditis
Systemic lupus erythematosus
IgA deficiency and multiple neoplasms
Other (nonthymic) cancers
Other autoimmune diseases

[1]Overall, approximately 40% of patients with thymoma have one of these conditions.

Thymomas may present as a consequence of the local effects of compression (trachea) or infiltration of adjacent structures, or they may produce "paraneoplastic syndromes," which are largely unexplained but show a close association with the presence of the thymoma (Table 30-6).

3. SEMINOMA & TERATOMA

Pure seminoma and seminoma admixed with other germ cell neoplastic elements occur rarely in the thymus as primary extragonadal neoplasms. Morphologically and behaviorally, they resemble the corresponding tumors of ovary or testis. It is important to distinguish these seminomas from epithelial thymomas, since seminomas, while highly malignant, are radiosensitive.

Immunohistologic techniques staining for keratin are valuable in recognizing the epithelial nature of thymoma—in contrast to seminoma. Additional monoclonal antibodies have recently become available that appear to be specific for thymic epithelial cells.

Section VII. Diseases of the Head & Neck

This section deals with diseases of the head and neck—but not the brain, which is covered in the nervous system section. The main rationale of including such diverse organs as the oral cavity, salivary glands, ear, nose, pharynx, and larynx in one section is that they are included in the surgical specialty of otolaryngology. Diseases of the teeth (dental pathology, Chapter 31) and eyes (ophthalmic pathology, Chapter 33) form the rest of this section. The oral cavity, nose, pharynx, and larynx form the common opening of the respiratory and gastrointestinal systems and are often collectively called the upper respiratory tract.

Viral infections of the upper respiratory tract which include coryza (the common cold) and pharyngotonsillitis are among the commonest infections of humans and are responsible for the loss of many man-hours of work throughout the world. The commonest neoplasms in this section are squamous carcinomas of the upper respiratory tract (Chapters 31 and 32) and salivary gland neoplasms (Chapter 31).

31 The Oral Cavity & Salivary Glands

STRUCTURE & FUNCTION

The oral cavity is lined by a mucosa composed of nonkeratinizing stratified squamous epithelium, continuous with the skin at the lips and with the pharyngeal mucosa posteriorly. Specialized structures in the oral cavity include the following:

(1) The **taste buds,** which are specialized nerve endings with afferents in the ninth (posterior tongue) and seventh (anterior tongue) cranial nerves.

(2) The **teeth,** which are embedded in the maxilla and mandible. That part of the mucosa that is reflected onto the bone in relation to the teeth is called the **gingiva (gum).**

(3) Three major pairs of **salivary glands,** plus numerous minor salivary glands. The **parotid glands** are composed almost entirely of serous cells and are situated in front of and below the ear. They secrete saliva through a duct (Stensen's duct) that opens in the cheek adjacent to the molar teeth. The seromucous submandibular gland lies beneath the mandible and opens by a duct (Warthin's duct) into the floor of the mouth. The sublingual gland, also seromucous in type, is situated in the floor of the mouth and empties through 10–20 small ducts.

(4) Lymphoid tissue, which guards the pharyngeal opening (Waldeyer's ring). The tonsils, which are situated between the faucial pillars and adenoids in the nasopharynx, are the largest collections of lymphoid tissue.

The function of the oral cavity is to accept food and begin the process of digestion. Mastication (by the grinding action of teeth), aided by the lubricant action of the saliva, converts the food into a bolus that is propelled back by the tongue muscles into the pharynx for swallowing. Saliva contains **(a) amylase,** which may initiate carbohydrate digestion; **(b) lysozyme,** which has bactericidal properties; and **(c) secretory IgA.** The salivary gland epithelium synthesizes the secretor piece, which complexes with IgA produced by plasma cells in the gland stroma.

MANIFESTATIONS OF DISEASES OF THE ORAL CAVITY

Pain

The oral cavity is richly supplied with sensory nerve endings, and pain is a feature of almost all diseases that affect the mucosa. Pain in diseases of the teeth occurs only when pain-sensitive fibers in the root of a tooth are involved.

Changes of the Oral Mucosa

Alterations of the mucosa include ulceration, vesicular lesions (blisters), and changes in color. Oral ulcers occur in many diseases, including infections, allergy, trauma, and neoplasms. Vesicular lesions occur in infections (eg, herpesvirus infections) and immunologic diseases such as pemphigus vulgaris and erythema multiforme that primarily affect the skin. White plaques on the mucosa (leukoplakia) occur in hyperplastic and neoplastic conditions, and melanin pigmentation occurs in many systemic diseases (Table 31–1).

Masses

Mass lesions may be solid or cystic and may be found in any part of the oral cavity. Mass lesions arising in structures outside the oral cavity (eg, bone of the mandible and maxilla) may involve the oral cavity by extension.

DISEASES OF THE TEETH

DENTAL CARIES

Etiology

Dental caries is a progressive decomposition of tooth substances caused by a wide variety of bacteria and fungi but most commonly *Streptococcus mutans*. The microorganisms proliferate in food residue on the teeth to form a hard adherent mass of calcified debris containing bacteria and desquamated epithelial cells (**plaque;** also called **tartar** and **calculus**). Enzymes and acids produced by the microorganisms cause proteolysis, decalcifica-

Table 31–1. Nonneoplastic diseases of the oral cavity.

Diseases	Symptoms	Causes
Infections		
Herpes simplex	See text	Herpes simplex
Herpangina	See text	Coxsackievirus A
Candidiasis	See text	*Candida albicans*
Aphthous stomatitis	See text	Unknown
Foot and mouth disease	Ulcers in mouth (common in animals, rare in man)	Virus
Vincent's angina (trench mouth)	Ulceration of gums (gingivitis)	Vincent's spirochete and fusiform bacilli
Tuberculosis	Ulcers, tongue or cheeks	*Mycobacterium tuberculosis*
Actinomycosis	Granuloma, ulcer, abscess	*Actinomyces israeli*
Syphilis	Chancre (primary), snail track ulcer (secondary), gumma (tertiary)	*Treponema pallidum*
Cancrum oris	Severe necrosis (gangrene), rare	Anaerobic streptococci
Measles	Koplik's spots (papules) on cheeks opposite molars	Measles virus
Diphtheria	Adherent "membrane" of fibrin and exudate on pharynx	*Clostridium diphtheriae*
Leishmaniasis (espundia)	Ulceration	*Leishmania*
Skin diseases associated with oral lesions		
Bullous pemphigoid	Blister type lesions	Chapter 61
Pemphigus vulgaris	Blister type lesions	Chapter 61
Erythema multiforme (Stevens-Johnson syndrome)	Blister type lesions	Chapter 61
Lichen planus	Flat "white lace" areas	Chapter 61
Oral manifestations of systemic disease		
Behçet's syndrome	Ulcers of mouth, conjunctiva, genitals	Unknown
Purpura	Involves mouth and skin	Chapter 27
Metal poisoning	Gingivitis and pigmentation (includes lead, silver, arsenic, gold, mercury)	Chapter 11
Phenytoin	Gingivitis, hypertrophied gums	...
Scurvy (vitamin C deficiency)	Gingivitis, bleeding from gums	Chapter 10
Vitamin B complex deficiency	Glossitis, cheilosis (inflammation of tongue and angles of mouth, respectively)	Chapter 10
Iron deficiency (Plummer-Vinson syndrome)	Atrophic glossitis and dysphagia	Chapter 37
Telangiectasia (Osler-Weber-Rendu)	Small vascular telangiectases of mucosa and lips	...
Addison's disease	Pigmentation of mucosa	Chapter 60
Hemochromatosis	Pigmentation of mucosa	Chapter 43
Peutz-Jeghers syndrome	Pigmentation of mucosa	Chapter 41

tion, and decay of first the enamel covering of the tooth, then the dentin, and finally the tooth pulp. Cavities are detectable with probes when there is a break in continuity of the enamel. There is an individual variation in the susceptibility of enamel to decay.

Several factors influence the risk of dental caries:

(1) Microorganisms are essential for formation of caries. Attempts to develop vaccines against common causative organisms have not proved successful. The use of antibiotics is not feasible because of the variety of microorganisms involved and the adverse effects of these drugs.

(2) Regular brushing prevents accumulation of food residue and clearly reduces the incidence of caries.

(3) Sugar, particularly in a form that sticks to the teeth, promotes dental caries because bacteria utilize carbohydrates for metabolism. The stickiness of plaque is caused by dextran, which is a product of sucrose fermentation by *Streptococcus mutans.*

(4) Once plaque has formed, it cannot be removed by simple brushing. Removal of plaque by regular use of dental floss or by scaling decreases the incidence of caries.

(5) Fluoride has a dual protective effect: It makes the enamel more resistant to bacterial degradation and has a weak microbicidal action.

(6) Saliva has a mechanical cleansing action and contains microbicidal substances (lysozyme, IgA). Any cause of decreased salivary secretion, such as Sjögren's syndrome or radiation, increases the risk of dental caries. Patients who undergo radiation treatment to the oral cavity need careful dental care to prevent "radiation caries."

Clinicopathologic Effects (Fig 31-1)

A. Early Caries: Early dental caries does not cause symptoms but can be recognized by clinical dental examination. Because caries is slowly progressive, regular dental examination permits effective treatment at an early stage.

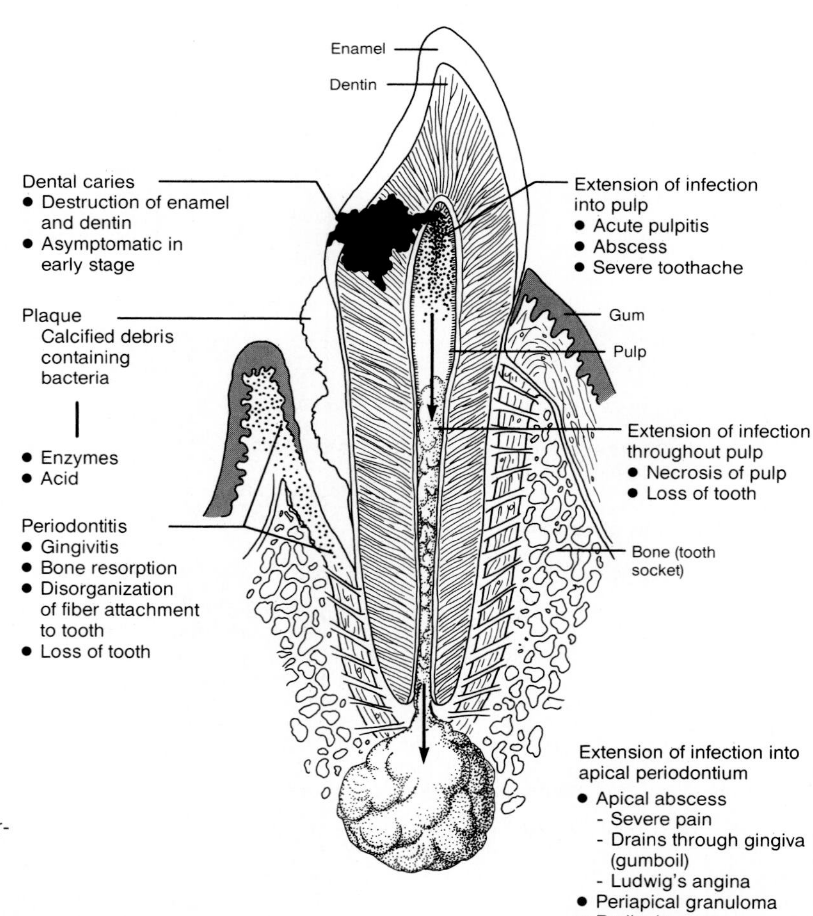

Figure 31-1. Dental caries, periodontitis, and their sequelae. The formation of plaque is the main etiologic factor for both conditions.

B. Pulp Infection: Deep caries that extends through the enamel and dentin layers into the tooth pulp permits the entry of microorganisms into the tooth pulp. Acute inflammation results, leading to the formation of a localized abscess or destruction of the entire pulp. Both are associated with severe pain (toothache) and swelling.

When there is a localized **pulp abscess,** simple drainage and antibiotic therapy may be sufficient treatment. Total destruction of the pulp requires clearance of the entire pulp cavity followed by replacement with an inert material and sealing (root canal therapy).

C. Periapical Infection: Extension of pulp infection to the apical periodontium results in an inflammatory lesion that progresses through several stages:

1. An **apical abscess** develops around the apex of the tooth and is intensely painful owing to the high tissue tension that develops in the bone. The abscess enlarges and eventually drains through the gingiva (parulis, gumboil). Rarely, the infection spreads in the floor of the mouth and neck along fascial planes, associated with extensive tissue necrosis (Ludwig's angina).

2. Periapical granuloma is a more chronic inflammatory response around the apex of the tooth, characterized by bone resorption and infiltration by lymphocytes, plasma cells, and histiocytes. Symptoms may be minor—typically mild pain when biting down or increased sensitivity of the tooth to heat and cold. X-ray reveals a well-demarcated lucent area in the bone at the apex of the tooth.

Periapical granulomas tend to undergo epithelialization from the periapical region to form a cystic structure lined by squamous epithelium and containing the fluid debris of inflammation. This is called a **radicular cyst**.

PERIODONTAL DISEASE

Periodontal disease is also a complication of plaque formation. Accumulation of **plaque** (see above) in the crevice between the gingiva and the tooth causes inflammation **(gingivitis),** which may progress to **periodontitis,** involving not only the gingival crevice but also the periodontal membrane, alveolar bone, and the outer layer of the tooth itself. The end result is instability of the tooth, resorption of the gingiva, purulent discharge from the gingival crevice (pyorrhea), and eventual tooth loss. Again, multiple bacteria are involved.

Gingival hyperplasia also occurs in pregnancy (often in localized areas, producing a "pregnancy" tumor), in some patients receiving phenytoin therapy, and in response to local gingival hemorrhage (in scurvy, leukemia, or thrombocytopenia). Fibrous thickening of the gingiva may also occur in chronic gingivitis resulting from low-grade chronic bacterial infection.

CYSTS OF THE JAW

Cysts of the jaw are very common. Many of them—eg, radicular cysts, follicular cysts, and odontogenic keratocysts—occur in relation to the teeth. Others, such as fissural and inclusion cysts, are not related to the teeth but enter the differential diagnosis.

Radicular cyst is the most common and is the result of epithelialization of a periapical granuloma.

Follicular cysts arise from the epithelium of the tooth follicle. They may be associated with failure of eruption of the involved tooth. If the unerupted tooth is present in the cyst wall, the term "dentigerous cyst" may be applied.

Odontogenic keratocysts are lined by a keratinized squamous epithelium and occur at the root of the tooth. They may be multiple, in which case they are frequently associated with basal cell carcinomas of the skin.

Fissural or inclusion cysts are derived from epithelial inclusions along lines of fusion of the embryologic facial processes; they are classified according to their site, eg, median palatine cyst, globulomaxillary cyst. A similar cyst arising in nasopalatine duct remnants is called a nasopalatine cyst. All of these are fluid-filled cysts lined by squamous or respiratory epithelium.

Bone cysts are discussed in Chapter 67.

NEOPLASMS OF TOOTH-FORMING (ODONTOGENIC) TISSUES

The commonest neoplasms in this region are those derived from bone (osteoma, osteosarcoma, etc) and soft tissues (neurofibroma, vascular neoplasms, etc). Ameloblastoma, though it is the most common odontogenic tumor, is rare, comprising 1% of cysts and tumors of the jaw. Other odontogenic neoplasms (cementomas, dentinomas, etc) are very rare.

Ameloblastoma occurs mainly in patients between 20 and 50 years of age, most often in the molar region of the mandible. It commonly is made up of both cystic and solid areas and arises from the epithelium of the dental lamina. It is a locally invasive neoplasm that does not metastasize, having a behavior and appearance similar to those of basal cell carcinoma of the skin. Because of its tendency to local invasion, it may recur after surgical removal.

DISEASES OF THE ORAL CAVITY (Table 31-1)

INFLAMMATORY LESIONS

HERPES SIMPLEX STOMATITIS

Herpes simplex type 1 is a common viral infection of the oral mucosa. The primary infection occurs in children or young adults as a widespread gingivostomatitis, characterized by multiple vesicles that rupture early to form ulcers. Systemic symptoms such as fever are present. Although locally severe, the disease is self-limited, and recovery is the rule.

Herpes simplex virus passes up the nerve trunks and infects the ganglia in the acute phase, where it remains dormant for long periods. Reactivation of the infection occurs repeatedly in some patients, the virus passing down the nerve to the oral mucosa to form isolated vesicular lesions and ulcers (herpes labialis—"fever blisters" and "cold sores"). Reactivation is often precipitated by a concurrent fever or common cold or by exposure to sunlight. About 20% of the population is affected.

HERPANGINA

Herpangina is an uncommon infection of the oral mucosa with coxsackievirus A. Vesicular lesions occur on the palate and posterior oral cavity and may be accompanied by skin lesions in the extremities (hand, foot, and mouth disease).

CANDIDIASIS (Oral Thrush)

Candida albicans is a normal commensal of the mouth. Clinical infection of the oral mucosa usually represents an opportunistic infection in a patient with increased susceptibility. Persons at risk are those with immunosuppression, eg, AIDS patients or those receiving cancer chemotherapy; newborn infants; patients with diabetes; and sick patients who must receive long-term antibiotic therapy.

Candida produces inflammation and edema of the epithelium, forming white patches that leave raw ulcerated lesions when they are rubbed off. The budding yeasts and pseudohyphae of *Candida* can be identified in smears, cultures, or biopsy specimens from the lesion.

APHTHOUS STOMATITIS

Aphthous stomatitis is a common disorder characterized by recurrent episodes of painful shallow ulcers ("canker sores") on the oral mucosa. The pathologic picture is of nonspecific acute inflammation. The cause is unknown—psychosomatic and allergic mechanisms have been suggested; no infectious agent has been identified. The disease is usually self-limited and is annoying but not ominous. Rarely, it is associated with genital and conjunctival ulcers and neurologic abnormalities (Behçet's syndrome).

RARE INFECTIONS OF THE ORAL CAVITY

Actinomyces israelii and *Actinomyces bovis* cause chronic suppurative inflammation in the mouth and jaw. Patients present with an indurated jaw mass that has multiple sinuses opening to the skin surface, which drain pus. The pus typically contains visible small colonies of the organism (sulfur granules). *Actinomyces* species are gram-positive filamentous bacteria that are part of the normal mouth flora, and actinomycosis usually follows dental extraction. The organism is sensitive to penicillin.

A wide variety of spirochetes and fusiform bacilli inhabit the mouth. In debilitated or malnourished individuals, they may cause severe ulcerative gingivitis (**Vincent's angina,** or trench mouth).

Syphilis may involve the mouth in all 3 stages. In primary syphilis, the chancre may be on the lips or tongue; in secondary syphilis, superficial mucous patches and "snail track" ulcers may be present; in tertiary syphilis, chronic inflammation may produce tongue ulcers or large granulomas (gummas). Congenital syphilis also produces scarring at the angles of the mouth (rhagades). Abnormalities in the permanent teeth—Hutchinson's incisors and Moon's ulcers—are described in Chapter 54.

SKIN DISEASES MANIFESTING IN THE MOUTH

The following skin diseases are frequently manifested in the mouth, with or without concurrent skin lesions: (1) lichen planus, (2) pemphigus vulgaris, (3) bullous pemphigoid, and (4) erythema multiforme (Stevens-Johnson syndrome). The histologic features of these lesions are characteristic and permit diagnosis (Chapter 61).

BENIGN "TUMORS" OF THE ORAL CAVITY

A large number of lesions present clinically as a mass in the oral cavity. Not all are neoplasms.

MUCOCELE (Mucus Escape Reaction)

Mucoceles represent a localized inflammatory reaction to the escape of mucus from a ruptured minor salivary gland or duct. They are usually small white cystic structures. More rarely, they become large and stretch the overlying mucosa. Large mucoceles of the floor of the mouth resulting from damage to the submandibular or sublingual salivary ducts are called ranulas. Mucoceles are distinct from mucous cysts, which contain mucus and are lined by columnar epithelium.

PYOGENIC GRANULOMA

Pyogenic granuloma is a common oral lesion that is the result of a reactive inflammatory proliferation of granulation tissue. It presents as a small, bright red nodule with ulceration of the overlying mucosa (Fig 31–2). Pyogenic granulomas occur commonly during pregnancy (pregnancy tumor). The cause is unknown. They resolve spontaneously.

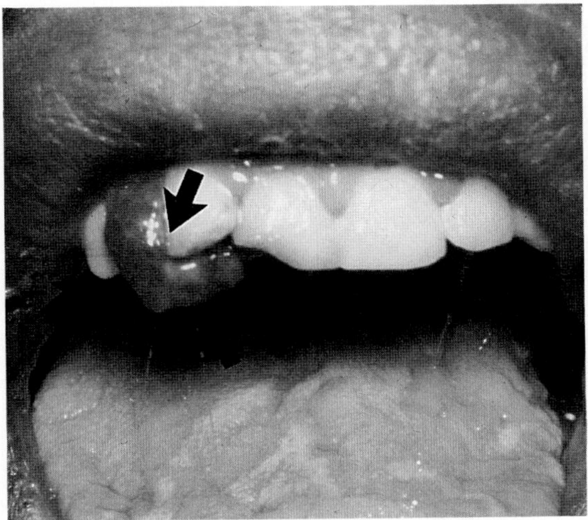

Figure 31–2. Pyogenic granuloma of upper gingiva. This appeared as a fleshy red mass projecting between 2 teeth (arrow).

EPULIS

The term epulis signifies a local reactive inflammatory lesion of the gum that presents as a mass. It includes pyogenic granuloma as well as a distinct lesion composed of multinucleated giant cells (giant cell epulis). A form of congenital epulis is characterized by the proliferation of large cells with abundant granular cytoplasm (granular cell epulis).

LINGUAL THYROID

Thyroid tissue at the root of the tongue is a rare condition that represents incomplete descent of thyroid tissue in the embryo. It usually coexists with a normal thyroid but in rare cases represents the individual's only thyroid tissue.

BENIGN NEOPLASMS OF THE ORAL CAVITY

Benign neoplasms in the oral cavity may arise from the squamous epithelium (squamous papilloma), from mesenchymal cells (fibroma, lipoma, neurofibroma), or from minor salivary glands (adenomas). One benign tumor that occurs commonly in the tongue is the granular cell tumor, probably a variant of a schwannoma in which the cells have abundant granular cytoplasm.

SQUAMOUS CARCINOMA OF THE ORAL CAVITY

Incidence & Etiology

Squamous carcinoma accounts for over 95% of malignant neoplasms in the oral cavity and 5% of all cancers in the United States. Cancers arising in the lower lip (40%), the tongue (20%), and the floor of the mouth (15%) account for the majority. Involvement of the upper lip, palate, gingiva, and tonsillar area (5% each) is less common. The mucosa of the cheek is rarely the primary site for squamous carcinoma.

Oral cancer is much more common in men than in women, and whites are affected more commonly than blacks. Etiologic factors include cigarette and pipe smoking, tobacco chewing, and alcohol.

Oral cancer is extremely common in Sri Lanka and parts of India, where chewing betel is common—betel is a green leaf that is mixed with areca nut, limestone, and tobacco to form a cud. The carcinogenic agent is believed to be in either the limestone or the tobacco. In parts of Italy where it is customary to smoke cigars with the lighted end inside the mouth, polycyclic hydrocarbons are believed to be the agents responsible for causing squamous carcinoma.

Clinical Features

Squamous cancer begins as a painless indurated plaque on the tongue or oral mucosa that commonly ulcerates to form a malignant ulcer. The lesion is usually readily visible, and diagnosis is made by biopsy. A significant number of patients with oral cancer present first with involved cervical lymph nodes. In very advanced local disease, there may be fixation of the tongue, interfering with speech and swallowing.

Pathology

The earliest lesion is squamous **epithelial dysplasia,** the most severe form of which is carcinoma in situ. At this stage there may or may not be visible whitish thickening (leukoplakia) of the epithelium (see below). However, most lesions are invasive to a variable depth at the time of diagnosis. The degree of differentiation varies; most tumors are well differentiated.

Oral cancer spreads primarily by lymphatics. Cervical lymph nodes are involved early. Bloodstream metastasis occurs late.

Leukoplakia is a term applied to visible flat, white lesions of the oral or genital mucous membranes. In most instances, it is due simply to hyperkeratosis (increased thickness of keratin layer) resulting from chronic irritation. However, in some instances, epithelial dysplasia is present, and the lesion is then considered precancerous. Persistent leukoplakia should therefore be biopsied.

Treatment & Prognosis

Treatment of oral squamous carcinoma is by radical surgery, radiotherapy, and chemotherapy. Squamous carcinoma of the oral cavity is sensitive to radiation therapy. The prognosis depends on the stage of the disease and is relatively good in the absence of cervical lymph node involvement.

OTHER MALIGNANT NEOPLASMS OF THE ORAL CAVITY

Rare malignant neoplasms in the oral cavity include malignant lymphomas and carcinomas of minor salivary gland origin. Malignant melanoma is very rare.

DISEASES OF THE SALIVARY GLANDS

INFLAMMATORY LESIONS OF THE SALIVARY GLANDS

SALIVARY DUCT CALCULI (SIALOLITHIASIS)

Calculi occur mainly in the duct of the submandibular gland, possibly related to the thicker mucoid secretion of this gland. Obstruction of a salivary gland duct produces acute inflammation (acute sialadenitis) followed by chronic inflammation, glandular atrophy, and fibrosis (chronic sialadenitis).

SJÖGREN'S SYNDROME

Sjögren's syndrome is an autoimmune disease in which there is immune-mediated destruction of the lacrimal and salivary glands. It is manifested clinically as dry eyes (keratoconjunctivitis sicca) and dry mouth (xerostomia) due to failure of gland secretion. It is commonly associated with other autoimmune diseases, notably rheumatoid arthritis. Patients with Sjögren's syndrome have an increased incidence of malignant lymphomas in the salivary gland.

About 75% of patients have rheumatoid factor in the blood, and 70% have antinuclear antibodies. Specific autoantibodies designated SS-A and SS-B have been identified in the serum of 60% of patients with Sjögren's syndrome.

Histologically, the lacrimal and salivary glands show marked lymphocytic and plasma cell infiltration with destruction of the glandular epithelium and fibrosis.

The diagnosis can be made by clinical tests to demonstrate absence of secretion of tears and by lip biopsy, which shows the typical histologic changes in the mucus glands of the lip (Fig 31–3).

INFECTIONS OF THE SALIVARY GLANDS

The parotid gland is the commonest site of involvement in **mumps virus** infection. The gland is painfully enlarged in the acute phase. Mumps is a self-limited illness.

Bacterial parotitis occurred commonly in the past in debilitated patients with dehydration and poor oral hygiene. It was characterized by painful enlargement of the gland, frequently complicated

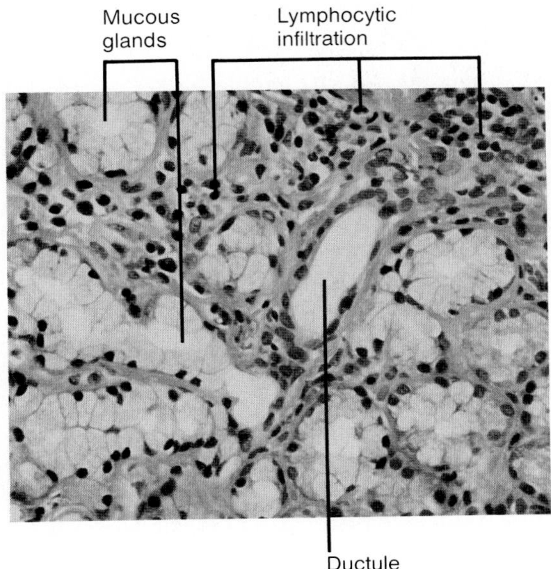

Figure 31-3. Lip biopsy in Sjögren's syndrome, showing infiltration by lymphocytes and plasma cells of minor salivary glands.

by abscess formation. Improvement in oral hygiene in patients at risk has made bacterial parotitis uncommon.

NEOPLASMS OF THE SALIVARY GLANDS (Table 31-2)

Salivary gland neoplasms are common and varied. About 80% occur in the parotids, 15% in the submandibular gland, and 5% in minor salivary glands. All present as a mass causing enlargement of the affected gland. Computerized tomography is helpful in assessment of the location and extent of salivary gland neoplasms. Diagnosis requires cytologic (fine-needle aspiration) or histologic examination.

BENIGN NEOPLASMS

Pleomorphic Adenoma (Mixed Tumor)

Pleomorphic adenoma accounts for over 50% of salivary gland tumors. Although the lesion is benign and well-circumscribed, encapsulation is incomplete, and simple enucleation is followed by a high rate of local recurrence due to regrowth of residual tumor. Wide excision is necessary for cure.

Pleomorphic adenoma is a firm, solid mass. Histologically, the tumor presents a greatly varied appearance. Uniform epithelial and myoepithelial

Table 31-2. Salivary gland neoplasms.

Neoplasm	Rate of Occurrence	Degree of Malignancy
Adenomas		
Pleomorphic adenoma (mixed parotid tumor)[1]	60%	Benign but tend to recur as a result of local extension
Adenolymphoma (Warthin's tumor)	10%	Benign
Monomorphic adenomas (various subtypes)	3%	Benign
Carcinomas		
Adenocarcinoma	5%	Variable degree of malignancy
Mucoepidermoid tumor	5%	Combined squamous and mucous cells, variable malignancy
Adenoid cystic carcinoma	3%	Malignant; marked tendency to invade locally; metastases occur late
Acinic cell carcinoma	3%	Low-grade[2]
Carcinoma in mixed tumor	3%	Variable degree of malignancy
Undifferentiated carcinoma	3%	Highly malignant[2]
Others[3]	Rare	

[1]Most of these tumors occur most often in the parotid gland, but any salivary gland may be involved.
[2]For highly malignant tumors, the 5-year survival rate is 20% or less; low-grade cancers have a 5-year survival rate of 80%.
[3]Others include lymphomas, squamous carcinomas.

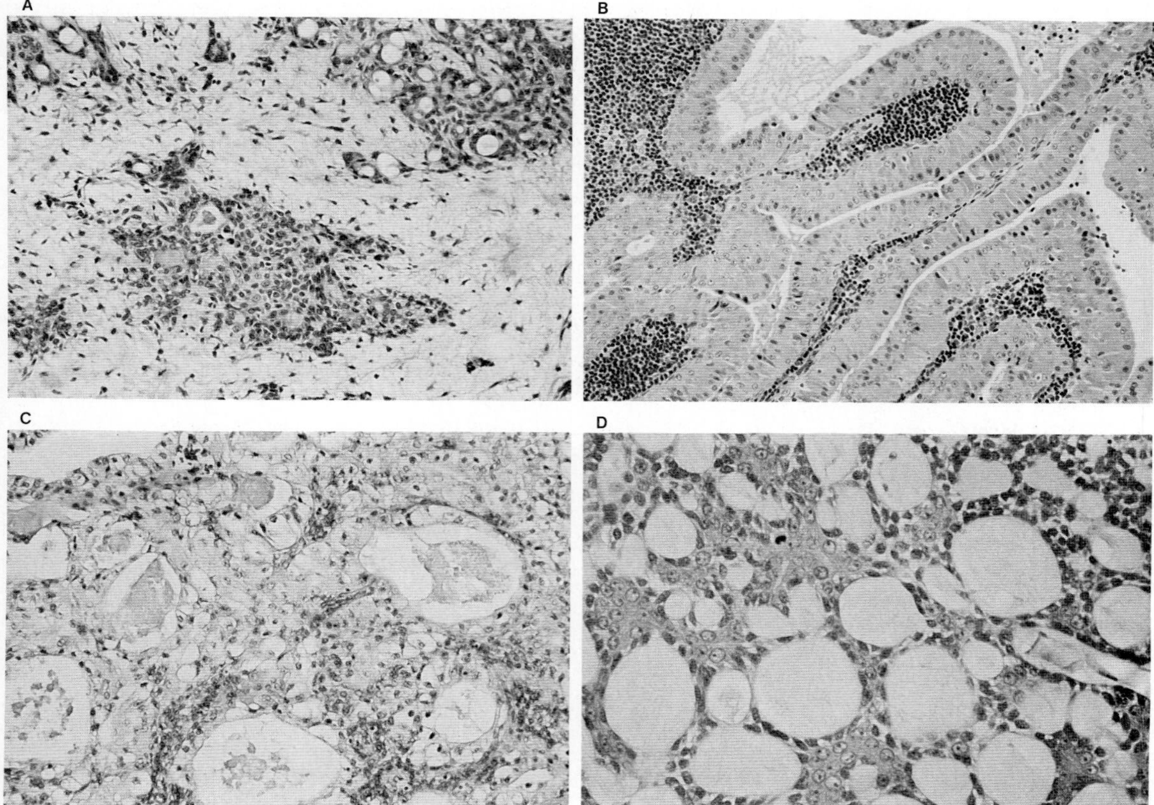

Figure 31–4. Neoplasms of salivary glands. **A:** Mixed tumor of salivary gland (pleomorphic adenoma) composed of small, uniform, polygonal cells forming sheets and small glands surrounded by abundant myxomatous intercellular material. **B:** Warthin's tumor, showing papillary structures lined by a double-layered epithelial lining composed of large cells with abundant granular cytoplasm (oncocytes) and lymphocytic infiltrate. **C:** Mucoepidermoid tumor of salivary gland, showing well-differentiated mucous cells lining glandular spaces and intervening solid epidermoid cells. **D:** Adenoid cystic carcinoma of salivary gland, characterized by small round epithelial cells forming round spaces containing basement membrane material.

cells are distributed in cords, nests, and strands within a matrix of mucoid material (Fig 31–4A), which frequently resembles cartilage (hence the mistaken notion that this was a mixed mesenchymal and epithelial tumor).

Warthin's Tumor (Adenolymphoma)

Most Warthin tumors occur in the parotid gland. They may rarely be multicentric and bilateral. The histologic appearance is distinctive (Fig 31–4B), with cystic spaces lined by a uniform double-layered epithelium that is frequently thrown into papillary folds. The neoplastic epithelial cells are large, with abundant pink cytoplasm, and surrounded by a dense lymphocytic infiltrate.

MALIGNANT SALIVARY GLAND NEOPLASMS

Malignant neoplasms of the salivary glands are of several different pathologic types (Table 31–2).

Most of these neoplasms are slow-growing. The exceptions are the rare undifferentiated carcinomas and the high-grade mucoepidermoid carcinomas. Low-grade mucoepidermoid carcinoma (Fig 31–4C) is a well-circumscribed neoplasm with variable solid and cystic areas that is cured in over 90% of cases by surgical removal. Adenoid cystic carcinoma (Fig 31–4D) is a highly infiltrative neoplasm with a tendency to invade along nerves. It is very rarely cured by surgery because of its invasiveness, and local recurrences and metastases often occur many (5–25) years after original treatment. Carcinomas arising in mixed tumors and acinic cell carcinoma have variable clinical courses.

The Ear, Nose, Pharynx, & Larynx 32

I. THE EAR

The ear (Fig 32–1) is divided into (1) the **external ear;** (2) the **middle ear,** which is separated from the external auditory meatus by the tympanic membrane and is in communication anteriorly with the pharynx via the auditory tube (eustachian tube) and posteriorly with the mastoid air cells; and (3) the **inner ear,** consisting of the semicircular canals, which are part of the vestibular system, and the cochlea, which is the hearing sense organ. The vestibular and auditory nerves arise in the inner ear and pass to the brain stem in the internal auditory meatus.

THE EXTERNAL EAR

The external ear consists of the pinna (or auricle) and the external auditory meatus. The pinna is composed of cartilage covered by skin. The meatus is lined by stratified squamous epithelium and contains wax-secreting ceruminous glands between the epithelium and the bony wall.

Preauricular Sinus & Cyst

This is a developmental anomaly associated with abnormal fusion of the facial folds. A blind-ending epithelium-lined tract opens as a small pit anterior to the meatus. Obstruction of the opening may lead to the development of an epidermal cyst; infection may cause an abscess and discharging sinus.

Otitis Externa

Inflammation of the external auditory canal is commonly caused by saprophytic fungi, commonly *Aspergillus* spp. This causes pain and a thick discharge. A foreign body or excessive exposure to water (swimmer's ear) predisposes to infection by low-grade pathogens.

Herpes Zoster

Herpes zoster involving the facial nerve ganglion (Ramsay Hunt syndrome) results in typical viral vesicles in the external ear, commonly associated with severe pain.

Lepromatous Leprosy

Lepromatous leprosy commonly involves the pinna of the ear, causing multinodular thickening of the skin and destruction of the cartilage.

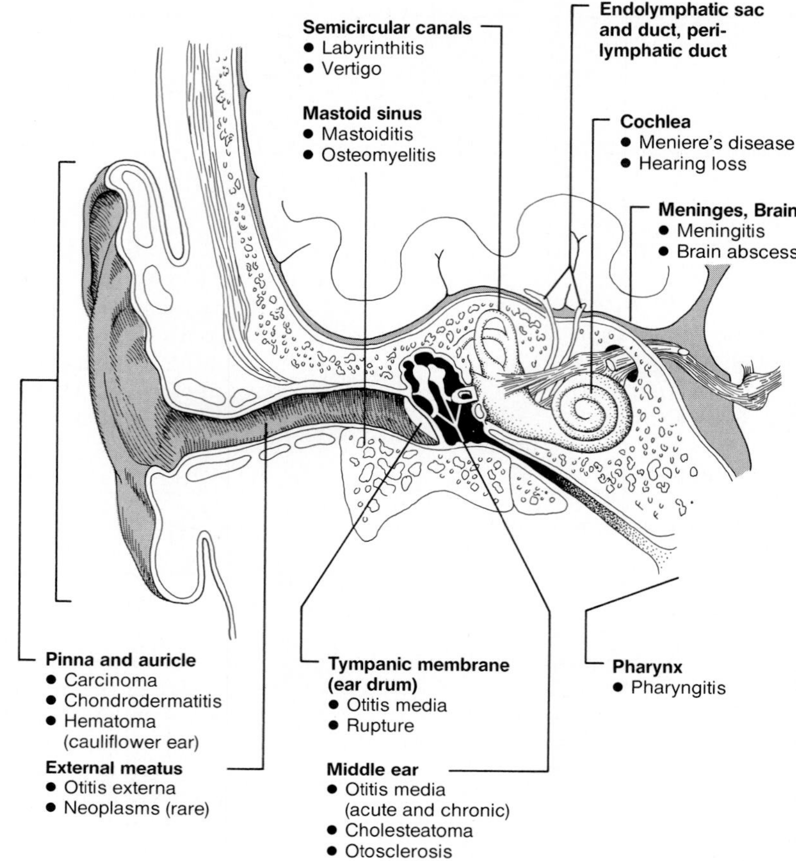

Figure 32-1. The structure of the ear and its principal diseases.

Chondrodermatitis Nodularis Helicis

This is a common lesion characterized clinically by the occurrence of a painful nodule in the helix. It is thought to result from trauma and is more common in males. Microscopically, there is ulceration of the skin and a chronic inflammatory infiltrate involving the perichondrium of the underlying cartilage. Surgical excision is curative.

Cauliflower Ear

This is the result of trauma and is most commonly seen in professional boxers. It is caused by thickening due to multiple organized and contracted hematomas.

Neoplasms of the External Ear

The skin of the external ear is a common site for basal cell and squamous carcinoma. Nevi and malignant melanoma also occur in the skin of the ear.

Neoplasms of the external auditory meatus, such as osteoma and ceruminous gland adenoma, are very rare.

THE MIDDLE EAR

OTITIS MEDIA

Incidence & Etiology

Otitis media is a common disease characterized by acute or chronic suppurative inflammation of the middle ear. Common causes are *Streptococcus pyogenes* and the pneumococcus. The middle ear is usually infected by pharyngeal organisms that reach the middle ear via the auditory tube. It usually occurs in children as a complication of viral and bacterial infections of the pharynx. Edema obstructing the pharyngeal opening of the auditory tube predisposes to infection.

Pathologic Features

In **acute otitis media,** the middle ear is filled with purulent exudate. The reddened tympanic membrane bulges into the external auditory meatus and may rupture, leading to a purulent discharge from the ear. Adequate and early treatment results in resolution with the middle ear reverting to normal.

In cases that are not properly treated, chronic suppuration occurs with fibrosis of the ossicles, leading to hearing loss. **Chronic otitis media** is associated with ingrowth of keratinizing squamous epithelium from the tympanic membrane, forming a pearly-white keratinized mass with acute and chronic inflammation known as a **choleastoma**.

Clinical Features

In **acute otitis media** there is earache and fever. The diagnosis is made by noting the outward-bulging, tense, reddened tympanic membrane. In cases where the membrane has ruptured, there is a purulent discharge from the ear. Impairment of hearing is common in these cases. Culture of the exudate is necessary to identify the causative bacterium.

Chronic suppurative otitis media may produce a chronic purulent ear discharge, commonly associated with hearing loss of varying degree. Systemic symptoms are usually not prominent. The tympanic membrane may show evidence of rupture. Granulation tissue in the middle ear may protrude from the external auditory meatus as a polypoid mass (''aural polyp''). A cholesteatoma may be present in the middle ear.

Complications

Complications usually result from spread of the infection:

A. Mastoiditis: The mastoid air cells often become involved, leading to both localized and extensive bone inflammation and necrosis (osteomyelitis).

B. Epidural Abscess, Meningitis, and Brain Abscess: Spread of infection through the thin roof of the middle ear may result in epidural abscess, meningitis, or brain abscess in the cerebellum or temporal lobes.

C. Thrombophlebitis of the lateral and sigmoid venous sinuses follows local spread. This is characterized by high fever, severe headache, and bacteremia. Septic embolization from affected sinuses may result in lung abscess.

OTOSCLEROSIS

Otosclerosis is a disease of uncertain cause characterized by sclerosis of the middle ear ossicles. The bone becomes abnormally vascular; abnormal trabeculae develop and lead to increased bone density, often with fusion of the foot process of the stapes. Bony ankylosis impairs transmission of sound waves to the cochlea, leading to deafness. The disease is usually bilateral and has a strong familial tendency, with about 40% of patients giving a positive family history. Autosomal dominant inheritance with variable penetrance appears likely.

Clinically, otosclerosis is characterized by progressive deafness, usually beginning in the third decade. Low tones are lost first, followed by failure of high tone perception.

GLOMUS JUGULARE TUMOR

The jugular glomus lies in the adventitia of the internal jugular vein at the base of the skull just below the bony floor of the middle ear. Glomus jugulare tumor is a **paraganglioma** that arises in this structure. It frequently erodes into the middle ear, forming a red nodular mass and causing conduction deafness. When large, it causes bulging under and then through the tympanic membrane into the external auditory meatus. Glomus jugulare tumors are extremely vascular and bleed profusely when handled. The diagnosis is established by histologic examination. Glomus jugulare tumors are locally aggressive but do not usually metastasize.

THE INNER EAR

ACUTE LABYRINTHITIS

Acute inflammation of the inner ear is a common cause of sudden unilateral hearing loss. It may also cause acute vertigo.

Viral infection is the commonest cause of acute labyrinthitis. It may be part of a systemic viral infection, as occurs in mumps and measles, or it may be an isolated infection of the inner ear. Viral labyrinthitis is usually a self-limited illness, but a significant number of patients have permanent hearing loss.

Bacterial labyrinthitis is a rarer, more serious infection which is usually due to extension of suppurative otitis media. It causes suppurative necrosis of the inner ear and commonly results in permanent deafness.

MENIERE'S DISEASE (Hydrops of the Labyrinth)

Meniere's disease is an uncommon lesion involving the cochlea. The cause is not known; infection, allergy and vascular disturbance have all been suggested. Meniere's disease occurs mainly in middle age, is more common in men than in women, and is bilateral in 20% of cases.

Pathology

Attacks of Meniere's disease are characterized by an imbalance in secretion and absorption of endolymphatic fluid that favors accumulation of fluid in the cochlea. This results in increased endolymphatic pressure in the cochlear duct. Initially, the process is reversible, but with repeated attacks there is degeneration of the cochlear hair cells that are the end organ for hearing.

Clinical Features

Clinically, Meniere's disease is characterized by fluctuating hearing loss and tinnitus, episodic vertigo, and a sensation of fullness in the ear. After several years, permanent and progressive hearing loss develops. No effective treatment is available. Treatment with diuretics is of value in some patients; otherwise, surgery may be used in an attempt to relieve the pressure.

II. THE UPPER RESPIRATORY TRACT

The upper respiratory tract includes the nose, the paranasal sinuses, the pharynx, and the upper part of the larynx above the level of the true vocal cords. It is concerned with ventilation and speech. The nasal cavity and sinuses are lined by respiratory epithelium, which is continuous with the skin at the anterior nares and with the squamous epithelium of the pharynx posteriorly.

THE NOSE, PARANASAL SINUSES, & PHARYNX

INFLAMMATORY DISEASES (Fig 32-2)

ACUTE RHINITIS (Coryza, Common Cold)

Acute infectious rhinitis (coryza) is almost always the result of viral infection and is one of the commonest infections of humans. It is caused by many different viruses, commonly rhinoviruses, influenza virus, myxoviruses, paramyxoviruses, and adenoviruses.

Acute inflammation of the nasal mucosa is accompanied by markedly increased mucous secretion (catarrhal inflammation). The watery nasal discharge may be accompanied by sore throat due to pharyngeal involvement, fever, and muscle aches. Coryza is a self-limited infection. Though it is an innocuous infection, the common cold is responsible for the loss of many hours in the work force with considerable economic loss.

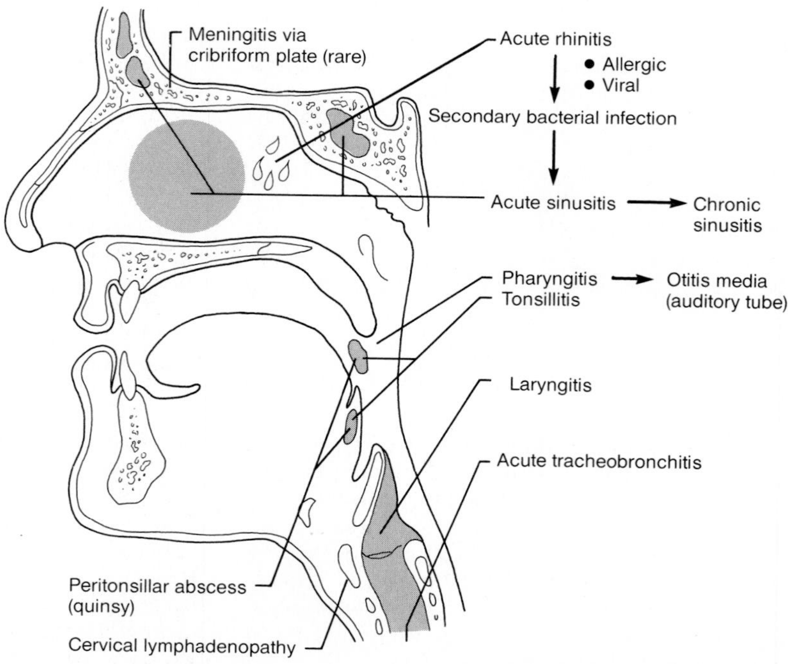

Figure 32-2. Inflammations of the upper respiratory tract.

ALLERGIC RHINITIS

Type I hypersensitivity (atopy) is also a common cause of acute rhinitis (hay fever). Susceptible patients are affected by a variety of allergens, most commonly pollens and dust. Patients who suffer from allergic rhinitis commonly have a positive family history and an increased frequency of developing other atopic diseases such as bronchial asthma and atopic dermatitis.

ACUTE PHARYNGOTONSILLITIS

Over 90% of cases of pharyngotonsillitis are the result of **viral infections;** influenza, parainfluenza, myxo- and paramyxoviruses, adenovirus, respiratory syncytial virus, and enteroviruses are the usual causes. Epstein-Barr virus (infectious mononucleosis) and cytomegalovirus produce pharyngotonsillitis as part of a distinctive systemic illness. **Bacterial infection,** most commonly with *Streptococcus pyogenes,* is responsible for less than 10% of cases. *Neisseria gonorrhoeae, Mycoplasma pneumoniae,* and *Corynebacterium diphtheriae* are rare causes.

Clinically, acute pharyngotonsillitis is characterized by hyperemia and erythema of the mucosa with pain **(sore throat).** Fever is commonly present. The various etiologic agents cannot be distinguished from one another clinically, and culture of a throat swab is essential for diagnosis. It is important to identify cases caused by bacteria because they require specific antibiotic therapy. Early treatment of streptococcal infections is important because it decreases the risk of poststreptococcal glomerulonephritis and acute rheumatic fever, which occur as complications of streptococcal pharyngotonsillitis. A quick (30-minute) nonculture test is now available for the rapid diagnosis of streptococcal sore throat.

Viral infections are usually self-limited. Bacterial infections may lead to suppuration, particularly around the tonsil to cause peritonsillar abscess (quinsy), which presents as a fluctuant red mass in the region of the tonsil that causes intense pain on swallowing and inability to open the mouth (trismus) due to spasm of the masseter. Abscesses may also occur in the retropharyngeal space and rarely involve the vertebral bone. Tonsils subject to recurring inflammation may be advantageously removed; otherwise, the enlarged tonsils and adenoids simply represent reactive hyperplasia of the lymphoid tissue of Waldeyer's ring, part of the body defense mechanism.

INFLAMMATORY & ALLERGIC NASAL POLYPS

Repeated episodes of acute rhinitis result in the development of nasal polyps. These common nasal "tumors" occur mainly in young adults and are usually multiple. Similar polyps may occur in the sinuses. Microscopically, they are composed of edematous stroma in which are found numerous neutrophils, eosinophils, lymphocytes, and plasma cells. Eosinophils are more numerous in allergic than inflammatory polyps. Nasal polyps may cause nasal obstruction and frequently need to be removed surgically.

CHRONIC RHINITIS

Chronic inflammation of the nasal cavity occurs in leprosy, leishmaniasis, and syphilis, with marked destruction of the nose. Nonspecific inflammation also occurs with cocaine sniffing, in which septal perforation may occur. Histologically, foreign body granulomas due to substances used to adulterate cocaine may be seen in the submucosa.

Nonspecific chronic bacterial infection of the nose often leads to atrophy of the nasal epithelium, accompanied by crusting and an offensive odor (**ozena,** or chronic atrophic rhinitis). The cause is unknown.

Rhinoscleroma is an uncommon infection in the United States but occurs more often in eastern Europe and Central America. It is caused by *Klebsiella rhinoscleromatis,* which multiplies in macrophages in the nasal mucosa. Accumulation of foamy macrophages (Mikulicz cells) filled with bacteria (see Chapter 13) and lymphoplasmacytic infiltration result in nodular polypoid masses and ulceration (Hebra nose). The diagnosis is made by demonstration of the organism in histologic sections and culture.

Rhinosporidiosis occurs in South India and Sri Lanka but is rare elsewhere. It is caused by the fungus *Rhinosporidium seeberi,* which appears in the nasal submucosa as large spherules containing endospores. The inflammation results in nasal polyps. The diagnosis is made by demonstrating the organism in histologic sections; *Rhinosporidium* cannot be cultured.

PARANASAL SINUSITIS

Inflammation of the maxillary, ethmoid, and frontal sinuses is a common complication of acute rhinitis and results from obstruction of the nasal openings of these sinuses by the nasal inflammatory edema. Chronic suppurative inflammation may occur. *Haemophilus influenzae* and *Strepto-*

coccus pneumoniae are the organisms found most commonly in chronic suppurative sinusitis.

Sinusitis causes **headache,** sometimes accompanied by fever and cervical lymph node enlargement. Extension of the inflammation to adjacent structures may lead to serious complications such as osteomyelitis, orbital cellulitis, cavernous sinus thrombophlebitis, meningitis, and brain abscess. These are rare.

FUNGAL INFECTIONS

Phycomycosis (mucormycosis) is an infection caused by fungi of the class Phycomycetes, most commonly Mucor species. *Mucor* (bread mold) is a saprophytic fungus commonly found in nature, and infection occurs only in a host with increased susceptibility. Patients with diabetic ketoacidotic coma and patients being treated for cancer with immunosuppressive anticancer drugs are those usually affected.

The fungus causes an acute nasal inflammation with extensive tissue necrosis due to invasion of blood vessels with thrombosis, frequently spreading to the adjacent orbit and the cranial cavity. Death is common unless emergent treatment is instituted. Irregularly branching nonseptate hyphae can be identified by microscopy and culture.

Aspergillus causes a similar necrotizing inflammation of the nasal cavity in immunocompromised patients. Aspergillus is distinguished from *Mucor* by culture and recognition of the thinner, dichotomously branching, septate hyphae.

Aspergillus spp may also cause a noninvasive infection in the nasal sinuses, particularly in the presence of chronic sinusitis. In these cases, the fungus forms an intracavitary mass (''fungus ball'').

WEGENER'S GRANULOMATOSIS

Wegener's granulomatosis is a rare disease which in its fully expressed form involves the upper and lower respiratory tract and the renal glomeruli (Chapters 35 and 48). Nasal and paranasal sinus lesions occur in 60% of patients and are characterized clinically by destructive granulation tissue masses in the nasopharynx. Biopsies of the nasal lesions may show necrotizing granulomas and a severe vasculitis.

LETHAL MIDLINE GRANULOMA

Lethal midline granuloma is a clinical term applied to a group of diseases characterized by a severe acute destructive ulcerative lesion of the middle of the face, including the nasal cavity (Fig 32–3). It may be caused by bacterial or fungal infections, Wegener's granulomatosis, or neoplasms. When these conditions have been excluded by culture and biopsy, the remaining cases of lethal midline granuloma often represent a progressive lymphoproliferative disease called **polymorphic reticulosis,** which is a form of malignant lymphoma. It is characterized by the presence of a polymorphous population of atypical lymphoid cells, accompanied by extensive necrosis. While the lymphoma is localized to this region initially, most cases develop systemic lymphoma.

NEOPLASMS

NEOPLASMS OF THE NASAL CAVITY

Nasal neoplasms are uncommon but display great variety (Table 32–1). They commonly present as polypoid masses obstructing the nasal cavity. Both benign and malignant tumors may ulcerate and bleed, producing epistaxis. The most common benign neoplasm is a squamous papilloma. A variant of squamous papilloma known as inverted papilloma has a locally infiltrative growth pattern (Fig 32–4) with a tendency to recur

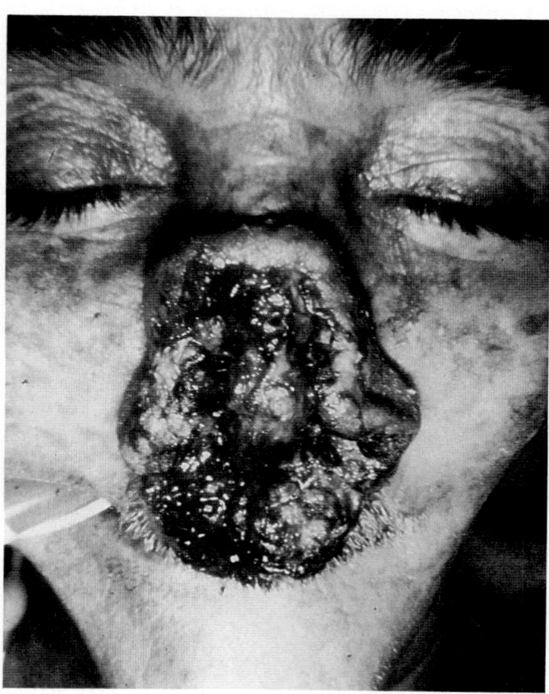

Figure 32–3. Lethal midline granuloma showing extensive nasal destruction.

Table 32-1. Neoplasms of the nasal cavity and paranasal sinuses.

Neoplasm	Location	Behavior	Histologic Appearance	Age and Sex
Juvenile angiofibroma	Roof of nasal cavity	Benign	Large blood vessels and fibrous stroma	Mainly in young adult males
Squamous papilloma	Nasal cavity, septum, sinuses	Benign	Papillary squamous epithelium	Adults
Inverted papilloma	Nasal cavity, lateral wall	Benign but may recur	Papillary epithelial growth; infiltrative	Adults
Extramedullary plasmacytoma	Nasal cavity	Malignant[1]	Diffuse sheets of abnormal plasma cells	Elderly
Malignant lymphoma	Nasal cavity, sinuses	Malignant	Monoclonal lymphoid proliferation	All ages
Nasal "glioma" (not a true neoplasm)	Roof of nasal cavity	Represents a herniation of normal brain through the cribriform plate		Newborn
Neoplasms of minor salivary glands	Sinuses	See Chapter 31		
Embryonal rhabdomyosarcoma (sarcoma botryoides)	Nasal cavity	Malignant	Primitive small cells; striated muscle differentiation	Children
Olfactory neuroblastoma (esthesioneuroblastoma)	Nasal cavity	Malignant	Primitive small cells; rosettes and neurofibrils	Children, adults
Squamous carcinoma	Nasal cavity, sinuses, nasopharynx, hypopharynx	Malignant	Infiltrative proliferation of atypical squamous epithelium	Adults
Malignant melanoma	Nasal cavity	Malignant	Infiltrative melanocyte proliferation	Adults

[1]Malignant plasmacytoma may occur as a solitary lesion or as part of multiple myeloma. Distinction from plasmacytosis in chronic inflammation is best achieved by demonstrating monoclonality in plasmacytoma (see Chapter 30).

locally after surgical excision. The malignant neoplasms, such as squamous carcinoma and embryonal rhabdomyosarcoma, infiltrate extensively and tend to metastasize via lymphatics to the cervical lymph nodes. Diagnosis of the specific type is made by biopsy.

Neoplasms of the paranasal sinuses (Table 32–1) tend to remain silent clinically until they are large.

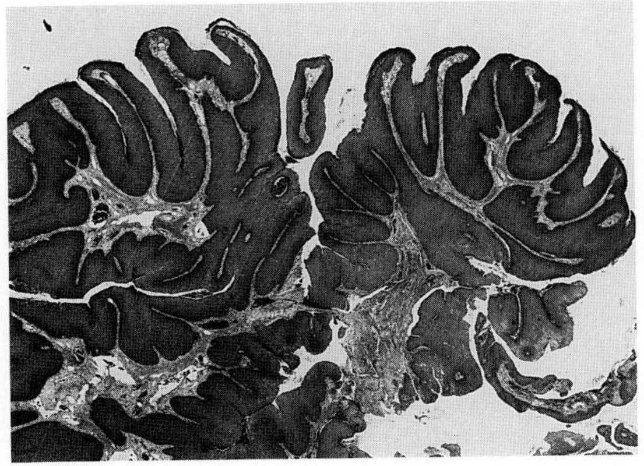

Figure 32-4. Inverted papilloma of the nasal cavity. Note the inverted, infiltrative growth pattern of the proliferating squamous epithelium.

CARCINOMA OF THE NASOPHARYNX

Carcinoma of the nasopharynx is of special interest because it has a striking geographic distribution, being very common in the Far East and eastern Africa, and because it has been linked etiologically to Epstein-Barr virus (EBV). Affected individuals show evidence of EBV infection, and the viral genome has been identified in the tumor cells. The mechanism of EBV carcinogenesis is unknown. Cigarette smoking is also an important etiologic factor, probably acting as a promoter (Chapter 18) in nasopharyngeal carcinoma. Nasopharyngeal carcinoma may occur at all ages but is particularly common in younger patients.

Nasopharyngeal carcinoma is a squamous carcinoma of varying differentiation. One subtype consists of poorly differentiated squamous carcinoma in an abundant associated lymphoid stroma (sometimes called lymphoepithelioma, though this designation is not favored because the lymphoid cells are not neoplastic). This variety occurs in younger patients, disseminates to lymph nodes at an early stage, and is more sensitive to radiation.

Nasopharyngeal carcinoma often presents with enlarged cervical lymph nodes resulting from metastasis. A few cases infiltrate the skull base, involving cranial nerves at the base of the brain. Obstruction of the opening of the auditory tube may result in otitis media. Only rarely is the primary tumor responsible for early symptoms. The diagnosis is made by examination of the nasopharynx and biopsy; in infiltrative lesions, "blind" biopsies may be positive even when no gross lesion is visualized.

MALIGNANT LYMPHOMA

The ring of lymphoid tissue in the oropharynx (Waldeyer's ring) is a common site for occurrence of extranodal malignant lymphoma. Most are of B cell origin; intermediate- and high-grade lymphomas are most common.

Malignant lymphoma presents as a nodular or ulcerative mass that resembles carcinoma grossly. Diagnosis is made by histologic examination with immunologic confirmation that the neoplastic cells bear lymphocytic markers such as common leukocyte antigen. Frozen sections stained for immunoglobulin light chains permit monoclonality of the lymphocytic proliferation to be established and are important in differentiating a malignant lymphoma from a reactive lymphoid proliferation.

THE LARYNX

The larynx is a specialized structure that is responsible for converting expired air into specific sounds during speech. It is encased in cartilage and lined by a stratified squamous epithelium that changes to respiratory columnar epithelium inferior to the true vocal cords.

INFLAMMATORY CONDITIONS

ACUTE LARYNGITIS

Acute laryngitis frequently accompanies viral and bacterial infections of the upper respiratory tract, causing pain and hoarseness. It is usually self-limited.

Acute epiglottitis is a common, important, and dangerous infection in very young children. It is caused either by *Haemophilus influenzae* or by viruses. The site of maximal involvement is the epiglottis, though in severe cases the entire larynx and trachea may be affected (acute laryngotracheobronchitis). The acute inflammation and its attendant swelling result in narrowing of the air passages, causing respiratory obstruction. Croup is acute respiratory difficulty with cyanosis in a child, due to epiglottitis, laryngeal spasm, or both.

DIPHTHERIA

Incidence

Diphtheria is caused by the gram-positive bacillus *Corynebacterium diphtheriae.* It has become rare in the United States and other developed countries because of effective immunization in childhood (the "D" in DPT vaccine represents diphtheria toxoid) but still occurs frequently in underdeveloped countries, where it is predominantly a disease of young children. In the United States, diphtheria is now seen in adults, who become infected as the effect of childhood immunization wanes, more commonly than in children.

Pathology (Fig 32–5)

Diphtheria is transmitted by droplet infection. Nasal, faucial, and laryngeal forms of diphtheria are recognized depending on the site of maximum involvement. Laryngeal diphtheria is the most common form as well as the most dangerous. The bacterium infects the mucosa, causing acute inflammation with exudation and necrosis. The necrotic mucosa and exudate remain adherent to the surface as a yellowish membrane (acute membranous inflammation), characteristic of diphtheria. Detachment of the membrane and impaction in the trachea may cause sudden death (Fig 32–6). Respiratory obstruction is a common cause of death in diphtheria and may require emergency tracheostomy.

The bacterium remains localized to the surface of the upper respiratory tract and does not invade deep tissues or the bloodstream. However, some strains produce an exotoxin that enters the bloodstream and causes myocardial and nerve damage (Fig 32–5).

Clinical Features & Treatment

Laryngeal diphtheria is characterized by pain and hoarseness. High fever and marked enlargement of cervical lymph nodes ("bull neck") is common. Physical examination reveals acute inflammation with the typical membrane. The diagnosis is made by clinical examination and culture (requires special media). Patients with nasal diphtheria may have a very mild illness, with nasal discharge only, and represent an important source of infection.

Treatment includes antibiotics to kill the organisms as well as high doses of antitoxin to neutralize any exotoxin that has been absorbed into the bloodstream. With adequate treatment, mortality rates of diphtheria are low.

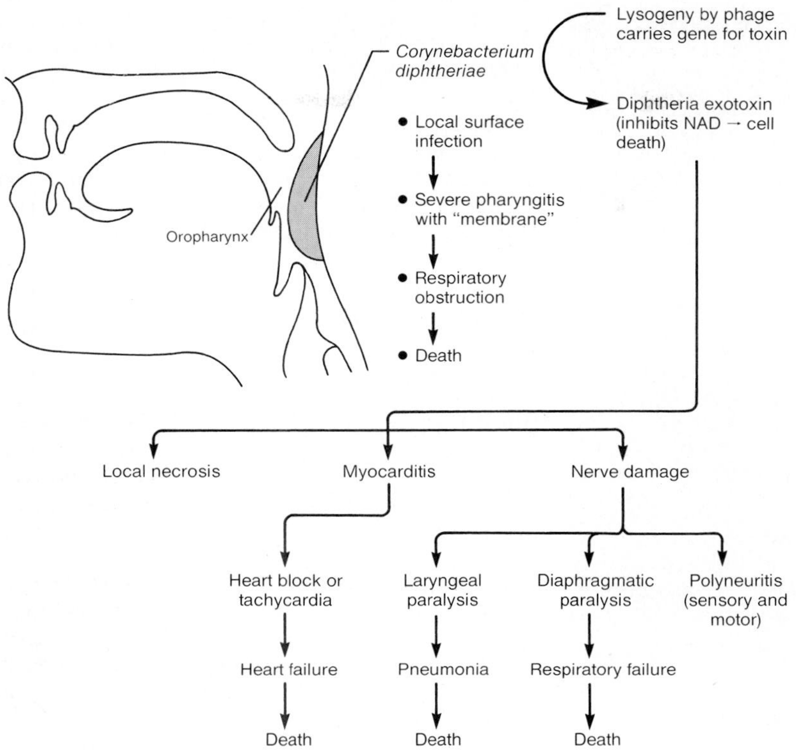

Figure 32-5. Diphtheria—local effects and remote effects due to exotoxin.

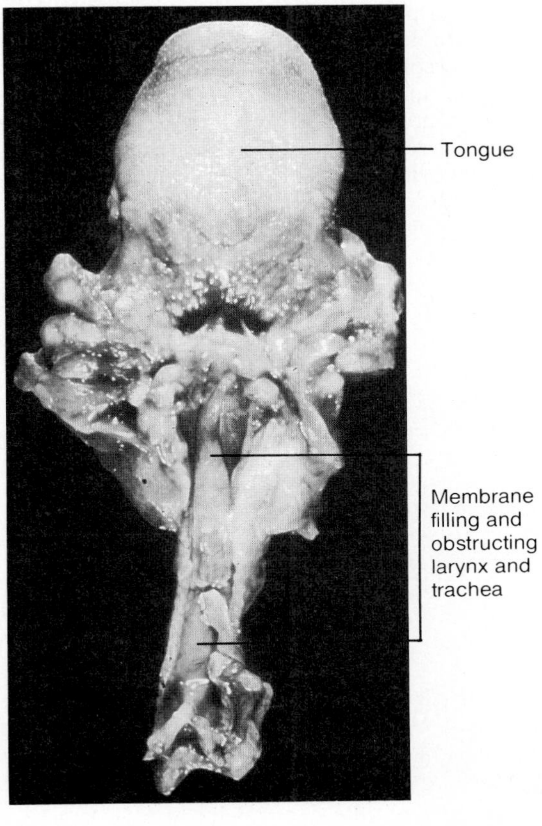

Tongue

Membrane filling and obstructing larynx and trachea

LARYNGEAL NODULE

Laryngeal nodule is a common lesion that occurs in the middle third of the true vocal cord. It is related to excessive use of the voice and occurs in singers ("singer's nodule"), teachers, and preachers. It is believed to be the result of trauma.

It appears grossly as a firm, rounded nodule covered by mucosa. Microscopically, dilated vascular spaces, fibrosis, and myxomatous degeneration are present to varying degrees.

Clinically, patients present with hoarseness and loss of ability to speak. Excision is curative. However, unless the patient stops overusing the voice, the lesion may recur.

Figure 32-6. Diphtheria. Larynx and trachea opened at autopsy showing detached, aspirated membrane filling the larynx and trachea, causing respiratory obstruction and death.

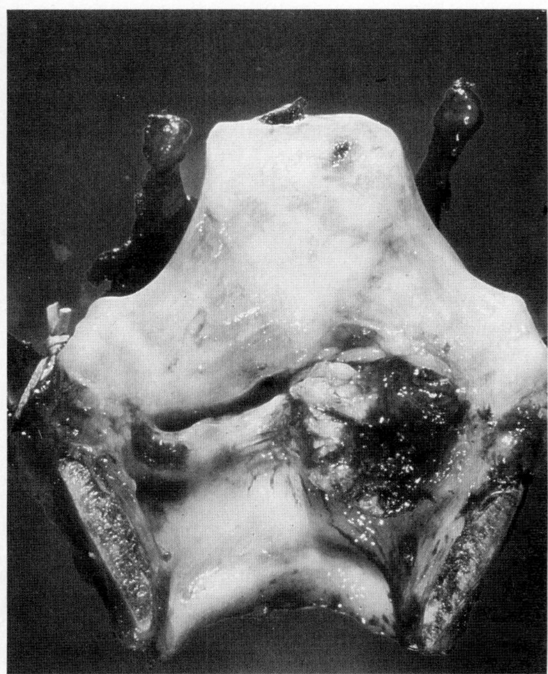

Figure 32-7. Ulcerative squamous carcinoma of the larynx involving vocal cord.

LARYNGEAL NEOPLASMS

SQUAMOUS PAPILLOMA

Laryngeal papilloma is a common benign neoplasm that usually presents with hoarseness. Laryngeal papillomas occur in 2 distinct forms: (1) solitary papillomas occurring in adults, cured by local excision; and (2) juvenile papillomatosis, which occurs mainly in children and is characterized by the development of multiple papillomas and a high incidence of local recurrence after surgical removal. Juvenile papillomatosis is caused by infection with papillomavirus. In many patients, the lesions regress after puberty. Very rarely, malignant transformation may occur.

SQUAMOUS CARCINOMA

Incidence & Etiology

Squamous carcinoma is the commonest malignant neoplasm of the larynx. Most cases occur after the age of 50 years. Men are affected 7 times more frequently than women. Cigarette smoking and exposure to asbestos have a statistical association with laryngeal carcinoma.

Pathologic Features

Laryngeal carcinomas are classified anatomically as (1) glottic (Fig 32–7), arising in the vocal cord; (2) supraglottic, arising in the aryepiglottic folds and epiglottis; and (3) subglottic, below the vocal cords.

Laryngeal carcinoma often begins as an area of squamous epithelial dysplasia progressing to carcinoma in situ before invasive carcinoma occurs. The noninvasive lesions appear as white areas of thickened plaquelike mucosa. Invasion is associated with nodularity and ulceration.

Microscopically, the majority are well-differentiated squamous carcinomas (Fig 32–8). A highly differentiated form of squamous carcinoma is characterized by a wartlike exophytic growth pattern with little invasion. This type, called verrucous carcinoma, is successfully treated by surgery.

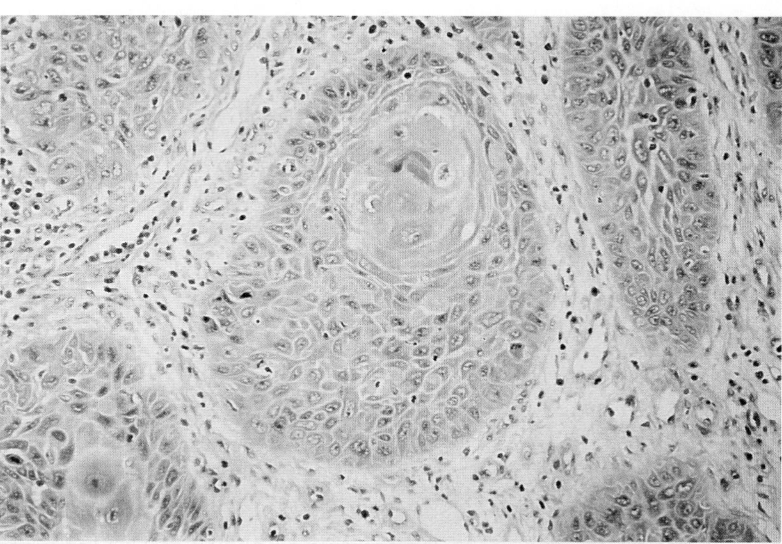

Figure 32-8. Invasive, well-differentiated squamous carcinoma of larynx.

Clinical Features

Laryngeal carcinoma commonly presents with hoarseness, and it is a good rule that carcinoma must be excluded in any patient with persistent hoarseness. Large masses may cause respiratory obstruction and hemoptysis. Metastasis to cervical lymph nodes occurs early. Distant metastases occur late. Diagnosis is established by laryngoscopy and biopsy. Surgical removal of laryngeal carcinoma is highly successful when the patient has an early neoplasm restricted to the vocal cord. When there is subglottic or supraglottic extension, total laryngectomy and removal of cervical lymph nodes is frequently necessary, and survival rates are much lower. Radiation therapy is effective, squamous carcinoma being a radiosensitive neoplasm.

33 The Eye

STRUCTURE & FUNCTION OF THE EYE

The eyes are complex vision receptors situated in a pair of bony cavities in the skull—the **orbits**—which open anteriorly to the exterior and posteriorly for the entry and exit of nerves and blood vessels. The main nerve—the **optic nerve**—carries visual impulses from the **retina** to the brain.

The anterior covering of the eyeball is the transparent **cornea,** which permits entry of light into the eyeball through the lens, which is the focusing mechanism (Fig 33–1). The cornea is continuous at the limbus with the **sclera.** The **conjuctiva** lines the inner surface of the eyelids (palpebral conjunctiva) and is reflected onto the sclera (bulbar conjunctiva). When the eyelids are closed, the conjunctiva forms a sac that is lubricated by **tears,** the secretion of the **lacrimal gland,** situated in the lateral part of the orbit.

The eyeball is separated from orbital bone by connective tissue, muscles, nerves, and blood vessels. The **eyelids,** which protect the front of the eye, are covered with skin on the outside and conjunctiva on the inside.

The function of the eye involves perception of images in the retina that are converted to electrical impulses that pass to the visual cortex for interpretation. The optic pathway includes the optic nerves, chiasm, lateral geniculate body, and optic radiation.

CLINICAL MANIFESTATIONS OF EYE DISEASE

Pain

Many different types of pain may occur in eye diseases. In conjunctival and corneal inflammation, burning or itching of the eye is commonly associated with increased sensitivity to light (photophobia). Deep aching pain occurs in angle-clo-

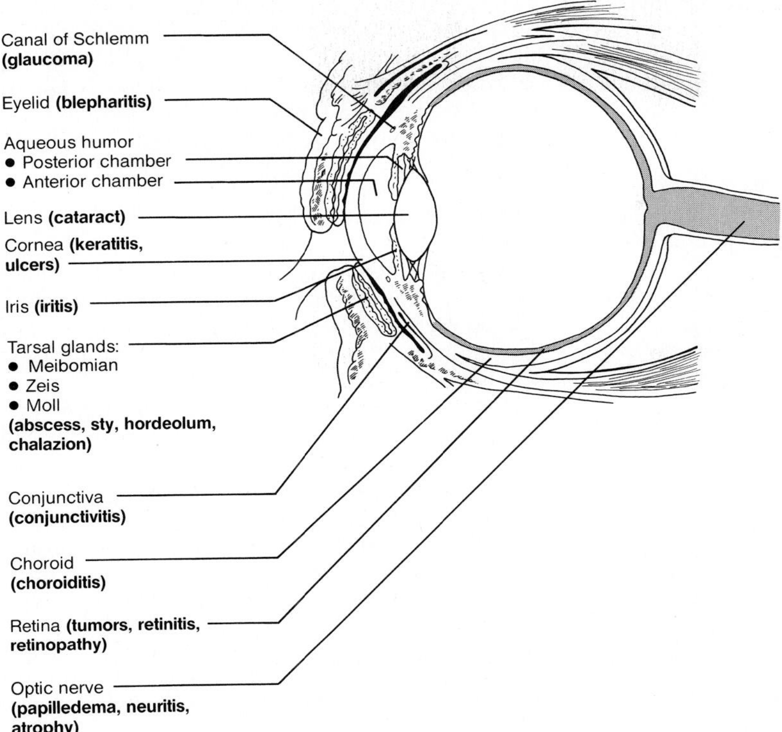

Figure 33-1. Structural components and principal diseases of the eye.

sure glaucoma and inflammation of the uveal tract. Pain in acute glaucoma may be so severe as to cause vomiting. Headache may accompany conditions of disturbed vision.

Visual Disturbances

Decreased visual acuity (amblyopia) is a feature of many ocular diseases. Spots and halos before the eyes occur in early cataract. Halos may also occur in glaucoma. Diminution of the visual field may signify disease of the retina, the optic disk, or the visual neural pathways, which include the optic nerve, chiasm, radiation, and visual cortex. Night blindness may result from vitamin A deficiency and retinal degenerative diseases. Double vision (diplopia) is a feature of eye muscle dysfunction.

Discharge

Eye discharge may represent increased tearing (eg, in allergy) or inflammation of the conjunctiva. Microscopic examination of the discharge with Giemsa's stain shows the type of inflammatory cells present and the presence of viral and chlamydial inclusions. The presence of numerous eosinophils is typical of allergic conjunctivitis, while neutrophils dominate in acute infectious conjunctivitis. Gram stain for bacteria and potassium hydroxide preparations for fungi are of value in some cases.

Change in Appearance

Inspection of the external eyes may disclose evidence of strabismus (muscle imbalance), hemorrhage, congestion, jaundice, swelling, displacements of the eye such as proptosis (forward displacement), and the presence of tumors. Ophthalmoscopic examination may reveal abnormalities of the anterior chamber (eg, hypopyon and hyphema—pus and blood, respectively, in the anterior chamber), lens (eg, early cataract, dislocation), vitreous (eg, hemorrhage), retina (eg, diabetic and hypertensive retinopathy, retinal degenerative diseases, detachment, hemorrhages, exudates, changes in retinal vessels), and optic disk (eg, optic atrophy, papilledema).

THE EYELIDS

The eyelids are covered by skin on the outside and conjunctiva on the inside. At the junction of the skin and conjunctiva are the eyelashes plus numerous modified skin adnexal glands.

The skin covering of the eyelids is subject to a wide variety of diseases, the most important of which is basal cell carcinoma. Low-grade inflammation of the lid margins is termed **blepharitis**. More specific diseases of the eyelids are discussed below.

STY (Hordeolum)

A sty is an acute suppurative inflammation of the hair follicle or associated glandular structures—the sebaceous glands of Zeis and the apocrine glands of Moll. It is usually caused by *Staphylococcus aureus* and produces a painful localized abscess (Fig 33–2), which is cured by rupture or extraction of the involved eyelash to effect drainage.

CHALAZION

A chalazion is a common chronic inflammatory process involving the meibomian glands. It is believed to be caused by duct obstruction, leading to retention of secretions, infection, and chronic inflammation with macrophages, lymphocytes, and plasma cells. Clinically, it produces an indurated mass that may be mistaken for a neoplasm.

XANTHELASMA

Xanthelasma, a small yellow plaque composed of collections of lipid-laden foamy macrophages in the subepithelial zone, occurs in some hyperlipidemic conditions and in diabetes. There are usually multiple lesions.

CYSTS

Several types of cyst occur in the eyelid. Congenital dermoid cysts occur along the lines of fusion of the facial skin folds, most often at the external angle of the upper eyelid. Microscopically, the cysts are lined by skin containing dermal glands. Acquired cysts arising in ducts of glands (eg, eccrine and apocrine hydrocystomas) and epidermal inclusions (epidermal cysts) are common.

MALIGNANT NEOPLASMS

Basal cell carcinoma is the commonest malignant neoplasm of the eyelid. It occurs much more commonly in the lower than in the upper lid. The skin about the eye is the most common location for basal cell carcinoma. These tumors begin as small nodules that grow and ulcerate, forming an enlarging ulcer with an elevated pearly margin (Fig 33–3). Microscopically, they are composed of nests of small hyperchromatic cells resembling basal cells. They invade locally and may extend deeply into the orbit, but they do not metastasize. **Squamous carcinoma** is uncommon in the eyelids.

Meibomian gland carcinoma (sebaceous carcinoma) occurs chiefly in the upper eyelid, which is the predominant location of meibomian glands. These tumors appear as slowly growing yellowish masses that may resemble a chalazion. Progression causes erosion of the lid margin or conjunctiva and the appearance of a large lobulated mass. Microscopically, the tumor resembles sebaceous glands, forming large invasive nests and sheets of cells with abundant cytoplasm. The diagnostic feature is the presence of large cells with vacuolated cytoplasm that contain lipid (demonstrable with lipid stains on frozen sections). Like other adenocarcinomas, meibomian gland carcinoma may spread laterally into the epidermis of the eyelid. Meibomian gland carcinoma is important to distinguish from squamous and basal cell carcinoma because it has a more aggressive biologic behavior. Lymph node metastasis is common.

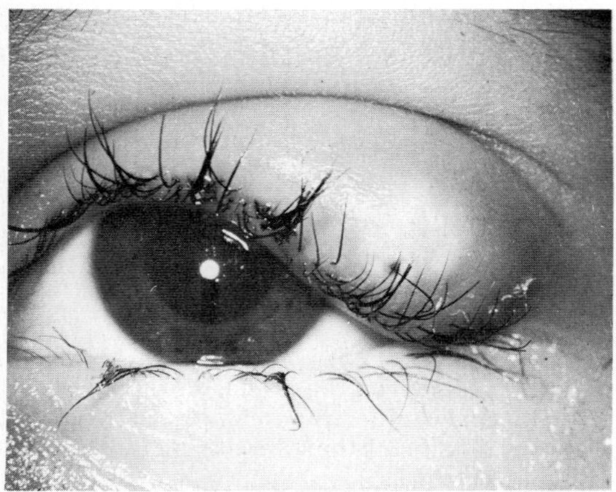

Figure 33–2. Internal hordeolum of the upper eyelid.

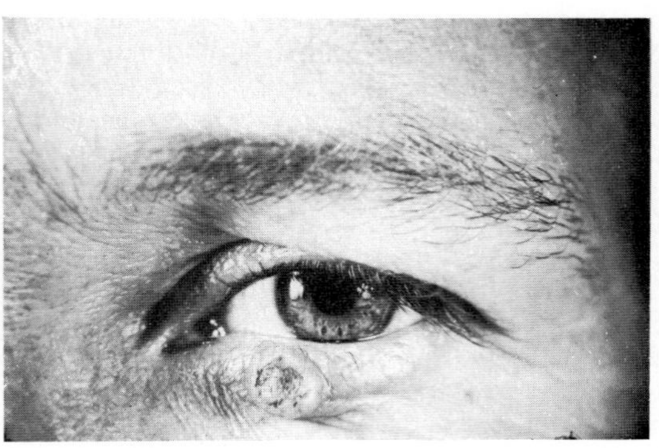

Figure 33–3. Basal cell carcinoma of the lower eyelid, showing an ulcer with raised edges. This is the commonest neoplasm of the eyelids and the commonest location for basal cell carcinoma.

THE CONJUNCTIVA & CORNEA

The conjunctiva is lined by a thin, transparent, nonkeratinizing stratified squamous epithelium in which are found scattered mucous cells. The cornea is composed of nonkeratinizing stratified squamous epithelium, Bowman's layer, an avascular stroma, Descemet's membrane, and an underlying endothelium lining the anterior chamber.

KERATOCONJUNCTIVITIS

Definition & Etiology

Inflammation of the conjunctiva is called **conjunctivitis** and inflammation of the cornea is called keratitis; when both are involved, as is frequently the case, the term **keratoconjunctivitis** is used.

Conjunctivitis is common and has many causes (Table 33–1).

Pathology & Clinical Features

Acute bacterial conjunctivitis is characterized by pain, hyperemia appearing as vascular injection **(red eye),** and a purulent discharge in which numerous neutrophils are present. *Neisseria* species, pneumococcus, and *Haemophilus aegyptius* infections are common. Ophthalmia neonatorum results from infection of the fetus with *Neisseria gonorrhoeae* during delivery through the birth canal. **Ulceration** occurs in severe cases, and when this involves the cornea visual impairment may occur.

Viral keratoconjunctivitis is most frequently caused by adenoviruses and herpes simplex virus (Fig 33–4).

Inclusion conjunctivitis (''swimming pool conjunctivitis'') is common worldwide, characterized clinically by acute inflammation with pain, red eye, and discharge and histologically by accumulation of lymphocytes in the conjunctiva. It is caused by **chlamydiae,** which may be demonstrated as cytoplasmic inclusions in infected cells in the exudate. The disease is transmitted via contaminated hands, shared towel, and infection of the fetus during delivery through an infected birth canal. It is self-limited, with recovery occurring in all cases after a few days of discomfort.

Trachoma is a much more serious chlamydial infection in which there is long-term destruction of the cornea, leading to blindness in cases not treated early. The acute conjunctival inflammation progresses to a chronic phase in which there may be epithelial hyperplasia, lymphocytic infiltration, and pannus formation—an inflamed mass of granulation tissue that replaces the superficial layers of the cornea and results in blindness. Trachoma is the commonest cause of blindness in underdeveloped tropical countries.

***Acanthamoeba* keratoconjunctivitis.** Recently, a serious epidemic of keratoconjunctivitis caused by amebae of the species *Acanthamoeba* occurred in users of soft contact lenses. The disease was traced to the use of contaminated lens cleaning fluids. Many patients developed permanent visual impairment due to keratitis.

Allergic conjunctivitis. Allergic conjunctivitis—also called vernal (''spring'') conjunctivitis—is typically seasonal in occurrence due to pollens in

Table 33–1. Causes of conjunctivitis and keratitis.

Infections
- Bacterial
  - *Haemophilus aegyptius,* staphylococci, pneumococci.
  - *Neisseria gonorrhoeae* (ophthalmia neonatorum) in babies born to mothers with active gonococcal cervicitis.
  - *Treponema pallidum;* interstitial keratitis in congenital syphilis.
- Viral
  - Especially severe in herpes simplex keratitis; occasionally herpes zoster, adenoviruses.
- Chlamydial
  - Trachoma.
  - Inclusion conjunctivitis.
- Protozoal
  - *Acanthamoeba* (grows in contact lens cleaning fluid).
- Filarial
  - *Onchocerca volvulus, Loa loa.*

Allergic conjunctivitis
- Includes seasonal or vernal conjunctivitis.

Chemical conjunctivitis
- Reaction to drugs, eye washes, makeup.

Solar conjunctivitis
- Ultraviolet light (snow blindness)

Trauma, foreign bodies

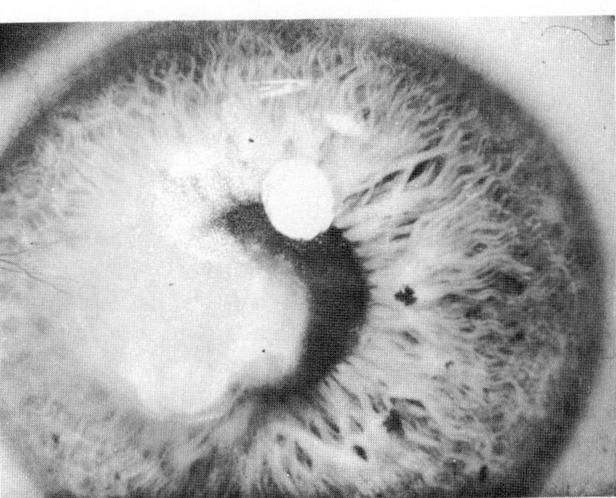

Figure 33–4. Corneal scar caused by recurrent herpes simplex keratitis.

the environment and is associated with hay fever. Histologically, it shows goblet cell hyperplasia and infiltration by lymphocytes and eosinophils.

Phlyctenular conjunctivitis is a delayed hypersensitivity response to antigens of bacteria such as *Mycobacterium tuberculosis* and *Staphylococcus aureus*. It is characterized by an elevated, hard, red triangular plaque at the limbus, which ulcerates and then heals in about 2 weeks. Corneal involvement may cause scarring and visual disturbances.

Diagnosis

The diagnosis of conjunctivitis can be made clinically based on the presence of conjunctival injection and discharge. Keratitis is diagnosed by examination; invisible epithelial lesions may be outlined by fluorescein staining. The etiologic agent is identified by culture and microscopic examination of conjunctival discharge and scrapings from corneal lesions. A finding of chlamydial and viral inclusions is diagnostic. Amebic trophozoites are present, often in large numbers, in *Acanthamoeba* keratoconjunctivitis.

DEGENERATIVE CONJUNCTIVAL & CORNEAL CONDITIONS

PINGUECULA

Pinguecula is a common degenerative disease caused by ultraviolet solar radiation and is similar to solar-induced changes in the skin, with epithelial atrophy, degeneration of collagen, and hyalinization of elastic tissue (see Chapter 61). The exposed interpalpebral part of the conjunctiva is chiefly affected. The atrophic epithelium may show precancerous dysplastic changes.

Pinguecula appears clinically as a thickened, yellowish area in the conjunctiva. It may become secondarily infected and ulcerate. The risk of squamous carcinoma is small.

PTERYGIUM

Pterygium is pathologically similar to pinguecula but differs in that it affects the sclerocorneal junction (limbus) and may extend into the cornea as a layer of vascularized connective tissue, producing corneal opacification and visual impairment. In the cornea, there is replacement of Bowman's layer by collagen and elastic tissue. Pterygia also have a greater tendency to recur after excision. The incidence of secondary infection, ulceration, and epithelial dysplasia is low.

SQUAMOUS METAPLASIA

In squamous metaplasia, the normally thin, transparent nonkeratinized squamous epithelium is replaced by a thick, opaque, keratinized squamous type. This appears as a pearly white plaque on the conjunctiva, sometimes called "leukoplakia." Areas of squamous metaplasia are more often subject to infection and ulceration but are not precancerous.

Squamous metaplasia may be caused by **(1)** insufficiency of tears, as occurs in **Sjögren's syndrome,** which causes frictional damage of the conjunctiva; **(2)** protrusion of the eyeball **(exophthalmos),** which prevents eyelid closure and results in excessive irritation; **(3) neuromuscular disorders** in which paralysis of the eyelid muscles is a feature (facial nerve paralysis), leading to inability to close the eyes, again increasing irritation; and **(4) vitamin A deficiency,** which causes a basic abnormality of squamous epithelium, leading to thickening. The areas of squamous metaplasia in vitamin A deficiency are called **Bitot's spots** and commonly extend to involve the cornea; they may become infected, causing softening of the cornea (keratomalacia) and visual impairment.

ARCUS SENILIS

Arcus senilis is a ring of fatty infiltration at the outer margin of the cornea, common in elderly individuals. A similar lesion occurs in younger patients with hyperlipidemia.

NEOPLASMS OF THE CONJUNCTIVA

BENIGN NEOPLASMS

Benign neoplasms such as squamous papilloma, melanocytic nevus, hemangioma, and neurofibroma occur rarely on the conjunctiva as small masses of various colors. Benign lymphoid hyperplasia may also occur, leading to a conjunctival mass.

SQUAMOUS CARCINOMA

Squamous carcinoma of the conjunctiva is also rare. Most cases are believed to be the result of exposure to ultraviolet radiation, complicating the actinic lesions pinguecula and pterygium. The neoplastic process progresses through increasing grades of dysplasia to carcinoma in situ and then invasive squamous carcinoma.

Conjunctival squamous carcinoma usually invades superficially and almost never metastasizes. It has an excellent prognosis and is treated by limited local excision.

Malignant Melanoma

Conjunctival malignant melanoma is rare. It may occur: (1) de novo, (2) in relation to a preexistent melanocytic nevus, or (3) in relation to an acquired melanocytic hyperplasia (lentigo). It presents clinically as a nodule that may or may not be pigmented. As with melanomas of the skin, the prognosis is related to depth of invasion. The more superficial lesions can be treated by local excision and have a good prognosis. With deeper invasion, lymphatic and vascular involvement commonly occurs, and the prognosis is guarded even following radical exenteration of orbital contents.

THE ORBITAL SOFT TISSUES

The orbital soft tissues are rarely the site of primary diseases but may be involved by extension of pathologic processes from surrounding structures (Fig 33–5).

INFLAMMATORY PSEUDOTUMOR

Inflammatory pseudotumor is characterized by forward protrusion of the eyeball (proptosis), pain, swelling, and restriction of ocular movement. Histologically, there is edema, hyperemia, and infiltration of the orbital soft tissue with neutrophils, eosinophils, lymphocytes, and plasmacytes. The diagnosis is usually made when orbital exploration in a patient suspected clinically of having a neoplasm shows only nonspecific inflammation. The cause is unknown.

GRAVES' DISEASE

Graves' disease (primary autoimmune hyperthyroidism) is commonly associated with exophthalmos as a result of edema and increased accumulation of mucopolysaccharides in the orbital soft tissues. The orbital muscles show marked myxoid change and weakness. The condition is usually bilateral and is believed to be caused by an autoantibody (exophthalmos-producing factor) that may persist even after the hyperthyroidism is treated (Chapter 58).

In all of these conditions—and in the neoplasms described below— the eyeball is displaced forward **(proptosis)**. Since the process is behind the conjunctival sac, special techniques are required to visualize and obtain tissue for diagnosis of these lesions.

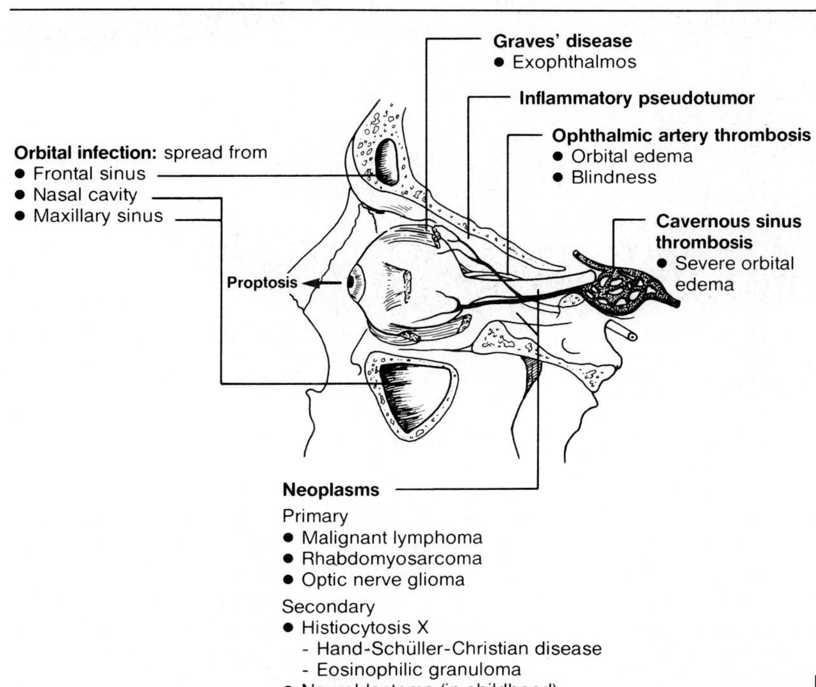

Figure 33–5. Diseases of the orbital soft tissues.

LACRIMAL GLAND

The lacrimal gland is situated in the lateral wall of the orbit and is rarely the site of pathologic processes. Sjögren's syndrome (see Chapter 31) is characterized by autoimmune destruction of the gland associated with dry eyes due to failure of tear production. The autoimmune process usually causes atrophy of the gland; more rarely, the lymphocytic infiltration may produce a mass lesion (benign lymphoepithelial lesion). Primary neoplasms of the lacrimal glands are very rare and are similar to salivary gland neoplasms.

PRIMARY NEOPLASMS OF THE ORBIT

MALIGNANT LYMPHOMA

Malignant lymphoma is the commonest malignant neoplasm of the orbit in adults. Most orbital lymphomas are low-grade B cell lymphomas (Chapter 29). An exception is Burkitt's lymphoma, an aggressive B cell lymphoma that occurs in children in Africa and often involves the orbit.

The diagnosis is established by histologic examination. Inflammatory lymphoid proliferations (pseudotumors) may be distinguished from lymphomas by immunologic methods (polyclonal versus monoclonal; Chapter 29); this usually requires preparation of frozen sections or living cell suspensions at the time of biopsy.

EMBRYONAL RHABDOMYOSARCOMA

Embryonal rhabdomyosarcoma is a rare orbital primary tumor, occurring mainly in children. It is highly malignant, with a rapid growth rate. The diagnosis is made by demonstrating an undifferentiated neoplasm in which primitive rhabdomyoblasts may be identified. Untreated, it is rapidly fatal. With chemotherapy and radiation, orbital embryonal rhabdomyosarcomas can be controlled and sometimes cured.

OPTIC NERVE GLIOMA

Optic nerve glioma is a rare neoplasm of the optic nerve, usually affecting the intraorbital part of the nerve. It is commonly a well-differentiated, very low grade, fibrillary astrocytoma that grows slowly over several years. Most cases occur in children, often in association with generalized neurofibromatosis (von Recklinghausen's disease).

NEOPLASMS OF BONE

Primary neoplasms of bone such as osteoma and histiocytosis X (Hand-Schüller-Christian disease and eosinophilic granuloma) and metastatic neoplasms such as neuroblastoma in children and metastatic carcinoma in adults may present as orbital masses.

THE EYEBALL

The eyeball itself is composed of several layers and compartments (Fig 33–1). The **retina** is the inner light-sensitive layer and is composed of modified neurons, the axons of which form the **optic nerve**. The **choroid,** which is pigmented, and the fibrous sclera are the outer layers of the eyeball.

The **lens** is attached to the sclera by the **ciliary muscle,** contraction of which controls the focal length of the lens. The lens and ciliary muscle separate the anterior part of the eyeball, filled with **aqueous humor,** from the posterior part, which is filled with **vitreous**. The **iris** projects into the aqueous humor in front of the lens, partially separating the anterior and posterior chambers. The iris, by its contraction, controls the amount of light entering the eye and also gives the eyes their color. The circular black opening in the center of the iris through which light passes into the eye is the **pupil**.

INFLAMMATORY CONDITIONS OF THE EYEBALL

Inflammations of the eye may involve one or more—or all—components of the eyeball or adnexa and are named accordingly (Fig 33–1 and Table 33–2).

BACTERIAL INFECTIONS

Pyogenic bacteria such as staphylococci gain entry into the eyeball following penetrating injuries to the eye or, less often, from orbital cellulitis or via the bloodstream from an infective focus elsewhere in the body. **Acute endophthalmitis** or **panophthalmitis** results, with swelling and a severe neutrophil infiltration. Untreated, there may be severe destruction with softening and collapse of the eyeball (phthisis bulbi). Both gonorrhea

Table 33-2. Terminology for inflammatory lesions of the eyeball.

Site of Inflammation	Term
Conjunctiva	Conjunctivitis
Cornea	Keratitis
Iris	Iritis
Ciliary body	Cyclitis
Iris and ciliary body	Iridocyclitis
Entire uveal tract	Panuveitis or uveitis
Sclera	Scleritis
Sclera and cornea	Sclerokeratitis
Choroid	Choroiditis
Retina	Retinitis
Choroid and retina	Chorioretinitis
Optic nerve	Optic neuritis
Optic nerve head in retina	Papillitis
Retina and optic nerve	Neuroretinitis
Anterior chamber (purulent exudate)	Hypopyon
Interior of eyeball	Endophthalmitis
Interior of eye and all layers	Panophthalmitis
Eyelid	Blepharitis
Lacrimal gland	Dacryoadenitis

and syphilis may produce iridocyclitis, usually in association with corneal disease. Tuberculosis produces chronic granulomatous uveitis.

TOXOPLASMA CHORIORETINITIS

Toxoplasma gondii infection involves the choroid and retina and occurs either as a congenital transplacental infection or as an acquired infection.

Congenital toxoplasmosis may cause neonatal or intrauterine death from encephalitis; survivors frequently show chorioretinitis, sometimes as the only manifestation of congenital toxoplasmosis. The organism persists in the choroid as pseudocysts, causing symptoms in childhood and early adult life.

Acquired toxoplasmosis occurs in adults. Ocular involvement is common, and the eye may be the only clinical site of involvement.

Pathologically, there is focal coagulative necrosis of the retina and choroid, with granulomatous inflammation and fibrosis. *Toxoplasma* can be identified as small crescent-shaped trophozoites and as larger pseudocysts.

OCULAR LARVA MIGRANS

Ocular larva migrans is usually caused by larvae of *Toxocara canis* (a dog nematode) that reach the interior of the eye through the uveal or retinal blood vessels. Children exposed to dog feces are chiefly affected. It causes a granulomatous endophthalmitis with large numbers of eosinophils around the larvae. Marked fibrosis frequently causes retinal detachment and visual loss.

NONINFECTIOUS INFLAMMATORY CONDITIONS

Sarcoidosis produces both an acute iridocyclitis, with fever and pain, and a chronic granulomatous disease, with corneal opacification and visual impairment.

Rheumatoid arthritis typically produces scleritis and uveitis, in which foci of necrotic collagen surrounded by palisading histiocytes resemble ill-defined rheumatoid nodules.

Both **ulcerative colitis** and **Crohn's disease** are associated with nonspecific chronic iritis.

Ankylosing spondylitis is associated with anterior uveitis in 20–50% of cases.

Sympathetic ophthalmia is an uncommon diffuse granulomatous uveitis that affects both eyes after a penetrating injury (or surgery) to one eye. It is believed to be the result of an immunologic reaction against antigens released or altered in some unknown way by the injury. The entire uveal tract is infiltrated by lymphocytes and plasma cells and may show ill-defined epithelioid cell granulomas. Severe visual loss commonly occurs.

Behçet's syndrome (uveitis plus oral and genital lesions) and **Reiter's syndrome** (conjunctivitis, uveitis, arthritis, and urethritis) probably represent postinfectious autohypersensitivity responses.

DEGENERATIVE CONDITIONS OF THE EYEBALL

CATARACT

Opacification of the lens, irrespective of cause (Table 33–3), is called a cataract (Fig 33–6). The lens is derived from surface ectoderm and consists of a mass of modified epithelial cells. It has no blood supply and derives its nutrition from the aqueous humor of the anterior chamber. Despite the fact that the oldest epithelial cells become compressed centrally throughout life, the lens normally remains transparent. Most individuals develop some lens opacification in later life (senile

Table 33-3. Principal types and causes of cataract.

Congenital, inherited (autosomal dominant), unilateral or bilateral.
Congenital, due to fetal infection, especially rubella.
Congenital, associated with chromosomal abnormalities: trisomy 13.
Galactosemia.
Hypoparathyroidism.
Radiation to the eye.
Trauma, including penetration and contusion.
Toxic, drug-induced: dinitrophenol, long-term steroids.
Senile (aggravated by solar radiation).
Diabetic (resembles accelerated senile cataract).

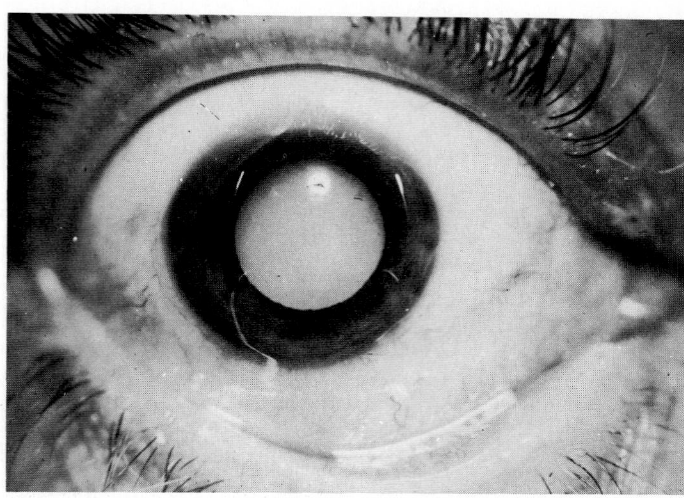

Figure 33-6. Mature senile cataract seen through a dilated pupil.

cataract). Whether this is an aging phenomenon or disease has not been elucidated.

Pathologically, visible cataracts may occur with minimal changes in water content of cortical cells. With advanced or mature cataracts, the epithelial cells break down, fragment, and undergo dissolution. In diabetes, high glucose levels cause excess production of sorbitol within the lens. Sorbitol is not diffusible and exerts a strong osmotic effect, leading to water imbibition and ultimately to cell degeneration. In galactosemia, galactose is metabolized in the lens to dulcitol, with similar results.

Clinically, cataracts cause progressive loss of visual acuity. Halos or spots in the visual field are early symptoms. Current treatment methods, which include extraction of the cataract and implantation of a prosthetic lens, are very successful.

GLAUCOMA

Glaucoma is defined as an increase in intraocular pressure sufficient to cause degeneration of the optic disk and optic nerve fibers. Normal intraocular pressure, measured by tonometry (which measures the pressure required to cause flattening of the cornea to a specified amount), is 10–20 mm Hg; elevations in pressure are thought to have a dual effect, inducing deformational changes in the optic disk plus decreased retinal blood flow. However, the correlation between intraocular pressure and optic nerve damage is not exact.

Glaucoma is the result of an abnormality in the dynamics of aqueous humor circulation. Aqueous humor production occurs at the ciliary body, partly by diffusion from plasma and partly by active secretion by the epithelium of the ciliary processes. The fluid passes from the posterior chamber through the pupil to the anterior chamber and then peripherally to the angle between the iris and cornea. Absorption of aqueous humor occurs at the iridocorneal angel by the trabecular meshwork and canal of Schlemm.

Glaucoma is a common disorder, with about 2% of all people over 40 years being affected. Visual loss is the most common effect. Of the many causes (Table 33–4), obstruction to the outflow of aqueous humor from the anterior chamber is most common (Fig 33–7). Glaucoma may occur as a complication of other diseases affecting the eye (secondary glaucoma) or as a primary disease.

Primary Open-Angle Glaucoma

Primary open-angle glaucoma, also called simple or chronic glaucoma, is a slowly progressive bilateral disease of insidious onset. It occurs in individuals over 40 years of age and is responsible for over 90% of cases of primary glaucoma. It is characterized by a slow rise in intraocular pressure with subtle microscopic abnormalities in the canal of Schlemm. There is progressive degeneration of the optic disk, an increase in size of the blind spot (scotoma), and peripheral visual field loss, ultimately causing blindness. Examination of the optic fundus shows deepening and enlargement of the optic cup. Patients usually present at a late stage with severe loss of vision.

Treatment with pupillary constrictors such as pilocarpine, which facilitate aqueous flow, is successful in lowering intraocular pressure in most cases. This halts the visual deterioration but does not reverse changes in the optic disk that are already established. Laser treatment of the trabecular meshwork (laser trabeculoplasty) produces a temporary improvement. Surgical treatment, which is indicated in severe cases, is successful in about 75% of cases in arresting visual loss.

Table 33-4. Glaucoma: Classification and causes.[1]

Congenital (rare)
- Primary: Defects in canal of Schlemm, congenital and infantile
- "Secondary": In association with other congenital anomalies: aniridia, Marfan's syndrome, neurofibromatosis, pigmentary glaucoma (degeneration of iris releases pigment that blocks outflow)

Primary (most common)
- Open (wide) angle glaucoma: Most common form, often familial
  - Due to degeneration of canal of Schlemm, age > 40 years
  - ?Due to primary vascular changes in optic nerve
- Closed (narrow) angle or angle closure glaucoma:
  - Blockage of the narrow anterior chamber by iris, especially when dilated at night; increase in lens size, causing further narrowing of anterior chamber

Secondary (common)
- Several mechanisms; usually act through obstruction outflow from anterior chamber
- Adhesions from uveitis (anterior synechiae)
- Adhesions from intraocular hemorrhage or trauma
- Dislocation of lens
- Retinal artery narrowing (or occlusion), especially in diabetes mellitus
- Arteriovenous fistulas (producing a direct increase in pressure)

[1]See also Fig 33–7.

Primary Angle-Closure Glaucoma

Angle-closure (closed-angle) glaucoma usually presents acutely. Many patients have a genetically determined anatomic variation that results in a shallow anterior chamber and a narrow anterior chamber angle (Fig 33–7). Increasing lens size, a normal occurrence with increasing age, causes forward displacement of the lens, further narrowing the angle. Acute attacks may be precipitated by dilatation of the pupil (as in preparation for funduscopy), which further narrows the angle by thickening the periphery of the iris during pupillary dilatation. Rapid increase of intraocular pressure causes severe pain, often accompanied by vomiting and rapid visual impairment. The optic disk is swollen, and complete blindness can occur within days.

Acute angle-closure glaucoma is an ophthalmologic emergency. Treatment with osmotic agents such as oral glycerin, intravenous mannitol, and pupillary constrictors such as pilocarpine is effective in reestablishing aqueous outflow and interrupting the acute attack. Peripheral iridectomy by laser is indicated whether or not the acute attack is controlled. This is effective both in the acute relief of symptoms and in preventing further episodes.

DISLOCATION OF THE LENS

The lens is connected to the ciliary body by a bundle of collagen fibers called the zonular liga-

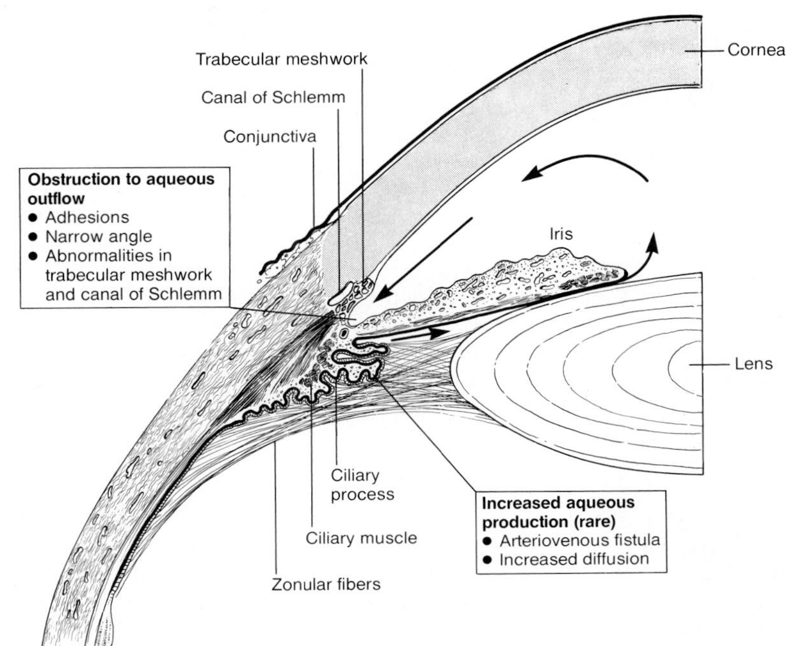

Figure 33-7. Circulation of aqueous humor, showing pathogenesis of glaucoma. Arrows indicate the direction of flow of aqueous humor.

ment and may be dislocated by trauma. Patients with abnormal collagen, as in Marfan's syndrome and homocystinuria, have weak zonular fibers that predispose to dislocation.

Anterior lens dislocation often causes obstruction to aqueous flow, leading to acute secondary glaucoma. Posterior dislocation of an intact lens does not cause severe symptoms except visual impairment. If the lens capsule is ruptured, lens protein may enter the bloodstream and stimulate antibody formation (lens protein contains antigens sequestered from the immune system during fetal life and is therefore regarded as foreign). This may result in immunologic endophthalmitis, with lymphocytic infiltration around the ruptured lens.

RETINITIS PIGMENTOSA Retina

Retinitis pigmentosa is a group of degenerative disorders with variable inheritance, most often recessive. Expression is variable, but retinal degeneration usually begins in early life and progresses slowly to blindness at age 50–60 years. The degeneration begins in the peripheral part of the retina, causing progressive loss of the peripheral visual field. Central vision, including macular vision, is spared until the very late stage.

Pathologically, there is disappearance of the rod and cone layer and loss of ganglion cells. Loss of night vision is an early symptom. The fundus becomes slate-gray in color because of an increase in pigment (Fig 33–8). There is no treatment at present. Occasional cases associated with betalipoproteinemia are arrested by large doses of vitamin A.

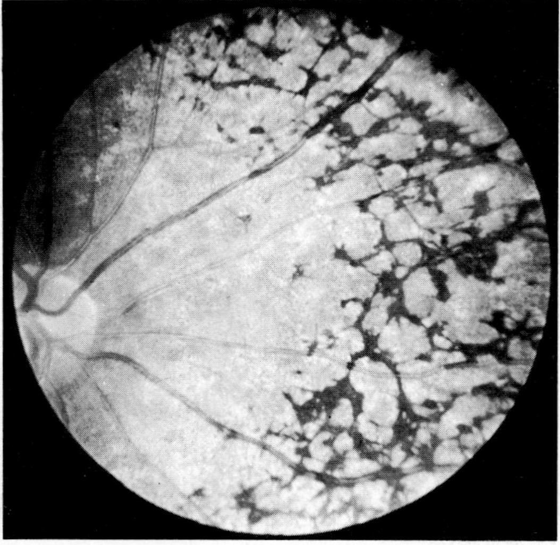

Figure 33–8. Retinitis pigmentosa, showing clumped, scattered pigmentation of retina.

RETROLENTAL FIBROPLASIA OF PREMATURITY

Retrolental fibroplasia is caused by excessive oxygen, usually given for therapy of respiratory distress syndrome in premature infants. The immature retina is exquisitely sensitive to increased partial pressure of oxygen, responding with vasospasm and proliferation of small retinal vessels into the vitreous. Edema and leakage of blood leads to organization, fibrous traction on the retina, retinal detachment, and blindness. Careful control of oxygen therapy in the newborn has reduced the incidence of retrolental fibroplasia.

VASCULAR DISEASES OF THE RETINA

The retina is commonly affected in diseases of small vessels such as the microangiopathy of diabetes mellitus (Chapter 46) and hypertension (Chapter 20).

Vascular lesions causing occlusion of the central artery of the retina result in pale retinal infarction. Hemorrhagic infarction occurs when the central vein of the retina is occluded. **Arterial emboli**—either cholesterol emboli, derived from atheromatous plaques in the carotid circulation, or septic emboli in septicemic states such as infective endocarditis—may produce microinfarcts in the retina.

RETINAL DETACHMENT

Detachment of the retina is separation of the neuroepithelial layer of the retina from the pigment layer, due either to fibrous contraction or to fluid collection between the 2 layers. Detachment deprives the neuroepithelial layer of its choroidal blood supply and causes degeneration within 4–6 weeks.

Retinal detachment may result from (1) extravasation of fluid from the choroid or retina in inflammations, neoplasms, and venous obstruction; (2) contraction of vitreous fibrous bands that have been formed by organization of vitreous hemorrhage, inflammation, or neovascularization (as occurs in retrolental fibroplasia and diabetic retinopathy); or (3) a hole in the retina, permitting passage of liquefied vitreous. Such holes are present in about 7% of individuals over 40 years. Trauma and severe myopia contribute to the occurrence of retinal detachment. Approximately 1% of myopic patients develop retinal detachment.

Clinically, retinal detachment causes sudden loss of part of the field of vision. The field defect depends on the site of detachment. Untreated, the detachment progresses, ultimately involving the entire retina and causing blindness. Laser treatment is effective in stopping the progression of retinal detachment and reversing the visual loss.

Eales's disease and **Coats's disease** are both rare causes of retinal detachment of unknown cause in young adults. In these conditions, recurrent retinal or vitreous hemorrhage leads to fibrosis and retinal detachment.

OPTIC ATROPHY

The term "optic atrophy" is applied to extreme pallor of the optic disk (optic nerve head). It usually reflects degeneration of optic nerve fibers and has many causes (Table 33–5). Primary optic atrophy—resulting from diseases of the optic disk—is distinguished from secondary optic atrophy, which is due to long-standing edema of the disk caused by raised intracranial pressure. Loss of vision follows unless the cause is treatable.

NEOPLASMS OF THE EYEBALL

MALIGNANT MELANOMA

Malignant melanoma occurs almost exclusively in white adults. In the United States and Europe, it is the commonest intraocular malignant neoplasm. It is uncommon in Asia, Africa, and South America.

Pathology

Intraocular malignant melanomas arise in the uveal tract (85% in the choroid, 10% in the ciliary body, 5% in the iris). They are composed of proliferating, invasive melanocytes, with several morphologic subtypes. **Spindle cell type A tumor,** composed of slender cells with elongated nuclei and no nucleoli, has the best prognosis (85% 10-year survival). **Spindle cell type B tumors,** composed of more ovoid spindle cells with nucleoli, have a slightly worse prognosis (80% 10-year survival). **Epithelioid cell tumors,** composed of large pleomorphic round cells with hyperchromatic nuclei, nucleoli, and a high mitotic rate, occur and have a bad prognosis (35% 10-year survival). Over 50% of melanomas of the uveal tract contain mixtures of the above cell types.

Clinical Features

Melanomas arising in the iris become visible as a black mass in the front of the eye and usually present at an early stage. Most melanomas of the iris are spindle cell type A tumors. The combination of early presentation and favorable histologic type gives iris melanomas a high survival rate (nearly 100%) after local surgical removal. Note that benign pigmented nevi also occur in the iris and are difficult to distinguish from melanoma clinically (Fig 33–9).

Melanomas arising in the ciliary body and choroid generally attain a large size before they are detected. They grow inward into the vitreous, producing detachment of the retina and visual impairment, the usual presenting feature. Such melanomas are usually treated by enucleation of the eye. Their prognosis depends mainly on the histologic type. In the epithelioid melanomas, death is commonly due to distant metastases.

Table 33–5. Causes of optic atrophy.

Optic neuritis
Viral infections: mumps, measles; leprosy; syphilis
Demyelinating diseases: multiple sclerosis and variants
Ischemia: arteriosclerosis, giant cell arteritis
Raised intracranial pressure: chronic low-grade
Metabolic disorders: nutritional (vitamin B_1, B_6, B_{12} deficiencies); tobacco-alcohol amblyopia; chemicals (eg, methyl alcohol)
Trauma to optic nerve
Familial and congenital forms

RETINOBLASTOMA

Retinoblastoma has a worldwide distribution and occurs in 2 forms: an inherited form (30%) and a sporadic form (70%). It occurs almost exclusively in children under 5 years of age, with a frequency of about 1:20,000.

Genetic Features (Chapter 18)

Inherited cases have an apparent autosomal dominant mode of inheritance and 90% penetrance. These patients commonly have bilateral

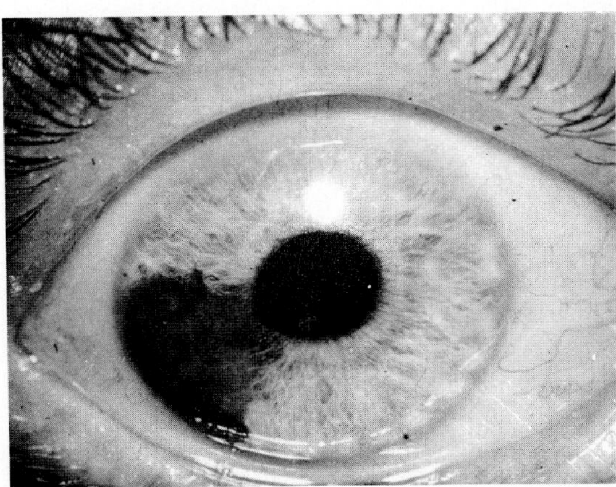

Figure 33–9. Pigmented lesion of the iris. Biopsy was necessary to determine whether this was a benign nevus (which it proved to be) or a malignant melanoma.

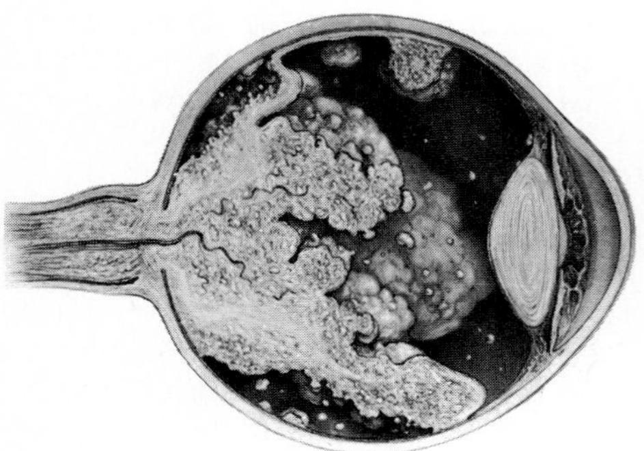

Figure 33-10. Retinoblastoma, showing a large retinal mass extending into the vitreous with multiple satellite nodules and optic nerve invasion.

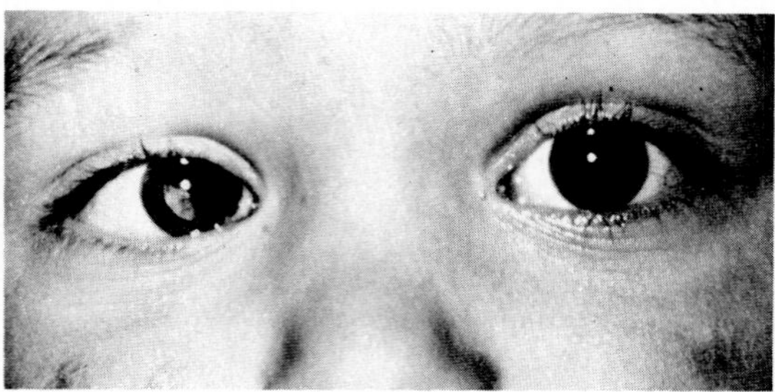

Figure 33-11. Retinoblastoma. Note the white spot in the right pupil resulting from reflection of light from the retinal tumor.

retinoblastoma. More than 90% of sporadic cases have unilateral disease. Retinoblastoma is associated with a constant karyotypic abnormality (deletion of 13q−). Recent molecular studies suggest that, in fact, a pair of recessive genes is involved, both of which must have undergone mutation to produce the disease. In the sporadic form of the disease, both mutations are acquired. In the hereditary form, one recessive gene is inherited in mutant form; the other suffers an acquired mutation, after which the tumor develops, mimicking incomplete penetrance of a dominant gene.

Pathology

Retinoblastoma arises in the retina from primitive neural cells in the retina and as such resembles neuroblastoma, which arises from neuroblasts elsewhere in the nervous system. It is an aggressive neoplasm, infiltrating the retina, extending into the vitreous (Fig 33–10) and along the optic nerve into the cranial cavity. Seeding of the cerebrospinal fluid may result in widespread dissemination in the subarachnoid space. Hematogenous spread also occurs. Microscopically, retinoblastoma is composed of undifferentiated small cells with a high nuclear:cytoplasmic ratio and hyperchromatic nuclei. Mitotic figures are frequent. The presence of Flexner-Wintersteiner rosettes composed of the neoplastic cells arranged in an orderly fashion around a central lumen is a diagnostic feature.

Clinical Features

The parent usually notices some peculiarity in the child's eye, commonly a white spot in the pupil (Fig 33–11; leukocoria—caused by the reflection of light entering the pupil by the retinal tumor). Increased size of the orbit due to the mass effect is a late sign. Fundal examination shows the presence of the neoplasm.

Without treatment, retinoblastoma causes rapid death in most cases. Treatment with radiation and chemotherapy has improved the prognosis somewhat. A significant number (1–2%) of retinoblastomas undergo spontaneous regression—being the most frequent human neoplasm to demonstrate this phenomenon. Regression is associated with cessation of proliferation of the neoplasm followed by fibrosis. Patients with inherited retinoblastomas that have regressed represent a source of transmission of the abnormal gene to the next generation. Examination of the parents of a child with the inherited form of retinoblastoma shows the presence of regressed tumor in one parent's retina.

Section VIII.
The Respiratory System

Lung cancer (Chapter 36) is responsible for more deaths (over 125,000 annually) in the USA than any other type of cancer. Chronic obstructive pulmonary disease (COPD, Chapter 35), which includes emphysema and chronic bronchitis, is the commonest type of lung disease. It is second only to ischemic heart disease as a cause of chronic disability. Both lung cancer and COPD are related to cigarette smoking, which is discussed in Chapter 12.

Pneumonia and tuberculosis (Chapter 34) have decreased in importance as a cause of death in developed countries but remain serious problems in developing countries. *Pneumocystis carinii* pneumonia is the commonest opportunistic infection in immunocompromised patients, including those with AIDS (Chapter 7). Pulmonary embolism (Chapter 35) is a life-threatening complication of many clinical states and is usually secondary to venous thrombosis (see Chapter 9).

34 The Lung: I. Structure & Function; Infections

Respiration is the process of gas exchange between an organism and its environment. Within the lungs, atmospheric oxygen is supplied to the blood in the alveolar capillaries, and waste carbon dioxide is removed.

STRUCTURE OF THE RESPIRATORY SYSTEM

THE AIR PASSAGES

The air passages—nasal cavity, pharynx, larynx, trachea, bronchi, and bronchioles—transmit air from the atmosphere to the alveoli (ventilation).

The bronchi divide dichotomously, becoming gradually smaller and more thin-walled as they progress away from the hilum toward the periphery. When the walls lose their cartilage, they are called bronchioles. Bronchioles are less than 2 mm in diameter, have smooth muscle walls, and terminate in the alveoli (Fig 34–1). The lining epithelium is ciliated columnar in the larger air passages and ciliated cuboidal in the distal bronchioles. Mucus-producing goblet cells are present, mainly in the larger bronchi. Scattered "small granule cells" are present in the bronchi on the basement membrane between epithelial cells; these are neuroendocrine cells that contain serotonin, bombesin, and other polypeptides. Small dome-shaped Clara cells in the terminal bronchioles secrete a protein that lines the small air passages.

THE LUNG PARENCHYMA

Two units of lung parenchyma are recognized. The **pulmonary lobule** is represented by the structures derived from a small bronchiole, composed of 5–7 terminal bronchioles and the structures distal to them (Fig 34–1). The lobule is separated from other lobules by connective tissue.

The **pulmonary acinus** is represented by the

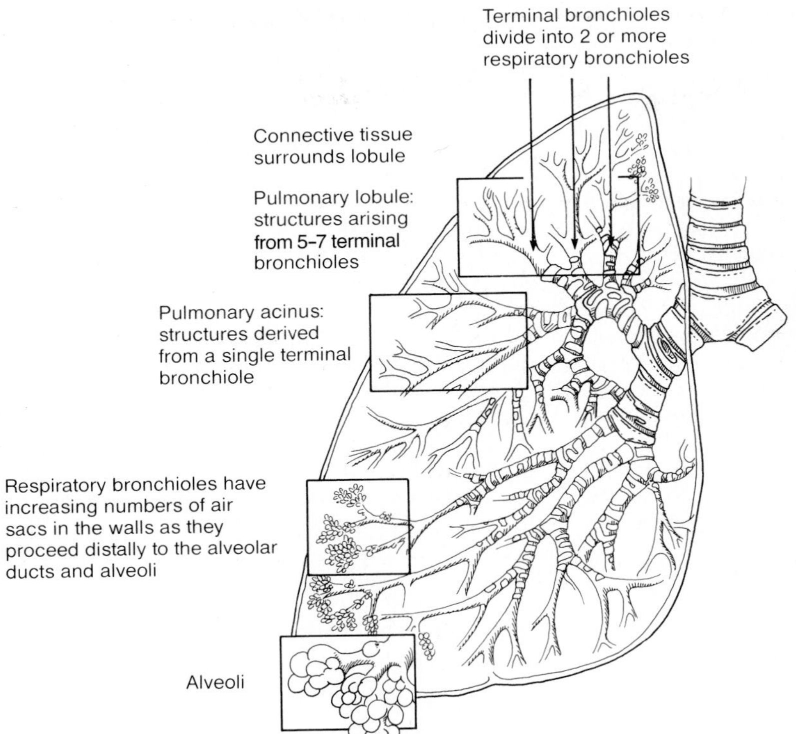

Figure 34–1. Structure of lung parenchyma.

structures arising from a single terminal bronchiole and consists of respiratory bronchioles and alveoli. Respiratory bronchioles are lined by simple cuboidal epithelium and participate in gas exchange. They lead into alveolar ducts. Alveolar sacs arise as saccular outpouchings from the alveolar ducts and respiratory bronchioles. The alveolar wall is 5–10 μm thick and covered by flat type I pneumocytes over 90% of the surface and by type II pneumocytes over the remainder. Type II pneumocytes are cuboidal cells with abundant cytoplasm that contains distinctive granules on electron microscopy. They produce surfactant and proliferate rapidly when there is alveolar injury.

THE PLEURA

The lung is encased by a layer of mesothelial cells, the visceral pleura, which becomes continuous with the internal lining of the chest wall (parietal pleura) at the lung hilum. The pleural cavity is lubricated by a small film of pleural fluid that permits movement of the lung in relation to the chest wall.

THE BLOOD SUPPLY

The lung has a dual blood supply. The bronchial arteriolar branches follow the bronchial tree and have a nutritive function. The pulmonary artery divides to produce a network of capillaries, the primary function of which is gas exchange.

EVALUATION OF THE INTEGRITY OF LUNG STRUCTURE

Though the lungs cannot be directly visualized without opening the chest wall, their structure may be assessed by several methods:

(1) Physical examination of the chest.

(2) Examination of sputum (coughed-up tracheal secretion) for the presence of specific microorganisms by culture and malignant cells by cytologic examination. Microbiologic interpretation requires care because sputum is almost invariably contaminated by saliva, which normally has a rich commensal flora, in the oropharynx. Less contaminated samples of sputum may be obtained by transtracheal aspiration.

(3) Radiologic examination, including chest x-ray, computerized tomography, bronchography (x-ray of the air passages after instilling radiopaque dye into the bronchus). Pulmonary arteriography displays the major arteries of the lung and is used in the diagnosis of pulmonary embolism.

(4) Laryngoscopy and bronchoscopy, which permit direct examination to the level of the large bronchi at the hilum but not farther. Bronchoscopy also permits biopsy both of the bronchial wall and the lung parenchyma (transbronchial lung biopsy).

(5) Percutaneous and open lung biopsy, which are other techniques of obtaining tissue from lung lesions. Percutaneous fine-needle aspiration under radiologic guidance is used for sampling mass lesions in the lung. Open lung biopsy is an effective method of obtaining representative tissue and is used mainly in diffuse lung disease; it requires a limited thoracotomy.

(6) Pleural diseases may be evaluated by needle biopsy of the pleura or aspiration of a pleural effusion, if one is present. Chemical examination of an effusion characterizes it as a transudate or exudate (see Chapter 3.) Microscopic examination may show inflammatory or neoplastic cells. Culture identifies microorganisms, normal pleural fluid being sterile. Needle biopsy of the pleura provides a sample of tissue for histologic examination.

FUNCTION OF THE LUNG

The function of the lung is gas exchange, supplying oxygen to and removing carbon dioxide from blood in the capillaries of the alveolar septa. The normal arterial partial pressure of oxygen (P_{O_2}) is 95 mm Hg and of carbon dioxide (P_{CO_2}) 40 mm Hg. Gas exchange involves **ventilation,** the flow of air through the air passages into the acini; **perfusion,** the flow of blood in the pulmonary circulation to the alveolar capillaries; and **diffusion,** the passage of oxygen and carbon dioxide from alveolar air to blood and vice versa. Interference with these processes may produce respiratory failure (Table 34–1).

VENTILATION

Ventilation is the process by which air from the atmosphere is brought to the pulmonary acini. The ventilation rate is controlled by the respiratory center in the brain stem, which is under the influence of arterial P_{CO_2} (acting directly) and P_{O_2} (acting via the chemoreceptors). The respiratory center controls the muscles of respiration, the diaphragm, and the intercostal muscles.

Ventilation may be quantitated as the volume of gas entering the alveoli per minute. This is equal to the total volume of inspired air minus the dead space volume (ie, the air in the trachea, bronchi, and bronchioles which is not available for gas exchange; see Fig 34–2).

Abnormal Ventilation

Impairment of total alveolar ventilation occurs by 2 mechanisms (Table 34–1):

A. Restrictive diseases, in which expansion of the lung does not occur normally. This may be due to (1) failure of chest wall expansion as a result of respiratory muscle failure (brain stem, nerve, and muscle diseases); or (2) intrinsic disease in the lung, such as pulmonary fibrosis, that prevents expansion.

B. Obstructive diseases, in which ventilation of the lung is impeded because of obstruction of the air passages. Decreased alveolar ventilation leads to hypoxemia (decreased P_{O_2}) and hypercapnia (increased P_{CO_2}).

Table 34–1. Classification of causes of respiratory failure.

Mechanism	Acute	Chronic
Reduced ventilation		
Restrictive		
Neuromuscular diseases (failure of respiratory muscles)	Tetanus, botulism, poliomyelitis, polyneuritis, spinal cord injury	Muscular dystrophy, myasthenia gravis
Chest wall diseases (failure of chest expansion)	Pneumothorax, flail chest (trauma)	Kyphoscoliosis, obesity, pleural effusion, mesothelioma, ankylosing spondylitis
Obstructive	Foreign bodies, epiglottitis, angioedema, diphtheria, bronchiolitis, bronchial asthma	COPD,[1] bronchiectasis
Abnormal perfusion	Pulmonary embolism, fat embolism	Recurrent emboli, vasculitis
Impaired diffusion		
Interstitial diseases	Shock, interstitial pneumonitis	Sarcoidosis, pneumoconiosis, interstitial pneumonitis, interstitial fibrosis
Pulmonary edema	Acute left ventricular failure, toxic gases, mitral stenosis	Chronic left ventricular failure

[1]COPD = chronic obstructive pulmonary disease.

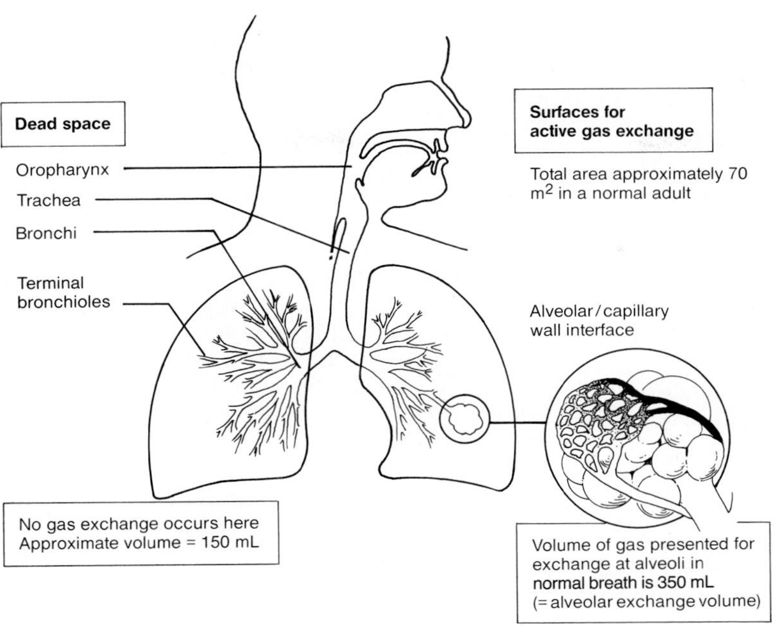

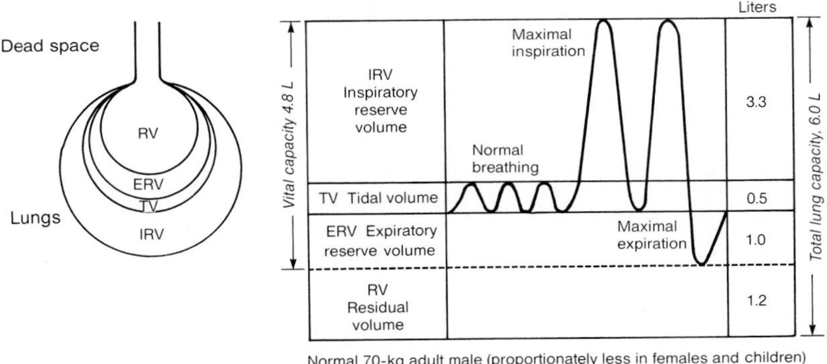

Figure 34–2. Air passages and ventilation of the lungs.

Increased alveolar ventilation caused by hyperventilation washes out carbon dioxide and causes hypocapnia (decreased P_{CO_2}). If the individual is breathing air at normal atmospheric pressure, the P_{O_2} does not increase with hyperventilation, since exchange in normal perfused lung already is maximal.

PERFUSION

Perfusion refers to the flow of pulmonary arterial blood to the alveolar capillaries for gas exchange. Failure of perfusion of part of the lung results in a decrease in the effective area available for gas exchange, thereby increasing the effective dead space volume. Partial loss of perfusion may be compensated by hyperventilation (increasing number and depth of breaths), which increases total ventilation; this response corrects the tendency to hypercapnia but not the hypoxemia unless the patient is breathing oxygen-enriched air.

Even in the normal lung, blood flow is not uniformly distributed, the basal regions receiving more blood than the apex. For proper gas exchange, ventilation and perfusion must be balanced. Mismatching of perfusion and ventilation results in (1) increased physiologic dead space if an area that is ventilated is not perfused and (2) right-to-left shunting of blood if an area that is perfused is not ventilated (Fig 34–3).

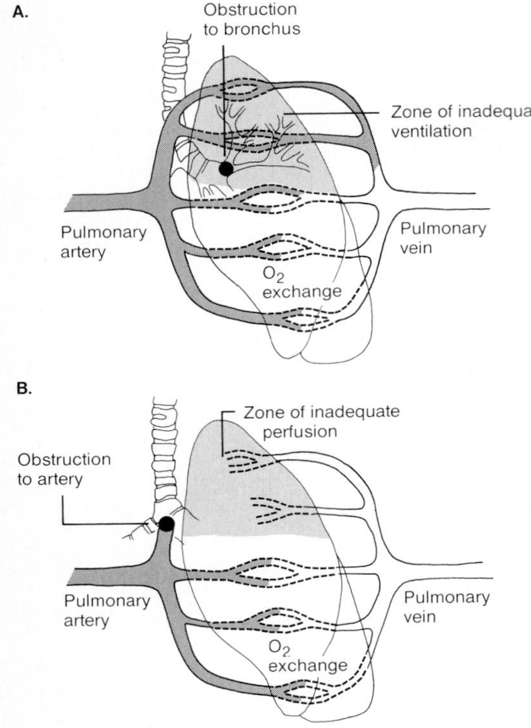

Figure 34–3. Effect of imbalance between ventilation and perfusion. **A:** Area of lung that is not ventilated but normally perfused. The blood is not oxygenated, producing a right-to-left shunt effect. **B:** Area of lung that is not perfused but ventilated normally. This area does not participate in gas exchange and acts as an area that is equivalent to dead space.

DIFFUSION

Diffusion of gases occurs through the alveolar diffusion membrane, which is composed of capillary endothelial cells, alveolar epithelial cells, and the fused basement membrane of these cells (Fig 34–4). The normal alveolar septum has a minimal amount of interstitial connective tissue containing collagen, elastin, and a few scattered lymphocytes and macrophages.

Abnormal diffusion of gases across the membrane usually causes hypoxemia. Carbon dioxide, which is much more diffusible than oxygen, is not affected. In diffusion defects, stimulation of the respiratory center by hypoxemia causes hyperventilation and hypocapnia (Table 34–2).

RESPIRATORY FAILURE

Respiratory failure is defined as a condition in which arterial P_{O_2} is decreased below or arterial P_{CO_2} is increased above its normal level. Normal P_{CO_2} is 40 ± 5 mm Hg and does not vary with age. Mean P_{O_2} varies with age and is derived from the following equation:

$$P_{O_2} = 100.1 - 0.323 \times \text{Age in years}$$

The normal range is the calculated value ± 5 mm Hg.

It is important to note that the diagnosis of respiratory failure is made by arterial blood gas analysis and not by clinical examination.

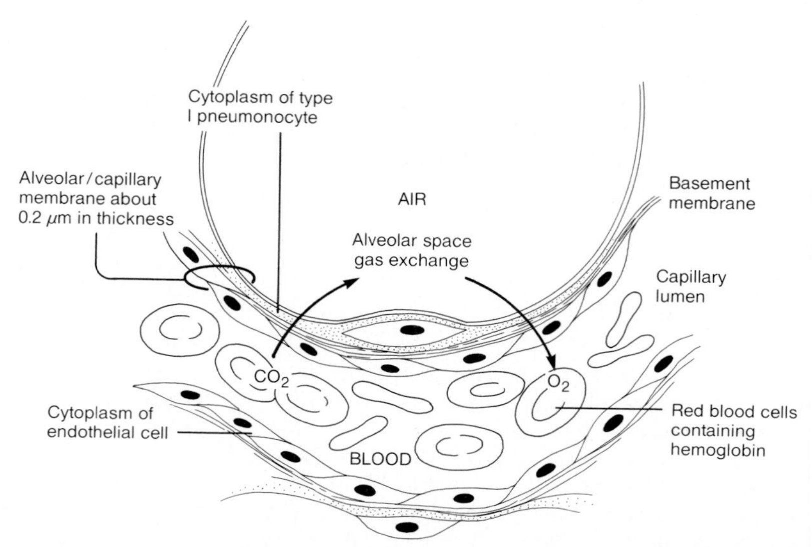

Figure 34–4. The alveolar diffusion membrane through which gas exchange occurs.

Table 34–2. Arterial blood gas changes in respiratory failure.

	P_{O_2}	P_{CO_2}	pH	Pathophysiology
Ventilation failure	Decreased	Increased	Decreased	Nonventilated lung is effectively right-to-left shunt, allowing venous type blood (low P_{O_2}, high P_{CO_2}) to pass directly to the left heart. Alveolar P_{O_2} is low, and P_{CO_2} is high in underventilated areas.
Perfusion failure	Decreased	Normal	Normal	Effective dead space is increased; hyperventilation of remaining lung may correct P_{CO_2} level, but oxygen exchange is already maximal and hyperventilation does not correct the fall in P_{O_2}.
Diffusion failure	Decreased	Decreased	Increased	Diffusion failure affects only exchange of oxygen, not CO_2; the resulting hypoxemia causes compensatory hyperventilation, washing out CO_2 and causing hypocapnia.

Respiratory failure may be acute or chronic and results from failure of ventilation, diffusion, or perfusion of the lungs (Table 34–1). The pattern of changes of blood gases may give an indication of the pathogenesis of respiratory failure (Table 34–2).

ASSESSMENT OF PULMONARY FUNCTION

ARTERIAL BLOOD GASES

Analysis of arterial blood for pH and partial pressures of oxygen and carbon dioxide is necessary to make the diagnosis of respiratory failure. Specific patterns of change occur in the different pathogenetic mechanisms (Table 34–2).

TESTS OF VENTILATORY FUNCTION

Spirometry permits measurement of different volumes of air involved in ventilation (Fig 34–2). **Total lung capacity** is the amount of air contained in the fully expanded lung. The maximum volume of air that an individual can exhale from total lung capacity is the **vital capacity,** and the amount of air remaining in the lung after maximum expiration is the **residual volume. Tidal volume** is the volume of air that enters the lung during a normal breath. Normal values for these lung volumes vary with age, sex, and height.

The dynamic properties of air movement in the lungs are most commonly expressed as the percentage of forced vital capacity (FVC) that is exhaled in the first second of a forced expiration (**FEV_1**). In health, the ratio of FEV_1 to FVC is over 75%.

On the basis of the FEV_1:FVC ratio, ventilatory disorders are classified as follows (Table 34–1): **(1) Restrictive ventilatory disorders,** due to failure of normal lung expansion, are characterized by decrease in vital capacity, total lung capacity, and residual volume but no decrease in the FEV_1:FVC ratio. **(2) Obstructive ventilatory disorders,** due to airway obstruction, are characterized by a marked reduction in FEV1 and the FEV_1:FVC ratio. Vital capacity may be normal or decreased; residual volume is usually increased because of air trapping in the lungs.

COMPLIANCE

Compliance is a measure of the work required to stretch the lungs and chest wall on inspiration. Surface tension forces are a significant factor at the beginning of inspiration, when the alveoli are empty and small. (Surface tension is greatest for small-diameter spaces—Laplace's law.) The production and release of **surfactant** from type II pneumocytes reduces these surface tension forces. Surfactant is a phospholipoprotein containing dipalmitoyl lecithin. Absence of surfactant inhibits expansion of alveoli on inspiration and is a major factor in hyaline membrane disease of the newborn (see below). Surfactant also has bactericidal properties and forms part of the fluid secretion that the cilia transport along the air passages.

Compliance is measured by observing incremental changes in lung volume that occur following changes in pressure in the major air passages.

MANIFESTATIONS OF RESPIRATORY DISEASE

DYSPNEA

Normal ventilation is a process that occurs subconsciously. Dyspnea is any alteration of this normal state and may therefore be a sensation of obstruction or pain associated with breathing or active awareness of the process of breathing. Dyspnea may result from a variety of causes (Table 34–3).

CYANOSIS

Cyanosis is a dusky, bluish discoloration of the skin and mucous membranes caused by the presence in the blood of increased amounts (over 5 g/dL) of reduced hemoglobin.

Table 34–3. Dyspnea: Principal causes.[1]

Large airway obstruction: often causes respiratory difficulty with coarse noise (stridor) on inhalation (as in laryngeal stridor).
Small airway obstruction: Produces an expiratory wheeze (as in asthma). The difficulty is greatest on expiration; small airways tend to collapse as intrathoracic pressure rises.
Fluid in the parenchyma or alveoli (as in left heart failure and pulmonary edema) produces decreased compliance and vital capacity.
Collapse and consolidation of lung parenchyma (as in pneumonia) reduce the vital capacity.
Destruction of lung tissue (as in emphysema) reduces vital capacity.
Diffuse pulmonary fibrosis: decreases compliance and produces diffusion abnormalities.
Hypoxemia and hypercapnia stimulate the respiratory center, increasing the ventilatory rate.
Painful lesions of chest or pleura (pleurisy and trauma) or restrictive chest diseases produce limited expansion.
Fluid or air (especially under pressure) in the pleural cavity, as in pleural effusion or pneumothorax, reduces expansion of the lung.
Pulmonary embolism and infarction produce perfusion defects and destruction of lung.

[1]Note that anxiety and exercise produce temporary "dyspnea" in normal individuals.

Two mechanisms may lead to cyanosis:

Central cyanosis is caused by admixture of deoxygenated venous blood with oxygenated arterial blood in the heart and lungs. Central cyanosis occurs in (1) congenital cyanotic heart disease where there is a right to left shunt, eg, Fallot's tetralogy, transposition of great vessels, and Eisenmenger's syndrome (see Chapter 21); (2) pulmonary arteriovenous fistula; and (3) extensive right-to-left shunting of blood in the lungs caused by lack of ventilation of adequately perfused alveoli.

Peripheral cyanosis is caused by increased delivery of oxygen to the tissues, resulting in excessive reduction of normally saturated hemoglobin. It usually results from slowing of blood flow, usually in the skin of the extremities, most commonly caused by cold and states of extreme cutaneous vasoconstriction such as shock.

Central cyanosis can be differentiated from peripheral cyanosis by the presence of blue discoloration of mucous membranes such as the tongue in addition to the skin; in peripheral cyanosis, the warm mucous membranes are normal in color.

CHEST PAIN

The lung parenchyma is not sensitive to pain, and most pulmonary diseases do not cause pain. The parietal pleura is sensitive, and diseases that cause inflammation of the parietal pleura, such as bacterial pneumonia and pulmonary infarction, cause chest pain. Pleural pain is characteristically related to ventilatory chest movement and often associated with a pleural friction rub that may be heard on auscultation.

COUGH

Cough is a common symptom of respiratory disease. It results from (1) stimulation of the cough reflex by the entry of foreign material into the larynx and (2) the accumulation of secretions in the lower respiratory tract. Cough may be dry (without sputum), as occurs typically in interstitial lung diseases, or productive of sputum in processes involving the air passages and alveoli.

SPUTUM PRODUCTION

Examination of sputum is very useful in the evaluation of patients with suspected lung disease. A purulent appearance or foul odor suggests bacterial infection; the presence of blood may indicate infarction, tuberculosis, or cancer, among other possibilities.

A Gram-stained smear of sputum and sputum culture are useful for assessing the presence of bacterial or fungal infections. Cytologic examination may reveal the presence of malignant cells.

HEMOPTYSIS

Coughing blood is a symptom of serious respiratory disease. Hemoptysis occurs in a variety of clinical conditions, including (1) left heart failure, due to rupture of pulmonary capillaries under increased hydrostatic pressure; (2) necrotizing parenchymal diseases such as infarcts, tuberculosis, and pneumonia; and (3) lung carcinoma.

CONGENITAL DISEASES OF THE LUNG

BRONCHOPULMONARY SEQUESTRATION

The lungs normally develop from buds that arise from the embryonic foregut. Occasionally, an additional segment of lung develops from an abnormal accessory lung bud. The bronchi in this sequestered segment may not communicate with the normal bronchial tree, causing accumulation of mucus secretion followed by infection with abscess formation, parenchymal fibrosis, and bronchial dilatation. Patients usually present with a mass in the lung, commonly in the left lower lobe or, more rarely, with accessory lung tissue in the mediastinum.

BRONCHOGENIC CYST

Bronchogenic cysts arise from accessory bronchial buds that lose communication with the tracheobronchial tree. The bud becomes dilated into a cyst by accumulation of mucoid fluid within it. The cyst is lined by respiratory epithelium and frequently has cartilage in its wall. Such cysts usually remain attached to the trachea. Rarely, they are found elsewhere in the mediastinum.

CONGENITAL CYSTIC ADENOMATOID MALFORMATION

This rare congenital malformation commonly presents in the newborn period. It usually involves one lobe, which is enlarged and composed of abnormal cystic cavities, lined by bronchiolar and columnar mucinous epithelium. The cystic mass may compress adjacent normal lung and displace the mediastinum, interfering with normal cardiac and lung function. Surgical removal of the involved lobe is curative.

TRACHEOESOPHAGEAL FISTULA

The presence of a fistula between the esophagus and the trachea usually is manifested by cyanosis and respiratory distress at the time of the first feeding, when milk enters the lung directly through the fistula. If feeding is continued, severe aspiration pneumonia occurs, causing death. Closure of the fistula is curative.

CONGENITAL ATELECTASIS

Failure of the lungs to expand at birth is termed atelectasis. It may be focal or may affect all of both lungs. Causes include inadequate attempts at respiration by the newborn (due to neurologic damage, severe anoxia), bronchial obstruction, or absence of surfactant (see Respiratory Distress Syndrome, below).

NEONATAL RESPIRATORY DISTRESS SYNDROME

Neonatal respiratory distress syndrome (RDS), also called hyaline membrane disease, is a common complication in premature infants—born before the lungs have attained maturity. RDS is also seen in babies born to diabetic mothers and occurs with a higher incidence in children delivered by cesarian section. Despite major improvements in the care of these infants, respiratory distress syndrome still accounts for about 7000 neonatal deaths every year in the United States.

Immaturity of the lungs is the major etiologic factor in RDS. The basic defect is deficient production of surfactant by type II pneumocytes. Surfactant normally reaches adequate levels after the 35th week of gestation. RDS occurs in 60% of babies born after less than 28 weeks of gestation, 40% of those born between 28 and 32 weeks, 20% of those born between 32 and 36 weeks, and less than 5% of those born after more than 36 weeks of gestation.

Surfactant reduces surface tension, decreasing the amount of pressure required to open the alveoli. In the immediate neonatal period, surfactant is important in maintaining expansion of the lung after the first few breaths. In surfactant deficiency, the alveoli tend to undergo collapse after initial expansion, causing failure of oxygenation, hypoxemia, alveolar damage, protein exudation, and alveolar hemorrhage. RDS has a mortality rate of about 25% even when treated with positive-pressure ventilation. In babies with a birth weight of less than 1000 g, the mortality rate is over 50%.

Grossly, the involved lung shows inadequate expansion and is heavy and purple as a result of fluid exudation and hemorrhage. Microscopically, there is severe diffuse damage, with intra-alveolar hemorrhage and coagulated protein lining the damaged alveoli and respiratory bronchioles; in tissue section, this protein lining appears as a hyaline membrane (Fig 34–5), leading to the alternative name **hyaline membrane disease** for RDS. It must be made clear that hyaline membranes are a nonspecific response to any type of acute alveolar damage; a similar "membrane" may be seen in acute viral, chemical, and allergic pneumonitis and in shock lung (adult respiratory distress syndrome). Babies that survive severe RDS—particularly if oxygen has been used in therapy—may progress to chronic lung disease with fibrosis, called **bronchopulmonary dysplasia**. (*Note:* The term "dysplasia" was inappropriately chosen at a time when this lesion was thought to be a congenital malformation rather than the end result of RDS.) The cause of bronchopulmonary dysplasia is believed to be a toxic effect of oxygen used in treatment of RDS rather than RDS per se.

Amniocentesis permits evaluation of lung maturity in premature babies by testing for the lecithin:sphingomyelin (L:S) ratio in amniotic fluid. In early pregnancy, sphingomyelin levels exceed lecithin levels. With lung maturity, there is a sharp increase in lecithin and a decline of sphingomyelin levels. When the L:S ratio reaches 2:1, the risk of RDS is very small.

INFECTIONS OF THE LUNG PARENCHYMA

Classification

Infections of the lung parenchyma are classified according to a variety of different criteria.

Hyaline membranes

Collapsed alveoli

Bronchiole

Figure 34–5. Neonatal respiratory distress syndrome, showing marked alveolar collapse and hyaline membranes.

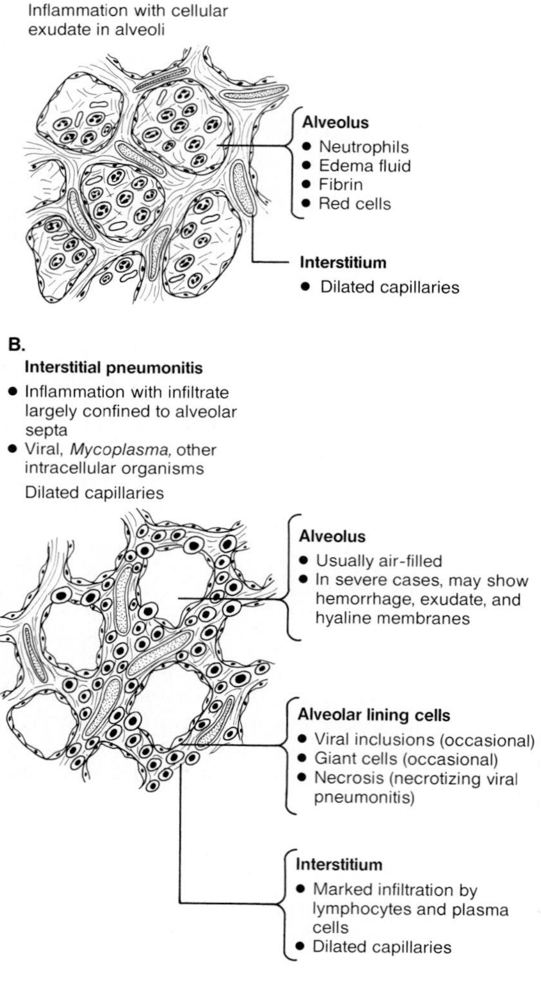

Figure 34–6. Pneumonia **(A)** as caused by bacteria characterized by intra-alveolar exudation and neutrophil emigration—contrasted with interstitial pneumonitis **(B),** where the inflammation is primarily mononuclear and involves the interstitium.

A. Acute Versus Chronic Infections:

1. **Acute infection** of the lung parenchyma producing an acute inflammatory response causes pneumonia or acute pneumonitis—"pneumonia" when there is alveolar involvement and consolidation, "pneumonitis" when the process is largely confined to the alveolar walls (see below).

2. **Chronic infections** produce chronic inflammatory responses associated with fibrosis and persistent suppuration or the formation of granulomas.

B. Alveolar Versus Interstitial Inflammation:

1. **Alveolar acute inflammation (pneumonia)** is usually caused by bacteria and is characterized by hyperemia of septal capillaries with exudation of fluid and neutrophil emigration into the alveolar spaces (Fig 34–6). The infection spreads to adjacent alveoli through interalveolar pores of Kohn; when large numbers of alveoli are filled by inflammatory cells, consolidation is said to be present. This type of inflammation is caused by infections with organisms, usually bacteria, that multiply extracellularly in the alveoli.

Alveolar acute inflammation is further classified as lobar pneumonia or bronchopneumonia. In **lobar pneumonia,** large confluent areas of lung are consolidated (eg, whole lobes; Figs 34–7 and 34–8); virulent organisms such as pneumococci and staphylococci are the usual cause. In **bronchopneumonia,** there is patchy consolidation of multiple small areas of lung adjacent to inflamed bronchioles (Figs 34–7 and 34–9). Bronchopneumonias are commonly caused by bacteria of lower virulence than those causing lobar pneumonia.

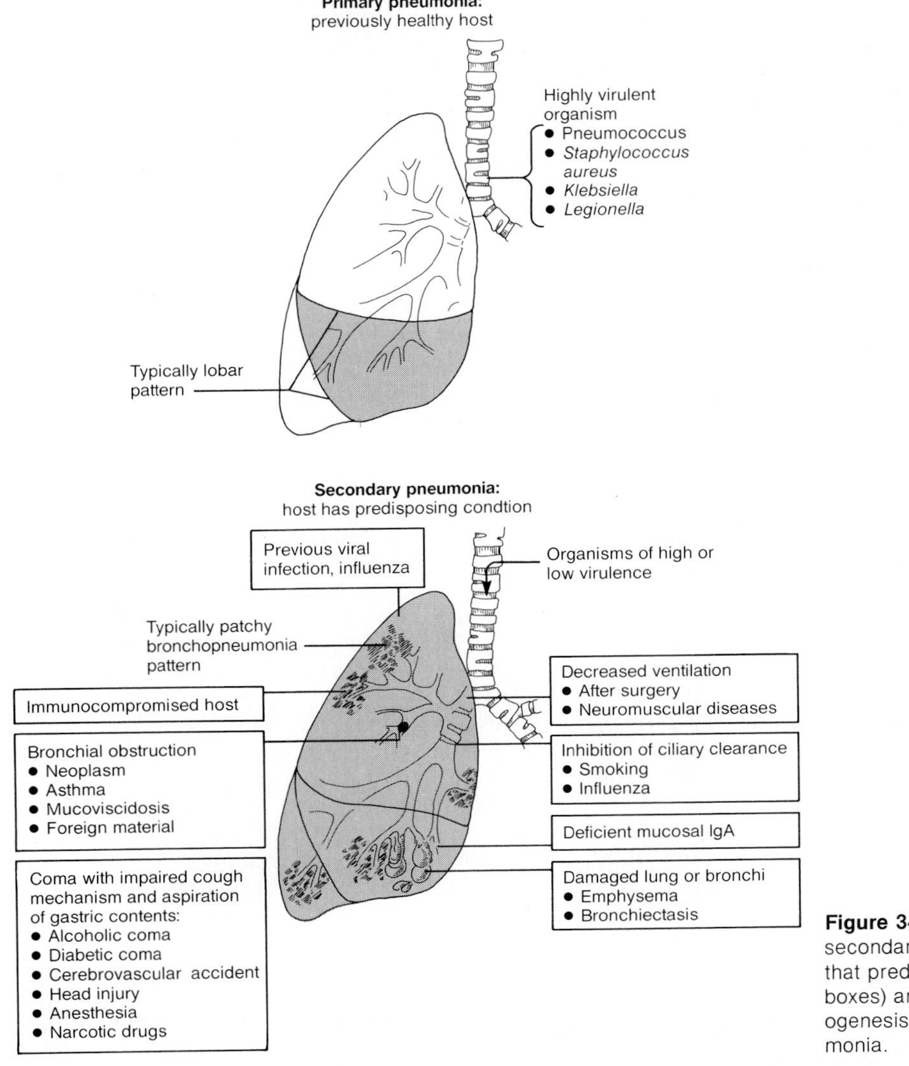

Figure 34–7. Primary versus secondary pneumonia. Note that predisposing diseases (in boxes) are important in the pathogenesis of secondary pneumonia.

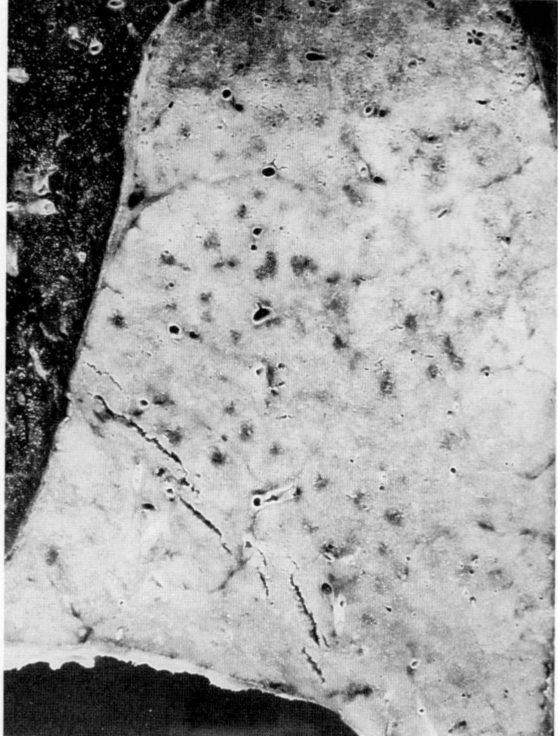

Figure 34-8. Lobar pneumonia. The lobe to the right of the interlobar fissure is pale and consolidated. The lobe to the left of the interlobar fissure is normal.

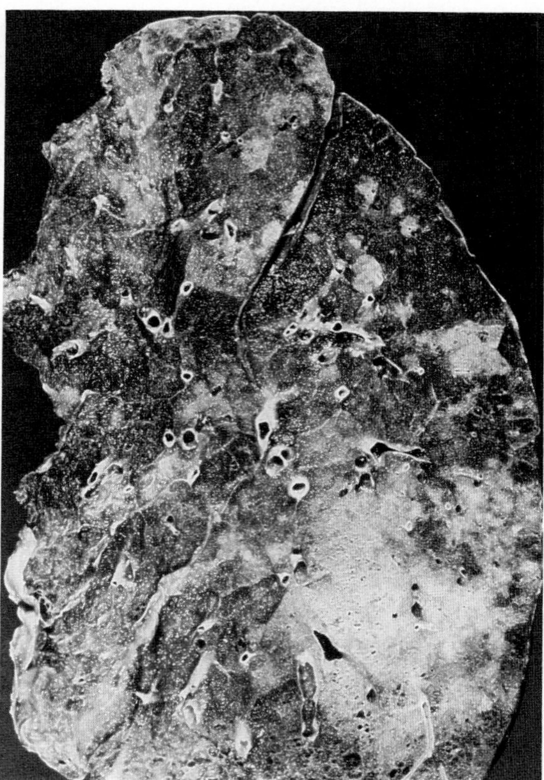

Figure 34-9. Bronchopneumonia. Note the small pale areas of patchy consolidation around bronchioles throughout the lung. There is a larger area of confluent bronchopneumonia at the base.

This distinction into lobar pneumonia and bronchopneumonia may be difficult to make in some cases of severe bronchopneumonia where areas of involvement become confluent, producing extensive consolidation (Fig 34-9).

2. Acute interstitial inflammation (pneumonitis) is characterized by expansion of the alveolar septa, hyperemia, and inflammatory cell infiltration, which often is predominantly lymphocytic (Fig 34-6). The alveolar spaces are usually spared except in severe infection, where alveolar epithelial damage and hemorrhage may occur. Acute interstitial pneumonitis occurs (1) in infections with obligate intracellular organisms—viruses, chlamydiae (psittacosis), and rickettsiae (Q fever); and (2) in *Mycoplasma pneumoniae* infection.

C. Primary Versus Secondary Pneumonia: (Fig 34-7.)

1. Primary pneumonias (usually lobar pneumonias) occur in previously healthy individuals. The causative agents are usually virulent bacteria such as *Streptococcus pneumoniae* (pneumococcus), *Staphylococcus aureus, Klebsiella pneumoniae,* and *Legionella pneumophila.* The pathogenesis of primary pneumonia is largely a function of microorganism virulence rather than decreased host resistance.

2. Secondary pneumonias occur when there is an underlying predisposition to infection of the pulmonary lobule. The lung normally resists such infection by a variety of defenses that include respiratory mucus, which traps bacteria; the mucosal cilia, which waft the mucus upward into the pharynx; immunoglobulin (mainly IgA) in the mucus; alveolar macrophages; and the laryngeal apparatus, acting mainly by the cough reflex. Abnormalities in any one of these defense mechanisms lead to increased susceptibility to pneumonia (Fig 34-7).

Secondary pneumonias tend to be bronchopneumonias and may be caused by virulent organisms such as the pneumococcus as well as by less virulent organisms such as *Haemophilus influenzae.* A mixed bacterial flora is frequently involved. Secondary pneumonias tend to be recurrent if the host factor leading to infection is one that persists. Correction of the underlying abnormality is therefore important in treatment.

D. Etiologic Classification: Identification of the causative organism is of great importance because the proper treatment of pneumonia is determined by the etiologic agent and its antibiotic sensitivity. A Gram-stained smear of sputum should be examined as the first step in identification: The presence of characteristic diplococci, gram-positive cocci, or gram-negative rods (Table 34–4) may serve to guide the choice of antibiotic while awaiting results of sputum culture and sensitivity assays.

LOBAR PNEUMONIA

Incidence & Etiology

Primary lobar pneumonia occurs in a healthy individual and classically is caused by the pneumococcus; a single lobe is involved and sharply demarcated from noninvolved lobes (Fig 34–8). While antibiotic therapy has decreased the mortality rate, lobar pneumonia still represents a serious and common infection, particularly in very ill hospitalized patients.

Pneumococci cause 90% of cases of lobar pneumonia. Other organisms include staphylococci, *Klebsiella, Pseudomonas,* and *Proteus.* The organisms are inhaled or aspirated into the alveoli, where their multiplication evokes an acute inflammatory response.

Pathology & Clinical Features

The natural course of pneumococcal pneumonia is rarely observed today because of the widespread availability of antibiotic therapy. When started early, antibiotics rapidly kill the bacteria and terminate disease progression. The natural history of *untreated* lobar pneumonia proceeds in 4 stages.

A. Acute Congestion: (Fig 34–10.) In this early stage, the bacteria are actively multiplying in the alveoli and spreading rapidly into contiguous alveoli. There is active dilatation of alveolar capillaries and fluid exudation into the alveoli. Clinically, the stage of acute congestion corresponds to the onset of illness, with high fever, bacteremia (positive blood culture is common), and cough productive of the exudate in the alveoli. Sputum is purulent and tinged with blood ("rusty") and will grow pneumococci on culture. Involvement of the pleura is common in this stage, causing chest pain, a pleural friction rub, and accumulation of effusion fluid.

B. Red Hepatization: Continued exudation and neutrophil emigration into the alveolar spaces cause the alveoli to become filled with fibrin and neutrophils (Figs 34–11). The involved area is consolidated (Fig 34–8) and appears grossly like liver ("hepatization"). The red color is due to continued hyperemia. Clinically, the illness is at its most severe stage, with high fever and cough. Physical signs of consolidation are present. The solid lung does not expand, and the sound of air entering the alveoli (vesicular breath sounds) is lost. Air movement in bronchi (bronchial breath sounds) is transmitted to the surface across the solid lung. Coarse, wet rales due to "bubbling" of the exudate in the air passages are present. Chest x-ray shows areas of consolidation as well-defined radiopaque zones.

C. Gray Hepatization: This is the early recovery phase. The organism has been controlled by the body defenses and antibiotic therapy, and the patient shows clinical improvement with defervescence. Hyperemia has disappeared because the chemical mediators are no longer generated once the organism is removed. The alveoli still contain the exudate, and the physical signs and radiologic evidence of consolidation are still present.

D. Resolution: The process by which the alveolar exudate is removed and the lung returns to normal is termed resolution. Resolution occurs because in the usual case, there is little destruction of lung tissue in spite of the apparent severity of acute inflammation. Complete resolution may take several weeks, during which radiologic abnormalities persist despite return of the patient's clinical state to normal.

Diagnosis & Treatment

Alveolar consolidation is demonstrated by clinical and radiologic examination, and *S pneumoniae* is identified in Gram-stained smears of sputum and by culture of sputum or blood. Penicillin is the drug of choice for pneumococcal pneumonia; in the case of strains with increased penicillin resistance as shown by in vitro antibiotic sensitivity testing, higher dosages are required.

Predisposing factors that may have favored establishment of the infection should be identified and controlled. Failure to do so may lead to failure of antibiotic therapy and recurrence of pneumonia.

Complications (Fig 34–12)

A. Disturbances of Ventilation and Perfusion: Lobar pneumonia interferes with gas exchange in the involved area of lung. There is no ventilation because the alveoli are filled with exudate, and perfusion of the consolidated area is also decreased. If both lungs are massively involved by the consolidation, respiratory failure may occur.

B. Involvement of the pleura with pleural inflammation and effusion is a common complication of lobar pneumonia. In most cases, this is a simple acute inflammation that resolves with the pneumonia. In a few cases, pleural inflammation becomes chronic, resulting in accumulation of pus in the pleural cavity **(empyema)**. Chronic empyema is associated with extensive fibrosis, which may restrict pulmonary expansion, causing ventilatory failure. Rarely, the infection spreads to involve the pericardium.

C. Bacteremia is the most serious complica-

Table 34-4. Usual laboratory findings in common lung infections.[1]

	Sputum	Sputum Culture	Blood Culture	White Blood Count	Chest X-Ray
Pneumococcus	Gram-positive diplococci	Positive	Often positive	10,000+	Lobar or bronchopneumonia
Staphylococcus aureus	Gram-positive clusters of cocci	Positive	Often positive	10,000+	Bronchopneumonia, abscesses
Group A streptococci	Gram-positive cocci	Positive	Often positive	20,000+	Bronchopneumonia
Haemophilus influenzae	Gram-negative short bacilli	Positive on chocolate agar in CO_2	Usually negative	10,000+	Bronchopneumonia
Klebsiella pneumoniae	Gram-negative short fat rods	Positive	Occasionally positive	20,000+	Broncho- or lobar-pneumonia; suppurative
Other enterobacteria: *Escherichia coli, Pseudomonas, Proteus*	Gram-negative large rods	Positive	Often positive late in course	10,000+	Bronchopneumonia; suppurative
Bacteroides	Gram-negative rods	Positive in anaerobic culture	Usually negative	10,000+	Bronchopneumonia; suppurative
Legionella	Gram-negative; silver and fluorescence stains positive	Positive in charcoal yeast agar	Negative	20,000+	Bronchopneumonia
Mycobacterium tuberculosis	Acid-fast bacilli	Positive but takes 6 weeks	Negative	May be normal	Bronchopneumonia; granulomas; cavities; fibrosis
Fungi: *Histoplasma, Coccidioides, Aspergillus, Cryptococcus, Candida*	Periodic acid-Schiff or silver stains show fungi	Sabouraud agar positive; growth is slow	Usually negative (except cryptococcus)	May be normal	Bronchopneumonia; granulomas; fibrosis; cavities
Viruses and *Chalmydia:* Influenza, measles, respiratory syncytial virus, adenovirus, varicella, psittacosis, Q fever	Not useful; show commensal flora	Not useful (long delay)	Negative	May be normal, or lymphocytosis	Interstitial infiltrates (pneumonitis)
Mycoplasma	Not useful	Positive on special media, but slow growth	Negative	Occasionally 10,000+	Pneumonitis or mild bronchopneumonia

[1]***Note:*** Many other organisms may cause lung infections; these are the more common ones.

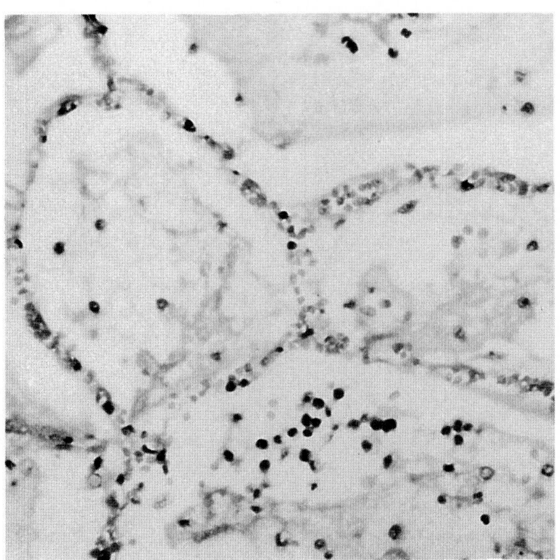

Figure 34-10. Lobar pneumonia. Early phase of acute congestion, showing marked hyperemia in alveolar septa with early exudation and neutrophil emigration into the alveoli.

tion of pneumococcal pneumonia. Its occurrence greatly increases the likelihood of death. Bacteremia may also lead to pneumococcal infections elsewhere in the body, most commonly meningitis and endocarditis.

D. Suppuration with abscess formation rarely occurs in pneumococcal pneumonia except with type 3 pneumococci, which produce a more severe infection than other types and a high incidence of suppuration, bacteremia, treatment failure, and death (see below). Suppuration is common in pneumonia caused by *Staphylococcus aureus* and gram-negative bacilli.

BRONCHOPNEUMONIA

As noted earlier, bronchopneumonias are usually secondary pneumonias occurring in patients with predisposing conditions. There are multiple small areas of peribronchiolar inflammation and consolidation involving all lobes of both lungs (Fig 34–9). Foci of bronchopneumonia may become confluent, causing consolidation of large areas of the lung. Liquefactive necrosis of the lung parenchyma may lead to frank abscess formation.

Etiology & Pathogenesis

Bronchopneumonia occurs in several clinical situations (Fig 34–7). It is a common finding at autopsy and contributes significantly to death in many patients, especially those with chronic diseases. Aspiration of pharyngeal secretions, either as a terminal event in a serious illness or due to abolition of the cough reflex in comatose states (termed aspiration pneumonia), plays an important role in pathogenesis. In most cases of bronchopneumonia, a mixed bacterial flora that includes many pharyngeal commensals is cultured from sputum. Pneumococci are present in 80% of cases. In seriously ill patients, gram-negative enteric bacilli are frequently the major causative

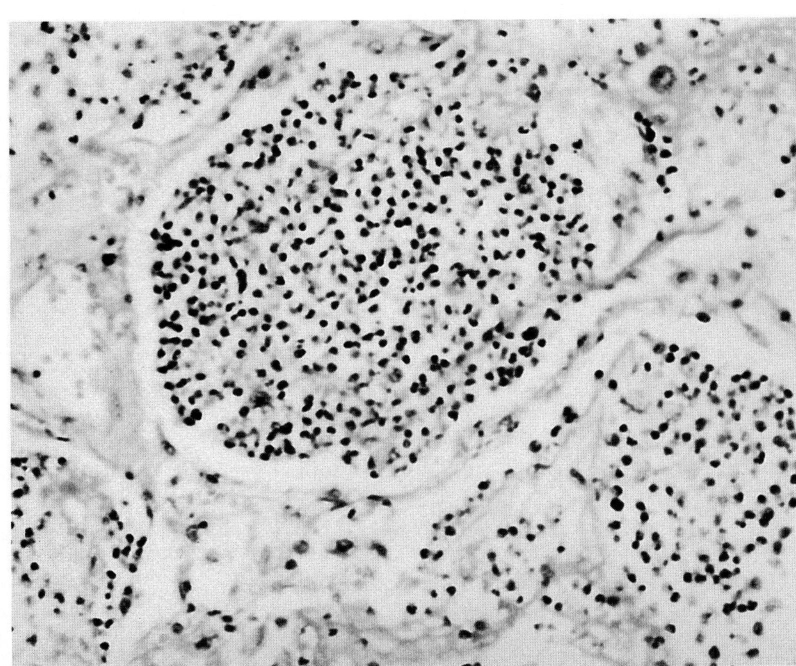

Figure 34-11. Lobar pneumonia—phase of hepatization. The alveoli are filled with exudate and large numbers of neutrophils.

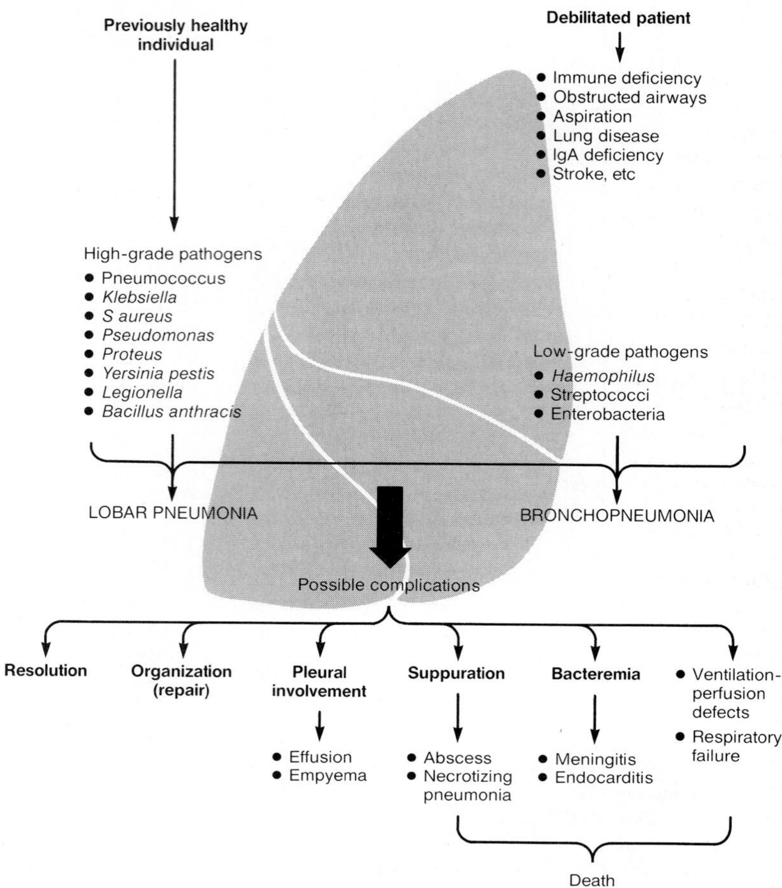

Figure 34–12. Common causes of bacterial pneumonia and possible complications.

organisms. Other organisms include *H influenzae* and streptococci other than *S pneumoniae.* In **aspiration pneumonia,** the inhaled pharyngeal secretions, gastric juice, and food debris may produce severe edema, foreign body-type reactions, and lipid pneumonia due to phagocytosis of fats and oils. When bronchopneumonia complicates a viral pneumonitis such as influenza or measles, S aureus is the most common pathogen. In immunosuppressed patients, organisms that generally do not cause disease may produce fatal pneumonia ("opportunistic infection"; see Chapter 14). Many of these hospital-acquired microorganisms show resistance to common antibiotics, complicating treatment.

Pneumocystis carinii **pneumonia** is an example of an opportunistic infection occurring in patients with AIDS, in malnourished children, and in patients undergoing chemotherapy for cancer. *P carinii* is a protozoan parasite that is commonly present in nature and has almost no virulence for humans with normal immune function.

The organism multiplies in the alveoli, which become filled with a pink, frothy mass (Fig 34–13A). Numerous crescent-shaped (2-μm) protozoa may be visualized by special stains (methenamine silver stain) (Fig 34–13B). The inflammatory response consists of plasma cells and lymphocytes in the alveolar septa. There is little exudation or neutrophil emigration into the alveoli. The mortality rate is over 50% despite the availability of effective antibiotics.

Bronchopneumonias caused by virulent organisms such as *S aureus,* type 3 pneumococci, and gram-negative organisms such as *K pneumoniae* are associated with severe acute inflammation with confluent consolidation, multiple abscesses, and bacteremia and have a high mortality rate.

Clinical Features

Bronchopneumonias have an extremely varied clinical presentation. Severe infections caused by virulent organisms present as an acute febrile illness with cough and dyspnea very similar to lobar pneumonia. Physical examination may show features of consolidation when large confluent areas are involved. In most cases of bronchopneumonia, however, chest auscultation reveals rales

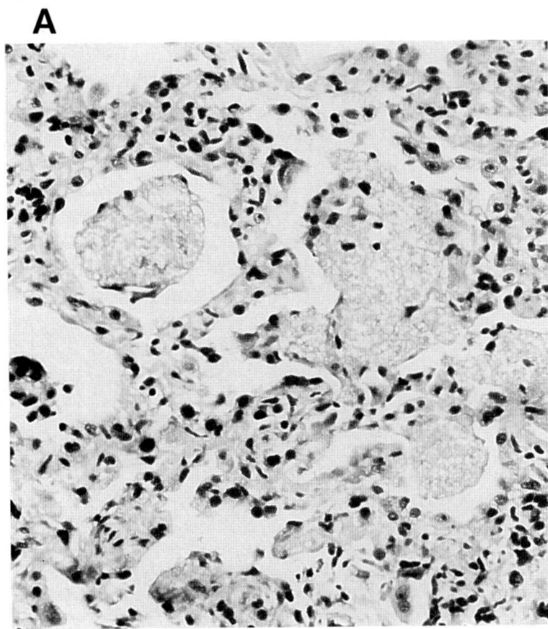

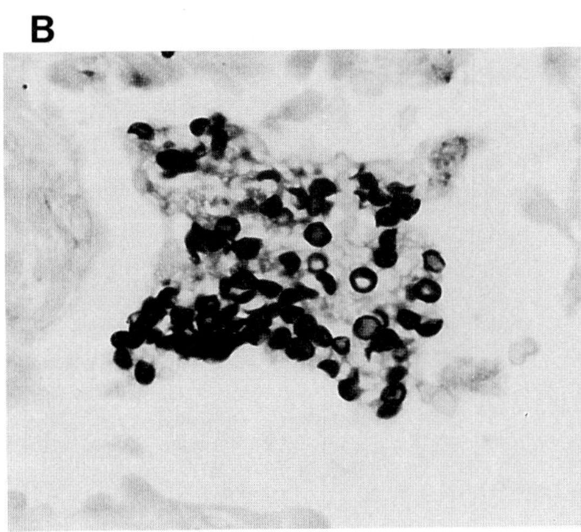

Figure 34–13. *Pneumocystis carinii* pneumonia. **A:** Routine hematoxylin and eosin stain showing frothy masses of organisms filling the alveoli associated with interstitial inflammation. **B:** Methenamine silver stain, showing the organisms in the frothy material in the alveolus.

without consolidation. X-rays show the patchy nature of the process. With less virulent organisms, bronchopneumonia may have a much less acute course, and clinical diagnosis can be difficult. In many patients in whom significant bronchopneumonia is present at autopsy, there is minimal pulmonary symptomatology during life. As in other lung infections, the specific etiologic diagnosis is made by identifying the organisms in sputum (Gram's stain and culture) or lung biopsy (*P carinii* pneumonia).

ACUTE NECROTIZING PNEUMONIAS

Acute necrotizing pneumonia is a severe acute pneumonia resulting from infection with highly virulent organisms. It is characterized clinically by a sudden onset and a severe course, often with rapid progression to death. Pathologically, there is extensive necrosis and intra-alveolar hemorrhage. The infections may cause death so rapidly that there is no time for an acute inflammatory response to develop.

Etiology

A. *Yersinia pestis* (Plague): Plague is a disease that wiped out entire populations in historical times up to the 19th century. The rat was the chief carrier of the organism. Today, Y pestis is still found in wild rodents, particularly squirrels, in many parts of the United States. Human infection due to contact with infected rodents now occurs rarely.

Bubonic plague is transmitted from rodents to humans by the bite of an infected flea (Fig 34–14). The site of the bite shows acute inflammation and ulceration. The organism spreads rapidly via lymphatics to the regional lymph nodes, which become markedly enlarged and necrotic. The enlarged lymph node mass is called a bubo, and this type of plague is called bubonic plague. From the lymph nodes, the plague bacilli enter the blood, causing a bacteremia that leads to infection of the lung and excretion of bacilli in sputum.

Pneumonic plague, a rapidly fatal necrotizing pneumonia, is the result of airborne spread of Y pestis from person to person.

B. *Bacillus anthracis* (Anthrax): Anthrax is most commonly a disease of the skin and is caused by inoculation of bacterial spores. In 5% of cases, anthrax spores are inhaled and lead to a severe necrotizing pneumonia with a high mortality rate.

C. Legionnaires' Disease: Legionnaires' disease is caused by *Legionella pneumophila,* a gram-negative bacillus. It may infect relatively healthy individuals in epidemic fashion (like the epidemic at the American Legion convention in Philadelphia in 1976 from which the disease was named) as well as sporadically. Legionnaires' disease has also become recognized as a common infection in immunocompromised hosts.

The bacillus of legionnaires' disease is widespread in nature. Infection has been traced to contamination of air conditioners, ventilation systems, and shower heads. Patient-to-patient transmission is less important than infection acquired from the environment.

Clinically, most patients develop a mild lobar pneumonia, with recovery within 2–3 weeks. In about 20% of cases, there is a severe necrotizing pneumonia with a high mortality rate. The infec-

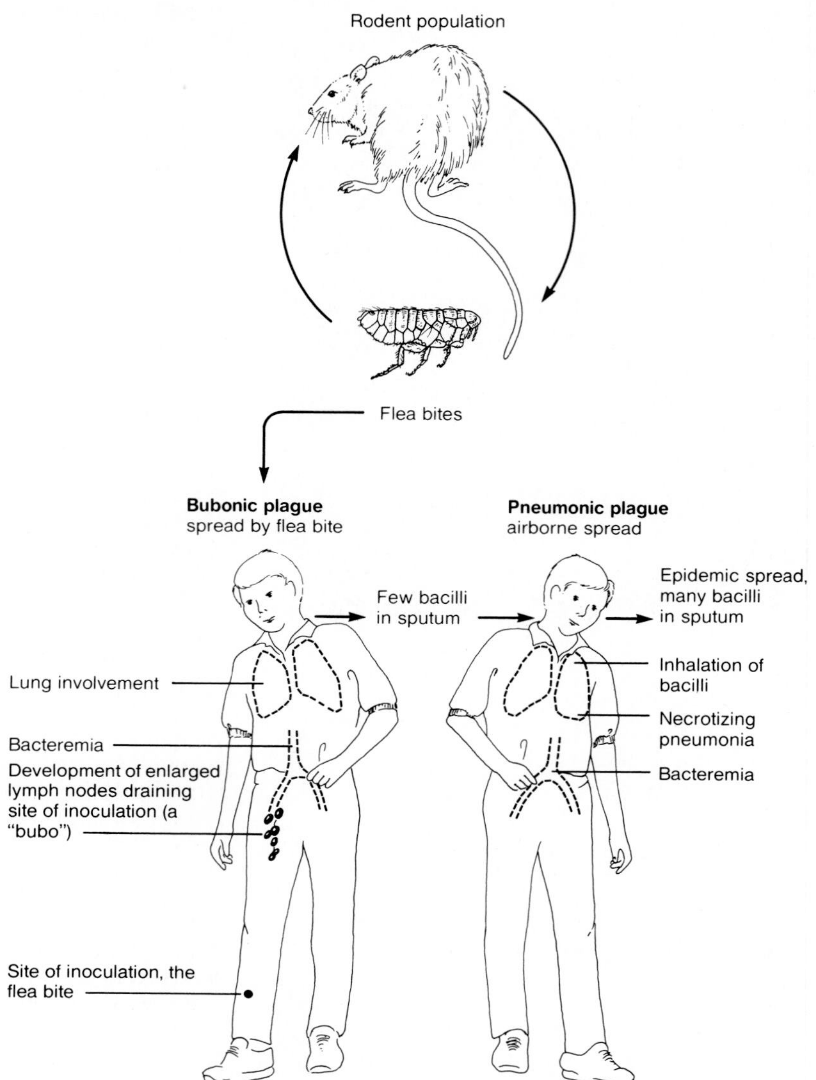

Figure 34–14. Epidemiology of plague.

tion tends to be necrotizing in immunocompromised patients.

The diagnosis can be made by demonstrating the organism in the alveolar exudate (sputum, bronchial washings, lung biopsy) using silver and acid-fast stains, electron microscopy, immunofluorescence techniques, or culture. Treatment with erythromycin is effective.

ACUTE INTERSTITIAL PNEUMONITIS

Acute interstitial pneumonitis is an acute inflammation characterized by infiltration of the alveolar septa by mononuclear cells (Fig 34–15). It may follow many different types of injury (see diffuse interstitial lung disease Chapter 35). Those conditions that are caused by infection will be considered here.

Etiology

Infectious agents producing an acute interstitial inflammation include obligate intracellular organisms such as the following: **(1) Viruses:** Influenza and parainfluenza virus, respiratory syncytial virus, adenoviruses, cytomegalovirus, herpesviruses, measles virus, echovirus, and coxsackieviruses. **(2) Chlamydiae:** *Chlamydia psittaci.* **(3) Rickettsiae:** *Coxiella burneti* (the agent of Q fever).

Mycoplasma pneumoniae is an exception in that it multiplies extracellularly. *Mycoplasma* is the commonest cause of acute interstitial pneumo-

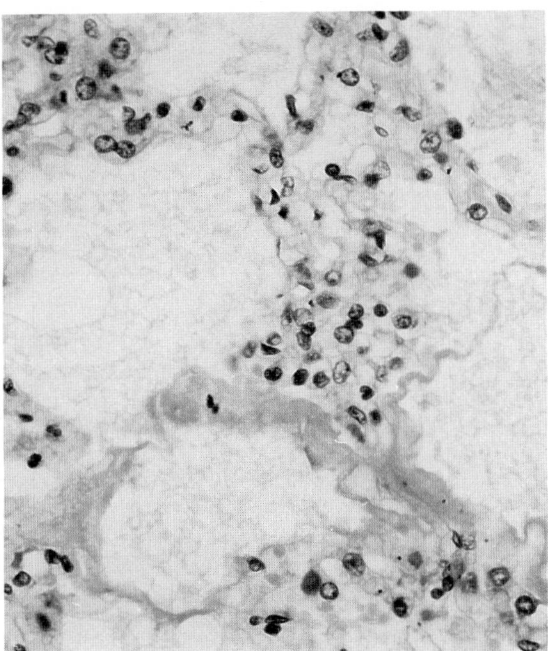

Figure 34-15. Acute interstitial pneumonitis in viral infection, showing expanded alveolar septa infiltrated with lymphocytes. Hyaline membranes and exudate are present in the alveoli, indicating severe pneumonitis.

nitis, followed by respiratory syncytial virus; in one-third of cases, no organism is identified.

Pathology

The pathologic features are those of interstitial pneumonitis with little alveolar involvement. The alveolar septa are expanded by hyperemia and a cellular infiltrate composed of plasma cells, lymphocytes, and macrophages (Figs 34-6 and 34-15). In many cases, the findings are nonspecific, and viral and chlamydial cultures are required for diagnosis.

In a few cases, there are additional cytopathic changes. **Necrosis of pneumocytes**—most commonly in influenza and adenovirus infections—causes denudation, intra-alveolar hemorrhage, and formation of a proteinaceous hyaline membrane on the surface. (This picture is sometimes called acute necrotizing viral pneumonia.) **Viral inclusion bodies** may be present with cytomegalovirus infection, herpes simplex infection, varicella, adenovirus infection, measles, influenza, and psittacosis. **Multinucleated giant cells** are found in measles and in respiratory syncytial virus infection.

Clinical Features

Acute interstitial pneumonitis is characterized by an acute onset of fever, cough, and dyspnea. The illness is usually mild (a clinical term is "walking pneumonia") and self-limited. Because of the absence of alveolar exudation and consolidation, there are few abnormal findings on physical examination. Scattered rales due to concomitant bronchiolitis are commonly the only findings.

Chest x-ray shows the pattern of interstitial inflammation, in contrast to the well-defined opacity of lobar pneumonia or the multiple patchy opacities of bronchopneumonia. Because of these differences, acute interstitial pneumonitis is sometimes called "primary atypical pneumonia."

INFLUENZA

Influenza is one of the most common causes of acute respiratory disease, including rhinitis, pharyngitis, laryngitis, tracheobronchitis, and pneumonitis, any of which may predominate.

Etiology & Epidemiology

Influenza virus is an RNA virus and a member of the myxovirus family related to measles, mumps, respiratory syncytial virus, and parainfluenza viruses (which are paramyxoviruses). Type A influenza virus is a major cause of epidemic disease, type B less so, and type C a rare cause. The virus has an outer envelope that shows frequent antigenic changes (antigenic drift), developing into new strains that are not affected by immune responses against strains of the virus previously encountered.

Influenza occurs endemically year-round with seasonal variation, peaking in the winter months. Epidemics occur not infrequently (3-4 years), and pandemics (worldwide epidemics) usually signify emergence of an antigenic strain that most of the population have not encountered previously. The newly emerged strain often represents reappearance of a strain that had been widespread 30-50 or more years previously. Thus, the 1947 epidemic was caused by strain A_1 (swine flu), the 1957 pandemic by A_2 (Asian flu), and the 1968 pandemic by A_3 (Hong Kong flu). The epidemic in the USA in 1976-1979 again resembled the A_1 strain (swine flu). Studies of antibody titers in the aged suggest that the 1918 pandemic was caused by A_1 and the pandemic of 1889 by A_2.

Pathology & Clinical Features

The incubation period is 2-3 days. The virus infects and multiplies in the respiratory epithelium; neuraminidase acts to thin the mucus and may promote spread. The effectiveness of the immune response is hampered by the tendency of the virus to infect the superficial cells in the respiratory epithelium. The inflammatory response is an interstitial pneumonitis characterized by active hyperemia, fluid exudation, and an infiltrate of lymphocytes and plasma cells. In severe cases, there is necrosis of alveolar epithelial cells, intra-alveolar hemorrhage and exudation, and formation of hyaline membranes.

The onset is abrupt, with fever, chills, malaise, headache, and muscle pains. Sputum is usually scanty but may be bloody. Purulent sputum is a sign of secondary bacterial infection.

Complications

Secondary bacterial infection is most important and is believed to have accounted for 10 million deaths worldwide in the 1918 epidemic; responsible organisms include *H influenzae,* staphylococci, pneumococci, and other streptococci. Less commonly, the influenza virus causes a severe necrotizing viral pneumonitis that progresses rapidly to respiratory failure and death. Other less common complications include myocarditis, encephalitis, polyneuritis, and Guillain-Barré syndrome. This last complication has occurred following use of some batches of influenza vaccine.

Reye's syndrome (acute encephalopathy with acute fatty degeneration of liver and kidney) complicates influenza, especially when high doses of salicylates are given to dehydrated children with infection.

Prevention

Vaccination may be successful against endemic influenza or in slowly developing epidemics when the antigenic characteristics of the strain are known. It is less effective in explosive pandemics that by definition represent an emergent new strain and require development of a new vaccine.

INFECTIONS CAUSING CHRONIC SUPPURATIVE INFLAMMATION

CHRONIC LUNG ABSCESS

Chronic lung abscess occurs commonly as a sequela of unresolved acute suppurative pneumonia. The area of suppuration becomes walled off by fibrosis, forming an abscess. Chronic lung abscesses occur in several clinical settings (Fig 34–16). Clinically, patients with chronic lung abscess present with low-grade fever, weight loss, and clubbing of fingers. The abscess commonly drains into a bronchus, leading to cough productive of a large volume of foul-smelling purulent sputum. Blood studies frequently show leukocytosis and increased serum immunoglobulin levels. The diagnosis is made by radiologic examination, which shows a cavitary lesion with an air-fluid level. Sputum culture usually grows multiple bacteria, commonly including anaerobes such as *Bacteroides* species.

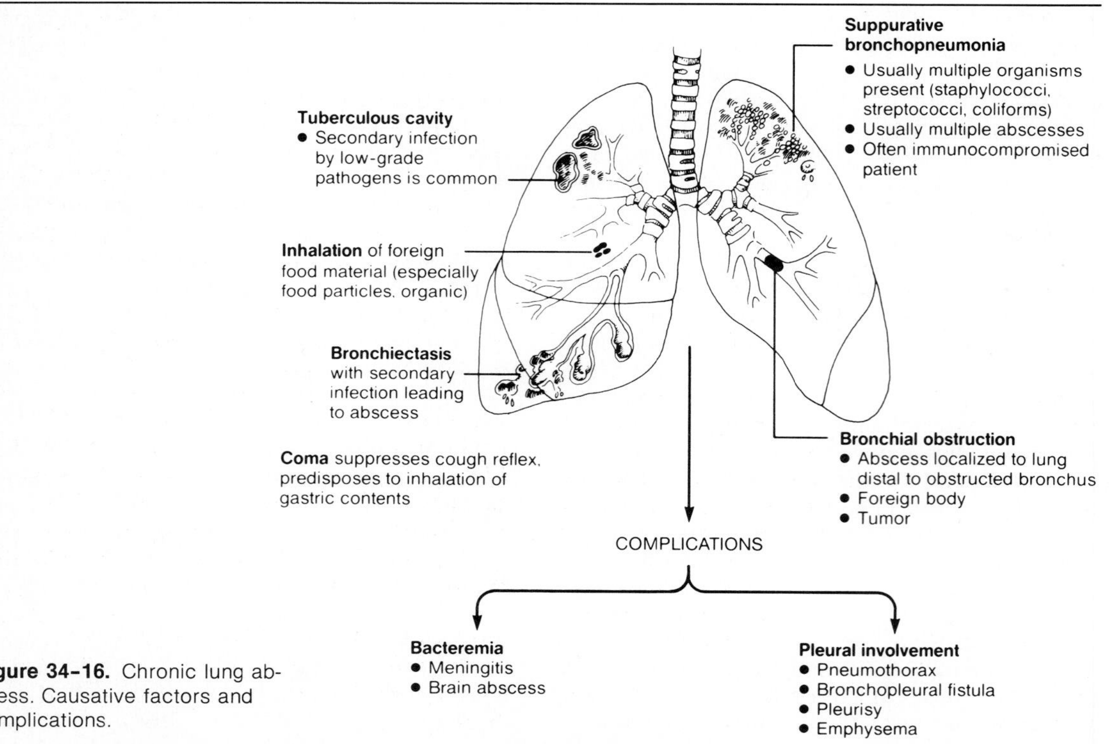

Figure 34–16. Chronic lung abscess. Causative factors and complications.

ACTINOMYCOSIS & NOCARDIOSIS

Actinomyces israelii and *Nocardia asteroides* are gram-positive filamentous bacteria that are rare causes of a chronic suppurative inflammation in the lung with extensive fibrosis. Multiple abscesses with colonies of organisms are present. The infection tends to spread by local extension and may produce chest wall abscesses that drain through the skin.

INFECTIONS CAUSING CHRONIC GRANULOMATOUS INFLAMMATION

Chronic granulomatous inflammation of the lung is caused by facultative intracellular organisms: (1) *Mycobacterium tuberculosis;* (2) atypical mycobacteria; and (3) fungi, commonly *Histoplasma capsulatum, Coccidioides immitis, Blastomyces dermatitidis, Paracoccidioides brasiliensis,* and *Cryptococcus neoformans.*

Pulmonary tuberculosis is the commonest of these infections and will be considered as the prototype. Many of the other infections have features in common with tuberculosis.

PULMONARY TUBERCULOSIS

Pulmonary tuberculosis is caused by *Mycobacterium tuberculosis.* The common human strain infects only humans and not animals. Patients with pulmonary tuberculosis who cough up bacilli in the sputum are the source of transmitted infections (Fig 34–17).

Tuberculosis has been fairly well controlled in most developed countries but still takes a heavy toll in underdeveloped countries or among malnourished people anywhere living in overcrowded conditions. In the United States, tuberculosis is emerging as a problem in crowded cities with a high concentration of immigrants, notably in Southern California, Texas, and Florida.

In the past, the bovine strain of *M tuberculosis* infected dairy herds, causing human infection via contaminated milk. Bovine tuberculosis has now been almost eradicated from dairy herds in most developed countries, and pasteurization of milk has further decreased the risk of human infection. Bovine tuberculosis typically involved the oropharynx or intestine, since the organism was ingested in milk and not inhaled. The primary focus would then be found in the gastrointestinal tract.

PRIMARY (CHILDHOOD) TUBERCULOSIS

Pathology

Primary pulmonary tuberculosis occurs when a child who has not been previously exposed to tubercle bacilli inhales the organism. The organism enters the alveoli and leads to the formation of the **primary (Ghon) complex** (Figs 34–17 and 34–18), which is composed of the Ghon focus and enlarged regional (hilar) lymph nodes. The Ghon focus is an epithelioid-cell granulomatous inflammation at the site of parenchymal infection. It is usually small and subpleural but may be large and located anywhere in the lung. Before immunity is established, tubercle bacilli survive in the macrophages that phagocytose them and are transported via lymphatics and the bloodstream throughout the body. This phase of relatively unhindered dissemination is called **preallergic lymphohematogenous dissemination.**

The development of an immune response against the tubercle bacillus results in (1) macrophage activation (by the lymphokine macrophage-activating factor), leading to destruction of tubercle bacilli; (2) inhibition of macrophage migration (by the lymphokine macrophage migration-inhibiting factor), which reduces further spread of bacilli in the body; and (3) delayed (type IV) hypersensitivity, which leads to caseous necrosis of granulomas in the Ghon focus and elsewhere in the body (Fig 34–18). Hypersensitivity is responsible for **tuberculin conversion**: The infected individual gives a positive reaction to intradermal injection of tuberculin (purified protein derivative of tubercle bacilli, or PPD).

Clinical Features

Primary pulmonary tuberculosis is usually asymptomatic or manifested as a mild flulike illness. In 95% of cases, immunity stops disease progression and healing occurs. The lesions heal by fibrosis and may calcify. There may or may not be radiologic evidence of healed primary infection.

Complications occur in 5% of cases of primary pulmonary tuberculosis. Locally progressive pulmonary disease, causing extensive caseous consolidation of the lung **(caseous pneumonia),** usually occurs only in malnourished or immunodeficient children. Erosion of a caseous granuloma into a bronchus may result in **tuberculous bronchopneumonia;** erosion into a blood vessel may cause severe bacteremia in which numerous small tuberculous granulomas are found all over the body **(miliary tuberculosis).**

Effects of Primary Tuberculosis

An individual who has recovered from primary tuberculosis shows the following evidence of infection:

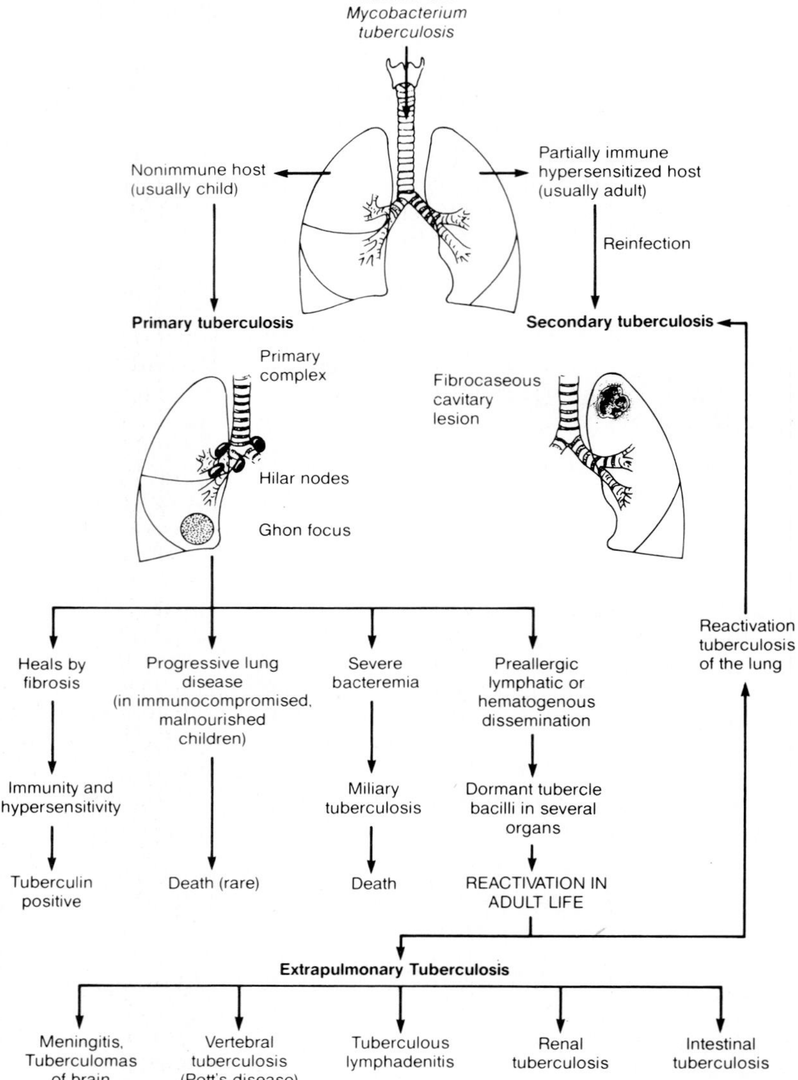

Figure 34-17. Pulmonary tuberculosis. Infection with *Mycobacterium tuberculosis* in the nonimmune host, usually in a child, causes primary tuberculosis. While most patients recover from this, many have subclinical lymphohematogenous dissemination of bacilli to many organs. These bacilli can remain dormant and become reactivated many years later, leading to secondary pulmonary and extrapulmonary tuberculosis. Secondary pulmonary tuberculosis may also result from reinfection in adult life. The pathologic features of reinfection and reactivation types of secondary pulmonary tuberculosis are identical. Note that extrapulmonary tuberculosis may occur in a patient without overt lung involvement.

(1) Tuberculin positivity. A positive skin test to tuberculoprotein may remain for a long period, often for several years.

(2) Partial immunity to tuberculosis. An individual who is tuberculin-positive requires a higher dose to be reinfected by tubercle bacilli.

(3) Presence of "dormant" tubercle bacilli—in the lungs, brain, meninges, bone, kidneys, lymph nodes, intestines, etc (Fig 34–17). Organisms are present in these tissues as a result of preallergic lymphohematogenous dissemination of bacilli. Not all of the bacilli in these foci are killed by the immune response, and some remain dormant for long periods within inactive caseous granulomas. Rarely, dormant granulomas are visible radiologically owing to the presence of calcification.

SECONDARY (ADULT) TUBERCULOSIS

Definition & Etiology

Secondary tuberculosis is occurrence of the disease in a patient who has had a prior primary infection. It usually occurs in an adult as a result either of reinfection or reactivation.

A. Reinfection: Because of partial immunity, the number of organisms that must be inhaled to reinfect such an individual is large; the source is usually a patient with active pulmonary tuberculosis discharging large numbers of organisms in sputum.

B. Reactivation: The mechanism that keeps dormant bacilli in check is uncertain, as are the rea-

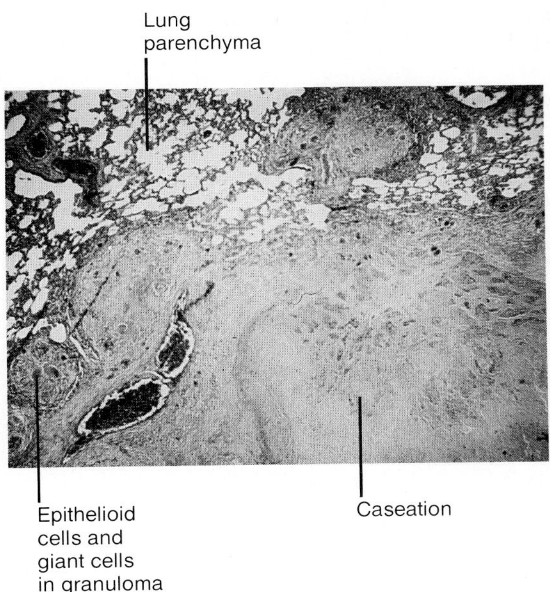

Figure 34–18. Pulmonary tuberculosis, showing multiple granulomas with a large area of caseous necrosis.

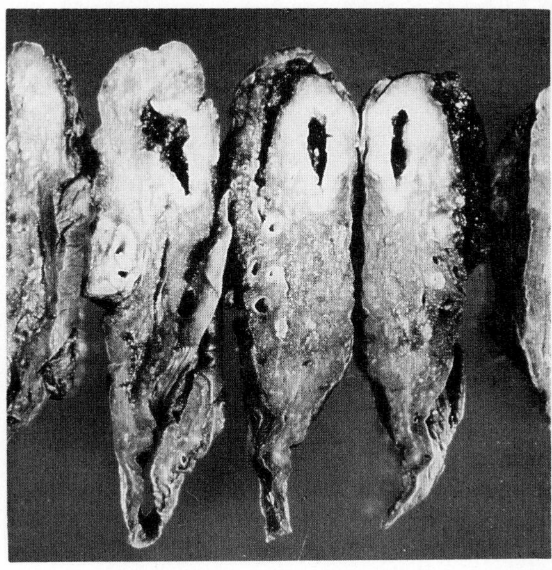

Figure 34–19. Secondary pulmonary tuberculosis, showing replacement of the lung apex by fibrosis, caseous necrosis, and cavitation. Three serial lung slices are shown.

sons why they become reactivated. Reactivation probably represents some breakdown of immunity and is believed to be a much more common pathogenetic mechanism for establishment of adult tuberculosis than reinfection. Reactivation of tuberculosis commonly occurs when an individual harboring tubercle bacilli (ie, a tuberculin-positive individual) is given immunosuppressive drugs such as corticosteroids. Such patients should be "covered" with antituberculous drugs.

Pathology

Multiplication of tubercle bacilli occurs in the presence of a rapidly developing secondary immune response, characterized by rapid lymphokine production by specifically activated T lymphocytes that limit dissemination of infected macrophages and localize the tubercle bacilli to the area of reactivation or reinfection. Enhanced delayed hypersensitivity produces a heightened local response with extensive caseous necrosis. The exact mechanism by which caseous necrosis is produced is unknown.

Secondary pulmonary tuberculosis may occur in any tissue (reactivation). The commonest site is the lung apex (Fig 34–19), due probably to the greater availability of oxygen in this better-ventilated zone of lung that favors multiplication of the aerobic tubercle bacilli.

The earliest lesions are small epithelioid cell granulomas characterized by caseous necrosis and fibrosis (see Chapter 5). These coalesce to form a large solid mass of fibrocaseous granulomatous inflammation called a tuberculoma. The caseous material is at first solid, but with continued multiplication of bacilli it undergoes liquefaction. The liquefied granuloma may open into a bronchus, leading to the following consequences: **(1) Infected sputum,** with coughing up of large numbers of tubercle bacilli. The patient is now highly infective. **(2) Cavitation** of the tuberculoma (Fig 34–19). The tuberculous cavity is lined by caseous granulomatous inflammatory tissue and associated with marked fibrosis ("cavitary fibrocaseous tuberculosis"). This is the typical lesion of secondary tuberculosis. **(3) Dissemination** via the bronchial tree, lymphatics, or bloodstream usually occurs late in the disease. With hematogenous spread, secondary granulomas may develop in any location in the body. Dissemination occurs early in the course of disease only in debilitated or immunologically incompetent patients.

Clinical Features

Secondary tuberculosis in the adult is almost always symptomatic. The commonest symptom is chronic cough, frequently with hemoptysis (due to erosion of a blood vessel in the wall of the cavity). Marked weight loss, low-grade fever, and night sweats are common.

Physical examination and chest x-ray show the changes of apical fibrosis and cavitation. The normal lung is replaced by an opacity caused by fibrosis and granulomatous inflammation. The occurrence of central cavitation is typical. Bronchopneumonia due to spread of bacilli in the bronchial tree may occur in elderly, debilitated, and immunodeficient patients.

Diagnosis

The diagnosis of tuberculosis must always be confirmed by microbiologic techniques.

A. Demonstration of Tubercle Bacilli in Smears of Sputum or in Tissue Sections: The ability of stained tubercle bacilli to withstand decolorization by acid (acid-fast reaction) is used for microscopic demonstration of the bacillus (Ziehl-Neelsen stain and auramine-rhodamine fluorescent technique). Only a few bacilli are usually seen, and failure to observe bacilli does not exclude a diagnosis of tuberculosis.

B. Culture of *M tuberculosis* From Sputum or Tissue: Culture of the slowly growing organism takes 4–6 weeks; the laboratory should be informed if atypical organisms (see below) are expected, since different culture conditions are necessary.

C. Tuberculin Test: Patients with tuberculosis usually give a strongly positive reaction to intradermal injection of tuberculin. Care is needed in the interpretation of a tuberculin test. A significant number of patients with active tuberculosis demonstrate immunologic anergy and give a false-negative tuberculin test. On the other hand, a positive tuberculin test may mean only past infection in a patient whose symptoms are caused by another disease.

Treatment & Prognosis

Many antituberculous drugs are available, the most effective of which are isoniazid (INH) and rifampin. The tubercle bacillus rapidly develops resistance to antimicrobial drugs; many strains are resistant to at least one drug, and most develop resistance rapidly if exposed to a single agent. It is therefore customary to start treatment of a new case with 3 drugs, one of which is isoniazid. When antimicrobial sensitivity test results become available after culture, the drugs are modified accordingly. Treatment must be continued for 12–18 months.

Asymptomatic patients who have recently become tuberculin-positive have a high likelihood of harboring dormant live tubercle bacilli and are advised to undergo chemoprophylaxis with an 18-month course of isoniazid.

Although the prognosis of tuberculosis has improved with the availability of effective drugs, tuberculosis continues to be a major cause of disease and death in endemic areas.

ATYPICAL MYCOBACTERIAL INFECTION

Atypical mycobacteria are commonly found in the soil but are less pathogenic for humans than *M tuberculosis* and cause disease less often. *Mycobacterium kansasii* may rarely infect normal individuals. *Mycobacterium avium-intracellulare* infection occurs in immunodeficient states and is one of the opportunistic infections commonly seen in patients with AIDS.

Pulmonary disease caused by atypical mycobacteria in the normal population is very similar to pulmonary tuberculosis and is distinguished only by culture. However, recognition is important because of differences in sensitivity to antituberculous drugs.

M avium-intracellulare infection occurring in the immunodeficient host takes the form that would be expected in the absence of effective cellular immunity. Organisms multiply freely within macrophages and disseminate widely in the body, probably due to the absence of lymphokines that activate and inhibit migration of macrophages. Caseous necrosis does not occur, and the granulomas are poorly formed, consisting of foamy macrophages that contain large numbers of mycobacteria.

FUNGAL GRANULOMAS OF THE LUNG

Fungi that are facultative intracellular organisms with the capability to survive and multiply in macrophages produce caseous granulomatous inflammation and pathologic lesions in the lung very similar to what is seen in tuberculosis. One major difference is that the source of infection is not an infected patient. Infection occurs after exposure to soil containing spores of fungi.

Etiology & Epidemiology

Histoplasmosis, caused by *Histoplasma capsulatum,* is common in the midwestern United States, with a very high incidence in the Mississippi Valley. **Coccidioidomycosis,** caused by *Coccidioides immitis,* is common in the Southwestern United States (San Joaquin Valley fever). **Blastomycosis** *(Blastomyces dermatitidis),* **paracoccidioidomycosis** *(Paracoccidioides brasiliensis),* and **sporotrichosis** *(Sporothrix schenckii)* are uncommon causes of pulmonary infection in the United States. *Cryptococcosis* is common and will be discussed separately below because it has some unique features.

HISTOPLASMOSIS, COCCIDIOIDOMYCOSIS, BLASTOMYCOSIS, PARACOCCIDIOIDOMYCOSIS, & SPOROTRICHOSIS

Pathology

The pathologic lesions are chronic granulomas with extensive caseation and fibrosis.

Clinical Features

Manifestations parallel those of tuberculosis.

A. Primary Infection: Primary infection is characterized by a parenchymal granulomatous focus and regional lymph node enlargement. The disease is usually asymptomatic, and recovery is the rule. About 90% of the population in the Mississippi Valley and 80% of people in the San Joaquin Valley in California have positive skin tests for histoplasmin and coccidioidin, respectively, indicating asymptomatic primary infection. Unlike tuberculosis, the level of immunity after a primary infection with these fungi is relatively low, so that reinfection is relatively common.

B. Progressive Primary Infection: Widespread dissemination of fungus in the body, similar to miliary tuberculosis, is common in malnourished or immunodeficient individuals.

C. Dormant Infection: Dormancy of fungi in inactive granulomas is common, and reactivation is responsible for many cases of pulmonary and all cases of secondary extrapulmonary fungal granulomas.

D. Secondary Infection: Secondary infection is very similar to that seen in tuberculosis, with large caseous granulomas that cause marked fibrosis and chronic cavitary lung disease.

Diagnosis

Precise diagnosis depends on identifying the

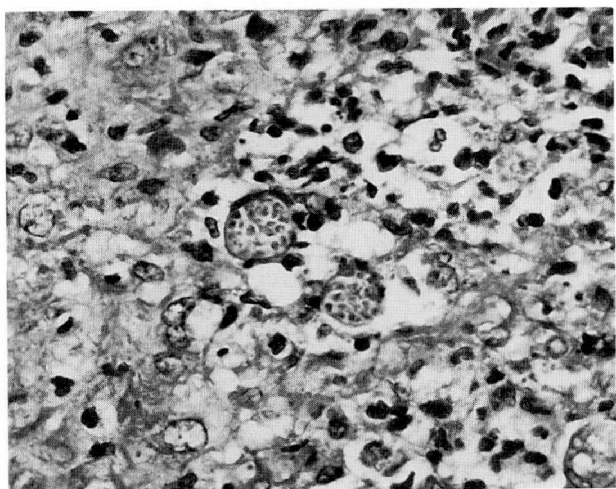

Figure 34–20. *Coccidioides immitis* spherules in a pulmonary granuloma.

2–4 μm group

Histoplasma capsulatum

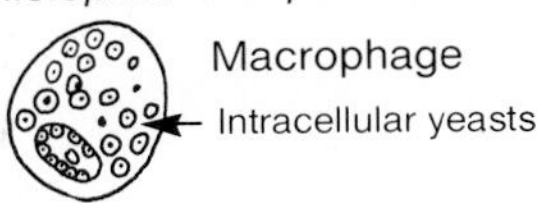

Sporothrix schenckii

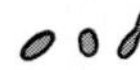

10–30 μm group

Cryptococcus neoformans

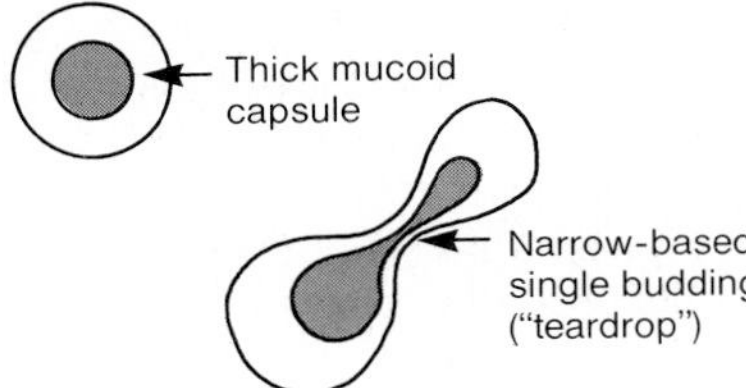

Blastomyces dermatitidis

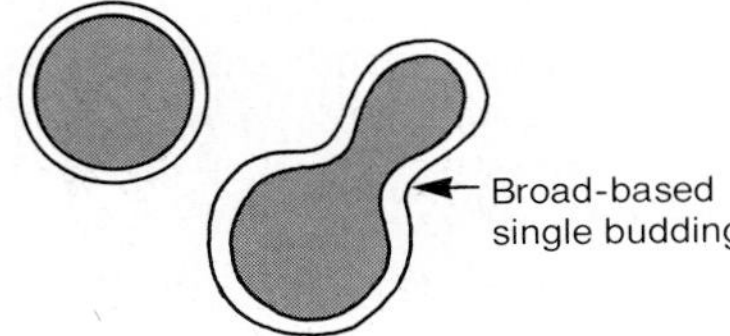

Paracoccidioides brasiliensis

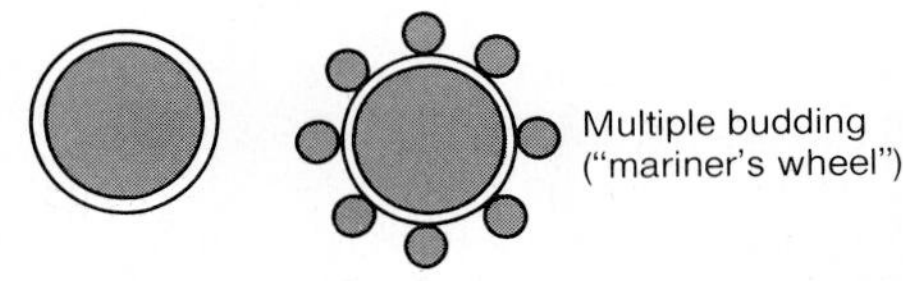

Over 30 μm

Coccidioides immitis

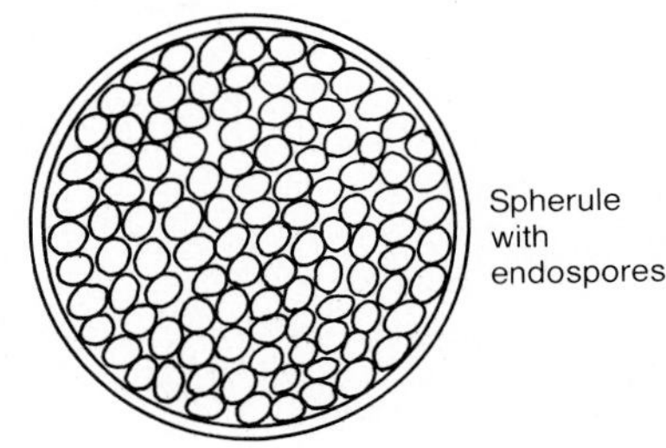

Figure 34–21. Morphologic features in tissue sections of the fungi that commonly cause granulomas.

fungus in sputum or in tissue by microscopy (Figs 34–20 and 34–21) or culture.

PULMONARY CRYPTOCOCCOSIS

Cryptococcus neoformans is a facultative intracellular yeast that may cause pulmonary disease both in healthy individuals (uncommon) and in immunodeficient patients (common). In individuals with a normal immune system, a chronic granulomatous inflammation occurs with formation of an inflammatory mass characterized by caseous necrosis and fibrosis. Differentiation from tuberculosis and other fungal granulomas depends on demonstrating cryptococci microscopically or by culture.

In the immunodeficient host, the yeast multiplies in the alveoli with little or no inflammatory reaction and spreads widely in the lung, producing an area of consolidation. Histologic examination of the consolidated lung shows alveoli filled with the yeasts. *Cryptococcus* is identified by its variability in size (10–25 μm), thick mucoid capsule, and narrow-based single budding.

Disseminated cryptococcal infection with meningeal involvement is common in the immunodeficient host. Cryptococcal antigens can be identified in the serum of patients with disseminated disease—the basis of a very useful diagnostic test.

PARASITIC INFECTIONS OF THE LUNG

DIROFILARIA IMMITIS INFECTION

Dirofilaria immitis is a filarial worm whose normal site of infection is the heart and pulmonary arteries of dogs (''dog heartworm''). Accidental infection of humans occasionally occurs, mainly in southeastern United States.

In human infections, the worm infects the pulmonary arteries; when the worm dies, it evokes an inflammatory reaction that causes fibrous occlusion of the vessel and pulmonary infarction. This causes chest pain and hemoptysis. A circumscribed opacity (''coin'' lesion) is seen on chest x-ray. The diagnosis is made by finding the worm in the pulmonary lesion.

TROPICAL PULMONARY EOSINOPHILIA

Hypersensitivity reactions to microfilariae in the lung are common in countries where filariasis *(Wuchereria bancrofti)* is prevalent. Clinically, this condition is characterized by fever, wheezing, weight loss, peripheral blood eosinophilia, hyperglobulinemia, and diffuse infiltrates seen on chest x-ray. Microfilariae are present in the blood. In the lungs, small lesions composed of microfilariae surrounded by eosinophils may be seen. The infection responds to treatment with antifilarial drugs.

OTHER PARASITIC LUNG INFECTIONS

Many other parasitic infections involve the lung, all rarely: hydatid cysts, cysticercosis, lung fluke *(Paragonimus westermani)* infection, and amebic *(Entamoeba histolytica)* lung abscess, usually secondary to transdiaphragmatic extension of an amebic liver abscess. Larval migration of Ascaris lumbricoides (roundworm) and Strongyloides stercoralis may also produce symptoms similar to those of pulmonary eosinophilia.

The Lung: II. Toxic, Immunologic, & Vascular Diseases

35

ACUTE DISEASES OF THE AIRWAYS

INFECTIONS OF THE AIR PASSAGES

ACUTE TRACHEOBRONCHITIS

Acute tracheobronchitis commonly complicates a severe upper respiratory tract infection, particularly *Haemophilus influenzae* infection of the larynx in young children and influenza in adults and children (see Chapter 32). Viral tracheobronchitis may also be complicated by secondary bacterial infection, most commonly with *Staphylococcus aureus.*

ACUTE BRONCHIOLITIS

Acute bronchiolitis is a common, often epidemic, infection of the small airways that occurs mainly in children under the age of 2 years. Most cases are mild, but 1–2% require hospitalization, and about 1% of these children die. Most cases are caused by respiratory syncytial virus; more rarely, parainfluenza virus and adenoviruses are responsible. The bronchioles show acute epithelial damage and lymphocytic infiltration of the walls. Their lumens are filled with mucus plugs, which cause distal alveolar air trapping. In patients who recover, the bronchiolar epithelium regenerates within 2 weeks. Patients present with acute-onset tachypnea and wheezing; fever is low-grade and may be absent. Cases caused by adenoviruses tend to have greater degrees of necrosis and a higher mortality rate.

WHOOPING COUGH (Pertussis)

Caused by *Bordetella* (formerly *Haemophilus*) *pertussis,* whooping cough is an extremely serious acute respiratory tract infection of the young.

Prior to immunization (the "P" of DPT), it accounted for 40% of all deaths in the first 6 months of life. Clinically, it is an acute tracheobronchitis, characterized by paroxysmal coughing and an inspiratory whoop (most often seen in older children). Otitis media, bronchitis, and bronchiectasis are serious complications. Tetracycline is effective in therapy.

BRONCHIAL ASTHMA

Bronchial asthma is characterized by acute narrowing of bronchioles due to smooth muscle contraction **(bronchospasm)**. Bronchospasm causes obstruction to air flow—maximal in expiration—and a high-pitched wheeze. Expiration is prolonged because of airflow obstruction. Attacks of asthma are usually of short duration and reverse completely. Rarely, they may be severe and prolonged (**"status asthmaticus"**), and may lead to acute ventilatory failure and even death.

Etiology & Classification

A. Extrinsic Allergic Asthma: Extrinsic allergic asthma is a reagin-mediated **type I hypersensitivity** (atopic) reaction. It is common in childhood and has a familial tendency. Many different antigens may be involved (Table 35–1). Serum IgE is increased, and skin tests against the offending antigens are positive.

Inhaled antigens combine with specific IgE on the surface of mast cells in the respiratory mucosa, releasing histamine (Fig 35–1). Secondary mediators such as leukotrienes and prostaglandins are produced in the area of reaction, prolonging the bronchoconstriction initiated by histamine.

B. Intrinsic (Nonallergic) Asthma: It has been suggested that patients with intrinsic asthma have **hyperreactive airways** that constrict in response to a variety of nonspecific stimuli, due in part to abnormal β-adrenergic responses. Aspirin, cold, exercise, and respiratory infections are common precipitants of attacks. Serum IgE levels are normal, and skin tests are negative. Intrinsic asthma occurs in older patients.

Table 35–1. Factors involved in asthma.

Allergens
Household dust
Contains waste products of house mite *Dermatophagoides pteronyssimus*
Other organic dusts
Includes allergic *Aspergillosis* in which the response is to antigens on fungi actually growing in the bronchi
Pollens
Especially grasses and trees; types vary in different geographic regions. This form of asthma usually is seasonal and often coexists with "hay fever" (allergic rhinitis)
Animal dander, fur
Cats, dogs, horses, birds; allergy is usually to fur and feathers; usually only one species (eg, cats, not dogs)
Food products
Ingested antigens may produce asthma after absorption and distribution in the bloodstream
Drugs
Ingested, act as haptens
Precipitating factors
Heat, cold, aerosols, chemicals, gases, cigarette smoke
Exercise
Infection
Emotional stress
Drugs, especially aspirin, may precipitate nonallergic asthma
In nonallergic asthma, bronchi are abnormally sensitive because of decreased beta-adrenergic responses

Pathology

Histologic changes are nonspecific (Fig 35–2). Inspissation of mucus leads to bronchiolar obstruction and focal collapse of alveoli. Obstruction that is less than complete permits entry of air but not its exit (because obstruction is maximal in expiration), leading to air trapping and distention of alveoli distal to the obstruction. Both FEV_1 and vital capacity are reduced during an attack.

The type I hypersensitivity reaction causes mild inflammation and edema in the bronchiolar wall. Numerous eosinophils are present owing to release of eosinophil chemotactic factor by mast cells, and there is peripheral blood eosinophilia. Sputum is scanty, thick, and viscous, forming casts of bronchioles (Curschmann's spirals); eosinophils are present along with Charcot-Leyden crystals (formed from degraded eosinophils). Infection may complicate prolonged attacks.

Clinical Features

Bronchial asthma is characterized by episodic attacks of dyspnea and wheezing. In severe attacks, there is frequently secondary bacterial infection. Allergic asthma occurs in childhood and tends to disappear as the child grows. Intrinsic asthma occurs in older individuals and tends to produce a more chronic disease.

Treatment & Prevention

Treatment of the acute attack is with bronchodilator drugs such as theophylline, epinephrine, and especially β_2-adrenergic agents like metaproterenol, which has minimal β_1 cardiovascular side effects. Corticosteroids are effective in severe cases. These drugs may be given as aerosol sprays.

Further treatment consists of control of secondary infection when it complicates a severe attack and identification of allergens followed by their avoidance. Skin testing to identify allergens may be followed by desensitization (hyposensitization), which involves serial injection of increasing

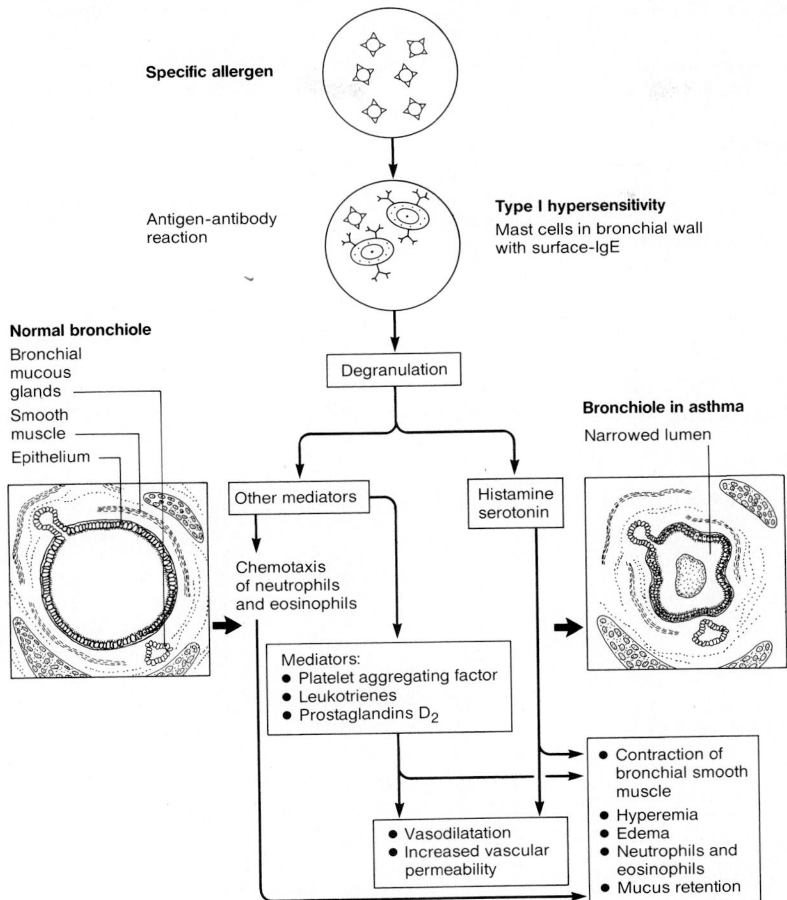

Figure 35–1. Pathogenesis of extrinsic allergic asthma.

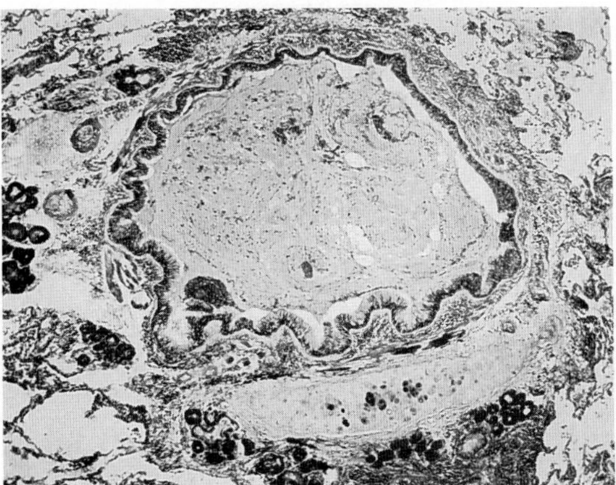

Figure 35–2. Bronchial asthma, showing a small bronchus filled with a plug of viscid mucus and inflammatory cells.

doses of the responsible antigen; IgG blocking antibodies probably form, and the severity of disease is reduced in about 20% of patients. Desensitization carries a risk of anaphylaxis, which may be fatal.

Disodium cromoglycate appears to stabilize mast cell membranes, reducing degranulation. It is used prophylactically.

ALLERGIC BRONCHOPULMONARY ASPERGILLOSIS

Allergic bronchopulmonary aspergillosis is a specific form of allergic asthma caused by inhalation of spores of *Aspergillus* species. The fungus grows in the bronchioles and evokes a hypersensitivity reaction (Table 35–2) that appears to be a combined type I (elevated serum IgE) and type III reaction (elevated serum levels of precipitating antibodies and an Arthus-type reaction in the lungs).

Clinically, the asthmatic attacks tend to be

Table 35-2. Immunologic hypersensitivity in lung disease.

Hypersensitivity Reaction	Clinicopathologic Effect
Type I IgE-mediated	Bronchial asthma Allergic bronchopulmonary aspergillosis
Type II Antibody against basement membrane	Goodpasture's syndrome Idiopathic pulmonary hemosiderosis
Type III Immune complex	Hypersensitivity pneumonitis Connective tissue diseases Allergic bronchopulmonary aspergillosis
Type IV Cell-mediated hypersensitivity	Tuberculous and fungal granulomas Some type of interstitial pneumonitis
Uncertain	Idiopathic interstitial pneumonitis Wegener's granulomatosis

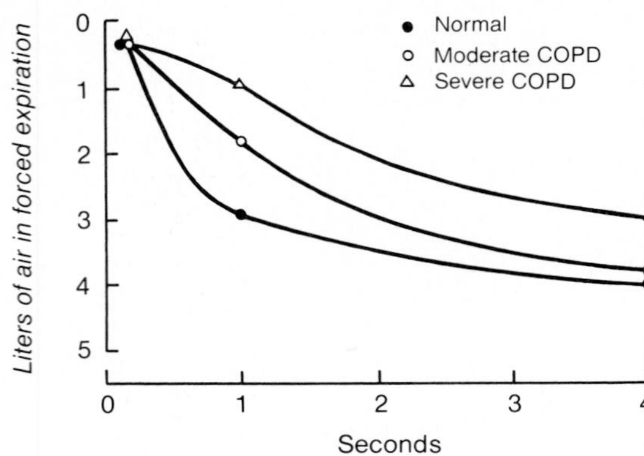

Figure 35-3. Mechanics of forced expiration in a normal person and in patients with chronic obstructive pulmonary disease. The FEV_1 is the volume of expired air at 1 second and the FVC is the terminal volume expired (at 4 seconds). As the severity of airway obstruction increases, there is a reduction in both FVC and FEV_1. The FEV_1/FVC ratio is 80% in a normal subject, 47% in moderate COPD, and 31% in severe COPD in the example shown.

more persistent, with infiltrates appearing on chest x-ray. Pulmonary fibrosis may occur.

CHRONIC OBSTRUCTIVE PULMONARY DISEASE (COPD)

COPD is characterized by features of chronic obstruction to air flow in the lungs. It is diagnosed by abnormalities in tests of ventilatory function. The FEV_1: FVC ratio (see Chapter 34) is the most widely used test. Normally, the FEV_1:FVC ratio is over 75%. In COPD, the ratio is decreased (Fig 35-3), the degree of reduction correlating well with disease severity and survival.

Incidence

COPD is a common disease second only to ischemic heart disease as a cause of chronic disability in older individuals. The incidence is increasing.

Pathology

COPD, as defined by the ventilatory abnormality, is associated with 2 distinctive pathologic conditions: chronic obstructive bronchitis and emphysema. These 2 conditions contribute in variable degree to COPD in individual patients.

A. Chronic Obstructive Bronchitis: Chronic bronchitis is defined clinically as the persistent presence of increased bronchial mucus secretion which leads to chronic cough productive of mucoid sputum. Pathologic examination shows hypertrophy of bronchial wall mucous glands associated with chronic inflammation and fibrous replacement of the muscular walls of small bronchioles (Fig 35-4). The Reid index—the ratio of mucous gland thickness to bronchial wall thickness—is increased above the normal value of 0.5.

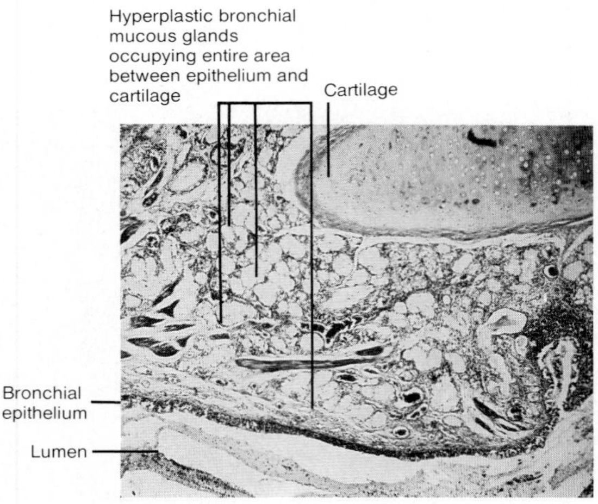

Figure 35-4. Chronic bronchitis, showing marked hyperplasia of the bronchial mucous glands. In this case, the glands occupy almost the entire area between the surface epithelium and cartilage, giving a Reid index of almost 1.

Fibrotic bronchioles tend to collapse in expiration under the influence of the positive intrathoracic pressure, resulting in ventilatory obstruction in expiration.

B. Emphysema in COPD: Emphysema is defined in pathologic terms as permanent dilatation of the air spaces distal to the terminal bronchiole, usually with destruction of lung parenchyma. To produce clinical COPD, large areas of the lung must be involved by emphysema. Two principal types of emphysema are recognized (Fig 35–5): **(1) centrilobular emphysema,** in which dilatation and destruction primarily involve the central part of the acinus formed by the respiratory bronchioles; and **(2) panacinar emphysema,** in which dilatation and destruction involve the entire acinus, including the alveoli and alveolar ducts as well as the respiratory bronchioles (Fig 35–5).

Accurate recognition of the gross and microscopic features of emphysema at autopsy requires fixation of the lungs in a state of inflation. This technique permits the gross demonstration of dilated air spaces and microscopic documentation of alveolar destruction (Fig 35–6). The detailed changes of emphysema are difficult to identify in routine autopsies, where the lung is not fixed while inflated.

C. Other Forms of Emphysema: Several other types of emphysema are recognized but are not usually associated with COPD (Table 35–3). These conditions fit the pathologic definition of emphysema—dilatation and destruction of the small airways and alveoli—but usually do not involve a large enough area of lung parenchyma to produce clinical effects.

Pathogenesis of Chronic Bronchitis (Table 35–3)

Chronic bronchitis is 5–10 times more common in heavy **cigarette smokers** than in nonsmokers, even after correction for other factors such as age, sex, place of residence, and occupation. Cigarette smoking acts as a local irritant, causing hypertrophy of bronchial mucous glands, increase in the number of mucous cells, hypersecretion of mucus, and increased numbers of neutrophils. Other inhaled irritants such as sulfur dioxide and oxides of nitrogen produce similar changes but are not present at high enough concentration in most environments to play a significant role.

The hypersecretion of mucus increases the susceptibility to bacterial infection. In cigarette smokers, this predisposition is further aggravated by interference with ciliary action that results from smoking. *Haemophilus influenzae,* pneumococci, and *Streptococcus viridans* are common pathogens. These organisms cause both a chronic low-

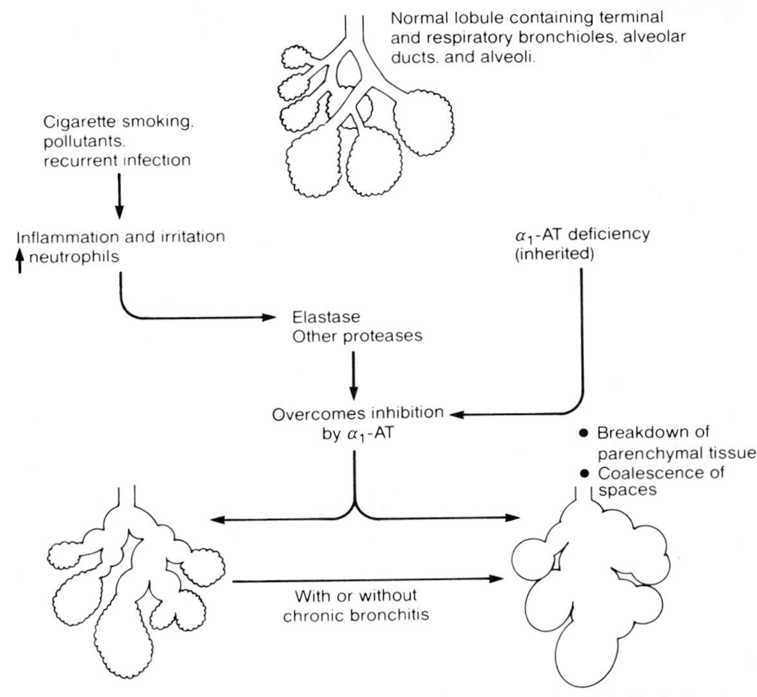

Figure 35–5. Pathogenesis and types of emphysema associated with chronic obstructive pulmonary disease. $\alpha_1 - AT = \alpha_1$-antitrypsin.

A

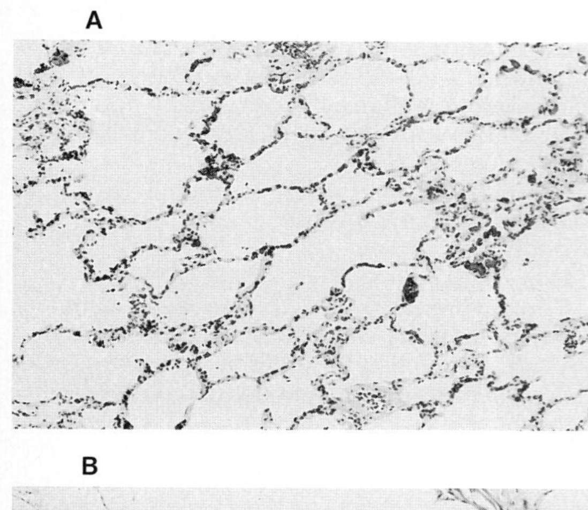

B

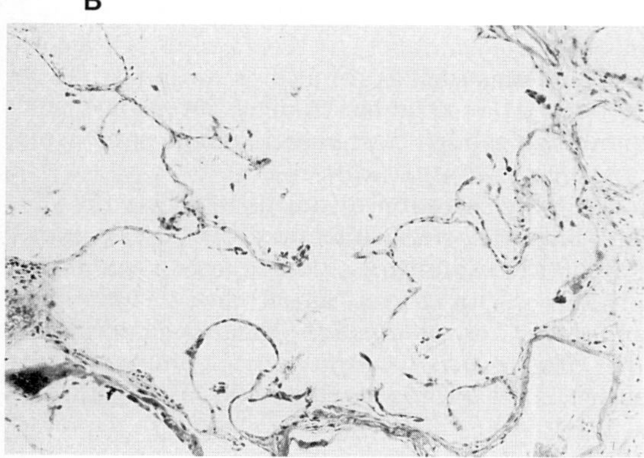

C

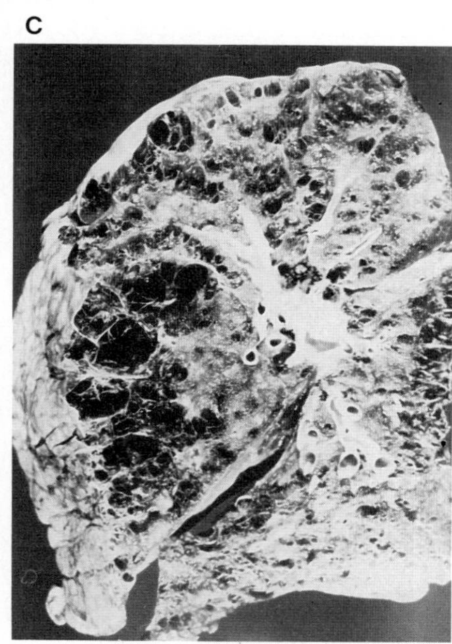

Figure 35-6. Normal lung **(A)** compared with emphysema **(B)** at equivalent magnification, showing destruction of lung parenchyma and marked dilatation of terminal air spaces in emphysema, both microscopically **(B)** and grossly **(C)**.

grade inflammation of the bronchiolar wall and acute exacerbations with suppuration manifested clinically as fever and expectoration of purulent sputum. Inflammation leads to progressive destruction of the muscle of the bronchiolar wall, with replacement by collagen.

In heavy smokers, the initial changes of chronic bronchitis are present from an early age, but COPD usually does not become clinically apparent until the fourth or fifth decade of life.

Pathogenesis of Emphysema (Table 35-3; Fig 35-5)

The destruction of lung parenchyma in emphysema is believed to be due the action of **proteolytic enzymes** (proteases, mainly elastase). One important source of these proteases is leukocytes associated with pulmonary inflammation. Normally, antiproteolytic substances such as antitrypsins in the plasma inactivate these proteolytic enzymes as they are released and thereby protect tissues from damage. However, lung destruction—and emphysema—occur in patients who either produce an excess of proteolytic enzymes (chronic neutrophil infiltration) or have too little antiproteolytic activity in the plasma (α_1-antitrypsin deficiency; see below). Hypersecretion of mucus in chronic bronchitis and emphysema favors inflammation and local leukocyte enzyme release.

Cigarette smoking is an important etiologic factor in emphysema. Chronic irritation resulting from smoking results in increased numbers of neutrophils, and cigarette smoke directly promotes elastase release from neutrophils. The chronic bacterial infection associated with chronic bronchitis in smokers also contributes to the increased levels of leukocyte-derived proteolytic enzymes. The lungs of heavy smokers show inflammation and destruction of the respiratory bronchioles, with centrilobular emphysema beginning at a relatively young age.

Alpha$_1$-antitrypsin deficiency predisposes to emphysema because α_1-antitrypsin is responsible for the major part of plasma antiproteolytic activity. The α_1-antitrypsin level in serum is determined by inheritance at a single (Pi, or protease inhibitor) locus. A normal individual has two M genes at this locus (PiMM). The **Z gene** is the commonest of several abnormal genes that may be inherited. PiZZ homozygotes have severe deficiency of α_1-antitrypsin and almost invariably develop panacinar emphysema by age 40 years.

PiZZ occurs with a frequency of 1:4000 and thus is a very rare cause of emphysema; it cannot account for most of the cases of COPD in the population. The heterozygous PiMZ state occurs in about 5% of the population in the United States and Europe and is potentially a factor in the genesis of the common type of COPD. The PiMZ state is associated with a moderate reduction in serum α_1-antitrypsin. While PiMZ has

Table 35-3. Chronic bronchitis and emphysema.

	Causal Factors	Clinical Effects
Destructive lung disease Chronic bronchitis, centrilobular emphysema, panacinar emphysema	Cigarettes Recurrent infection ?Pollutants Alpha$_1$-antitrypsin deficiency	Chronic obstructive pulmonary disease (COPD)
Senile emphysema	Aging	Asymptomatic
Paraseptal emphysema (paracicatricial)	Associated with any cause of collapse or fibrosis (scars [paracicatricial])	Rarely sufficient to produce symptoms
Bullous emphysema	Unknown	Asymtomatic, but rupture leads to pneumothorax
Nondestructive disease Compensatory emphysema (dilatation without destruction)	Removal or collapse of part of lung; remaining lung expands	Asymptomatic
Focal dust emphysema (dilatation without destruction)	Various dust diseases, pneumoconioses, eg, coal miners's lung	Usually insufficient to produce symptoms
Dilatation distal to obstruction; no destruction	Acute bronchial asthma: air trapping	Symptoms of asthma

been associated with emphysema in some families, general population studies have not confirmed a causal association between emphysema and the PiMZ genotype.

Clinical Features (Fig 35–7)

Patients with COPD are asymptomatic in the early stages of the disease because of pulmonary reserve; however, the FEV$_1$:FVC ratio is decreased, as is vital capacity and maximal ventilatory volume. The total lung capacity and residual volume are often increased as a result of air trapping in the distended air spaces.

In the later symptomatic phase, COPD patients present with a spectrum of symptoms, the 2 extremes of which are sometimes designated types A and B. In most cases, features of both type A and type B are present.

Type A patients present with chronic cough—either dry or productive of mucoid sputum—progressive dyspnea, and wheezing. They hyperventilate, and often sit hunched forward (to bring accessory respiratory muscles into action) with

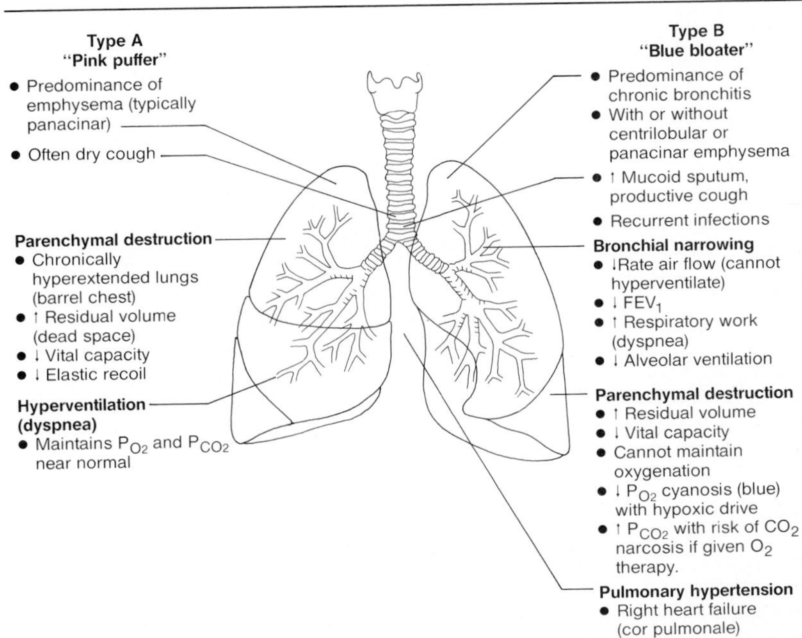

Figure 35–7. Clinical effects and types of chronic pulmonary obstructive disease.

mouth open and nostrils dilated in an attempt to overcome the ventilatory difficulty. Their lungs are overinflated, with increased anteroposterior diameter of the chest ("barrel chest") and flattened diaphragm on chest x-ray. These patients successfully maintain oxygenation of the blood by hyperventilation. Patients with type A COPD are sometimes called "pink puffers."

Type B COPD patients have marked chronic obstructive bronchitis and cannot hyperventilate. There is decreased oxygenation of blood (cyanosis) and increased arterial carbon dioxide content. They also have pulmonary hypertension caused by changes in the microvasculature of the lung parenchyma. This leads to right ventricular hypertrophy and failure **("cor pulmonale")**, and peripheral edema due to right heart failure is a dominant clinical feature. Type B patients are sometimes called "blue bloaters."

The correlation between these clinical types and pathologic changes is inexact. Type A patients frequently have dominant emphysematous changes, while type B patients usually have dominant chronic obstructive bronchitis. Most patients, however, have varying mixtures of both pathologic changes and clinical features.

Changes in blood gases in patients with COPD are variable. In the early stages, blood gases are normal at rest, but hypoxemia develops during exercise due to the decreased pulmonary reserve. Blood gas changes result from decreased alveolar ventilation and imbalanced ventilation and perfusion, the latter being the dominant effect in many cases.

In type B patients with chronic hypercapnia (elevated P_{CO_2}), the respiratory center becomes insensitive to the P_{CO_2} stimulus and is driven by the hypoxemia. Administration of oxygen in these patients can remove the respiratory center drive and cause carbon dioxide retention and death ("carbon dioxide narcosis").

BRONCHIECTASIS

Bronchiectasis is abnormal and irreversible dilatation of the bronchial tree proximal to the terminal bronchioles—in contrast to emphysema, which involves the bronchial tree distal to the terminal bronchioles.

Etiology

Bronchiectasis is the result of chronic infection with resulting parenchymal destruction, fibrosis, and abnormal permanent dilatation of damaged bronchi. Several causes act singly or in concert.

A. Long-standing bronchial obstruction, as occurs in bronchial tumors and stenosis. Stagnation of mucus is followed by bronchopneumonia distal to the obstruction, progressing to localized fibrosis and bronchiectasis.

B. Mucoviscidosis (Fibrocystic Disease of the Pancreas): (See Chapter 45.) In this condition, mucus is abnormally thick and viscous; it plugs the smaller bronchi, causing obstruction and predisposing to recurrent infection.

C. Bronchopneumonia, particularly following childhood infections such as measles and whooping cough, which in the past were common antecedents of bronchiectasis. Bronchiectasis occurs today in immunodeficient children who are susceptible to recurrent pulmonary infections.

D. Kartagener's Syndrome: Kartagener's syndrome is due to a congenital defect in ciliary motion caused by absence of the dynein arms of cilia. The lack of ciliary action interferes with clearance of mucus and bacteria in the bronchi, predisposing to bronchopneumonia and therefore bronchiectasis. Chronic infection of the paranasal sinuses also results in absence of the frontal sinuses in this condition. In the male, absence of dynein arms in the microtubules of the sperm tail leads to loss of sperm motility and infertility. Dextrocardia (location of the heart on the right side) completes the syndrome.

Kartagener's syndrome is inherited as an autosomal recessive gene and has an incidence of 1:20,000.

E. Intralobar Sequestration of the Lung (Congenital): In this condition, also rare, a part of the lung receives either no pulmonary arterial supply or no communication with the bronchial tree. The sequestered lobe maintains nutrition via its bronchial arterial supply. The bronchi within the area, however, have no drainage and therefore undergo infection and dilatation.

Pathology (Figs 35–8 and 35–9)

Bronchiectasis usually has a patchy distribution, depending on the extent of bronchial obstruction. The dilated bronchi and bronchioles may be cylindric, fusiform, or saccular and are made more conspicuous by extensive destruction and fibrosis of the intervening lung parenchyma. An important diagnostic feature is the finding of large bronchi near the pleura.

The walls of the distended bronchi show inflammation and fibrosis. The mucosa may be ulcerated, and the lumen is commonly filled with pus.

Clinical Features (Fig 35–8)

Bronchiectasis is a chronic illness with cough, usually productive of a large volume of foul-smelling sputum, and episodic fever. The chronic

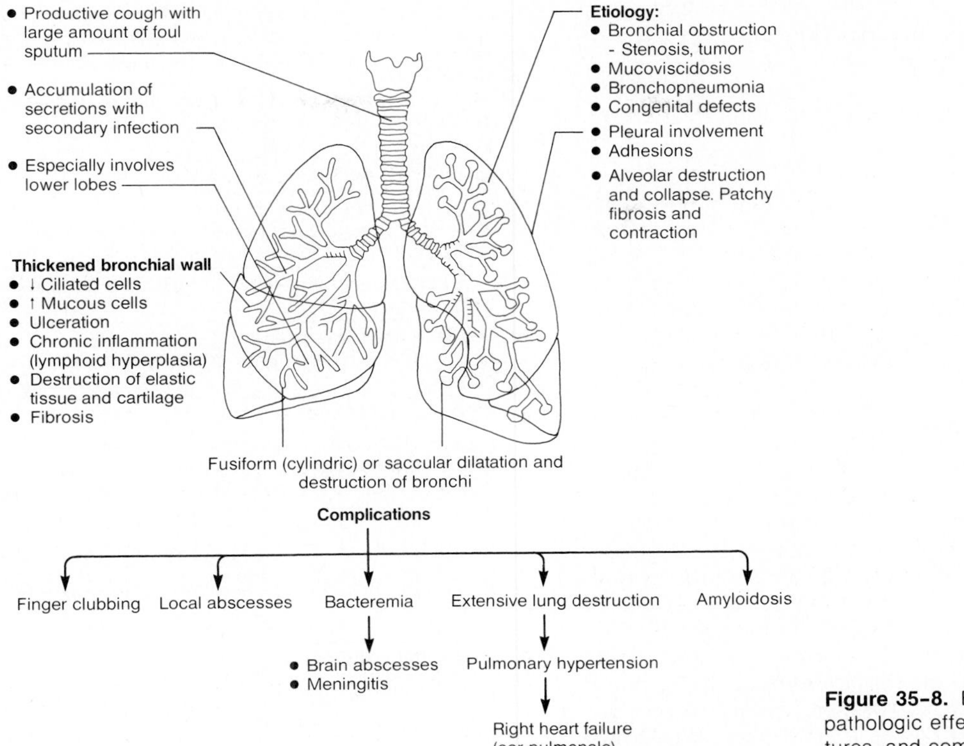

Figure 35-8. Bronchiectasis—pathologic effects, clinical features, and complications.

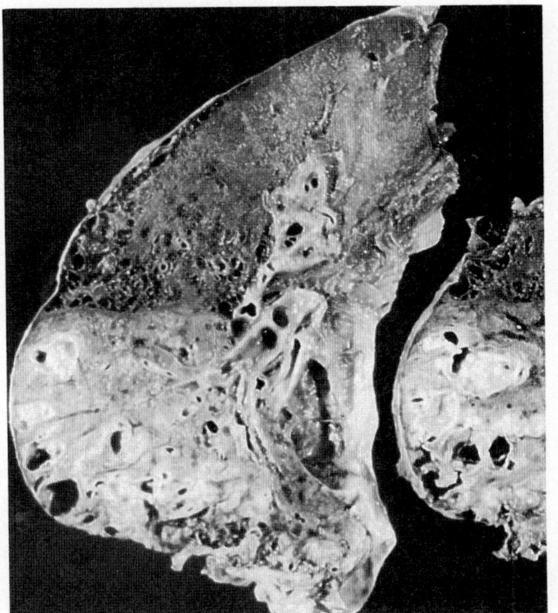

Figure 35-9. Bronchiectasis, showing fibrosis and dilatation of bronchi in the lower lobe. Note the dilated bronchi immediately beneath the pleura, a feature of diagnostic value.

infection commonly causes clubbing of fingers and hyperglobulinemia and may cause secondary amyloidosis.

Common bacteria cultured from bronchiectatic cavities include *Staphylococcus aureus, Staphylococcus epidermidis;* streptococci of all types, including pneumococci; *Haemophilus influenzae;* enteric gram-negative bacilli; and anaerobes. Several of these organisms can usually be grown at any one time.

Treatment

The treatment of bronchiectasis consists of control of infection with antibiotics and removal of predisposing causes such as bronchial obstruction by surgery, when possible. Surgical removal of bronchiectatic areas is important because the permanently dilated bronchi represent foci of almost continuous infection.

CHRONIC DIFFUSE INTERSTITIAL LUNG DISEASE

Chronic diffuse interstitial lung diseases are noninfectious disorders characterized by diffuse inflammation and fibrosis involving the interstitium of the alveolar septum (Fig 35–10). The end stage is associated with extensive parenchymal destruction, fibrosis, and often the formation of abnormal cystic spaces (honeycomb lung).

General Clinical & Pathologic Features

Patients with diffuse interstitial lung disease present with dyspnea, tachypnea, and cyanosis. Pulmonary function abnormalities are of the restrictive type, with reduced vital capacity but no airway obstruction. The FEV_1:FVC ratio is normal. Thickening of the alveolar membrane affects diffusion of oxygen, leading to hypoxemia. This stimulates the respiratory center, resulting in increased ventilation. Carbon dioxide, being much more diffusible than oxygen, is washed out, resulting in lowered P_{CO_2} levels. Chest x-ray shows a characteristic reticulonodular pattern of interstitial involvement.

Etiology

Diffuse infiltrative lung disease has many causes (Table 35–4). While all produce the general picture described above, some have individual features that permit specific diagnosis.

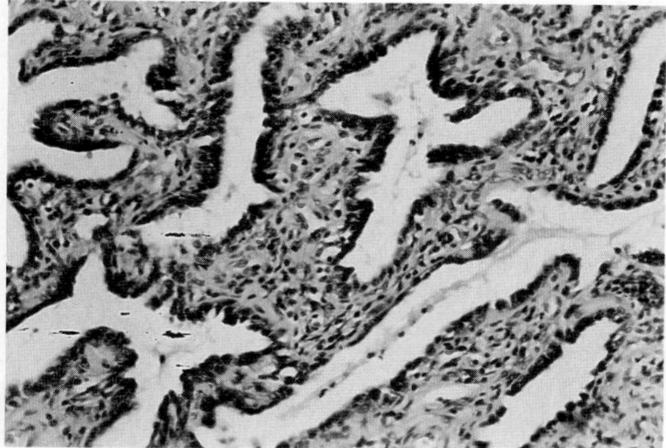

Figure 35–10. Chronic diffuse interstitial fibrosis of the lung, showing chronic inflammation and fibrosis of the interstitium and abnormal air spaces lined by cuboidal cells ("honeycomb lung").

Table 35–4. Causes of chronic diffuse interstitial lung disease.

Cause
Immunologic injury
"Idiopathic": Usual interstitial pneumonitis, desquamative interstitial pneumonitis, lymphocytic interstitial pneumonitis
Hypersensitivity pneumonitis
Connective tissue diseases (systemic lupus erythematosus, progressive systemic sclerosis, rheumatoid arthritis)
Goodpasture's syndrome and idiopathic pulmonary hemosiderosis
Physical and chemical agents
Inhaled mineral dusts (pneumoconioses): Silica, asbestos
Inhaled gases: Oxygen toxicity
Ingested toxins and drugs: Paraquat (a herbicide); cancer chemotherapeutic agents such as bleomycin, methotrexate, busulfan, and cyclophosphamide; nitrofurantoin (a urinary antiseptic)
Radiation
Intravenous drug (heroin) abuse
Uncertain etiology
Sarcoidosis
Eosinophilic granuloma
Wegener's granulomatosis
Lymphomatoid granulomatosis
Vascular
Chronic left heart failure: Passive venous congestion
Multiple small pulmonary emboli
Prior infections
Following recurrent pneumonitis
Following recurrent bronchopneumonia

IMMUNOLOGIC INTERSTITIAL PNEUMONITIS & FIBROSIS

IDIOPATHIC INTERSTITIAL PNEUMONITIS (Fibrosing Alveolitis, Hamman-Rich Syndrome)

Idiopathic interstitial pneumonitis is actually a group of diseases characterized by diffuse interstitial fibrosis occurring without recognized cause. About half of cases of chronic diffuse interstitial lung disease fall into this category. Though the cause is unknown, the presence of circulating immune complexes, immunoglobulin deposition in the interstitium in many patients, and the response of early disease to treatment with steroids strongly suggest an immunologic basis.

Clinically, patients present with progressive dyspnea and cough, and ventilatory failure of the restrictive type. A defect in oxygen diffusion across the abnormal alveolar membrane may also contribute. The rate of progression is quite variable; a rapidly progressive variant that may cause death in 1–2 years is sometimes called Hamman-Rich syndrome.

Idiopathic interstitial pneumonitis is classified according to the histologic appearance of the lung, as discussed below.

Usual Interstitial Pneumonitis (UIP)

This accounts for the majority of cases. In the acute phase, there is interstitial infiltration with lymphocytes, plasma cells, and macrophages; pulmonary edema; acute alveolar damage; and proteinaceous hyaline membranes. The damaged alveoli are lined by type II pneumocytes, which can appear so atypical cytologically as to mimic the appearance of an adenocarcinoma. In the acute phase, the disease may respond to treatment with immunosuppressive agents such as corticosteroids. The acute phase is followed by proliferation of fibroblasts and laying down of collagen in the alveolar interstitium (Fig 35–10). The rate of fibrosis is variable, but the occurrence of fibrosis represents irreversibility.

The course is characteristically protracted, with respiratory failure occurring many years after onset. When interstitial fibrosis (honeycomb lung) is present, the clinical response to steroids is poor.

Desquamative Interstitial Pneumonitis (DIP)

The desquamative form is similar to the foregoing except for the aggregation of desquamated cells in alveoli—a variable mixture of macrophages and type II pneumocytes. Controversy exists about whether this is a variant of usual interstitial pneumonitis or a completely different disease. The course is similar to that of slowly progressive usual interstitial pneumonitis.

Lymphocytic Interstitial Pneumonitis (LIP) (Pseudolymphoma)

Lymphocytic interstitial pneumonitis is characterized by extensive infiltration of the interstitium with lymphocytes and plasma cells. It may be diffuse or may involve a single area of lung, producing a mass lesion ("pseudolymphoma"). The disorder is associated with an increased incidence of primary pulmonary malignant lymphoma; in some cases, the process appears to be a primary low-grade lymphoma.

HYPERSENSITIVITY PNEUMONITIS (Extrinsic Allergic Alveolitis)

Hypersensitivity pneumonitis results from inhalation by susceptible individuals of small organic particles (antigens), most commonly spores of thermophilic fungi. These fungi grow best at 50–60 °C in decaying vegetation such as hay and sugar cane or in heated water in air-conditioning and heating systems.

Individuals working in a variety of occupations are at risk, and the disease frequently bears the name of these occupations (see Chapter 8). Thermophilic actinomycete spores occur in moldy hay (farmer's lung), moldy sugar cane residue (bagassosis), and compost for mushroom growing (mushroom worker's disease). In urban areas, the spores are most frequently found in contaminated forced air heating and air-conditioning systems. Antigenic products are also found in bird droppings (bird-fancier's lung), dead wood (maple bark stripper's disease), and barley malt used in brewing (malt worker's lung).

Pathogenesis

Hypersensitivity pneumonitis is caused by a combination of **type III hypersensitivity** associated with precipitating IgG antibodies, which are present in the serum of 70% of patients, producing a local Arthus type immune complex reaction with complement deposition in the lung; and **T lymphocyte-mediated type IV hypersensitivity,** leading to the formation of small, noncaseating epithelioid cell granulomas in the alveolar septa.

Pathology

Hypersensitivity pneumonitis is characterized by an acute interstitial pneumonitis. The alveolar septa are expanded by neutrophils, lymphocytes, and plasma cells. Poorly formed alveolar granulomas with giant cells are typically present. Fibrous obliteration of bronchioles (bronchiolitis obliterans) is a common change.

If the disease is recognized early and the patient removed from the source of antigen, the disease is reversible. With continued exposure, diffuse interstitial fibrosis occurs, leading to end-stage honeycomb lung. As fibrosis becomes more advanced, the disease becomes irreversible.

Clinical Features

Patients present with acute dyspnea, fever, and cough 4–6 hours after exposure to the antigen. Initially, these symptoms subside spontaneously in 12–18 hours. As pulmonary fibrosis ensues, the disease goes into its chronic phase, with all the features of diffuse interstitial lung disease.

INTERSTITIAL PNEUMONITIS IN CONNECTIVE TISSUE DISEASES

Diffuse interstitial pneumonitis with fibrosis leading to honeycomb lung indistinguishable from usual interstitial pneumonitis occurs in progressive systemic sclerosis (scleroderma) and rheumatoid arthritis. Systemic lupus erythematosus may also be complicated by immune complex deposition in the alveoli, transient patchy lung infiltrates, vasculitis, and acute alveolar damage.

GOODPASTURE'S SYNDROME

Goodpasture's syndrome is a rare disease characterized by a combination of hemoptysis and pulmonary infiltrates, glomerulonephritis, and the presence of anti-basement membrane antibodies in the circulation. There is a striking male predominance.

Pathology

The circulating anti-basement membrane antibody, which is thought to be an autoantibody, fixes onto the basement membrane of pulmonary alveoli and renal glomeruli, causing a complement-mediated **type II hypersensitivity** reaction (Table 35–2). Immunofluorescence shows linear deposition of IgG and complement in the alveoli, a finding that is diagnostic of Goodpasture's syndrome. In the lung, hemorrhage into the alveoli is the dominant feature; hemosiderin-containing macrophages may be found in the sputum.

Grossly in the acute phase, the lungs are consolidated, heavy, and hemorrhagic. In the chronic phase, the lung is firm because of marked interstitial fibrosis, brown because of hemosiderin, and may show changes of honeycomb lung.

Clinical Features

Onset is most frequently in the second or third decade of life. Patients present with recurrent hemoptysis. Massive pulmonary hemorrhage occurs rarely.

In the chronic phase, there is progressive dyspnea, cough, and right heart failure due to pulmonary fibrosis. Iron deficiency anemia may result from chronic blood loss. Chest x-ray shows pulmonary infiltrates due to intra-alveolar hemorrhage. Changes of increasing pulmonary fibrosis dominate chronic disease.

Patients almost invariably have evidence of glomerulonephritis, most frequently microscopic hematuria. In many cases of Goodpasture's syndrome, the renal disease dominates the clinical picture and generally determines the prognosis, which is poor. Renal changes are described in Chapter 48. Treatment by plasmapheresis (to remove the antibody) and steroids has proved effective in a minority of cases.

IDIOPATHIC PULMONARY HEMOSIDEROSIS

Idiopathic pulmonary hemosiderosis is morphologically identical to Goodpasture's syndrome and considered by some to be a variant of Goodpasture's without renal involvement. It differs from Goodpasture's syndrome in that it tends to affect a younger age group; there is no male preponderance; and anti-basement membrane antibodies cannot be demonstrated in the blood, though they are present on the alveolar membranes.

PNEUMOCONIOSES (Inorganic Dust Diseases)

The term pneumoconiosis literally means "dust in the lungs" and denotes pulmonary disease secondary to inhalation of various inorganic dusts (Table 35–5). Changes that occur in the lung vary with the type and amount of dust inhaled and the presence of other lung diseases, most importantly those associated with cigarette smoking. Genetic factors play an uncertain role in susceptibility. Some dusts such as coal dust do not evoke a fibrous response **(noncollagenous pneumoconioses)**, whereas others such as silica do **(collagenous pneumoconioses)**. In some patents, inhalation of several different kinds of dust results in mixed disease (eg, anthracosilicosis).

There is a variable latent period between exposure to dust and onset of clinical disease that may be as long as 20–30 years. Rarely, acute disease develops within weeks after a massive exposure.

COAL WORKER'S PNEUMOCONIOSIS (Anthracosis)

Anthracosis results from exposure to coal (carbon) dust and is seen in its most extensive form in coal miners and workers in old coal-burning railways. Lesser degrees of anthracosis occur in almost all urban dwellers.

The basic pathologic lesion is the coal dust macule, which is a collection of carbon-laden macrophages around the respiratory bronchiole (Fig 35–11). This dust accumulation induces only a very small amount of delicate fibrosis. There may also be insignificant dilatation of the respiratory bronchiole (focal dust emphysema). There are usually no symptoms and no detectable abnormalities in lung function.

Rarely, coal workers develop **progressive massive fibrosis** when heavy exposure is coupled with a complicating factor such as infection with *Mycobacterium tuberculosis* (found in 40% of patients with massive fibrosis), significant silica contamination (silica induces fibrosis), or development of allergic responses to various proteins that have passively adsorbed onto the coal dust. Progressive massive fibrosis is characterized by the presence of multiple irregular, firm, homogeneous black fibrous masses in both lungs.

Table 35-5. Different types of pneumoconioses in humans.

Disease	Inorganic Dust	Occupations
Anthracosis	Coal dust[1]	Coal mining, railroad work
Silicosis	Crystalline silica	Mining, sandblasting, stone masonry, foundry work; glass, tile, brick, and pottery manufacture
Silicate pneumoconiosis Abestosis	Asbestos	Asbestos mining and milling, shipyard workers, welders, pipe fitters, boilermakers, insulators, brake lining manufacturers, "tearing-out" of old asbestos insulation
Talcosis	Talc	Often found with asbestos
Kaolin pneumoconiosis	Kaolin or porcelain clay	Ceramics manufacture
Fuller's earth pneumoconiosis	Fuller's earth	Oil refining, foundry work
Diatomaceous earth pneumoconiosis	Diatomaceous earth	Water filtration
Mica pneumoconiosis	Mica	Rare
Graphite pneumoconiosis	Graphite[1]	Graphite mining
Berylliosis	Beryllium	Fluorescent lights
Aluminum pneumoconiosis	Aluminum oxide	"Shaver's disease"
Tungsten carbide pneumoconiosis	?Cobalt	Battery manufacture
Stannosis	Tin[1]	Rare

[1]These dusts in pure form tend not to cause fibrosis (noncollagenous pneumoconioses) and have minimal clinical effects. Other dusts, especially silica and asbestos, may lead to severe fibrosis (collagenous pneumoconioses).

There is also a peculiar relationship between coal workers' pneumoconiosis and rheumatoid arthritis. When coal miners develop rheumatoid arthritis, they tend to develop large rheumatoid nodules in the lung (Caplan's syndrome).

SILICOSIS

Silicosis is caused by inhalation of crystalline silicon dioxide (silica) dust particles in the 1- to 3-μm range. Silica exists in nature as quartz, chrystobalite, and tridymite. Occupations at increased risk for silicosis are hardrock, gold, tin, and copper mining; sand blasting; and iron, steel, and granite working. More than 1 million workers in the United States are at risk for developing silicosis. Significant pulmonary disease usually occurs with 10–15 years of exposure but may rarely occur after as little as 1 year. Silicotic lesions may be found long after exposure has been terminated.

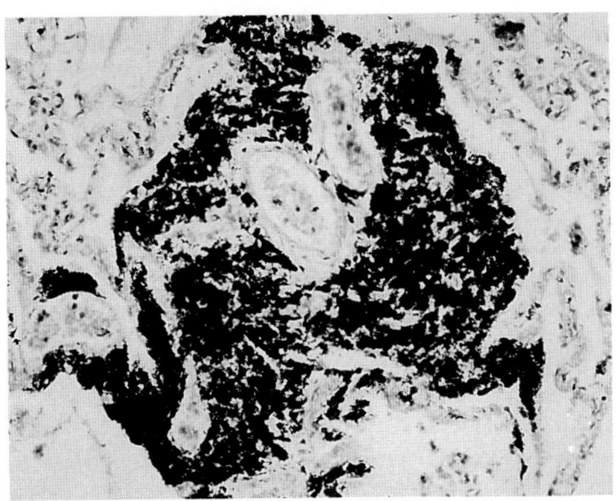

Figure 35-11. Anthracosis of the lung, showing a coal dust macule. There is little or no associated fibrosis.

Pathology

Small silica crystals, when inhaled, reach the lung acinus. Larger crystals (> 3 μm) are caught in the bronchial mucus layer and wafted upward by the ciliary action to be expelled; particles less than 1 μm remain airborne and are exhaled.

In the alveoli, the silica crystals are phagocytosed by macrophages. Silica is toxic to the internal organelle membranes of the macrophages and causes phagolysosomal disruption, cell death, and liberation of free silica particles. Inflammation and fibrosis follow, leading to formation of a nodule composed of hyalinized collagen around the crystals (Fig 35–12). Silica crystals are also carried in lymphatics to the hilar lymph nodes, where similar silicotic nodules form. One theory suggests that fibrosis is the result of a fibroblast-stimulating factor liberated by macrophages upon phagocytosis of silica particles. A second theory attributes fibrosis to a lymphokine produced by silica-activated T lymphocytes.

Grossly, the silicotic nodule is gray-black (due to associated carbon pigment), hard, and brittle and has concentric rings of hyalinized collagen in cross section. Nodules are found mainly along

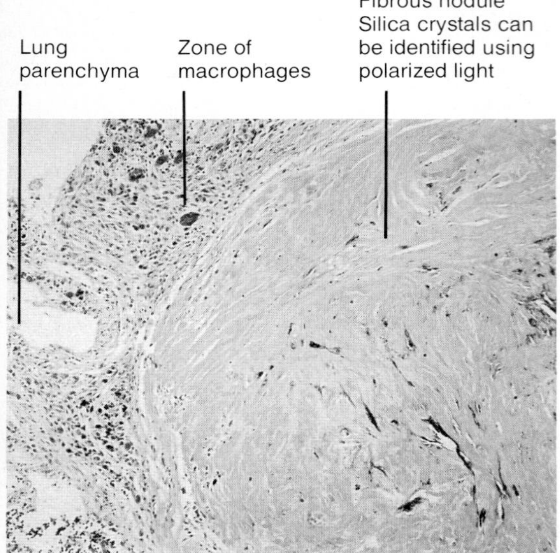

Figure 35-12. Pulmonary silicosis, showing a large fibrotic nodule surrounded by macrophages.

lymphatic pathways, especially around the hilum and in the upper lobes. Microscopically, the nodules are composed of a solid mass of macrophages, fibroblasts, and collagen (Fig 35-12). Silica particles are recognized as birefringent needle-shaped crystals in the nodules when examined by polarized light.

Clinical Features

Silicosis is often asymptomatic, being found incidentally at chest x-ray or histologic examination of lungs and hilar lymph nodes removed for an unrelated reason. Rarely, when patients are exposed to massive amounts of dust, acute lung disease may occur, with alveolar thickening and accumulation of proteinaceous material in the alveoli (acute silicotic proteinosis). More often, there is chronic pulmonary fibrosis with a mild restrictive ventilatory defect, decreased compliance, slowly progressive dyspnea, and pulmonary hypertension (cor pulmonale).

Complications

Progressive massive fibrosis may complicate chronic silicosis, particularly when the level of exposure to dust is high. The disorder is characterized by confluence of silicotic nodules into large masses of fibrous tissue that cause obliteration of vessels and bronchioles. Central necrosis and cavitation may occur in these masses as a result of ischemia. Progressive massive fibrosis commonly involves the upper lobes and is associated with a significant ventilatory defect and respiratory failure.

Patients with silicosis have a greatly increased incidence of **tuberculosis,** believed to be due to the adverse effects of silica dust on macrophage function. Tuberculosis causes extensive necrosis in the nodules, and large numbers of tubercle bacilli can be found in such lesions.

Silicosis is also associated with an increased incidence of autoimmune disease, especially progressive systemic sclerosis.

ASBESTOSIS

Asbestos is a fibrous silicate found in nature as the minerals chrysotile, amosite, and crocidolite. It is present in such diverse components of the modern environment as insulation, flame retardants, flooring and roofing materials, water and sewage pipes, and brake linings in vehicles, making low-grade exposure almost universal among urban dwellers. It is estimated that up to 11 million workers in the United States have had significant asbestos exposure since 1940.

Asbestos-related disease was first recognized in those with the highest levels of exposure, ie, workers in shipyards and the construction industry. Approximately 40% of World War II shipyard pipe fitters now have evidence of asbestosis. It is becoming clear, however, that lower levels of exposure are also associated with significant risk. Asbestos-related neoplasms occur in families of shipyard workers—due presumably to the presence in the home of contaminated clothing—and in communities with asbestos-based industries (air pollution by asbestos dust). It is estimated that about 10,000 deaths every year in the United States are due to asbestos-related diseases.

Pathology

One of the commonest changes associated with asbestos exposure is thickening of the parietal pleura by a plaquelike deposition of hyalinized collagen, maximal in the lateral and diaphragmatic pleura. This change on chest x-ray provides epidemiologic evidence of significant asbestos exposure. Pleural fibrosis does not cause symptoms and does not fall within the definition of asbestos pneumoconiosis since it does not involve lung parenchyma.

Asbestos fibers, when inhaled into the alveoli, are taken up by macrophages and evoke a diffuse interstitial fibrosis. The mechanism of stimulation of pulmonary fibrosis by asbestos is poorly understood. Asbestos, unlike silica, is not cytotoxic to macrophages; there is evidence of activation of macrophages by asbestos. Asbestos, when added to in vitro cultures of fibroblasts, stimulates increased collagen synthesis by these cells. Initially, fibrosis occurs around bronchioles but eventually extends into the alveolar interstitium. Advanced asbestosis causes end-stage fibrosis (honeycomb lung).

Microscopically, asbestos fibers are visible as ferruginous bodies ("asbestos bodies") composed of a thin central asbestos fiber 5–10 μm long encased in an iron-containing glycoprotein coat which is brown and typically beaded ("shish kebab" appearance; Fig 35–13). Ferruginous bodies are best seen in sections that have been stained for iron with Prussian blue. While ferruginous bodies are most commonly seen in asbestosis, they are not diagnostic, since a similar iron-glycoprotein coat may form on other types of inhaled fibers.

Asbestos fibers that do not have the iron-glycoprotein coat are not visible microscopically, but they outnumber coated fibers 10:1. The amount of asbestos in the lung thus cannot be accurately estimated by microscopy. A quantitative evaluation of asbestos in the body is best made by chemical analysis of lung tissue.

Clinical Features

Asbestos-induced lung disease presents with the features of diffuse interstitial lung disease, ie, chronic cough, progressive dyspnea, a diffuse infiltrative pattern on chest x-ray, decreased vital capacity with no obstructive element, decreased compliance, and blood gas changes of restrictive lung disease (hypoxemia with a normal or reduced arterial P_{CO_2}). Asbestosis rarely causes sufficient lung destruction to result in respiratory failure.

The most significant effect of asbestos exposure is the greatly increased risk of malignant neoplasms. **(1) Bronchogenic carcinoma** is the commonest neoplasm associated with asbestosis. Cigarette smoking has a profound additive effect to asbestos exposure in causing bronchogenic carcinoma. **(2) Malignant mesothelioma** of the pleura, peritoneum, and pericardium, although less common than bronchogenic carcinoma, represents the most specific neoplasm associated with asbestos exposure; most patients with mesotheliomas give a history of asbestos exposure. Malignant mesothelioma has a 100% mortality rate, and 90% of patients die within 2 years after diagnosis.

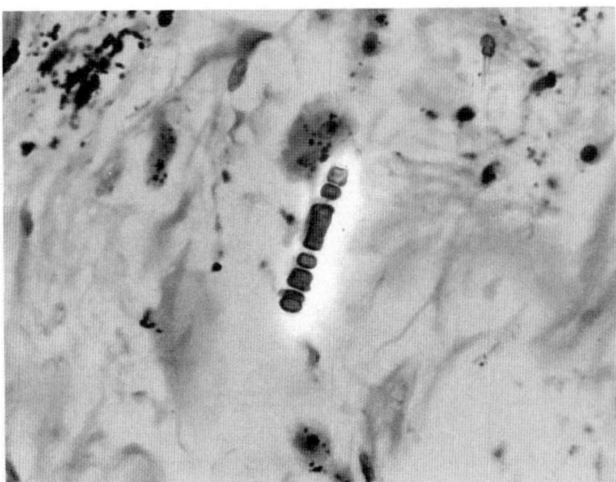

Figure 35–13. Ferruginous body in asbestosis, showing "shish-kebab" appearance of the iron-containing glycoprotein deposit around the linear asbestos fiber. Note that the asbestos fiber at the center of the ferruginous body cannot be seen in routine histologic sections.

BERYLLIOSIS

Berylliosis is rarely seen today because beryllium use has declined. Beryllium was used in the past in fluorescent lights and in the aerospace industry.

Acute exposure to beryllium results in a nonspecific acute pneumonitis. Chronic exposure is characterized by pulmonary fibrosis and the formation of noncaseating epithelioid cell granulomas resembling those of sarcoidosis. Beryllium can be demonstrated in these lesions as refractile crystalline material using polarized light. The formation of granulomas suggests a T cell reaction. It is postulated that beryllium forms antigenic complexes with host proteins.

The diagnosis is made by a history of exposure and confirmed by chemical analysis of lung tissue.

IATROGENIC DRUG-, CHEMICAL-, OR RADIATION-INDUCED INTERSTITIAL FIBROSIS

A large number of drugs—notably the **anticancer drugs** bleomycin, busulfan, melphalan, methotrexate, and cyclophosphamide—cause diffuse interstitial pulmonary disease with fibrosis. The pulmonary changes are usually dose-related. Lung fibrosis occurs insidiously, often appearing several months after treatment. The fibrosis progresses even after the drug is withdrawn and may cause death if excessive dosages of the drug have been used.

Paraquat, a commonly used herbicide, causes a severe toxic reaction in the lung when ingested or inhaled. In the acute phase there is pulmonary edema, hemorrhage, and interstitial inflammation. This progresses rapidly to interstitial pulmonary fibrosis, often leading to respiratory failure and death.

Radiation pneumonitis may complicate cancer therapy if the lungs are included in the field of radiation. High doses cause acute radiation pneumonitis, characterized by necrosis of epithelial cells, intra-alveolar hemorrhage, and formation of hyaline membranes. With lower doses, chronic pulmonary fibrosis occurs.

Toxic gases (mustard gas, 100% oxygen) also produce diffuse fibrosis that may be severe. The pulmonary fibrosis that complicates **intravenous drug abuse** by addicts may be more a response to impurities in the injected material than to the heroin itself. Foreign body granulomas are commonly present in the thickened alveolar septa in addicts who use intravenous drugs.

INTERSTITIAL DISEASES OF UNCERTAIN ETIOLOGY

SARCOIDOSIS

Sarcoidosis is a systemic disorder of uncertain cause that is commonly manifested in the lungs. Although the cause is unknown, immunologic mechanisms have been implicated, and abnormalities of the immune system are usually present: **(1) Depressed cell mediated immunity** is manifested by decreased numbers of T cells in the peripheral blood and by anergy (failure of delayed hypersensitivity to antigens injected in intradermal skin tests). The presence of numerous granulomas suggests a perverted type IV hypersensitivity reaction. **(2) Hyperactive humoral immunity** is probably the result of removal of T suppressor activity. There is an increased number of B lymphocytes in the peripheral blood, and most patients have hyperimmunoglobulinemia.

Pathology

The hallmark of sarcoidosis is the presence of small, noncaseating epithelioid cell granulomas (Fig 35–14). The granulomas contain Langhans type giant cells and are associated with fibrosis. Several types of inclusions may be present, but although characteristic of sarcoidosis they are not pathognomonic. Schaumann (conchoidal) bodies are round, calcified, laminated bodies in the cytoplasm of giant cells. Asteroid bodies are smaller and have a central pink zone surrounded by a clear halo that is traversed by fine radial pink lines.

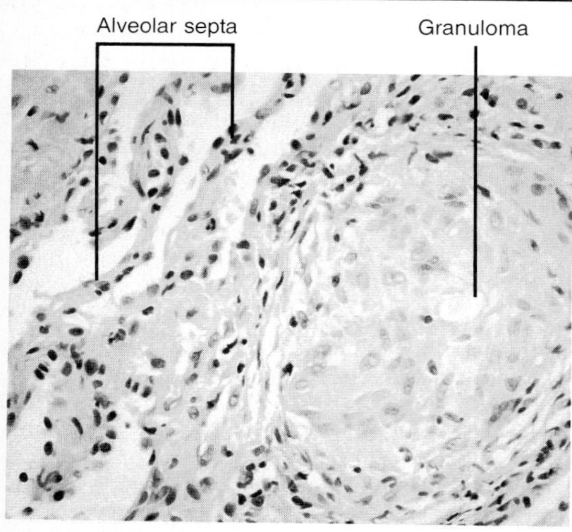

Figure 35–14. Lung in sarcoidosis, showing noncaseating epithelioid cell granuloma in the alveolar septum.

In the lung, granulomas are found in the alveolar septa (Fig 35–14) and along the pulmonary lymphatics in the bronchial wall. Granulomas are associated with interstitial inflammation and fibrosis. Chronic disease progresses to end-stage honeycomb lung. Granulomas may also be found in lymph nodes, liver, spleen, skin, and many other organs.

The diagnosis of sarcoidosis is made on clinical grounds. A finding of noncaseating epithelioid granulomas on histologic examination of biopsies provides confirmatory evidence when cultures of these tissues do not grow out mycobacteria and fungi. The cells in the granuloma release angiotensin-converting enzyme into the serum; the detection of elevated levels of this enzyme in serum (seen in 60% of patients) is a useful test for sarcoidosis. High serum levels of angiotensin-converting enzyme indicate activity of sarcoidosis and, when present, provide an important method of monitoring the course of disease.

Clinical Features (Fig 35–15)

In the United States, sarcoidosis occurs 10 times more frequently in blacks than in whites. Women are more commonly affected, and the most common age at onset is between 20 and 35 years. In Europe, sarcoidosis is more common in the Scandinavian countries.

An abnormality in the chest x-ray is present in over 90% of patients with sarcoidosis. Bilateral hilar lymphadenopathy is the commonest finding. Pulmonary infiltrates due to interstitial pneumonitis may also be present.

Sarcoidosis has a variable course. About 65% of patients with hilar adenopathy alone undergo spontaneous remission. Pulmonary parenchymal involvement usually signifies progressive chronic disease. Disability and death from pulmonary fibrosis occur in a minority of patients. Steroids are effective in controlling the disease and are indicated when there is symptomatic lung involvement, ocular lesions, cardiac disease, or neurologic disease.

WEGENER'S GRANULOMATOSIS

Wegener's granulomatosis is a disease of unknown cause, though a hypersensitivity reaction to an unknown antigen has been postulated. It is characterized by necrotizing vasculitis of small arteries. The inflammatory reaction around the affected vessel is granulomatous, with scattered neutrophils, eosinophils, and lymphocytes.

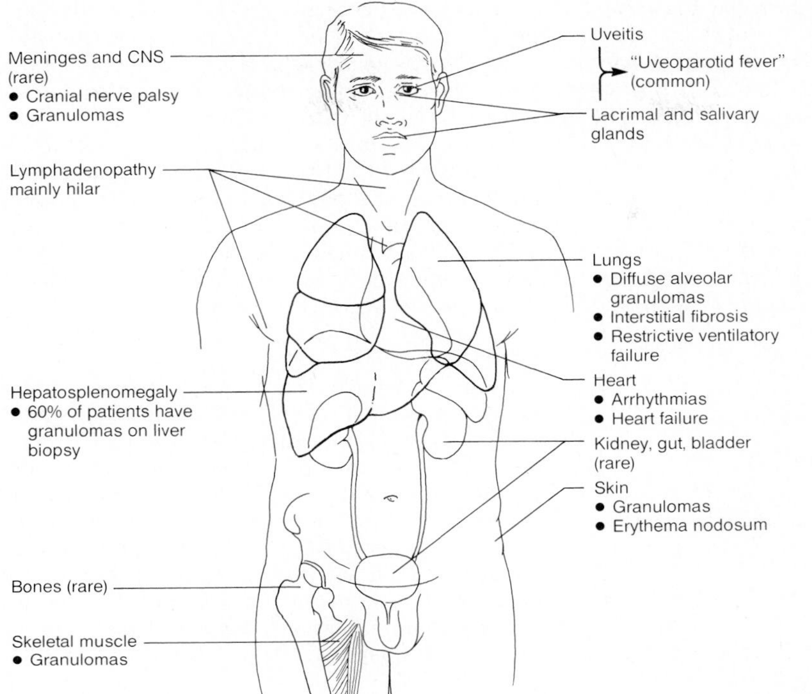

Figure 35–15. Clinical manifestations of sarcoidosis.

The classic form of the disease involves (1) the nose, paranasal sinuses, and nasopharynx; (2) the lungs; and (3) the kidneys. Variants with involvement of other organs or sparing of one or 2 of the classic sites also occur.

Pulmonary involvement is characterized by a rapidly expanding infiltrate that tends to be bilateral, with multiple nodular mass lesions which tend to cavitate. The renal disease is a necrotizing glomerulitis that frequently progresses to crescentic glomerulonephritis and renal failure. Nasal lesions are usually ulcerating granulomas.

Clinical progression is rapid, with death from either the renal or pulmonary lesions in the majority of cases. Immunosuppressive drugs such as cyclophosphamide have prolonged survival, though the ultimate prognosis is still very poor.

LYMPHOMATOID GRANULOMATOSIS

Lymphomatoid granulomatosis is a poorly defined entity of uncertain cause. It is a systemic disorder affecting the lung, nervous system, kidney, skin, and many other organs. Histologically, there are necrotizing granulomas in the lung which are infiltrated by atypical lymphocytes resembling immunoblasts. Lymphomatoid granulomatosis is a premalignant lesion with a high risk for pulmonary malignant lymphoma; some authorities hold that the process is an indolent form of lymphoma from the outset. The prognosis is poor.

BRONCHOCENTRIC GRANULOMATOSIS

Bronchocentric granulomatosis is a disease of uncertain cause characterized by granulomatous inflammation centered around the airways. The walls of the airways are destroyed, and their lumens are filled with necrotic material. No infectious agent can be isolated. Patients present with dyspnea, wheezing, and the consequences of bronchial obstruction such as pneumonia, lung abscess, and bronchiectasis.

PULMONARY ALVEOLAR PROTEINOSIS

Though traditionally included with infiltrative lung diseases, pulmonary alveolar proteinosis is neither an interstitial pneumonitis nor is it associated with fibrosis. It is characterized by filling of the alveolar spaces with a homogeneous, proteinaceous, lipid-rich material thought to be composed of surfactant and cellular debris. Few or no inflammatory cells are present.

The cause is unknown. Increased production or

decreased clearance of surfactant has been suggested as the cause.

Patients with alveolar proteinosis present with dyspnea and dry cough. The chest x-ray shows consolidation first affecting the lung bases. The infiltrates have a typical ground-glass appearance on chest x-ray. Hypoxemia is common and often severe.

While a few deaths have been reported, alveolar proteinosis is usually a benign disease, with most patients undergoing spontaneous remission. There is a good clinical response to treatment with pulmonary lavage.

PULMONARY VASCULAR DISORDERS

PULMONARY EDEMA

Edema fluid may enter the alveolar septa and alveolar spaces as a result of (1) changes in the permeability of the lung capillaries (in acute inflammation) or (2) increased capillary blood pressure in acute left heart failure. Acute edema, if extensive, interferes with respiratory gas exchange and is a medical emergency. Histologically, alveoli contain pale pink fluid. The pathophysiology is discussed in Chapter 2.

ADULT RESPIRATORY DISTRESS SYNDROME (ARDS; "Shock Lung")*

ARDS is an acute diffuse alveolar injury that occurs commonly in seriously ill patients. It is most frequently seen (1) with severe hypovolemic shock, most commonly following trauma ("Viet Nam lung"); (2) with sepsis, particularly that associated with gram-negative organisms; (3) with acute pancreatitis; (4) following inhalation of toxic gases such as chlorine and sulfur dioxide, including oxygen therapy; (5) with fat embolism; or (6) with disseminated intravascular coagulation. An estimated 150,000 patients in the United States develop ARDS annually.

Pathogenesis

The mechanisms by which ARDS occurs are complex and varied. In patients with hypovolemic shock, the acute alveolar injury is secondary to prolonged vasoconstriction that occurs as a compensatory phenomenon; the vasoconstriction results in ischemic injury to the alveolar epithelium. In gram-negative bacteremia, alveolar damage is caused by endotoxins. In acute pancreatitis, the acute alveolar injury is caused by enzymes liberated into the bloodstream from the injured pancreas. These phospholipases damage alveolar epithelium and antagonize the action of surfactant. With toxic gas inhalation, the alveolar damage is direct; with oxygen at toxic levels, the damage is caused by oxygen-based free radicals.

Pathology

ARDS is characterized by acute diffuse alveolar damage leading to necrosis and loss of type I pneumocytes. Endothelial damage also occurs, leading to exudation of protein-rich fluid into the alveoli and resulting in pulmonary edema, hemorrhage, and formation of hyaline membranes. Hyaline membranes are composed of a pink proteinaceous material that lines the alveoli in any condition where there is acute loss of alveolar lining epithelium. They are composed of fibrin together with coagulated cell debris from necrotic cells.

Grossly, the lungs are purple, heavy, and solid. Hemorrhagic fluid exudes from the cut surface.

If the patient recovers, the alveolar epithelium regenerates, initially with hyperplasia of the type II pneumocytes. Residual interstitial fibrosis is present in severe cases.

Clinical Features

Patients with ARDS are often seriously ill with some other disease, and the features of ARDS are superimposed. The respiratory symptoms of ARDS are rapidly increasing dyspnea, hypoxemia, and cyanosis. These usually occur 1–2 days after the onset of acute injury or disease that has become complicated by ARDS. Chest x-ray shows diffuse interstitial or alveolar edema but may be normal in the early stages. ARDS is commonly the terminal event in many of these patients. Where the underlying cause is reversible, the recognition of ARDS and its aggressive management may reduce the frequency of death.

PULMONARY EMBOLISM (See Chapter 9)

Pulmonary embolism causes over 50,000 deaths per year in the United States and occurs as a complication in as many as 30% of hospitalized patients.

Pulmonary emboli originate from deep leg vein thrombi in over 90% of cases. Thrombi in pelvic veins are second in frequency. Deep vein thrombosis and pulmonary embolism occur most commonly (1) after surgery; (2) after childbirth; (3) in

*Respiratory distress syndrome of the newborn (hyaline membrane disease) has many features in common with ARDS and is discussed in Chapter 34.

patients who are immobilized for any reason; (4) in patients with cardiovascular diseases, such as myocardial infarction and congestive heart failure; and (5) in patients receiving oral contraceptives. The risk of thromboembolism with oral contraceptives is less with newer pills containing small amounts of estrogen. The mechanisms leading to deep vein thrombosis and pulmonary embolism have been considered fully in Chapter 9.

Effects of Pulmonary Embolism

A. Sudden Death: Sudden death may occur with a large embolus that becomes impacted in the right ventricular outflow tract or main pulmonary artery ("saddle embolus"), effectively obstructing the circulation of blood. When circulatory obstruction is incomplete, the patient may survive long enough for emergency surgical removal of the thromboembolus from the pulmonary artery.

B. Pulmonary Infarction: Pulmonary infarction occurs when a medium-sized embolus obstructs a peripheral pulmonary artery in a patient whose bronchial arterial circulation is also impaired (patients with left heart failure and pulmonary hypertension).

Pathologically, pulmonary infarcts are hemorrhagic (red) and have a wedge shape with the base at the pleura and the apex directed toward the occluded vessel. Microscopically, alveolar necrosis and hemorrhage are present in the infarcted area. Pulmonary infarcts heal by fibrosis, leading to a subpleural scar.

Clinically, patients present with pleuritic chest pain, dyspnea, fever, and hemoptysis. A hemorrhagic pleural effusion may be present.

C. Pulmonary Hypertension: Isolated small emboli lodging in small pulmonary arterial branches produce no immediate effect, the bronchial artery supply being sufficient for oxygenation of tissues. Multiple small emboli over a long period may cause diffuse alveolar fibrosis and pulmonary hypertension.

PULMONARY HYPERTENSION

Pulmonary hypertension is elevation of the mean pulmonary arterial pressure.

Most patients with pulmonary hypertension have a recognizable cause for the elevated pressure **(secondary pulmonary hypertension)** (Table 35–6). In a small number of patients, there is no recognizable cause; this is called **primary (idiopathic) pulmonary hypertension** and occurs mainly in young women in the second and third decades. Primary pulmonary hypertension is frequently associated with immunologically mediated collagen diseases such as rheumatoid arthritis.

Table 35–6. Pulmonary hypertension.

Causes
Idiopathic (primary)
Secondary
Mitral valve disease
Left ventricular failure
Congenital heart (valve) disease with left-to-right shunt
Atrial septal defect
Ventricular septal defect
Patent duct arteriosus
Chronic pulmonary disease (cor pulmonale)
Emphysema
Chronic bronchitis
Diffuse interstitial fibrosis
Multiple recurrent pulmonary emboli
Results
Hypertrophy of muscular pulmonary arteries
Fibrous thickening of pulmonary arteries
Pulmonary atherosclerosis
Progressive increase in pulmonary artery blood pressure
Right ventricular hypertrophy
Right heart failure

Pathology

The pathologic features of both primary and secondary pulmonary hypertension are similar. There is fibrous thickening of pulmonary arteries of all sizes, with medial hypertrophy and atherosclerosis in the large pulmonary arteries. Atherosclerosis occurs in the pulmonary circulation only in patients with pulmonary hypertension. Abnormal plexiform arteriolar structures may be present in the lungs.

Clinical Features

The elevated mean pulmonary arterial pressure causes **right ventricular hypertrophy** and a loud pulmonary valve closure sound with increased separation from the sound of aortic valve closure (split S_2). Pulmonary valve closure is delayed because right ventricular output is prolonged. **Right ventricular failure** with peripheral edema ensues and is the common presenting feature.

Primary pulmonary hypertension is irreversible and slowly progressive. Few patients survive 10 years after diagnosis. In some, disease progression is more rapid. In patients with secondary pulmonary hypertension, treatment of the cause—eg, surgical replacement of a diseased mitral valve—if it is undertaken early enough, may halt progression of the hypertension.

36 The Lung: III. Neoplasms

- Carcinoma of the Lung (Bronchogenic Carcinoma)
  - Squamous (Epidermoid) Carcinoma
  - Adenocarcinoma
  - Small Cell Undifferentiated Carcinoma
  - Large Cell Undifferentiated Carcinoma
  - Mixed Types
- Other "Tumors" of the Lung
- Metastatic Neoplasms of the Lung
- Diseases of the Pleura
  - Pleural Effusion
  - Chylothorax
  - Pneumothorax
  - Neoplasms of the Pleura
    - Primary Mesothelial Neoplasms
    - Secondary Pleural Neoplasms

CARCINOMA OF THE LUNG
(Bronchogenic Carcinoma)

Incidence

Lung carcinoma is one of the major problems of modern society. In the United States, it causes about 120,000 deaths annually; in England and Wales, it accounts for 40,000 deaths annually—about one-third of total cancer deaths and almost one-tenth of all deaths from any cause. The incidence has increased markedly since 1950 (approximately 5-fold) and continues to increase. Rates of lung cancer vary greatly in different countries, principally due to differences in smoking habits.

Lung carcinoma is more common in males; the male:female ratio was 7:1 in 1960 but has fallen to about 2.5:1 in 1987. Lung cancer has recently overtaken breast cancer as the leading cause of death by cancer in women. It is a disease of older individuals, being rare under 40 years of age.

Etiology

A. Cigarette Smoking: Cigarette smoking is the main cause of lung carcinoma (Chapter 12). Heavy cigarette smokers (over 40 cigarettes a day) have a 20-fold increase in incidence compared to nonsmokers. Cessation of smoking decreases the risk: 10 years after stopping smoking, the risk falls to that of a nonsmoker. The risk is only slightly less with "low-tar" filter cigarettes. Cigar smoking and pipe smoking carry a much lower risk (probably because of less smoke inhalation).

The mechanism by which smoking causes lung carcinoma is not clear. A large number of potent carcinogens are present in cigarette smoke, including polycyclic hydrocarbons, aromatic amines, and heavy metals such as nickel. Any or all of these may be involved in human carcinogenesis (Chapter 18). However, "experimental" cigarette smoking at levels comparable to the exposure endured by heavy smokers does not produce lung carcinoma in animals. This failure of smoking to produce lung carcinoma in animals may be due to species differences or to insufficient duration of smoking in most experiments.

Cigarette smoking produces changes in the respiratory epithelium of humans. There is loss of cilia and progression from squamous metaplasia through all degrees of dysplasia to carcinoma in situ. Squamous metaplasia alone is not premalignant, but dysplasia is. Dysplasia is very uncommon in nonsmokers. In patients with lung carcinoma, the respiratory epithelium away from the neoplasm frequently shows dysplasia and carcinoma in situ.

Cigarette smoking is most strongly associated with squamous carcinoma and small cell undifferentiated carcinoma and to a lesser degree with adenocarcinoma.

B. Industrial Carcinogens: The best-known occupational lung carcinogen is asbestos, exposure to which increases the risk of lung carcinoma as documented among World War II shipyard workers (Chapter 35). The risk of lung cancer following asbestos exposure is compounded by cigarette smoking.

Mining of many different heavy metals (uranium, nickel, chromate, gold) is also associated with an increased risk of lung cancer.

C. Radiation: Historically, the miners of Jáchymov in Czechoslovakia and Schneeberg in Germany were described as developing "mountain sickness" for 4 centuries before it was realized that the sickness was lung carcinoma from exposure to natural radioactive elements in the mines.

D. Urban Pollution: The common urban pollutants are ozone and oxides of nitrogen and sulfur. While there is great concern, most studies to date have failed to demonstrate a significant association between lung carcinoma and urban pollutants.

E. "Scar Cancer": There is a slightly increased incidence of lung carcinoma—especially peripherally located adenocarcinoma—in areas of scarring due to prior infarcts, granulomas, or diffuse fibrosis.

Classification (Figs 36-1 and 36-2)

The International Classification of Lung Carcinoma introduced by the World Health Organization recognizes 4 major and several minor types.

A. Squamous (Epidermoid) Carcinoma: Squamous carcinoma arises in metaplastic squamous epithelium of the bronchi. It is characterized by marked cytologic pleomorphism, intercellular bridges (desmosomes) between tumor cells, and keratinization of the cytoplasm (Fig 36–2A). Squamous carcinoma is strongly associated with cigarette smoking and accounts for 40–60% of all lung cancers. There may be a preceding phase of dysplasia and carcinoma in situ. Squamous carcinoma tends to remain localized more than the other types, resulting in large masses in the lung. Central cavitation is common.

B. Adenocarcinoma: Adenocarcinoma of the lung, as elsewhere, shows formation of glands or secretion of mucin by the tumor cells (Fig 36–2B). Several different forms of adenocarcinoma are recognized: (1) adenocarcinoma arising centrally in large bronchi, (2) adenocarcinoma arising

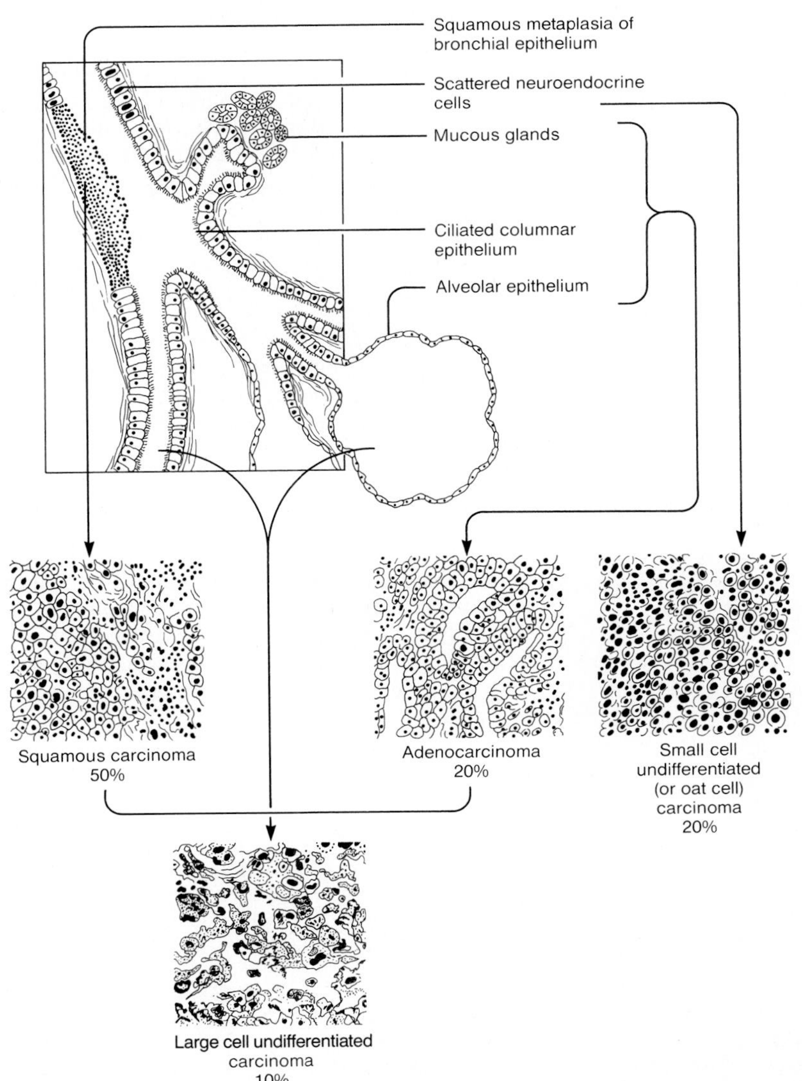

Figure 36–1. Histogenetic classification of bronchogenic lung carcinoma.

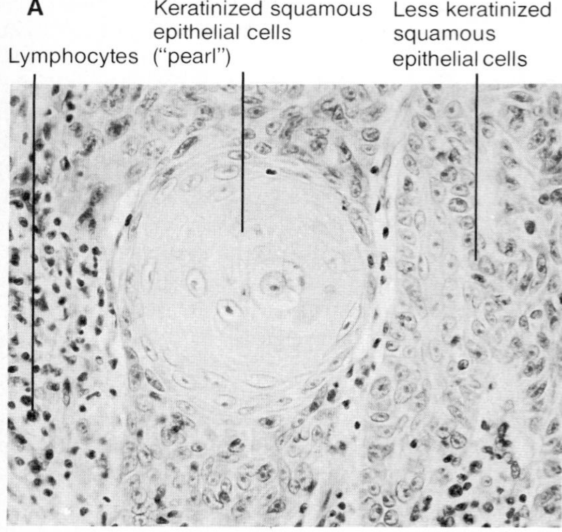

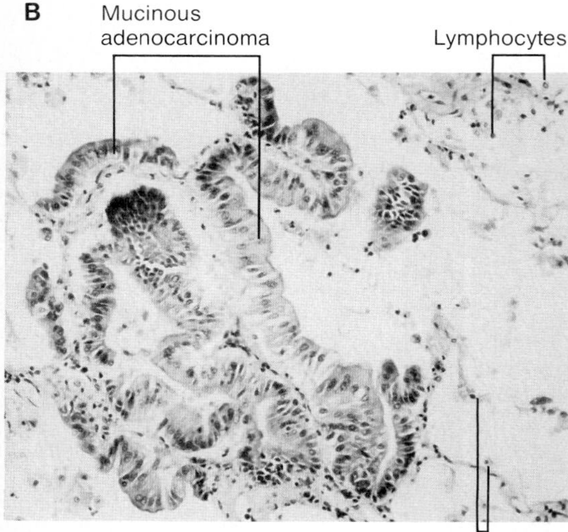

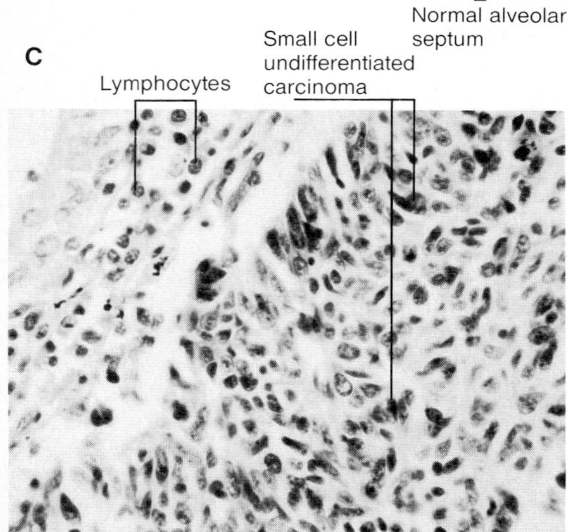

in peripheral scars in the lungs ("scar carcinoma"), and (3) bronchiolo-alveolar carcinoma arising in small bronchioles or alveoli, probably from the surfactant-producing Clara cells or from type II pneumocytes. The tumor cells typically line intact alveoli, producing a striking histologic appearance (Fig 36–2B). Bronchiolo-alveolar carcinoma may be solitary (good prognosis) or multiple (bad). The histologic appearance of bronchiolo-alveolar carcinoma may be mimicked by metastatic adenocarcinoma, especially from the pancreas or ovary. Adenocarcinoma constitutes 10–25% of lung carcinomas, has an equal sex incidence, and is associated with cigarette smoking though not as strongly as squamous carcinoma and small-cell undifferentiated carcinoma.

C. Small-Cell Undifferentiated ("Oat Cell") Carcinoma: Small-cell undifferentiated carcinoma is composed of small round to oval cells with scant cytoplasm, a high nuclear:cytoplasmic ratio, and hyperchromatic nuclei that do not have prominent nucleoli (Fig 36–2C). Small-cell undifferentiated carcinoma is believed to arise from neuroendocrine cells in the bronchial mucosa (Fig 36–1); it stains positively with neuroendocrine immunologic markers such as chromogranin and neuron-specific enolase and has neurosecretory granules in the cytoplasm on electron microscopy. Small-cell undifferentiated carcinoma is highly malignant. Bloodstream metastasis occurs early in the course of the neoplasm.

Small-cell undifferentiated carcinomas account for 10–25% of lung carcinomas and are strongly associated with smoking. They almost always occur in the large bronchi near the hilum of the lung (Fig 36–3).

D. Large Cell Undifferentiated Carcinoma: This tumor type comprises 5–20% of lung carcinomas and is composed of large cells that show no squamous or glandular differentiation on light microscopy. In some cases, immunohistochemical or electron microscopic examination is able to detect early glandular and squamous differentiation. Pleomorphic giant-cell carcinoma is a highly malignant variant with numerous multinucleated giant cells.

Figure 36–2. Common microscopic types of lung carcinoma. **A:** Squamous carcinoma showing squamous epithelial pearl with keratinization. **B:** Adenocarcinoma, bronchiolo-alveolar type, showing malignant glandular epithelium growing along the alveolar basement membrane. **C:** Small cell undifferentiated ("oat cell") carcinoma, showing small oval cells with hyperchromatic nuclei and scant cytoplasm. Note that these pictures are at different magnifications. The best guide to the size of malignant cells is to compare them with lymphocytes present in all 3 photographs.

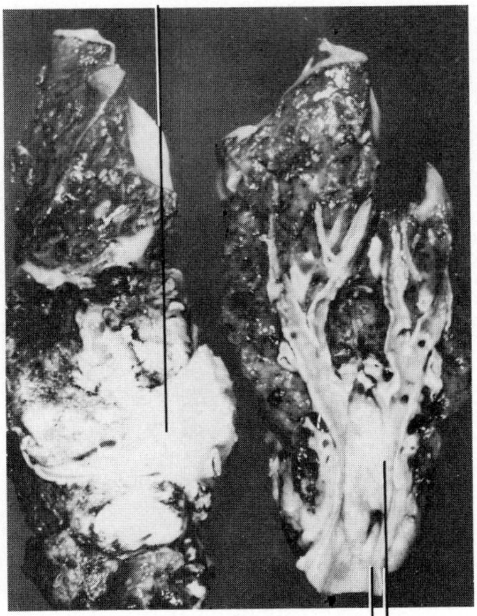

Invasive mass

Bronchial origin of the carcinoma

Bronchial region of resected lung

Figure 36-3. Bronchogenic carcinoma, showing the neoplasm in 2 slices of lung. The lung slice at the right shows the origin of the tumor, seen as an intrabronchial mass; the lung slice at left shows the invasive mass in the adjacent lung.

E. Mixtures of the above histologic types are common (eg, adenosquamous carcinoma), leading to the hypothesis that lung carcinoma arises from a primitive cell that has the capability to differentiate in several directions.

Pathology

Two distinct gross types of lung carcinoma can be distinguished.

A. Central (Bronchogenic) Carcinoma (75%): "Central" carcinomas arise in the first-, second-, or third-order bronchi near the hilum of the lung (Fig 36-3) and tend to be hidden in chest x-rays during their early growth phase. They can, however, be seen and biopsied at an early stage by bronchoscopy. All histologic types occur, but the majority are squamous or small-cell undifferentiated carcinomas.

The earliest lesion is carcinoma in situ, which on bronchoscopy may produce no visible change or simply a plaquelike mucosal thickening. However, cytologic examination of sputum shows malignant cells. The term "stage 0 carcinoma" is used for patients with positive sputum cytology in whom no tumor can be demonstrated by chest radiography and bronchoscopy.

From its mucosal origin, the neoplasm grows into the bronchial lumen (causing ulceration, bleeding, or obstruction) and infiltrates the bronchial wall and adjacent lung parenchyma. Infiltration tends to occur very early. Rarely, tumor growth is mainly endobronchial; in most cases, there is extensive invasion of the bronchial wall and lung parenchyma, forming a large hilar mass with areas of necrosis and hemorrhage.

B. Peripheral Lung Carcinoma (25%): Peripheral carcinomas arise in relation to small bronchi, bronchioles, or alveoli. These neoplasms are visible on chest x-ray at an early stage as a circumscribed mass but cannot be seen by bronchoscopy.

Peripheral lung carcinomas tend to be adenocarcinomas. Small-cell undifferentiated carcinoma rarely occurs in the periphery.

Spread of Lung Carcinoma (Fig 36-4)

A. Local Invasion: With central lung carcinomas, invasion involves vital mediastinal structures such as the superior vena cava and pericardium. Peripheral lung carcinomas tend to extend locally in the lung, with involvement of the pleura occurring early.

B. Lymphatic Metastasis: Lymphatic metastasis to lymph nodes occurs early in all types of lung carcinoma, being commonest in oat cell carcinoma and least frequent in well-differentiated squamous carcinoma. Involvement of the hilar and scalene lymph nodes (Fig 36-4) is present in 50% of cases at presentation.

Retrograde permeation of pleural lymphatics (pleural lymphatic carcinomatosis) occurs in advanced lesions, leading to multiple pleural nodules, pleural effusion, and a typical reticular appearance on chest x-ray.

C. Bloodstream Metastasis: Hematogenous metastasis also occurs early, and patients with lung carcinoma frequently present with a distant metastasis. In small-cell undifferentiated (oat cell) carcinoma, distant metastases are almost invariably present at the time of diagnosis. Hematogenous metastases occur later in the course of non-small-cell carcinomas.

Common sites of metastasis of lung carcinoma are the adrenals (50%), liver (30%), brain (20%), bone (20%), and kidneys (15%).

Staging of Lung Carcinoma

The TNM (T = tumor, N = node, M = metastases) staging system has been recommended for classification of lung carcinoma (Table 36-1). Using this system, lung carcinoma is divided into 3 stages. **Stage I** lesions are confined to the lung and are either large (> 3 cm) without node involvement, or small (< 3 cm) with local nodal involvement only; **stage II** lesions are large (> 3 cm) and confined to the lung, with only local nodal involvement; and **stage III** includes all other lesions.

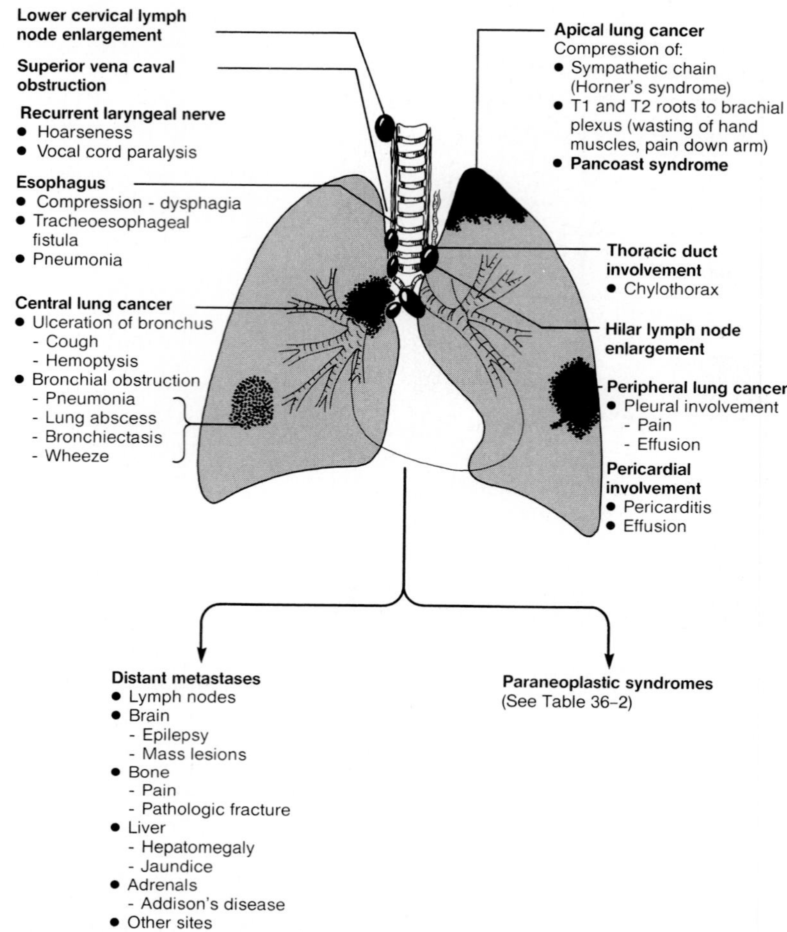

Figure 36-4. Clinical features and spread of lung carcinoma.

This system is commonly used in clinical practice and correlates well with prognosis.

Clinical Features (Fig 36-4)

The earliest symptoms of bronchogenic carcinoma are cough, hemoptysis, dyspnea, chest pain, and weight loss. Unfortunately, these occur at a relatively advanced stage. A minority of cases of lung carcinoma are detected at an asymptomatic stage by routine chest x-ray.

A. Bronchial Obstruction: A few patients with central lesions present with features of bronchial obstruction, including unresolving pneumonia, lung abscess, and bronchiectasis.

B. Local Invasion: Patients with lung carcinoma may also have symptoms due to local invasion of nearby structures by the neoplasm. Direct invasion of the pleura and pericardium results in pleural and pericardial effusion. The finding of carcinoma cells in aspirated effusion fluid is one method of diagnosis of lung carcinoma. Involvement of the thoracic duct at the lung hilum may result in chylothorax, and superior vena caval obstruction causes edema and congestion of the face and brain ("superior vena caval syndrome"). Large hilar neoplasms may invade the esophagus, causing dysphagia and tracheoesophageal fistula.

C. Pancoast's Syndrome: This is a specific clinical presentation of lung carcinoma resulting from an apical lung carcinoma (usually squamous) that invades the apical pleura. The tumor causes destruction of the T1 intercostal nerve and leads to a T1 motor and sensory deficit—weakness and wasting of small muscles of the hand and numbness on the medial side of the arm—and the cervical sympathetic trunk, causing Horner's syndrome—ptosis of the eyelid, pupillary constriction, and absent sweating on the side of the lesion.

D. Distant Metastases: A significant number of patients with lung carcinoma present with evidence of lymph node or hematogenous metastases. Cervical lymph node enlargement, pathologic fractures due to bone metastasis, and brain masses are common presenting features.

E. Paraneoplastic Syndromes: A minority

Table 36–1. Staging of lung cancer using the TNM system.[1]

Primary tumor
- T_x Malignant cells in sputum but no demonstrable primary
- TIS Carcinoma in situ
- T_1 Tumor < 3 cm, confined to lung
- T_2 Tumor > 3 cm, confined to lung (or visceral pleura)
- T_3 Tumor any size but with invasion of mediastinum or parietal pleura or within 2 cm of carina

Regional nodes
- N_0 No demonstrable nodes involved
- N_1 Ipsilateral bronchial or hilar nodes involved
- N_2 Mediastinal nodes involved

Metastases
- M_0 No distant metastases
- M_1 Distant metastases

Staging according to TNM categories	5-Year Survival[2] Rates
Stage I = TIS, N_0, M_0; T_1, N_0, M_0; T_1, N_1, M_0; and T_2, N_0, M_0	50%
Stage II = T_2, N_1, M_0	20%
Stage III = all T_3; all N_2; all M_1, irrespective of other factors	5%

[1]TNM: Tumor, nodes, metastases.
[2]With aggressive surgery, radiotherapy, and chemotherapy.

Table 36–2. Paraneoplastic syndromes in lung carcinoma.

Ectopic hormone syndromes	
Adrenocorticotropic hormone	Small-cell undifferentiated carcinoma; causes bilateral adrenal hyperplasia and Cushing's syndrome
Antidiuretic hormone	Small-cell undifferentiated carcinoma; causes hyponatremia
Parathyroid hormone (PTH)	Squamous carcinoma; causes hypercalcemia
5-Hydroxytryptamine	Carcinoid syndrome
Gonadotropins	Gynecomastia
Finger clubbing and pulmonary hypertrophic osteoarthropathy	
Dermatomyositis and polymyositis	
Migratory thrombophlebitis	
Neuromuscular syndromes	
Peripheral neuropathy	
Myopathy	
Myasthenic syndrome (Eaton-Lambert syndrome)	
Cerebellar degeneration	
Leukoencephalopathy	
Skin rashes	

of patients present with a variety of signs or symptoms that cannot be attributed to the direct effects of destruction by primary or metastatic tumors; these conditions are referred to as paraneoplastic syndromes (Table 36–2). These include the effects of secretion of hormones by the neoplasm (ectopic hormone syndromes). The mechanisms that cause many of the other paraneoplastic syndromes are largely unknown, though autoimmune phenomena have been postulated.

Diagnosis

Lung carcinoma must be considered a possibility when a patient presents with any of the protean clinical manifestations described above. This is particularly so if there is a strong smoking history. Chest x-ray and computerized tomography are effective for demonstrating the presence of a mass in the lung, but they do not predict the pathologic diagnosis and have a significant failure rate in detection of small hilar lesions.

The diagnosis of lung carcinoma must in every case be substantiated by pathologic examination. In addition to cytologic examination of sputum for malignant cells, bronchoscopy is useful for visualization of central lung cancers, direct biopsy, recovery of brush specimens for cytologic examination, and taking of transbronchial needle biopsies from peripheral lung masses. Percutaneous needle aspiration biopsy may be done under radiologic guidance when a mass lesion is visible on chest x-ray or CT scan. Open lung biopsy may rarely be necessary for diagnosis, especially in peripheral lesions. Biopsy of metastatic lesions in other organs frequently provides the first evidence of a previously undiagnosed lung carcinoma. Aspiration of pleural effusions and biopsy of enlarged cervical lymph nodes and brain masses are examples.

With all of these techniques, both cytologic and histologic examinations provide not only the diagnosis but also the classification of lung carcinoma.

Treatment & Prognosis

The overall 5-year survival rate of patients with lung cancer is a dismal 10–20%. Recent chemotherapeutic regimens combined with aggressive surgery have shown an improving trend.

Small-cell undifferentiated carcinoma is treated primarily by chemotherapy, which has improved median survival from less than 6 months to about 2 years. Surgery is contraindicated because this type of tumor is almost invariably stage III at the time of presentation. Few patients survive 5 years.

Non-small-cell carcinoma (squamous carcinoma, adenocarcinoma, and large-cell undifferentiated carcinoma) tend to remain localized to the lung for longer periods, and surgical resection is possible in about 30% of cases. Five-year survival rates are as follows: patients with surgically resected stage I tumors, 50%; patients with surgically resected stage II tumors, 20–30%; patients with stage III tumors, 5–10%.

The prognosis is similar for squamous carcinoma, adenocarcinoma, and large-cell undifferentiated carcinoma, which all have overall 5-year survival rates of about 20–30%. Bronchioloalveolar carcinoma has a better prognosis, with a 60% survival rate at 5 years. Chemotherapy for squamous carcinoma and adenocarcinoma is largely palliative.

OTHER "TUMORS" OF THE LUNG

While the term "lung cancer" commonly denotes the types of lung carcinomas described above, one should bear in mind that many other benign or malignant neoplasms as well as inflammatory lesions may present as a mass in the lung.

The term **bronchial adenoma** was used in the past for a group of neoplasms that include **bronchial carcinoid tumor, mucoepidermoid tumor,** and **adenoid cystic carcinoma.** These arise in the bronchi, usually near the hilum of the lung, and are slowly growing neoplasms that infiltrate locally but have a very low incidence of metastasis. They therefore behave like low-grade malignant neoplasms, which is why the term "adenoma"—traditionally used to denote benign epithelial neoplasms—was discarded. Bronchial carcinoid tumors arise from neuroendocrine cells and resemble carcinoid tumors of the intestine (Fig 36–5). Rarely, they secrete sufficient amounts of serotonin to cause the carcinoid syndrome (see Chapter 41). Mucoepidermoid carcinoma and adenoid cystic carcinoma are probably derived from bronchial mucous glands and resemble the corresponding tumors in the salivary glands (see Chapter 31).

Other tumors of the lung include sclerosing hemangioma and chondroid hamartoma (Fig 36–6). **Chondroid hamartoma** is a benign hamartomatous lesion composed of a disorganized mass of cartilage, fat, and spaces lined by bronchial epithelium. Pulmonary blastoma and carcinosarcoma are malignant neoplasms involving the lung parenchyma. Inflammatory lesions such as infectious granulomas (Chapter 34), plasma cell granuloma, and inflammatory pseudotumor may all present with mass lesions in the lung. All these lesions are rare and have specific types of biologic behavior. They are mentioned here merely to emphasize that the diagnosis of a mass lesion of the lung requires histologic examination.

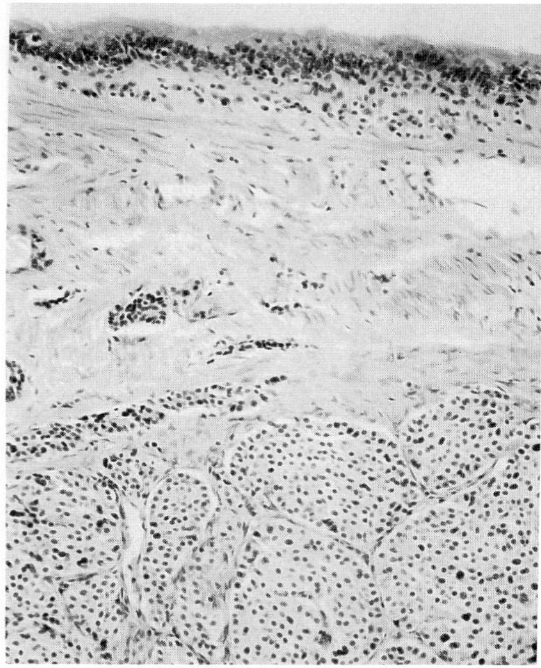

Figure 36–5. Bronchial carcinoid tumor, showing nests of small, round, uniform cells. Bronchial epithelium and muscle are seen in the upper half of the figure.

METASTATIC NEOPLASMS TO THE LUNG

Metastatic neoplasms occur commonly in the lung, which acts as the first capillary bed in the systemic circulation for entrapment of tumor em-

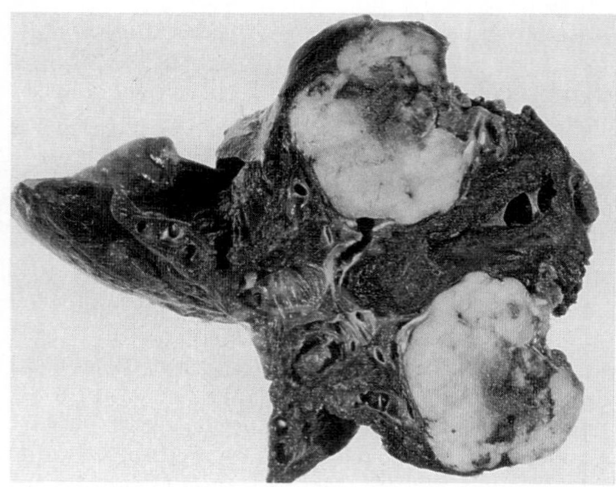

Figure 36–6. Chondroid hamartoma of the lung. The resected lung segment and tumor have been bisected, showing the well-circumscribed cartilaginous mass.

boli. It is often difficult to distinguish metastatic from primary lung neoplasms on the basis of histologic examination alone; a full clinical evaluation of the patient is necessary to make a diagnosis of metastatic carcinoma. Carcinomas, sarcomas, melanomas, and almost any other malignant neoplasm may give rise to lung metastases.

DISEASES OF THE PLEURA

PLEURAL EFFUSION

A pleural effusion is a collection of fluid in the pleural cavity. Simple accumulation of small amounts of fluid in the pleural cavity does not cause any symptoms. Large effusions interfere with lung expansion during inspiration, causing a reduction in vital capacity. The presence of a large pleural effusion can be detected clinically by the absence of chest wall movement, shift of mediastinal structures to the opposite side, decreased breath sounds, and dullness to percussion over the effusion. Small pleural effusions cannot be detected clinically and require radiologic examination. When more than 300 mL of fluid is present in the pleural cavity, it can be seen on an upright chest x-ray.

Once the presence of an effusion has been established, aspiration of fluid is helpful to identify its cause. Low specific gravity, low protein concentration, and lack of inflammatory cells identify a transudate. Exudates have a specific gravity over 1.015, a protein level of over 1.5 g/dL, and many inflammatory cells. Bacterial infection commonly produces a frankly purulent exudate (empyema). Hemorrhagic exudates occur in malignant effusions, tuberculosis, uremia, and pulmonary infarction. Cytologic examination of effusion sediment for malignant cells is frequently positive when malignant neoplasia is the cause of the effusion (Table 36–3).

Pleural biopsy provides a core of pleural tissue for histologic examination and is useful in the diagnosis of tuberculosis or cancer.

Table 36–3. Causes of pleural effusion.

Transudates
- Cardiac failure
- Hypoalbuminemic states, including nephrotic syndrome, protein malnutrition, chronic liver disease, protein-losing enteropathy

Exudates secondary to pleural inflammation
- Bacterial pneumonias
- Tuberculosis
- Fistulous opening of abscess cavities (lung abscess, amebic liver abscess) into the pleural cavity
- Collagen diseases: systemic lupus erythematosus and rheumatoid arthritis
- Uremia
- Pulmonary infarction

Malignant neoplasms affecting the pleura
- Malignant mesothelioma
- Lung carcinoma
- Metastatic carcinoma from extrathoracic sites
- Malignant lymphoma involving the pleura

Chylothorax
- Thoracic duct injuries: trauma, surgery, malignant neoplasms of the mediastinum

CHYLOTHORAX

Chylothorax is a specific kind of pleural effusion characterized by accumulation of chyle in the pleural cavity. Chyle is a milky fluid of high fat content that is normally present in the thoracic duct. Chylothorax may be differentiated from other turbid pleural effusions by the presence of chylomicrons and a high triglyceride content. The presence of chylothorax is evidence of an abnormal communication between the thoracic duct and the pleura. This may result from injuries to the thoracic duct by trauma and surgery or by infiltration of the thoracic duct by malignant neoplasms.

PNEUMOTHORAX

Pneumothorax is the presence of air in the pleural cavity. Pneumothorax may result from trauma, air being sucked in through a chest wall defect or entering via a laceration of the lung surface; or from spontaneous rupture of a bulla on the lung surface into the pleural cavity. Spontaneous pneumothorax may complicate many lung diseases such as bronchial asthma, emphysema, and tuberculosis, or it may occur in healthy, young, muscular individuals and may be recurrent. In this instance, rupture of subpleural blebs is believed to be responsible.

Patients with pneumothorax present with acute onset of chest pain and dyspnea, directly proportionate to the amount of air that accumulates in the pleural cavity. When the pneumothorax is progressive, dyspnea rapidly worsens. Physical examination reveals an absence of chest expansion, mediastinal shift to the opposite side, decreased breath sounds, and a tympanic sound on percussion. The diagnosis may be confirmed by chest x-ray.

In most cases, the air in the pleural cavity is reabsorbed, with reexpansion of the collapsed lung. Occasionally, a valvelike effect develops, producing a "tension" pneumothorax, or spontaneous resorption occurs so slowly that the collapsed lung begins to undergo fibrosis. In these cases, insertion of a chest tube is essential.

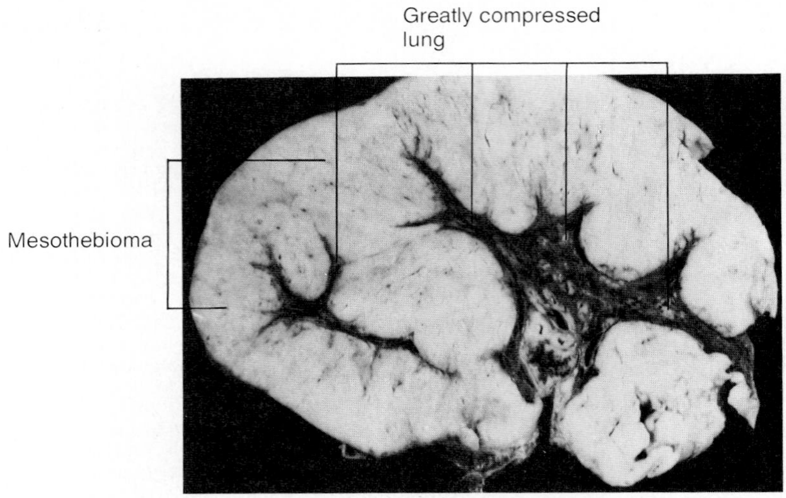

Greatly compressed lung

Mesothebioma

Figure 36–7. Malignant mesothelioma, showing diffuse encasement and marked compression of the lung by the neoplasm.

NEOPLASMS OF THE PLEURA

1. PRIMARY MESOTHELIAL NEOPLASMS

Benign Fibrous Mesothelioma

Fibrous mesothelioma is a rare benign neoplasm of the pleura, usually discovered incidentally on routine chest x-ray. It appears grossly as a localized growth of firm, dense fibrous tissue on the visceral pleura, often attached to the lung surface by a pedicle. Most fibrous mesotheliomas are small; rarely, they may reach large size. Microscopically, they are composed of fibroblastlike spindle cells and collagen. They do not invade, and the prognosis after surgical excision is excellent.

Malignant Mesothelioma

Malignant mesothelioma is a rare neoplasm strongly related etiologically to asbestos exposure; many cases have occurred in World War II exposure in shipyard workers.

Malignant mesothelioma commonly occurs in the over-50 age group. Clinical presentation is with dyspnea and features of pleural effusion. Grossly, the tumor diffusely involves the pleura, encasing large areas of lung as a firm, grayish, gelatinous mass (Fig 36–7). Invasion of both lung parenchyma and chest wall occurs frequently. Microscopically, the tumor is biphasic, with a sarcomatoid spindle cell component and epithelial elements that form tubular and papillary structures. When the epithelial component predominates, differentiation from adenocarcinoma may be difficult.

The prognosis is very poor, with 50% of patients dead within 1 year after diagnosis and few survivals of more than 2 years.

2. SECONDARY PLEURAL NEOPLASMS

Secondary involvement of the pleura by malignant neoplasms is much more common than mesothelioma. Direct involvement of the pleura by lung carcinoma is the commonest secondary pleural neoplasm. Metastases from distant sites such as the breast, colon, kidney, and thyroid also occur. Involvement of the pleura by malignant lymphoma is common.

Secondary pleural neoplasms cause dyspnea and effusion. On x-rays, nodular pleural masses may be identified. The diagnosis may be established by identifying malignant cells in aspirated pleural fluid. The differentiation of secondary pleural neoplasms from malignant mesothelioma on the basis of cytologic features may be difficult. Immunoperoxidase techniques may be helpful, carcinoma being positive for keratin and frequently for carcinoembryonic antigen, while mesothelioma is positive for keratin and negative for carcinoembryonic antigen.

Section IX. The Gastrointestinal System

Colorectal cancer is the second commonest type of cancer in the USA after lung cancer and is responsible for about 50,000 deaths annually in the United States (Chapter 41). Gastric cancer is less common in the USA but has a high prevalence in Japan and South America (Chapter 38). Cancer of the esophagus (Chapter 37) also has a marked geographic variation, being much more common in China than in the USA. These geographic variations provide insights into causes of cancer (see Chapter 18).

Gastrointestinal infections (Chapter 40) are very prevalent in developing countries where poor sanitary conditions favor fecal-oral transmission of infection (see Chapter 14). Acute appendicitis (Chapter 40) is the commonest surgical emergency. Peptic ulcer disease (Chapter 38) is common all over the world. Inflammatory bowel disease (ulcerative colitis and Crohn's disease, Chapter 40) is common in the USA and Europe, but uncommon in tropical Asia and Africa.

37 The Esophagus

STRUCTURE & FUNCTION

The esophagus is a muscular tube 25 cm long that extends from the neck down the posterior mediastinum and diaphragm to the stomach (Fig 37–1). It is lined by nonkeratinizing stratified squamous epithelium that transforms abruptly to gastric epithelium at the gastroesophageal junction. The junction is usually 37–40 cm from the incisor teeth and may be identified endoscopically by a change in appearance from the white squamous mucosa to the tan glandular mucosa.

The esophagus has physiologic high-pressure zones at either end that act as sphincters. There is no anatomic sphincter at either end. The upper cricopharyngeal sphincter prevents entry of air and pharyngeal contents into the esophagus except during swallowing, and the lower "cardiac" or gastroesophageal sphincter prevents reflux into the esophagus of acid gastric juice.

Deglutition (swallowing) is a reflex that is initiated when a bolus of food stimulates nerve endings in the mucosa of the posterior pharyngeal wall (Fig 37–1). Efferent impulses from the deglutition center in the brain stem cause pharyngeal muscle contraction and relaxation of the cricopharyngeal sphincter, permitting entry of food into the esophagus and initiating peristalsis.

Peristalsis consists of successive waves of contraction preceded by relaxation of the esophageal muscle, which propels food down the esophagus. Peristaltic action is coordinated by the myenteric plexus of nerves. Three types of peristaltic wave are recognized: (1) primary waves, which originate in the lower pharynx and pass down the entire esophagus; (2) secondary waves, which originate in the mid esophagus and pass down to the stomach; and (3) tertiary waves, which are irregular contractions of segments of the wall. Primary and secondary waves are propulsive; tertiary waves are nonpropulsive. The lower esophageal sphincter relaxes when a propulsive peristaltic wave (either primary or secondary) reaches the lower esophagus, permitting food to enter the stomach.

CLINICAL EFFECTS OF ESOPHAGEAL DISEASE

Dysphagia simply means difficulty in swallowing. The patient often complains that food "gets stuck" without passing down normally. The term odynophagia is used when there is pain during deglutition. Most diseases of the esophagus cause dysphagia (Table 37–1).

Retrosternal pain ("heartburn") unassociated with deglutition commonly occurs when acidic gastric juice refluxes into the esophagus across an incompetent lower esophageal sphincter.

Hematemesis (vomiting of blood) may be due to acute hemorrhage into the lumen of the esophagus or stomach. Peptic ulcer disease and rupture of esophageal varices are the most common causes of hematemesis (Table 37–2). Slower, more sustained bleeding produces melena (tarry black stools containing blood altered by the action of gastric acid) or iron deficiency anemia with occult

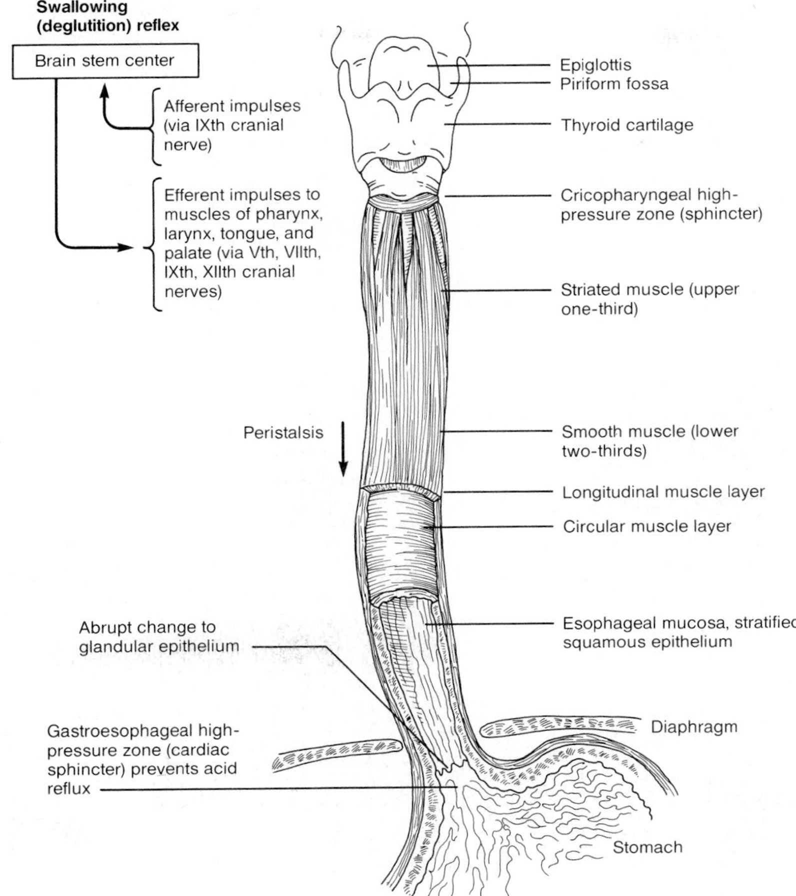

Figure 37–1. Structure and function of the esophagus.

blood in the stools. ("Occult" blood is blood not grossly visible but detectable by chemical testing.)

METHODS OF EVALUATING THE ESOPHAGUS

Clinical Examination

The esophagus is inaccessible for physical examination, most of its course being in the posterior mediastinum.

Radiology

Chest x-ray may in some cases show extreme esophageal dilatation. The only condition that commonly produces esophageal enlargement sufficient to be seen on chest x-ray is achalasia of the cardia ("megaesophagus").

Swallowing barium permits visualization of the passage of dye down the esophagus. This provides information regarding propulsive peristalsis, the presence of any obstructive lesions, and mucosal abnormalities.

Computerized tomography of the chest permits evaluation of lesions in the wall of the esophagus and is a good technique for evaluating spread of esophageal neoplasms.

Esophagoscopy

Passage of a fiberoptic endoscope into the esophagus permits direct visualization and biopsy of mucosal lesions of the esophagus.

Manometry & pH Measurement

The passage of a manometer and pH meter down the esophagus permits measurement of pressures and pH in different parts of the esophagus. This is useful in the evaluation of esophageal peristalsis and competence of the lower esophageal sphincter.

Table 37-1. Esophageal causes of dysphagia.[1]

Functional: Failure of deglutition reflex without mechanical obstruction of the esophagus
- Neurologic diseases affecting the lower cranial nerves (cranial polyneuritis), medulla oblongata (poliomyelitis), upper motor neuron (bilateral cerebral ischemia, motor neuron disease, hysteria)
- Muscular dystrophies may affect the striated muscle of the upper esophagus
- Myasthenia gravis may interfere with neuromuscular transmission
- Plummer-Vinson syndrome
- Progressive systemic sclerosis (scleroderma) due to replacement of esophageal muscle by fibrosis, causing failure of peristalsis
- Achalasia of the cardia
- Aging: abnormalities of peristalsis occur in the elderly (presbyesophagus)

Mechanical: Physical obstruction of the esophagus
- Intraluminal obstruction
  - Foreign bodies
  - Webs (in some cases of Plummer-Vinson syndrome)
- Intramural obstruction
  - Strictures, following reflux esophagitis, peptic ulceration, or ingestion of lye (a corrosive alkali)
  - Neoplasms of the esophagus
    - Benign (rare)
    - Malignant (carcinoma of the esophagus is the most important cause)
- Extrinsic compression (uncommon)
  - Abnormal arteries: dysphagia lusoria
  - Enlarged left atrium (mitral stenosis) and pericardial effusion
  - Aortic aneurysms
  - Hypertrophic vertebral osteophytes
  - Mediastinal cysts and neoplasms

[1]Oropharyngeal abnormalities may also cause dysphagia: pharyngeal diverticula (Zenker's); oropharyngeal tumors; and inflammatory lesions (see Chapter 31). The most common single cause of dysphagia is pharyngotonsillitis.

Table 37-2. Causes of hematemesis.[1,2]

Esophageal causes
- *Esophageal varices in portal hypertension
- *Carcinoma of the esophagus
- *Mallory-Weiss syndrome
- Peptic ulcer and reflux esophagitis
- Esophageal perforation
  - Traumatic, postendoscopic
- Other neoplams of the esophagus
  - Leiomyosarcoma, malignant lymphoma

Gastric causes
- *Chronic gastric ulcer
- Postgastrectomy marginal ulcer
- *Acute gastric ulcer and acute gastritis
  - Stress ulcers (burns, postsurgical)
  - Drug-induced gastritis
    - Aspirin (salicylates), indomethacin, phenylbutazone, ibuprofen, corticosteroids
  - Alcoholic gastritis
- Benign polyps of the stomach
  - Inflammatory, adenomatous, hyperplastic
- *Gastric malignant neoplasms
  - Carcinoma, lymphoma, leiomyosarcoma
- Pancreatic pseudocyst perforating into the stomach

Duodenal causes
- *Chronic duodenal ulcer
- *Acute duodenal ulcer
  - Stress ulcers
- Duodenal neoplasms
  - *Periampullary carcinoma
  - Benign neoplasms
    - Brunner's gland adenoma, adenomas (Gardner's syndrome), paraganglioma

Generalized diseases
- *Hereditary hemorrhagic telangiectasia
- Scurvy
- Congenital diseases of collagen synthesis
  - Pseudoxanthoma elasticum, Ehlers-Danlos syndrome, blue rubber bleb nevus syndrome
- Henoch-Schönlein purpura
- Polyarteritis nodosa
- Amyloidosis
- Kaposi's sarcoma (in AIDS)

[1]More common causes are marked with asterisk.
[2]Hematemesis usually occurs when there is rapid bleeding into the gastrointestinal tract above the duodenojejunal junction. Exceptions to this rule are uncommon.

CONGENITAL ESOPHAGEAL ANOMALIES

TRACHEOESOPHAGEAL FISTULA

Tracheoesophageal fistula is the commonest congenital anomaly of the esophagus. Several clinical types exist (Fig 37–2B–D), some associated with varying degrees of atresia (failure of development) of the esophagus. The most dangerous types of fistula are those in which swallowed material (the first milk meal of the newborn) passes into the trachea, causing severe acute respiratory distress with cyanosis and aspiration pneumonia.

OTHER ANOMALIES

Other congenital anomalies are rare. Esophageal atresia (Fig37–2A) causes narrowing (stricture) of a part of the esophagus. In congenital short esophagus (uncommon), the gastroesophageal junction is above the diaphragm; it must be carefully distinguished from Barrett's esophagus. Also uncommon is the congenital occurrence of ectopic gastric mucosa in the esophagus.

INFLAMMATORY LESIONS OF THE ESOPHAGUS

REFLUX ESOPHAGITIS (Peptic Esophagitis)

Reflux of acid gastric juice into the lower esophagus occurs several times a day even in nor-

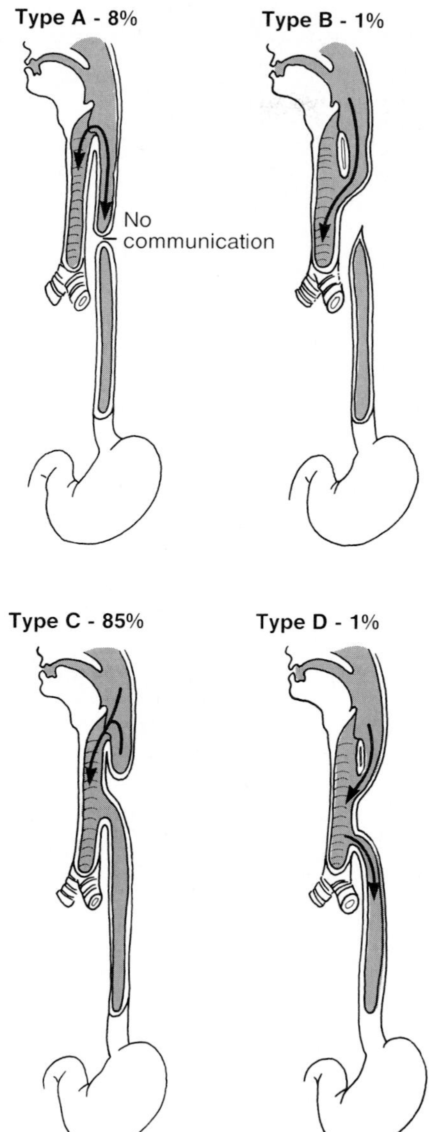

Figure 37–2. Congenital anomalies of the esophagus. **Type A (8%):** Atresia of the esophagus without tracheoesophageal fistula. Collection of food and fluid in the upper esophagus may result in aspiration into the larynx. **Type B (1%):** Atresia of the esophagus with fistula between the blind upper segment and the trachea. **Type C (85%):** Atresia of the esophagus with fistula between the trachea and distal segment. **Type D (1%):** Esophageal atresia with fistulous communication between both segments and the trachea. In **type E** (**5%,** not shown), there is a fistula between a normal esophagus and the trachea. Those children in whom the defect causes milk to enter the trachea, either directly **(B, D,** and **E)** or by reflux **(A** and **C)**, present with coughing and cyanosis during feeding; aspiration bronchopneumonia may follow. Those anomalies in which the trachea communicates with the lower esophagus **(C, D,** and **E)** are associated with gastric dilatation due to ''swallowed'' air.

mal individuals without producing symptoms or inflammation. Symptomatic esophagitis is believed to occur when there is excessive reflux, both in number of episodes and in volume, or when the normal mechanisms for clearing the lower esophagus are impaired. In a normal individual, any fluid regurgitated into the lower esophagus is rapidly returned to the stomach by peristalsis. Impairment of peristalsis permits prolonged exposure of the mucosa to acid. The composition of the refluxed gastric juice may also be an important determinant of reflux. The levels of acid and pepsin, as well as the presence of bile and pancreatic enzymes refluxed from the duodenum—all may play a part. When bile reflux is present, esophagitis may occur even when the refluxed gastric juice is alkaline (''alkaline reflux'').

The relationship of reflux to **hiatal hernia** is not clear. A hiatal hernia is defined as protrusion of part of the stomach through the diaphragmatic hiatus (Fig 37–3). Reflux occurs most often in sliding type hernias, probably because obliteration of the cardioesophageal angle renders the lower esophageal sphincter incompetent. However, most patients with reflux esophagitis do not have a detectable hiatal hernia, and most patients with a demonstrable hernia do not have symptoms of reflux esophagitis despite increased reflux, suggesting a role for other factors such as clearing of the lower esophagus by peristalsis.

Pathology (Fig 37–3)

Reflux esophagitis can be recognized endoscopically as reddening and superficial erosion of the lower esophagus. It may progress to peptic ulceration and fibrous narrowing of the esophagus (stricture).

Histologically, early reflux esophagitis can be diagnosed in an esophageal biopsy by the presence of hyperplasia of the basal cells of the squamous epithelium, elongation of submucosal papillae, and the presence of neutrophils in the epithelium.

Clinical Features

Reflux of acid gastric juice into an inflamed esophagus causes a low retrosternal sensation of burning pain (''heartburn''), typically when the patient lies flat. In chronic cases, pain may be constant and dysphagia may occur as a result of fibrous stricture formation.

Complications

A. Barrett's Esophagus: (Fig 37–4.) Prolonged reflux esophagitis commonly leads to metaplasia of the epithelium of the esophagus from squamous to glandular (Barrett's esophagus). Three types of glandular epithelium occur: (1) a cardiac type, resembling gastric cardiac mucosa; (2) a fundic type, resembling gastric fundus with acid-secreting cells; and (3) an intestinal type,

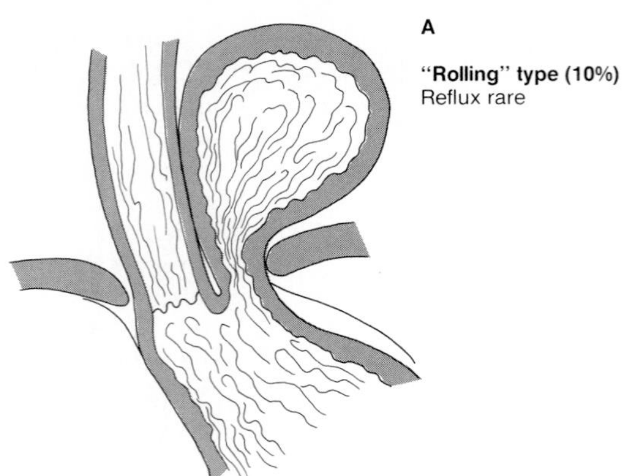

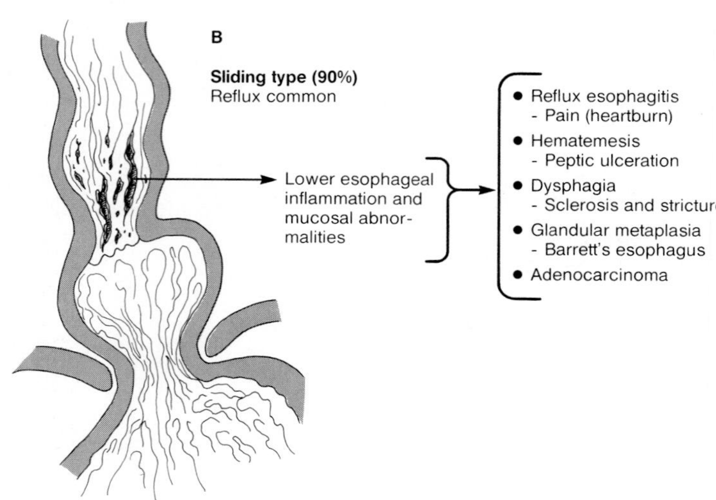

Figure 37-3. Hiatus hernia. **A:** Rolling type (10%) characterized by herniation of the gastric cardia into the thorax through the diaphragmatic hiatus alongside the normal esophagus. Note that the normal cardioesophageal angle is maintained; reflux is rare. **B:** Sliding type (90%) characterized by shortening of the esophagus and entry of the gastroesophageal junction and proximal stomach into the thorax. The normal cardioesophageal angle is lost, and reflux of gastric juice is common. Complications of reflux of gastric juice include reflux esophagitis, peptic ulceration, fibrosis and stricture formation, and Barrett's esophagus.

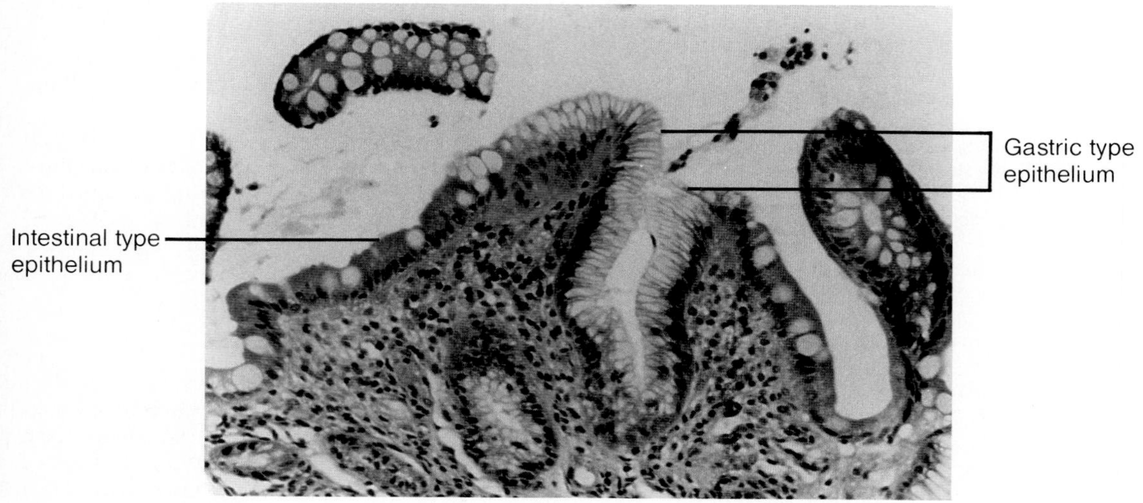

Figure 37-4. Barrett's esophagus, showing the characteristic specialized columnar epithelium composed of a mixture of gastric and intestinal type epithelial cells.

which resembles small intestine, with villi and goblet cells. Most primary adenocarcinomas of the lower end of the esophagus arise in Barrett's esophagus—particularly the intestinal type, which therefore is a precancerous lesion. The glandular epithelial cells pass through progressive dysplastic changes that permit histologic recognition of imminent change to cancer.

B. Peptic Ulceration and Fibrous Strictures: Severe reflux leads to chronic peptic ulcers in the lower esophagus. Subsequent fibrosis leads to esophageal stricture and dysphagia.

INFECTIOUS ESOPHAGITIS

Infections are rare in the esophagus except in immunocompromised patients, notably in AIDS.

1. *CANDIDA ALBICANS* ESOPHAGITIS

Esophageal candidosis is one of the common opportunistic infections in patients receiving cancer chemotherapy and those with AIDS. The yeast infects the superficial layers of the squamous epithelium, forming grossly visible adherent white plaques. The main symptom is odynophagia. The diagnosis is made by identifying the fungus in smears, cultures, or biopsy specimens taken from the lesions.

2. VIRAL ESOPHAGITIS

Herpes simplex esophagitis is common in AIDS and can be recognized in biopsies by the presence of Cowdry type A intranuclear inclusions and herpetic giant cells and by the immunologic demonstration of herpes simplex antigen.

Cytomegalovirus is also a common cause of esophagitis in AIDS. CMV infects submucosal endothelial cells, causing focal ischemia, hemorrhage, inflammation, and ulceration. Typical enlarged cells with large intranuclear inclusions and granular cytoplasmic inclusions are present.

Esophageal involvement may rarely occur in severe attacks of chickenpox, where vesiculation of infected epithelium is followed by ulceration.

TRAUMATIC & CHEMICAL ESOPHAGITIS

Prolonged feeding through a nasogastric tube frequently causes mucosal inflammation, often with ulceration.

Ingestion of corrosives such as phenol, strong acids, and mercuric chloride leads to chemical esophagitis. The strongly alkaline chemical known as lye, which is swallowed in some parts of the world in suicide attempts, causes severe esophagitis with mucosal denudation in the acute phase. Marked fibrous scarring in survivors often requires repeated dilatation of the esophagus to overcome resulting obstruction. Lye ingestion is also associated with a greatly increased risk (1000 times normal) of development of squamous carcinoma of the esophagus.

FUNCTIONAL CAUSES OF DYSPHAGIA (Table 37-1)

PLUMMER-VINSON SYNDROME

Plummer-Vinson syndrome consists of severe iron deficiency anemia, koilonychia, atrophic glossitis, and dysphagia. It is common in Scandinavian countries and uncommon in the United States. The disease has a marked female preponderance owing to the frequency of negative iron balance in women as a result of menstrual blood loss.

The dysphagia is corrected when the iron deficiency is treated. Dysphagia results from (1) atrophy of the pharyngeal mucosa, caused by iron deficiency, which is believed to interfere with the afferent arc of the deglutition reflex; and (2) weblike mucosal folds present in the upper esophagus in some patients, causing mechanical obstruction.

There is a greater than normal risk of developing squamous carcinoma of the upper esophagus, oropharynx, and posterior tongue.

PROGRESSIVE SYSTEMIC SCLEROSIS (Scleroderma)

The esophagus is commonly involved in systemic sclerosis, and dysphagia is a common symptom. Involvement takes the form of submucosal and muscular vasculitis with muscle wall degeneration and fibrosis. Smooth muscle loss leads to failure of peristalsis and dysphagia.

ACHALASIA OF THE CARDIA

Achalasia (Gk "unrelaxed") of the cardia is a common disease resulting from loss of ganglion cells in the myenteric plexus of the esophagus. Ganglion cell loss is present throughout the body of the esophagus and is not restricted to the cardia. The cause is unknown in most cases; a few cases are caused by *Trypanosoma cruzi* infection

(South American trypanosomiasis; Chagas' disease).

The myenteric plexus abnormality leads to failure of propulsive peristaltic waves without which the cardiac sphincter does not relax, creating a zone of high pressure that obstructs the passage of food into the stomach. The esophagus dilates massively above the cardia and becomes elongated and tortuous (Fig 37–5). The mucosa is usually normal but may show areas of superficial inflammation and ulceration.

Patients present with dysphagia. Nutrition is maintained reasonably well until the late stages of the disease, when obstruction becomes complete. With collection of food in the esophagus, the hydrostatic pressure therein increases and becomes sufficient to physically overcome the sphincter, permitting the intermittent entry of food into the stomach.

An important complication of achalasia is aspiration of the contents of the dilated esophagus into the trachea, leading to recurrent attacks of aspiration pneumonia.

Treatment by intraluminal dilatation or by surgical myotomy is effective, but many patients need repeated dilatations. Achalasia imposes a minimal or no increased risk of carcinoma and should not be regarded as a premalignant lesion.

ESOPHAGEAL DIVERTICULA

Diverticula (outpouchings of the lumen of a viscus outside the wall of that viscus) are not common, but if large they may cause dysphagia or local inflammation. Pulsion diverticula are believed to occur when internal pressure forces an epithelial sac through a weakened or defective muscle wall. Traction diverticula are due to external inflammatory lesions resulting in fibrosis and traction force that pulls out the full thickness of the esophageal wall as a diverticulum.

ESOPHAGEAL VARICES

Gastroesophageal varices (Fig 37–6) occur in the lower esophagus and gastric fundus at the site of portosystemic venous anastomoses in patients

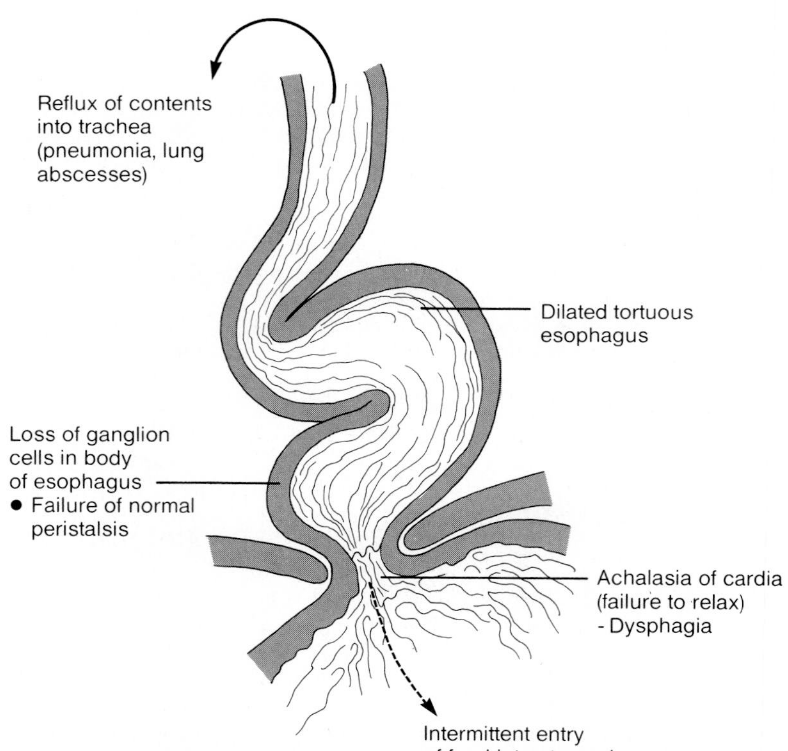

Figure 37–5. Achalasia of the cardia. The primary defect is a failure of normal peristalsis due to loss of ganglion cells in the body of the esophagus. This leads to failure of relaxation (achalasia) of the lower esophageal sphincter (cardia).

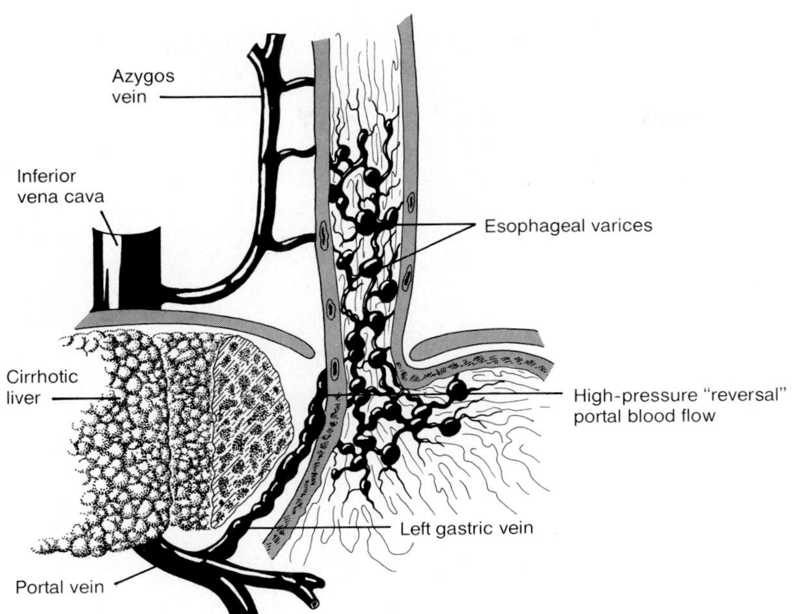

Figure 37-6. Esophageal varices resulting from portal venous hypertension caused by cirrhosis of the liver.

with portal hypertension due to any cause. The dilated, tortuous veins at increased hydrostatic pressure are mainly submucosal, and their rupture causes severe hemorrhage (hematemesis and melena).

MALLORY-WEISS SYNDROME

Prolonged vomiting is common in alcoholics and pregnant women. Violent retching may produce a longitudinal tear in the mucosa of the lowest part of the esophagus. Severe hemorrhage with hematemesis occurs.

NEOPLASMS OF THE ESOPHAGUS

CARCINOMA OF THE ESOPHAGUS

Incidence

Esophageal carcinoma accounts for over 95% of neoplasms of the esophagus and about 1% of cancers involving the gastrointestinal tract. It is highly lethal and causes about 2% of all cancer deaths in the United States (about 9000 per year). It is a disease of older people (over 50 years) and is more common in males and blacks. Cancer of the esophagus is much more common in the Far East (notably China) and in certain parts of Africa and Iran. In Iran, there is an unusual female preponderance of the disease.

Etiology

In the United States, chronic alcoholism increases the risk of esophageal carcinoma 20- to 30-fold. Cigarette smoking increases the risk 10- to 20-fold. Smoking and alcoholism are less often factors in the epidemiology of esophageal cancer in China, Africa, and Iran. The cause of esophageal cancer in the high-incidence areas of the world is unknown. Hot rice and tea, nitrosamines and aflatoxins in food, contaminants in locally brewed beer, and smoked fish have all been suggested as causative factors—all without proof.

Many premalignant conditions are associated with an increased risk of esophageal carcinoma. These include lye strictures (squamous carcinoma), Plummer-Vinson syndrome (squamous carcinoma), and Barrett's esophagus (adenocarcinoma).

Pathology

In the United States, 50% of esophageal cancers arise in the middle third, 30% in the lower third, and 20% in the upper third of the organ. In Scandinavia, where Plummer-Vinson syndrome is common, upper esophageal cancer is more frequent.

The early lesion is a plaquelike thickening of the mucosa (Fig 37–7). From its mucosal origin, carcinoma may extend (1) into the lumen as a polypoid, fungating mass that may break down to form a malignant ulcer with raised everted edges (Fig 37–8); (2) transversely in the submucosa, to involve the whole circumference of the esophagus; or (3) into the wall of the esophagus. A marked desmoplastic (fibrotic) response causes fibrosis with esophageal narrowing (malignant stricture). The exact appearance of the carcinoma depends on which of these growth patterns predominates.

Microscopically, over 90% of esophageal carcinomas are squamous carcinomas. Adenocarcinoma (arising in esophageal glands or in Barrett's esophagus) and undifferentiated carcinomas account for the rest. Most adenocarcinomas occur in the lower third of the esophagus.

Spread (Fig 37–9)

Local invasion through the esophageal wall to involve adjacent cervical and mediastinal structures occurs early. Invasion of the bronchial wall may rarely result in tracheoesophageal fistula, commonly complicated by necrotizing pneumonia. Invasion of the aorta may lead to massive hemorrhage. Recurrent laryngeal nerve involvement leads to vocal cord paralysis (hoarseness).

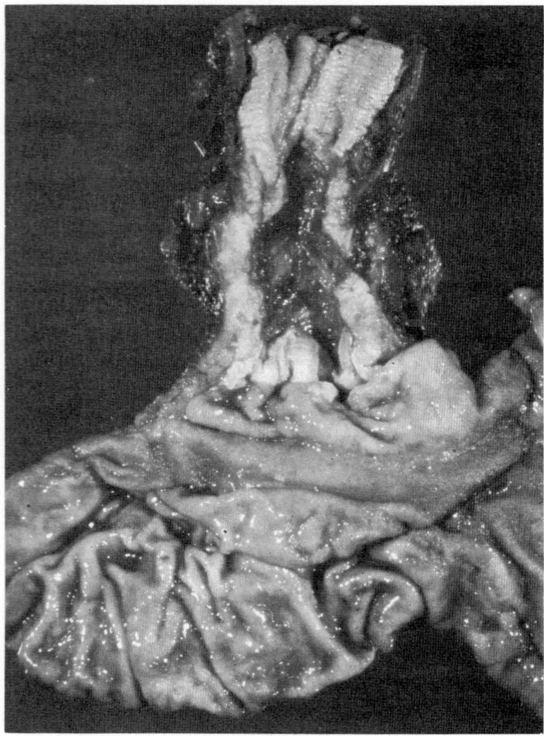

Figure 37–8. Carcinoma of the esophagus, immediately superior to the gastroesophageal junction, showing a large ulcer with everted edges.

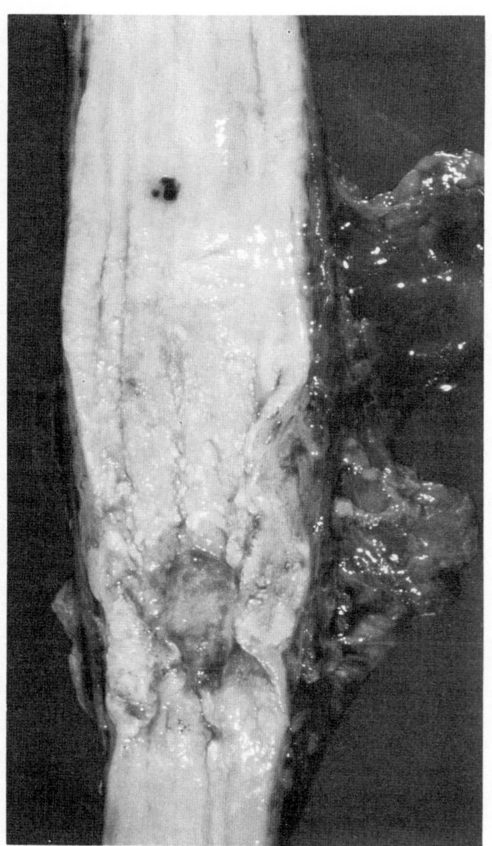

Figure 37–7. Carcinoma of the esophagus, showing ulceration and circumferential involvement of the mucosa.

Lymphatic spread occurs early, and lymph node metastases are usually present at the time of diagnosis. Bloodstream spread with metastases to liver and lung also occurs early.

Clinical Features & Diagnosis

Most patients present with dysphagia and severe weight loss, and most have large unresectable tumors at this stage. Less often, presentation is with anemia, hematemesis, or melena. The diagnosis is best established by endoscopic visualization of the tumor followed by biopsy.

Cytologic examination of a brush specimen of esophageal mucosa has been used as a screening method in high-incidence areas such as China; it is not cost-effective for use in the United States because of the relative infrequency of the disease.

Treatment & Prognosis

Most patients with esophageal cancers have unresectable tumors at the time of presentation. Ra-

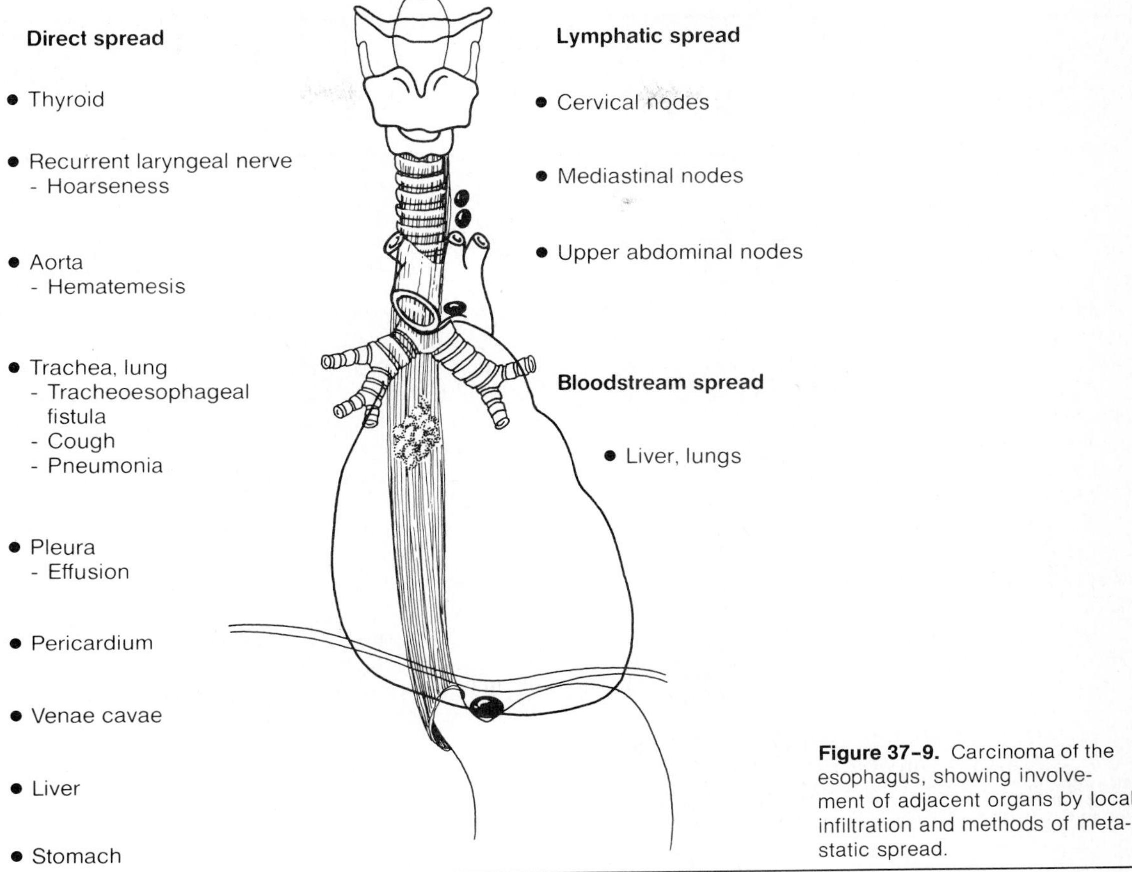

Figure 37-9. Carcinoma of the esophagus, showing involvement of adjacent organs by local infiltration and methods of metastatic spread.

diotherapy may cause some regression of tumor but is not curative. Chemotherapy is not very effective, though new regimens are starting to provide a glimmer of hope.

The overall prognosis is very poor, 70% of patients being dead within 1 year after diagnosis and fewer than 10% surviving 5 years. Often the aim of treatment is palliation to relieve pain and permit swallowing.

OTHER NEOPLASMS OF THE ESOPHAGUS

Neoplasms other than carcinomas are rare in the esophagus. Leiomyoma is the commonest benign neoplasm, but it rarely causes symptoms. Leiomyosarcoma, malignant lymphoma, malignant melanoma, and carcinoid tumors have been reported.

38 The Stomach

STRUCTURE & FUNCTION

The stomach lies in the epigastrium and is composed of mucosa, submucosa, a thick muscle layer, and serosa. The mucosa of the stomach is thrown into regular folds, or rugae. The serosa on the lesser and greater curvatures is continuous with the lesser and greater omentum.

The Gastric Mucosa (Fig 38–1)

The epithelial lining of the mucosa is composed of uniform mucous cells without goblet cells. Simple tubular glands open on the surface at epithelial pits. The glands vary in structure in different parts of the stomach: (1) In the cardiac region near the gastroesophageal junction, the glands are composed mainly of mucous cells. (2) In the body and fundus, the glands contain parietal (oxyntic) cells that secrete acid and chief (zymogen, or peptic) cells that secrete pepsin. The parietal cells also probably secrete intrinsic factor. (3) In the pyloric antrum, the glands contain mainly mucous cells.

Neuroendocrine cells are present in the mucosa of the stomach just as they are throughout the remainder of the intestinal tract. These cells are present throughout the mucosa and produce a variety of biogenic amines and peptide hormones. Neuroendocrine cells in the pyloric antral region (G cells) represent the source of gastrin and may be stained by immunohistologic methods using antigastrin antibodies.

Gastric Mucosal Resistance to Acid

The secretion of acid by the stomach is a continuous process, occurring at a basal rate during fasting and increasing markedly in response to a meal. Acid secretion during a meal has 3 phases: cephalic, gastric, and intestinal (Fig 38–2). Histamine plays an important yet uncertain role in acid release; drugs that are histamine H_2 receptor antagonists (eg, cimetidine) are extremely effective in reducing gastric acid secretion. Intestinal hormones also provide negative feedback on acid secretion via secretin, enteroglucagon, vasoactive intestinal polypeptide (VIP), and gastric inhibitory peptide (GIP).

The gastric mucosa is protected by a variety of mechanisms from the erosive effect of gastric acid:

(1) The anatomic integrity of the mucosa. The mucosal cells have tight intercellular junctions that prevent back-diffusion of acid.

(2) Gastric mucus, which coats the mucosal cells and acts as a barrier. The mucus represents an alkaline layer that prevents direct action of acid on the mucosa.

(3) Prostaglandins (E series), which are synthesized and secreted by gastric mucosal cells and have a cytoprotective effect on the gastroduodenal mucosa, acting to increase bicarbonate secretion, gastric mucus production, mucosal blood flow, and the rate of mucosal cell regeneration.

(4) Mucosal blood flow. Ischemia of the mucosa decreases mucosal resistance.

Functions of the Stomach

The main function of the stomach is to serve as a reservoir for meals, presenting food to the duodenum in small regulated amounts. The acid gastric juice contains the proteolytic enzyme pepsin and initiates digestion. The acidity also has an

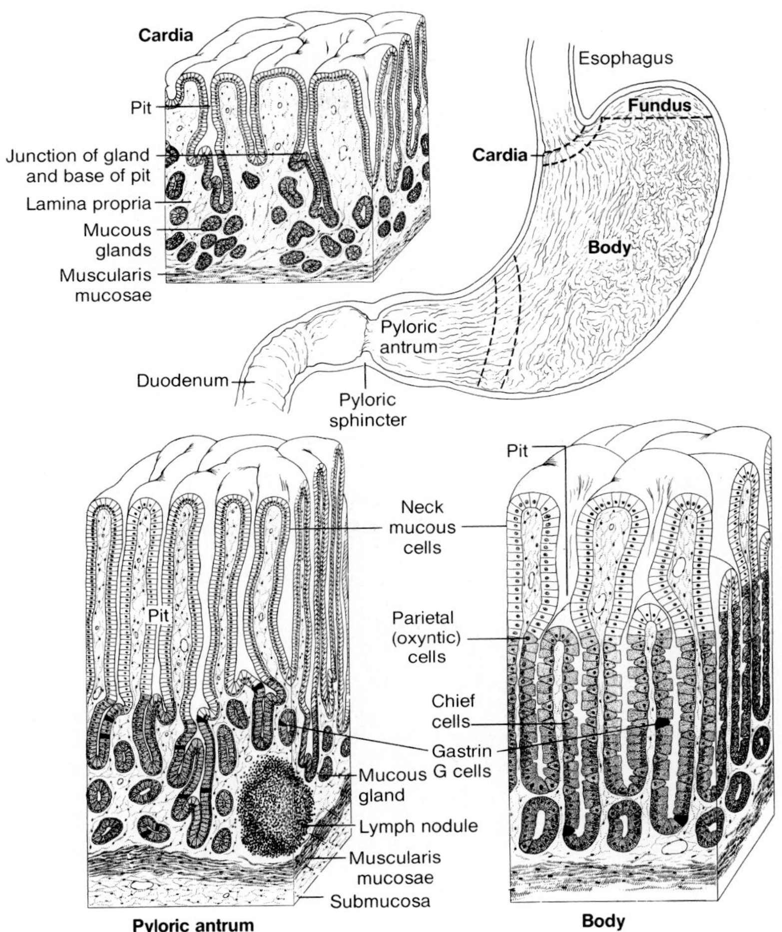

Figure 38–1. Regions of the stomach and their histologic structure.

antibacterial action. Simple molecules such as iron, alcohol, and glucose may be absorbed from the stomach.

The stomach has 2 sphincters. A physiologic sphincter at the cardioesophageal junction prevents reflux of acid gastric juice into the esophagus. The distal or pyloric sphincter is an anatomic thickening of the muscle that controls the rate of gastric emptying and prevents reflux of bile into the stomach.

CLINICAL MANIFESTATIONS OF GASTRIC DISEASE (Fig 38–3)

Pain & Dyspepsia

Pain is a feature of acute gastritis and peptic ulcer disease. It is epigastric, burning in nature, and is related to intake of food. Pain of gastric origin is often accompanied by nausea and vomiting. Dyspepsia may include pain but is also manifested by bloating, distention, and eructation.

Loss of Appetite

A loss of desire for food (anorexia) occurs in gastritis and gastric carcinoma. This must be distinguished from a fear of eating because it precipitates pain (as occurs with peptic ulcer) and from early satiety (feeling of fullness), which occurs in conditions where gastric volume is decreased (commonly neoplasms).

Bleeding

Bleeding into the gastric lumen is a common manifestation of gastric disease, occurring in any disease where the mucosal surface becomes eroded. The clinical manifestations depend on the severity and rate of bleeding. When bleeding is severe and rapid, the patient vomits bright red blood (hematemesis). When bleeding is less rapid, the blood is altered by gastric acid and passes

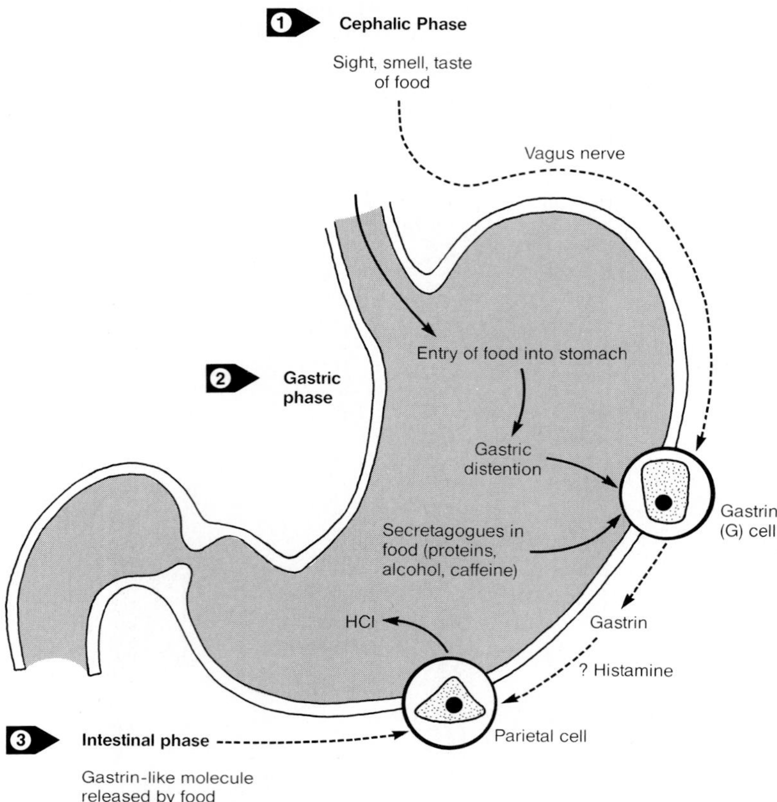

Figure 38-2. Secretion of acid in the stomach.

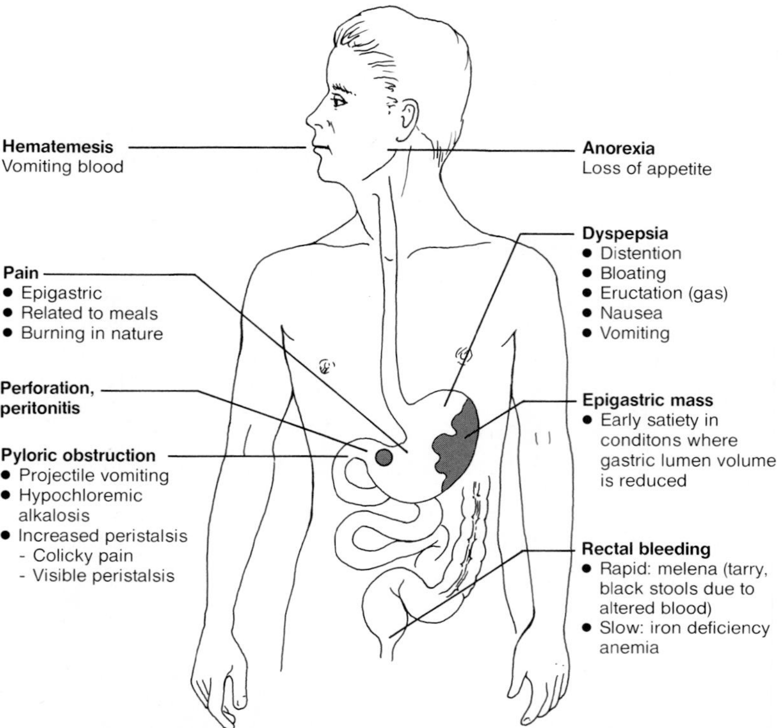

Figure 38-3. Clinical manifestations of gastric disease.

through the intestines, forming tarry black stools (melena). With chronic slow bleeding, the patient commonly presents with iron deficiency anemia and the fecal occult blood test is positive.

Gastric Mass

Neoplasms of the stomach may produce a palpable mass in the epigastrium. In most cases, radiologic examination is required to confirm the gastric origin of an epigastric mass.

Gastric Outlet Obstruction (Pyloric Stenosis)

Obstruction at the pylorus leads to dilatation of the stomach and active peristalsis, which may be visible. Vomiting is a feature and is often profuse. The loss of large volumes of gastric juice in vomiting leads to hypokalemic alkalosis.

Pyloric stenosis may occur as a congenital anomaly (see below) or may be associated with peptic ulcer disease or gastric neoplasms, mainly carcinoma.

METHODS OF EVALUATING THE STOMACH

The mucosal structure of the stomach can be assessed by x-rays taken after a meal of radiopaque material, such as barium, or by gastric endoscopy. Endoscopy also permits photography and biopsy of suspicious areas.

Abdominal ultrasound and computerized tomography permit assessment of the stomach wall, being particularly useful in the detection of mass lesions.

Gastric function tests include the following: (1) tests to determine secretion of acid under a variety of conditions, including resting acid secretion and maximum secretion after histamine or pentagastrin stimulation; (2) Schilling's test for absorption of vitamin B_{12}, which gives information about secretion of intrinsic factor; (3) measurement of the serum gastrin level, which is useful in evaluation of peptic ulcer disease and certain rare neoplasms; and (4) detection of antibodies in serum against parietal cell components and intrinsic factor, which may aid in diagnosis of autoimmune gastritis (pernicious anemia).

CONGENITAL PYLORIC STENOSIS

Pyloric stenosis is one of the most common congenital disorders of the gastrointestinal tract, occurring in 1:500 live births. It is 4 times more common in males than in females and tends to affect the first-born. There is a familial tendency, but no clear inheritance pattern has been demonstrated.

Marked hypertrophy of the muscle at the pyloric sphincter results in obstruction to gastric emptying. Symptoms of gastric outlet obstruction typically appear 1–2 weeks after birth. Projectile vomiting is accompanied by visible enlargement of the stomach in the epigastric region. Peristalsis can be observed in the dilated stomach, and in most cases the hypertrophied pylorus can be palpated as a firm ovoid mass.

Treatment consists of surgical splitting of the hypertrophied muscle to the level of the mucosa (myotomy). This procedure is successful in most cases.

INFLAMMATORY LESIONS OF THE STOMACH

ACUTE GASTRITIS (Fig 38–4)

Acute gastritis is a common pathologic finding in autopsies and in gastric biopsies. It is characterized by hyperemia, edema, and neutrophilic infiltration of the lamina propria. The lesion may involve the stomach diffusely or may be localized to one region of the mucosa. Affected areas show diffuse reddening of the mucosa with multiple small erosions and ulcers. Severe cases are characterized by hemorrhage into the mucosa (acute hemorrhagic gastritis), multiple erosions of the mucosa (acute erosive gastritis), and the occurrence of small mucosal ulcers (acute stress or peptic ulceration; Fig 38–5); an erosion is a partial denudation of the surface epithelium and differs from an ulcer, which involves the full thickness of the mucosa.

Etiology & Pathogenesis

Many factors have been implicated in acute gastritis (Fig 38–4); however, in individual cases the exact mechanism is often obscure.

A. Direct infection of the stomach with agents such as viruses and *Salmonella* causes cell

CAUSES
Corrosive chemicals
Alcohol
Heavy smoking
Corticosteroids
Anticancer drugs
Radiation
Uremia
Bile reflux

Infection
- Viral gastroenteritis (rota virus)
- Hepatitis virus
- Salmonellosis (food poisoning)
- *Campylobacter pylori*
- Staphylococcal entero-toxin

Severe stress
- Burns (Curling's ulcers)
- Intracranial lesions (Cushing's ulcers)
- Shock
- Myocardial infarction

Mucosal edema, hemorrhage, and inflammation
Diffuse mucosal hyperemia
Multiple erosions and ulcers

Figure 38-4. Acute gastritis. Causes and pathologic features.

loss and inflammation. *Campylobacter pylori* is a recently described bacterium commonly found in the gastric mucosa in patients with gastritis. *C pylori* is believed to cause the histologic changes of acute gastritis in those cases where the organism is present. It may be demonstrated in gastric biopsies by histologic examination or culture.

B. Direct toxicity by chemicals such as ethyl alcohol and bile produces cell damage. Alcoholic gastritis is characterized by hemorrhage in the lamina propria.

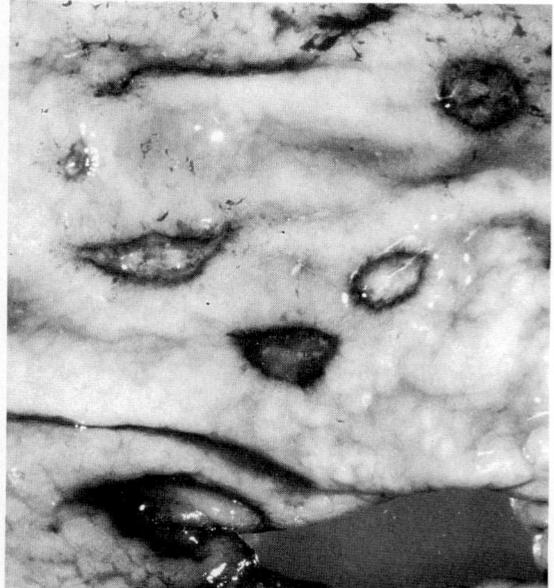

Figure 38-5. Acute gastritis showing multiple small ulcers in the mucosa.

C. Decreased mucosal resistance to acid is believed responsible for most other cases of gastritis. Decreased resistance permits back diffusion of acid into the mucosa, resulting in injury and acute inflammation; the level of acid secretion itself is usually normal in these patients. Mucosal resistance may decrease for the following reasons:

1. Inhibition of prostaglandin secretion by aspirin or other anti-inflammatory agents. Smoking also inhibits synthesis of prostaglandin E.

2. Interference with mucosal epithelial regeneration by antimitotic drugs results in loss of an effective anatomic mucosal barrier.

3. Ischemia-Decreased mucosal blood supply is believed to play a role in the gastritis associated with shock. Cigarette smoking may also decrease perfusion due to the vasoconstrictive action of nicotine.

Clinical Features

Mild acute gastritis causes no symptoms. Epigastric pain, nausea, vomiting, and anorexia occur in moderate and severe gastritis. The correlation between symptoms, endoscopic changes, and histologic changes is poor. Acute gastric hemorrhage causing hematemesis and melena occurs mainly with drug-induced (aspirin is the chief offender) and stress-induced gastritis. Hemorrhage in these cases may rarely be so severe as to threaten life.

Treatment of acute gastritis depends on recognizing the cause. Symptomatic treatment, mainly reducing acid secretion with cimetidine, may be required for the more severe cases. Antibiotics (eg, erythromcycin) and bismuth compounds are effective for *Campylobacter* gastritis.

CHRONIC GASTRITIS (Fig 38–6)

Chronic gastritis is defined as an increase in the number of lymphocytes and plasma cells in the gastric mucosa. The correlation between these changes and endoscopic and clinical features is poor. Several different degrees of chronic gastritis are recognized. The mildest is chronic superficial gastritis, in which there is a lymphocytic infiltrate in the superficial lamina propria. More severe cases involve the full thickness of the mucosa and may be associated with atrophy of the glands.

Etiology & Classification

A. Chronic Atrophic Gastritis of Pernicious Anemia: Pernicious anemia is an autoimmune disease in which there is a constant association between anemia, vitamin B_{12} deficiency, and chronic atrophic gastritis (Chapter 24). Three different autoantibodies may be present in the serum: (1) anti-parietal cell antibody (also called parietal canalicular antibody) in 90%; (2) intrinsic factor-blocking antibody (interferes with intrinsic factor binding to vitamin B_{12}) in 75%; and (3) intrinsic factor-binding antibody (binds with both intrinsic factor and intrinsic factor-B_{12} complex, preventing absorption of the latter) in 50%. The antibodies against intrinsic factor are also found in gastric juice. A minority of pernicious anemia patients lack these antibodies; a T cell-mediated response against parietal cells has been postulated but not proved. There is an association with autoimmune disease of the adrenals and thyroid.

The immune reaction manifests as a lymphoplasmacytic infiltrate in the mucosa around parietal cells, which progressively decrease in number. The fundal and body mucosa decreases in thickness, and the glands become predominantly lined by mucous cells. The gastric epithelium frequently shows intestinal metaplasia, characterized by the appearance of goblet cells in the surface epithelium and Paneth cells in the glands. In the end stage of the disease, the mucosa is atrophic, with absent parietal cells. Since the target of the immune response has been completely destroyed, the immune cells decrease in number. This end stage is sometimes called simple gastric atrophy.

The end results are failure of secretion of acid (hypochlorhydria) and failure of absorption of vitamin B_{12}, due either to defective secretion of intrinsic factor (lack of parietal cells), blockage of intrinsic factor combination with vitamin B_{12} (blocking antibody), or prevention of absorption of the intrinsic factor-vitamin B_{12} complex (binding antibody). Failure of vitamin B_{12} absorption causes megaloblastic anemia, which is the main manifestation of the disease (see Chapter 24).

Patients with pernicious anemia have an increased incidence of development of gastric carcinoma—ie, autoimmune chronic atrophic gastritis is a premalignant lesion. The epithelial cells pass through increasing degrees of dysplasa before cancer develops. Recognition of these changes in biopsies is an indication for partial gastrectomy.

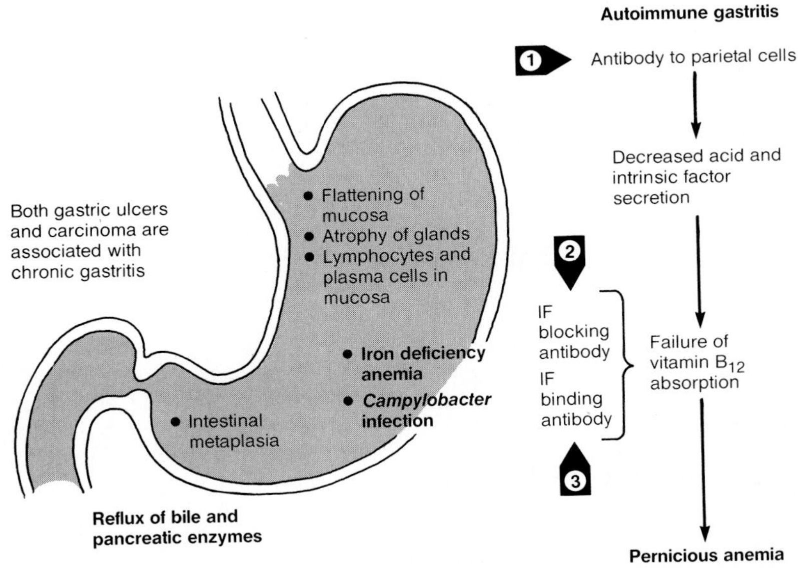

Figure 38–6. Chronic gastritis. Autoimmune gastritis that causes pernicious anemia is an uncommon but specific form of chronic gastritis. The failure of vitamin B_{12} absorption may be caused by failure of synthesis due to destruction of parietal cells by antibody **(1)** or sensitized T cells, intrinsic factor blocking antibody **(2),** or intrinsic factor binding antibody **(3).** Chronic gastritis not associated with autoimmune gastritis has many causes, including *Campylobacter pylori* infection, bile reflux, and iron deficiency anemia. Chronic gastritis occurs commonly in association with gastric ulcers and carcinoma.

The risk of gastric carcinoma in these patients persists even after treatment of pernicious anemia with vitamin B_{12}.

B. Chronic Atrophic Gastritis Not Associated With Pernicious Anemia: Gastric mucosal changes histologically identical with those seen in pernicious anemia may occur in the fundus and body in elderly patients without clinical pernicious anemia. Over half of such patients have serum antibodies against parietal cells or a family history of pernicious anemia. However, these patients do not have antibodies against intrinsic factor, and vitamin B_{12} absorption is normal.

C. Atrophic Gastritis of Iron Deficiency: Iron deficiency anemia typically is associated with gastric mucosal atrophy and hypochlorhydria. Autoantibodies are not present, and the mechanism is unknown.

D. Chronic Antral Gastritis: Chronic inflammation of the pyloric antrum is a completely different disease. The antrum is infiltrated by lymphocytes and plasma cells, and there is intestinal metaplasia of the pyloric epithelium with the appearance of goblet cells and Paneth cells. The fundus and body mucosa is normal, and there is no parietal cell loss or decreased secretion of intrinsic factor. Acid secretion may be reduced owing to loss of antral gastrin-producing G cells (anti-G cell antibodies are present in some cases).

Multiple etiologic factors are involved. Bile acids and lysolecithin have been suggested as the active injurious agents, and antral gastritis is associated with chronic gastric ulcer and gastric carcinoma by an uncertain mechanism. *Campylobacter pylori* is commonly present in biopsies and cultures in antral gastritis and is believed to be causally related.

Clinical Features

Most patients with chronic gastritis—even severe atrophic gastritis—are asymptomatic. Mild epigastric discomfort and pain, nausea, and anorexia may occur, particularly when acute gastritis is superimposed. The diagnosis is suspected upon demonstration of hypochlorhydria and is confirmed by biopsy. Vitamin B_{12} deficiency due to intrinsic factor deficiency is present in cases associated with pernicious anemia.

MENETRIER'S DISEASE (Hypertrophic Gastritis; Rugal Hypertrophy)

Menetrier's disease is a rare condition of unknown cause that occurs mainly in males over 40 years of age. It is characterized by greatly thickened gastric rugal folds (Fig 38–7) that are visible both radiologically and endoscopically. Hyperplasia and cystic dilatation of mucous glands, together with proliferation of the smooth muscle of the muscularis mucosae, suggest that this may be a hamartomatous lesion. Most patients with Menetrier's disease have reduced or normal acid secretion. Overproduction of gastric mucus leads to increased protein loss in the intestine. In the original description of the disease, protein-losing enteropathy was a constant feature.

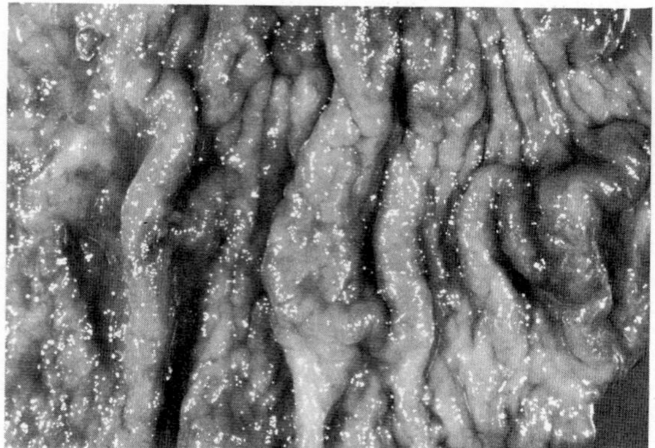

Figure 38–7. Hypertrophic gastritis (Menetrier's disease), showing thickened gastric rugal folds.

Enlarged gastric mucosal folds may also occur in gastric neoplasms, notably malignant lymphoma and gastric carcinoma; in Zollinger-Ellison syndrome, in which hyperplasia of parietal cells is associated with hypersecretion of acid; and in eosinophilic gastroenteritis.

EOSINOPHILIC GASTROENTERITIS

This is a rare disease believed to be due to immunologic hypersensitivity. The gastric and intestinal mucosa is infiltrated by chronic inflammatory cells and numerous eosinophils. The deeper parts of the intestinal wall may be affected, causing thickening of the intestine. Rarely, epithelioid granulomas and a small-vessel vasculitis may be present.

PEPTIC ULCER DISEASE

Peptic ulcers are ulcers occurring in any part of the gastrointestinal tract exposed to the action of acid gastric juice. They occur principally in the duodenum (duodenal ulcer) and stomach (gastric ulcer) (Table 38–1). Peptic ulcer disease is common all over the world. It has been estimated that 5–10% of individuals in the United States suffer from peptic ulcers during their lifetime. Duodenal

Table 38-1. Sites in which peptic ulcers occur.

Site	Comment
Duodenum (first part)	75% of peptic ulcers
Stomach	20% of peptic ulcers, mainly in lesser curvature and pyloric antrum
Lower esophagus	Associated with acid reflux
Stomal (marginal) ulcer	At the stoma of a gastro-enterostomy
Meckel's diverticulum	Associated with the presence of heterotopic gastric mucosa
Distal duodenum, jejunum	In addition to gastric and first-part duodenal ulcers, in patients with Zollinger-Ellison syndrome
Ileum, colon	Very rare; associated with presence of heterotopic gastric mucosa

ulcer is 2–3 times more frequent in males, particularly those under the age of 50 years.

Peptic ulcers occur at all ages; the most common age at onset is 20–40 years. A familial tendency exists for duodenal ulcers but not gastric ulcers. Duodenal ulcers are associated with blood group O, absence of blood group antigens in saliva (''nonsecretors''), and HLA-B5 histocompatibility antigen.

Pathogenesis (Fig 38–8)

A. Hypersecretion of Acid: Acid is necessary for peptic ulcers to form, and ulcers do not occur in achlorhydric states. The cornerstone of treatment of peptic ulcer is to decrease secretion of acid; histamine H_2 receptor antagonists (eg, cimetidine) are highly effective.

However, the exact causal role played by the acid is uncertain. Patients with duodenal ulcers have increased acid secretion with heightened responses to normal stimuli, but patients with gastric ulcers frequently have normal or low acid production. Gastric ulcers most commonly form in the transitional zone between the acid-secreting mucosa of the body and the pyloric antral mucosa. The location of this zone varies greatly in different individuals. Hypersecretion of acid is thus a vital factor but not the complete explanation for peptic ulcer disease.

A marked increase in acid secretion occurs in patients with Zollinger-Ellison syndrome, caused by a gastrin-producing neoplasm of the pancreas. The high gastrin levels stimulate continuous maximal acid secretion by parietal cells. These patients have severe intractable peptic ulcers affecting the stomach, duodenum, and jejunum. In Zollinger-Ellison syndrome, high acid output is the primary cause of peptic ulceration.

B. Decreased Mucosal Resistance to Acid: Decreased resistance of the mucosa to acid is believed to be the primary cause of most gastric ulcers. **Prostaglandin E_2** levels in gastric juice have been shown to be consistently decreased in patients with peptic ulcer. PGE levels rise during the healing phase and remain low in patients whose ulcers do not heal. Inhibitors of prostaglandin synthesis such as aspirin, ibuprofen, and indomethacin—and cigarette smoking—are known to

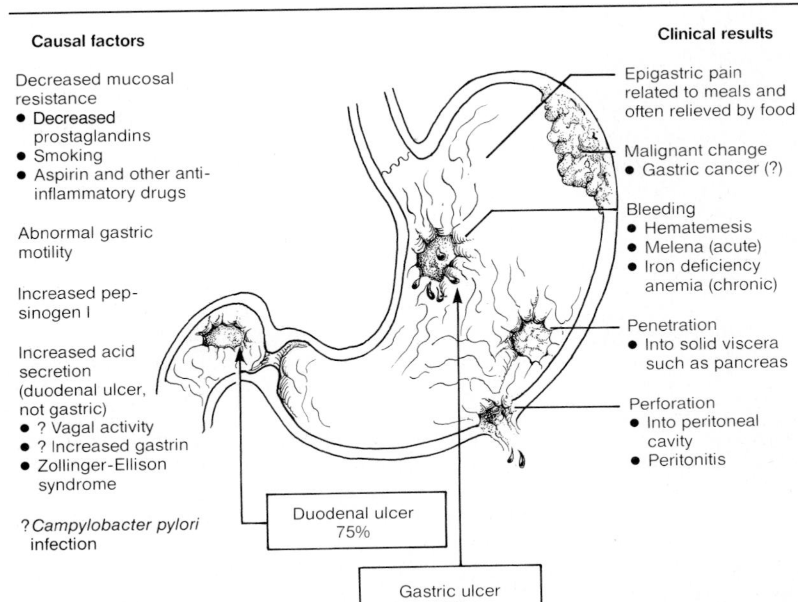

Figure 38–8. Chronic peptic ulcer disease. Causal factors and clinical effects.

have an adverse effect on peptic ulcer healing. Synthetic PGE analogues like misoprostol accelerate healing in experimental studies.

C. Abnormal Gastric Motility: Patients with duodenal ulcer show increased rates of gastric emptying. The precipitous entry of gastric contents may exceed the ability of the duodenum to neutralize the acid, leading to peptic ulceration.

D. Pepsinogen: Increased levels of pepsinogen occur in some ulcer-prone families. However, in the majority of patients with peptic ulcer disease, pepsinogen secretion is unchanged.

Pathology

Chronic peptic ulcers are usually solitary, often large (over 1 cm, rarely larger than 5 cm), and round-to-oval with a punched-out appearance (Fig 38–9). The margins are either flush with the mucosal surface or slightly raised because of edema. The floor of the ulcer is smooth, and its base is thick and firm because of fibrosis. The mucosa around the ulcer is either normal or—in the stomach—shows changes of chronic gastritis. The mucosal folds around the ulcer appear to radiate outward from the ulcer, an effect of fibrous contraction of the base of the ulcer.

Chronic peptic ulcer differs from acute stress ulcer in its etiologic factors and in the size, number, and distribution of lesions (Table 38–2). Acute peptic ulcers tend to be small (< 1 cm), multiple, and distributed throughout the stomach, whereas chronic ulcers are large, solitary, and usually found on the lesser curvature or pyloric antrum (Fig 38–9).

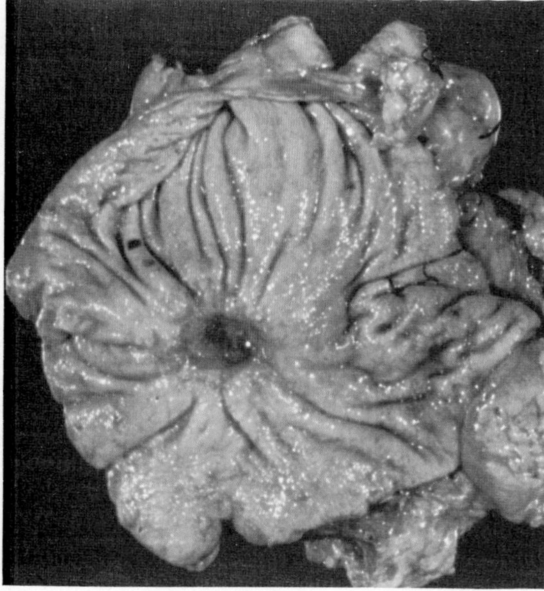

Figure 38–9. Chronic peptic ulcer, showing a large punched-out ulcer below the level of the mucosa. The ulcer edge is flat and flush with the mucosal surface. Note gastric folds radiating from the ulcer.

Microscopically, the base of a chronic peptic ulcer is composed of a surface layer of necrotic, acutely inflamed debris below which is a zone of granulation tissue. Chronic peptic ulcers typically have extensive fibrosis of the base, with extension of fibrosis into the muscle wall. The muscle wall is commonly drawn up into the ulcer base. The epithelium at the edge of the ulcer shows regenerative hyperplasia, which frequently demonstrates marked cytologic atypia, mimicking neoplastic change.

Clinical Features

Peptic ulcer disease is chronic, with remissions and relapses of symptoms, associated with healing and activation of the ulcer disease. Relapses may be precipitated by emotional stress, by drugs such as aspirin, ibuprofen, and steroids, and by cigarette smoking. Few patients with peptic ulcer die of their disease.

Burning or gnawing epigastric pain related to meals is the characteristic symptom of chronic peptic ulcer. Ingestion of food leads to an immediate reduction in pain because the food neutralizes the acid. However, acid secretion is stimulated by the meal, and eating therefore leads to recurrence of pain at a variable time after a meal.

The diagnosis is best established by endoscopy, including biopsy to rule out carcinoma in gastric ulcers. Radiology is also a very effective diagnostic method but is rarely necessary if endoscopy is available. The differentiation of benign and malignant ulcers by radiology is not completely accurate.

Complications (Fig 38–8)

A. Bleeding: Bleeding is the result of erosion of a blood vessel by the ulcer and occurs in about 30% of patients with peptic ulcer. If slow, it causes occult blood loss in feces, leading to iron deficiency anemia. When bleeding is brisk, as occurs when a large artery like the gastroduodenal artery is eroded, hematemesis or melena occurs. Peptic ulcer disease is the commonest cause of hematemesis. Hemorrhage is responsible for 10% of deaths from peptic ulcer disease.

B. Perforation: Perforation occurs in about 5% of peptic ulcer patients, being most common with anterior duodenal ulcers. The entry of gastric juice into the peritoneal cavity results in chemical peritonitis with sudden onset of abdominal pain and boardlike rigidity of the abdominal muscles. Perforation is responsible for over 70% of deaths due to peptic ulcer.

C. Pyloric Obstruction: The fibrosis associated with an ulcer in the pyloric canal or first part of the duodenum may result in gastric outlet ob-

Table 38-2. Differences between acute ulcers, chronic peptic ulcers, and ulcerative gastric carcinoma.

	Acute Ulcer	Chronic Peptic Ulcer	Carcinoma
Etiology	Alcohol, drugs, stress	Hyperacidity, decreased mucosal resistance	Carcinogens (unknown)
Location	Stomach (any part), first part of duodenum	Pyloric antrum, lesser curvature; first part of duodenum	Pyloric antrum; rest of stomach, both lesser and greater curvatures; duodenum spared
Size and form	Small	1-5 cm; may be larger; deep; flat margins	Commonly over 5 cm; may be smaller, polypoid, diffuse, or ulcer with raised margins
Number	Multiple	One or 2	Solitary
Rest of mucosa	Acutely inflamed	Chronic gastritis	Chronic gastritis
Complications	Hemorrhage, perforation	Hemorrhage, perforation, pyloric stenosis, carcinoma (gastric)	Hemorrhage, pyloric stenosis, metastasis
Result	Healing	Healing, recurrence	Usually fatal

struction. Severe vomiting with hypochloremic alkalosis results.

D. Penetration: The ulcerative process may extend through the full thickness of the gut wall into adjacent organs. The fibrotic base of the ulcer is intact in such slow penetration, and there is no perforation. Penetration into the pancreatic substance occurs with posterior ulcers and may lead to constant back pain.

E. Malignant Transformation: Patients with gastric ulcers are at increased risk—probably small (1–3%)—to develop gastric carcinoma. Duodenal ulcers are not associated with an increased risk of malignant transformation.

Treatment

Symptomatic treatment includes diet in the form of frequent small meals and avoidance of cigarette smoking, coffee, and alcohol, the use of antacids and anticholinergic drugs to block vagal stimulation, and cimetidine to block histamine H_2 receptors. Cimetidine (and other histamine H_2 receptor antagonists) is the most effective form of treatment. Surgical treatment includes removal of the ulcer and procedures to decrease gastric acid secretion such as vagotomy to reduce vagal stimulation, and pyloric antrectomy to remove the gastrin-producing region of the stomach.

If a gastric ulcer does not heal with nonsurgical treatment, it should be reexamined by endoscopy and biopsied to exclude the presence of cancer.

Complications of treatment. Hypercalcemia (milk-alkali syndrome) was seen following intensive antacid (diet) therapy. Removal of part of the stomach by surgery may produce "dumping syndrome" due to rapid gastric emptying and postprandial hypoglycemia (due to insulin "overshoot" following rapid entry of glucose into duodenum).

NEOPLASMS OF THE STOMACH

BENIGN NEOPLASMS

MUCOSAL POLYPS

Epithelial polyps are rare in the stomach. Two types occur: adenomatous (10%) and hyperplastic (90%). Both types are usually pedunculated and impose a slightly increased risk of carcinoma—smaller with hyperplastic than with adenomatous polyps. With hyperplastic polyps, cancer frequently occurs in the adjacent mucosa, not in the polyp itself, and removal of the polyp does not remove the risk.

The risk of carcinoma in gastric adenomatous polyps was greatly exaggerated in the past; though adenomatous polyps are to be regarded as premalignant lesions, only a very small number of gastric carcinomas arise in adenomatous polyps.

MESENCHYMAL NEOPLASMS

Mesenchymal neoplasms are uncommon. They include leiomyomas and neurofibroma. Also presenting as a gastric tumor is heterotopic pancreas (also called choristoma) which is not a true neoplasm (see Chapter 17). All of these present as intramural or submucosal nodules that rarely cause symptoms.

MALIGNANT NEOPLASMS

GASTRIC ADENOCARCINOMA

Incidence & Etiology (Table 38-3)

Adenocarcinoma accounts for over 90% of malignant neoplasms of the stomach. The incidence of gastric carcinoma is 5–10 times higher in Japan than in the United States. The incidence is also high in Iceland and Chile. In the United States, the incidence has declined since 1950; presently, about 14,000 individuals die of gastric carcinoma per year (American Cancer Society Statistics, 1984).

Studies in Japanese immigrants to the United States show a decreased incidence from generation to generation, strongly suggesting that some environmental factor causes gastric cancer in Japan. It has been postulated that polycyclic hydrocarbons in smoked fish may be responsible.

The declining incidence of gastric carcinoma in the United States has been attributed to better refrigeration of meat, thereby decreasing the need for preservatives, mainly nitrites. Nitrites are converted to nitrosamines, which have been shown to cause gastric carcinoma in experimental animals.

Gastric carcinoma is statistically commoner in individuals with blood group A. There is no significant familial tendency.

Precancerous Lesions

Gastric carcinoma occurs with increased frequency (1) in patients with chronic atrophic gastritis associated with pernicious anemia (high risk); (2) in those with chronic atrophic gastritis not associated with pernicious anemia, particularly when there is intestinal metaplasia (uncertain risk); (3) in those with adenomatous and hyperplastic polyps (low risk); and (4) in those with chronic gastric ulcer (very low risk). Following subtotal gastrectomy, the residual gastric stump is believed to be at increased risk, though a recent study casts serious doubt on this.

Table 38-3. Gastric carcinoma: Risk factors and presentation.

Increased risk
Sex: Male > female
Race: Japan, Chile, Iceland (probably environmental rather than genetic)
Family history: Blood group A = 20% increase in risk
Age: 50 plus
Precancerous lesions:
Pernicious anemia (atrophic gastritis)
Adenomatous polyp
?Intestinal metaplasia
?Previous partial gastrectomy
?Chronic gastric ulcer (slight risk)
Clinical presentation
Weight loss (asthenia)
Anorexia
Dyspepsia
Early satiety
Anemia (iron deficiency)
Hematemesis
Left supraclavicular lymph node enlargement

Pathology

A. Gross Appearance:

1. Early gastric cancer (defined as gastric carcinoma restricted to the mucosa and submucosa) is being increasingly recognized. In Japan, where the incidence is high, population screening for gastric cancer is carried out, and early gastric cancer accounts for 30% of cases. In the United States, the incidence is much lower, and screening is not attempted; consequently, less than 5% are detected at this early stage. Early gastric cancer appears as a small, flat mucosal thickening that may have a minimal polypoid and ulcerative component (Fig 38–10). It is thought that there may be a long period (months to years) before invasion of the muscle occurs.

2. Late gastric cancer (defined as a gastric carcinoma that has invaded the muscle wall) is the stage at which the tumor is commonly diagnosed in the United States. It may present in various ways: (1) as a fungating mass that protrudes into the lumen; (2) as a malignant ulcer with raised, everted edges (Fig 38–11); (3) as an excavated ulcer resembling a chronic peptic ulcer; or (4) as a diffusely infiltrating lesion that causes thickening and contraction of the stomach wall with relatively little mucosal involvement (linitis plastica, or leather-bottle stomach). Differentiation of benign peptic ulcer and ulcerative carcinoma may be difficult without histologic examinatin (Fig 38–12).Any gastric ulcer that does not heal as expected should be biopsied to rule out carcinoma.

B. Microscopic Appearance: Gastric carcinomas are adenocarcinomas of varying differentiation. The most common form is poorly differentiated, with cells distended by intracellular mucin (**signet ring cell carcinoma**; Fig 38–13). Well-differentiated adenocarcinoma is less common. A reactive fibrosis is commonly present in relation to the neoplastic cells.

C. Spread: (Fig 38–14.) Gastric carcinoma infiltrates the submucosa and invades through the muscle wall into the omental fat. Involvement of the serosa leads to spread of tumor cells in the peritoneal fluid (transcoelomic spread). Such metastasis occurs to the ovary (Krukenberg tumor) and rectovesical pouch. Involvement of submucosal lymphatics by tumor results in microscopic satellite nodules, often some distance from the main mass. Microscopic examination of frozen sections of the resection margins is therefore very important at the time of surgical removal of tumor. Lymphatic involvement also leads to metastasis to lymph nodes around the stomach. Later, exten-

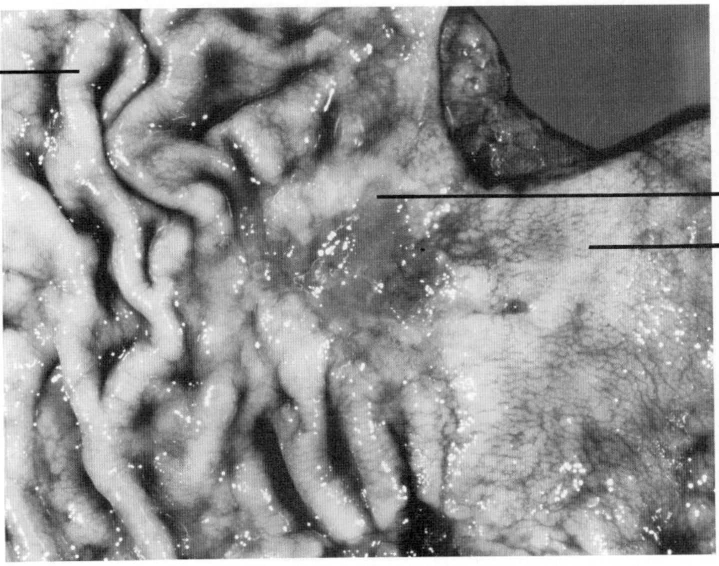

Figure 38-10. Early gastric cancer, showing shallow ulceration of mucosa. Note the difference between the flat mucosa of chronic gastritis (to the right of the carcinomatous ulcer) and normal gastric rugal folds to the left of the ulcer.

sion of tumor up the thoracic duct may lead to involvement of the left supraclavicular node (Virchow's node). Lymph node metastases are present in about 50% of cases at the time of diagnosis. Bloodstream spread to the liver and lungs also occurs early.

Clinical Features

Gastric carcinoma is asymptomatic in its early stages and can be detected only by screening of high-risk populations. A few patients with early gastric cancer have symptoms resembling chronic peptic ulcer. Biopsy of a nonhealing gastric ulcer is essential, because some of these patients prove to have carcinoma.

Late gastric cancer presents with anorexia, anemia (due to blood loss), and weight loss. Early satiety may occur in a patient with a large mass or a contracted (linitis plastica) stomach. Hematemesis and melena may occur. Tumors near the pylorus may cause gastric outlet obstruction.

Diagnosis may be established by endoscopy and biopsy, which provides a histologic diagnosis; and by radiologic examination—particularly computerized tomography—which provides information about the extent of spread and surgical resectability. Note that radiologic diagnosis of carcinoma must always be confirmed by endoscopic biopsy.

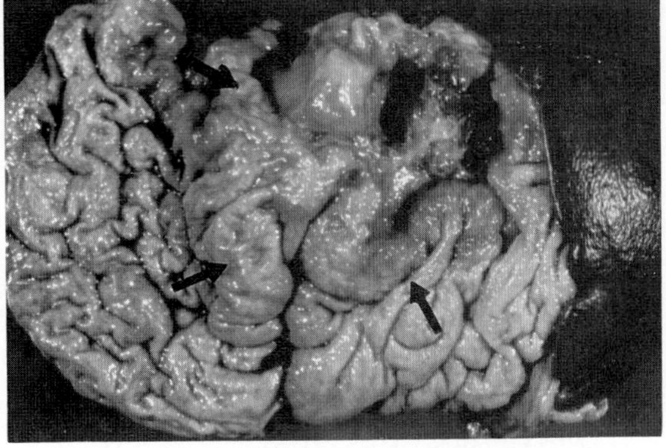

Figure 38-11. Advanced gastric cancer, showing large ulcer in the fundus (arrows). The ulcer has raised, everted edges. The spleen is present in the specimen because the carcinoma infiltrated the splenic hilum.

Prognosis

The prognosis depends almost entirely on the depth of invasion of the neoplasm. Early gastric cancer restricted to the mucosa and submucosa has a 5-year survival rate of about 85%. Tumors that have invaded the muscle wall (late gastric cancer) but have not involved lymph nodes have only a 30% 5-year survival rate. When there is extension of tumor through the full thickness of the wall and lymph node involvement is present, the 5-year survival rate drops to about 5%.

Histologic features and degree of differentiation are of little prognostic importance.

MALIGNANT LYMPHOMA

Gastric lymphoma accounts for about 3% of malignant tumors of the stomach. Most are ag-

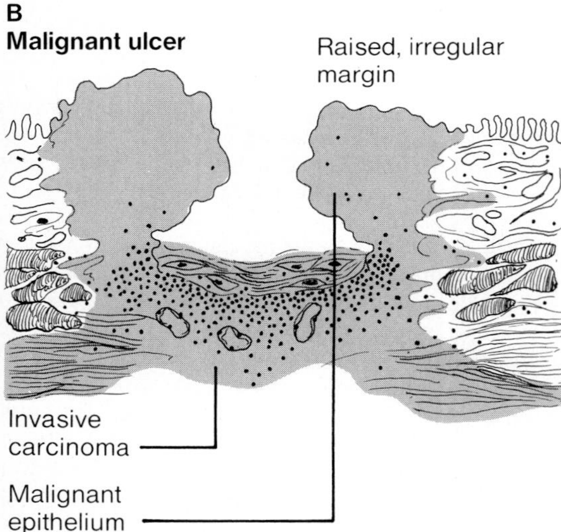

Figure 38–12. Comparative features of benign versus malignant gastric ulcers. **A:** Chronic peptic ulcer. showing the flat, punched-out ulcer with regenerating epithelium at the edges. **B:** Carcinomatous ulcer with raised edges composed of malignant epithelial cells. The shaded gray areas in the base and at the edges of the ulcer represent malignant epithelial cells.

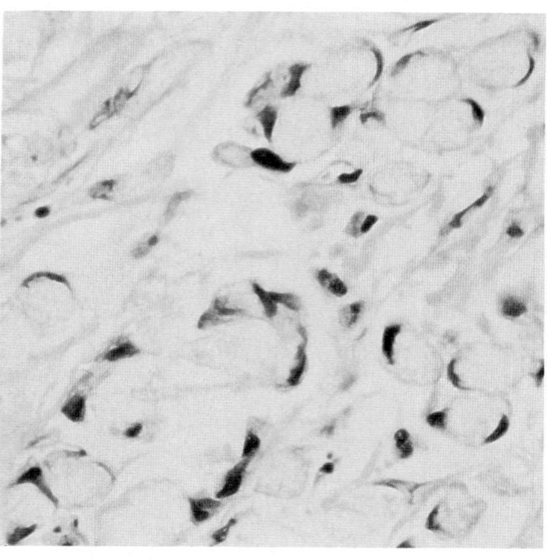

Figure 38–13. Gastric adenocarcinoma, showing signet ring cells.

gressive B cell non-Hodgkin's lymphomas, B-immunoblastic sarcoma being the commonest histologic type.

Gastric lymphomas present as polypoid masses, ulcers, thickened mucosal folds, and large intramural masses (Fig 38–15). The diagnosis is difficult on clinical grounds. Histologic examination of endoscopic biopsies shows a proliferation of large lymphoid cells, which may be difficult to distinguish from poorly differentiated carcinoma. The lack of mucin and keratin—plus the presence of B lymphocyte antigens in the lymphoma cells—permits diagnosis.

Gastric lymphoma responds well to chemotherapy. The 5-year survival rate is around 50–60% for disease localized to the stomach.

GASTRIC LEIOMYOSARCOMA

Malignant smooth muscle neoplasms, although they are the commonest mesenchymal neoplasm in the stomach, account for only 2% of gastric malignancies. They present as large masses that originate in and involve the wall, usually protruding both into the mucosa and out as an extragastric mass. Mucosal ulceration and cavitation of the central part of the tumor occur commonly. Though it forms a large mass, the tumor has less tendency to infiltrate and metastasize than gastric carcinoma. Surgical resection is therefore more successful than with carcinoma.

Microscopically, leiomyosarcoma is composed of a cellular mass of smooth muscle cells showing increased mitotic activity and areas of necrosis and hemorrhage.

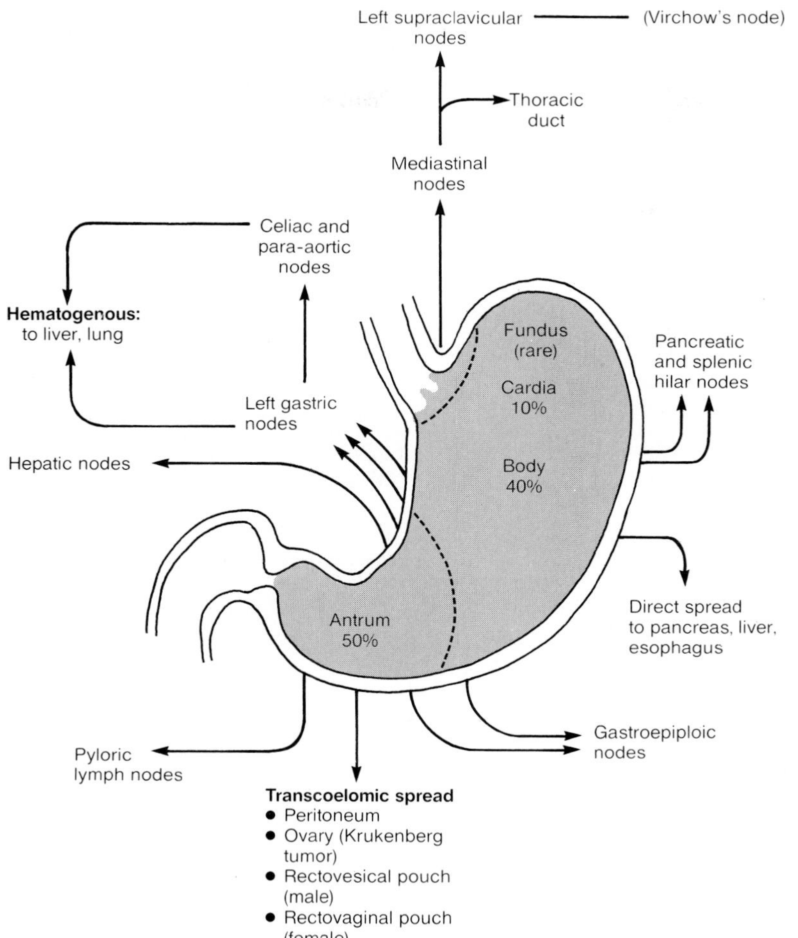

Figure 38-14. Gastric carcinoma—distribution of lesions and spread.

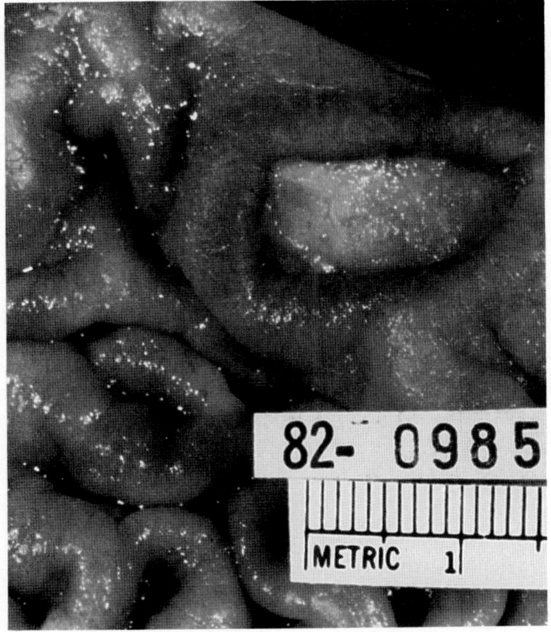

Figure 38-15. Malignant lymphoma of the stomach, showing thickened rugal folds and ulceration. Biopsy is required to differentiate this from a gastric carcinoma.

Patients present with bleeding, blood loss anemia, or a palpable mass. The diagnosis is usually suggested by radiologic appearances. Endoscopic biopsy of the intramural mass is frequently negative for tumor, which is located deep to the submucosa. With surgical resection, over 50% of patients survive for 5 years. Failures may be due either to local recurrence or to distant metastases.

CARCINOID TUMORS

Carcinoid tumors of the stomach are discussed along with other intestinal carcinoid tumors in Chapter 41.

39 The Intestines: I. Structure & Function; Malabsorption Syndrome; Intestinal Obstruction

STRUCTURE & FUNCTION

The intestine begins at the pylorus and ends at the anorectal junction. It is divided into small and large intestine, which are separated by the ileocecal valve. The small intestine is composed of the duodenum, jejunum, and ileum and is about 6 meters long; the large intestine is composed of the cecum, ascending, transverse, descending, and sigmoid colon and the rectum, totaling about 1.5 meters in length.

The intestinal wall has 4 layers:

(1) Mucosa, which is lined by glandular epithelium. The small intestine is characterized by the presence of villi and crypts (Fig 39–1). The villi increase the surface area for absorption. The colonic mucosa has no villi and is composed only of crypts. The crypts contain proliferating cells that continually divide to replace lost surface epithelial cells.

(2) Submucosa, which contains blood and lymphatic vessels and the submucosal nerve plexus.

(3) Muscularis externa, which is composed of 2 layers in the small intestine. In the large intestine, the longitudinal muscle is attenuated to form the taenia coli. The muscle is responsible for propulsive peristalsis. The myenteric plexus of nerves is situated between the 2 muscle layers and provides the neural impetus to peristalsis.

(4) Serosa, which is the peritoneal lining in those parts of the intestine that lie in the peritoneal cavity.

The intestine digests and absorbs essential components from ingested food, eliminating the waste at defecation. Digestion is effected in the upper small intestine by enzymes contained in the secretions of intestinal juice, pancreatic juice, and bile. The small molecules resulting from digestion—monosaccharides, amino acids, and fatty acids—are absorbed in the small intestine. The colon absorbs water from the liquid ileal effluent to form solid feces.

CLINICAL MANIFESTATIONS OF INTESTINAL DISEASE

Malabsorption

See p 586.

Intestinal Obstruction

Mechanical obstruction may result from (1) lesions outside the intestine that compress or constrict the intestine, eg, fibrous adhesions in the

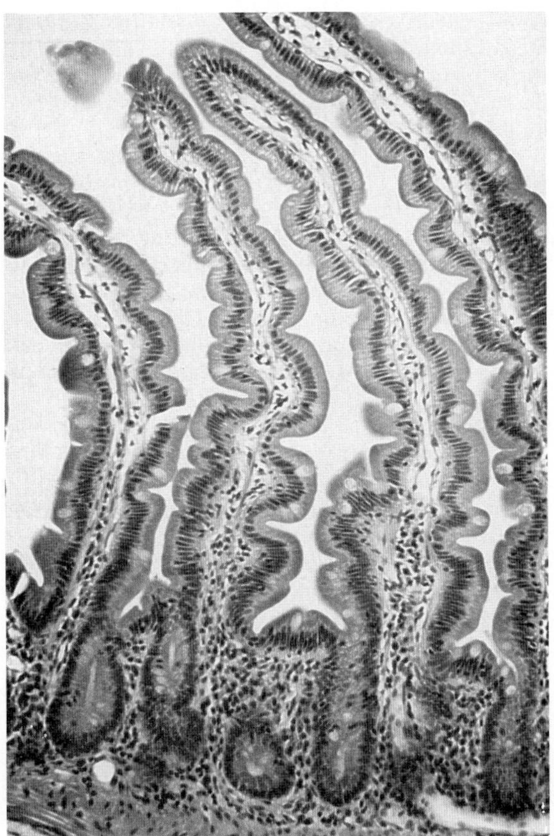

Figure 39–1. Normal small intestinal mucosa, showing tall, fingerlike villi which are more than 3–4 times the length of the crypts.

peritoneal cavity and hernial sacs; (2) intramural lesions such as fibrous strictures and neoplasms; (3) volvulus of the intestine (see p 595); (4) intussusception (see p 595); and (5) intraluminal foreign bodies.

Failure of peristalsis may be the result of paralysis of the intestinal smooth muscle (paralytic ileus) or abnormalities of the myenteric plexus, eg, congenital megacolon (Hirschsprung's disease), or smooth muscle diseases, eg, familial visceral myopathy. Paralysis occurs after abdominal surgery, in patients with peritoneal inflammation, and in severe acute intestinal inflammation (eg, toxic megacolon).

Intestinal obstruction has the following physiologic consequences:

(1) Failure of propulsive movement of intestinal contents, leading to constipation and absence of flatus.

(2) Accumulation of food and fluid secretions in the intestine proximal to the obstruction. This leads to dilatation of bowel loops, which become filled with fluid, food, and gas; hypovolemia and electrolyte imbalance; abdominal distention; and vomiting.

(3) Increased peristalsis when the obstruction is mechanical, resulting in colicky abdominal pain and increased bowel sounds on abdominal auscultation. In cases where intestinal obstruction is due to muscle paralysis, pain does not occur and bowel sounds are absent.

Intestinal Perforation

Complete disruption of the bowel wall permits leakage of luminal contents into the peritoneal cavity. When perforation occurs in a part of the intestine whose wall is not covered by serosa, eg, the posterior wall of the descending colon and rectum, the luminal contents leak into the pericolic fat, causing pericolic abscess.

Many diseases may lead to free perforation into the peritoneal cavity. The effect of intestinal perforation depends on the site of the perforation. Perforation of a duodenal ulcer produces chemical peritonitis due to the acid content. Perforation of the intestine distal to the first part of the duodenum leads to bacterial peritonitis due to the intestinal bacterial flora. In all of these types of perforation, gas enters the peritoneal cavity and can be detected under the diaphragm on x-ray.

Intestinal Hemorrhage

Bleeding into the lumen of the intestines may be manifested in several ways: (1) Bright red blood per rectum occurs with rapid bleeding and when the source of bleeding is near the rectum. (2) Passage of dark stools containing altered blood admixed with stools occurs with bleeding originating in the proximal colon and small intestine. (3) Passage of tarry black stools occurs when bleeding is in the stomach and duodenum and the blood is altered by the action of acid. (4) Iron deficiency anemia may develop with chronic slow bleeding and is associated with occult blood in stools.

Protein Loss in the Intestine (Protein-Losing Enteropathy)

Increased loss of protein in the intestine may result in hypoproteinemia and edema.

Diarrhea

Diarrhea is the passage of fluid feces and occurs when the rate of movement of intestinal contents is increased, so that complete digestion and absorption of fluid in the intestine fails to occur. The volume of feces is usually greatly increased in diarrhea, leading to increased frequency of evacuation and increased loss of water and electrolytes.

The mechanisms in the production of diarrhea are summarized in Table 39–1. Diarrhea may result from (1) increased fluid secretion into the intestine (secretory diarrhea); (2) the presence of increased amounts of osmotically active substances in the intestinal lumen; (3) inflammation of the

Table 39–1. Mechanisms in the production of diarrhea.

Secretory diarrhea
- Associated with cAMP increase
  - Enterotoxin of *Vibrio cholerae*
  - Enterotoxin of *Escherichia coli*
  - Vasoactive intestinal polypeptide (from pancreatic islet cell neoplasms)
  - Bile acids
- Not associated with cAMP
  - Enterotoxin of *Staphylococcus aureus*
  - Enterotoxin of *Clostridium perfringens*
  - Some laxatives (bisacodyl, phenolphthalein)
  - AIDS (unknown mechanism)
- Mucosal injury
  - Infections: Viral and *Salmonella* gastroenteritis, *Shigella, E coli, Campylobacter* colitis
  - Inflammatory bowel disease
- Neoplasms
  - Gastrinoma (gastrin)
  - Carcinoid syndrome (serotonin, prostaglandins)
  - Villous adenoma

Osmotic diarrhea
- Disaccharidase deficiency (lactose or sucrose intolerance)
- Postgastrectomy
- Postvagotomy
- Laxatives (lactulose, magnesium salts)

Motility disorders
- Irritable bowel syndrome
- Autonomic neuropathy (diabetes mellitus)
- Laxatives

intestine—mainly the small intestine; (4) increased peristalsis, eg, resulting from stimulation of smooth muscle by serotonin in carcinoid syndrome and in irritable bowel syndrome; or (5) failure of colonic water absorption, eg, after surgical removal of the colon.

Steatorrhea is a specific form of diarrhea defined by the presence of excessive fat (> 6 g/d) in the feces. Most patients with steatorrhea have diarrhea. Steatorrhea is a typical clinical manifestation of maldigestion or malabsorption of fat.

Dysentery

Dysentery is a specific type of diarrhea characterized by the passage of small amounts of bright red blood and mucus at frequent intervals. The volume of feces is usually small. Dysentery is the characteristic symptom of acute colonic inflammation. When the rectum is inflamed, dysentery is accompanied by a constant and painful desire to defecate **(tenesmus)**.

METHODS OF EVALUATING THE INTESTINE

Endoscopy

Upper endoscopy permits evaluation of the duodenum up to the ligament of Treitz. Sigmoidoscopy permits evaluation of the rectum and sigmoid colon. Colonoscopy permits evaluation of the entire colon and, in some cases, the terminal ileum. The rest of the small intestine is inaccessible to direct examination by endoscopy.

Radiography

Administration of barium and visualization of its passage through the small intestine by fluoroscopy permits evaluation of the mucosal pattern of the small intestine. Barium enema permits examination of the colonic mucosa. Computerized tomography of the abdomen is very effective in detecting mass lesions of the intestinal wall.

Biopsy

Endoscopic biopsies may be obtained from any lesion that is detected at endoscopy. Biopsy of the jejunum, which is important for the diagnosis of malabsorption, may be performed by means of a biopsy capsule that is swallowed. The capsule has a spring mechanism that cuts off a piece of jejunal mucosa when activated.

MALABSORPTION SYNDROME

NORMAL ABSORPTION IN THE SMALL INTESTINE

Absorption of Fat (Fig 39–2)

A. Luminal Phase: Fifty to 100 g of fat is ingested daily by an adult, mainly as long-chain triglycerides. Pancreatic lipase hydrolyzes triglycerides to fatty acids and monoglycerides. The fatty acids and monoglycerides, along with fat-soluble vitamins, are complexed with bile salts to form a globular structure called a micelle.

B. Cellular Phase: The micelles dissociate at the surface of the intestinal mucosal cell, and the fatty acids, monoglycerides, and fat-soluble vitamins move into the cell while the bile salts remain in the lumen. The bile salts are finally reabsorbed in the terminal ileum and pass to the liver for reexcretion (the enterohepatic circulation of bile salts).

Fat absorption occurs mainly in the upper jejunum, and about 100 cm are required for normal fat absorption. In the intestinal cells, monoglycerides are further hydrolyzed by mucosal cell lipase. The fatty acids are then reconverted to triglycerides in the endoplasmic reticulum and complexed with protein, phospholipid, and some cholesterol to form chylomicrons. Chylomicrons exit the cell at the antiluminal border of the mucosal cell, en-

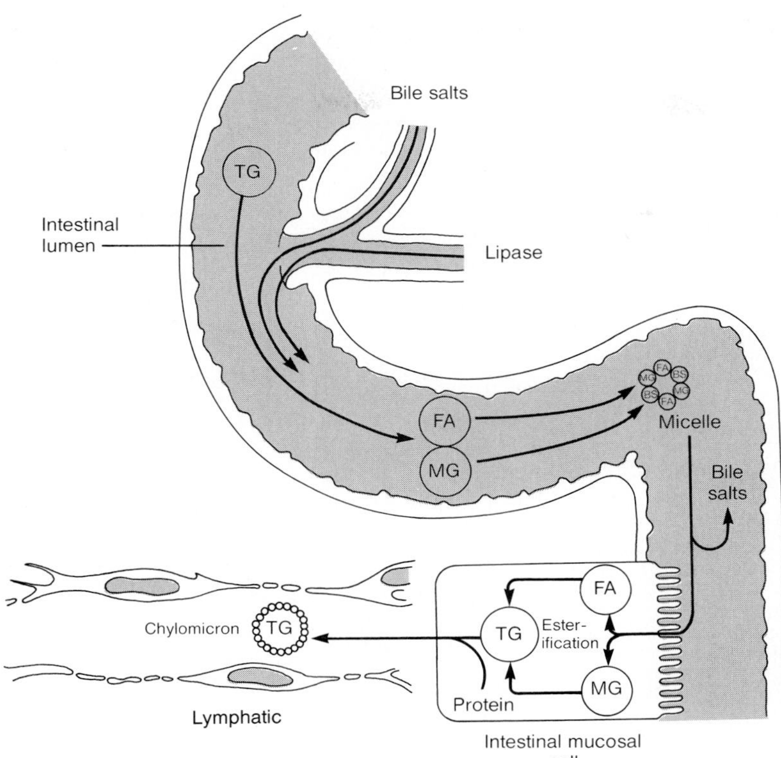

Figure 39-2. Absorption of dietary triglycerides (long-chain). TG = triglycerides, FA = fatty acids, MG = monoglycerides, BS = bile salts.

ter intestinal lymphatics, and pass to the jugular vein via the thoracic duct.

Medium-chain triglycerides (containing 6–10 fatty acids), which normally form a small component of fat in the diet, are handled differently. They are better absorbed because they are more completely hydrolyzed and form micelles more readily than long-chain triglycerides. Limited absorption (30% of an oral dose) is also possible without formation of micelles, the medium chain triglycerides passing directly into the mucosal cell, where they are hydrolyzed by cellular lipase into fatty acids. Medium-chain fatty acids can also pass directly into the portal circulation without re-esterification and formation of chylomicrons. For these reasons, medium-chain triglycerides are useful in the treatment of some patients with malabsorption syndrome.

Absorption of Protein & Carbohydrate

Proteins and carbohydrates are hydrolyzed by enzymes in saliva (amylase), gastric juice (pepsin), pancreatic juice (amylase, trypsin, and chymotrypsin), and intestinal juice (disaccharidases, carboxypeptidases) into amino acids and monosaccharides. Because they are hydrophilic molecules, these substances are absorbed into the mucosal cells and pass into the portal venous radicals.

DEFINITION OF MALABSORPTION SYNDROME

Malabsorption syndrome is a clinical syndrome characterized by increased fecal excretion of fat (steatorrhea) and the systemic effects of deficiency of vitamins, minerals, protein, and carbohydrates (Table 39–2). The complete clinical syndrome of malabsorption may not be present in all patients. Some patients have malabsorption of specific types of dietary constituents.

Steatorrhea is passage of soft, yellowish, greasy stools containing an increased amount of fat. The presence of steatorrhea is established when fat excretion exceeding 6 g/d is demonstrated in a 72-hour stool sample. The high fat content of the stool makes it float in water, and flushing it down the toilet may be difficult—a feature that is highly suggestive of steatorrhea.

PATHOPHYSIOLOGY OF MALABSORPTION (Table 39–3)

Deficiency of Pancreatic Enzymes

Pancreatic juice contains numerous enzymes. Pancreatic lipase is essential for complete fat digestion, and its absence leads to steatorrhea. Pan-

Table 39-2. Systemic effects of malabsorption.

Dietary Substance	Clinical Effect
Total calories (fat, carbohydrate)	Weight loss, general weakness
Protein	Muscle wasting (increased gluconeogenesis) Osteoporosis Decreased pituitary hormone output (causes amenorrhea) Hypoproteinemia, edema
Calcium	Hypocalcemia Tetany, paresthesias Secondary hyperparathyroidism Osteomalacia, osteitis fibrosa cystica Bone pain
Magnesium	Hypomagnesemia, tetany
Iron	Hypochromic microcytic anemia Glossitis, koilonychia
Folic acid	Macrocytic megaloblastic anemia
Vitamin B_{12}	Macrocytic megaloblastic anemia Peripheral neuropathy Subacute combined degeneration of the spinal cord
Vitamin B complex	Cheilosis, angular stomatitis, glossitis
Vitamin K	Hypoprothrombinemia Hemorrhagic diathesis
Vitamin D	Hypocalcemia Osteomalacia
Vitamin A	Night blindness Bitot's spots, xerophthalmia

Table 39-3. Mechanisms and causes of malabsorption syndrome.

Inadequate digestion
Postgastrectomy
Deficiency of pancreatic lipase
Chronic pancreatitis
Cystic fibrosis
Pancreatic resection
Zollinger-Ellison syndrome (high acid inhibits lipase)
Deficient bile salt concentration
Obstructive jaundice
Bacterial overgrowth (leading to bile salt deconjugation)
Stasis in blind loops, diverticula
Fistulas
Hypomotility states (diabetes, scleroderma, visceral myopathy)
Interrupted enterohepatic circulation of bile salts
Terminal ileal resection
Crohn's disease
Precipitation of bile salts
Neomycin, cholestyramine
Primary mucosal abnormalities
Celiac disease
Tropical sprue
Whipple's disease
Amyloidosis
Radiation enteritis
Inadequate small intestine
Intestinal resection
Crohn's disease
Mesenteric vascular disease with infarction
Jejunoileal bypass
Lymphatic obstruction
Intestinal lymphangiectasia
Malignant lymphoma

creatic amylase and trypsin are important for carbohydrate and protein digestion, but their function can be taken over by other enzymes in intestinal juice.

Absence of pancreatic lipase is usually the result of primary pancreatic disease, commonly chronic pancreatitis. Rarely, lipase secretion is normal but its activity is decreased, either because of increased gastric acidity (eg, Zollinger-Ellison syndrome) or because rapid gastric emptying dilutes pancreatic enzymes.

Deficiency of Bile Salts

Bile salts deficiency occurs when bile does not enter the intestine, as in biliary obstruction, or as a result of bile salt deconjugation in the intestinal lumen resulting from overgrowth of bacteria. The small intestine is free of bacteria in about 50% of individuals; in the remainder, small numbers of bacteria (up to 1000 organisms per gram of luminal contents) are present. The small intestine becomes colonized with bacteria when there is stasis of luminal contents from any cause.

A third mechanism of bile salt deficiency is failure of reabsorption of bile salts in the terminal ileum, due either to absence or disease of that segment of intestine.

Deficiency of bile salts results in failure of micelle formation, interfering with absorption of fat and fat-soluble vitamins. Medium-chain triglycerides, proteins, and carbohydrates are absorbed normally.

Abnormalities in the Absorptive Mucosa

Quantitative and qualitative abnormalities in the absorptive mucosa are a common cause of malabsorption. Quantitative abnormalities occur (1) when there is a reduction in the length of small intestine due to extensive surgical resection; or (2) when the surface area of villi decreases, as occurs in villous atrophy (Fig 39–3) (celiac disease, tropical sprue, giardiasis, radiation, etc) or when the villous surface is abnormal, as in severe giardiasis.

Qualitative abnormalities of the villi such as amyloidosis and Whipple's disease also result in malabsorption.

Decreased Intestinal Transit Time

Digestion and absorption require a certain minimum amount of time. In conditions where there is increased intestinal motility such as carcinoid syndrome (serotonin stimulates smooth muscle) and after gastrectomy, there may be malabsorption.

Failure of Removal of Intestinal Triglyceride

Triglycerides formed in the mucosal cell must be complexed with a carrier protein to form chylomicrons before they can enter the intestinal lymphatics. This fails in abetalipoproteinemia, a rare autosomal recessive inherited disease characterized by decreased serum betalipoprotein levels and abnormal erythrocytes. The triglyceride accumulates in the intestinal mucosal cell (fatty change), which can be seen on intestinal biopsy.

Synthesized chylomicrons pass from the intestine into the lymphatics. Obstruction of lymphatics, as in intestinal lymphangiectasia and extensive intestinal lymphomas, may cause malabsorption.

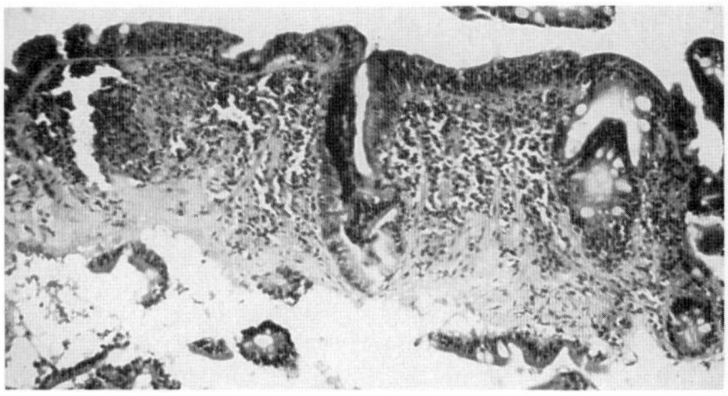

Figure 39–3. Total villous atrophy in a case of celiac disease. Note the flat surface epithelium without villi. The surface epithelium also appears more cuboidal, with less cytoplasmic mucin than is normal. The hypercellular appearance of the surface epithelium is due to the presence of numerous intraepithelial lymphocytes (visible only at higher magnification).

DISEASES CAUSING MALABSORPTION

CELIAC DISEASE (Nontropical Sprue; Gluten-Induced Enteropathy)

Celiac disease is caused by the action of acidic peptides contained in the gliadin fraction of the wheat protein gluten on the intestinal mucosa. The exact mechanism of damage is not certain, but immunologic hypersensitivity seems most likely. Serum contains IgA antibodies to gliadin in most patients, and antibody titers fall when these patients are maintained on a gluten-free diet. The possibility that the disease is a direct toxic effect of gliadin on the mucosal cells has not been ruled out.

Susceptibility to gluten-induced intestinal damage is rare and has a familial tendency; 80–90% of patients have the histocompatibility antigen HLA-B8 or HLA-DR3.

Celiac disease occurs commonly in children. When it occurs in adult life, the term idiopathic steatorrhea may be used.

Pathology (Fig 39–3)

The changes of celiac disease are restricted to the small intestinal mucosa. The basic abnormality is thought to be an increased rate of loss of epithelial cells. The crypt cell shows increased activity but cannot keep pace with the loss of cells, resulting in progressive decrease in height of villi (villous atrophy). The epithelial cells show decreased cytoplasm and mucus, appearing cuboidal. There is associated lymphocytic infiltration of the epithelium, suggesting that cell-mediated immunologic mechanisms may have a part in the genesis of the lesion. Immunologic studies show the presence of anti-gliadin IgA antibodies in the mucosa.

Intestinal biopsy shows a decrease in the villus:crypt ratio. Normally (Fig 39–1), the villi are 3–4 times the height of the crypts (ratio of 3–4:1); in celiac disease, the ratio decreases progressively (partial, subtotal, and total villous atrophy). The shortened villi are also wider than normal (''spadelike'' rather than ''fingerlike'') and infiltrated by chronic inflammatory cells. In severe celiac disease, the villi are completely atrophic (ratio of 0:1, or total villous atrophy; Fig 39–3). The crypts are normal or even hyperplastic.

Villous atrophy is a nonspecific abnormality resulting from increased loss of epithelial cells due to any cause. Total villous atrophy rarely occurs except in celiac disease.

Clinical Features & Diagnosis

Celiac disease presents with severe malabsorption syndrome. The diagnosis may be suggested by an abnormal mucosal pattern on small bowel follow-through radiologic studies and confirmed by the findings of total villous atrophy and epithelial abnormalities on jejunal biopsy.

Withdrawal of gluten from the diet produces dramatic improvement in both clinical symptoms and histologic changes in the small intestine. The ultimate diagnostic test is the demonstration of reversal of histologic changes after the patient has been on a gluten-free diet for 6 months.

Complications

Celiac disease is now regarded as a premalignant condition that imposes an increased risk of malignant lymphoma of the intestine. It is not known whether removal of gluten from the diet removes this risk.

TROPICAL SPRUE

Tropical sprue is an acquired disease that is commonly seen in the Caribbean, Far East, and India. It is thought to result from chronic bacterial infection of the small intestine, because treatment with broad-spectrum antibiotics is often successful.

Tropical sprue occurs in adults and is characterized by a severe malabsorption syndrome in which folic acid deficiency is often a dominant feature. Treatment with folic acid may also produce improvement in the disease, including a decrease in the degree of steatorrhea, suggesting a possible etiologic role for folate deficiency.

Jejunal biopsy shows villous atrophy that is usually partial. Total villous atrophy is rare. The correlation between the degree of villous atrophy and malabsorption is poor.

WHIPPLE'S DISEASE (Intestinal Lipodystrophy)

Whipple's disease is a rare disease characterized pathologically by distention of the lamina propria of the small intestine by macrophages with abundant pale foamy cytoplasm (Fig 39–4). The macrophages contain large numbers of bacilli (seen on electron microscopy) which produce a fine granular staining with periodic acid-Schiff (PAS) reagent. Infiltration of the mucosa by these cells results in a gross increase in size of the villi, which gives the mucosal surface a coarse appearance resembling the pile of a shaggy rug.

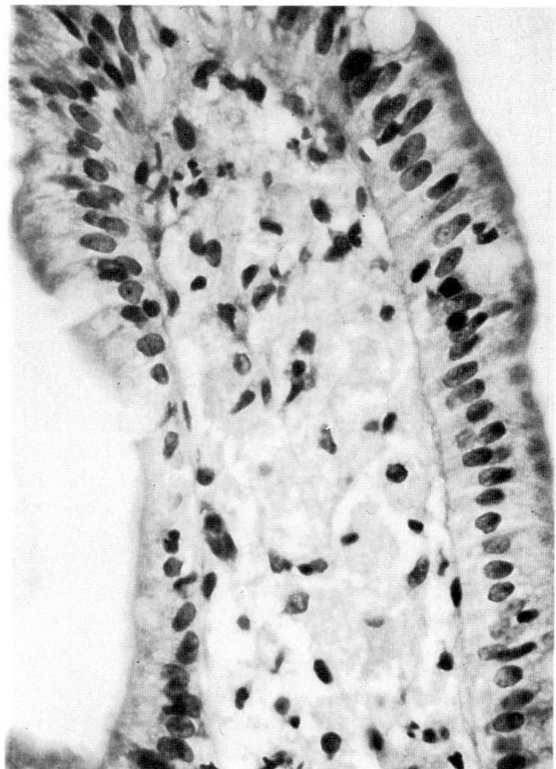

Figure 39–4. Whipple's disease, showing the lamina propria of the small intestinal villi distended with large histiocytes characterized by abundant foamy cytoplasm.

Treatment with antibiotics causes improvement of symptoms as well as disappearance of the bacillary bodies, suggesting that this is also a form of bacterial infection. The specific organism or organisms responsible have not been identified.

The disease occurs mainly in males over 30 years of age. Presentation is with severe malabsorption syndrome. The diagnosis may be made by demonstration of the typical macrophages on jejunal biopsy.

Forty percent of patients have the abnormal macrophages in tissues other than the small intestine—usually lymph nodes, commonly mesenteric; rarely, the spleen, liver, kidney, lungs, heart, and brain may be affected. Fever is present in 30% of patients, and polyarthritis and polyserositis (pleural effusion and ascites) are common. Extraintestinal Whipple's disease may sometimes occur in the absence of intestinal symptoms.

CONGENITAL DISEASES OF THE INTESTINE

INTESTINAL ATRESIA

Atresia is a rare disorder consisting of failure of development of the lumen in one part of the intestine. The jejunum and ileum are most commonly affected, and multiple bowel segments may be affected. Atresia presents with intestinal obstruction in the first week of life. Surgical correction is curative.

IMPERFORATE ANUS

Imperforate anus is a common congenital abnormality that results from failure of the entodermal hindgut to open at the anal dimple. Varying degrees of abnormality result, sometimes associated with fistulous communications with the bladder, urethra, and vagina.

MALROTATIONS

The intestine rotates in a specific manner during development. Malrotation is characterized by failure of the cecum to reach its normal position in the right lower quadrant. The importance of malrotation is that the abnormal mobility of the cecum predisposes to twisting (volvulus) and intestinal obstruction.

MECKEL'S DIVERTICULUM

Meckel's diverticulum is persistence of the intestinal end of the omphalomesenteric duct. It is present in 2% of the population (the commonest congenital anomaly of the gastrointestinal tract), is found within 2 feet (1 m) of the ileocecal valve, and is usually 2 inches (5 cm) long.

The diverticulum is usually lined by small intestinal mucosa. About 40% of cases have heterotopic gastric mucosa or pancreatic tissue (Fig 39–5). Peptic ulceration may occur when there is gastric mucosa. Bleeding from an ulcerated Meckel diverticulum is an important cause of chronic intestinal blood loss, resulting in iron deficiency anemia. Other complications include infection (Meckel's diverticulitis), which presents a clinical picture very similar to that of acute appendicitis and may result in perforation and peritonitis. Volvulus may occur in relation to Meckel's diverticulum, especially when it is attached to the umbilicus by the obliterated omphalomesenteric duct. Rarely, the diverticulum inverts into the ileum and acts as the apex of an intussception.

CONGENITAL MEGACOLON (Hirschsprung's Disease)

Hirschsprung's disease is caused by failure of development of ganglion cells in the myenteric and submucosal plexuses of the colon. The aganglionic segment usually starts at the anorectal junction and extends proximally for a variable distance. In 90% of cases, aganglionosis is restricted to the rectum. Rarely, the aganglionic segment is longer, and in exceptional cases the entire colon lacks ganglion cells.

The absence of ganglion cells in the myenteric plexus results in failure of peristalsis in the affected segment. This segment remains narrow and spastic and represents a zone of functional intestinal obstruction. The colon proximal to the aganglionic segment dilates—often massively—leading to abdominal distention (Fig 39–6).

Most affected children present soon after birth with failure to pass meconium followed by distention and vomiting. In a few cases, the onset is delayed. Without treatment, death occurs from fluid and electrolyte imbalance or from perforation of a massively dilated cecum.

The diagnosis may be made by demonstrating absence of ganglion cells in the submucosa of an adequate rectal biopsy. Absence of ganglion cells in the submucosa correlates well with absence of ganglion cells in the myenteric plexus. Treatment consists of surgical removal of the aganglionic segment. Because aganglionosis may extend from the narrow segment to involve part of the dilated segment, confirmation of the presence of ganglion cells by frozen section examination is necessary at surgery to make certain that the entire aganglionic segment has been removed.

VASCULAR DISEASES OF THE INTESTINES

Blood Supply to the Intestine

The intestine is supplied by 3 major arteries that arise from the aorta: (1) the celiac artery, which supplies the stomach, duodenum, liver, and pancreas; (2) the superior mesenteric artery, which supplies the rest of the small intestine and the ascending and transverse colon; and (3) the inferior mesenteric artery, which supplies the distal colon to the level of the rectum. The lowest part of the rectum receives its arterial supply from pelvic arteries.

The small intestine is entirely dependent on the mesenteric arteries for its blood supply; the colon receives a supplementary supply from retroperitoneal arteries and is much less susceptible to infarction, but more commonly it shows chronic ischemic damage of the mucosa (ischemic colitis).

The main mesenteric arteries supply a large segment of bowel, and their sudden occlusion causes infarction in a large area. Beyond the initial branches there is an extensive collateral circulation via the arterial arcades at the mesenteric border of the intestine, which is why obstruction of a secondary branch of a mesenteric artery usually does not cause infarction. From the arterial arcades, small arteries penetrate the intestinal wall; these are functional end-arteries, and their occlusion results in small areas of intestinal infarction.

Slow occlusion of the main mesenteric arteries, particularly the inferior mesenteric artery, does not produce infarction, since adequate collaterals can develop. Generally, extensive arterial disease must be present before there is evidence of ischemia if the arterial disease causes slowly progressive narrowing.

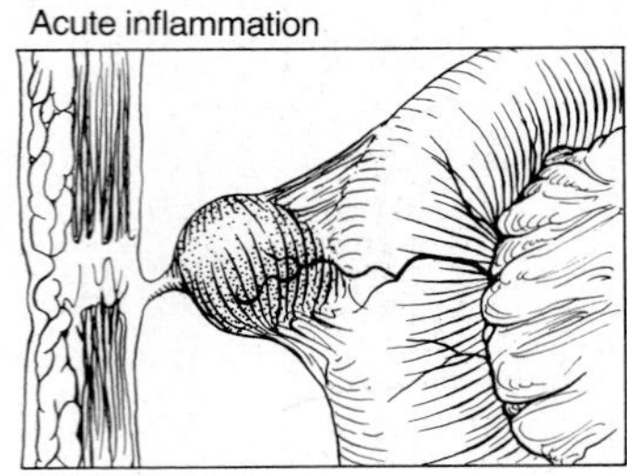

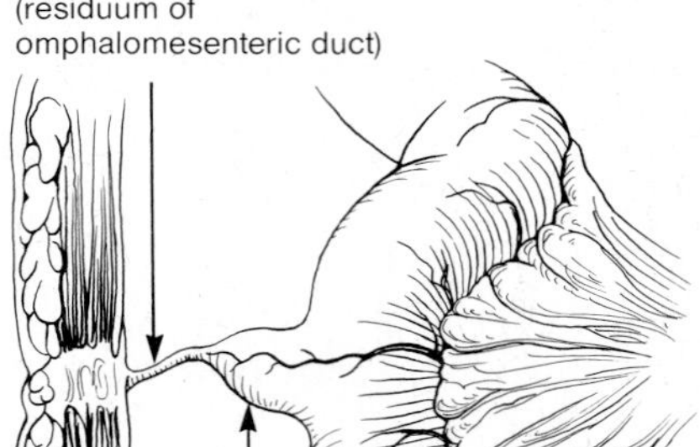

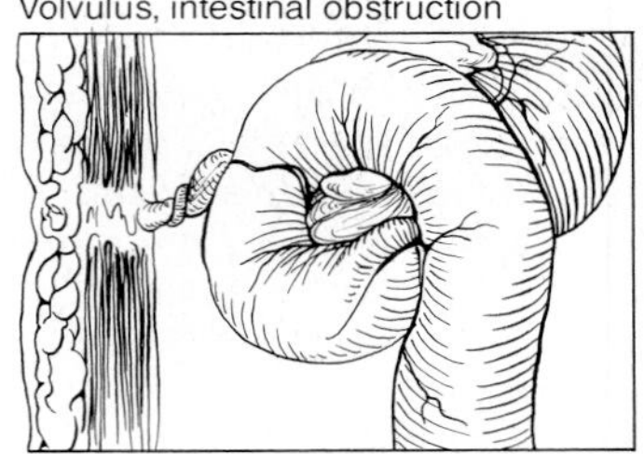

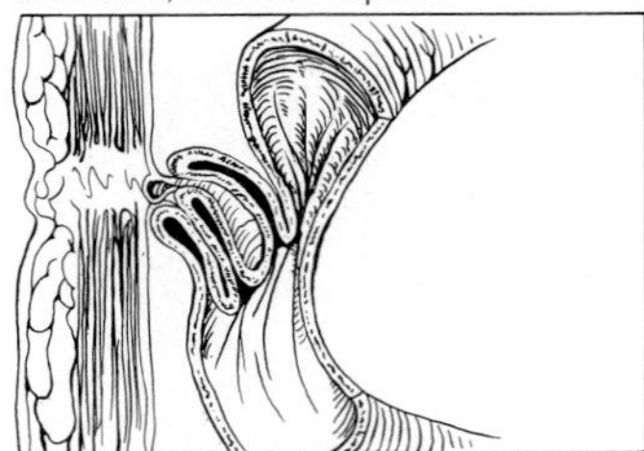

Figure 39-5. Meckel's diverticulum. In the example shown, the diverticulum is connected to the umbilicus by the fibrous residuum of the omphalomesenteric duct. Most cases do not have such a connection. Complications associated with Meckel's diverticulum include acute inflammation, peptic ulceration, perforation, volvulus, and intussusception.

ACUTE SMALL INTESTINAL INFARCTION

Etiology

A. Sudden Occlusion of the Superior Mesenteric Artery: (50% of cases.) This is due to atherosclerosis in over 90% of cases. Other causes of superior mesenteric artery occlusion include (1) vasculitis—most commonly polyarteritis nodosa, which commonly affects the branches of the main artery; (2) aortic dissection; (3) embolism from mural cardiac thrombi and valvular vegetations in patients with cardiac disease; and (4) fibromuscular dysplasia of mesenteric arteries.

B. Nonocclusive Infarction: (25% of cases.) Intestinal infarction may occur without physical obstruction of the mesenteric arteries in severe shock, where there is prolonged vasoconstriction in the intestinal arterial circulation.

C. Mesenteric Vein Occlusion: (25% of cases.) Intestinal infarction due to venous occlusion may be caused by (1) obstruction of the superior mesenteric vein as a result of thrombosis (in hypercoagulable states such as polycythemia vera

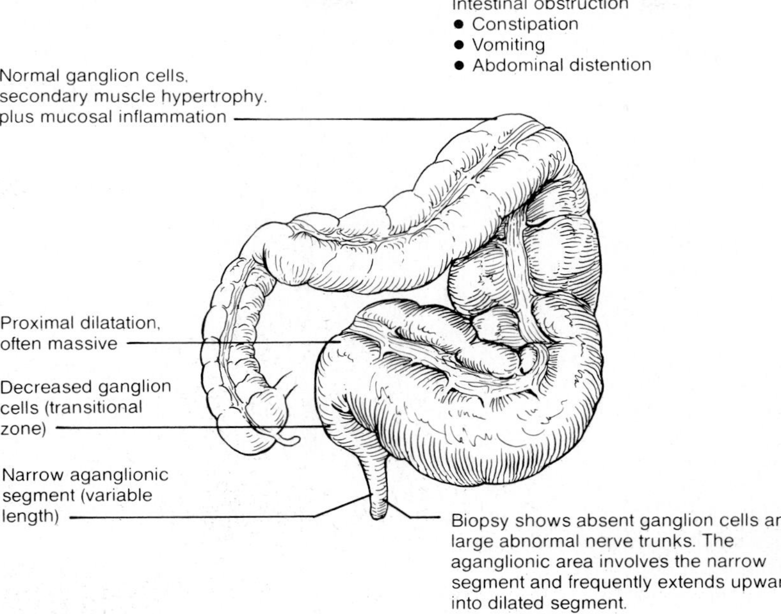

Figure 39–6. Hirschsprung's disease. The aganglionic narrow segment involves the rectum and is of varying length. It causes functional obstruction and dilatation of proximal colon. The dilated segment usually has ganglion cells. The transitional zone between the ganglionic and aganglionic segments varies in length.

and with oral contraceptive use) or (2) infiltration by malignant neoplasms.

Pathology

Intestinal infarction due to obstruction of the main superior mesenteric artery or vein at the root of the mesentery involves a large part of the small intestine (Fig 39–7). Affected bowel loops are hemorrhagic, appearing purple to black. The demarcation of viable and nonviable bowel on gross examination at surgery may be difficult.

Microscopically, there is transmural necrosis of the intestinal wall. This is rapidly followed by bacterial infection from the lumen and acute inflammation, leading to wet gangrene. The distinction between arterial and venous infarction cannot be

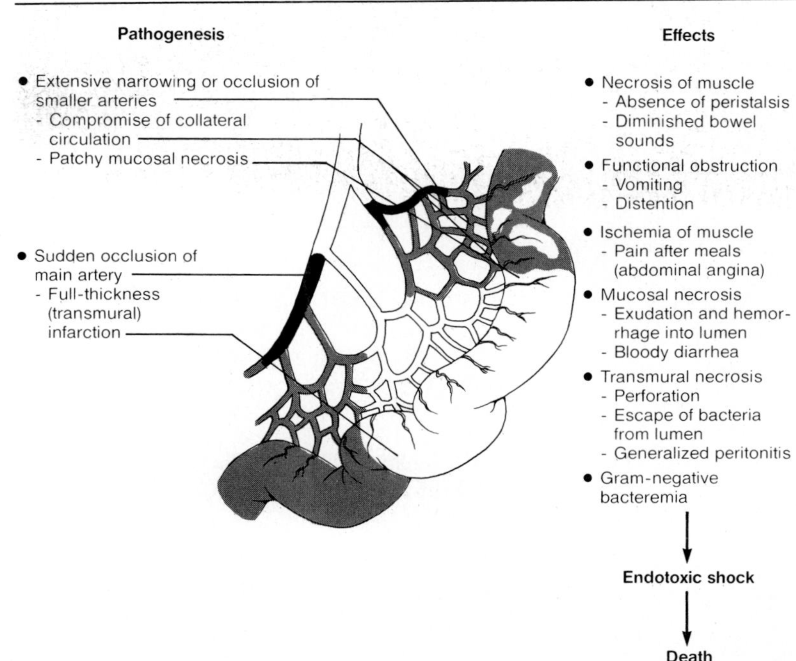

Figure 39–7. Pathogenesis and clinical features of small intestinal infarction and ischemia.

made on examination of the bowel; it is necessary to dissect the vessels at the root of the mesentery or to have angiographic evidence of arterial occlusion.

Intestinal infarction associated with vasculitis and nonocclusive infarction characteristically causes multiple discontinuous areas of intestinal necrosis. Commonly the mucosa, which is the layer most sensitive to ischemia, is selectively involved by the necrosis. Transmural necrosis does not usually occur.

Clinical Features

Intestinal infarction occurs most often in elderly individuals with severe atherosclerosis. Embolism occurs in patients with cardiac diseases in which valve vegetations (infective endocarditis) or mural thrombi occur (myocardial infarction, mitral stenosis, atrial fibrillation).

In a few patients, infarction may be preceded by the syndrome of intestinal ischemia (called "abdominal angina"). This is characterized by abdominal pain 15–30 minutes after a meal—when intestinal oxygen demand is greatest. This may result in a fear of eating and weight loss. Identification of this syndrome may permit arterial reconstruction and prevent the occurrence of intestinal infarction.

Infarction is characterized by a sudden onset of severe abdominal pain accompanied by fever, vomiting, and abdominal distention. There is functional intestinal obstruction with absent bowel sounds. Bloody diarrhea may be present in some patients as a result of sloughing of the necrotic mucosa. The disease progresses very rapidly, with shock and peritonitis due to bacterial permeation of the necrotic bowel wall occurring within 1–2 days after onset of symptoms. Without treatment, there is a 100% mortality rate because the dead intestinal wall cannot regenerate and rapidly perforates. Even with emergency surgery, the mortality rate remains high (50–75%).

Nonocclusive infarction occurs in shocked patients and is characterized by abdominal pain and bloody diarrhea. Treatment is by correction of the shock state, with restoration of intestinal perfusion. Since only the mucosa is necrotic in most of these cases, regeneration is possible, and the bowel returns to normal.

ISCHEMIC COLITIS

Ischemic colitis is caused by extensive atherosclerotic narrowing of the inferior mesenteric artery and the collateral arteries that supply the colon. The splenic flexure and rectosigmoid area are most commonly involved.

Ischemic colitis is characterized by patchy mucosal necrosis in the affected region, the mucosa being most susceptible to ischemia. Necrosis is accompanied by acute inflammation and ulceration. The condition is usually self-limited, with healing by fibrosis and epithelial regeneration. Rarely, fibrosis may be so extensive as to cause narrowing (stricture) of the colon.

Clinically, patients present with an acute onset of fever, left-sided abdominal pain, and bloody diarrhea. Colonoscopy and histologic examination of biopsies show nonspecific necrosis, inflammation, and ulceration. The differentiation from other inflammatory lesions of the colon (infections, idiopathic inflammatory bowel disease) is difficult.

ANGIODYSPLASIA

Angiodysplasia has been recently recognized as a common and important cause of intestinal bleeding. It occurs in elderly patients, probably as an acquired degenerative change. It commonly involves the right side of the colon but may occur anywhere in the gastrointestinal tract.

Angiodysplasia is characterized by the presence of numerous dilated, tortuous, thin-walled blood vessels in the mucosa and submucosa of the colon. Rupture of these vessels causes painless bleeding, which can be sudden and severe. The diagnosis is best made by angiography, which shows the vascular malformation bleeding into the lumen. Surgical resection of the involved segment of colon is usually necessary to control the bleeding.

Pathologic demonstration of angiodysplasia requires injection of silicone rubber into the mesenteric arteries to distend the vessels before the specimen is fixed. If this is not done, the dilated vessels collapse after removal from the body and cannot be identified microscopically.

MISCELLANEOUS DISEASES OF THE INTESTINE

ABDOMINAL HERNIAS

An abdominal hernia is the protrusion of a sac of peritoneum through a defect or weakness in the abdominal wall. Hernias occur (1) through the internal inguinal ring (indirect inguinal hernia; Fig 39–8), (2) through the posterior wall of the inguinal canal (direct inguinal hernia), (3) into the femoral canal (femoral hernia), (4) around the umbilicus (periumbilical hernia), (5) through areas weakened by surgical scars (incisional hernia), (6) in the posterior abdominal wall (lumbar hernia), and (7) through the diaphragm (diaphragmatic hernias).

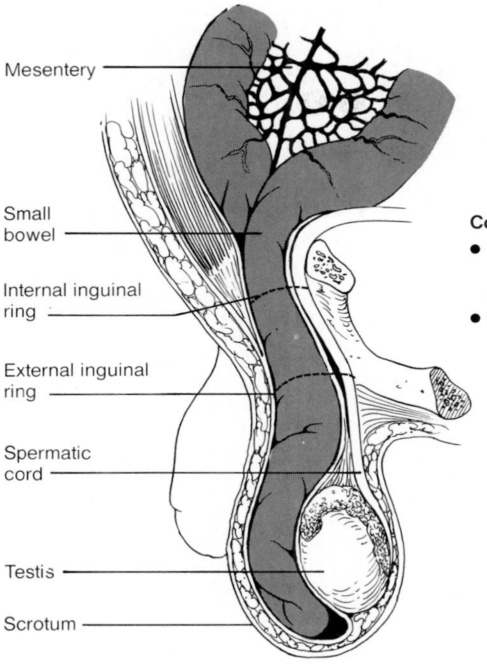

Complications of hernia
- Constriction of blood vessels in mesentery produces ischemia and infarction ("strangulation")
- Constriction of bowel lumen produces intestinal obstruction

Figure 39-8. Indirect inguinal hernia, showing a loop of small intestine herniating through the inguinal canal into the scrotum.

Abdominal hernias are common, especially inguinal, umbilical, and incisional types. The peritoneal sac of a hernia may contain a variety of abdominal tissues, commonly omentum and intestine and more rarely bladder. When intestine constitutes part of the contents, intestinal obstruction ("obstructed hernia") may occur as well as strangulation—occlusion of venous drainage and arterial supply to the segment because of constriction at the neck, causing infarction and gangrene (Fig 39–8).

INTUSSUSCEPTION

Intussusception is telescoping of one segment of bowel into another (Fig 39–9). Once the intussusception begins, peristalsis pushes the intussusceptum farther distally. The common location for an intussusception is the terminal ileum.

Intussusception occurs in weaning infants and in adults with polypoid tumors, commonly lipomas or leiomyomas. During weaning, exposure to new antigens or infectious agents is believed to cause hypertrophy of lymphoid follicles in the terminal ileum. The hypertrophied follicles are pushed into the lumen as the apex of an intussusception. In adults it is the tumor that acts as the apex.

Intussusception causes intestinal obstruction. The blood supply to the intussusceptum (the segment of bowel that telescopes into the distal segment), which must pass along its outer wall, frequently becomes constricted at the neck, leading to hemorrhagic infarction and gangrene.

Clinical presentation is with abdominal pain, vomiting, and passage of blood per rectum. The intussuscepted bowel may be palpable as a sausage-shaped mass in the abdomen.

VOLVULUS

A volvulus is a twisting of the intestine about the axis of its mesentery or around an abnormal fibrous band. Abnormal fibrous bands usually result from previous local peritonitis followed by formation of fibrous adhesions between loops of bowel during repair. Complete twisting leads to intestinal obstruction and often strangulation of the vascular supply, causing infarction.

Volvulus commonly occurs in the sigmoid colon in elderly individuals. Cecal volvulus occurs in younger people who have developmental malrotation of the bowel.

DIVERTICULOSIS

A diverticulum is an outpouching of the mucosa of the intestine. Diverticula are classified as true or false. The walls of **true diverticula** have all the layers of the intestine; congenital diverticula such as Meckel's diverticula are true diverticula. **False diverticula,** which are really mucosal herniations through a weakened intestinal wall, often

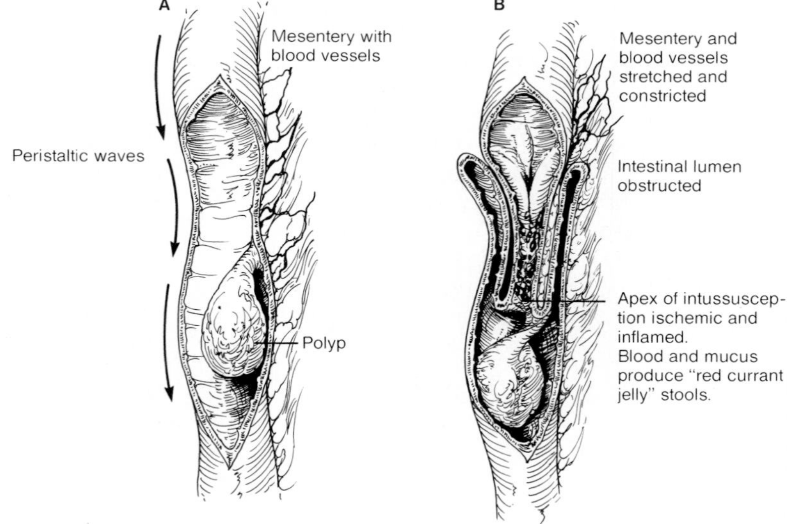

Figure 39–9. Intussusception. In the example shown, intussusception has been precipitated by a mucosal polyp **(A)** that acted as the apex of the intussusception **(B).** Note that the intussuscepted intestine becomes swollen and obstructs the intestinal lumen.

at a point of deficiency in the muscularis externa, are lined by mucosa and fibrous tissue and do not have muscle (Fig 39–10). Most acquired diverticula are false diverticula. Meckel's diverticulum is discussed on p 591. Other intestinal diverticula are discussed below.

Jejunal Diverticulosis

This disease is relatively uncommon and is characterized by the presence of multiple diverticula in the jejunum. Bacterial overgrowth in the static contents of the diverticula causes bile salt deconjugation and malabsorption.

Colonic Diverticulosis (Fig 39–10)

Colonic diverticulosis is common in developed countries, being present in over 50% of patients over the age of 60 years. The sigmoid colon is most commonly involved. The diverticula are false diverticula which occur in a double vertical row along the antimesenteric taenia coli.

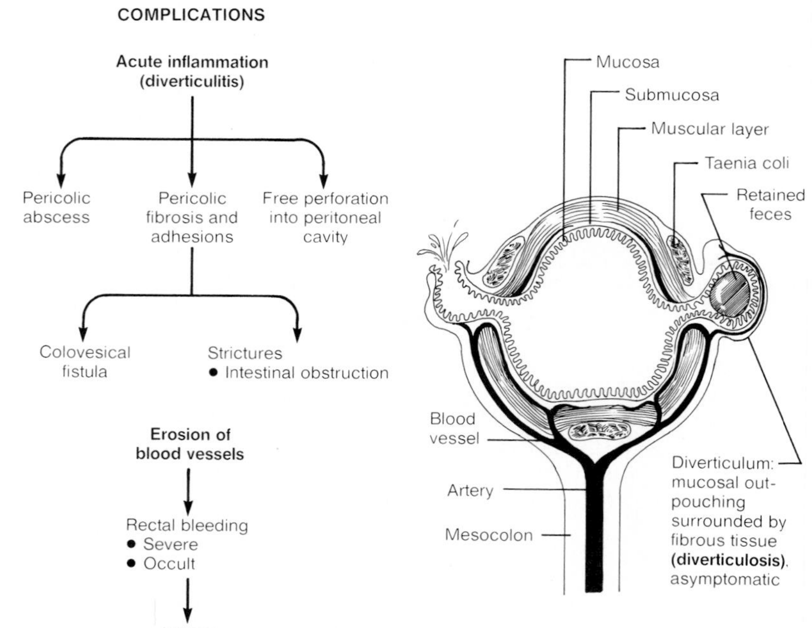

Figure 39–10. Cross section of sigmoid colon, showing diverticulosis. Complications associated with diverticulosis are shown on the left side.

The rarity of diverticula in underdeveloped countries has led to the suggestion that they are the result of a diet deficient in fiber. Such a diet produces a stool that is small and hard, which requires a high luminal pressure for evacuation. With high-fiber diets, the stool is soft and bulky, and defecation occurs with relatively low intraluminal pressures. High intraluminal pressure causes the mucosa to herniate at the point of greatest weakness, which is the point of penetration of the muscle wall by the arteries along the antimesenteric taenia coli.

Most cases of sigmoid diverticulosis are asymptomatic, but the following complications may occur: Infection (diverticulitis) causes fever, leukocytosis, and left lower quadrant abdominal pain ("left-sided appendicitis"). Extension of inflammation to the pericolic fat may occur, resulting in pericolic abscesses or rupture into the peritoneal cavity. Intestinal obstruction may occur as a result of marked pericolic fibrosis resulting from healed diverticulitis. Fistulas occur most commonly between the sigmoid colon and the urinary bladder. Hemorrhage may occur as a result of erosion of blood vessels in the wall of the diverticulum, causing the passage of bright red blood per rectum or slower occult bleeding, causing iron deficiency anemia. Diverticulitis is second only to hemorrhoids as a cause of rectal bleeding in elderly patients.

40 The Intestines: II. Infections; Inflammatory Bowel Diseases

I. INFECTIONS OF THE INTESTINE

Classification

Intestinal infections can be divided into 3 broad groups (Table 40–1):

(1) Enterotoxin-mediated, where the disease is caused by a bacterial exotoxin; the organism does not invade the tissues and in some cases does not even enter the body (staphylococcal toxin, botulism), the exotoxin being preformed in food.

(2) Invasive infections, where the organism invades the intestinal mucosa.

(3) Noninvasive infections, where the organism exists in the intestinal lumen and does not invade the tissues.

Most intestinal infections are transmitted by fecal contamination of food or drinking water. They are common in parts of the world where public health sanitary measures such as disposal of feces and purification of water supplies are not adequate.

Clinically, infections that involve the small intestine result in profuse watery diarrhea, while those that involve the colon produce dysentery (frequent small-volume diarrhea with blood and mucus). Fever is present in most invasive infections but is often absent in enterotoxin-mediated diseases.

Diagnosis (Table 40–2)

Diagnosis of intestinal infection is largely by stool culture (eg, *Shigella, Salmonella, Campylobacter, Escherichia coli*) or by observation of organisms in smear preparations of stool (eg, *Entamoeba, Giardia, Cryptosporidia, Isospora*). Serologic diagnosis is of value in certain instances (eg, rising titers of antibody to lipopolysaccharide cell wall "O" antigens in *Salmonella* infections). In diseases produced by toxins, identification of the toxin is often the only means of diagnosis (eg, *Clostridium difficile* enterocolitis).

With intestinal worm infections, stool specimens may reveal whole worms, body segments, larvae, or eggs depending upon the species.

ENTEROTOXIN-MEDIATED DISEASES

CHOLERA

Cholera is caused by *Vibrio cholerae.* The original classic strain has been supplanted by the El Tor variant, which is presently endemic in several Southeast Asian countries and occurs also in the southeastern United States. Infection occurs when

Table 40-1. Infections of intestines.

Organism	Source of Toxin or Infectious Agent	Clinical Illness
Toxin-mediated *Vibrio cholerae*	Contaminated water	Severe diarrhea
Escherichia coli, toxigenic	Food, water	Traveler's diarrhea
Staphylococcus aureus toxin	Toxin in food	Food poisoning
Clostridium perfringens	Reheated foods	Food poisoning
Bacillus cereus	Reheated foods	Food poisoning
Vibrio parahaemolyticus	Shellfish	Diarrhea and dysentery
Clostridium botulinum	Neurotoxin in food	Botulism
Invasive infections Viral Rotaviruses and adenoviruses	Person to person	Infantile diarrhea
Parvoviruses	Person to person	"Stomach flu"
Cytomegalovirus	Person to person	Enterocolitis (mainly in immunocompromised patients)
Bacterial *Salmonella* species	Food, milk, or water	Food poisoning
Salmonella typhi	Food, water	Typhoid
Shigella species	Food, water	Dysentery
Enteropathogenic *E coli*	Mostly person to person	Diarrhea and dysentery
Campylobacter fetus	Animals, infected persons, food	Childhood diarrhea
Yersinia species	Infected persons, food	Mesenteric adenitis, diarrhea
Mycobacterium tuberculosis	Infected person or milk	Chronic disease
Atypical mycobacteria	Infected person, soil	Chronic diarrhea (mainly in immunodeficient patients)
Protozoal *Entamoeba histolytica*	Fecal contamination (cysts)	Amebic colitis
Metazoan parasites (see Table 40–3)		
Noninvasive infections *Giardia lamblia*	Contaminated water	Giardiasis
Cryptosporidium, Isospora	Contaminated food, water	Diarrhea (mainly in immunocompromised patients)
Metazoan parasites (see Table 40–3)		

the organism is ingested with fecally contaminated food or water.

The organism multiplies in the intestinal lumen and produces an exotoxin that binds irreversibly to ganglioside receptors on the surface membranes of small intestinal mucosal cells (Fig 40–1). Toxin binding results in activation of adenylate cyclase and increased cAMP synthesis in the cell. cAMP is a stimulus for increased secretion of fluid and electrolytes by the cell into the intestinal lumen and causes secretory diarrhea. The toxin acts for about 24 hours but does not permanently damage the cell. Pathologic examination reveals a normal small intestinal mucosa on gross, light microscopic, and electron microscopic examination even in fatal cases.

Clinically, there is a severe secretory diarrhea, often without abdominal pain or fever. Patients become rapidly dehydrated, hypovolemic, and electrolyte-depleted. Shock and death may occur within 24 hours. The diagnosis is made by demonstrating the vibrio in a stool sample.

Cholera is theoretically easy to treat. The diarrhea subsides when the organism has been killed (tetracycline is highly effective) and when the cells bearing bound toxin have been replaced by regenerating cells. Correction of dehydration with fluid therapy is vital in the acute phase. Glucose-containing fluids can be administered orally because the mucosal cell retains the ability to absorb fluid and electrolytes in the presence of glucose; this is important in underdeveloped regions of the world, where intravenous fluid therapy may not be available. The mortality rate in epidemics of cholera is high, partly because of the rapidity with which dehydration occurs and partly because epidemics commonly occur in regions where medical facilities are inadequate.

Table 40-2. Laboratory diagnosis of intestinal infections.

Visual examination of feces	Large volume, watery ("rice water") stool indicates severe secretory diarrhea. Seen in toxin-mediated small intestinal infections (eg, cholera).
	Moderate volume, liquid brown or green ("pea soup") stool. Seen in many small bowel infections (eg, gastroenteritis, typhoid fever).
	Small volume stool composed largely of blood and mucus ("red currant jelly stool"). Seen in colonic diseases with mucosal ulceration.
Microscopic examination for neutrophils	Neutrophils absent: toxigenic bacteria, viruses, protozoa.
	Neutrophils present: invasive bacterial infections (*Shigella, Salmonella, Yersinia, Campylobacter,* pathogenic *Escherichia coli*). Also seen in noninfectious inflammatory bowel disease.
Direct examination for organisms	Hanging drop technique (*Vibrio cholerae*).
	Gram stain (*Staphylococcus aureus* in staphylococcal pseudomembranous enterocolitis).
	Electron microscopy for viruses.
	Fresh wet mount for *Entamoeba, Giardia,* helminth ova.
	Acid-fast stain for mycobacteria, *Cryptosporidium, Isospora.*
Stool culture	Routinely for *Shigella, Salmonella, Yersinia,* and *Campylobacter* (selective media).
	Vibrios can be cultured (thiosulfate-citrate-bile salt agar).
Blood culture	Typhoid fever (positive blood culture in 90% of cases).
	Usually negative in other intestinal infections; rarely, *Shigella* bacteremia may occur.
Serologic tests	*Salmonella* H, O, Vi antibodies in diagnosis of typhoid fever.
	Antibodies against *Entamoeba histolytica* useful in diagnosis of extraintestinal amebiasis.
Demonstration of enterotoxin	*Clostridium difficile* cytotoxin in stool and blood; heat-labile enterotoxin of *V cholerae* and *E coli.*

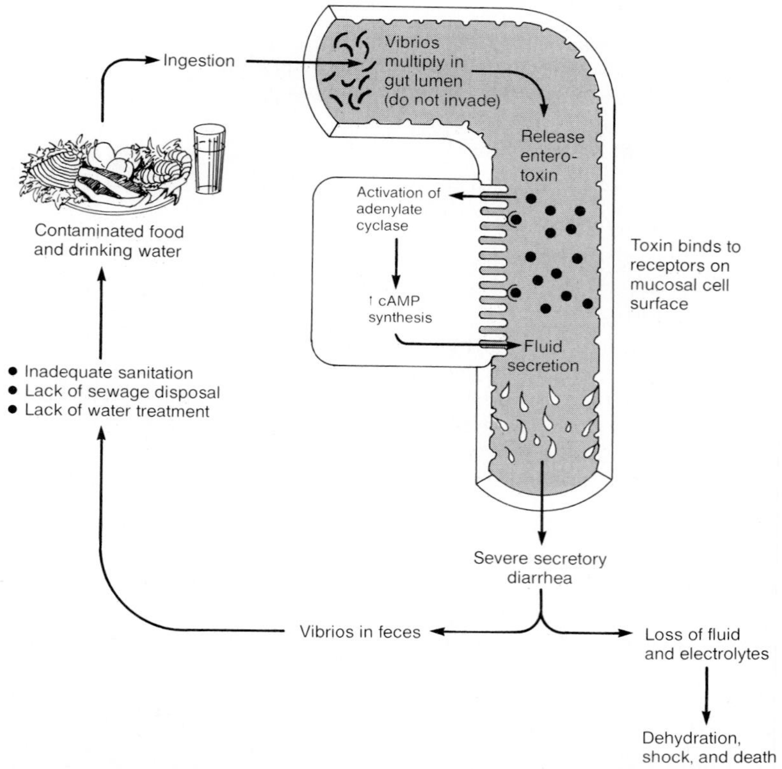

Figure 40–1. Cholera—mode of infection and pathogenesis.

TOXIGENIC *ESCHERICHIA COLI* INFECTION

Certain strains of *E coli* produce a heat-labile enterotoxin similar to cholera toxin in its mode of action. The ability to produce toxin is plasmid-induced and may therefore be transferred to other organisms. Toxigenic *E coli* causes **(1) traveler's diarrhea** in adults exposed to toxigenic strains of the bacillus against which they have no immunity and **(2) diarrhea epidemics** in neonatal units.

The disease is usually mild, though in neonates diarrhea may result in dangerous fluid and electrolyte depletion. The diagnosis is difficult to establish. *E coli* is a normal commensal in the colon and is present in normal stools. Though specific serotypes of *E coli* have been reported as being toxigenic, the correlation between serotypes and toxigenicity is not completely accurate. Techniques using tissue culture systems for identifying the heat-labile toxin of *E coli* are not widely available.

STAPHYLOCOCCAL FOOD POISONING

Staphylococcal food poisoning is a common form of epidemic food poisoning all over the world. It is caused by enterotoxin-producing strains of *Staphylococcus aureus* (Table 40–3). The organism multiplies in food that has been prepared and kept without refrigeration for several hours before it is eaten, leading to accumulation of the enterotoxin. Heating the food before ingestion destroys staphylococci but not the heat-stable toxin. The toxin causes severe nausea and vomiting of short duration, usually accompanied by abdominal cramps and diarrhea. The disease is self-limited. Death almost never occurs.

CLOSTRIDIUM DIFFICILE PSEUDOMEMBRANOUS ENTEROCOLITIS

Pseudomembranous enterocolitis complicates treatment with certain antibiotics—most commonly clindamycin, ampicillin, or tetracycline—that alter the intestinal bacterial flora, permitting the overgrowth of *C difficile,* which produces a powerful exotoxin that binds to and has a cytotoxic effect on mucosal epithelial cells, resulting in superficial necrosis and acute inflammation of the intestinal mucosa. The necrotic mucosa and exudate remain adherent to the mucosal surface as yellow plaques or membranes. The colon is usually most severely involved.

Clinically, there is an acute severe diarrhea with blood and mucus, accompanied by fever and an elevated white blood count. The disease progresses rapidly and is frequently fatal in the absence of prompt treatment. The diagnosis is based on the endoscopic and histologic features (Fig 40–2) and demonstration of *C difficile* exotoxin in blood and stool. Stool culture shows decreased numbers of commensal organisms; the finding of *C difficile* is difficult to interpret, since the organism is a normal commensal. Vancomycin is effective in treatment; cholestyramine is of immediate value in that it binds with and neutralizes the toxin.

Approximately 90% of cases of pseudomembranous enterocolitis are caused by *C difficile.* The causes in the other cases are unknown. Very rarely, invasive *S aureus* infection causes a severe pseudomembranous enterocolitis associated with the presence of large numbers of gram-positive cocci in a gram-stained smear of feces.

Table 40–3. Food poisoning.

Organism	Mechanism of Disease	Incubation	Illness
Staphylococcus aureus	Preformed heat-stable toxin, pies, non-refrigerated dairy products	2–4 hours	Vomiting, diarrhea
Bacillus cereus	Heat-stable toxin formed in food or gut, especially reheated fried rice	2–14 hours	Vomiting, diarrhea
Escherichia coli (toxin)	Organisms produce toxin in gut	24–72 hours	Mild traveler's diarrhea in adults; severe diarrhea in neonates
Clostridium perfringens	Organisms ingested in poorly cooked or reheated food; produces enterotoxin	8–14 hours	Diarrhea
Vibrio parahaemolyticus	Organism in poorly cooked shellfish; produces toxin in gut	8–96 hours	Vomiting, diarrhea, mild fever
Salmonella species (*typhimurium, enteritidis, newport,* etc)	Ingested organisms in food (especially shellfish) or water; invasive infection	8–24 hours	Fever, vomiting, diarrhea
Clostridium botulinum	Toxin in inadequately processed canned food or sausage	24–96 hours	Vomiting rare; diplopia, dysphagia, respiratory difficulty

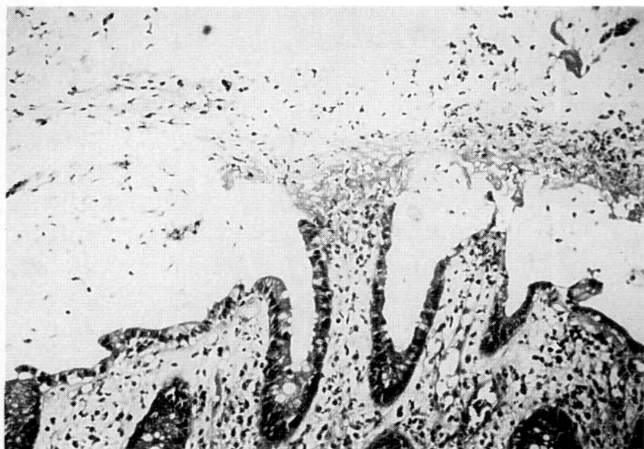

Figure 40-2. Pseudomembranous colitis caused by *Clostridium difficile,* showing superficial necrosis of the mucosa and the adherent mushroom-shaped pseudomembrane composed of necrotic tissue and inflammatory exudate.

OTHER ENTEROTOXIC DISEASES

Clostridium perfringens and *Bacillus cereus* also produce toxins that give a clinical picture of food poisoning similar to staphylococcal food poisoning (Table 40–3). *Vibrio parahaemolyticus,* often ingested in uncooked shellfish, multiplies in the intestine much like *V cholerae.* The mechanism of action of the enterotoxin is not known. The disease is mild and self-limited and is characterized by abdominal pain and diarrhea. In **botulism,** the toxin of *C botulinum* is present in inadequately processed food (commonly sausage or home-canned food). The toxin is destroyed by heating for 20 minutes at 100 °C, which is achieved in commercial canning operations. Though classified as a form of "food poisoning," botulism rarely causes diarrhea and usually presents with neuromuscular paralysis due to the systemic action of the exotoxin (see Chapter 13).

INVASIVE VIRAL & BACTERIAL INFECTIONS

VIRAL GASTROENTERITIS

Viral gastroenteritis ("stomach flu") is one of the commonest infections of humans. It is most often caused by rotaviruses and parvoviruses, of which the best known is the Norwalk agent.

The viruses infect the small intestinal epithelial cells, causing acute inflammation. The villi become blunted and infiltrated with lymphocytes and plasma cells.

Clinically, patients present with fever, acute diarrhea, vomiting, and abdominal pain. The illness is self-limited and mild, lasting 3–4 days. Diagnosis may be made by demonstrating the virus in stools or detecting a rise in antibody titer.

CYTOMEGALOVIRUS ENTEROCOLITIS

Cytomegalovirus is an important cause of intestinal infection in immunocompromised patients and is common in persons with AIDS. The virus infects the entire intestinal tract, producing a severe chronic diarrhea that may cause death, and infects mucosal epithelial cells as well as vascular endothelial cells. Cytomegalovirus vasculitis may result in focal ischemic necrosis of the wall; rarely, perforation of the intestine results. The diagnosis is established by demonstrating infected cells—greatly enlarged and containing large intranuclear inclusions and granular cytoplasmic inclusions—in biopsy specimens taken endoscopically.

SALMONELLA GASTROENTERITIS

Salmonella species other than *Salmonella typhi* are a common cause of bacterial "food poisoning" all over the world (Table 40–3). Infection results when food, water, and dairy products are contaminated with infected human or animal feces. Pasteurization of milk has decreased the incidence of this disease.

Infection causes acute inflammation of the small intestine, with diffuse mucosal hyperemia, swelling, focal superficial ulceration, and neutrophil infiltration.

Patients present with an acute onset of fever, abdominal pain, and diarrhea 1–3 days after infection. The disease is usually mild. Rarely, a more severe illness with bacteremia may occur.

TYPHOID FEVER

Typhoid fever is caused by *Salmonella typhi; Salmonella paratyphi* may produce a similar illness. The organism infects only humans, and infection results from contamination of food and water with feces from a case or carrier of typhoid. Typhoid is uncommon in the United States but is still prevalent in Third World countries.

Pathology & Clinical Features

The ingested bacillus invades the small intestinal mucosa, where it is taken up by macrophages and transported to regional lymph nodes. *S typhi* is a facultative intracellular organism and multiplies in the intestinal lymphoid tissue during the 1- to 3-week incubation period (Fig 40–3).

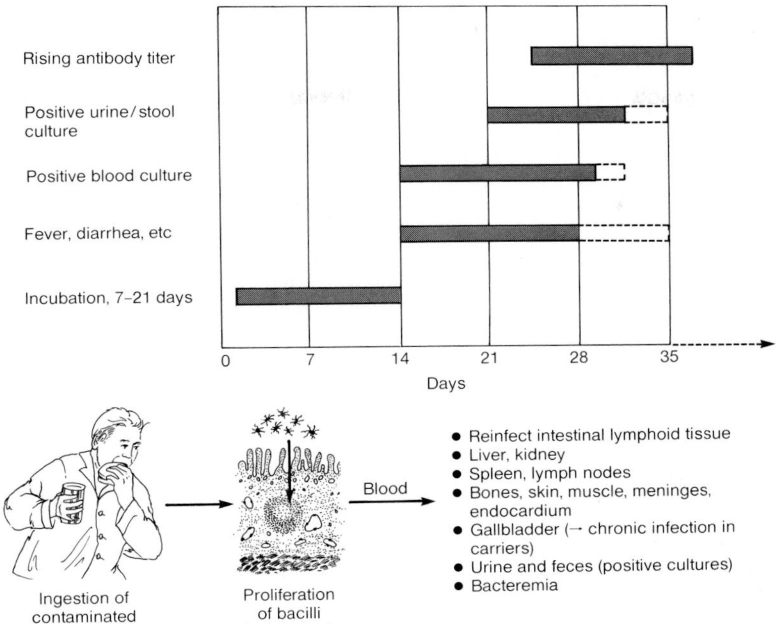

Figure 40–3. Typhoid fever—course and diagnostic tests. In the example above, the incubation period is 14 days (range, 7–21 days).

At the end of the incubation period, the bacilli enter the bloodstream (bacteremic phase), resulting in fever, headache, and muscle aches. Many tissues, including liver, heart, kidney, lungs, meninges, and bone, may be infected during this phase.

The diagnosis of typhoid fever is suggested by the following in a patient with continued fever: (1) splenomegaly; (2) a petechial skin rash (rose spots); (3) bradycardia, which is unusual in other febrile illnesses; and (4) peripheral blood neutropenia. All of these findings are present toward the end of the first week of clinical illness. The diagnosis is established at this time by blood culture, which is positive in 95% of cases.

In the second week of illness, *S typhi* reenters the intestinal lumen by way of biliary excretion (intestinal phase). The organism reinfects lymphoid tissue in the small intestine and colon in large numbers, causing acute inflammation, necrosis, and ulceration. Necrosis is the result of direct invasion plus endotoxin released by the bacillus, together with delayed hypersensitivity, which has developed by this time. The mucosal ulcers tend to take the shape of the underlying lymphoid follicles and typically occur as longitudinal ulcers overlying the Peyer patches in the ileum (Fig 40–4).

Microscopic examination shows edema and acute inflammation. The cellular infiltrate in typhoid is deficient in neutrophils and composed of macrophages, lymphocytes, and plasma cells. Necrosis and ulceration follow.

Clinically, the intestinal phase is characterized by diarrhea and continued fever. The diagnosis can be established by stool and urine culture (Fig 40–3), which is positive at this stage. Blood culture is still positive in about 60% of patients.

Complications

Bacteremia is common and often fatal if the patient is not treated. Hemorrhage may occur from the intestinal ulcers, and perforation may lead to peritonitis.

There may be evidence of skin infection ("rose spots") or, rarely, of meningitis, endocarditis, chondritis, osteomyelitis, or widespread focal necrosis of muscle (Zenker's degeneration).

After clinical recovery, 5% of patients continue to excrete bacilli in urine or feces; this carrier state is believed to be due to persistent low-grade infection in the kidney and gallbladder. Carriers represent a public health hazard, particularly if they are involved in handling food.

SHIGELLA COLITIS (Bacillary Dysentery)

Bacillary dysentery is caused by *Shigella* species. *Shigella sonnei* and *Shigella flexneri* are the common species and cause a relatively mild illness. *Shigella boydii* is uncommon. *Shigella dysenteriae* type I (Shiga's bacillus) produces a severe illness and is endemic in Central America and

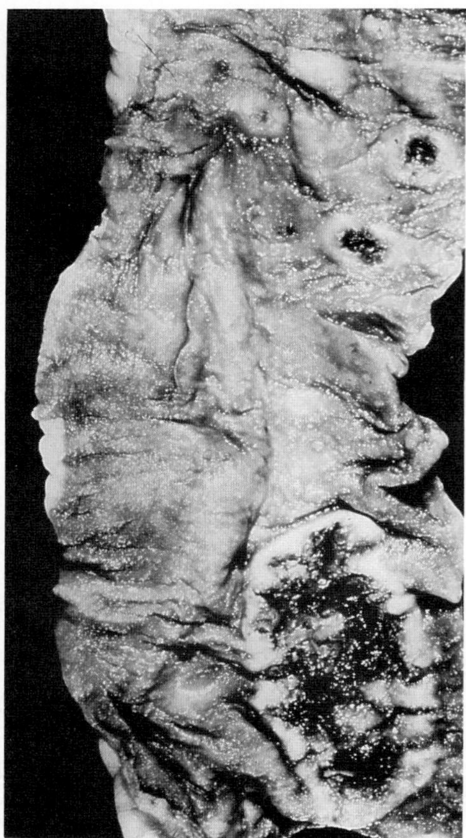

Figure 40–4. Typhoid fever, showing ulceration of lymphoid patches in the terminal small intestine. The longitudinal ulcer, which takes the shape of Peyer's patches, is typical of typhoid fever.

parts of Asia. Shigella dysentery is common in the United States.

Shigella species affect the colon, producing an acute inflammation with diffuse hyperemia, edema, and multiple superficial ulcers. Neutrophils are the dominant cells. Bacteremia is rare. *S dysenteriae* type I produces an exotoxin that is absorbed into the bloodstream and causes endothelial damage, leading to disseminated intravascular coagulation.

Clinically, bacillary dysentery is an acute illness characterized by high fever, severe diarrhea with blood and mucus in the stool, and neutrophilic leukocytosis. Passage of 10–40 stools per day is usual; individual stools are of small volume and often composed entirely of blood, mucus, and the inflammatory exudate. Diagnosis is made by stool culture.

ENTEROINVASIVE *ESCHERICHIA COLI* INFECTION

Some strains of *Escherichia coli* have the ability to invade the intestinal mucosa and cause epidemics of **necrotizing enterocolitis** in neonates or **invasive intestinal infections** in older children and adults. Extensive necrosis of the mucosa often causes death in neonates. The disease in children and adults simulates either salmonellosis, when the small intestine is maximally involved, or *Shigella* dysentery when colitis predominates. Children who recover may develop fibrous strictures. The identification of serotypes of *E coli* that are invasive is very difficult.

CAMPYLOBACTER FETUS INFECTION

Campylobacter fetus is a curved bacterium recognized recently as being a common cause of enterocolitis and responsible for about 10% of cases of bacterial diarrhea in children. The disease is acquired from infected humans and animals.

Both small intestine and colon are affected, causing diarrhea and dysentery. The disease is usually mild. Diagnosis is by stool culture. Treatment with antibiotics is effective.

YERSINIA ENTEROCOLITICA & *YERSINIA PSEUDOTUBERCULOSIS* INFECTION

These two *Yersinia* species cause fever, diarrhea, and marked painful enlargement of mesenteric lymph nodes **(mesenteric adenitis)**, with right lower quadrant abdominal pain. Differentiation from acute appendicitis can be difficult.

Diagnosis is made by stool culture.

INTESTINAL TUBERCULOSIS

Primary Intestinal Tuberculosis

Primary tuberculous infection of the intestine has become rare as a result of pasteurization of milk and eradication of bovine tuberculosis in dairy herds. It is characterized by a small focus in the intestine and large mesenteric lymph nodes, analogous to the primary complex in the lung.

Secondary Intestinal Tuberculosis

This form of tuberculosis still occurs as a result of swallowing of infected sputum by patients with active pulmonary disease or reactivation of a dormant intestinal focus, usually in the terminal ileum or cecum.

Typical caseous granulomas form. The organisms spread locally in the intestinal lymphatics, resulting in ulcers that are transverse because the intestinal lymphatics pass circumferentially. Fibrosis leads to strictures (Fig 40–5). Involvement of the serosa results in fibrous adhesions between loops of intestine. Fistula formation may occur.

Clinically, intestinal tuberculosis is a chronic illness characterized by low-grade fever and diarrhea, which may be tinged with blood. A mass may be palpable in a few cases (hyperplastic cecal tuberculosis). The diagnosis is made by culturing tubercle bacilli from the stools.

Complications of intestinal tuberculosis include intestinal obstruction, caused by strictures, fistulas, and tuberculous peritonitis.

ATYPICAL MYCOBACTERIOSIS

Intestinal infection with *Mycobacterium avium-intracellulare* occurs in elderly or immunocompromised patients. *M avium-intracellulare* enteritis is one cause of severe chronic diarrhea in patients with AIDS. The organisms accumulate in large numbers in macrophages in the mucosa, and there is little or no inflammation. Spread to lymph nodes is common. The diagnosis may be established by biopsy or identification of the organism in stools by direct examination (using acid-fast stain) or culture.

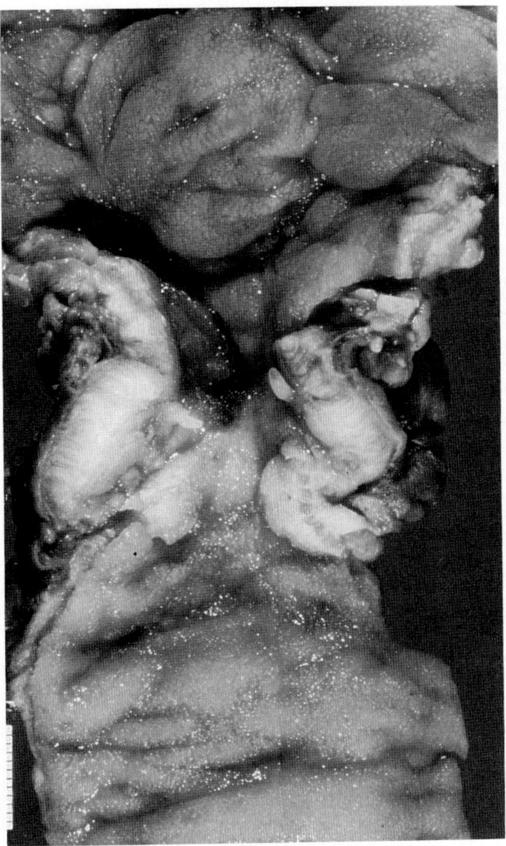

Figure 40–5. Intestinal tuberculosis, chronic phase, showing formation of a stricture secondary to fibrosis of the circumferential ulcers. The intestine proximal to the stricture is dilated secondary to intestinal obstruction.

ACUTE APPENDICITIS

Acute appendicitis is the commonest surgical emergency. It occurs at all ages, with a peak incidence in young adulthood.

In most cases, inflammation of the appendix is preceded by obstruction of the appendiceal lumen (Fig 40–6) by a fecalith (hardened mass of feces), by kinking of the wall, or by submucosal lymphoid hyperplasia. Stagnation distal to the obstruction permits multiplication of colonic bacterial flora, including potential pathogens such as *Escherichia coli, Streptococcus faecalis,* and anaerobic bacteria. These bacteria then invade the mucosa and appendiceal wall, causing acute inflammation.

Pathology

Acute inflammation of the mucosa is followed by ulceration and inflammation of the entire wall. Neutrophils are the dominant cells. Suppuration commonly occurs. Grossly, the inflamed appendix appears swollen and red, with a surface that has lost its normal shiny appearance and frequently is covered by a fibrinopurulent exudate. In a minority of cases, the external appearance is normal, and the diagnosis is confirmed only on histologic examination.

Clinical Features

Patients present with acute onset of fever, abdominal pain, and vomiting. Pain is initially periumbilical (referred pain) but becomes localized to the right lower quadrant when the pain-sensitive parietal peritoneum is involved. Tenderness and guarding (reflex muscle spasm during palpation) are commonly present. The peripheral blood shows neutrophilic leukocytosis. The diagnosis must be made on the basis of the clinical features, since laboratory and radiologic features are nonspecific. Surgical treatment (appendectomy) is curative.

Complications

Local extension of the inflammatory process may involve the periappendiceal tissues and result in an inflammatory mass ("phlegmon") in the right lower quadrant or appendiceal abscess. Perforation into the peritoneal cavity may result in acute peritonitis, and distant abscesses may form—commonly in the rectovesical pouch or subphrenic region. Infection of the portal venous radicals—very rare—causes portal vein thrombo-

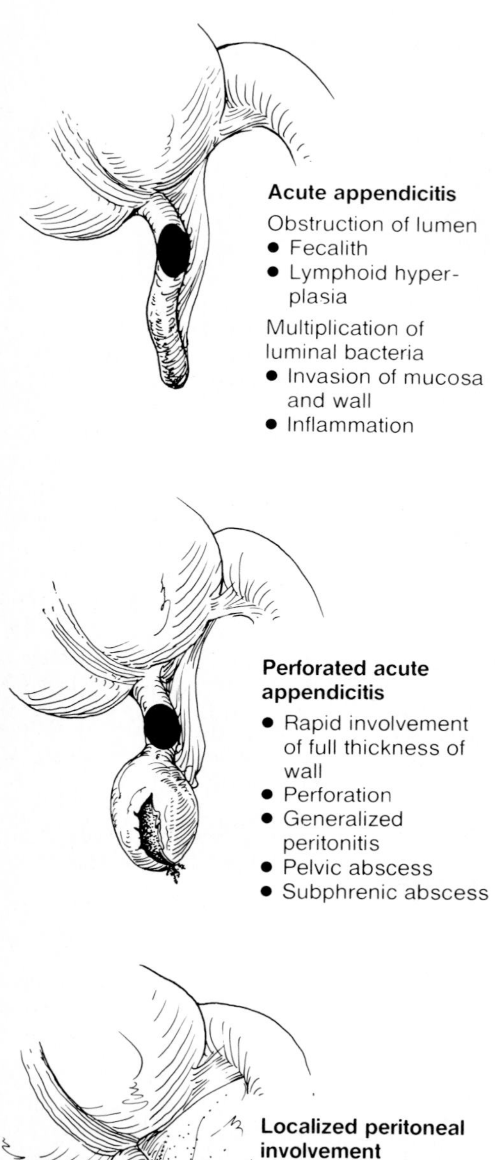

Figure 40-6. Pathogenesis and complications of acute appendicitis.

phlebitis with multiple liver abscesses (pylephlebitis suppurativa).

PROTOZOAL INFECTIONS

AMEBIASIS

Entamoeba histolytica is a common pathogen of the colon in underdeveloped countries. In the United States it occurs mainly in cities with high immigrant populations.

Infection occurs by ingestion of cysts in food and water contaminated with feces. Ingested cysts release active amebas (trophozoites) that invade the large intestinal mucosa and enter the submucosa, which is the site of maximum involvement. The amebas cause multiple areas of enzymatic necrosis of tissue and acute inflammation, leading to "flask-shaped" submucosal abscesses throughout the colon (Fig 40–7). The mucosal surface—as seen at colonoscopy—shows multiple ulcers separated by healthy-appearing mucosa which is, however, undermined by the submucosal abscesses. Amebas are found in the walls of the ulcers (Fig 40–8) The trophozoites typically contain phagocytosed erythrocytes in their cytoplasm.

Infection is usually localized to the submucosa and mucosa. Rarely, necrosis involves the muscle, leading to intestinal perforation. Hemorrhage and toxic megacolon may also occur with severe infection, and venous spread to the liver may occur (Chapter 42).

Clinically, patients with amebic colitis present with bloody and mucous diarrhea accompanied by low-grade fever. The illness is less severe than *Shigella* colitis but tends to be more persistent. The diagnosis is made by the finding of trophozoites of *E histolytica* in the stools or in a biopsy specimen. Amebicidal drugs such as metronidazole are highly effective in treatment.

GIARDIASIS

Giardiasis is a common infection caused by the protozoan flagellate *Giardia lamblia.* Infection is by ingestion of cysts in food and water contaminated with feces. After ingestion, excystment and release of trophozoites occurs in the duodenum.

Giardia attaches itself to the surface of the small intestinal mucosal cells by its ventral sucker. The duodenum is involved most heavily. In heavy infections, a large part of the mucosal surface area may be occupied by parasites, causing mechanical interference with absorption. Giardiasis also causes partial villous atrophy, which contrib-

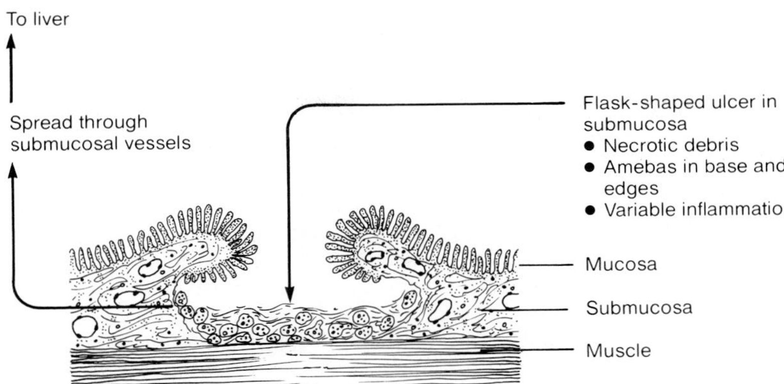

Figure 40-7. Amebic colitis, showing typical flask-shaped ulcers with maximal involvement of the submucosa.

utes to malabsorption. The organism does not invade tissues.

Clinically, infected individuals develop cramping abdominal pain, with diarrhea and steatorrhea due to malabsorption. The diagnosis is made by identifying the organism in stools, duodenal aspirates (Fig 40-9), or duodenal biopsies.

INTESTINAL CRYPTOSPORIDIOSIS & ISOSPORIASIS IN AIDS

Two protozoa belonging to the *Cryptosporidium* and *Isospora* species have been identified as common causes of chronic watery diarrhea in patients with AIDS. Diarrhea is severe and chronic and not uncommonly causes death.

The parasites may rarely infect healthy individuals, causing a mild self-limited acute diarrhea. In AIDS, multiplication proceeds unimpeded, leading to massive infection of the small intestine and colon, and severe diarrhea. *Cryptosporidium* is present in large numbers, usually attached to the surface of the epithelial cell. The diagnosis is established by identifying the organism in stool smears stained with acid-fast stains. *Cryptosporidium* is 2–4 μm in diameter, round, and seen only in acid-fast stained smears. *Isospora* is larger and may be seen in both unstained wet mounts and acid-fast stained smears.

INTESTINAL HELMINTHIASIS

Intestinal helminthiasis is extremely common in underdeveloped countries and has been estimated as afflicting about 25% of the world population.

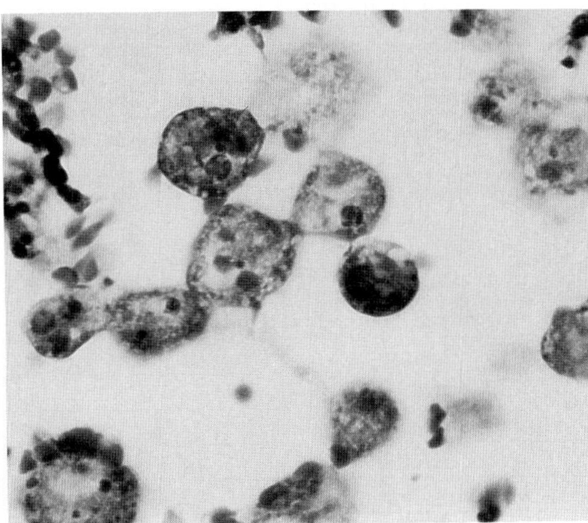

Figure 40-8. Amebic colitis. High-magnification photograph of the edge of an ulcer, showing trophozoites of *Entamoeba histolytica*. Note the presence of ingested erythrocytes that characterize tissue forms.

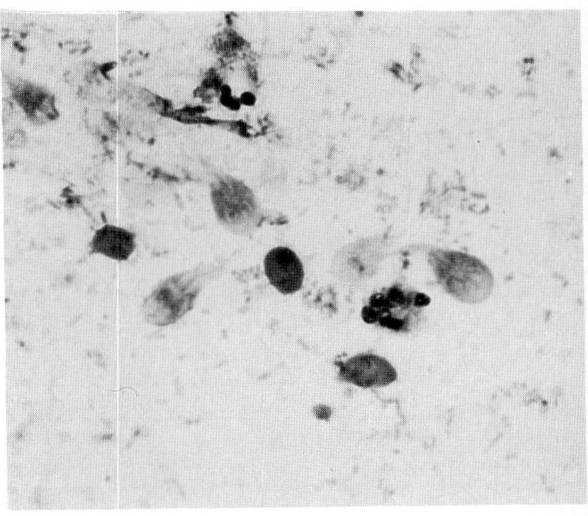

Figure 40-9. *Giardia lamblia* trophozoites in a duodenal aspirate.

In many of these diseases, the worm lives in the lumen without causing major symptoms; in others, significant clinical manifestations occur (Table 40–4).

II. IDIOPATHIC INFLAMMATORY BOWEL DISEASE

The term idiopathic inflammatory bowel disease is used for 2 diseases—Crohn's disease and ulcerative colitis. Though their causes are still not unclear, the 2 diseases probably have an immunologic hypersensitivity basis. They are recognized as distinct entities with distinct clinical and pathologic features (Table 40–5).

In about 10% of patients with idiopathic inflammatory bowel disease affecting the colon, it is difficult to differentiate between Crohn's disease and ulcerative colitis because features of both are present. These cases are characterized as indeterminate idiopathic inflammatory bowel disease. Because such "mixed" cases occur and because both Crohn's disease and ulcerative colitis have similar geographic distributions and occur in similar ethnic and age groups—or even in single families—it has been suggested that both may represent one disease process. However, there are so many differences that it is probably best to regard them as 2 diseases until their cause is determined.

CROHN'S DISEASE

Crohn's disease is a chronic inflammatory disorder that most commonly affects the ileum and colon but has the potential to involve any part of the gastrointestinal tract from the mouth to the anus. It is characterized by involvement of discontinuous segments of intestine ("skip areas"), noncaseating epithelioid cell granulomas, and transmural (full-thickness) inflammation of the affected parts (Fig 40–10).

Incidence

Crohn's disease occurs mainly in Western Europe and the United States and is uncommon in Asia and South America. The incidence appears to be increasing. In the United States, Crohn's disease affects chiefly whites; blacks, Native Americans, and Hispanics are less frequently affected. The highest incidence is in Jews.

Both sexes are affected equally. The disease can occur at any age but has its highest incidence in young adults. It is uncommon in young children. Crohn's disease has a familial tendency, with 20–30% of patients giving a positive family history. There is no inheritance pattern, and the familial tendency is likely to be the result of sharing a common environment.

Table 40–4. Helminthic infections of the intestine.

Parasite	Site	Clinical Effects
Ascaris lumbricoides (roundworm)	Small intestine	Intestinal obstruction by worm mass; migration up bile duct (cholangitis, gallstones) and pancreatic duct
	Lung (larval migration)	Cough, wheezing (Löffler's syndrome)
Enterobius vermicularis (pinworm)	Cecal region	Anal pruritus; migration up vagina, urethra (rare)
Trichuris trichiura (whipworm)	Colon	Bloody diarrhea, rectal prolapse (rare; only in heavy infestations)
Ancylostoma duodenale and *Necator americanus* (hookworm)	Small intestine	Iron deficiency anemia caused by sucking of blood by worm (common)
Strongyloides stercoralis	Small intestine	Bloody diarrhea
	Lung (larval migration)	Hyperinfection in immunodeficient patients
Trichinella spiralis	Small intestine	Abdominal pain and diarrhea
	Parasitemia	Myositis, myocarditis, encephalitis
Taenia solium	Small intestine	Asymptomatic
	Larval migration	Cysticercosis
Taenia saginata	Small intestine	Asymptomatic
Diphyllobothrium latum	Small intestine	Vitamin B_{12} deficiency
Schistosoma mansoni	Colon	Bloody diarrhea; portal hypertension
Schistosoma japonicum	Small intestine	Diarrhea; portal hypertension
Fasciolopsis buski	Small intestine	Abdominal pain, diarrhea (with heavy infestations)

Table 40–5. Differences between ulcerative colitis and Crohn's colitis.

	Ulcerative Colitis	Crohn's Colitis
Clinical features		
Rectal involvement	Over 90%	Rectum spared in > 50%
Distribution of lesions	Continuous	Skip lesions
Mucosal appearance	Friable, purulent, diffusely involved	Aphthous, linear ulcers with cobblestoning
Associated ileal disease	10%, mild, terminal ileal inflammation	50% have combined ileal and colonic involvement
Perianal abscess, fistulas	Rare	Common
Intestinal strictures and obstruction	Not seen	Common
Intestinal fistulas	Not seen	Common
Fissures (radiologic)	Not seen	Common
Intestinal perforation	Rare	Rare
Intestinal hemorrhage (severe)	Common	Rare
Pathologic features		
Depth of inflammation	Mucosal (submucosal rarely)	Transmural
Creeping mesenteric fat	Not seen	Common
Fibrous thickening of wall	Not seen	Common ("lead pipe")
Crypt abscesses	Common	Common
Pseudopolyps	Common	Common
Granulomas (epithelioid, noncaseating)	Not seen	Common
Fissures (microscopic)	Not seen	Common
Dysplasia	Common	Rare
Carcinoma	10%	Rare

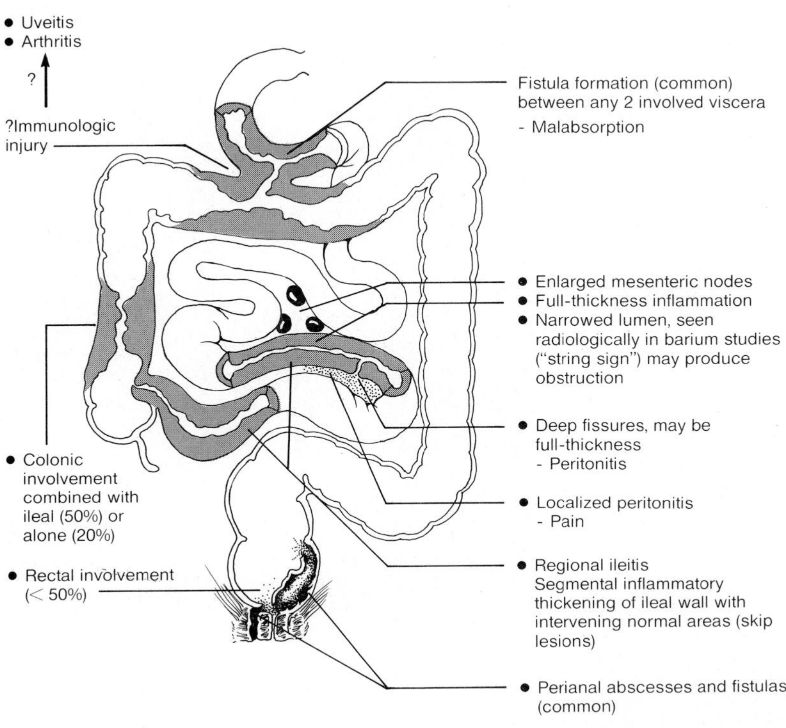

Fig 40–10. Pathologic features of Crohn's disease.

Etiology

The cause of Crohn's disease is unknown. Despite extensive search, no infectious agent has been found.

There is strong but not conclusive evidence that Crohn's disease is the result of some immunologic injury. Antibodies with activity against intestinal epithelial cells have been identified in the serum and lymphocytes of patients with Crohn's disease. These antibodies may be autoantibodies (making Crohn's disease an autoimmune disease), or they may represent an immune response to an intestinal epithelial injury due to other causes. Patients with active Crohn's disease frequently have T cell dysfunction (anergy to tuberculin and mumps antigen, low peripheral blood T cell count).

Pathology (Fig 40-10)

A. Sites of Involvement: Combined ileal (most commonly terminal ileum) and colonic disease is most common (50%). The ileum alone is involved in 30% of patients and the colon alone in 20%. Crohn's disease of the colon is also called granulomatous colitis. Involvement of the oral cavity, larynx, esophagus, stomach, and perineum are rare.

Patients with Crohn's disease commonly (in 75% of cases) have perianal lesions such as abscesses, fistulas, and skin tags. Perianal disease occurs in both ileal and colonic disease and is not dependent on the presence of rectal involvement.

B. Gross Appearance: Involvement is typically segmental, with skip areas of normal intestine between areas of involved bowel. Normal and affected intestine are sharply demarcated from one another.

In the acute phase, the intestine is swollen and reddened. The mucosa shows diffuse hyperemia, acute inflammation, and ulceration. In the chronic phase, the affected segment is greatly thickened and rigid ("lead pipe" or "garden hose" appearance; Fig 40-11). Marked fibrosis causing luminal narrowing, with intestinal obstruction, is common. The serosa is dull and granular. In involved ileal segments, the mesenteric fat creeps from the mesentery to surround the bowel wall ("creeping fat"). The mucosal surface shows longitudinal serpiginous ulcers separated by irregular islands of edematous mucosa. This results in the typical "cobblestone" effect (Fig 40-12). Fissures (deep and narrow ulcers that look like stabs with a knife that penetrate deeply into the wall of the affected intestine) and fistulas (communications with other viscera) may be present.

C. Microscopic Features: Crohn's disease is characterized by distortion of mucosal crypt architecture, transmural inflammation (Fig 40-13), and the presence of epithelioid granulomas on histologic examination (Fig 40-14); granulomas are present in about 60% of patients. Numerous other

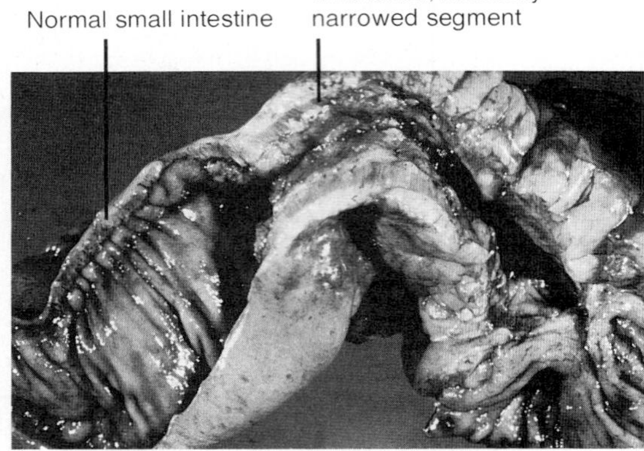

Figure 40-11. Crohn's disease of the terminal ileum, showing marked segmental narrowing and thickening ("lead pipe" or "garden hose" appearance).

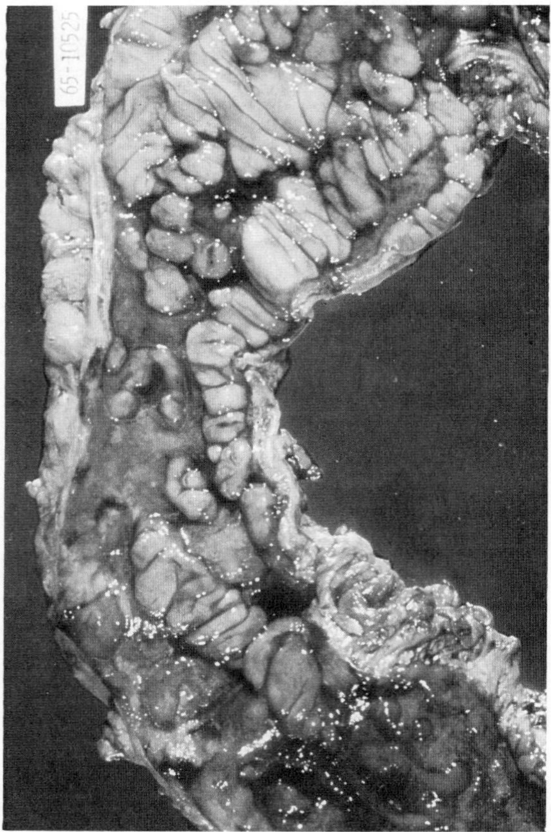

Figure 40-12. Crohn's disease of the colon, showing typical cobblestone appearance of the mucosa with longitudinal ulceration and intervening islands of less affected mucosa.

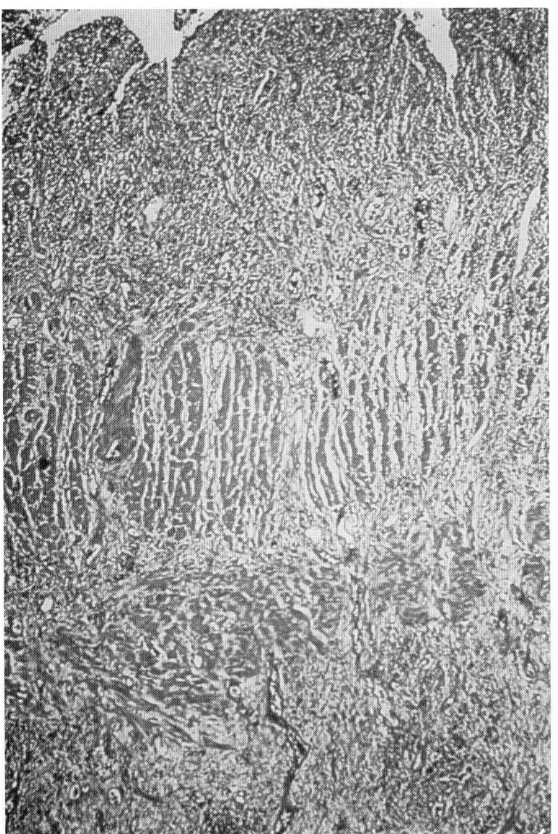

Figure 40-13. Crohn's disease. Low-power microscopic appearance, showing transmural inflammation. The ulcerated, inflamed mucosa is at the top; the muscle fibers in the wall at center are separated by the inflammatory cell infiltrate.

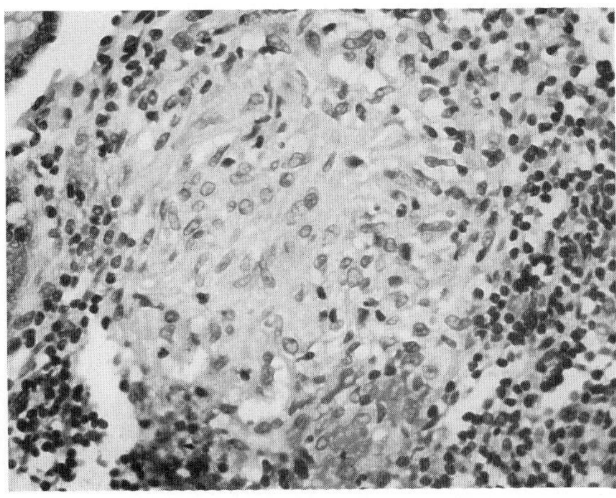

Figure 40-14. Crohn's disease. Noncaseating epithelioid cell granuloma in the mucosa.

histologic changes occur in Crohn's disease, but none are of great diagnostic use. These features include lymphedema of the submucosa, lymphoid follicles at all levels of the bowel wall, and marked fibrosis. Fissure-ulcers and fistulas can be seen microscopically.

The regional mesenteric lymph nodes are frequently enlarged and may contain noncaseating granulomas.

Clinical Features

Presentation is extremely variable. In the acute phase, fever, diarrhea, and right lower quadrant pain may mimic acute appendicitis.

Chronic disease is characterized by remissions and relapses over a long period of time. Asymptomatic periods may last several months. With the passage of time, weight loss and anemia appear. Thickening of the intestine may produce an ill-defined mass in the abdomen.

Diagnosis

Diagnosis is based on a combination of clinical, radiologic, and pathologic findings. In the active phase of the disease, the erythrocyte sedimentation rate and white blood cell count may be elevated, but these are nonspecific findings.

Complications

Crohn's disease may be complicated by intestinal obstruction or by fistula formation between involved loops of bowel and adjacent viscera. Fistulas between the ileum and the colon result in malabsorption as a result of colonization of the ileum with colonic bacteria; those between ileal loops may short-circuit the bowel, again resulting in malabsorption. Enterovesical fistulas lead to urinary infections and passage of gas and feces with urine. Enterovaginal fistulas produce a fecal vaginal discharge.

Malabsorption syndrome may also follow disease in the terminal ileum, in which there may be failure of absorption of vitamin B_{12} and bile salts, resulting in megaloblastic anemia and fat malabsorption. Iron deficiency anemia may occur as a result of chronic occult bleeding, and protein-losing enteropathy as a result of loss of protein from the inflamed mucosa.

Extraintestinal manifestations are common in Crohn's disease and include arthritis and uveitis. The mechanisms are unknown.

Crohn's disease carries a slightly increased risk of development of carcinoma of the colon—much less than in ulcerative colitis.

ULCERATIVE COLITIS

Ulcerative colitis is an inflammatory disease of uncertain cause. It has a chronic course characterized by remissions and relapses.

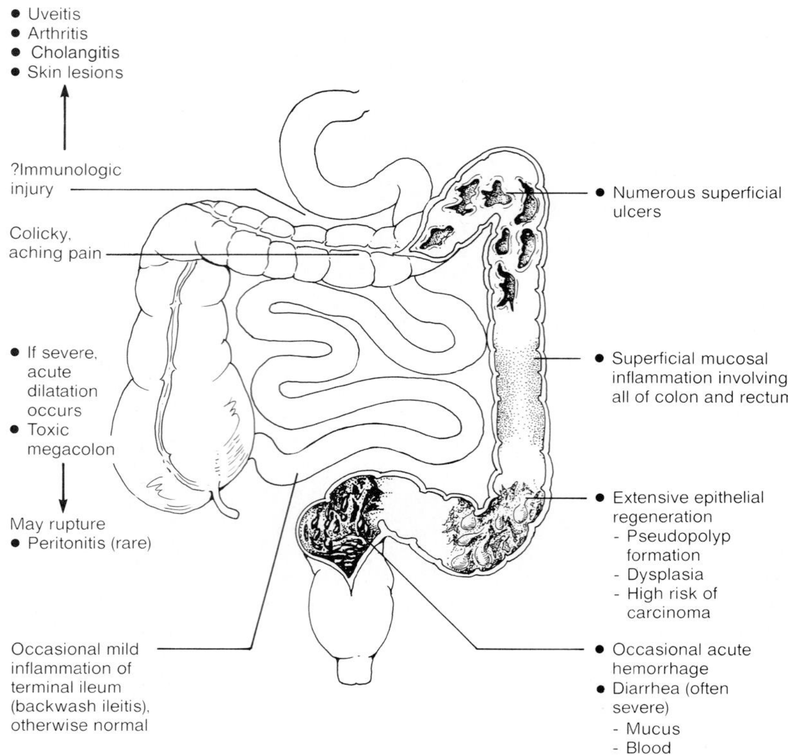

Figure 40-15. Pathologic features of ulcerative colitis.

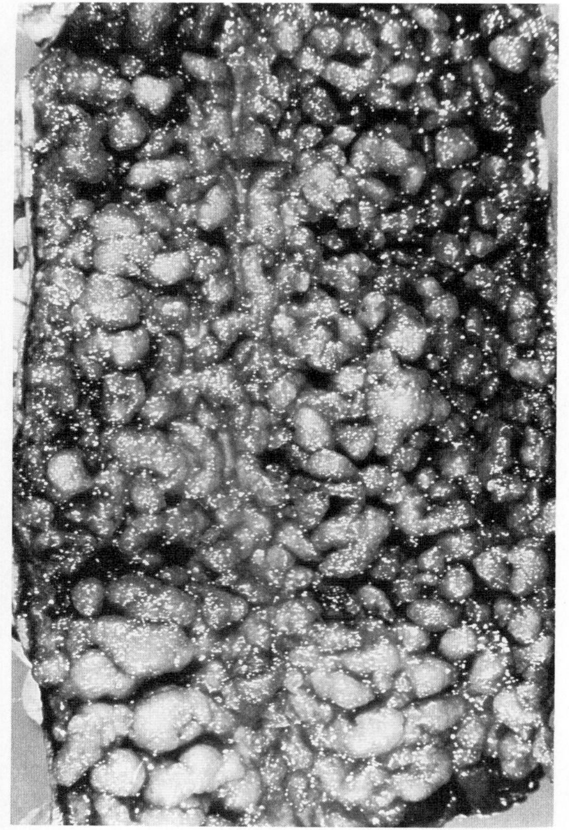

Figure 40-16. Acute ulcerative colitis, showing diffuse erythema and edema of the colonic mucosa. The extensive ulceration of the mucosa is masked by the pseudopolypoid appearance of the inflamed surviving mucosa.

Incidence

In the United States, about 400,000 patients suffer from ulcerative colitis, and there are about 25,000 new cases every year. The disease is common in the 20- to 30-year age group but may occur at any age. The incidence is slightly higher in females than in males. In the United States, whites are more often affected than blacks, and Jews more often than non-Jews. Worldwide, the disease is most prevalent in North America and Western Europe and less prevalent in Asia, Africa, and South America.

Etiology

The cause is unknown; no infectious agent has been identified. Antibodies that cross-react with intestinal epithelial cells and certain serotypes of *Escherichia coli* have been demonstrated in the serum of some patients with ulcerative colitis. Allergy to food proteins has been suggested as a possible cause but without proof.

Psychologic stress frequently precipitates ulcerative colitis, leading to the suggestion that the disease has a psychosomatic basis.

Pathology (Fig 40–15)

A. Sites of Involvement: Ulcerative colitis is a disease of the rectum, which is involved in almost all cases and in some patients remains the only site of disease, and the colon. The disease tends to extend proximally from the rectum in a continuous manner without skip areas. Total colonic involvement is not uncommon. The appendix is involved in about 30% of cases. The ileum is not involved as a rule; 10% of cases show mild nonspecific mucosal inflammation for a few centimeters proximal to the ileocecal valve ("backwash ileitis").

B. Gross Appearance: Ulcerative colitis involves mainly the mucosa. Even in severe disease, the external appearance of the affected colon shows nothing other than mild hyperemia. There is rarely any thickening of the wall. In very rare cases of severe acute ulcerative colitis, toxic dilatation (megacolon) occurs.

The mucosal surface shows diffuse hyperemia with numerous superficial ulcerations in the acute phase. The rough, red, velvety appearance on colonoscopy is characteristic though not specific (Fig 40–16). In the chronic phase of the disease during remission, the mucosa appears flat and atrophic due to reepithelialization of the ulcers. The regenerated or nonulcerated mucosa may appear polypoid (inflammatory "pseudopolyps") in contrast with the atrophic areas or ulcers (Fig 40–17).

C. Microscopic Appearance: In the acute phase, the mucosa shows marked inflammation with neutrophils, lymphocytes, and plasma cells. Neutrophils are present in both lamina propria and in glands (crypt abscesses). In the chronic phase, the crypts are decreased in number (crypt atrophy) and show distorted architecture due to abnormal branching (Fig 40–18). There are numerous chronic inflammatory cells in the lamina propria. Most cases have both acute and chronic features.

The inflammation is usually restricted to the mucosa. In severe cases with extensive ulceration, the superficial part of the submucosa may be involved, but the muscle wall is not affected (Fig 40–19).

Clinical Features

In the acute phase and during relapse, the patient has fever, leukocytosis, lower abdominal

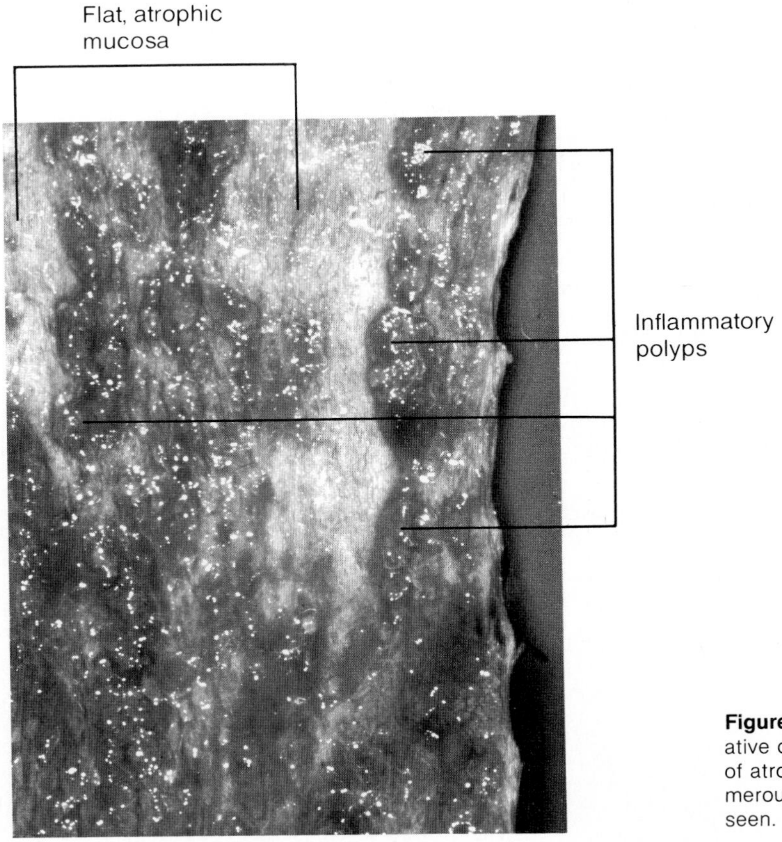

Figure 40–17. Chronic ulcerative colitis, showing flat areas of atrophic mucosa in which numerous inflammatory polyps are seen.

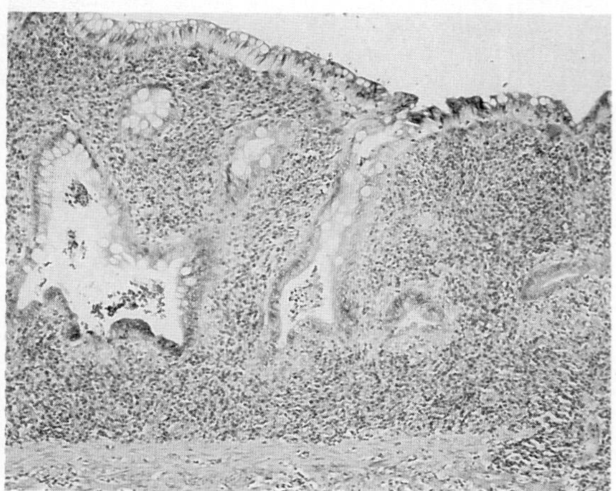

Figure 40-18. Colonic mucosal changes of chronic idiopathic inflammatory bowel disease, showing marked atrophy and distortion of crypts with increased numbers of chronic inflammatory cells in the lamina propria. Note that these changes are present in both ulcerative colitis and Crohn's disease.

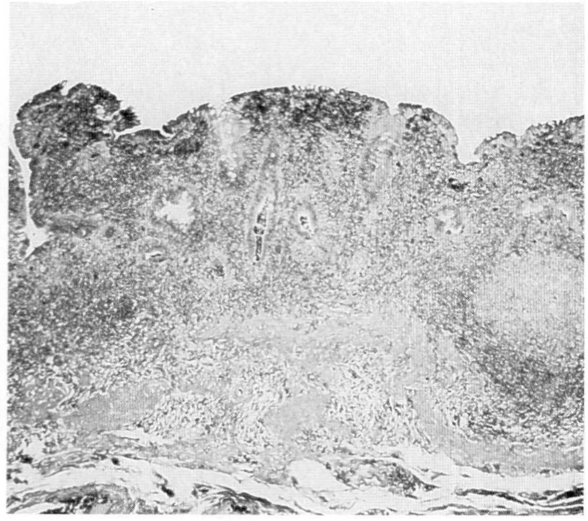

Figure 40-19. Chronic ulcerative colitis, showing inflammation restricted to the mucosa. The muscularis externa is seen at the bottom. At right is shown a lymphoid follicle.

pain, and diarrhea with blood and mucus in the stool. The disease usually has a chronic course, with remissions and exacerbations; in some cases, the patient has chronic continuous disease with mild diarrhea and bleeding.

Diagnosis

The diagnosis of ulcerative colitis is based on a combination of clinical, radiologic, and pathologic findings. The erythrocyte sedimentation rate and white blood count are elevated during the acute phase.

Mucosal biopsies taken at endoscopy are useful in diagnosis. The presence of crypt atrophy, distortion of crypt architecture, and an increased number of lymphocytes and plasma cells in the lamina propria are helpful in differentiating ulcerative colitis from other causes of acute colitis. However, these mucosal changes can be seen in both ulcerative colitis and Crohn's disease (Fig 40-18). The only finding on mucosal biopsy that reliably differentiates ulcerative colitis and Crohn's disease is the presence of noncaseating epithelioid granulomas in the latter (Table 40-5).

Complications

Severe bleeding may occur as a complication in the acute phase. Toxic megacolon in severe acute disease is characterized by dilatation of the colon, with functional obstruction and, rarely, perforation. It carries a high mortality rate and requires emergency colectomy.

Extraintestinal manifestations occur more commonly in ulcerative colitis than in Crohn's disease. They include arthritis, uveitis, skin lesions (a necrotic skin lesion in the extremities known as pyoderma gangrenosum is typical), and sclerosing pericholangitis (fibrosis around bile ducts), leading to obstructive jaundice.

Patients with chronic ulcerative colitis have an increased risk of developing colon carcinoma. The overall risk is about 10%. The risk increases progressively with disease duration beyond 7 years, with the length of colon involved—greatest with involvement of the entire colon—and the age at onset of disease—the earlier the onset, the greater the risk. Carcinomas occurring in ulcerative colitis tend to be poorly differentiated, infiltrative, and aggressive neoplasms with a poor prognosis.

Epithelial dysplasia precedes carcinoma in most cases. The presence of severe dysplasia in mucosal biopsies in patients with total colitis of over 10 years' duration imposes a high risk of cancer and is an indication for total colectomy to prevent the occurrence of cancer.

The Intestines: III. Neoplasms

41

I. PRIMARY EPITHELIAL TUMORS

Many different pathologic processes involving the epithelium result in mucosal tumors that produce polyps that project into the lumen of the intestine. Intestinal polyps may be foci of epithelial hyperplasia, epithelial neoplasms, hamartomas, or retention polyps. Not all polyps are associated with epithelial proliferation. Inflammation (inflammatory polyps), lymphoid hyperplasia (lymphoid polyps), and mesenchymal neoplasms (lipoma, leiomyoma) may also result in polyps (Table 41-1).

BENIGN NEOPLASMS

COLONIC ADENOMA

Adenomas of the colon are present in 20–30% of all individuals over the age of 50 years. They are of 2 major types: tubular and villous (Fig 41-1).

1. TUBULAR ADENOMA (ADENOMATOUS POLYP; POLYPOID ADENOMA)

Tubular adenomas account for over 90% of colonic adenomas. They are commonly multiple, 10–20 lesions being present in some patients, and are pedunculated with a well-defined stalk (Figs 41-1B and 41-2).

Histologically, a tubular adenoma is composed of benign neoplastic glands bunched together above the muscularis. The epithelial cells are hyperchromatic and stratified and show loss of normal mucin content (Fig 41-3)—sometimes termed "adenomatous change." The proliferating epithelium may be composed of tubular glands (tubular adenoma) or a mixture of tubular and villous structures (tubulovillous adenoma). A benign adenoma shows no evidence of invasion and has a clearly defined stalk (Fig 41-1).

Tubular adenomas are **premalignant lesions.** Though the risk of cancer is small (1–3%), the frequency of these polyps in the population makes them the most important precancerous colonic lesion. The development of carcinoma is preceded by increasing epithelial dysplasia. The risk of developing carcinoma increases with increasing size and number of polyps.

The only means of differentiating a tubular adenoma from a polypoid adenocarcinoma is histologic examination of the completely excised polyp. Pedunculated polyps can be safely removed at colonoscopy. The risk that a colonic polyp is a polypoid carcinoma increases with the size of the polyp. Polyps over 2 cm in diameter

Table 41-1. Intestinal tumors: Types and relative frequency.

	Duodenum	Jejunum	Ileum	Colon	Rectum	Appendix
Benign neoplasms						
Adenomatous polyp	+	+	+	+++	++	+
Villous adenoma	+	Rare	Rare	++	+++	+
Leiomyoma	+	+	+	+	+	Rare
Others[1]	Rare	Rare	Rare	Rare	Rare	Rare
Nonneoplastic tumors						
Hamartomatous polyp	+	++	+	+	+	Rare
Hyperplastic polyp	Rare	Rare	Rare	+++	+++	++
Juvenile retention polyp	Rare	Rare	Rare	+	+++	Rare
Lymphoid polyp	+	+	++	++	++	+
Inflammatory polyp	+	+	+	+	+	+
Malignant neoplasms						
Carcinoma	+[2]	Rare	Rare	+++	+++	+
Carcinoid tumor	+	+	++	+	++	+++
Malignant lymphoma	+	+	++	+	+	+
Leiomyosarcoma	+	+	+	+	+	Rare

Rare = almost never occurs; + = occurs uncommonly; ++ = common; +++ = very common and characteristic location.
[1]All rare; include neurofibroma, schwannoma, granular cell tumor, lipoma, hemangioma, lymphangioma.
[2]Most duodenal carcinomas occur in the periampullary region.

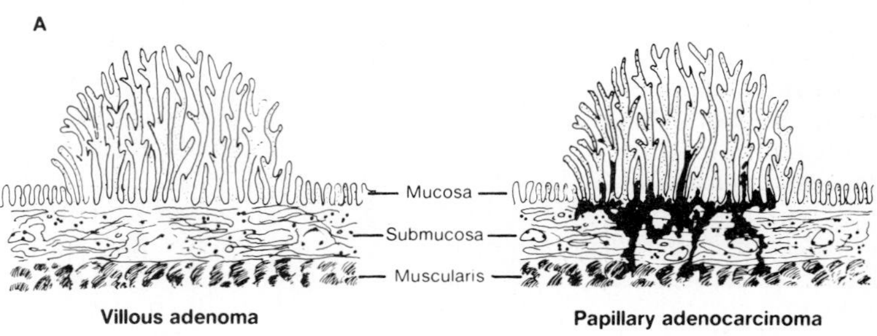

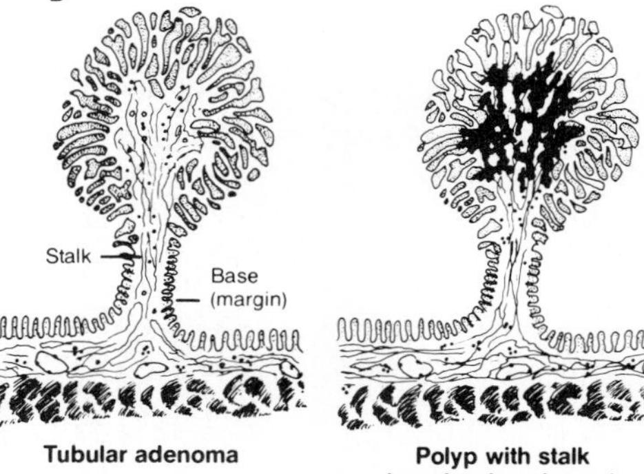

Figure 41-1. Villous adenoma **(A)** and tubular adenoma **(B)** of the colon, with their malignant counterparts. Dark areas represent invasive carcinoma.

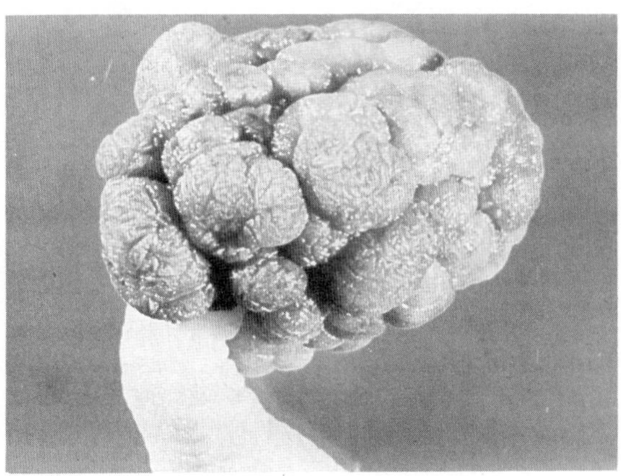

Figure 41-2. Pedunculated adenomatous polyp of the colon. Microscopic examination of the polyp and stalk is necessary to evaluate the presence of malignant change.

should be considered highly suspicious. Malignancy of a polyp is most reliably determined by the presence of stalk invasion (Fig 41-1), which gives the neoplastic cells access to the lymphatics and predisposes to metastasis. The risk of lymph node involvement in a cancerous polyp with tumor confined to the upper part of the stalk (Fig 41-1B) is only about 1-2%. Simple removal of such a malignant polyp with stalk invasion is therefore curative in 98-99% of cases. When the invasion by cancer cells involves the base of the polyp (Fig 41-1B), the patient is not cured by endoscopic removal of the polyp and needs colon resection to remove residual cancer.

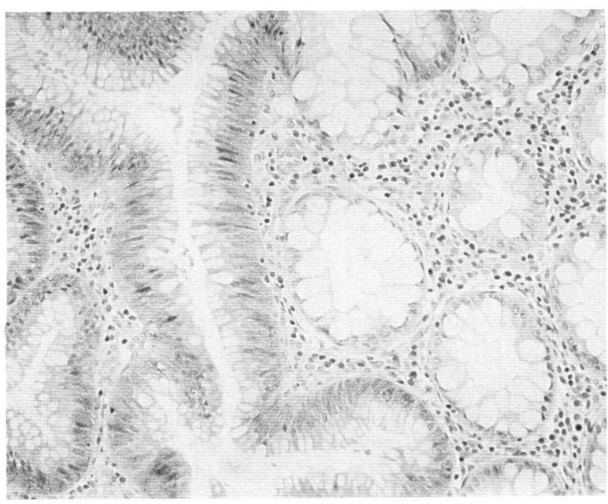

Figure 41-3. Edge of an adenomatous polyp, showing adenomatous change (left), compared with normal mucosal glands (right). Adenomatous change is characterized by increased size and stratification of nuclei and loss of cytoplasmic mucin. Note arrangement of nuclei of the adenoma perpendicular to the basement membrane (polarity).

Clinically, most patients with tubular adenomas are asymptomatic. A few will present with overt rectal bleeding; most will have occult blood in the stools if multiple samples are taken. The diagnosis is made by colonoscopic visualization and biopsy. The recognition of colonic adenomas has become important because it is believed that their removal may decrease the incidence of colon carcinoma.

2. VILLOUS ADENOMA

Villous adenomas are uncommon, comprising less than 10% of colonic adenomas. They commonly occur in older individuals as a solitary large, sessile lesion—ie, have a broad base of attachment to the mucosal surface without a defined stalk (Fig 41-1A). The most common location is the rectum.

Villous adenomas appear grossly as soft, velvety, papillary growths that project into the lumen (Fig 41-4). Their consistency is so soft that even large growths may be difficult to feel on digital rectal examination. They are usually 1-5 cm in diameter but may be larger. Patients with villous adenomas frequently present with rectal bleeding or mucous discharge. The diagnosis may be made by colonoscopy and biopsy.

Histologically, villous adenoma is composed of neoplastic proliferation of colonic epithelial cells organized into long fingerlike papillary or villous processes (Fig 41-5). Cancer in a villous adenoma (papillary adenocarcinoma) is most reliably determined by the presence of invasion of the muscularis mucosae at the base of the lesion (Fig 41-1A).

Villous adenomas have a 30-70% incidence of carcinoma. For this reason—and because they cannot be excised endoscopically—treatment usually consists of excision of the segment of colon harboring the lesion.

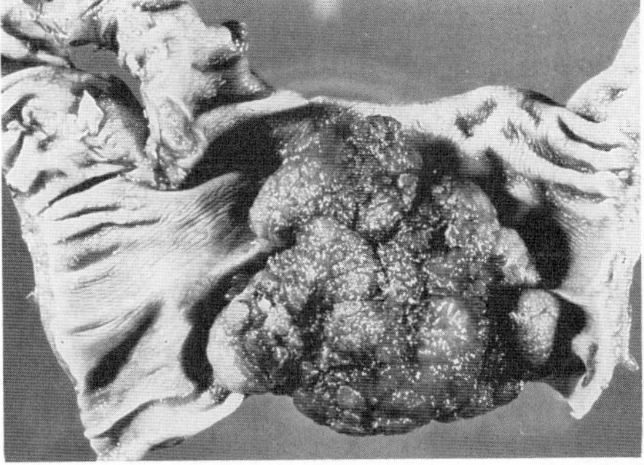

Figure 41-4. Villous adenoma of the colon. Examination of the base of the sessile polyp is necessary to evaluate the presence of infiltrating carcinoma.

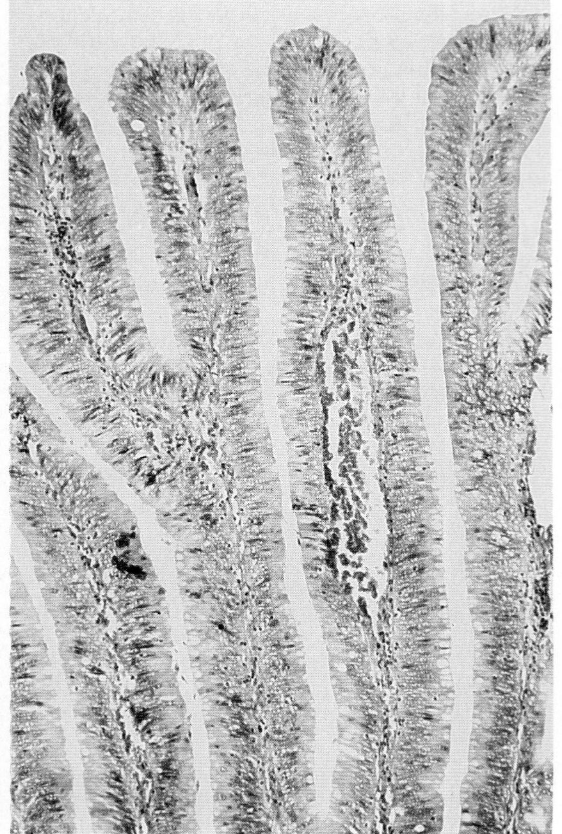

Figure 41-5. Villous adenoma. Note fingerlike papillary processes and adenomatous change of the epithelium.

NONNEOPLASTIC EPITHELIAL TUMORS

INTESTINAL HAMARTOMAS

Hamartomas are uncommon lesions in the intestinal mucosa and present as polyps. They can be found as isolated lesions anywhere in the intestine and as familial hamartomatous polyposis in Peutz-Jeghers syndrome (see below). Hamartomas are composed of a proliferating mass of different kinds of benign cells—including intestinal epithelium, various intestinal glands, and smooth muscle—arranged in a disorganized manner. All of the constituent tissues are histologically normal. The epithelial cells do not show adenomatous change. Hamartomatous polyps are not associated with an increased risk of carcinoma.

HYPERPLASTIC POLYPS

Hyperplastic polyps are very common in the colonic mucosa. They are commonly small (usually < 5 mm in diameter) and appear as small sessile polyps in the mucosa. They are composed of hyperplastic colonic epithelial cells with basal nuclei and markedly increased cytoplasmic mucin content; the lumens of glands containing increased numbers of these cells have a typical serrated appearance. Hyperplastic polyps do not imply an increased risk of cancer.

It is important to recognize **mixed hyperplastic and adenomatous polyps**. These may be larger, resembling tubular adenoma grossly, and do carry an increased risk of carcinoma.

JUVENILE RETENTION POLYPS

Juvenile retention polyps are also common, occurring mainly in the rectum in children and young adults. They are characterized by the presence of cystically dilated mucous glands lined by flat epithelium surrounded by a stroma that commonly shows marked inflammation. The epithelial cells do not show adenomatous change, and juvenile polyps are not associated with an increased risk of carcinoma.

FAMILIAL POLYPOSIS SYNDROMES

The familial polyposis syndromes are a group of inherited diseases characterized by the presence of multiple polyps in the intestine. Several different types exist (Table 41-2).

FAMILIAL POLYPOSIS COLI

Polyposis coli is the commonest of the familial polyposis syndromes. It has an autosomal dominant inheritance pattern. The number of polyps exceeds 100 in all cases and frequently reaches several thousand (Fig 41-6).

Polyps are not present at birth but begin to appear at about 10–20 years of age. Polyps are manifested by rectal bleeding. The diagnosis is made by demonstration of numerous adenomas by colonoscopy and biopsy.

Colon carcinoma supervenes in 100% of cases. The mean age at development of carcinoma is 35–40 years. Total colectomy to prevent cancer is absolutely indicated.

Table 41–2. Familial polyposis syndromes.

Syndrome	Type of Polyp	Locations	Cancer Risk	Inheritance[1]	Other Features
Polyposis coli	Adenoma	Colon	100%	AD	
Gardner's syndrome	Adenoma	Colon, small intestine	100%	AD	Bone and soft tissue lesions; ampullary cancer common
Turcot's syndrome	Adenoma	Colon	100%	?AR	Nervous system neoplasms
Peutz-Jeghers syndrome	Hamartoma	Jejunum, rest of intestine	Slight increase	AD	Pigmentation in mouth; theca or granulosa cell tumors of ovary
Juvenile polyposis[2]	Retention	Colon	Slight increase	AD	

[1]AD/AR = autosomal dominant/recessive.
[2]Canada-Cronkite syndrome is a nonfamilial juvenile polyposis syndrome.

GARDNER'S SYNDROME

Gardner's syndrome is similar to polyposis coli in inheritance pattern, appearance of the colon, and risk of carcinoma but differs in that there are polyps elsewhere in the intestine also and in the presence of extraintestinal lesions such as osteomas in the jaw bones, epidermal cysts, fibromas in the skin, and fibromatosis of soft tissues. The incidence of periampullary (duodenal) carcinoma is increased in patients with Gardner's syndrome. It has been postulated that familial polyposis coli and Gardner's syndrome result from the presence of the same abnormal gene and that the latter is merely a more complete expression of the gene than the former.

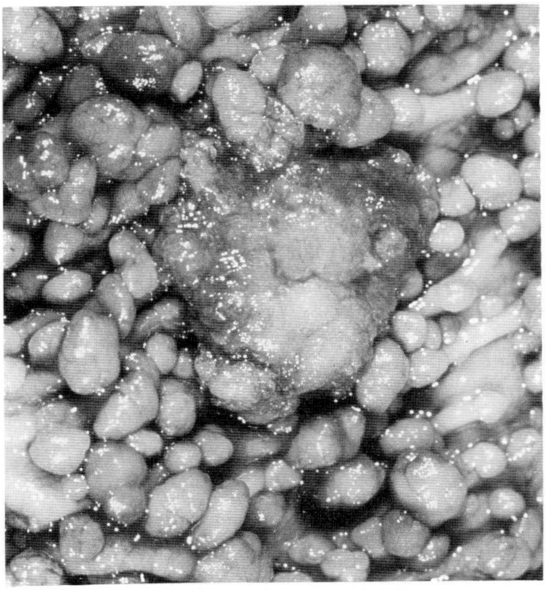

Figure 41–6. Familial polyposis coli, showing innumerable adenomatous polyps. The central area of ulceration represents an adenocarcinoma. Note that there is hardly any normal mucosa.

TURCOT'S SYNDROME

This extremely rare polyposis syndrome is inherited as an autosomal recessive but carries a risk of colon carcinoma at an earlier age. The syndrome is characterized by the association of multiple colonic adenomas with central nervous system neoplasms (usually glioblastoma multiforme).

PEUTZ-JEGHERS SYNDROME

Peutz-Jeghers syndrome is second in frequency to polyposis coli among the familial syndromes discussed here. It is characterized by hamartomatous polyps throughout the intestine, with maximum density in the jejunum. Patients have pigmented macules in the circumoral skin and buccal mucosa. There is a slightly increased risk of colon carcinoma.

JUVENILE POLYPOSIS SYNDROME

This is a very rare syndrome characterized by the presence of multiple juvenile retention polyps in the colon. There is a slightly increased risk of colon carcinoma.

MALIGNANT NEOPLASMS

Malignant epithelial neoplasms (ie, carcinomas) account for 95% of intestinal malignancies. Most of these occur in the colon and rectum. Considering the length of the small intestine, its massive epithelial surface area, and the rate of cell turnover, carcinomas of the small intestine are remarkably uncommon. This is believed due to the rapid movement of fluid luminal contents through the small intestine. Slower passage of the more solid feces in the colon permits more prolonged contact with dietary carcinogens, accounting for the high incidence of epithelial neoplasms there.

CARCINOMA OF THE COLON & RECTUM

Incidence

Colorectal carcinoma accounts for over 90% of malignant neoplasms of the intestine and is second only to lung cancer as a cause of cancer deaths—over 50,000 a year—when both sexes are considered together. Colorectal carcinoma is common in North America and Europe and uncommon in Asia, Africa, and South America. About 110,000 new cases occur every year in the United States.

Colorectal carcinoma occurs mainly in older individuals; 90% of cases are in the over-50 age group. Females show a 2:1 preponderance of colon cancer; rectal cancer is slightly more common in males. There is no genetic basis, but high-risk families have been described in which several members have developed colon carcinoma.

Etiology

The cause of colorectal carcinoma is unknown. The high incidence in developed countries is thought to be due to the intake of a diet rich in animal fat and low in fiber content. Such a diet produces a small, hard stool with slow movement through the colon, permitting carcinogenic agents to remain in contact with the mucosa for a longer period of time.

Premalignant Lesions

Most colon carcinomas are believed to arise in premalignant lesions, only a few arising de novo in previously normal mucosa.

The greatest risk for carcinoma is in the heredofamilial adenomatous polyposis syndromes, where the risk is 100%. Villous adenomas also have a high incidence of malignant transformation. In these conditions, colonic resection is justified to prevent carcinoma.

The risk is somewhat less (10% overall) in chronic ulcerative colitis, but prophylactic colectomy is justified when there is total colonic involvement, disease over 10 years in duration, and epithelial dysplasia on biopsy.

Tubular adenomas have a low risk of carcinoma, but because they are so common they are believed to be the most frequent precursor lesion for colon carcinoma. Aggressive detection and removal of polypoid adenomas may decrease the incidence of colon carcinoma in the future.

Pathology

The rectosigmoid region accounts for about 50% of colon carcinomas, the remainder being distributed throughout the colon (Fig 41–7). Multiple carcinomas are present in 5% of cases.

Carcinomas in the right side of the colon tend to be large polypoid masses that project into the lumen (Fig 41–7). Left-sided cancers tend to involve the whole circumference and often constrict the lumen (''napkin ring'' or ''apple core'') (Fig 41–8). Rectal carcinomas are most commonly malignant ulcers with raised everted edges (Fig 41–9).

Microscopically, most colon carcinomas are adenocarcinomas of varying differentiation. The majority are well or moderately differentiated (Fig 41–10).

Clinical Features (Table 41–3)

Colon carcinoma is asymptomatic in its early stages. It is recommended that all individuals over the age of 40 years undergo regular examination by sigmoidoscopy or colonoscopy to exclude early colon carcinoma. Asymptomatic rectal carcinomas are detected by rectal examination, which should be part of every routine physical examination.

The earliest detectable abnormality is the presence of occult blood in the stools. Examination of

Table 41–3. Colorectal cancer: Presentation and risk factors.

Sex	Colon F > M 2:1; rectum M > F 3:2
Racial and geographic	All races but much more common in developed countries
Age	50 plus
Family history	High-risk families and polyposis syndromes
Premalignant lesions	Familial polyposis syndromes, colonic adenoma, chronic ulcerative colitis
Associated diseases	Acanthosis nigricans, sensory neuropathy
Presentation	Obstruction, left-sided lesion Occult bleeding leading to iron deficiency anemia; right-sided lesion Frank hemorrhage, bleeding per rectum Perforation and peritonitis Fistula (other parts of intestine, bladder, vagina) Weight loss Pain Abdominal mass Diarrhea Change in bowel habits

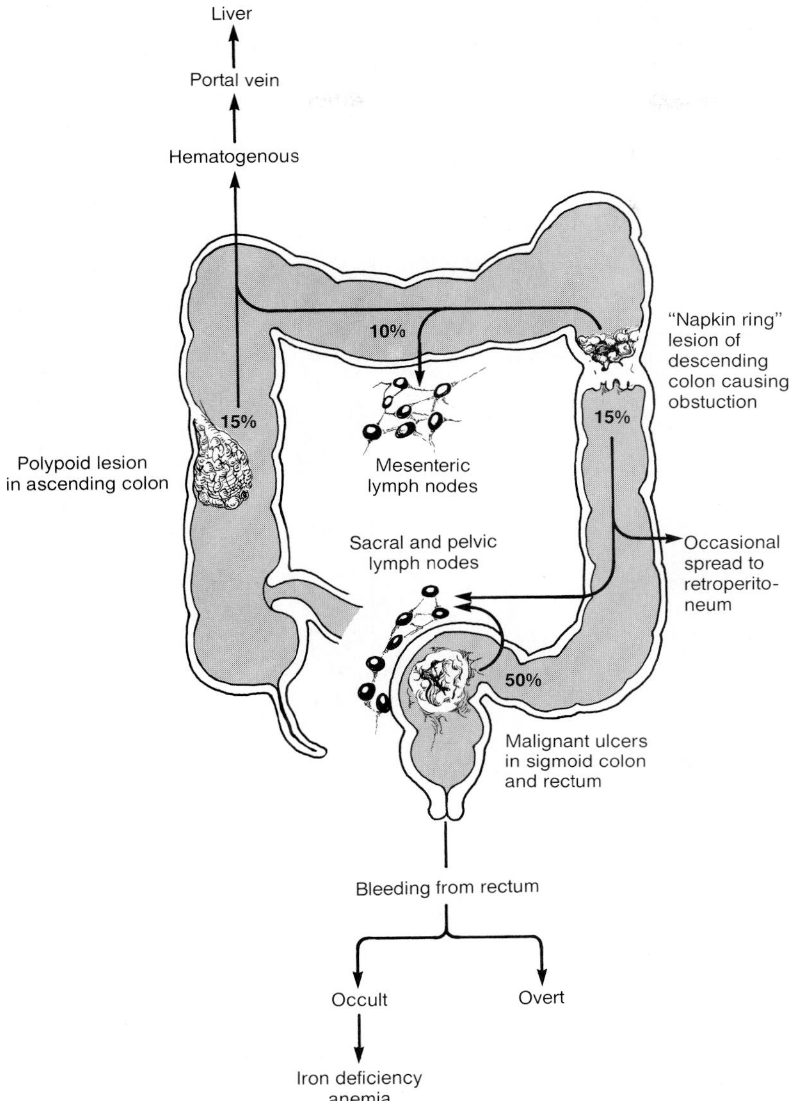

Figure 41-7. Colon carcinoma—sites, gross appearances, and spread.

stools for occult blood is the only cost-effective means of detecting early colon carcinoma. Chronic intestinal blood loss causes iron deficiency anemia. All patients with iron deficiency anemia must be evaluated for intestinal cancer.

Symptoms in colon carcinoma are any change in bowel habits, including constipation and diarrhea, and bleeding per rectum. Blood is bright red in rectosigmoid cancers and admixed with feces and altered in more proximal lesions.

Left-sided colon cancers commonly present with intestinal obstruction because they tend to be constricting lesions in a narrow part of the colon where the feces are solid. In contrast, right-sided carcinomas rarely present with intestinal obstruction because they are polypoid masses in a more capacious part of the colon where the feces are still semiliquid. Right-sided colon carcinoma commonly presents with abdominal pain, weight loss, anemia, and a palpable abdominal mass is frequently present.

Diagnosis & Treatment

Both colonoscopy and barium enema examination are accurate in detecting colon carcinoma; the former permits biopsy and pathologic diagnosis before surgery. Surgical resection of the involved segment of colon is the mainstay of treatment of colon cancer. Neither radiotherapy nor chemotherapy is effective in curing patients who fail surgical treatment, though they may prolong life.

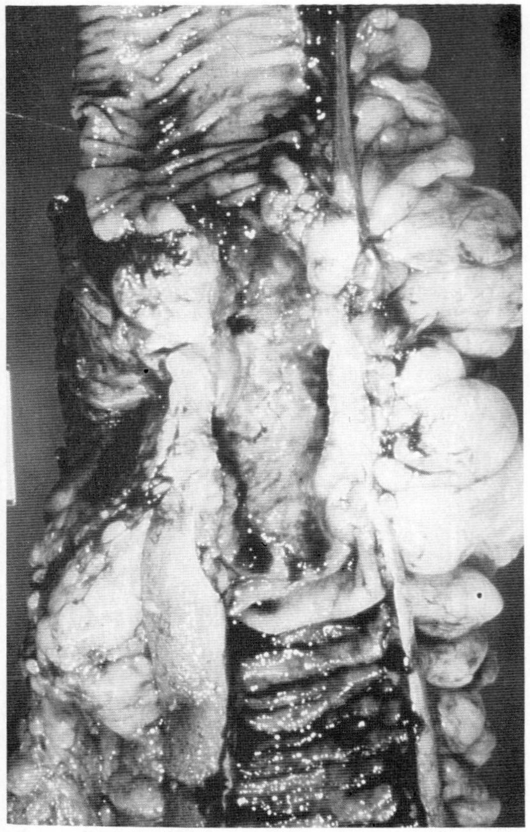

Figure 41-8. Colon carcinoma, showing the circumferential, stenosing type of carcinoma ("apple core" lesion) that is typically seen in the left side of the colon.

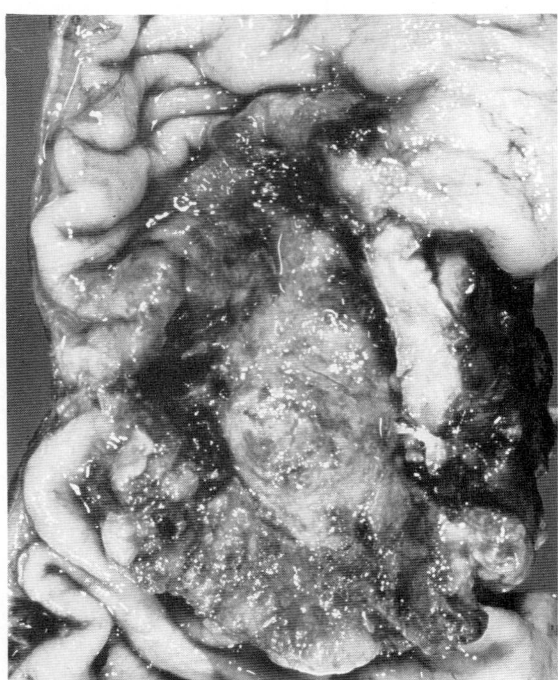

Figure 41-9. Rectal carcinoma, showing the typical malignant ulcer with raised, everted edges.

Prognostic Factors

A. Clinicopathologic Stage: The clinicopathologic stage of the disease—assessed by microscopic examination of the resected colon—is the most important prognostic factor. The most commonly used staging system in the United States is the modified Dukes system (Table 41-4).

B. Histologic Grade: The histologic grade is a numerical expression of the degree of differentiation of the adenocarcinoma. This is a minor prognostic factor. Poorly differentiated (grade III) neoplasms and those with large amounts of extracellular mucin (mucinous carcinoma) have a worse prognosis than well-differentiated (grade I) carcinoma.

C. Vascular invasion is a minor adverse prognostic factor.

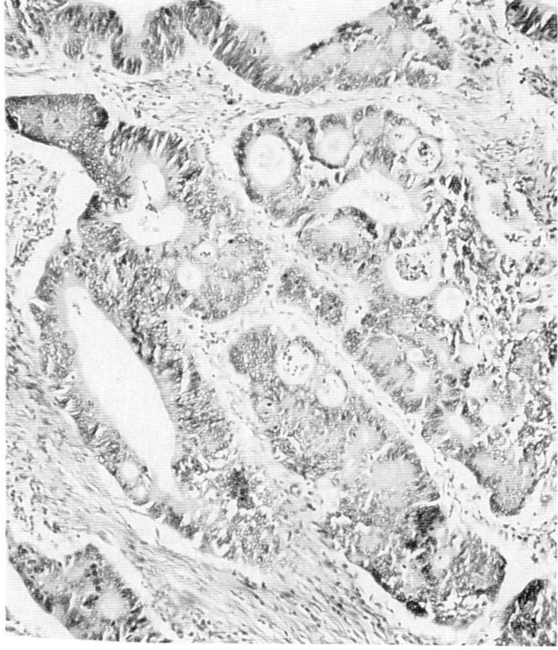

Figure 41-10. Adenocarcinoma of the colon, showing malignant, infiltrating glands. The glandular architecture is complex, with cribriform spaces. The nuclei are arranged irregularly with loss of polarity.

CARCINOMA OF THE ANAL CANAL

Anal canal carcinoma is rare but is being seen with increasing frequency in anoreceptive male homosexuals. Sexual transmission of a virus—

Table 41-4. Astler-Coller modification of Dukes staging system for colon carcinoma.

Dukes Stage	Invasion of Colonic Wall	Lymph Node Metastases	Distant Metastases	Five-Year Survival Rate
A	Mucosa and submucosa[1]	No	No	> 90%
B1	Partial muscle wall thickness	No	No	67%
B2	Full thickness of muscle wall	No	No	55%
C1	Partial muscle wall thickness	Yes	No	40%
C2	Full thickness of muscle wall	Yes	No	20%
D	Any	Yes or no	Yes	< 10%

[1]Involvement of the submucosa is not addressed in the original Astler-Coller classification, and is placed in stage A arbitrarily. Some authorities place submucosal lesions in stage B1.

probably a papilloma virus—is strongly suspected of causing this neoplasm.

Pathologically, there is an infiltrative mass in the anal canal. The most common histologic type is squamous carcinoma. The less differentiated basaloid (or cloacogenic) carcinoma is a specific subtype believed to arise in the transitional zone at the anorectal junction.

Clinically, patients present with rectal discomfort, discharge, bleeding, or a mass. Treatment by radiation and chemotherapy in combination with surgery has improved survival rates considerably.

ADENOCARCINOMA OF THE SMALL INTESTINE

Despite the length and massive surface epithelial area of the small intestine, carcinoma of that organ accounts for less than 1% of malignant gastrointestinal neoplasms (Table 41-1). The reason for this low incidence is unknown but may relate to the rapid movement of small intestinal contents, which does not permit carcinogenic agents to remain in contact with the mucosa. Patients with Crohn's disease have about a 4-fold increased risk of small intestinal carcinoma.

The most common location for small intestine carcinoma is the periampullary region of the duodenum (Fig 41-11). The pathologic features, staging scheme, and prognosis are similar to those of colon carcinoma.

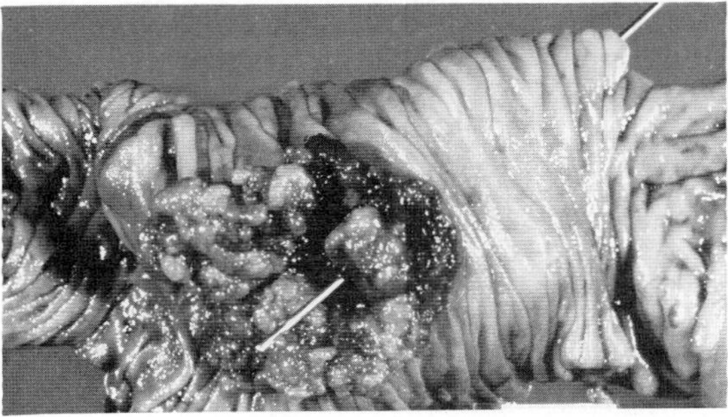

Figure 41-11. Periampullary carcinoma of the duodenum, showing a papillary mass obstructing the terminal bile duct. A metal probe has been passed through the ampulla into the common bile duct.

MUCINOUS NEOPLASMS OF THE APPENDIX

Mucinous neoplasms occur rarely in the appendix; most are benign (mucinous cystadenoma) or low-grade malignant (mucinous cystadenocarcinoma). They produce dilatation of the lumen of the appendix, which is filled with mucin and lined by the neoplastic mucinous epithelium. Extension of the neoplasm through the wall may lead to extensive seeding of the peritoneum and mucinous peritonitis, characterized by nodular masses of mucin in which are found nests of mucus-producing adenocarcinoma cells (pseudomyxoma peritonei).

II. PRIMARY NONEPITHELIAL NEOPLASMS

MALIGNANT LYMPHOMA

The intestine is a common site of primary extranodal malignant lymphoma, most often non-Hodgkin's lymphomas of B cell type. Patients with AIDS have an increased incidence of intestinal lymphomas. Lymphomas may occur in any part of the intestine; the ileocecal region is a favored site for Burkitt's lymphoma. An increased incidence of intestinal lymphoma is seen in lymphoproliferative states associated with alpha heavy chain disease (see Chapter 30). Lymphomas also occur with increased frequency in patients with celiac disease.

SMOOTH MUSCLE NEOPLASMS

Leiomyoma and leiomyosarcoma are the commonest mesenchymal neoplasms of the intestine.

They may form submucosal polypoid masses that precipitate intussusception or may form large mural masses (Fig 41–12). Ulceration with bleeding and intestinal obstruction are common presenting features. A mass may be palpable.

The distinction between benign and malignant smooth muscle tumors of the intestine is difficult. Large size, the presence of necrosis, and a high mitotic rate suggest malignancy. Even leiomyosarcomas tend to be well-circumscribed, and surgical removal has a 60% 5-year survival rate.

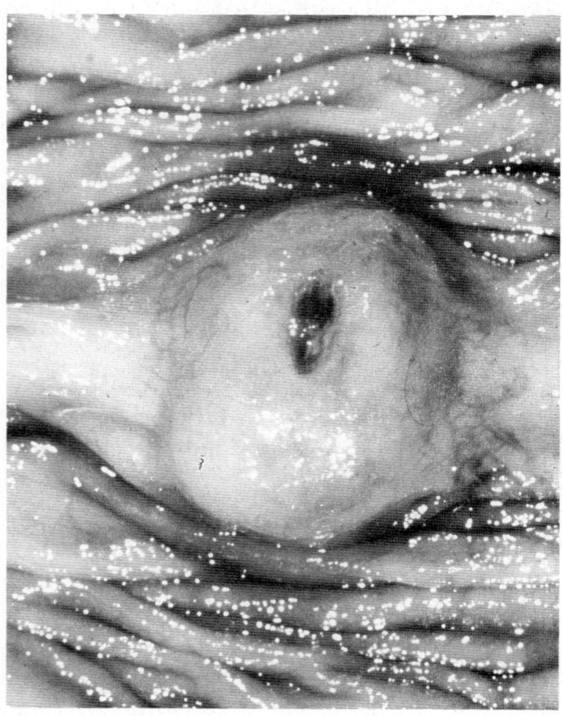

Figure 41–12. Smooth muscle tumor of the colon, showing the submucosal mass covered by mucosa except at the central area of ulceration.

CARCINOID TUMORS

Origin & Sites of Occurrence

Carcinoid tumors arise from neuroendocrine cells present in the mucosa throughout the gastrointestinal tract. Such cells formerly were termed argentaffin cells, APUD (amine precursor uptake and decarboxylation) cells, or Kulchitsky cells (Table 41–5). The normal neuroendocrine cells produce polypeptide hormones and biogenic amines; the tumors may do likewise.

The tip of the appendix is the most common site for carcinoid tumor (Table 41–6). Appendiceal carcinoids are usually incidental findings at appendectomy, are almost always less than 2 cm in diameter, and are benign in over 95% of cases. Only those rare tumors that are over 2 cm in diameter have potentially malignant behavior.

The ileum is the next most frequent site. Ileal carcinoids tend to be malignant in about 60% of cases. Most malignant ileal carcinoids are over 1 cm in diameter. Rectal carcinoids are intermediate

Table 41–5. The intestinal neuroendocrine system.

Designation	Product	Stomach	Small intestine	Colon and rectum
A (alpha)	Glucagon (like)			
D (delta)	Somatostatin			
G	Gastrin			
D_1 (delta)	VIP (like)			
E	Serotonin			
I	Cholecystokinin			
P	Bombesin			
PP	Pancreatic polypeptide			

Table 41-6. Incidence and risk of cancer of intestinal carcinoids.

Site	Incidence	Percentage Malignant
Appendix	40%	1%
Ileum	25%	60%
Rectum	20%	15%
Stomach	5%	?High
Colon	10%	?High

in malignant potential between appendiceal and ileal carcinoids (15% are malignant).

Pathology

Grossly, carcinoid tumors are firm and yellow. They arise in the submucosa, elevating and ulcerating the mucosa and locally infiltrating the wall. Multiple lesions are present in 25% of cases. Carcinoid tumors may be associated with marked fibrosis and distortion of the intestine.

Microscopically, carcinoid tumors are composed of nests and cords of small, uniform round cells separated by vascular channels (Fig 41–13). Local muscle and blood vessel invasion is common in all carcinoid tumors but is not evidence of malignant behavior. Malignancy in a carcinoid tumor is certain only when metastases occur.

Histologic diagnosis can be confirmed (1) by noting the affinity of carcinoid cells for silver stains (argentaffin and argyrophil staining reactions); (2) by immunoperoxidase staining for neuron-specific enolase or chromogranin, markers for cells of neuroendocrine derivation; and (3) by electron microscopy, which demonstrates the presence in the cytoplasm of membrane-bound dense-core neurosecretory granules.

Carcinoid tumors commonly secrete amines, notably 5-hydroxytryptamine (serotonin) and histamine—or polypeptide hormones.

Clinical Features

The average age at presentation for carcinoid tumors is 55 years; they are rare in the teens and increase in frequency thereafter. They are much less common than carcinomas. Most are asymptomatic and are incidental findings at appendectomy and autopsy.

The most common clinical presentation of carcinoid tumor is intestinal obstruction. **Carcinoid syndrome** is another mode of presentation resulting from the release of serotonin into the systemic circulation. Serotonin secretion by an intestinal carcinoid does not cause carcinoid syndrome because the serotonin produced is inactivated to 5-hydroxyindoleacetic acid in the liver. Carcinoid syndrome occurs only when a malignant intestinal carcinoid has metastasized to the liver. Serotonin

A

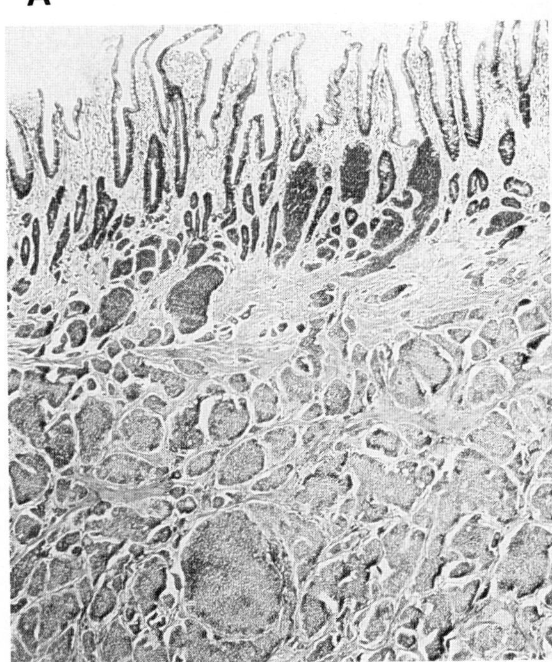

B

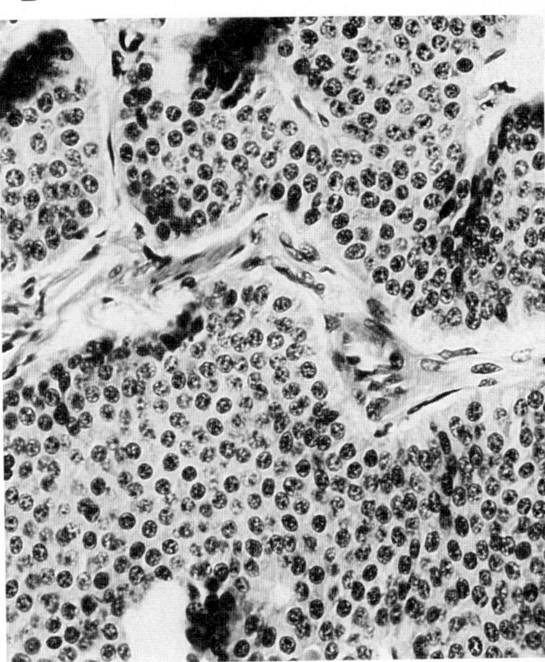

Figure 41–13. Carcinoid tumor of the ileum. **A:** Nests of cells in the submucosa and deep mucosa. **B:** The cell nests are composed of small uniform round cells and are separated by blood vessels.

produced by the hepatic metastases now reaches the systemic circulation.

Carcinoid syndrome is characterized by smooth muscle stimulation by serotonin, which causes abdominal cramps, diarrhea, and bronchospasm; vasodilatation in the skin, causing episodic flushing, thought to be due to vasoactive amines such as histamine secreted by the tumor; and cardiac valve fibrosis, an effect of serotonin. Pulmonary and tricuspid valve stenosis are the common lesions occurring in carcinoid syndrome.

III. METASTATIC NEOPLASMS

Metastases to the intestine occur rarely. The most common are lung carcinoma and malignant melanoma. Direct invasion of the colon by neoplasms in adjacent structures is common and may result in fistulous tracts. Carcinomas of the urinary bladder and cervix not uncommonly invade the colon.

Section X.
The Liver, Biliary Tract, & Pancreas

All kinds of viral hepatitis (Chapter 42) are very common throughout the world, though the prevalence of Virus A hepatitis is greatest in developing countries. Chronic Virus B infection is most common in Far East Asia and Africa. Ethyl alcohol abuse is a worldwide problem (see Chapter 12); in the United States, it is estimated that 10% of the population are affected by alcoholism. Liver and pancreatic disease are major complications of alcoholism (Chapter 43 and 45). Gall stone disease (Chapter 44) is common, particularly in middle-aged women.

The endocrine pancreas is discussed in this section rather than in the endocrine section because neoplasms of the islet of Langerhans enter the differential diagnosis of pancreatic tumors (Chapters 45 and 46). Diabetes mellitus (Chapter 46) is a very common disease; affecting an estimated 2% of the population of the USA.

42 The Liver: I. Structure & Function; Infections

STRUCTURE OF THE LIVER

The liver is situated under the right diaphragm in the lower part of the right rib cage. The left lobe of the liver is in the epigastrium, not protected by the rib cage. The normal liver is firm and has a smooth surface.

The liver parenchyma is divided into functional units called **lobules** (Figs 42–1 and 42–2). Each lobule is 1–2 mm in diameter and is made up of a mazelike arrangement of interconnected plates of hepatocytes separated by endothelium-lined sinusoids (Fig 42–2). The liver cell plates are arranged radially around the central vein; the liver cells that surround a portal tract comprise the **limiting plate**. Liver cell plates are normally one hepatocyte in thickness. Individual hepatocytes are large, with a central round nucleus, a prominent nucleolus, and abundant granular cytoplasm.

The **liver cells** are separated from the sinusoids by a narrow space (space of Disse) that contains connective tissue and represents the scant interstitial compartment of the liver. The hepatic sinusoids are lined by a fenestrated endothelium that permits free fluid exchange between the blood in the lumen and the interstitium. Specialized cells of the macrophage system (Kupffer cells) are present in the sinusoids scattered among the endothelial cells.

The **biliary system** begins at the biliary canaliculi, which are small channels lined by the complex microvilli of surrounding liver cells. The biliary canaliculi form the intralobular bile ductules (canals of Hering), which drain into the bile ducts in the portal tract. The bile ducts pass toward the hilum, forming the right and left main hepatic ducts, the common hepatic duct, and, after union with the cystic duct, the common bile duct.

FUNCTIONS OF THE LIVER

The normal liver has a huge reserve functional capacity. When the liver is normal, about 80% of it can be removed without compromising function. The liver has synthetic, excretory, and metabolic functions.

Synthetic Functions

The liver is the source of plasma albumin; many plasma globulins, including α_1-antitrypsin; and many proteins of the coagulation cascade.

Excretory Functions

Many substances are excreted by the liver in bile. The main component of bile is bilirubin.

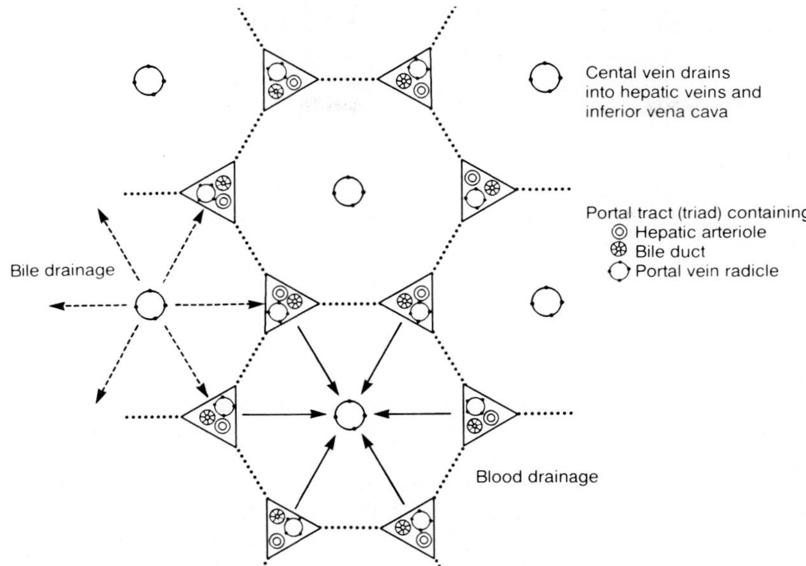

Figure 42–1. Liver lobular architecture, showing blood and bile flow. The sinusoids receive blood from branches of the portal vein and hepatic artery and drain into the central vein (solid arrows). Bile drainage is in the opposite direction, toward the portal tracts (dotted arrows).

Cholesterol, urobilinogen, and bile salts are also present in bile.

Metabolic Functions

The liver plays a central role in the metabolism of fat, carbohydrates, and protein and in detoxification.

A. Fat Metabolism: Free fatty acids from adipose tissue and medium- or short-chain fatty acids absorbed in the intestine are brought to the liver. Triglycerides, cholesterol, and phospholipids are synthesized in the liver from the fatty acids and complexed with specific lipid acceptor proteins to form **lipoproteins** that enter the plasma.

B. Carbohydrate Metabolism: The liver is the main source of plasma **glucose**. Following a meal, glucose is derived from intestinal absorption. In the fasting state, glucose is derived from glycogenolysis and gluconeogenesis in the liver. The liver is the main body storage site for glycogen. When there is a glucose deficiency, the liver metabolizes fatty acids to form ketone bodies, which represent an alternative energy source for many tissues.

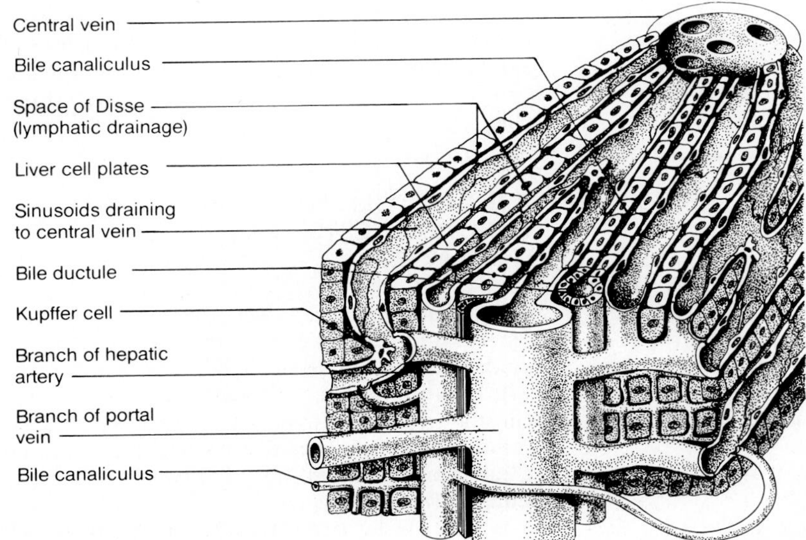

Figure 42–2. Detailed structure of the liver lobule, showing blood and bile flow.

C. Protein Metabolism: In addition to its synthetic function, the liver is the central organ in protein catabolism and synthesis of urea. Urea is secreted by the liver into the plasma for excretion in the kidney.

D. Detoxification: The liver also plays a vital role in detoxifying noxious nitrogenous compounds derived from the intestine and many drugs and chemicals.

METHODS OF EVALUATING THE LIVER

The structure of the liver can be assessed by physical examination, radiography, liver biopsy, and liver function tests.

An enlarged liver can usually by palpated below the costal margin. Any alteration in its normally smooth surface may then also be assessed.

Ultrasonography, computerized tomography, and magnetic resonance imaging disclose mass lesions in the liver or dilatation of the biliary system. Hepatic blood flow can be investigated by arteriography and isotope scans.

Liver biopsy is a relatively safe method of obtaining tissue for histologic examination (Table 42–1). Blind biopsy using a cutting needle is indicated for diffuse lesions of the liver. Radiologically directed fine needle aspiration biopsy is indicated when it is necessary to examine a localized lesion.

Liver function tests are summarized in Table 42–2.

Table 42–1. Needle biopsy of the liver.[1]

Indications
Investigation of:
Hepatomegaly
Jaundice
Hepatitis
Cirrhosis
Persistently abnormal liver function tests
Liver masses:[2] primary tumor, metastases, abscess
Liver involvement in sarcoidosis, brucellosis, tuberculosis, systemic lupus erythematosus, amyloidosis, hemochromatosis
Pyrexia of unknown origin
Contraindications
Bleeding diathesis[3]
Massive ascites
Difficult patient, lack of blood transfusion support
Suspected hydatid cyst
Complications
Hemorrhage; rarely severe enough to cause death
Bile leakage, peritonitis
Pain, shock

[1]The use of a "cutting" needle provides a core of liver tissue for histologic examination.
[2]Radiologically guided biopsy using a fine-needle aspiration technique gives the best results.
[3]Prothrombin and bleeding times should be checked prior to biopsy.

MANIFESTATIONS OF LIVER DISEASE (Table 42–3)

PAIN

Pain is an uncommon symptom of liver disease and occurs only in conditions such as acute hepatitis and right ventricular failure when rapid enlargement of the liver occurs. Pain—commonly constant in the lower right chest region—is the result of stretching of the liver capsule. Pain may be referred to the right shoulder.

ALTERATION IN LIVER SIZE

Most liver diseases are associated with hepatomegaly. When the liver enlarges, its inferior edge becomes palpable below the right costal margin. Enlargement is usually diffuse but may be localized if due to a focal lesion such as neoplasm or abscess. When the liver is palpable, changes in its consistency and surface can be appreciated. The enlarged liver of heart failure is firm, tender, and has a smooth surface. That of cirrhoses has an increased firmness (hard) and a nodular surface.

Shrinkage of the liver occurs in massive liver necrosis and some forms of cirrhosis. A shrunken liver recedes further under the right lower ribs. It can be detected clinically by a decrease in the area of liver dullness on percussion of the right lower chest.

ABNORMAL LIVER FUNCTION TESTS (Table 42–2)

An abnormality in a liver function test detected on routine blood examination is a common method of presentation of liver disease. Patients with asymptomatic chronic liver disease (eg, chronic hepatitis, cirrhosis) may show decreased serum albumin, increased enzyme levels, or an increased prothrombin time. Patients with mass lesions in the liver or partial bile duct obstruction may have an elevated alkaline phosphatase level in serum. As the frequency of routine blood testing

Table 42-2. Liver function tests.

Test[1]	Functional Significance
*Serum bilirubin levels Indirect (unconjugated)	↑ in hemolysis or defective bilirubin uptake
Direct (conjugated)	↑ in hepatocellular failure and biliary obstruction
*Urine bilirubin	↑ in biliary obstruction
*Urine urobilinogen	↓ in biliary obstruction ↑ hemolysis, hepatocellular failure
Dye excretion tests (rose bengal, Bromsulphalein)[2]	↓ in hepatocellular damage and biliary obstruction
*Serum alkaline phosphatase	↑ in biliary obstruction, mass lesions of liver
*Serum aspartate and alanine aminotransferase[3]	↑↑↑ in liver cell necrosis ↑ in obstruction
*Serum albumin (albumin:globulin ratio)[4]	↓ albumin in hepatocellular failure; globulin levels ↑ in chronic liver disease
Serum ammonia (NH_3)	↑ in hepatocellular failure
Serum cholesterol	↓ in hepatitis and cirrhosis ↑ in biliary obstruction
*Prothrombin time (one stage)	prolonged in biliary obstruction and liver damage; reflects ↓ synthesis of prothrombin, coagulation factors V, VII, and X
Plasma glucose	↓ in acute liver failure
*Serum alpha-fetoprotein	↑ in hepatocellular carcinoma (also some cases of cirrhosis with active regeneration)
*Serum α_1-antitrypsin	↓ in α_1-antitrypsin deficiency
Serum ceruloplasmin	↓ in Wilson's disease
Serum free copper (or liver cell copper)	↑ in Wilson's disease (lesser increases in primary biliary cirrhosis)
Serum iron	↑ in hemochromatosis

[1]Asterisk indicates most commonly used tests.
[2]Dye excretion tests are largely obsolete; BSP (sulfobromophthalein, Bromsulphalein) is sensitive but may produce hypersensitivity reactions.
[3]Liver enzymes; aspartate aminotransferase (AST), formerly known as GOT (glutamate oxaloacetic transferase); and alanine aminotransferase (ALT), formerly known as GPT (glutamate pyruvate transferase) are most commonly used. Lactate dehydrogenase and isocitrate dehydrogenase are also used to detect liver cell necrosis.
[4]Various flocculation tests reflected these changes in serum albumin and globulin but are now obsolete.

increases, more patients with abnormal tests such as these will need to be evaluated for asymptomatic liver disease.

JAUNDICE

Jaundice (hyperbilirubinemia) is an increase in the plasma bilirubin above its normal upper limit of 0.8 mg/dL. Bilirubin is derived from breakdown of hemoglobin in the reticuloendothelial system (see Chapter 1). Jaundice may be classified according to the type of bilirubin that accumulates—conjugated or unconjugated hyperbilirubinemia; or according to cause—hemolytic, hepatocellular, or obstructive.

Table 42-3. Manifestations of liver disease.

Pain
Alteration in size
Abnormal liver function tests
Jaundice
Hepatocellular failure
Portal hypertension
Hepatic encephalopathy
Hepatorenal syndrome
Hepatocellular necrosis

Etiology (Table 42-4)

A. Hemolysis: (Increased red cell breakdown.) Excessive hemolysis leads to increased production of bilirubin, and jaundice results when the load exceeds the capacity of the liver for conjugation (this usually signifies a severe degree of hemolysis). The bilirubin that accumulates in the plasma is unconjugated (not water-soluble), complexed with albumin, and does not appear in urine ("acholuric jaundice"). Increased amounts of bilirubin are excreted into the intestine, resulting in

Table 42-4. Causes of jaundice.

Hemolysis See Chapter 25.
Hepatocellular disease Defective uptake: Gilbert's syndrome
Defective conjugation
Neonatal and prematurity
Crigler-Najjar syndrome
Drugs: Novobiocin
Hepatocellular damage: Viral Hepatitis, toxic chemicals, drugs, cirrhosis
Obstruction or deficient excretion Defective excretion: Dubin-Johnson and Rotor syndromes
Intrahepatic cholestasis (small bile duct obstruction): Viral hepatitis, alcoholic liver disease, drugs, pregnancy, primary biliary cirrhosis
Extrahepatic cholestasis (large bile duct obstruction): Gallstones, bile duct stricture, carcinoma of head of pancreas, biliary atresia, sclerosing cholangitis

increased amounts of urobilinogen in feces and urine (Table 42-5). The causes of hemolytic jaundice are discussed in Chapter 25.

B. Hepatocellular Abnormality:

1. Defective hepatic uptake of bilirubin–Unconjugated bilirubin in the plasma is carried into the liver cell by intracellular transport proteins. Absence of these proteins results in failure of bilirubin uptake, leading to unconjugated hyperbilirubinemia (Table 42-5). The commonest cause is **Gilbert's syndrome,** inherited as an autosomal dominant trait and characterized by transient episodes of mild jaundice, usually precipitated by intercurrent illness. There is no structural abnormality, and patients have a normal life expectancy.

2. Abnormal conjugation of bilirubin–Conjugation of bilirubin to bilirubin glucuronide is effected by UDP-glucuronyl transferase. Deficiency of this enzyme results in unconjugated hyperbilirubinemia (Table 42-5).

a. Neonates (neonatal or physiologic jaundice)–Mild jaundice in the first few days after birth is common and is the result of immaturity of the liver enzyme system. The enzyme deficiency is more extreme with increasing degrees of prematurity, and neonatal jaundice can reach dangerous levels in very premature babies.

b. Crigler-Najjar syndrome–This is a very rare autosomal recessive disease characterized by complete absence of the enzyme in the homozygous patient (type A disease). It causes severe jaundice with kernicterus and death in early life. A less severe form of Crigler-Najjar syndrome (type B) in which the enzyme deficiency is partial is compatible with more prolonged survival.

c. Drugs–Drugs may interfere with this enzyme system. Novobiocin is an example.

3. Hepatocellular damage–Acute or chronic hepatocellular damage leads to jaundice when the number of liver cells is reduced enough so that bilirubin metabolism becomes abnormal. Jaundice is generally more severe in acute liver failure than chronic liver failure. Patients with jaundice due to hepatocellular damage commonly have cholestasis superimposed on the failure of conjugation, producing a mixed conjugated and unconjugated hyperbilirubinemia.

C. Obstruction or Impaired Excretion of Bilirubin:

1. Defective excretion–After conjugation, bilirubin is excreted by the liver cell into the biliary canaliculus, and from there it passes to the bile ducts and the intestine. Failure of transfer of bilirubin glucuronide from the liver cell into the canaliculus occurs as an inherited disease in **Dubin-Johnson syndrome** and **Rotor's syndrome.** The defect is usually partial. Dubin-Johnson syndrome is characterized by conjugated hyperbilirubinemia (Table 42-5) and accumulation of pigment (probably lipofuscin) in the hepatocytes, imparting a dark brown to black color to the liver. There is no obvious cholestasis in the liver. Rotor's syndrome is identical except for the absence of pigment. These diseases are usually mild and are compatible with a normal life span.

2. Obstruction at the intrahepatic level (cholestasis)–Obstruction to the flow of bile in the intralobular biliary canaliculi is called intrahepatic cholestasis. Bile accumulates in the lobule within dilated biliary canaliculi and hepatocytes. The bile ductules in the portal tract and the larger bile ducts are normal. The cause is unknown, but many cases show abnormalities in the actin cytoskeleton of the hepatocyte microvilli bordering the biliary canaliculi.

Intrahepatic cholestasis occurs (1) in viral hepatitis; (2) in alcoholic liver disease; (3) as a toxic reaction to drugs, including androgens (methyltestosterone), anabolic steroids, oral contraceptives, and phenothiazines; (4) in benign familial cholestatic jaundice, a rare familial disease in which recurrent attacks of cholestatic jaundice represent the only abnormality; and (5) during pregnancy (recurrent jaundice of pregnancy), most commonly in the last trimester. Spontaneous reversal of cholestasis occurs after delivery, and the disorder is probably due to increased sex hormone levels in pregnancy affecting susceptible individuals.

In general, all of these causes of cholestasis are associated with severe jaundice, which usually reverses spontaneously and is not associated with liver failure.

3. Extrahepatic obstruction–To cause jaundice, obstruction must involve both main hepatic ducts, the common hepatic duct, or the common bile duct. Obstruction of a smaller duct in one lobe of the liver does not cause jaundice, because the normally draining lobe can compensate by in-

Table 42-5. Laboratory findings in the differential diagnosis of jaundice.

Type of Jaundice	Blood						Stools	Urine	
	Hct	Unconjugated Bilirubin (Indirect)	Conjugated Bilirubin (Direct)	Alkaline Phosphatase	Aminotransferases	Cholesterol	Color	Bilirubin	Urobilinogen
Hemolytic	↓	↑↑	N	N	N	N	N	0	↑
Hepatocellular									
Gilbert's syndrome	N	↑	N	N	N	N	N	0	N or ↓
Abnormal conjugation	N	↑	N	N	N	N	N	0	N or ↓
Hepatocellular damage	N	↑	↑	↑	↑↑	N	N	↑	↑
Obstructive									
Defective excretion	N	N	↑	N	N	N	N	↑	N
Intrahepatic cholestasis	N	N	↑	↑	N	N or ↑	Pale	↑	↓
Extrahepatic biliary obstruction	N	N	↑	↑↑	N or ↑	↑	Pale	↑	↓

creasing the excretion of bilirubin. Partial biliary obstruction may result in an elevated serum alkaline phosphatase level.

Complete obstructive jaundice prevents entry of bilirubin into the intestine, producing pale clay-colored or chalky stools. Absence of bilirubin in the gut also results in absence of fecal and urinary urobilinogen (Table 42-5). Regurgitation of conjugated bilirubin into the plasma produces conjugated hyperbilirubinemia, which in turn leads to excretion of a dark brown urine containing bilirubin.

Histologically, large bile duct obstruction produces dilatation of bile ductules, which are plugged with bile and frequently rupture, leading to "bile lakes" in the lobule. Stagnant bile commonly becomes infected, leading to cholangitis with neutrophil infiltration and progressive fibrosis around the dilated bile ducts in the portal areas. In chronic cases, fibrosis may be so marked as to produce fine granularity of the liver ("secondary biliary cirrhosis").

Effects of Jaundice

Jaundice is diagnosed clinically by yellow discoloration caused by deposition of bilurubin pigment in elastic fibers of the interstitial tissues, most easily seen in the scleras. Jaundice must always be confirmed by serum bilirubin measurement because other pigments such as carotene may cause yellow discoloration of skin and eyes.

Deposition of bilirubin by itself does not cause symptoms. However, patients with cholestasis and obstructive jaundice frequently have intense pruritus believed to be caused by bile acids, which are also present in elevated levels in the plasma.

Bilirubin is dangerous when it crosses the blood-brain barrier because it has a toxic effect on brain cells, causing **kernicterus**. Kernicterus occurs only when there is an increased level of free unconjugated bilirubin (not complexed to plasma proteins) in plasma during the neonatal period (see Chapter 1).

HEPATOCELLULAR FAILURE (Fig. 42-3)

Because of its tremendous functional reserve, liver failure occurs only when there is extensive liver disease destroying over 80% of the organ.

Acute Liver Failure

Acute liver failure most commonly results from acute **massive liver cell necrosis** caused by viral hepatitis and toxic drugs and chemicals but may also follow acute fatty change of the liver (see Chapter 1). **Reye's syndrome** is a disease of uncertain causation occurring mainly in children and characterized by acute liver failure with encephalopathy. There is acute fatty change in many organs, including the liver, kidney, and heart. Reye's syndrome has been linked to the administration of aspirin to children with acute viral illnesses such as chickenpox and influenza. **Acute fatty liver of pregnancy** in the last trimester is characterized by microvacuolar acute fatty change and acute liver failure. High-dosage intravenous **tetracycline** therapy was a cause of acute fatty liver in the past.

Acute liver failure is characterized by (1) jaundice; (2) hypoglycemia; (3) a bleeding tendency due to disseminated intravascular coagulation and failure of synthesis of clotting factors in the liver; (4) electrolyte and acid-base disturbances (hypokalemia is the most dangerous); (5) hepatic encephalopathy; (6) hepatorenal syndrome; and (7) elevation of serum enzymes (LDH, AST, ALT; see Table 42-2) in cases associated with extensive necrosis of liver cells.

Acute liver failure has a very high mortality rate. Patients who recover usually do so completely, with regeneration of liver in cases of massive necrosis and rapid reversal of the fatty change in acute fatty liver.

Chronic Liver Failure

Chronic liver failure usually results from cirrhosis, which is associated with progressive necrosis of liver cells, fibrosis, and nodular regeneration.

The effects of chronic liver failure can be listed as follows:

(1) Decreased synthesis of albumin, leading to low serum albumin levels, edema, and ascites.

(2) Decreased levels of prothrombin and of factors VII, IX, and X, resulting in a bleeding tendency.

(3) Portal hypertension (see below).

(4) Hepatic encephalopathy (see below).

(5) Hepatorenal syndrome (see below).

(6) Endocrine changes caused by disordered metabolism of certain hormones. Accumulation of estrogens causes gynecomastia, testicular atrophy, and small vascular telangiectasias in the skin (spider angiomas). Failure of aldosterone metabolism causes sodium and water retention and contributes to edema. Failure of metabolism of antidiuretic hormone contributes to inappropriately high serum levels of ADH in some cases, causing hyponatremia.

(7) Fetor hepaticus—a breath like that of "a freshly opened corpse"—believed to be due to deficient methionine catabolism.

PORTAL HYPERTENSION (Fig 42-4)

Portal hypertension is elevation of portal venous pressure above the upper limit of normal of

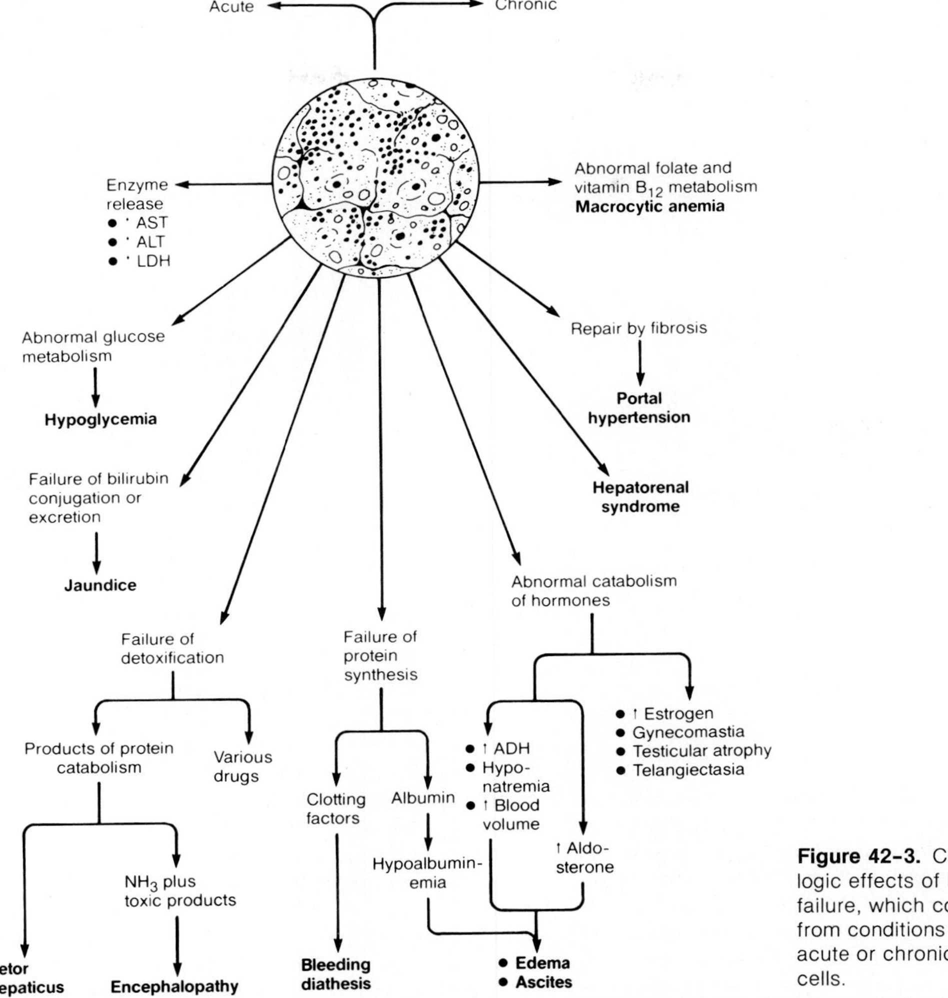

Figure 42–3. Clinical and pathologic effects of hepatocellular failure, which commonly results from conditions associated with acute or chronic necrosis of liver cells.

12 mm Hg. Most cases result from obstruction to the outflow of blood from the portal system. More rarely, portal hypertension results from transmission of arterial pressure to the portal circulation through arteriovenous fistulas, or, in some cases of massive splenomegaly, through dilated splenic sinusoids.

Classification

Portal hypertension resulting from obstruction may be classified according to the level of obstruction.

A. Presinusoidal: Presinusoidal portal hypertension may be caused by obstruction of the extrahepatic portal vein by thrombosis, neoplasms, or inflammation; or by obstruction of intrahepatic portal venous radicals, as occurs in schistosomiasis, biliary cirrhosis, and congenital hepatic fibrosis. Idiopathic portal hypertension is also presinusoidal, but the mechanism is unknown.

B. Sinusoidal: Sinusoidal portal hypertension accounts for over 90% of cases and is caused by cirrhosis of the liver in which fibrosis and distortion restrict the portal circulation and lead to establishment of hepatic arterioportal venous anastomoses.

C. Postsinusoidal: Postsinusoidal portal hypertension occurs when the hepatic venous radicles are obstructed by thrombosis (Budd-Chiari syndrome) or neoplasm, commonly hepatocellular carcinoma. Right ventricular failure and constrictive pericarditis also produce functional postsinusoidal obstruction.

Effects of Portal Hypertension

A. Splenomegaly: Splenic enlargement is caused by passive venous congestion.

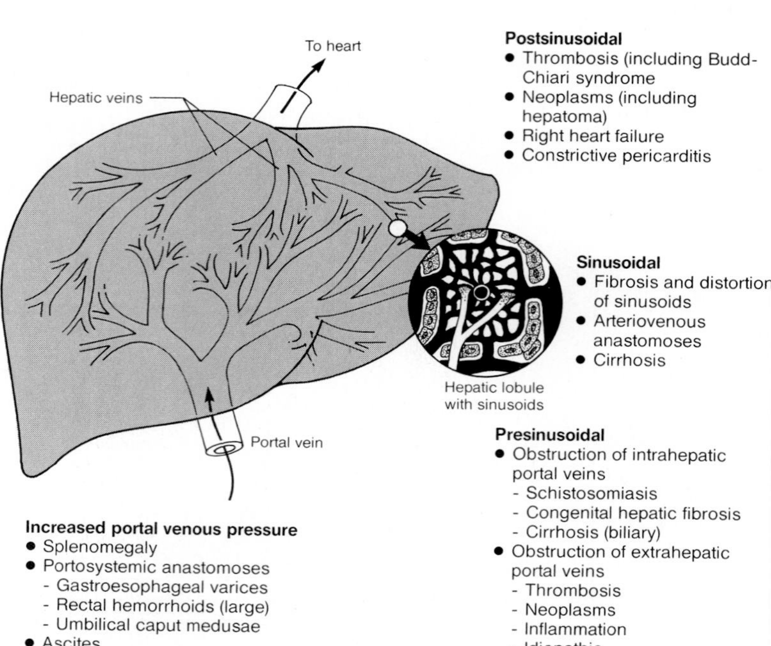

Figure 42–4. Pathogenesis and clinical effects of portal hypertension.

B. Development of Portosystemic Venous Anastomoses, Bypassing the Obstructed Portal Circulation: Venous anastomoses occur wherever the portal and systemic venous drainages commingle, resulting in dilated, tortuous veins at the following sites: (1) in the lower esophagus and stomach (gastroesophageal varices)—these frequently rupture, causing severe upper gastrointestinal bleeding (see Chapter 37); (2) in the rectum (hemorrhoids); and (3) around the umbilicus, where the collateral veins radiate outward in the abdominal wall (“caput medusae”).

Entry of portal venous blood into the systemic circulation through these collateral channels may result in **hepatic encephalopathy** because blood bypassing the liver eludes detoxification. Portacaval anastomoses created surgically to relieve portal hypertension may have the same effect.

C. Ascites: Ascites is due to increased transudation of fluid across the peritoneal membrane, particularly over the surface of the liver. The major factor leading to severe ascites in chronic liver disease is a decrease in serum albumin level, with portal hypertension playing only a contributory role.

HEPATIC ENCEPHALOPATHY

Hepatic encephalopathy is characterized by cerebral dysfunction (hypersomnia, delirium, “flapping” tremors of the hands) leading to convulsions, coma, and death. It may occur in both acute and chronic liver disease and is usually accompanied by other evidence of liver failure. In patients with extensive portosystemic venous anastomoses, hepatic encephalopathy may occur in isolation.

The pathogenesis of hepatic encephalopathy is unclear, but it is believed that nitrogenous products of intestinal bacteria accumulate in the systemic blood, having bypassed the liver through portosystemic anastomoses or having undergone deficient detoxification by the failing liver cells. These nitrogenous products then cross the blood-brain barrier, causing edema and neuronal degeneration.

Substances suspected of being involved in the pathogenesis of hepatic encephalopathy are (1) ammonia, which is present in high plasma and cerebrospinal fluid concentrations in patients with liver failure; and (2) amides like octopamine, which act as false neurotransmitters.

HEPATORENAL SYNDROME

Hepatorenal syndrome is the occurrence of acute renal failure in a patient with liver disease.

The mechanism by which renal failure occurs is uncertain. There are no pathologic changes in the kidneys, and when these kidneys are transplanted into normal individuals, they function normally. Renal failure has features similar to those of "prerenal" failure occurring in hypovolemic shock, with production of a small volume of concentrated urine. This has led to the hypothesis that hepatorenal syndrome is the result of an alteration in distribution of blood flow in the kidneys, caused perhaps by the effect of false neurotransmitters on the sympathetic nervous system.

The occurrence of hepatorenal syndrome is an ominous sign in a patient with liver disease.

HEPATOCELLULAR NECROSIS

Liver cell necrosis is a common manifestation of many liver diseases. If severe, it causes acute or chronic liver failure. In many diseases, however, necrosis is subclinical and revealed only by elevations of liver enzyme concentrations in serum (Table 42–2) or by histologic changes in a liver biopsy. If chronic or recurrent, cell necrosis may lead to cirrhosis.

Different liver diseases cause different patterns of liver cell necrosis. Recognition of these patterns is useful in diagnosis (Fig 42–5).

Focal Necrosis

Focal liver cell necrosis is randomly occurring necrosis of single cells or small clusters of cells in all areas of liver lobules. Not all lobules are involved. Its presence is recognized in biopsies by (1) acidophilic (Councilman) bodies, which are necrotic liver cells with pyknotic or lysed nuclei and coagulated pink-staining cytoplasm; and (2) areas of lysed liver cells surrounded by collections of Kupffer cells and inflammatory cells.

Focal necrosis is commonly seen in viral hepatitis, toxic damage, and bacteremic infections.

Zonal Necrosis

Zonal liver cell necrosis is necrosis of liver cells occurring in identical regions in all liver lobules. The causes differ according to the zone involved. Centrizonal necrosis, which involves the cells around the central hepatic vein, occurs in viral hepatitis, carbon tetrachloride and chloroform toxicity, and anoxic states such as cardiac failure and shock. Midzonal necrosis is uncommon and occurs in yellow fever. Peripheral zonal necrosis, which involves liver cells around the portal tracts, occurs in eclampsia and phosphorus poisoning.

Submassive & Massive Necrosis

Submassive necrosis is the occurrence of liver cell necrosis that extends across lobular boundaries, often bridging portal areas and central veins ("bridging necrosis"). The most severe form is massive liver necrosis, in which large confluent areas of liver undergo necrosis, leaving only small islands of viable liver cells intact. Massive necrosis is characterized by sudden decrease in size of the liver, which appears soft, yellow, and flabby, with a wrinkled capsule (sometimes called "acute yellow atrophy"). Areas of residual viable liver are seen as mottled dark brown areas contrasting with the necrotic yellow zones.

Massive liver necrosis is commonly caused by hepatitis viruses (B and non-A, non-B). It is less commonly due to drugs (halothane, acetamino-

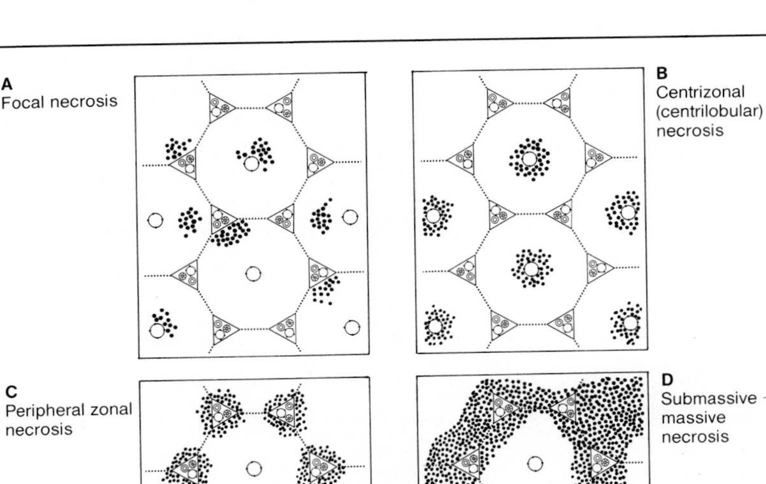

Figure 42–5. Patterns of liver cell necrosis. **A:** Focal necrosis is a patchy necrosis involving lobules haphazardly. **B and C:** Zonal necrosis is a necrosis of liver cells in a constant part of every liver lobule. **D:** Submassive and massive necrosis is extensive necrosis of cells involving multiple adjacent lobules in a contiguous manner.

phen, isoniazid, methyldopa) or toxic chemicals (*Amanita phalloides* mushrooms, chlorinated hydrocarbon insecticides, chloroform, carbon tetrachloride).

Patients with submassive and massive liver necrosis present with acute liver failure of variable severity. Serum enzyme levels are greatly elevated. The mortality rate is high, but those who recover show regeneration of a normal liver.

CONGENITAL DISEASES OF THE LIVER

Congenital defects in bilirubin uptake, conjugation, or excretion have already been considered (see Jaundice, above). Congenital anomalies of the bile ducts are described later along with biliary tract disease (Chapter 44).

CONGENITAL HEPATIC FIBROSIS

Congenital hepatic fibrosis is uncommon and is usually associated with polycystic renal disease. It is characterized by fibrosis connecting adjacent portal tracts. It is not true cirrhosis, because the basic liver lobular architecture is intact, with central veins being present in the center of the nodules demarcated by fibrosis.

There is usually also an abnormal proliferation of bile ducts that appear grossly as microcystic structures (bile duct hamartomas; Meyenberg complexes). Larger cysts lined by biliary epithelium may occur; when cysts are conspicuous, the condition is termed congenital polycystic disease of the liver.

Congenital hepatic fibrosis usually presents as an incidental finding in a patient with polycystic renal disease. Rarely, portal fibrosis causes a presinusoidal type of portal hypertension associated with ascites and esophageal varices.

VASCULAR LESIONS OF THE LIVER

CHRONIC HEPATIC VENOUS CONGESTION

Chronic venous congestion of the liver occurs in right heart failure and is most marked in patients with tricuspid incompetence and constrictive pericarditis. The liver is enlarged; the increased systemic venous pressure is transmitted to the central hepatic vein, and there is congestion of the centrilobular sinusoids. With prolonged congestion, the liver cells around the central vein undergo necrosis. The periportal areas are normal or show fatty change (Fig 42–6).

Grossly, the regular alternation of the red congested central area and the normal (brown) or fatty (yellow) periportal zone produces a characteristic mottled appearance that resembles the cut surface of a nutmeg (''nutmeg liver''). Prolonged congestion leads to fibrosis around the central vein, producing a finely granular liver (''cardiac sclerosis'' or, incorrectly, ''cardiac cirrhosis'').

Clinically, passive congestion is characterized by tender enlargement of the liver. Mild abnormalities in liver function are common, but liver failure almost never occurs.

INFARCTION OF THE LIVER

Because of the liver's dual blood supply from the portal vein and hepatic artery, either of which can independently sustain the liver, infarction rarely occurs. Infarction may occur when the hepatic artery becomes suddenly occluded beyond the origin of the gastroduodenal and right gastric arteries. Occlusion may be caused by thrombosis, atherosclerosis, polyarteritis nodosa, or accidental ligation at surgery. Portal vein occlusion usually does not cause infarction.

BUDD-CHIARI SYNDROME

This rare clinical syndrome is caused by extensive occlusion of hepatic venous radicles by fibrosis, thrombosis, or neoplasm. The changes in the liver are those of severe chronic venous congestion, characterized by the presence of erythrocytes in the sinusoids and space of Disse in the centrizonal region. This is associated with extensive fibrosis and nodular regeneration. Clinically, patients present with an enlarged liver and portal hypertension; ascites is commonly a prominent feature.

INFECTIONS OF THE LIVER

VIRAL HEPATITIS

1. ETIOLOGY

Viruses that primarily infect the liver include hepatitis A, hepatitis B, hepatitis non-A, non-B,

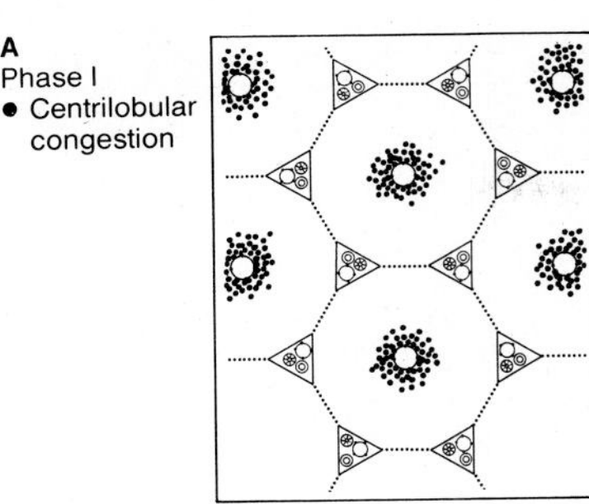

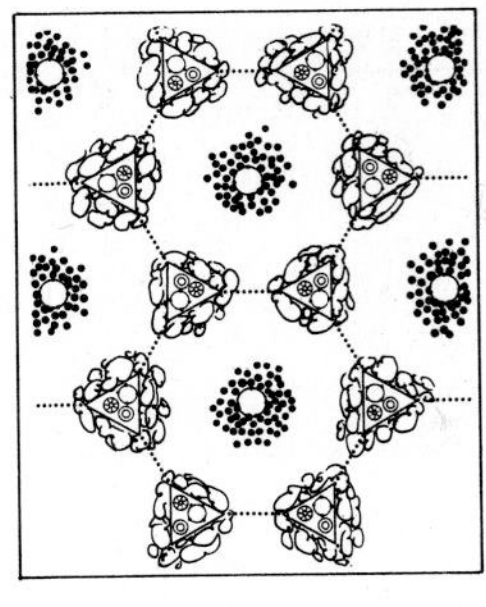

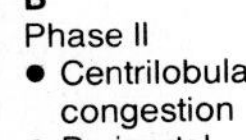

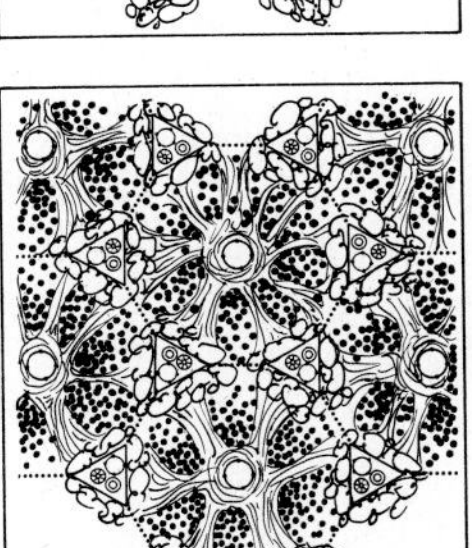

Figure 42–6. Hepatic venous congestion and centrizonal sclerosis. This occurs commonly in chronic right heart failure and is called cardiac sclerosis.

and delta hepatitis viruses. Hepatitis also occurs as part of systemic viral infection in yellow fever (uncommon in the United States; common in parts of Africa and South America), infectious mononucleosis (Epstein-Barr virus), cytomegalovirus infection, herpes simplex, and varicella-zoster infection.

The 4 hepatitis viruses and their broad clinical and epidemiologic features are described in the following sections, followed by a discussion of the clinical syndromes that may result from infection with these viruses.

Hepatitis A (Infectious Hepatitis)

Hepatitis A is caused by an RNA enterovirus measuring 27 nm that has been identified in the stools of patients and infected volunteers and in the liver of marmosets (the animal model for the disease). It is usually transmitted via the fecal-oral route and has a short incubation period (2–6 weeks). Explosive epidemics have been recorded after fecal contamination of water, milk, and shellfish (where untreated sewage spills into coastal waters). Parenteral transmission is rare, occurring only in the transient acute viremic phase.

Hepatitis A has a global incidence, highest in low socioeconomic populations where fecal-oral transmission is greatest.

Hepatitis A is usually a mild acute illness with recovery occurring in a few weeks. It is rarely fatal, does not progress to chronic hepatitis, and there is no carrier state. IgM antibodies appear early in the acute phase, rise rapidly, and wane during the convalescent period. IgG antibodies appear later in the illness, rise rapidly, and remain elevated throughout life (Fig 42–7). The presence of IgG antibody against hepatitis A virus is evidence of previous infection. More than 30% of the United States population have antibodies but give no history of hepatitis, suggesting that subclinical infection is common.

Hepatitis B (Serum Hepatitis)

Hepatitis B is caused by a DNA virus (Fig 42–8) composed of (1) an inner core synthesized in the hepatocyte nucleus and containing the hepatitis B core antigen (HBcAg), hepatitis B e antigen (HBeAg), DNA, and DNA polymerase; and (2) an outer envelop that is synthesized in the hepatocyte cytoplasm and contains the hepatitis B surface antigen (HBsAg). The entire particle measures 42 nm and is called the **Dane particle**. There is excess production of the envelope, free forms of which appear in the blood; these measure 22 nm and have a spherical or tubular structure. These envelope particles were first discovered in the blood of an Australian aborigine with serum hepatitis (HBsAg is therefore also called Australia antigen). HBsAg itself is not infective, the core of the virus being required for infection.

Hepatitis B is usually transmitted in blood or blood products from an individual with active disease or a carrier. Transfer may occur with shared needles, mainly among drug abusers (most hospitals now use disposable needles), during sexual intercourse, by accidental spillage of specimens in the laboratory, and by transfusion of blood prod-

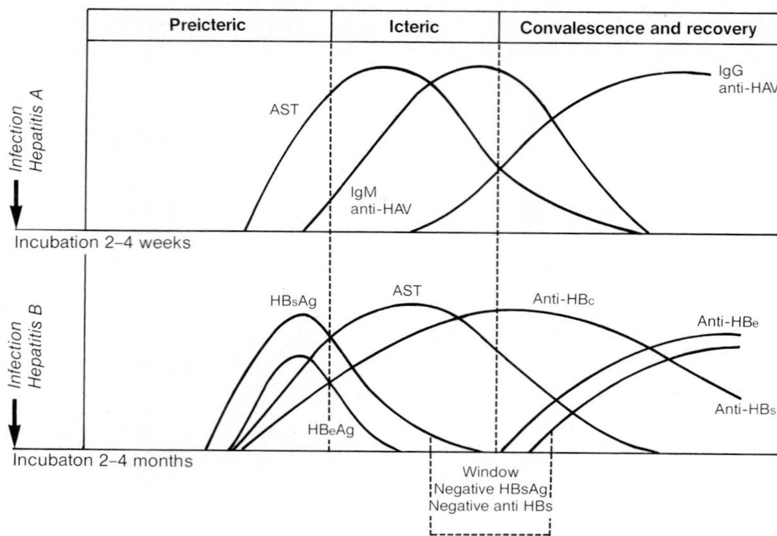

Figure 42–7. Serum antibody and antigen levels in hepatitis A and hepatitis B.

ucts. Routine screening of blood products for hepatitis B coupled with a trend away from use of paid blood donors has greatly reduced the incidence of hepatitis B transmission via blood transfusion. Several epidemics of hepatitis B infection have occurred among patients and staff of renal dialysis units.

Hepatitis B has a long (6 weeks to 6 months) incubation period. Illness is of varying severity and often subclinical. However, the risk of a complicated course, death, chronic disease, and a carrier state is much greater than in hepatitis A.

The appearance of the various hepatitis B antigens and antibodies (Fig 42–7) is important from a diagnostic standpoint. HBsAg appears first, late in the incubation period, and is followed by HBeAg. The presence of HBeAg and hepatitis B-DNA in the serum correlate well with the presence of the infective Dane particles in the blood and are indications of infectivity. In patients who recover, both HBsAg and HBeAg disappear at the onset of clinical recovery. The first antibody to appear is anti-HBc during the acute illness, followed by anti-HBe and anti-HBs. The presence of anti-HBe in the blood indicates absence of the infective Dane particle; such patients are usually not infec-

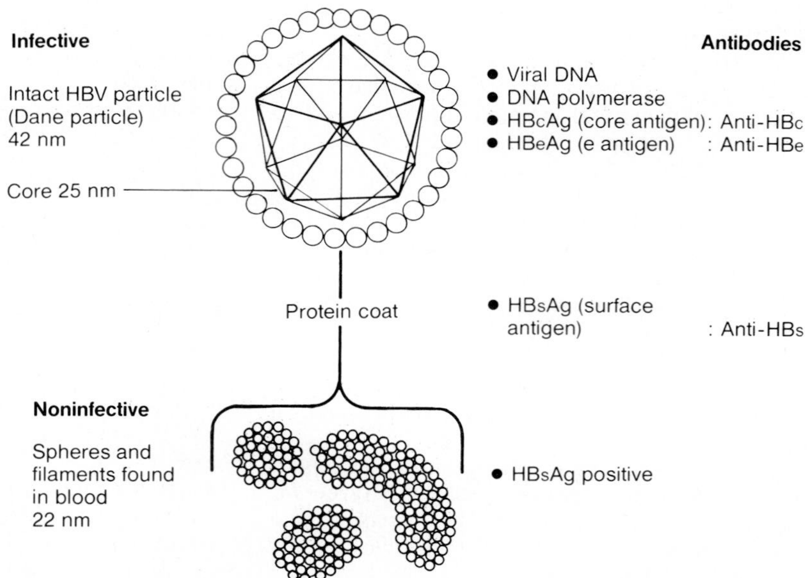

Figure 42–8. Hepatitis B virus. The antibodies that are commonly detected in serum for diagnosis are shown on the right.

tive. Testing for all antigens and antibodies permits diagnosis at all stages of the illness. If the testing includes only HBsAg and anti-HBs, there is a "window" during the recovery phase when both of these are negative and the diagnosis may be missed.

Hepatitis B-infected hepatocytes may be identified (1) in biopsy material by the presence of hepatocytes with ground-glass cytoplasm (Fig 42–9A); (2) by Shikata orcein stain, which selectively stains hepatitis B-infected cells; and (3) by immunoperoxidase stains using labeled antibodies against HBsAg (Fig 42–9B). The last method is the most specific.

Hepatitis Non-A, Non-B

Hepatitis non-A, non-B is caused by a yet unidentified virus (or viruses). It is now responsible for over 90% of cases of hepatitis associated with transfusion of blood products in the United States. The disease also occurs among drug abusers, in transplant recipients, and in renal dialysis units. The incubation period varies between 2 weeks and 6 months, with 2 peaks suggesting that 2 different viruses are involved.

Hepatitis non-A, non-B has clinical features almost identical to those of hepatitis B except for a higher incidence of chronic hepatitis. There is no serologic test for diagnosis or detection of the carrier state.

Delta Hepatitis

The delta hepatitis agent is an RNA virus that has the envelope of hepatitis B virus but an antigenically distinct core of delta antigen; it appears to be a "defective" virus that uses hepatitis B virus as a "helper." It is incapable of causing infection in the absence of hepatitis B virus. Transmission is parenterally, by blood transfusions or intravenous drug abuse. Delta hepatitis is uncommon in the United States but has been reported more frequently in Europe.

Delta hepatitis occurs (1) as an acute disease along with hepatitis B or (2) as acute or chronic hepatitis in a chronic carrier of HBsAg. The diagnosis is made by demonstration of the antigenically unique delta agent in the blood or in liver cells.

2. CLINICOPATHOLOGIC SYNDROMES (Fig 42–10)

The clinicopathologic features of viral hepatitis are considered here as a group (Table 42–6). It is important to note that hepatitis A is a mild disease associated with few deaths and no chronic phase. The other viruses cause much more severe illness with a chronic phase and carrier state.

A

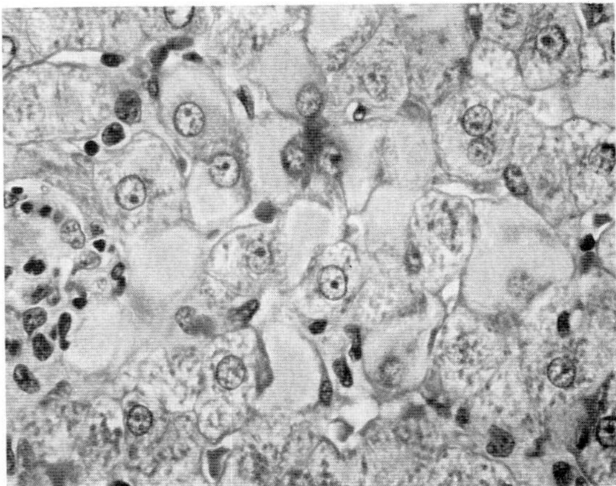

B

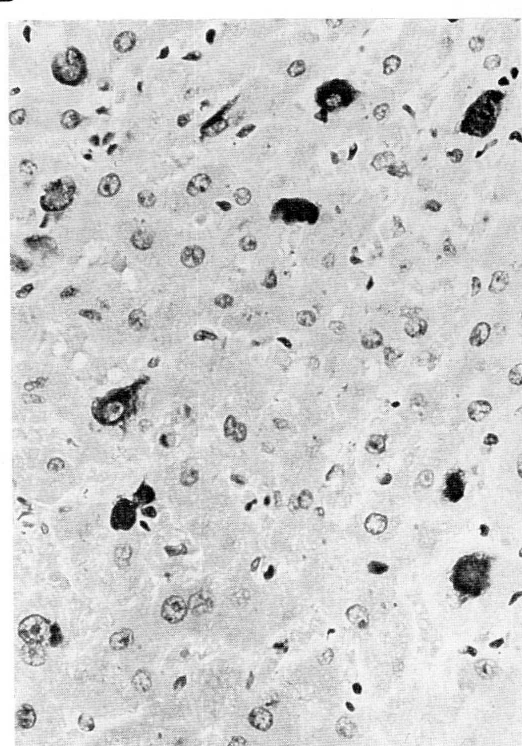

Figure 42–9. **A:** Hepatocytes infected with hepatitis B virus show a ground-glass appearance that contrasts with the coarsely granular cytoplasm of uninfected hepatocytes. **B:** Hepatitis B antigens demonstrated in infected hepatocytes by the immunoperoxidase technique (positive cells show black cytoplasmic staining).

Table 42-6. Hepatitis viruses and the different clinicopathologic forms of liver disease.[1]

	Subclinical	Acute Hepatitis	Fulminant Hepatitis (Massive Necrosis)	Subacute Necrosis (Impaired Regeneration)	Chronic Persistent Hepatitis	Chronic Active Hepatitis	Cirrhosis	Hepatocellular Carcinoma
Hepatitis A	+	+	–	–	–	–	?	–
Hepatitis B	+	+	+	+	+	+	+	+
Non-A, non-B (NANB) hepatitis	+	+	+	+	+	+	+	?
Delta hepatitis	+	+	?	?	+	+	?	?

[1]The outcome in any given patient is dependent on age, immunologic status, "dose" of virus, and interaction of viruses such as that between hepatitis B virus and delta virus.

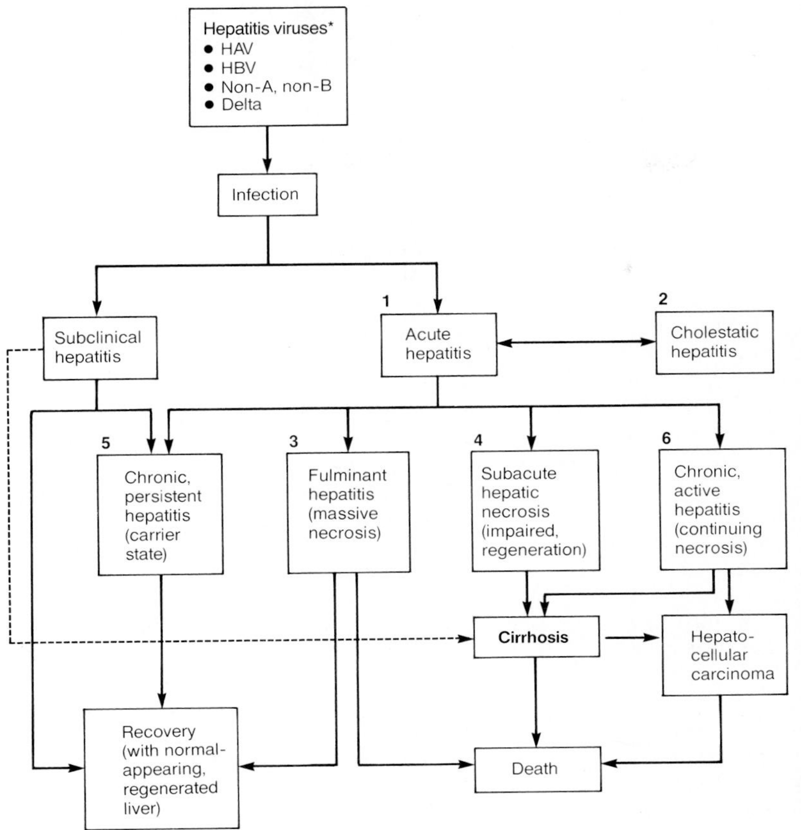

Figure 42–10. Clinical syndromes associated with viral hepatitis. The commonest clinical syndrome is acute hepatitis **(1),** which is sometimes associated with intrahepatic cholestasis **(2).** Fulminant hepatitis **(3)** is associated with massive necrosis and is associated with a high mortality rate. Subacute hepatic necrosis **(4)** is rare but progresses to death in many cases. Chronic viral hepatitis may be persistent **(5)** or active **(6).** Chronic active hepatitis commonly progresses to cirrhosis of the liver.
*Note that the different viruses have greatly differing tendencies to cause these various clinical syndromes.

Acute Viral Hepatitis

All the hepatitis viruses, replicating within the cell, cause damage, either as a direct effect or via an immunologic response against cells bearing viral antigens. Damaged cells show diffuse swelling ("ballooning"; Fig 42–11). Focal or centrizonal necrosis follows. Single necrotic liver cells have coagulated pink cytoplasm and show pyknosis or karyolysis (Councilman body). There is a lymphocytic and plasma cell infiltrate in the portal tracts (Fig 42–11).

Acute hepatitis is associated with sudden onset of fever, loss of appetite, vomiting, jaundice, and tender enlargement of the liver. Jaundice is caused by a combination of liver cell dysfunction and cholestasis. Bile is present in the urine in most cases, and urinary urobilinogen levels are increased (Table 42–5). Liver enzymes (aminotransferases and lactate dehydrogenase) enter the bloodstream from the necrotic cells, appearing early in the course of illness. A few patients develop extrahepatic manifestations such as lymph node enlargement, skin rashes, and joint pains that probably result from circulating immune complexes.

Acute viral hepatitis is frequently subclinical or

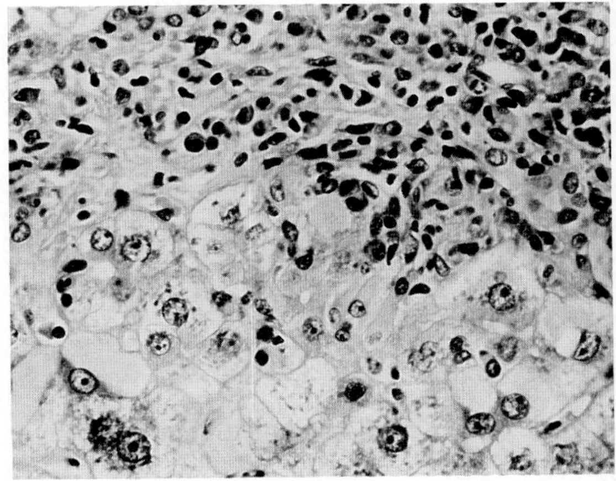

Figure 42–11. Acute viral hepatitis, showing marked edema of hepatocytes and lymphocytic infiltration of the portal areas.

associated with a flulike illness ("anicteric hepatitis"). It can then be diagnosed only by liver function tests (elevated liver enzymes, increased urinary urobilinogen) or hepatitis antibody testing. Antibody testing is the only means of identifying the specific virus.

Clinical recovery occurs within 2–3 weeks in most cases. Return of biochemical abnormalities to normal may take months. Recovery is associated with liver cell regeneration.

Cholestatic Viral Hepatitis

A clinical variant of acute viral hepatitis is characterized by severe intrahepatic cholestasis, with deep jaundice, bilirubin in the urine, and absence of urobilinogen in urine and feces. The chances of complete recovery are not reduced by this complication.

Fulminant Viral Hepatitis

A fulminant course characterized by acute liver failure associated with massive or submassive liver cell necrosis occurs in about 1% of cases of hepatitis B and non-A, non-B. The mortality rate is high. Survivors regenerate a normal liver and do not have chronic liver disease.

Subacute Hepatic Necrosis (Impaired Regeneration Syndrome)

In hepatitis B and non-A, non-B, there is rarely a protracted illness lasting several months with increasing liver dysfunction and a high mortality rate. Patients who survive progress to cirrhosis of the liver.

Pathologically, this condition shows submassive necrosis, with areas of necrosis bridging portal areas and central veins and traversing lobular boundaries. The diagnostic hallmark is an absence of regenerative activity.

Chronic Persistent Viral Hepatitis

Persistent hepatitis is a more common clinical syndrome due to infection with hepatitis B and non-A, non-B viruses. The patient usually has mild symptoms or only slight abnormalities in liver function tests lasting for 6 months or more. (*Note:* Six months is an arbitrarily defined period to exclude cases of acute viral hepatitis that have a protracted recovery phase.) Chronic persistent hepatitis is a benign self-limited disease that may last for several years but does not progress to cirrhosis. It is important because it represents the **chronic carrier state**. Hepatitis B virus or the agent of non-A, non-B hepatitis is present in the blood, and the patient is infective. Chronic persistent hepatitis tends to occur frequently in immunocompromised patients, notably those with chronic renal failure and Down's syndrome. The carrier state is also observed in patients who inherit the virus in the genome (vertical transmission), a common situation in Southeast Asia and in Africa, where the carrier rate for hepatitis B is 30–40%. Patients who inherit the genome have immunologic tolerance to the viral antigens. In addition, integration of hepatitis B virus DNA into the host cell genome may account for the oncogenic action of hepatitis B virus (see below).

Histologically, persistent hepatitis shows increased numbers of lymphocytes and plasma cells confined to the portal tracts, and the limiting plate of hepatocytes is intact. There is no active necrosis of liver cells. In those cases caused by hepatitis B virus, the liver cells in tissue sections stain positively for HBsAg.

Chronic Active Viral Hepatitis

Chronic active viral hepatitis is caused by hepatitis B, non-A, non-B, and delta agent. An identical clinicopathologic syndrome occurs as a toxic reaction to certain drugs (oxyphenisatin, methyldopa, isoniazid) or with α_1-antitrypsin deficiency, Wilson's disease, and an autoimmune disease called "lupoid hepatitis." Cases caused by hepatitis B and delta agent can be identified by immunologic studies. Non-A, non-B hepatitis is inferred if the hepatitis followed transfusion of blood products. Antinuclear autoantibodies are present in the serum of patients with autoimmune chronic active hepatitis.

Clinically, chronic active hepatitis is characterized by a chronic illness associated with marked elevation of liver enzymes. Episodes of acute hepatitis may be superimposed, and portal hypertension may develop. Chronic active hepatitis progresses to cirrhosis (Chapter 43) and chronic liver failure. It has a bad prognosis.

Histologically, the hallmark is continuing focal necrosis of liver cells. The portal tracts show widening due to lymphocytic and plasma cell infiltration and fibrosis (Fig 42–12). The inflammation extends into the liver lobule, disrupting the limiting plate of hepatocytes, with entrapment and necrosis of liver cells in the periphery of the lobule ("piecemeal necrosis").

Patients with chronic hepatitis B, both chronic active hepatitis and chronic persistent hepatitis, have an increased incidence of hepatocellular carcinoma (see Chapter 43).

3. PREVENTION OF VIRAL HEPATITIS

Preventive measures against viral hepatitis may be necessary (1) for individuals with known exposure to hepatitis A virus-contaminated food or water; (2) for hospital employees exposed to blood products, who are at risk for developing hepatitis B and hepatitis non-A, non-B infections; and (3) for patients receiving transfused blood and blood products, again at risk for hepatitis B and hepatitis non-A, non-B infection.

Hyperimmune gamma globulin provides pas-

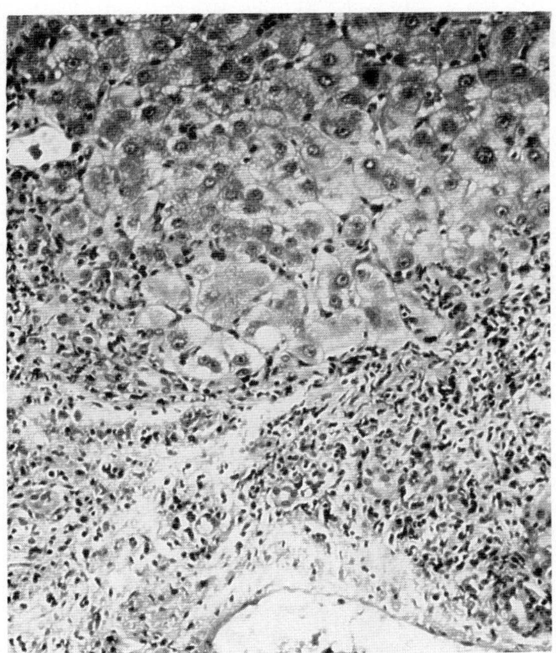

Figure 42–12. Chronic active hepatitis, showing marked lymphocytic infiltration and fibrosis of the portal areas. The lymphocytes extend into the peripheral part of the lobule through the limiting plate. There is ongoing necrosis of hepatocytes in the peripheral part of the lobule (piecemeal necrosis).

sive protection against hepatitis A but not hepatitis B and can be used to prevent a clinical attack of hepatitis A after exposure to the virus. The use of pooled hyperimmune gamma globulin (a blood product) itself carries a risk of hepatitis B and non-A, non-B transmission.

A vaccine containing formalinized (killed) HBsAg-positive material is effective in preventing hepatitis B infection and has been recommended for high-risk groups such as hospital employees who have contact with patients' blood and tissues. An attenuated live vaccine is being developed but is not yet available.

Screening of blood donors for hepatitis B antigens has virtually eradicated hepatitis B viral transmission via blood transfusion. There is no method yet of detecting non-A, non-B in blood donors, and this infection is still a serious problem in blood transfusions.

BACTERIAL INFECTIONS OF THE LIVER

1. NONSUPPURATIVE INFECTIONS

Nonsuppurative bacterial infections of the liver occur as a result of bacteremia associated with any systemic bacterial infection. Liver involvement may provide a means of diagnosis, such as finding caseous granulomas in a liver biopsy specimen from a patient with miliary tuberculosis. Systemic infections such as typhoid fever, brucellosis, and leptospirosis may produce focal necrosis and inflammation in the liver. Apart from minor abnormalities in liver function tests (eg, slight elevation of transaminases, bilirubin, or alkaline phosphatase), these nonsuppurative infections do not usually cause any clinical features. Leptospirosis is an exception, since it commonly causes jaundice.

2. PYOGENIC LIVER ABSCESS

In areas where *Entamoeba histolytica* is not prevalent, most liver abscesses are caused by pyogenic organisms. Many different bacteria may be involved, most commonly *Escherichia coli,* other gram-negative bacilli, anaerobic bacilli, *Staphylococcus aureus,* and streptococci. Culture of pus is necessary for etiologic diagnosis and often reveals a mixed flora.

Bacteria may reach the liver in the course of a systemic bacteremia in the hepatic artery or from the intestine along the bile duct or portal vein (Fig 42–13). Liver abscesses are walled-off collections of pus with liquefactive necrosis of liver cells and neutrophil accumulation. About 50% of cases have multiple abscesses.

Clinically, patients present with high fever, right-sided upper abdominal pain, and hepatomegaly. Pyogenic abscess is a focal lesion and not usually associated with abnormalities in liver function tests except elevation of serum alkaline phosphatase. Treatment consists of drainage of the abscess followed by antibiotic therapy directed by culture and antibiotic sensitivity of the bacteria isolated from the pus.

PARASITIC INFECTIONS OF THE LIVER

1. HEPATIC AMEBIASIS

Hepatic amebiasis is caused by the entry of amebic trophozoites into portal venous radicles in the colonic submucosa, whence they are carried to the liver. Hepatic infection usually occurs in patients with subclinical or chronic intestinal amebic infection and very rarely during an attack of acute amebic colitis. About half of patients with hepatic amebiasis give no history suggestive of preceding amebic colitis.

When they reach the liver, the amebas cause focal enzymatic necrosis of hepatocytes. In the early stage of the disease, there are multiple microabscesses throughout the liver (***Note:*** Though the

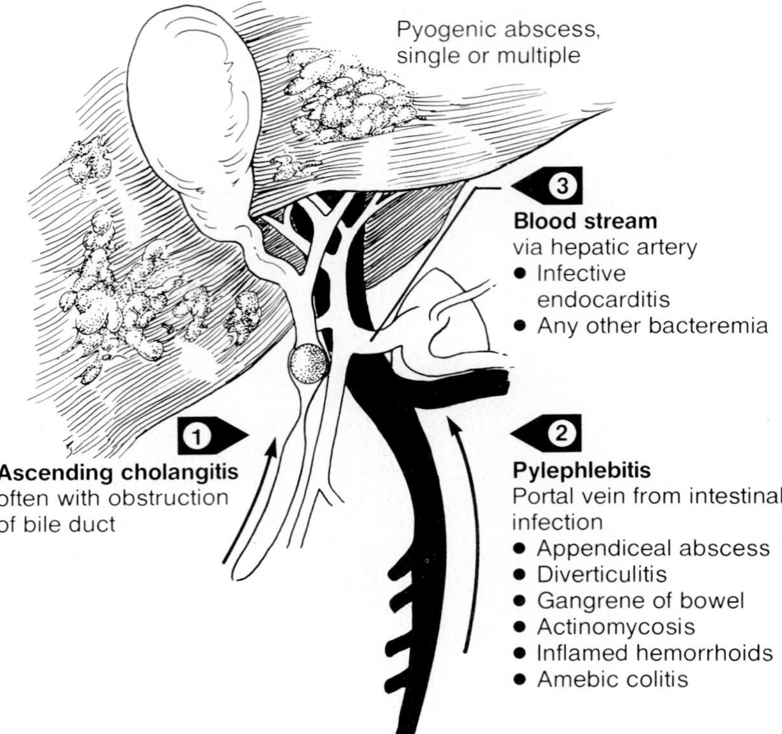

Figure 42–13. Pathogenesis of pyogenic liver abscess, showing the 3 main routes of bacterial infection, via the bile duct **(1),** the portal vein **(2),** and the systemic circulation **(3).**

term "abscess" is used, amebic liver abscesses are not true abscesses because they contain few neutrophils, being composed of liquefied liver cells.) The patient presents at this stage with high fever, right upper abdominal pain, and tender hepatomegaly. This stage of the disease is sometimes called amebic hepatitis. With progression, the microabscesses coalesce to form larger abscesses.

Grossly, amebic abscesses are large, lined by an irregular wall, and contain amebic "pus," which has the typical reddish-brown hue (likened to anchovy paste) of liquefied liver (Fig 42–14). Trophozoites of *Entamoeba histolytica* may be found in the abscess wall.

Diagnosis is based on clinical findings, which include fever, pain in the lower right chest, with hepatomegaly and marked tenderness. Chest x-ray, ultrasonography, CT scan, elevated serum titers of amebic antibodies, and the finding of trophozoites in aspirated pus are useful for confirmation. Liver function tests are usually normal except for an elevated serum alkaline phosphatase level.

Without treatment, amebic liver abscess has a high mortality rate. Deaths are due to (1) rupture into the free peritoneal cavity; (2) rupture into the pleural cavity and lung; (3) rupture into the pericardial sac (in left lobe abscesses), causing acute pericardial tamponade; and (4) systemic spread of trophozoites, resulting in amebic abscesses in the brain and lung.

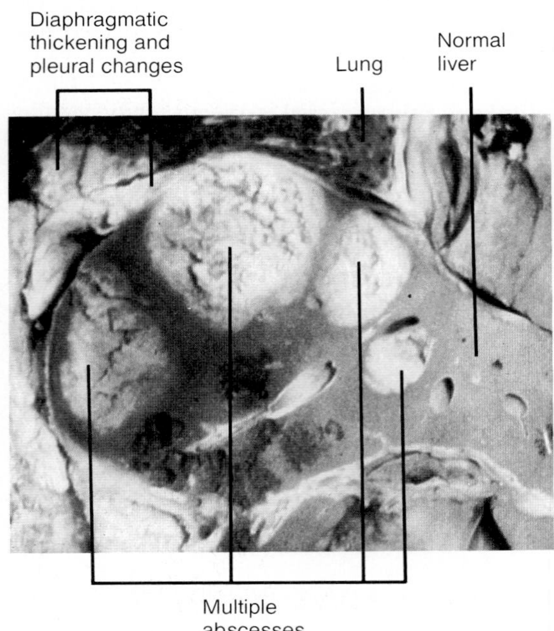

Figure 42–14. Amebic liver abscesses.

Treatment is with the highly effective amebicidal drug metronidazole. Drainage is required for large abscesses.

2. HEPATIC SCHISTOSOMIASIS

Schistosomiasis of the liver complicates intestinal schistosomiasis. *Schistosoma mansoni,* which cause colonic infection in the Middle East, and *Schistosoma japonicum,* which causes small intestinal infection in the Far East, are the species involved. The adult worms live in the intestinal venous plexuses and produce eggs that are carried via the portal vein to the liver, where they are deposited in the portal areas. They produce granulomas in the acute phase followed by "pipestem fibrosis" of the portal areas in the chronic phase. The finding of schistosome ova in the fibrous portal tracts is diagnostic.

Hepatic schistosomiasis causes portal hypertension and ascites and is an important cause of these conditions in endemic areas. The distribution and life cycle of schistosomiasis has been considered in Chapter 14.

3. HYDATID CYST

Hydatid cysts occur in humans as a result of accidental infection by ova of *Echinococcus granulosus.* The liver is the most common site for hydatid cysts, which may reach a large size and may be multiple. Histologic examination shows a thick, acellular laminated eosinophilic wall with an inner surface lined by the germinal epithelium of the larva. The cysts are filled with a granular fluid that is characterized by numerous small larval capsules containing scoleces ("brood capsules").

Patients present with a cystic mass in the liver. The diagnosis is made by the typical radiologic appearance (calcified wall). During surgical removal, care must be taken to avoid spillage of cyst contents into the peritoneal cavity, since the cyst fluid is highly antigenic and may lead to anaphylactic shock.

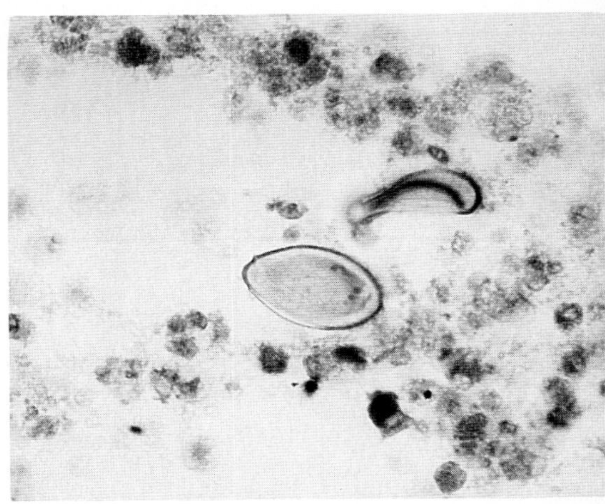

Figure 42–15. Aspirate of bile in oriental cholangiohepatitis, showing ova of *Clonorchis sinensis.*

4. ORIENTAL CHOLANGIOHEPATITIS

Infection of the bile ducts with Clonorchis sinensis is common in eastern Asia. The fluke attaches with its sucker to the bile duct wall and causes inflammation and strictures of the bile ducts and fibrosis of the surrounding liver. The dilated bile ducts proximal to the narrowed segments contain numerous crumbling black calculi. Numerous flukes and ova may be found (Fig 42–15). Patients present with episodes of fever and right upper abdominal pain. The diagnosis is usually made by the radiologic appearance. Surgical resection of the affected areas may be necessary.

43 The Liver: II. Toxic & Metabolic Diseases; Neoplasms

ALCOHOLIC LIVER DISEASE

Incidence & Pathogenesis

Chronic alcoholism is a major problem in almost every society (see also Chapter 12). In developed countries, it has been estimated that about 10% of the population consume potentially harmful amounts of ethyl alcohol. The habit begins in the teen years and continues throughout life. The incidence is increasing, and in developed countries chronic liver disease and accidents associated with alcoholism are among the 10 most common causes of death. Alcoholic liver disease is most common in middle-aged men, but there is an increasing incidence among women and in the young.

The greater the amount and the longer the duration of alcohol consumption, the greater the risk of liver disease. Most patients with chronic alcoholic liver disease have consumed about 150 g or more of ethyl alcohol daily for over 10 years (a standard 750-mL bottle of 80-proof whisky contains about 300 g of alcohol).

Not all heavy drinkers develop liver disease. About 50% of alcoholics have no detectable liver disease, 30% have alcoholic hepatitis, and 20% develop cirrhosis. Prediction of liver disease in individual cases is uncertain.

Alcohol is metabolized in the hepatocyte cytoplasm by the NADH-dependent enzyme alcohol dehydrogenase into acetaldehyde. Acetaldehyde or a related substance is believed to exert a toxic effect on liver cells. Malnutrition, which frequently coexists with alcoholism, may aggravate the liver injury.

Clinicopathologic Syndromes

Alcoholic liver disease may be manifested as fatty liver, alcoholic hepatitis, or alcoholic cirrhosis (Fig 43–1). These lesions may coexist.

A. Fatty Liver: (See Chapter 1.) Fatty liver is a common early manifestation of alcohol injury. It is the result of decreased fatty acid oxidation, increased synthesis of triglycerides, and impaired secretion of lipoproteins by the liver cell. Fat accumulates first as small globules that coalesce, increasing in size and pushing the hepatocyte nucleus to one side.

Clinically, fatty liver causes diffuse liver enlargement. Liver function is normal even when there is severe fatty change. Fatty liver is reversible if the patient stops drinking at this stage.

B. Acute Alcoholic Hepatitis (Acute Sclerosing Hyaline Necrosis of the Liver): Acute alcoholic hepatitis is characterized pathologically by (1) focal lytic necrosis of hepatocytes, causing an increase in serum enzyme levels; (2) cholestasis with jaundice; (3) neutrophilic infiltration of the sinusoids and around necrotic liver cells; (4) sclerosis around the central venule, initially as fine fibrils in the space of Disse and later as coarse fibrosis that may obliterate central veins; and (5) the presence of eosinophilic waxy "alcoholic" hyalin—Mallory bodies—in the cytoplasm of liver cells (Fig 43–2). Hyalin is a fibrillar material derived from the cell's cytoskeleton; it stains positively for cytokeratin by the immunoperoxidase technique. Hyalin is not specific for alcoholic liver

A
Fatty change

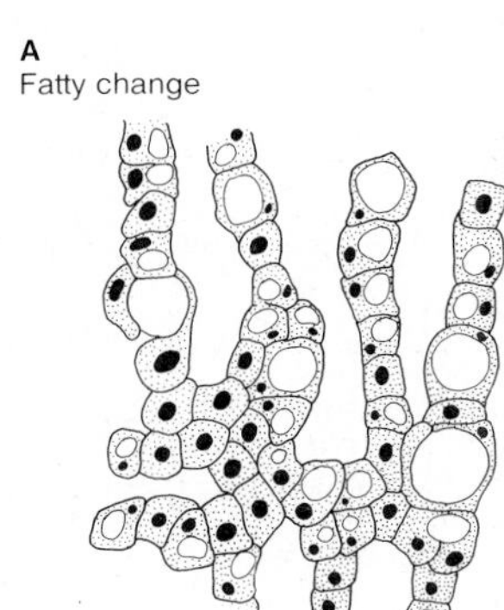

- Chronic, macrovacuolar
- Reversible

B
Acute sclerosing hyaline necrosis

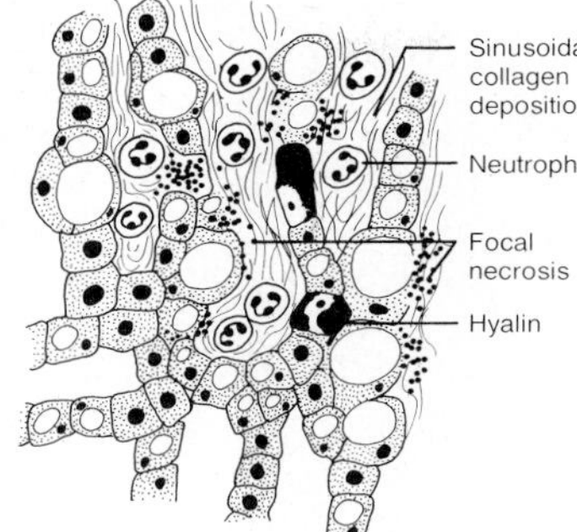

- Focal necrosis with neutrophils
- Cholestasis → jaundice
- Alcoholic hyalin (Mallory bodies)
- Sinusoidal fibrosis
- Reversible unless severe

C
Chronic alcoholic liver disease

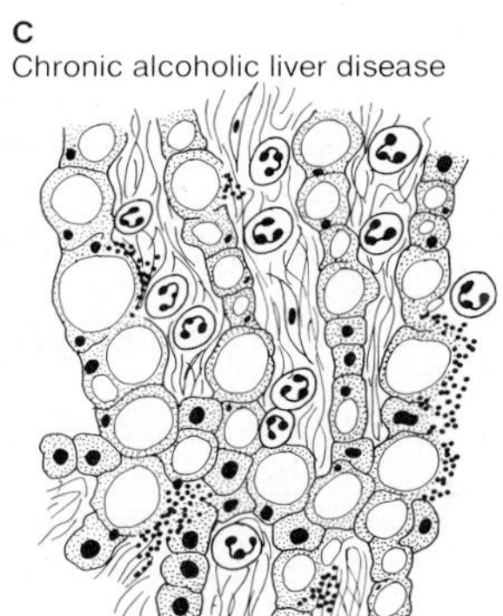

- Ongoing focal necrosis
- Centrilobular and sinusoidal fibrosis
- Some regeneration conserving normal architecture
- ? Irreversible
- ? May not be progressive

D
Alcoholic cirrhosis

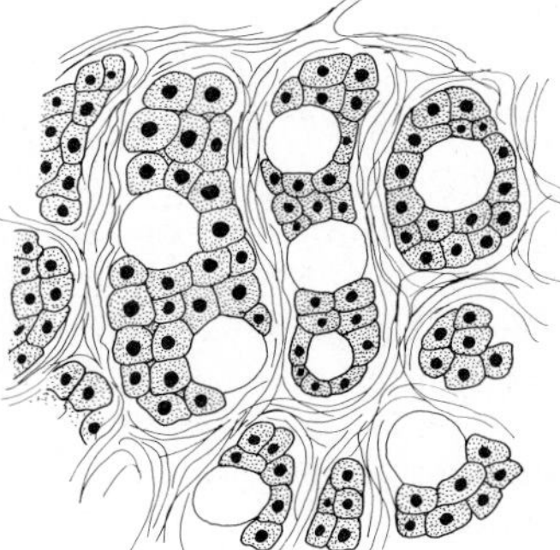

- Ongoing focal necrosis
- Extensive fibrosis
- Regenerative nodules
- Loss of normal architecture
- Progressive and irreversible

Figure 43–1. Alcoholic liver disease. **A:** Fatty change. **B:** Acute alcoholic hepatitis (acute sclerosing hyaline necrosis). **C:** Chronic alcoholic liver disease, precirrhotic. **D:** Alcoholic cirrhosis.

injury, being found also in biliary cirrhosis, Indian childhood cirrhosis, Wilson's disease, and liver cell carcinoma.

Clinically, patients present with an acute onset of fever, jaundice, tender enlargement of the liver, and ascites, commonly after a recent bout of heavy drinking. With severe alcoholic hepatitis, encephalopathy and death may occur. Symptoms and most of the pathologic features resolve with cessation of drinking, but the fibrosis increases progressively with each episode.

C. Chronic Alcoholic Liver Disease: Chronic ingestion of alcohol is associated with progressive fibrosis in the centrizonal region of the liver and distortion of liver architecture by fibrous bands that may connect portal areas and central veins; this differs from cirrhosis in the absence of true regenerative nodules. Progression may slow or come to a halt if alcohol ingestion is discontinued.

D. Alcoholic Cirrhosis: Cirrhosis of the liver is discussed on p 652 and alcoholic cirrhosis on p 654.

CHEMICAL- & DRUG-INDUCED LIVER DISEASE

Many drugs and other chemical substances cause liver damage by a variety of mechanisms (Table 43–1).

Predictable (Dose-Related) Toxicity

Agents in this group cause liver cell necrosis in

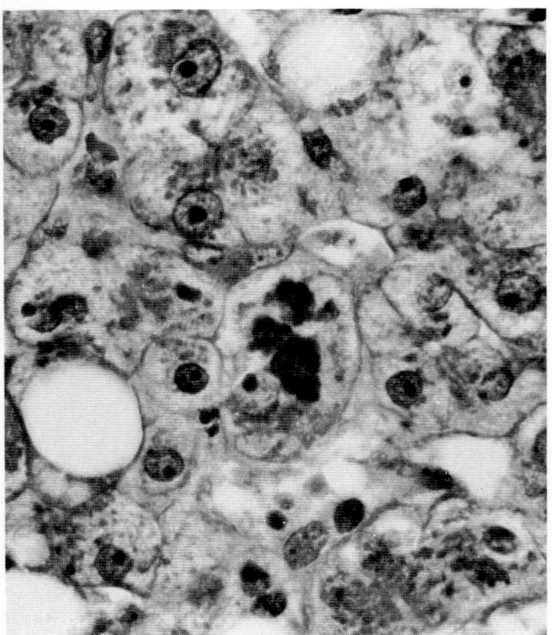

Figure 43–2. Alcoholic hyalin in the cytoplasm of the cell in the center.

all individuals at a predictable dose level. **Acetaminophen,** which is normally metabolized by the glutathione reductase system, is an example of this phenomenon. In overdosage, the glutathione becomes exhausted, and alternative metabolic pathways yield toxic products. Salicylates in high doses and cytotoxic anticancer drugs such as methotrexate also cause liver cell necrosis. Carbon tetrachloride and chloroform, which are used in industry, also cause liver cell necrosis (Fig 43–3).

Tetracycline in high intravenous dosages has been reported to cause acute microvacuolar fatty change in the liver, with liver failure and a high mortality rate.

Unpredictable (Idiosyncratic) Toxicity

Some hepatotoxic drugs cause liver injury in an unpredictable manner, usually unrelated to dose and in only a small percentage of susceptible individuals. Injury is manifested in a variety of ways.

A. Massive Hepatocellular Necrosis: Isoniazid, halothane, and methyldopa may cause submassive or massive liver necrosis, with acute liver failure. Lesser degrees of liver necrosis have been reported following exposure to other antituberculous drugs and antidepressants.

Isoniazid-induced necrosis is important because of the recommendation that this drug be used for chemoprophylaxis in all patients who give a positive tuberculin skin test. Massive necrosis occurs in only 0.1% of patients taking isoniazid; the risk

Table 43–1. Chemical and drug-induced liver disease.

Type of Injury	Drugs or Chemicals
Dose-related ("predictable") reactions	
Hepatocellular necrosis	Mushroom (*Amanita phalloides*) poisoning Aflatoxin Phosphorus Carbon tetrachloride, chloroform, benzene Cytotoxic drugs (eg, methotrexate) Acetaminophen Salicylates Vitamin A (toxic levels)
Acute fatty liver	Tetracycline (intravenous)
Idiosyncratic reactions	
Hepatocellular necrosis (massive)	Halothane, isoniazid, methyldopa
Cholestasis	Phenothiazines, oral contraceptives, anabolic steroids, oral antidiabetic agents
Acute hepatitis-like	Isoniazid, phenytoin, salicylates
Fatty change	Methyldopa, oxyphenisatin, methotrexate
Granulomatous hepatitis	Phenylbutazone, hydralazine, allopurinol
Focal nodular hyperplasia	Oral contraceptives
Liver cell adenoma	Oral contraceptives, anabolic steroids
Angiosarcoma of the liver	Vinyl chloride, thorium dioxide (Thorotrast)
Hepatocellular carcinoma	Aflatoxin

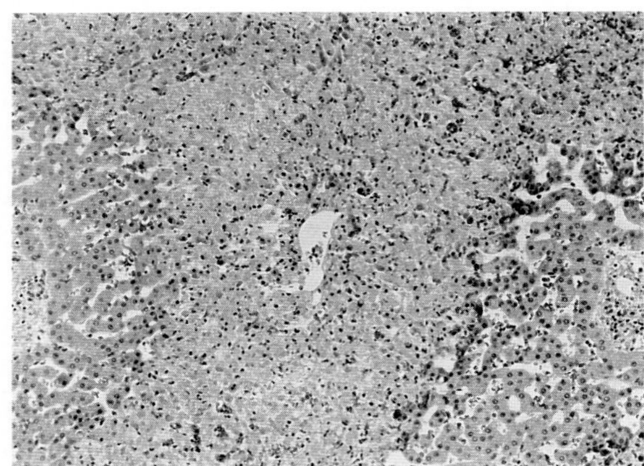

Figure 43–3. Centrizonal necrosis secondary to inhalation of chloroform. Note the large pale zone around the central vein composed of necrotic liver cells. The surviving cells in the peripheral zone have dark cytoplasm.

is insignificant in individuals under 30 years of age and rises after that.

Halothane is an anesthetic agent that causes massive necrosis in a small number of patients. More than one exposure is usually necessary.

B. Cholestasis is caused by anabolic steroids, oral contraceptives, phenothiazines, and oral antidiabetic drugs. Clinically, patients present with deep jaundice of the obstructive type. Liver biopsy shows cholestasis with minimal inflammation and necrosis. The bile ducts in the portal areas are normal, and radiologic studies show lack of dilatation of the intrahepatic biliary system.

C. Acute hepatitis indistinguishable clinically and pathologically from viral hepatitis has been reported as a complication of isoniazid (in about 1% of patients taking the drug), phenytoin, and salicylates.

D. Fatty change occurs as an idiosyncratic effect of methyldopa, oxyphenisatin, and methotrexate.

E. Chronic hepatitis of a type that is very difficult to distinguish clinically and pathologically from viral and autoimmune chronic active hepatitis occurs with methyldopa and oxyphenisatin. The disease may progress to cirrhosis.

F. Granulomatous hepatitis: Noncaseating epithelioid cell granulomas occur with a variety of drugs. Distinction from sarcoidosis is possible only by clinical means.

G. Mass lesions in the liver, including liver cell adenoma and focal nodular hyperplasia, have been attributed to oral contraceptives and anabolic steroids. A few cases of liver cell carcinoma have been reported in oral contraceptive users, but a causal relationship has not been established. Vinyl chloride and thorium dioxide (Thorotrast—a radiologic dye used in the past) are associated with angiosarcoma of the liver.

NUTRITIONAL LIVER DISEASE

Malnutrition (kwashiorkor) is associated with fatty liver and nutritional cirrhosis. Indian childhood cirrhosis is now thought to be the result of malnutrition. The exact mechanism by which undernutrition causes cirrhosis is uncertain.

At the other extreme, obese patients treated with ileoileal bypass (no longer performed) developed liver disease characterized by fatty change and sclerosing hyaline necrosis very similar to alcoholic liver disease. The mechanism of liver injury after ileal bypass is uncertain.

IMMUNOLOGIC DISEASES OF THE LIVER

The role of immunologic hypersensitivity in liver disease is difficult to evaluate. Immune injury probably contributes to the changes seen in viral hepatitis and in several types of drug-induced liver injuries. There is strong evidence that nonviral chronic active hepatitis and primary biliary cirrhosis are the result of injuries mediated by immune mechanisms.

CHRONIC ACTIVE HEPATITIS ("Lupoid Hepatitis")

Immune-mediated and viral chronic active hepatitis have identical clinical and pathologic features. However, patients with immune-mediated disease are hepatitis B-negative and have no history of transfusion of blood products to suggest non-A, non-B virus infection. Anti-smooth muscle antibody and antinuclear antibodies are frequently present in the serum, and the LE cell test is positive (hence "lupoid" hepatitis). Immune-mediated chronic active hepatitis has no relationship to systemic lupus erythematosus.

In contrast to its viral counterpart, immune-mediated chronic active hepatitis occurs more frequently in women. The disease has a bad prognosis, progressing to cirrhosis in the majority of cases. Corticosteroids are sometimes of value in treatment.

PRIMARY BILIARY CIRRHOSIS

Primary biliary cirrhosis occurs predominantly (over 90% of cases) in middle-aged women. The exact cause is uncertain, but immunologic injury is strongly suspected. Primary biliary cirrhosis is associated with other immunologic diseases such as progressive systemic sclerosis and Sjögren's syndrome and is characterized by the presence in serum of several autoantibodies, the most specific of which is antimitochondrial antibody; when present in the serum in a titer in excess of 1:160, it is diagnostic of primary biliary cirrhosis.

Histologically, the diagnostic changes are in the portal tracts. Lymphocytes and plasma cells surround, infiltrate, and appear to actively destroy the walls of the bile ductules. Epithelioid cell granulomas with Langhans' giant cells occur in 30% of cases. Initial bile duct proliferation is followed by progressive destruction. In the final stage of the disease, bile ducts are absent from the portal tracts, which show marked fibrosis. Even in the terminal phase, primary biliary cirrhosis shows only moderate fibrosis. It does not show nodular regeneration of the liver and is therefore not a true cirrhosis despite its name.

Hepatic parenchymal changes are nonspecific and consist of cholestasis and Kupffer cell hyperplasia. Hyalin may be present in the peripheral zonal liver cells.

Clinically, patients present with slowly progressive biliary obstruction. The onset is insidious; pruritus is the most common first symptom, resulting from accumulation of bile salts in the blood. Serum alkaline phosphatase is elevated early, but jaundice occurs later, usually 6–18 months after onset. Most patients have elevated serum triglyceride and cholesterol levels, and many develop xanthomas in the skin. There is an increased risk of atherosclerosis. Portal hypertension and liver failure may occur 5–15 years after onset.

CIRRHOSIS OF THE LIVER

Cirrhosis of the liver is a pathologic entity characterized by (1) necrosis of liver cells, slowly progressive over a long period and ultimately causing chronic liver failure and death; (2) fibrosis, which involves both central veins and portal areas; (3) regenerative nodules, the result of hyperplasia of surviving liver cells; (4) distortion of normal hepatic lobular architecture; and (5) diffuse involvement of the whole liver. A regenerative nodule is an abnormal mass of liver cells without a normal cord pattern or central venule and surrounded completely by fibrosis (Fig 43–4).

Pathology

Grossly, the liver is enlarged in the early stages, but later it becomes smaller because of cell loss and fibrous contraction. It is much firmer than normal. Nodularity is the most characteristic feature (Fig 43–5). Depending on whether the nodules are more or less than 3 mm in size, cirrhosis is classified as macronodular, micronodular, or mixed.

Histologically, regenerative nodules are characteristic. They are composed of hyperplastic liver cells organized into irregular plates that are often several hepatocytes thick. Liver cells often show enlargement, with atypical nuclei—a picture sometimes called "dysplasia" because of the suspicion that such changes are a precursor of liver cell carcinoma.

The vasculature of the liver is greatly distorted. The fibrous bands obstruct the portal venous radicles and lead to abnormal fistulous communications between portal veins and hepatic arterioles, resulting in portal hypertension.

Clinical Features

Cirrhosis is manifested clinically by features of chronic liver failure and portal hypertension (Fig 43–6). Common presenting symptoms include hematemesis due to rupture of gastroesophageal varices and ascites. Cirrhosis is an irreversible and progressive disease that ultimately causes death. The rate of progression is variable.

Cirrhosis is a premalignant lesion. The risk of hepatocellular carcinoma is greatest in cirrhosis caused by hemochromatosis, virus-induced cirrhosis, "cryptogenic" cirrhosis, and alcoholic cirrhosis, in order of decreasing hazard.

A

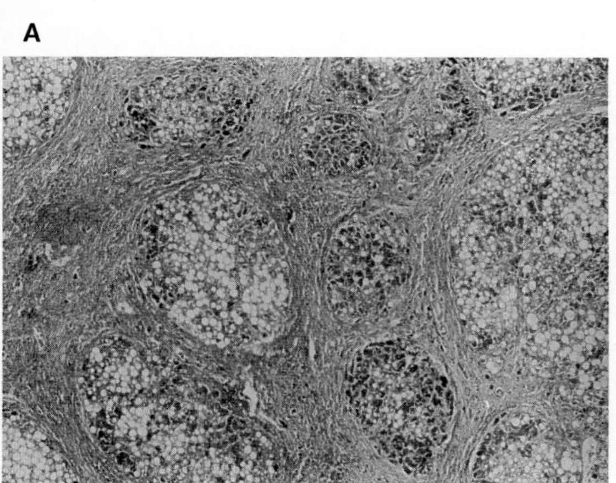

B

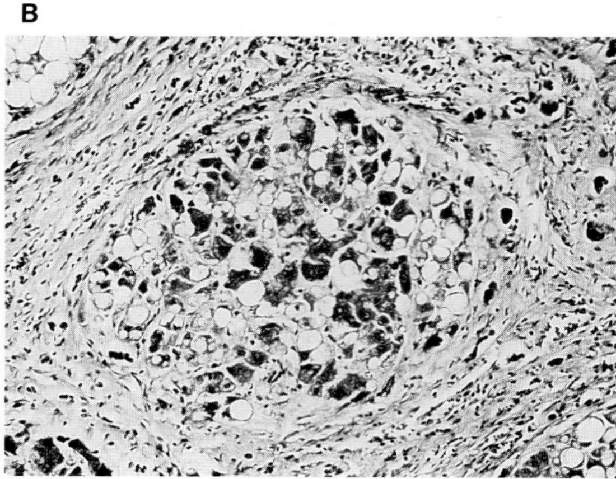

Figure 43–4. Alcoholic cirrhosis of the liver. **A:** Small regenerative nodules are separated by coarse bands of collagen in which are found blood vessels, bile ducts, and inflammatory cells. **B:** The regenerative nodule is composed of a disorganized mass of liver cells showing fatty change. There is no central hepatic vein in the nodule.

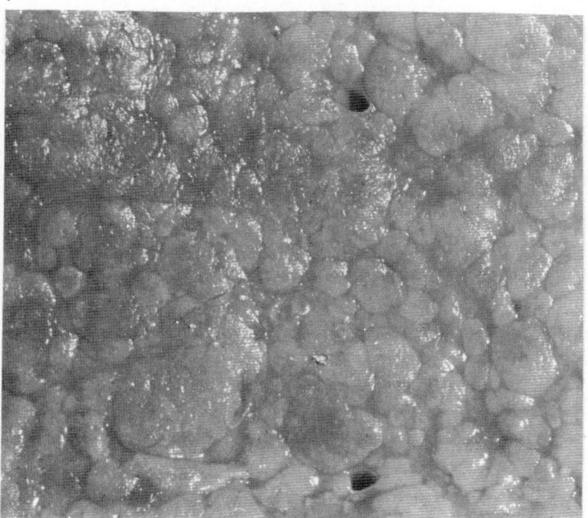

Figure 43-5. Cirrhosis of the liver (cut surface), showing diffuse nodularity.

Etiologic Types of Cirrhosis (Table 43-2)

The terminology of this disorder is confusing and unsatisfactory. Characterizing cirrhosis as "micronodular" and "macronodular" according to the size of the nodules is of little value, since the size of nodules does not correlate with etiology. The terms "portal cirrhosis" and "Laennec's cirrhosis" are no longer used; both denoted micronodular cirrhosis of the alcoholic type. The term "postnecrotic cirrhosis" should no longer be used, because all forms of cirrhosis are associated with necrosis of liver cells and are therefore postnecrotic.

Cirrhosis is most usefully classified according to its causes. All etiologic classifications include a group called cryptogenic cirrhosis (of unknown cause). The incidence of cryptogenic cirrhosis depends on how diligently the cause is sought and how rigorous the criteria are for assigning specific causes to individual cases.

CRYPTOGENIC CIRRHOSIS

Hepatic cirrhosis is said to be cryptogenic when complete evaluation of the patient has failed to

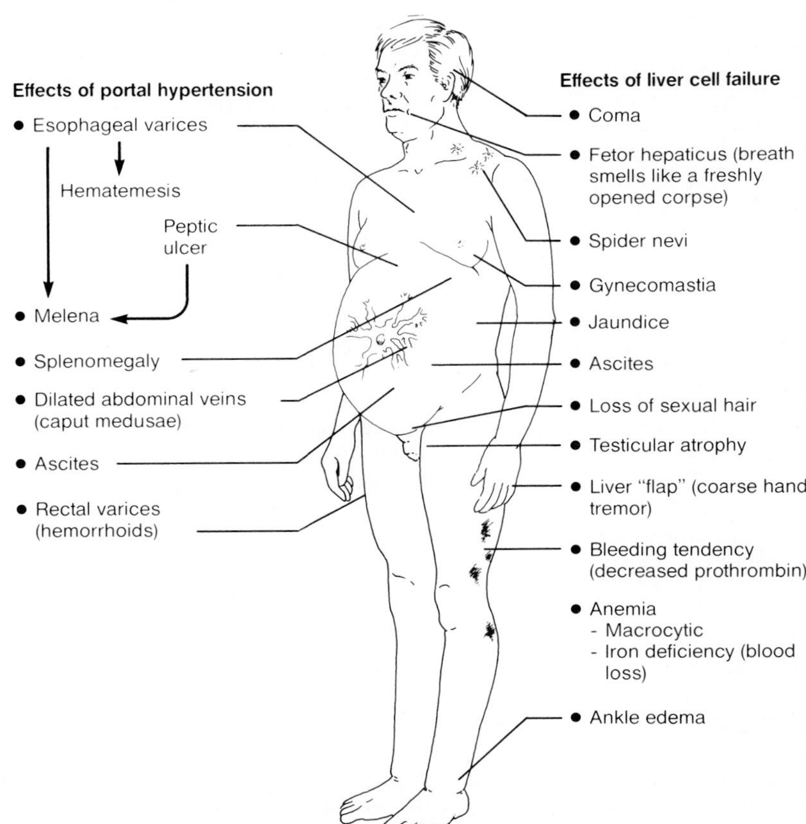

Figure 43-6. Clinical effects of cirrhosis of the liver.

Table 43–2. Etiologic classification of cirrhosis.

Type of Cirrhosis	Relative Frequency[1]
Cryptogenic (cause not established)	10–30%
Alcoholic	30–60%
Virus-induced (B and non-A, non-B [NANB])	10–30%
Biliary cirrhosis Primary[2] Secondary	10%
Immune-mediated chronic active hepatitis	?10%
Hemochromatosis	5%
Wilson's disease	Rare
Alpha$_1$-antitrypsin deficiency	Rare
Galactosemia	Rare
Cardiac cirrhosis[2]	Rare

[1]The frequency of these etiologic types of cirrhosis differs greatly in different countries. The commonly quoted figures for the USA are given here. In the UK, the incidence of cryptogenic cirrhosis is higher.
[2]Although traditionally termed cirrhosis, not all of the definitional features are present in these conditions.

identify a cause. Cryptogenic cirrhosis may include cirrhosis following immune-mediated chronic active hepatitis; following hepatitis due to non-A, non-B hepatitis virus; or following injury due to drugs or chemicals—because there is no way to identify these causes with certainty. A history of blood transfusion in the distant past may suggest non-A, non-B viral infection, but such a history is not sufficient to ascribe the cause of cirrhosis to the infection. Many patients with cirrhosis give a history of drug ingestion, but it is difficult to establish a causal role for the drugs.

ALCOHOLIC CIRRHOSIS

Alcoholic cirrhosis is frequently associated with evidence of fatty change or acute alcoholic hepatitis. Alcoholic cirrhosis is typically a fatty micronodular cirrhosis (Fig 43–4). In patients who stop drinking, the nodules are not infrequently larger and fat is absent.

Alcoholic cirrhosis tends to have a slow rate of progression, particularly if the patient stops drinking. The disease is irreversible and causes death.

VIRUS-INDUCED CIRRHOSIS

Cirrhosis may follow chronic active hepatitis resulting from infection with hepatitis B and non-A, non-B viruses. Patients who present with cirrhosis may or may not give a history of hepatitis. Typically, virus-induced cirrhosis is macronodular. Features of chronic active hepatitis may coexist. Virus-induced cirrhosis tends to progress rapidly, with death due to chronic liver failure, portal hypertension, or hepatocellular carcinoma.

Cirrhosis caused by hepatitis B virus may be identified by the presence of HBsAg in the serum and in liver cells; orcein stains and immunoperoxidase stains for HBsAg are positive. The diagnosis of non-A, non-B cirrhosis is presumptive, based upon the history of transfusion of blood products. When a patient with cirrhosis gives a history of a single transfusion in the distant past, it is probably more correct to regard the cirrhosis as cryptogenic.

The relationship of delta hepatitis agent to cirrhosis has not been completely evaluated, but this agent can also be demonstrated in liver cells by immunoperoxidase techniques.

BILIARY CIRRHOSIS

Primary biliary cirrhosis causes portal fibrosis, but the changes fall short of the definition of cirrhosis because regenerative nodules are usually absent (Fig 43–7).

Secondary biliary cirrhosis occurs in patients with prolonged large bile duct obstruction (gallstones, stricture, tumor, cholangitis). Marked cholestasis causes liver cell necrosis, and prolonged cholangitis leads to portal fibrosis (Fig 43–7). Biliary cirrhosis causes a fine nodularity (micronodules). Features of chronic liver failure and portal hypertension occur late.

HEMOCHROMATOSIS

Hemochromatosis results from iron overload in the body as demonstrated by increased serum iron, ferritin, and saturation of iron-binding protein; increased iron stores in the bone marrow; and the presence of iron in liver cells.

Etiology

A. Idiopathic Hemochromatosis: This is a familial disease with autosomal recessive inheritance of an abnormal gene located on chromosome 6 in close linkage with HLA-A3. The disease occurs in homozygotes; heterozygotes show slightly elevated serum iron levels. The mechanism by which the abnormal gene causes iron overload is not certain but is believed to involve increased intestinal iron absorption.

B. Secondary Hemochromatosis: Secondary hemochromatosis is the occurrence of iron overload due to recognizable causes such as the following:

1. Increased dietary intake of iron–This occurs in the Bantu tribe of Africa, who use iron cooking utensils ("Bantu siderosis"). The exces-

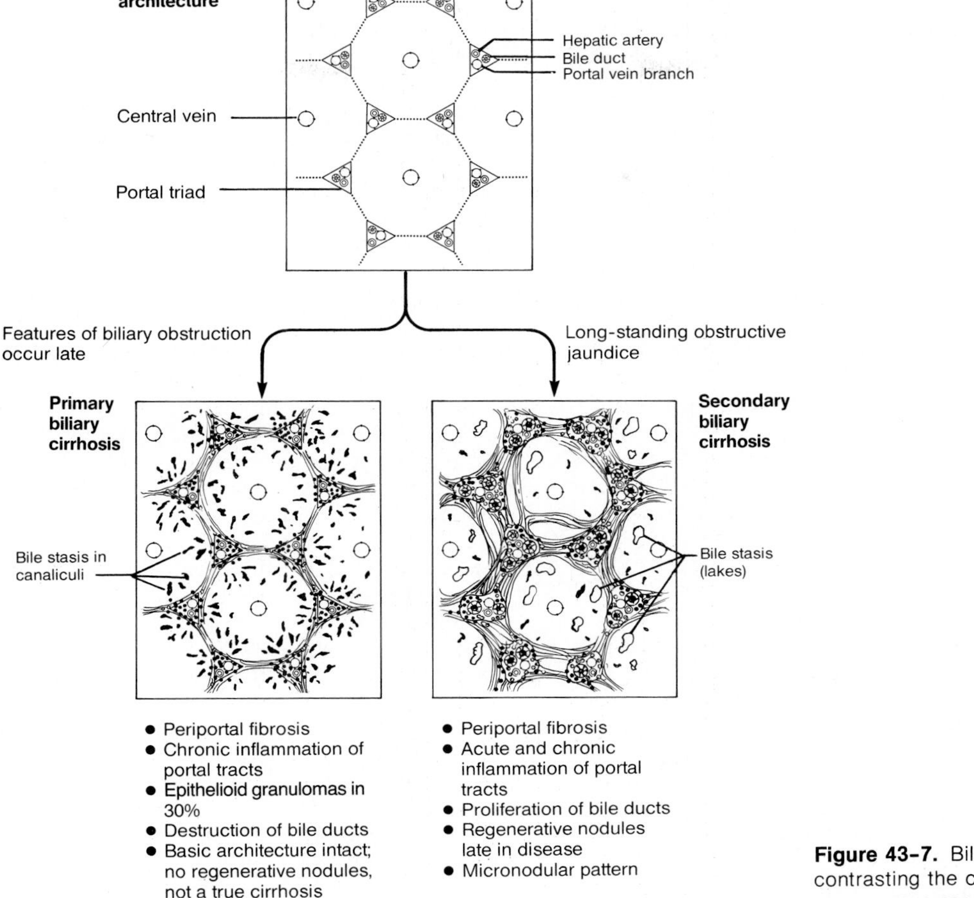

Figure 43-7. Biliary cirrhosis, contrasting the changes of primary versus secondary disease.

sive use of iron-containing drugs and iron-rich wine and beer may also cause iron overload.

2. **Iron infusions-**Usually in the form of repeated blood transfusions for chronic anemias.

3. **Liver disease-**Particularly alcoholic cirrhosis, which is associated with increased iron absorption. The resulting iron deposition in liver cells may contribute to further liver cell damage.

4. **Chronic hemolytic anemias-**Thalassemia is the commonest cause of secondary hemochromatosis. Iron overload is due to repeated blood transfusions and stimulation of intestinal iron absorption by erythroid hyperplasia in the bone marrow.

Liver Changes in Hemochromatosis

Iron is deposited as hemosiderin in the cytoplasm of Kupffer cells and hepatocytes. Hemosiderin appears as golden brown granules in routine microscopic sections (see Chapter 1). The Prussian blue stain for iron produces an intense blue color.

Accumulation of iron in hepatocytes causes cellular degeneration, functional impairment, and clinical disease. This occurs early in idiopathic hemochromatosis and later in secondary forms of hemochromatosis. The mechanism by which stored iron causes cell damage is uncertain. It is believed that free iron accumulates in the cytoplasm when the capacity for storage as ferritin and hemosiderin is exhausted. Free ferric iron undergoes reduction, causing abnormal electron transfers and the formation of toxic oxygen-based free radicals.

Initially, the liver is slightly enlarged. Over a long period of time, there is progressive loss of liver cells accompanied by fibrosis—leading to cirrhosis, which is commonly macronodular. Hepatic hemochromatosis progresses rapidly and may be complicated by hepatocellular carcinoma.

Changes in Extrahepatic Tissues

Iron deposition occurs in many other tissues: The pancreas, myocardium, skin, endocrine glands, and joints are commonly affected, producing the extrahepatic clinical manifestations of hemochromatosis (Fig 43–8). Increased pigmentation of the skin and pancreatic islet destruction result in "bronze diabetes," which is an alternative name for hemochromatosis.

WILSON'S DISEASE

Wilson's disease is an autosomal recessive disorder characterized by (1) defective excretion of copper into bile; (2) increase in total body copper, resulting from unchanged absorption in the face of decreased biliary excretion; (3) accumulation of copper in the cytoplasm of liver cells, complexed to an abnormal protein; (4) decreased ceruloplasmin level in plasma; and (5) increased "free" copper in plasma, causing increased urinary excretion of copper and deposition of copper both in cells and in connective tissue. The primary defect is in the liver cell and is corrected by liver transplantation.

Liver Changes in Wilson's Disease

Liver involvement is responsible for the dominant clinical features. Intracellular copper produces an injury manifested as a progressive microvacuolar fatty change and focal liver cell necrosis. It may present, usually in late childhood, as acute hepatitis clinically resembling viral hepatitis. With continuing liver cell necrosis, it progresses to fibrosis and finally to cirrhosis with chronic liver failure. Increased copper levels in the liver can be demonstrated biochemically. Histochemical methods (rubeanic acid stain) are not always positive, because of the abnormal protein binding of the copper in liver cells.

Extrahepatic Changes in Wilson's Disease

Copper deposition in the **brain** involves the basal ganglia (particularly the lenticular nucleus), thalamus, red nucleus, and dentate nucleus of the cerebellum, all of which show atrophy, slight brown discoloration, and cavitation. Microscopically, the neurons are decreased in number, representing chronic cell necrosis. Reactive astrocytic proliferation is present. These changes produce clinical features of extrapyramidal dysfunction. Wilson's disease is also called **hepatolenticular degeneration**.

Deposition of copper in Descemet's membrane at the **sclerocorneal junction** is important for clin-

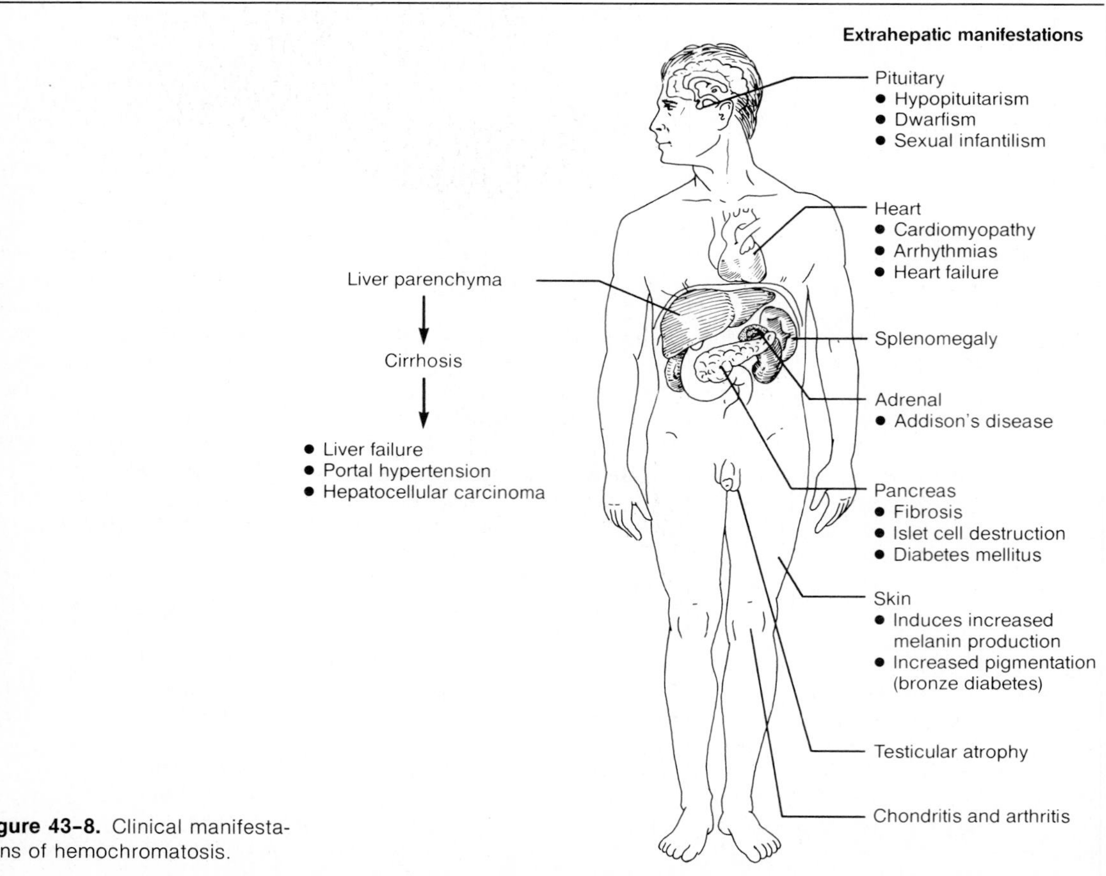

Figure 43–8. Clinical manifestations of hemochromatosis.

ical diagnosis, producing a characteristic greenish-brown ring (Kayser-Fleischer ring) at the corneal edge. This is not seen with the naked eye until a late stage of the disease but can be recognized early by slit-lamp examination. Copper deposition in the eye does not cause visual impairment.

ALPHA$_1$-ANTITRYPSIN DEFICIENCY (See also Chapter 35.)

Severe α_1-antitrypsin deficiency occurs in homozygous PiZZ individuals and is a rare cause of cirrhosis, usually with onset during childhood. The abnormal gene results in hepatic synthesis of an abnormal α_1-antitrypsin molecule that accumulates in the liver cell cytoplasm, appearing as eosinophilic globules. These globules are present in liver cells in the peripheral part of the lobule and stain positively with periodic acid-Schiff (PAS) stain. They also stain by immunoperoxidase methods using antibody against α_1-antitrypsin. The demonstration of these globules establishes the diagnosis, which can be further confirmed by absence of α_1-antitrypsin in the blood.

GALACTOSEMIA

Galactosemia is a rare inherited disease caused by deficiency of galactose-1-phosphate uridyl transferase. Galactose metabolites accumulate in the liver, causing injury. Affected patients present in early infancy following feeding of milk (which contains lactose, a disaccharide of glucose and galactose). Cholestasis, fatty change, and cirrhosis progress rapidly to liver failure. Galactosemia is also associated with cataracts and mental retardation.

Galactosemia is routinely looked for in neonatal screening tests. Diagnosis in a neonate followed by administration of a diet that contains no milk products prevents liver damage.

NEOPLASMS OF THE LIVER

BENIGN NEOPLASMS

Benign neoplasms of the liver are not uncommon as incidental findings at autopsy and are becoming increasingly important because modern radiologic imaging procedures are now able to detect small tumors, raising the question of whether such tumors are benign or malignant, primary or secondary.

Cavernous Hemangioma

Hemangiomas are common incidental findings at surgery, radiologic examination, and autopsy. Histologically, they are composed of large endothelium-lined spaces filled with blood.

Peliosis Hepatis

Peliosis hepatis is a rare degenerative condition associated with multiple blood-filled spaces in the liver, many of which lack an endothelial lining. It may be associated with use of anabolic steroids.

Sclerosing Bile Duct Adenoma

Bile duct adenoma is uncommon and usually presents as an incidental finding at surgery. It appears as a firm, gray-white nodule situated beneath the capsule. Over 90% are less than 1 cm in diameter. Histologically, adenoma is composed of irregular glands surrounded by collagen. Distinction from metastatic adenocarcinoma can be difficult.

Liver Cell Adenoma

Liver cell adenoma is a rare benign neoplasm that occurs mainly in women taking oral contraceptives and athletes taking anabolic steroids; some tumors have regressed when these drugs were withdrawn.

The tumors may be multiple and large and may have foci of hemorrhage and necrosis. Microscopically, liver cell adenomas are composed of cytologically benign hepatocytes arranged in thickened cords. Bile ducts and portal tracts are absent. The distinction from a well-differentiated hepatocellular carcinoma may be difficult.

Clinically, patients may present with a mass, sudden pain due to infarction, or hemorrhage due to rupture through the liver capsule.

Focal Nodular Hyperplasia

Focal nodular hyperplasia is another mass lesion of the liver that has been etiologically related to oral contraceptives. It is not a true neoplasm; the mechanism by which it arises is unknown.

Focal nodular hyperplasia most frequently presents as a solitary solid mass lesion, usually subcapsular, well-circumscribed, and only rarely larger than 5 cm. On cut section, it is gray-white and typically has a central scar with bands of fibrosis radiating to the periphery.

Microscopically, nodules of liver tissue are separated by fibrous bands in which portal tracts containing bile ductules can be identified. The lesion resembles a neoplasm grossly and localized cirrhosis microscopically.

MALIGNANT NEOPLASMS

Malignant neoplasms may arise in the liver from (1) hepatocytes (hepatocellular carcinoma),

(2) intrahepatic bile ductules (cholangiocarcinoma), and (3) mesenchymal elements such as blood vessels (angiosarcoma and hemangioendothelioma).

1. HEPATOCELLULAR CARCINOMA (Hepatoma)

Incidence

Hepatocellular carcinoma (sometimes called hepatoma) has a marked geographic variation in incidence, being common in the Far East and certain parts of Africa (Chapter 17; Table 43-3), where in some areas it is the most common type of cancer. It is uncommon in Western Europe and North America (about 8000 cases a year in the United States).

Etiology

The cause is unknown, but several factors have been implicated. **(1) Aflatoxin,** a product of the fungus *Aspergillus flavus,* which grows on improperly stored grain and nuts (including peanuts), is toxic to liver cells. It is present in high levels in grain in Africa and Asia, leading to the suggestion that chronic ingestion of aflatoxin may be responsible for the high incidence of liver cell carcinoma in these areas. **(2) Hepatitis B virus infection** is strongly suspected of causing hepatocellular carcinoma. Africa and Far East countries where hepatocellular carcinoma is common have high rates of hepatitis carriers, probably with vertical transmission of the virus from generation to generation.

Over 80% of patients who develop hepatocellular carcinoma have **cirrhosis of the liver.** The increased cell turnover in regenerative nodules of cirrhosis is associated with cytologic abnormalities that have been interpreted as being premalignant dysplastic changes. While all types of cirrhosis may be complicated by carcinoma, the association is greatest with hemochromatosis, virus-induced cirrhosis, and alcoholic cirrhosis.

Pathology

Grossly, hepatocellular carcinoma may present as a large solitary mass (Fig 43-9), as multiple nodules, or as a diffusely infiltrative lesion. Microscopically, the neoplasm is composed of abnormal liver cells of variable differentiation. The better-differentiated tumors are composed of cells resembling liver cells arranged in cords separated by sinusoids (Fig 43-10). The cells have enlarged nuclei that show prominent nucleoli and hyperchromatism and may contain bile in the cytoplasm. The less well differentiated tumors have sheets of anaplastic cells. Invasion of hepatic venous radicles is a typical feature that permits differentiation from adenoma. It may be difficult to distinguish a poorly differentiated hepatocellular carcinoma from metastatic carcinoma. Rarely, venous involvement is so extensive as to produce Budd-Chiari syndrome. Even more rarely, a tumor thrombus extends along the hepatic vein into the inferior vena cava and up into the right atrium.

Immunohistochemical stains may show the presence of **alpha-fetoprotein (AFP)** in the neoplastic cells. Hepatocellular carcinoma also secretes AFP into the blood; elevated levels are present in 90% of patients, making serum AFP assay an important diagnostic test. (*Note:* AFP levels

Table 43-3. Presentation and risk factors: Hepatocellular carcinoma, cholangiocarcinoma, carcinoma of gallbladder or biliary tract.

	Hepatocellular Carcinoma	Cholangiocarcinoma	Carcinoma of Gallbladder and Biliary Tract
Sex	M > F-3:1 in HBV endemic areas; 9:1 elsewhere	F > M 2:1	F > M 4:1
Racial/geographic distribution	High-Asia, Africa Low-Europe, USA	High-Far East Low-Europe, USA	High in Native Americans and in South America (Mexico); relatively low in Africa, Asia
Age	30-50 years in HBV-endemic areas; 60+ elsewhere	60+	50+
Medical history	Hepatitis B infection; alcoholism; hemochromotosis; cirrhosis	*Clonorchis sinensis* infection; Thorotrast exposure	Gallstones; chronic cholecystitis
Presentation	Weight loss, anorexia; tender hepatomegaly; fever; abdominal distention (ascites, peritoneal hemorrhage, large liver)	Weight loss, anorexia; tender hepatomegaly; abdominal distention	Weight loss, anorexia; enlarged gallbladder; jaundice
Alpha-fetoprotein (AFP)	Elevated in 90%	Normal	Normal
Other secretory products	Erythropoietin (polycythemia), insulin-like polypeptide (hypoglycemia)	None	None

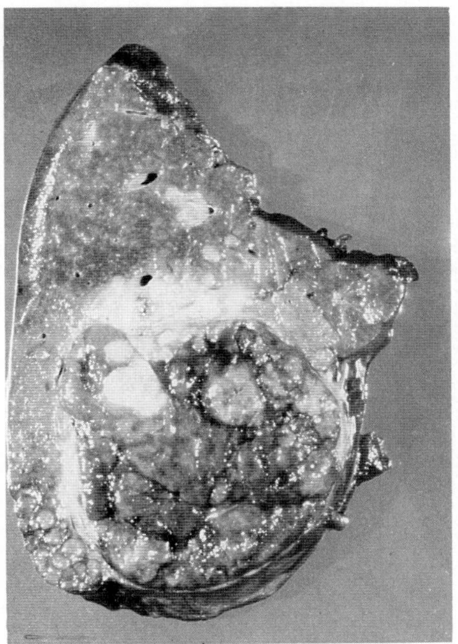

Figure 43-9. Hepatocellular carcinoma, showing a large solitary nodule that is grossly encapsulated except in one area.

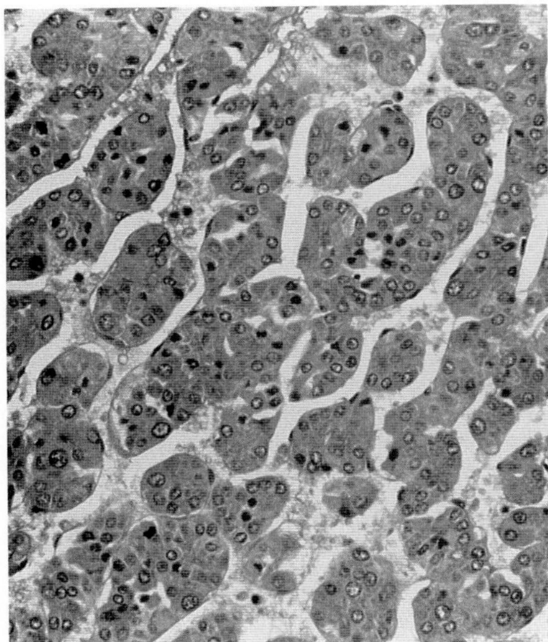

Figure 43-10. Well-differentiated hepatocellular carcinoma, showing trabeculae of malignant hepatocytes separated by sinusoidal spaces. This is characterized by absence of portal areas and greatly expanded trabeculae composed of several layers of malignant hepatocytes.

may be slightly elevated in some cases of hepatitis and cirrhosis as well as in some germ cell neoplasms of the gonads.)

Hepatocellular carcinoma tends to metastasize early via the bloodstream to produce lung metastases. Metastases to other sites occur terminally.

Clinical Features (Fig 43-11)

Hepatocellular carcinoma should be suspected when a patient with known cirrhosis presents with any new symptom such as pain, loss of weight, fever, increasing liver size, or increasing ascites. About 20% of patients present with intraperitoneal hemorrhage. Rarely, hepatocellular carcinoma may secrete an ectopic hormone, causing hypoglycemia (insulinlike polypeptide), polycythemia (erythropoietin), and hypercalcemia (parathyroid hormone-like polypeptide).

Surgical resection is rarely undertaken for the treatment of hepatocellular carcinoma, and chemotherapy and radiotherapy are not very effective. Progression is extremely rapid, and most patients are dead within 1 year. The median survival after diagnosis is 2 months; the 5-year survival rate is less than 1%.

2. CHOLANGIOCARCINOMA

Cholangiocarcinoma arises in the intrahepatic bile ductules. It is uncommon in the United States and Europe but has a relatively high incidence in the Far East, where infection with the liver fluke, *Clonorchis sinensis,* is thought to be a predisposing factor. Cholangiocarcinoma is not associated with cirrhosis.

Grossly, cholangiocarcinoma presents features indistinguishable from those of hepatocellular carcinoma. Histologically, it is an adenocarcinoma that shows mucin secretion. The presence of cytoplasmic mucin permits differentiation from hepatocellular carcinoma, which does not secrete mucin. Marked sclerosis is common. Differentiation from metastatic adenocarcinoma is almost impossible on histologic grounds alone. Serum alpha-fetoprotein levels are normal.

The clinical presentation is with a liver mass. The progress of disease is often slow, but bloodstream spread ultimately occurs, and the prognosis is poor.

3. MALIGNANT VASCULAR NEOPLASMS

Angiosarcoma

Hepatic angiosarcoma is a highly malignant rare neoplasm that has been linked etiologically to **polyvinyl chloride,** which is used extensively in the plastics industry; and to **Thorotrast,** a thorium dioxide-containing radiographic dye that was used

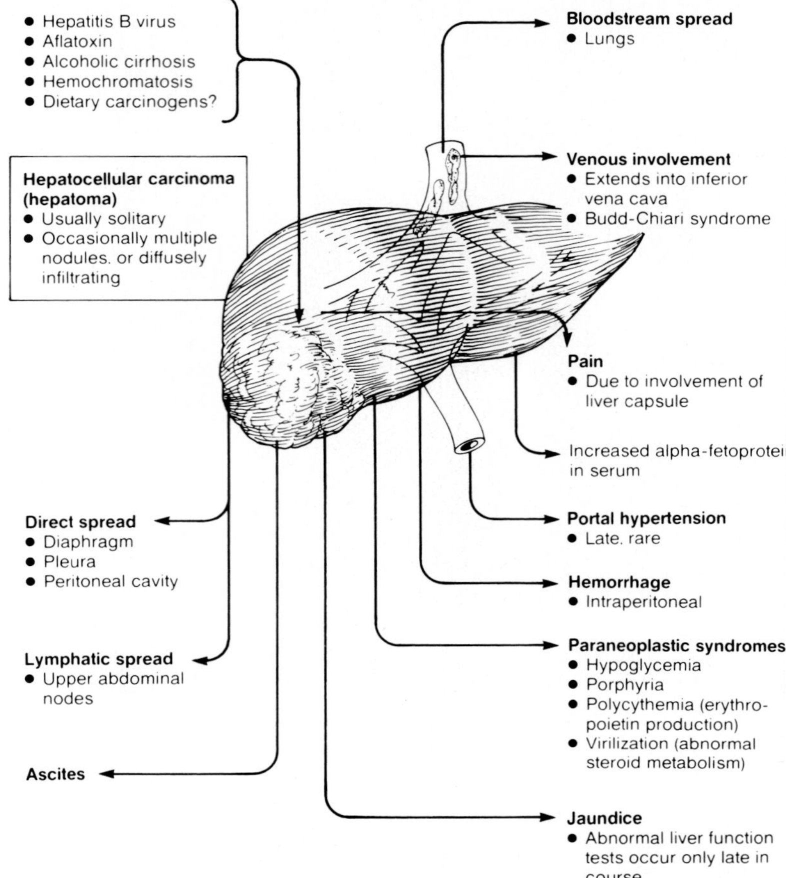

Figure 43–11. Clinical and pathologic effects of hepatocellular carcinoma.

several decades ago. Thorium was deposited as refractile crystals in the portal tracts and acted as a carcinogen.

Patients present with rapid liver enlargement. The tumor appears as a solid, often very large hemorrhagic mass composed histologically of intercommunicating vascular spaces lined by malignant endothelial cells.

Epithelioid Hemangioendothelioma

This rare malignant neoplasm of endothelial cells has a slower rate of progression than angiosarcoma. It produces a diffusely infiltrative mass with marked fibrosis. Metastases occur late, and death occurs 10–15 years after diagnosis.

METASTATIC NEOPLASMS

Metastases account for most neoplasms involving the liver. Virtually any malignant neoplasm in the body can metastasize to the liver; those from the gastrointestinal tract (via the portal vein), breast, and lung and malignant melanoma are most common.

Metastatic carcinoma characteristically produces massive liver enlargement with multiple nodules (Fig 43–12). However, differentiation of hepatocellular carcinoma from metastatic carcinoma is sometimes very difficult. The following features are helpful: (1) Grossly, the nodules of metastatic carcinoma often show central necrosis and umbilication. (2) The presence of cirrhosis favors hepatocellular carcinoma. (3) The demonstration of alpha-fetoprotein in tumor cells or in the blood is almost pathognomonic of hepatocellular carcinoma. (4) Invasion of hepatic veins favors hepatocellular carcinoma.

If metastatic spread is from an adenocarcinoma, distinction from primary cholangiocarcinoma of the liver may be impossible unless a primary adenocarcinoma is found elsewhere in the body.

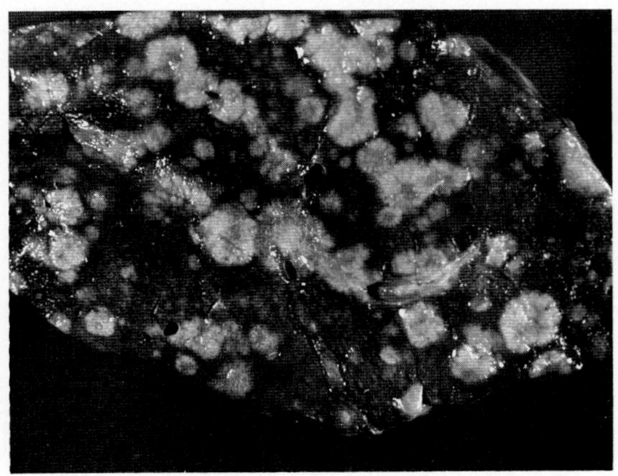

Figure 43-12. Metastatic carcinoma in the liver, showing multiple nodules some of which have central necrosis and umbilication. The patient had a primary carcinoma in the pancreas.

LIVER NEOPLASMS IN INFANCY

Several rare neoplasms have been described as occurring in the liver in infancy.

Infantile hemangioendothelioma is a benign neoplasm of endothelial cells characterized by anastomosing vascular spaces. It is often large and tends to shunt blood from the arterial to the venous side, acting as an arteriovenous fistula and leading to a hyperdynamic circulation; the usual presentation is heart failure in infancy.

Mesenchymal hamartoma also produces a mass—often a large mass—in the liver. It is solid, with areas of cystic change; microscopically, mesenchymal hamartoma is composed of bile duct-like structures admixed with disorganized mesenchymal elements. It is benign. Surgical removal is curative.

Hepatoblastoma is a malignant neoplasm composed of primitive cells that resemble fetal liver cells. Mesenchymal elements such as bone are present in most cases. Alpha-fetoprotein is present both in tumor cells and in the blood. This tumor commonly presents as marked liver enlargement in infancy. It has a poor prognosis.

44 The Extrahepatic Biliary System

STRUCTURE & FUNCTION

The extrahepatic biliary system is composed of the bile ducts and the gallbladder (Fig 44–1). In 70% of patients, the common bile duct and pancreatic duct join at the ampulla of Vater and have a common duodenal opening. In the other 30%, the pancreatic and bile ducts open separately. The common bile duct has a luminal diameter of 0.5–0.7 cm in the adult.

Histologically, the entire biliary tract is lined by mucus-secreting columnar epithelium. In the gallbladder, the epithelium is thrown up into delicate folds, and mucous glands are buried deeply in the smooth muscle wall (Aschoff-Rokitansky sinuses). The biliary tract is covered by peritoneum except for the surface of the gallbladder that lies on the liver bed and the intrapancreatic portion of the common bile duct.

The biliary system stores and delivers the bile secreted by the liver into the duodenum, the gallbladder acting as a reservoir in which the bile is stored and concentrated (from about 1000 mL/d down to 50 mL/d). The gallbladder is not required for adequate functioning of the system. Bile is an alkaline fluid that contains the excretory bilirubin pigments, bile acids and bile salts, cholesterol, inorganic ions, and mucus. Cholesterol, which is insoluble in water, is maintained in solution by the formation of complexes with the hydrophilic bile salts and lecithin.

MANIFESTATIONS OF BILIARY TRACT DISEASE

Pain

Several types of pain occur in diseases of the extrahepatic biliary system. **Biliary colic** is severe intermittent pain in the right upper abdomen that radiates to the back and right shoulder. It is caused by increased muscular contraction of the bile duct and occurs when there is bile duct obstruction. Vague **epigastric pain ("dyspepsia"),** which may be aggravated by ingestion of fatty foods, is common in patients with gallstones and chronic cholecystitis. The mechanism of this pain is unknown. Constant **right upper abdominal pain,** often severe, occurs in acute cholecystitis when the inflammation extends to involve the pain-sensitive parietal peritoneum.

Obstructive Jaundice (Fig 44–2)

Obstruction of the common bile duct results in obstructive jaundice. The biliary system undergoes dilatation proximal to the obstruction, and bile backs up in the liver (cholestasis). The gallbladder undergoes enlargement when it is normal; in patients who have gallstones and fibrotic thickening of the gallbladder wall, gallbladder enlargement does not occur (Courvoisier's law).

Fever

Fever occurs in acute cholecystitis and in patients with obstructive jaundice in whom infection of the static column of bile commonly occurs (acute cholangitis). Intestinal bacteria are the agents usually responsible, and bacteremia is common.

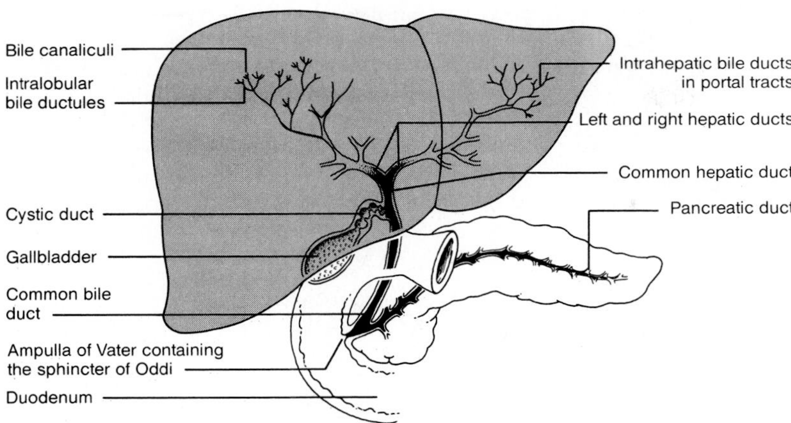

Figure 44-1. Anatomy of the biliary system.

ASSESSMENT OF THE BILIARY TRACT

Cholecystography & Cholangiography

The biliary tract may be outlined by a radiopaque dye, permitting evaluation of its anatomy. The dye may be given orally or intravenously, to be excreted in bile. Oral cholecystography and intravenous cholangiography have a high failure rate in patients with obstructive jaundice because the dye is not excreted in adequate amounts in the bile. Dye may also be injected into the common bile duct through an endoscope in the duodenum (endoscopic retrograde cholangiopancreatography, ERCP) or directly into the dilated intrahepatic ducts in patients with obstructive jaundice

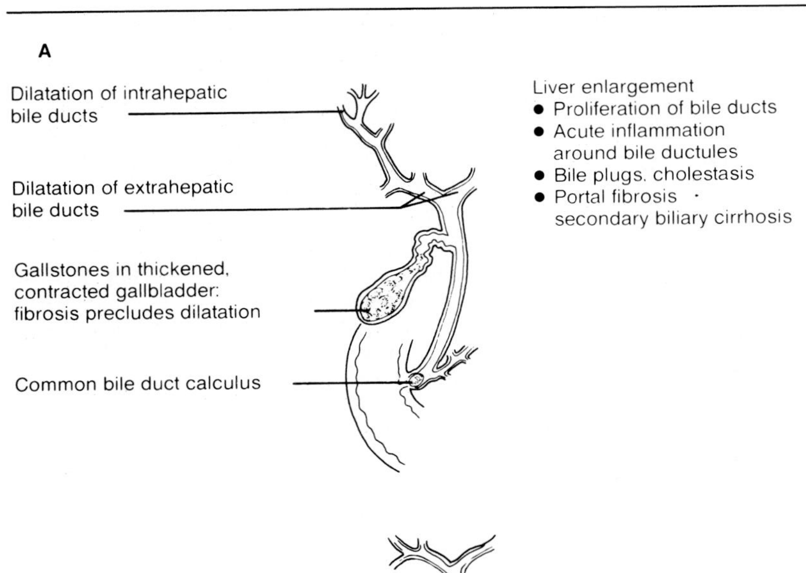

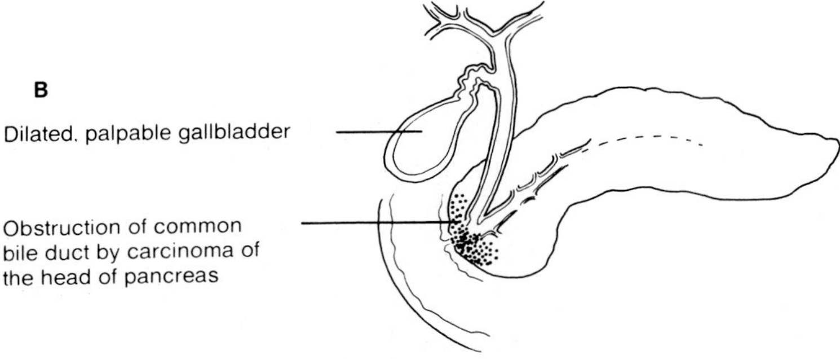

Figure 44-2. Courvoisier's law. **A:** When obstructive jaundice is caused by a calculus in the common bile duct, there is no enlargement of the gallbladder. **B:** When obstructive jaundice is caused by anything other than gallstones, the gallbladder is enlarged. Note that many exceptions exist to this rule.

(transhepatic cholangiography, THC). ERCP also permits the taking of biopsy specimens from the terminal part of the common bile duct and samples of bile for cytologic study.

Other Radiologic Techniques

Ultrasonography and computerized tomography are extremely accurate in detecting dilated bile ducts, calculi in the biliary system, and masses in the head of the pancreas and bile ducts. When a mass is present, a fine needle may be passed into it under radiologic guidance and material aspirated for cytologic diagnosis (fine-needle aspiration biopsy).

Functional Evaluation

Tests to evaluate obstructive jaundice have been considered in Chapter 42. Chemical examination of bile is of little clinical diagnostic value and is rarely performed.

CONGENITAL MALFORMATIONS

ANATOMIC VARIATIONS OF THE BILIARY SYSTEM

Minor variations in the way in which the common hepatic, cystic, and common bile ducts connect are very common and frequently associated with varying distributions of the arteries supplying the biliary system and liver. Recognition of these normal variations is important at cholecystectomy in order to prevent accidental ligation of ducts and blood vessels.

Anatomic abnormalities of the gallbladder include absence, duplication with the presence of 2 gallbladders, intrahepatic location, and floating gallbladder surrounded by peritoneum and connected to the inferior surface of the liver by a pedicle. A peculiar abnormality is a focal concentric narrowing of the body of the gallbladder, producing an expanded fundus (''phrygian cap'' gallbladder).

BILIARY ATRESIA

Biliary atresia is the most common cause of neonatal obstructive jaundice. Atresia is failure of development of the lumen in the epithelial cord that ultimately becomes the bile ducts; this failure may be complete or incomplete. The cause of atresia is controversial; some authorities believe it is the result of an intrauterine infection. Atresia commonly involves the extrahepatic bile ducts only; more rarely, the intrahepatic ducts are involved. Complete atresia involving the entire system is associated with a high mortality rate. The liver shows the features of severe large bile duct obstruction with secondary biliary cirrhosis.

Without treatment, death occurs in infancy. Surgical treatment may be successful in cases where atresia is partial. In cases where atresia involves intrahepatic ducts, liver transplantation represents the only hope of survival.

CHOLEDOCHAL CYST

Choledochal cyst, though uncommon, is the most frequent cause of obstructive jaundice in older children. Choledochal cysts are caused by focal dilatation, often massive, of the common bile duct. The wall is thick and fibrotic, and the cavity contains bile. Rarely, dilatation of intrahepatic bile ducts (Caroli's disease) may coexist.

Women are more commonly affected. Clinical presentation is with pain, jaundice, and a cystic mass in the right upper quadrant.

CHOLELITHIASIS

Most gallbladder diseases are associated with the formation of gallstones (cholelithiasis). Gallstones are usually formed in the gallbladder and rarely in the common bile duct.

Etiology & Incidence (Table 44–1)

A. Cholesterol-based gallstones (pure, mixed, and combined) are common and are formed when the concentration of cholesterol is increased or when bile salts are decreased. (Bile salts keep cholesterol in solution.) Women are more apt to be affected. Middle age, obesity, and multiparity (''fat, fertile females of forty and fifty'') increase the risk to as high as 20%. Oral contraceptives increase biliary cholesterol excretion and predispose to gallstones. Three-fourths of Native American women develop gallstones. The incidence is also high in South American and Mexican women.

In patients with terminal ileal disease such as Crohn's disease or those who have undergone ileal resection and ileal bypass surgery, failure of bile salt reabsorption in the terminal ileum is associated with decreased bile salt levels in bile and formation of gallstones.

Patients with diabetes mellitus also have an increased incidence of cholesterol gallstones, probably related to increased cholesterol levels in bile.

B. Pigment (bilirubin) stones are uncommon

Table 44-1. Types of gallstones.

Type	Frequency	Chemical Composition	Gross Appearance
Mixed	80%	Cholesterol, calcium carbonate, calcium bilirubinate	Multiple, small, faceted; variable in size and shape; smooth surface, yellow; laminated on cut section.
Pure cholesterol	5%	Cholesterol	Solitary, large, oval, white; rough surface; cut section: radiating crystalline structure
Combined	10%	Pure cholesterol center, mixed shell	Solitary or 2 stones; oval or barrel-shaped, yellow; smooth surface
Pigment	Rare	Calcium bilirubinate	Multiple, very small, faceted, black
Calcium	Very rare	Calcium carbonate	Multiple, amorphous; small grains, rarely large

and occur (1) in patients suffering from chronic hemolytic anemias such as sickle cell disease and thalassemia, in whom bilirubin excretion is greatly increased; and (2) in patients with parasitic infestations, most commonly *Clonorchis sinensis,* in whom the parasite ova form a nidus for pigment stones (see Oriental Cholangiohepatitis, Chapter 42).

Clinicopathologic Syndromes (Fig 44-3)

A. Asymptomatic Gallstones: Thirty percent or more of patients with gallstones have no symptoms, and gallstones are frequently found incidentally at radiologic examination. Only about 25% of gallstones contain sufficient calcium to be visible on plain x-rays, but ultrasonography and computerized tomography are highly effective at detecting gallstones. The presence of asymptomatic gallstones is not an indication for surgical removal.

B. Acute Cholecystitis: Acute cholecystitis rarely occurs in the absence of gallstones. In 80% of cases, a stone is found obstructing the cystic duct, leading to stasis of bile in the gallbladder. The residual bile becomes highly concentrated and causes a chemical acute inflammation. The damaged gallbladder is then susceptible to infection by bacteria; *Escherichia coli* and other gram-negative bacilli are cultured from the bile in 80% of cases.

Pathologically, the gallbladder shows congestion, thickening of the wall by edema, mucosal ul-

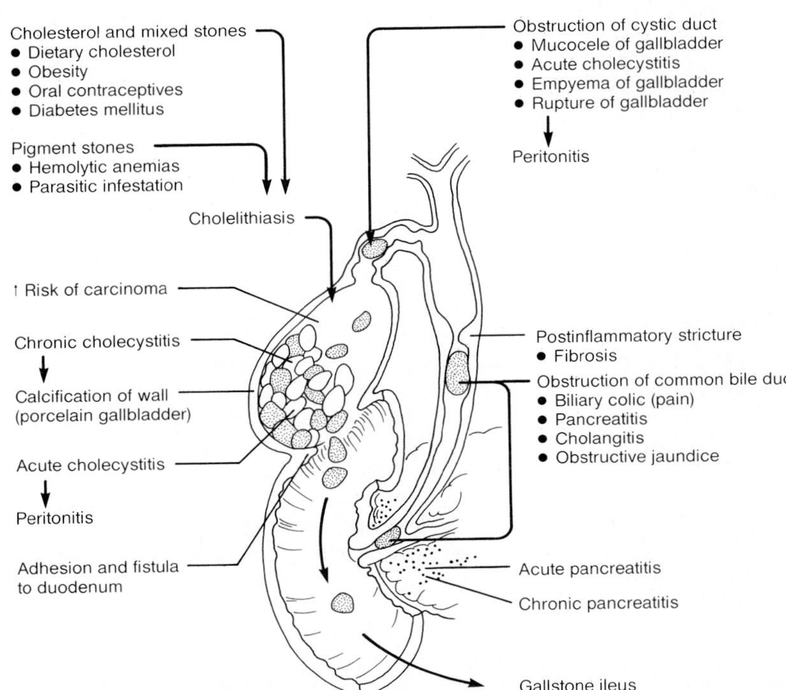

Figure 44-3. Clinical and pathologic effects of cholelithiasis.

ceration, and fibrinous exudation. Large numbers of neutrophils are present. The gallbladder may become filled with pus ("empyema of the gallbladder"). In severe cases, necrosis of the wall occurs, with greenish-black discoloration (gangrenous cholecystitis). Perforation may lead to local abscess formation or to generalized peritonitis.

Clinically, acute cholecystitis produces acute onset of fever and right upper quadrant pain. An enlarged, tender gallbladder is palpable in 40% of cases; mild jaundice may be seen in about 20%. Treatment is with antibiotics and surgical drainage or cholecystectomy.

C. Chronic Cholecystitis: Chronic cholecystitis almost never occurs without gallstones. Pathologically, the gallbladder is contracted and its wall thickened by fibrosis (Fig 44–4), with infiltration by lymphocytes, plasma cells, and macrophages. Calcification may occur in the wall; when extensive, the gallbladder is outlined on abdominal x-ray ("porcelain gallbladder"). The mucosa of the gallbladder may be near normal, or thinned by pressure of a stone, or may show yellow flecks due to accumulation of cholesterol-filled foamy macrophages in the mucosa (cholesterolosis).

Symptoms are usually vague; abdominal pain, often related to the ingestion of fatty foods, is the commonest feature. Biliary colic—severe inter-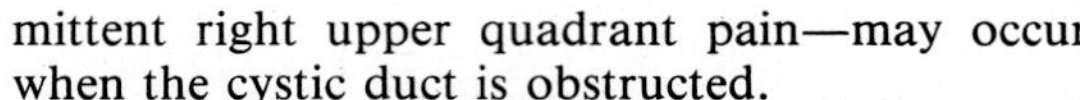mittent right upper quadrant pain—may occur when the cystic duct is obstructed.

D. Movement of Gallstones: Migration of gallstones from the gallbladder may cause obstruction or fistula formation.

1. Cystic duct obstruction is characterized by distention of the gallbladder with watery bile (hydrops) or mucus (mucocele). Acute cholecystitis also complicates duct obstruction.

2. Common bile duct obstruction may be intermittent, with attacks of biliary colic, jaundice, and high fever due to cholangitis (Charcot's triad of symptoms). Less commonly, obstruction is complete, leading to deep jaundice. In patients with obstructive jaundice resulting from stones, the presence of chronic cholecystitis prevents dilatation of the gallbladder (Courvoisier's law; see Fig 44–2). Impaction of a gallstone in the ampulla of Vater may obstruct the pancreatic duct, leading to acute pancreatitis.

3. Fistulous tracts develop rarely between the gallbladder and intestine due to the chronic inflammation. A large gallstone may then pass directly through such a cholecystoenteric fistula into the intestine, causing intestinal obstruction **(gallstone ileus).**

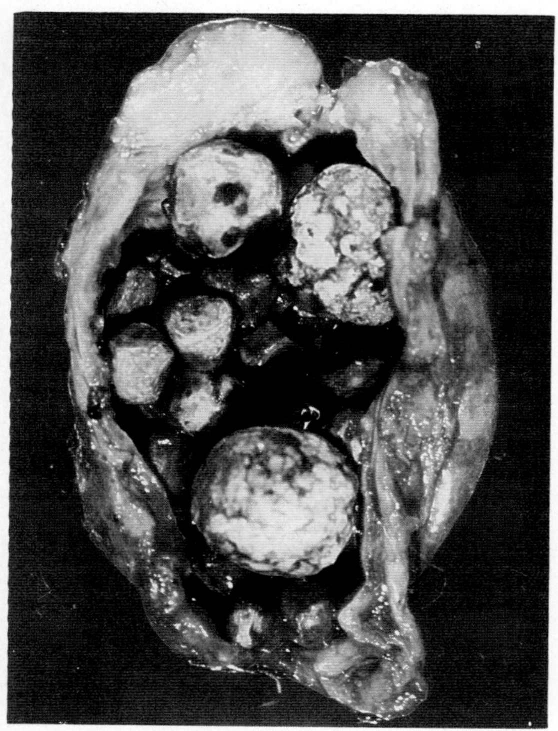

Figure 44–4. Gallbladder filled with multiple mixed gallstones. The wall shows diffuse thickening due to fibrosis.

FIBROUS STRICTURES OF THE COMMON BILE DUCT

Fibrous strictures of the common bile duct are an important cause of obstructive jaundice. They occur (1) after biliary surgery, most frequently cholecystectomy; (2) after external trauma (rarely); and (3) following inflammation, either caused by a gallstone in the bile duct or chronic pancreatitis.

Sclerosing cholangitis is a rare specific disease that occurs in patients with chronic ulcerative colitis. Its cause is unknown, but immunologic injury is thought to be involved. The large bile ducts both within and outside the liver undergo irregular fibrosis with narrowing, leading to obstructive jaundice. Sclerosing cholangitis is difficult to distinguish from bile duct carcinoma.

Fibrous strictures of the biliary system, both intrahepatic and extrahepatic, occur in *Clonorchis sinensis* infection. Multiple strictures of the bile duct are associated with irregular dilation of the biliary system and the presence of numerous pigment stones and sludge containing parasites and ova.

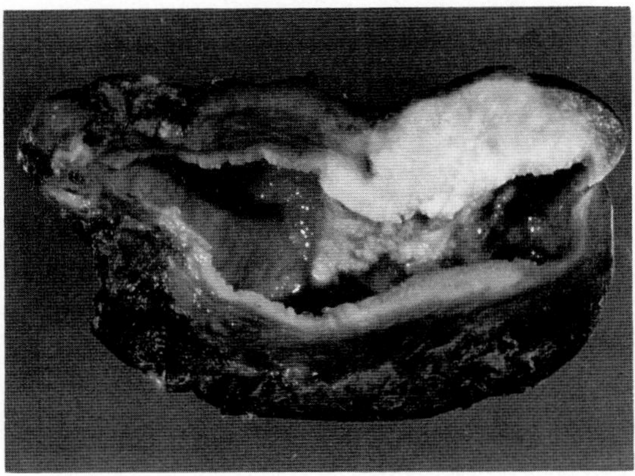

Figure 44-5. Carcinoma of the gallbladder, showing a large mass in the fundus that projects into the lumen and has infiltrated the wall.

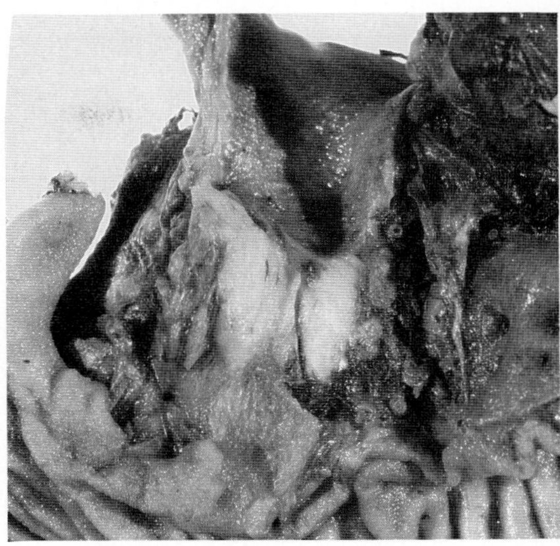

Figure 44-6. Neoplastic stricture of the terminal portion of the common bile duct, causing biliary obstruction. The bile duct proximal to the tumor is markedly dilated. This is the typical appearance of carcinoma of the bile duct.

NEOPLASMS OF THE EXTRAHEPATIC BILIARY SYSTEM

BENIGN NEOPLASMS

Benign neoplasms are rare in the biliary system. Papillary adenoma, which may occur at the ampulla of Vater or in the gallbladder, presenting as a polyp, is the most common type.

The biliary tract is a site in which granular cell tumors occur. Granular cell tumors are believed to be variants of schwannomas and are composed of large cells containing an abundance of granular cytoplasm. Though rare, these neoplasms are important because they cause stenosis of the common bile duct and resemble bile duct carcinoma.

CARCINOMA OF THE GALLBLADDER

Carcinomas of the gallbladder and biliary tree are relatively uncommon—less than 1% of causes of cancer in the United States. Gallbladder carcinoma is much more common in women, following the sex distribution of gallstones (80% of gallbladder carcinomas are associated with gallstones), and occurs with high frequency among Native Americans and Mexicans. Chronic cholecystitis with extensive calcification of the wall (porcelain gallbladder) is associated with a 25% incidence of carcinoma.

Grossly, gallbladder carcinoma presents as a polypoid mass that projects into the lumen, with infiltration of the wall (Fig 44-5). In some cases, the infiltrative component dominates, producing thickening of the wall. Histologically, it is an adenocarcinoma of variable differentiation frequently associated with marked fibrosis and a tendency to perineural invasion.

Most cases of gallbladder carcinoma are found in patients being evaluated for gallstones. In advanced disease, there is weight loss, a palpable mass, or evidence of metastases. The prognosis depends on the stage. Tumors confined to the gallbladder have a good prognosis. When there is extension through the wall of the gallbladder into the liver or peritoneum with or without evidence of metastatic disease, the 5-year survival rate is close to zero.

CARCINOMA OF THE BILE DUCTS

Though uncommon, bile duct carcinoma represents an important cause of obstructive jaundice in adults. Tumors may involve the hepatic ducts at the hilum of the liver (Klatskin tumor) or common bile duct, most commonly at its terminal portion (at the ampulla of Vater; Fig 44-6).

Bile duct carcinoma tends to cause obstructive jaundice at an early stage. Histologically, these tumors are usually well-differentiated and associated with marked sclerosis.

Bile duct carcinoma grows slowly, with local extension along the biliary system and neighboring structures. Lymph node involvement is early, but blood stream metastasis usually occurs late. The ultimate prognosis is poor, though many patients have a long survival.

45 The Exocrine Pancreas

STRUCTURE & FUNCTION

The pancreas is situated retroperitoneally in the upper abdomen. It is divided into the **head,** which lies in the curve of the duodenum; the **body,** which is situated horizontally in the upper retroperitoneum; and the **tail,** which extends to the left to the hilum of the spleen.

The pancreas has 2 components: exocrine and endocrine.

(1) The **exocrine pancreas** contains acini that secrete a variety of enzymes into the pancreatic ducts. The main pancreatic duct opens at the duodenal papilla and in 70% of patients joins with the terminal common bile duct at the ampulla of Vater. An accessory (minor) pancreatic duct usually opens independently into the duodenum proximal to the papilla.

(2) The **endocrine pancreas** is composed of the islets of Langerhans, distributed throughout the pancreas with a maximum density in the tail and containing several different hormone-producing cells (Chapter 46).

MANIFESTATIONS OF PANCREATIC DISEASE

Pain

Acute or chronic inflammation of the pancreas is associated with pain, often severe and constant, situated deep in the epigastric region and frequently radiating to the back.

Failure of Exocrine Secretion

Failure of exocrine pancreatic function leads to maldigestion of fat (lack of lipase), which results in steatorrhea. Lack of pancreatic proteolytic enzymes, though important in protein digestion, can be compensated for by gastric and intestinal proteases.

Changes in Pancreatic Hormone Production

See Chapter 46.

METHODS OF EVALUATING THE PANCREAS

Assessment of Structure

The pancreas is not easily evaluated clinically, becoming palpable only when it contains a large mass. Plain abdominal x-ray is useful for demonstration of pancreatic calcification, which is a prominent feature of chronic pancreatitis. Ultrasonography and computerized tomography permit visualization of the pancreas and detection of mass lesions. It is also possible to cannulate the pancreatic duct via an endoscope in the duodenum and inject dye to permit evaluation of the duct system (endoscopic retrograde cholangiopancreatography, ERCP).

Pancreatic biopsy with a large-bore cutting needle is dangerous even at surgery, since it carries a risk of pancreatic fistula. Percutaneous fine-needle aspiration biopsy under radiologic control is a safe method of obtaining cytologic material for diagnosis of mass lesions of the pancreas.

Assessment of Function

Elevated serum levels of amylase and lipase provide evidence of necrosis of pancreatic cells, as in acute pancreatitis. It is more difficult to test the adequacy of secretion of enzymes by the pancreas into the duodenum, and failure of exocrine secretion is usually deduced by the occurrence of maldigestion (steatorrhea). Assays for hormones secreted by the pancreatic islets are useful in diseases of the endocrine pancreas.

CONGENITAL DISEASES

ECTOPIC PANCREATIC TISSUE

Ectopic pancreatic tissue is present in about 2% of persons, usually discovered as an incidental finding at autopsy. In descending order of frequency, ectopic pancreas is found in the stomach, duodenum, jejunum, and Meckel's diverticula. Because ectopic pancreatic tissue is a developmental mass composed of disorganized pancreatic acini, ducts, and muscle that do not belong in these locations, the term "choristoma" may be used.

MALDEVELOPMENT OF THE PANCREAS

Pancreatic developmental abnormalities are uncommon. The most important is a rare malformation of the head of the pancreas, which results in a complete collar of pancreatic tissue around the second part of the duodenum (annular pancreas); this may result in duodenal constriction and obstruction.

CYSTIC FIBROSIS (Mucoviscidosis; Fibrocystic Disease)

Cystic fibrosis is a common congenital disease that is inherited as an autosomal recessive trait and affects one in 2000 Caucasian infants. It is rare in blacks and Orientals. About 2–5% of the population of the United States are heterozygous carriers of the abnormal gene.

The disease is characterized by abnormally viscous secretion of exocrine glands throughout the body. The basic defect has not been identified. Among the numerous biochemical abnormalities that have been recognized in abnormal secretions are (1) increased sodium and chloride content, resulting from inhibition of sodium reabsorption in the ducts; (2) increased calcium, resulting from hypersecretion, which increases the permeability of mucus to water and causes it to become dehydrated and abnormally viscous; and (3) the presence of abnormal glycoproteins.

The pathologic changes in cystic fibrosis are the result of obstruction of ducts of exocrine glands by the viscid mucus (hence the alternative name "mucoviscidosis") (Fig 45–1). **Pancreatic abnormalities** are present in 80% of patients. Pancreatic ducts are plugged with mucus, leading to chronic inflammation, with atrophy of acini, fibrosis, and dilatation of ducts (hence the term "fibrocystic disease"). Lack of pancreatic lipase in the intestine causes maldigestion of fat, leading to **steatorrhea.**

Pulmonary changes (see Chapter 35) are the most serious manifestation of cystic fibrosis. Bronchial mucus plugs lead to collapse of the lung, recurrent infections—including lung abscess—and ultimately fibrosis and bronchiectasis.

Increased amounts of viscid intestinal mucus in the lumen may result in intestinal obstruction in the neonatal period **(meconeum ileus)**. Bile duct obstruction may result in jaundice; changes in the vas deferens and seminal vesicles may cause infertility in the male.

The diagnosis is established by determination of electrolyte levels in sweat. A sweat sodium level in excess of 60 meq/L is diagnostic in a patient with clinical features of cystic fibrosis. Most patients with cystic fibrosis die of pulmonary complications. Twenty years ago, survival beyond infancy was unusual; today, most individuals survive to adulthood, though life expectancy is still much less than normal.

INFLAMMATORY LESIONS OF THE PANCREAS

ACUTE PANCREATITIS

Acute pancreatitis is a clinical syndrome resulting from the escape of activated pancreatic digestive enzymes from the duct system into the parenchyma. It is associated with extensive destruction of pancreatic and peripancreatic tissue and acute inflammation.

Acute pancreatitis is a common and important

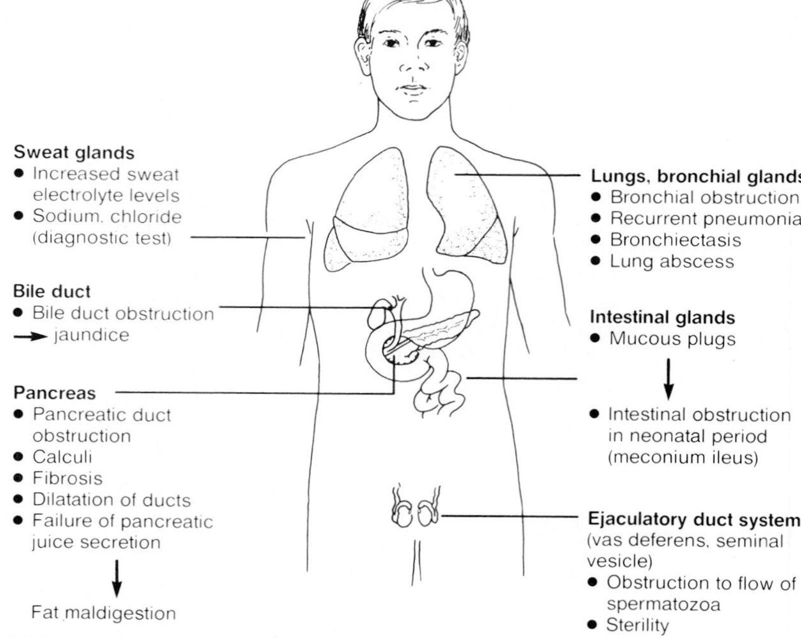

Figure 45-1. Clinical features of cystic fibrosis. Many of the features of this disease are caused by obstruction of exocrine ducts due to the increased viscosity of secretions.

medical emergency, accounting for about one in every 500 admissions to general hospital emergency rooms.

Etiology

In about 25% of cases of acute pancreatitis, no etiologic factor can be identified. Infectious agents are usually not involved, though mild nonnecrotizing acute pancreatitis occurs in association with some viral diseases—commonly mumps and cytomegalovirus infection.

Factors associated with acute pancreatitis are shown in Fig 45-2 and discussed briefly below.

A. Biliary Tract Calculi: Biliary tract calculi are present in about 50% of cases and may obstruct the terminal bile duct. Reflux of bile or infected duodenal contents into the pancreatic duct has been suggested as a mechanism leading to pancreatitis in bile duct disease. Obstruction of the pancreatic duct may occur when a calculus becomes lodged in the ampulla of Vater. Acute pancreatitis complicating gallstones is chiefly a disorder of women because of the female preponderance of gallstone disease.

B. Alcoholism: Alcoholism as a cause of acute pancreatitis occurs with varying frequency in different parts of the world. It is common in the United States, being involved in 65% of cases of acute pancreatitis; in Europe, the incidence is 5-20%. Acute pancreatitis commonly occurs after a bout of heavy drinking. A direct toxic effect of alcohol on pancreatic acinar cells has been postulated.

C. Hypercalcemia: Hypercalcemia, as occurs in primary hyperparathyroidism, is complicated by acute pancreatitis in about 10% of cases. A high plasma calcium concentration is thought to stimulate activation of trypsinogen in the pancreatic duct.

D. Hyperlipidemias: The hyperlipidemias—particularly those types associated with increased plasma levels of chylomicrons—are complicated by acute pancreatitis. It is postulated that free fatty acids liberated by the action of pancreatic lipase produce acinar injury.

E. Shock and Hypothermia: In shock and hypothermia, decreased perfusion of the pancreas may lead cellular degeneration, release of pancreatic enzymes, and acute pancreatitis.

F. Drugs and Radiation: Thiazide diuretics, corticosteroids, anticancer agents, and other drugs may also cause acute pancreatitis. Radiation to the retroperitoneum for treatment of malignant neoplasms is an uncommon cause of acute pancreatitis.

Pathogenesis

The pathologic changes in acute pancreatitis are the result of the action of pancreatic enzymes on the pancreas and surrounding tissues (Fig 45-3). Trypsin and chymotrypsin activate phospholipase and elastase as well as kinins, complement, the coagulation cascade, and plasmin, leading to acute inflammation, thrombosis, and hemorrhage. Elastase contributes to vascular injury. Phospholipases act on cell membranes, causing cell injury.

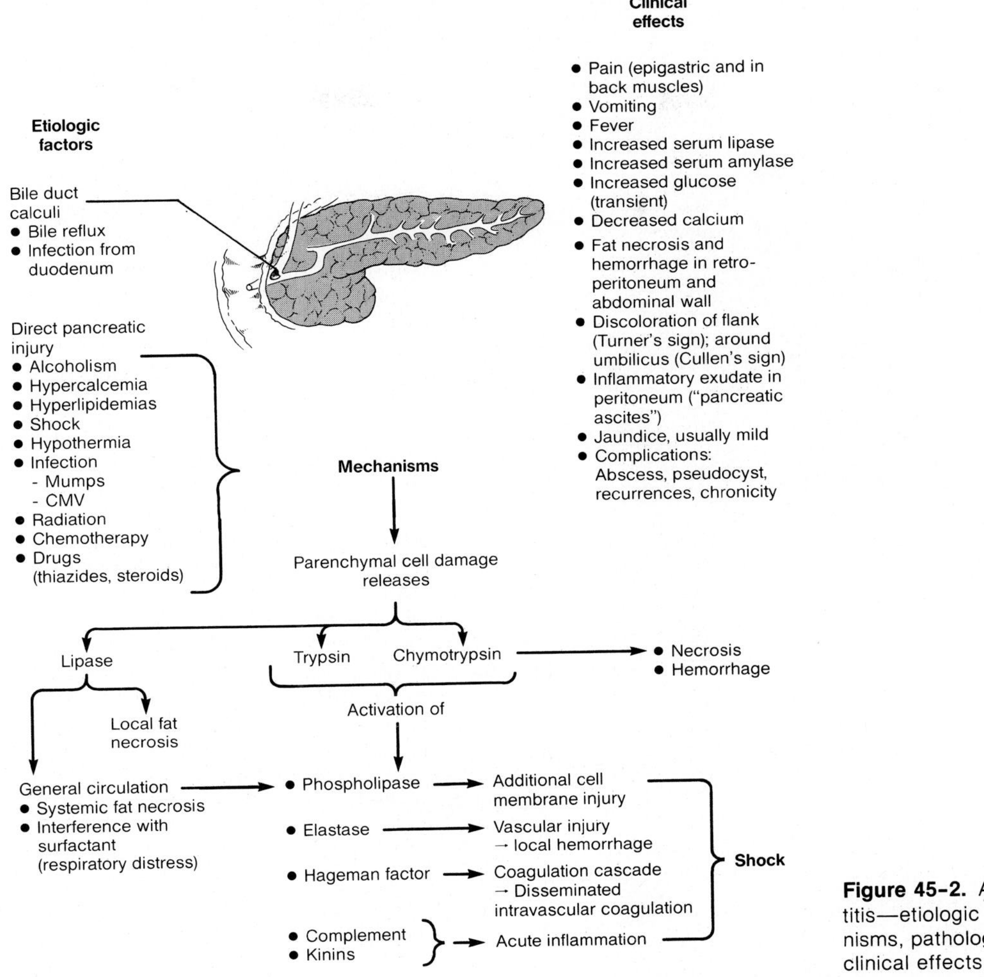

Figure 45-2. Acute pancreatitis—etiologic factors, mechanisms, pathologic changes, and clinical effects.

Pancreatic lipase acts on surrounding adipose tissue, causing enzymatic fat necrosis (see Chapter 1).

In addition to a local action, pancreatic enzymes enter the bloodstream. Circulating amylase does not contribute to cell injury; however, phospholipases are thought to contribute to the production of adult respiratory distress syndrome by interfering with the normal function of pulmonary surfactant. Rarely, high serum lipase levels are associated with fat necrosis at sites distant from the pancreas.

Pathology

Acute pancreatitis is characterized by widespread necrosis in tissues subjected to the effect of extravasated pancreatic enzymes. Necrosis of pancreatic parenchyma is initially coagulative but the necrotic cells rapidly undergo liquefaction. Vascular necrosis and disruption result in hemorrhage. Fat necrosis appears as chalky white foci that may be calcified, usually in and around the pancreas, omentum, and mesentery (Fig 45–3). Rarely, fat necrosis extends down the retroperitoneum and into the mediastinum. In severe cases, massive liquefactive necrosis of the pancreas occurs, resulting in a pancreatic abscess.

In very severe cases, death may occur before an adequate inflammatory response can be mobilized. Neutrophils predominate when the inflammation becomes established.

The peritoneal cavity often contains a brownish serous fluid (**"pancreatic ascites"**). This fluid contains altered blood, fat globules ("chicken broth"), and very high levels of amylase.

Clinical Features

Acute pancreatitis usually presents as a medical emergency. Patients develop severe constant epigastric pain, frequently referred to the back, accompanied by vomiting and shock. Shock is caused by peripheral circulatory failure resulting from hemorrhage and the entry of kinins into the

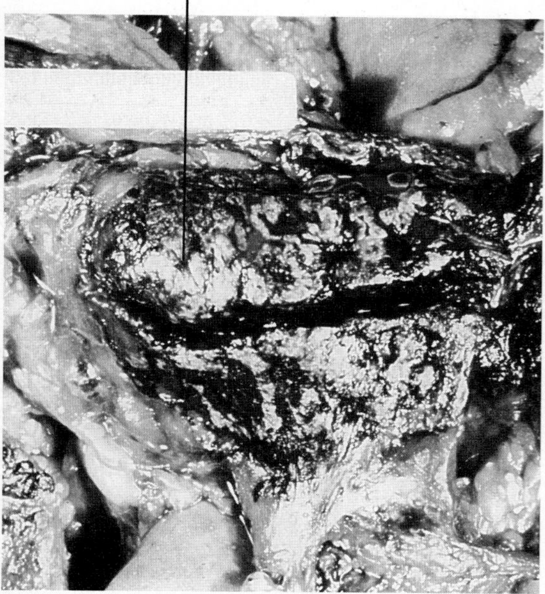

Figure 45-3. Acute pancreatitis, showing marked hemorrhagic necrosis in the upper retroperitoneum around the pancreas.

bloodstream (Fig 45-2). Mild jaundice may be present. In severe pancreatitis, there is discoloration due to hemorrhage in the subcutaneous tissue around the umbilicus (Cullen's sign) and in the flanks (Turner's sign). Activation of the plasma coagulation cascade may lead to disseminated intravascular coagulation.

Laboratory Studies

There is an almost immediate (within hours) elevation of the serum amylase, often to 10-20 times the normal upper level; amylase levels return to normal in 2-3 days. Serum lipase is increased later, usually after 72 hours. Hypocalcemia is present in severe cases and is a bad prognostic sign. Transient glycosuria is present in the acute stage in about 10% of cases as a result of islet dysfunction. Permanent diabetes mellitus almost never follows a single attack of acute pancreatitis.

Complications

Most patients recover from the acute attack with proper supportive care, and the pancreas regenerates and returns almost to normal, with mild residual scarring. In severe cases, death may occur as a consequence of pancreatic abscess, severe hemorrhage, shock, disseminated intravascular coagulation, or respiratory distress syndrome.

Pancreatic pseudocyst (see below) may follow weeks to months after recovery from an acute attack.

CHRONIC PANCREATITIS

Chronic pancreatitis is a chronic disease characterized by progressive destruction of the parenchyma with chronic inflammation, fibrosis, stenosis and dilatation of the duct system, and eventually impairment of pancreatic function.

Etiology

Chronic alcoholism and biliary tract calculi are the 2 main conditions that are associated with chronic pancreatitis. In the United States, alcoholism is believed to be implicated in about 40% of cases and biliary tract disease in 20%. In 30-40% of cases, no etiologic factors are identified. Some cases follow recurrent acute episodes; cystic fibrosis is a specific type of chronic pancreatitis described earlier.

Pathology (Fig 45-4)

Chronic pancreatitis is characterized by shrinkage of the pancreas as a result of fibrosis and atrophy of acinar structures. The changes usually involve the gland diffusely; more rarely, a firm, localized mass forms that is difficult to distinguish grossly from carcinoma.

The pancreatic ducts show multiple areas of stenosis with irregular dilatation distally. Ducts are filled with inspissated secretions that may undergo calcification to form calculi (Fig 45-5). Diffuse calcification imparts a rock-hard consistency to the gland.

Microscopically, there is acinar loss with marked fibrosis. At the end stage there are almost no recognizable acini, and the gland is composed of dilated ducts separated by collagen. Islets tend to withstand destruction better than acini. A variable lymphocytic infiltrate is present.

Clinical Features

Pain is the dominant symptom. It may be constant or intermittent and can be so severe as to lead to narcotic dependence. In many cases, pain is associated with acute exacerbations. When pain is caused by dilatation of the duct system, surgical correction by draining the dilated duct system may provide relief.

Pancreatic exocrine insufficiency due to failure of secretion of pancreatic juice leads to steatorrhea, malabsorption of fat-soluble vitamins, and weight loss. Endocrine insufficiency (diabetes mellitus) occurs in about 30% of cases.

The course is variable. Many patients have recurrent attacks of severe pain, vomiting, and elevation of serum amylase, due probably to re-

Etiologic factors

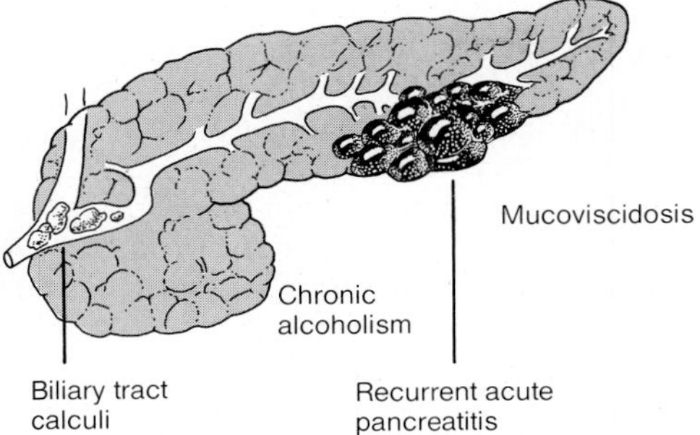

Pathologic changes

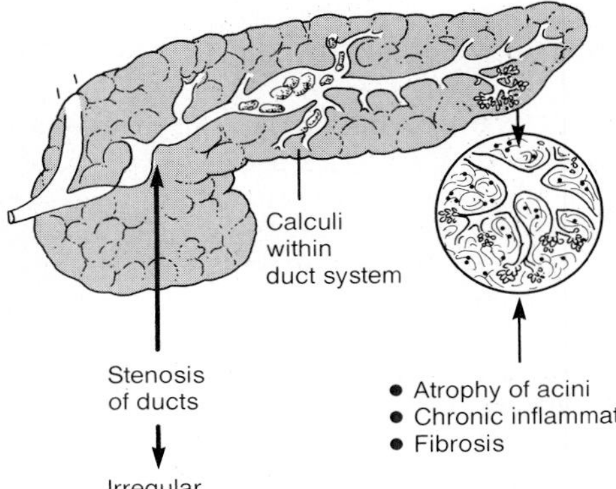

Clinical effects

- Pain (severe)
- Maldigestion (steatorrhea)
- Diabetes mellitus
- Obstructive jaundice due to stenosis of common bile duct

Figure 45-4. Chronic pancreatitis—etiologic factors, pathologic changes, and clinical effects.

peated acute episodes (chronic relapsing pancreatitis). Acute attacks may be followed by formation of pancreatic pseudocysts (see below).

In about 5% of patients with severe sclerosing chronic pancreatitis affecting the head of the pancreas, obstruction of the common bile duct leads to deep jaundice. This condition is difficult to differentiate from jaundice due to pancreatic carcinoma.

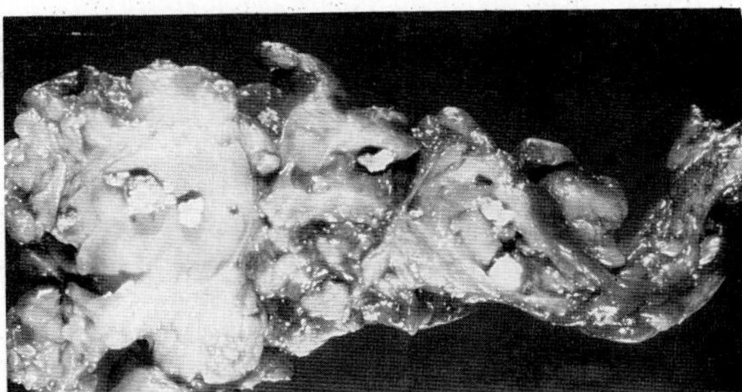

Figure 45-5. Chronic pancreatitis, showing markedly dilated ducts containing calculi. The pancreatic parenchyma between the ducts has undergone marked atrophy and fibrous contraction.

The diagnosis of chronic pancreatitis is made on clinical grounds. There are no specific laboratory tests, but the presence of calcification on x-ray provides supportive evidence. In chronic disease, the amount of residual pancreatic tissue may be insufficient to cause elevation of serum amylase.

Treatment & Prognosis

Treatment of chronic pancreatitis consists of management of the pain, malabsorption, and diabetes. When pain cannot be controlled by drugs, surgery to drain the pancreatic duct (by creating an opening between the duct and a loop of jejunum, ie, pancreaticojejunostomy) often has good results. Malabsorption and diabetes mellitus can be controlled by dietary supplements and insulin if necessary. The complications of diabetes mellitus represent the main threat to life.

PANCREATIC CYSTS

A variety of lesions enter into the differential diagnosis of pancreatic cysts revealed by computerized tomography.

PANCREATIC PSEUDOCYST

Pancreatic pseudocyst is the most common type of cyst found in the pancreas. A pseudocyst is usually a solitary fluid-filled unilocular structure of variable size lined by a wall composed of collagen and inflamed granulation tissue. It is called a pseudocyst because it does not have an epithelial lining. Pseudocysts usually occur after an attack of acute necrotizing pancreatitis or during chronic relapsing pancreatitis and probably represent the end result of hemorrhagic necrosis, the liquefied material being walled off by granulation tissue and fibrosis. They contain brownish serous fluid composed of pancreatic juice with a high enzyme content and altered blood. Most pseudocysts occur in and around the pancreas; rarely, when pancreatic enzyme leakage produces necrosis away from the pancreas, pseudocysts may occur at a considerable distance from the pancreas (eg, in the right iliac fossa).

Patients with pseudocysts present with an abdominal mass, and most give a history of abdominal pain suggestive of acute or chronic pancreatitis. Other patients give only a history of alcoholism.

Treatment consists of establishing surgical drainage of the cyst either into the stomach or into a loop of jejunum.

Complications of pancreatic pseudocyst include (1) acute rupture of the cyst into the intestine, most commonly the stomach and transverse colon, producing intestinal hemorrhage, which may be severe; (2) secondary infection, leading to the formation of an abscess; and (3) compression of the common bile duct, causing obstructive jaundice.

CONGENITAL CYSTS

Rarely, maldevelopment of parts of the pancreatic duct system produces multiple cysts ranging in size from very small to 5 cm in diameter. These are true cysts, lined by epithelium and filled with serous fluid.

Congenital pancreatic cysts are often associated with polycystic renal disease and congenital hepatic fibrosis. Congenital pancreatic cysts also occur in von Hippel-Lindau disease (see Chapter 62).

NEOPLASTIC CYSTS

1. SEROUS CYSTADENOMA

Serous cystadenoma is a rare solitary, benign cystic neoplasm of the pancreas. It may reach large size but rarely causes symptoms, being most commonly an incidental finding at abdominal surgery or radiography. It consists of multiple small locules lined by cuboidal epithelium, the cells of which contain abundant glycogen (also called microcystic, serous, and glycogen-rich cystadenoma). With very rare exceptions, it does not undergo malignant change.

2. MUCINOUS CYSTADENOMA & CYSTADENOCARCINOMA

Mucinous cystic neoplasms are more common than serous cystadenoma. They are usually solitary, unilocular, and often very large. The cysts are lined by tall columnar epithelium and contain a glairy mucinous fluid. The malignant counterpart shows cytologic atypia, stratification of cells, and invasion of the capsule. Mucinous cystadenocarcinoma behaves like a slowly growing low-grade malignant neoplasm. The 5-year survival rate after complete surgical removal is about 70%.

CARCINOMA OF THE PANCREAS

Carcinoma of the pancreas is understood to involve the exocrine pancreas; islet cell neoplasms are classified separately.

Incidence & Etiology

Approximately 20,000 patients annually in the United States die from pancreatic carcinoma, accounting for 6% of cancer deaths; the incidence is slightly higher in men than in women and is increasing. Pancreatic carcinoma occurs mainly after age 50 years.

The etiology is unknown. There is a 6-fold increased risk in diabetic women but not in diabetic men. A large number of dietary factors have been proposed, most recently decaffeinated coffee and high-fat diets. Cigarette smokers show a 5-fold increase in incidence.

Pathology (Fig 45-6)

Carcinomas occur throughout the pancreas: 70% in the head, 20% in the body, and 10% in

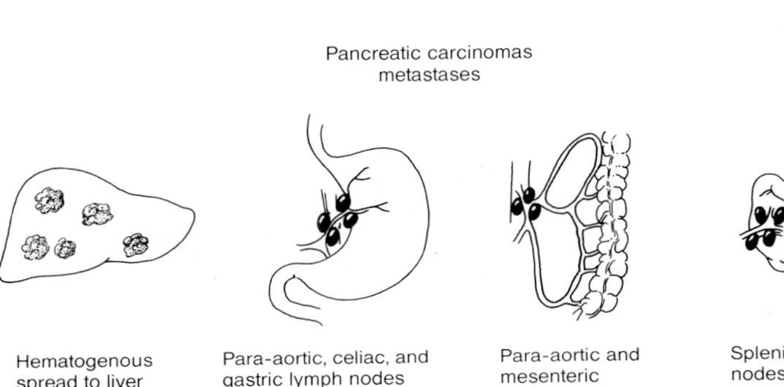

Figure 45-6. Neoplasms of the pancreas. Figures indicate frequency of carcinoma (top) and islet cell neoplasms (bottom) in the head, body, and tail of the pancreas. Note that 20% of pancreatic carcinomas involve the gland diffusely. Islet cell neoplasms are more commonly adenomas than carcinomas. Ten percent of patients with islet cell adenomas have multiple tumors. Both pancreatic carcinoma and islet cell carcinoma have similar patterns of metastasis.

the tail; 99% take origin from the ducts (Fig 45–7) and the remainder from the acini.

Grossly, pancreatic carcinoma presents as a hard infiltrative mass (Fig 45–8) that obstructs the pancreatic duct, frequently causing chronic pancreatitis in the distal gland. Carcinomas of the head tend to obstruct the common bile duct early in their course and present at a stage when the tumor is small. Tumors in the body and tail tend to present late and be very large. Pancreatic carcinoma frequently evokes marked fibrosis; it may distort the duodenal loop, producing a typical "inverted 3" appearance on barium x-ray studies.

Microscopically, over 90% of cases are well-differentiated adenocarcinomas, associated with marked fibrosis. Perineural invasion is common (Fig 45–9). The remaining 10% include adenosquamous carcinomas, anaplastic carcinomas—which contain spindle cells and pleomorphic giant cells (sarcomatoid and pleomorphic carcinomas)—and acinar cell carcinomas. Rarely, acinar cell carcinomas secrete lipase into the bloodstream and cause fat necrosis in the subcutaneous tissue and bone marrow throughout the body.

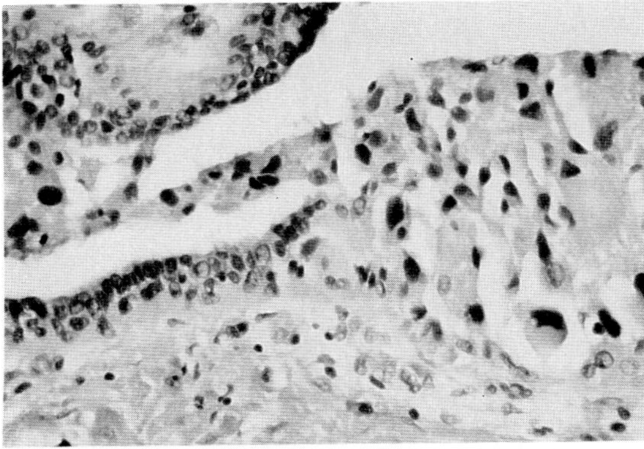

Figure 45-7. Carcinoma of the pancreas, showing the origin from a pancreatic duct. Contrast the normal ductal epithelial cells on the left with the greatly enlarged and pleomorphic carcinoma cells on the right and in the lumen.

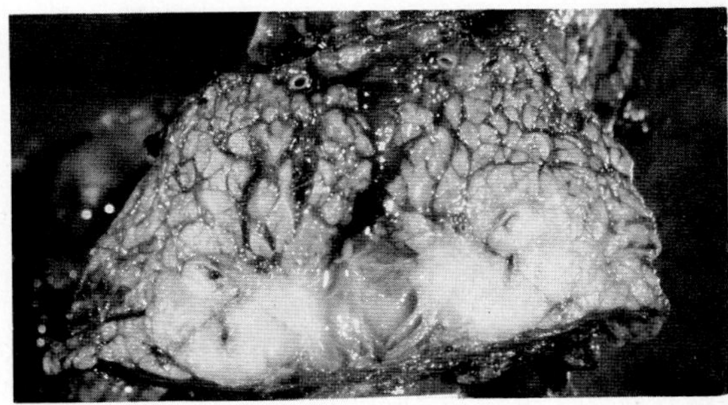

Figure 45-8. Carcinoma of the head of the pancreas, showing the typical hard infiltrative mass.

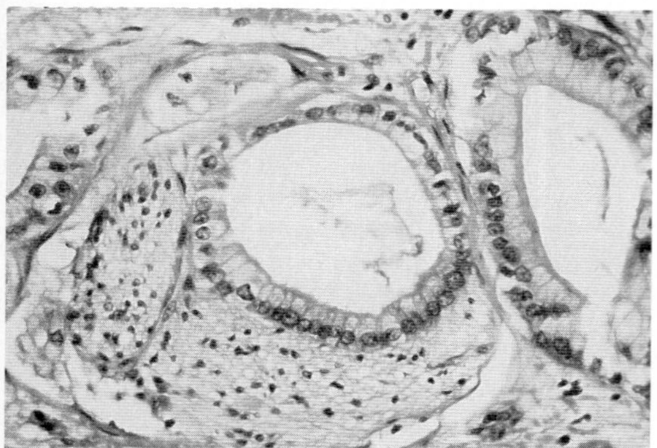

Figure 45-9. Well-differentiated carcinoma of the pancreas, showing perineural invasion (the nerve is at the bottom center of this photograph). The carcinoma cells show minimal cytologic abnormality.

Spread

The tumor tends to infiltrate into surrounding structures. Spread along the perineural fascial spaces is a typical feature. Lymphatic involvement occurs early, with metastasis to regional lymph nodes. Bloodstream spread also occurs early, with the liver being the commonest site of secondary deposits.

Clinical Features

Carcinoma of the head of the pancreas presents with common bile duct obstruction. (Courvoisier's law: Obstructive jaundice in the presence of a dilated gallbladder usually indicates carcinoma of the head of the pancreas). Carcinoma of the body and tail presents at a late stage with an abdominal mass, severe weight loss, and anemia. A high proportion of patients present with evidence of metastatic disease, most often in the liver. Skin rashes and lytic bone lesions due to fat necrosis may be present in lipase-secreting acinar cell carcinomas.

Carcinoembryonic antigen levels in the serum are elevated in some cases; this is not a specific finding, since colon, lung, and other cancers may also show elevated levels. The presence of a more specific pancreatic oncofetal antigen has been reported recently in a high proportion of cases, but data are preliminary. Computerized tomography is effective in establishing the presence of a solid mass. Percutaneous fine-needle aspiration of the mass under radiologic guidance provide tissue for cytologic examination and is an excellent method of making the diagnosis.

A common **paraneoplastic manifestation** in patients with carcinoma of the pancreas is superficial thrombophlebitis in the leg veins (Trousseau's sign). Rarely, patients with pancreatic carcinoma develop disseminated intravascular coagulation, due probably to thromboplastic substances present in the mucinous product of the adenocarcinoma.

Treatment & Prognosis

Most pancreatic carcinomas are inoperable at presentation. Small carcinomas confined to the head of the pancreas may be cured by total pancreaticoduodenectomy (Whipple procedure). Chemotherapy and radiotherapy are ineffective. The prognosis is dismal: Mean survival is 6 months after diagnosis, and the overall 5-year survival rate is less than 5%.

46 The Endocrine Pancreas (Islets of Langerhans)

STRUCTURE & FUNCTION

The islets of Langerhans are microscopic structures 50–250 μm in diameter. They are scattered throughout the pancreas, with a maximum density in the tail. The islets appear to have a great reserve capacity; islet dysfunction is not a major problem even after 90% of the pancreas is removed in a distal pancreatectomy. The islets are not connected to the exocrine duct system; the hormonal products are secreted directly into the bloodstream.

Microscopically, the islets are composed of small uniform cells arranged in a nestlike or trabecular pattern. The cells have round nuclei and scant cytoplasm. Routine microscopy does not permit differentiation of the various types of cells contained within the islets; this requires immunohistochemistry or electron microscopy (Table 46–1 and Fig 46–1).

The most important hormone secreted by the pancreas is **insulin.** The beta cells of the islets are the only source of insulin in the body, and failure of secretion of adequate amounts of insulin results in diabetes mellitus.

Glucagon, secreted by the alpha cells, also plays a role in glucose metabolism. The role of glucagon is a less vital one, and absence of glucagon has not been shown to cause clinical disease. The physiologic functions of **pancreatic polypeptide (PP)** and **vasoactive intestinal polypeptide (VIP)** have not been elucidated, and the amount of somatostatin and gastrin normally secreted by the pancreatic islets is thought to be too small to be of any physiologic significance. However, excessive secretion of any of these hormones by pathologic islets causes specific clinical syndromes.

Assessment of islet structure is very difficult because of their small size and scattered distribution in the pancreas. Only large islet cell neoplasms are distinguishable on computerized tomography. The main tests of islet function are serum assays of the various hormones secreted by the islets.

DIABETES MELLITUS

Diabetes mellitus is a chronic disease characterized by relative or absolute deficiency of insulin, resulting in glucose intolerance. It occurs in 4–5 million persons in the United States (approximately 2% of the population). The incidence varies with age: 0.1% of persons under age 20 years, 2% of those between 20 and 44 years, 4% of those between 45 and 64 years, and 8–10% of those over 65 years have diabetes mellitus.

Normal Insulin Metabolism

Insulin is a polypeptide composed of an A chain, with 21 amino acids, and a B chain, with 30 amino acids (Fig 46–2). It is released from the beta cell by a variety of stimuli (Fig 46–2), the most important of which—from a physiologic standpoint—is glucose. Amino acids and drugs of the sulfonylurea group also stimulate insulin release. Calcium is required for insulin release by the beta cell. Insulin is transported in the plasma with the alpha and beta globulins; no specific transport protein has been identified.

Insulin release occurs in 3 phases: (1) Basal secretion is responsible for the fasting level of insulin in serum; (2) initial rapid secretion after a meal is due to release of stored insulin in the beta cells within 10 minutes after eating; and (3) delayed re-

Table 46-1. Cell types in the islets of Langerhans.

Cell Type	Frequency	Secretion[1]	Electron Microscopic Granule Appearance
Beta (B)	60–70%	Insulin	Irregular, crystalline; surrounded by a halo
Alpha (A)	10–20%	Glucagon	Dark center, gray halo
Delta (D)	2–8%	Somatostatin	Large, uniformly gray
PP	1–5%	Pancreactic polypeptide	Small, uniformly dark
D_1	Rare	Vasoactive intestinal polypeptide	No specific granule
G	Rare	Gastrin	No specific granule

[1]Demonstrable by immunostaining methods using the appropriate antibody.

lease after meals is due to stimulation of insulin synthesis in response to glucose.

Insulin interacts with target cells that have insulin receptors on their plasma membranes (Fig 46–3). Important target cells are liver, muscle, and fat, though receptors have been demonstrated in many other cells. The number of insulin receptors on individual cells is variable, and the affinity of the receptor to insulin also varies.

The binding of insulin to receptors triggers a chain of events in the cell that mediates the action of the hormone; it is believed that small peptides act as second messengers to activate insulin-dependent enzyme systems.

Metabolic Actions of Insulin (Fig 46–3)

The major biochemical function of insulin is to regulate the transfer of glucose from the plasma into the cytoplasm of cells.

After a large meal, high insulin levels in the blood induce the tissues to take up and store glucose. Glycogenesis is stimulated in the liver and in skeletal muscle, and lipogenesis increases in adipose tissue. In this state, free glucose represents the major source of immediate energy for muscle cells.

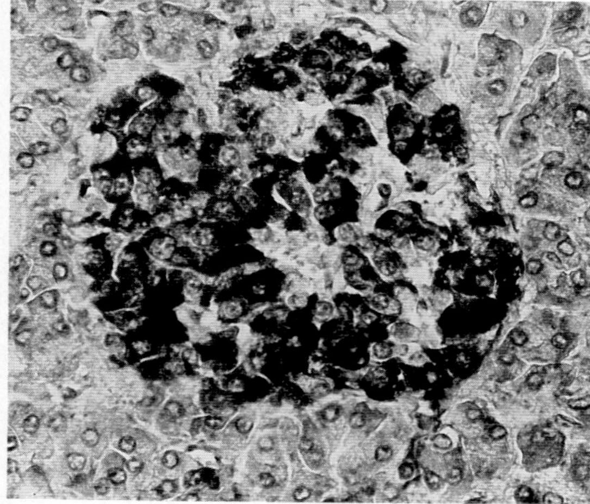

Figure 46–1. Pancreatic islet stained by immunoperoxidase technique with antibody against insulin, showing beta cells in the islet that stain darkly. The nonbeta cells of the islet and the pancreatic acini around the islet remain unstained.

In the fasting state, low levels of insulin result in mobilization of body stores to satisfy energy needs of the body. Glycogenolysis and proteolysis in liver and skeletal muscle provide glucose; lipolysis in adipose tissue produces free fatty acids, which enter the circulation and are metabolized to ketone bodies in the liver. The cells of the body, with the exception of brain cells, utilize fatty acids and ketone bodies for energy in states of low insulin secretion. Brain cells are dependent on a continuous supply of glucose for metabolic needs; in the fasting state, this is supplied mainly by gluconeogenesis from amino acids.

Etiology of Diabetes Mellitus (Table 46–2)

Diabetes mellitus is caused by a relative or absolute deficiency of insulin. In **primary diabetes** (95% of cases), there is no underlying disease process that might explain insulin deficiency. Primary diabetes is of 2 types, I and II (see below and Table 46–3). The remaining 5% of cases of **secondary diabetes** are due either to pancreatic destruction or to the presence of increased levels of hormones that antagonize the action of insulin.

There is an absolute deficiency of insulin in type I primary diabetes and in those cases of secondary diabetes associated with destruction of the pancreas. In type II primary diabetes—and in the presence of increased levels of antagonistic hormones—the insulin deficiency is relative, and serum insulin levels are usually normal and may even be elevated.

A. Type I Diabetes Mellitus: Type I diabetes mellitus **(insulin-dependent diabetes mellitus, IDDM)** is due to destruction of pancreatic beta cells. Plasma insulin levels are low, and there is a tendency to ketoacidosis. Such patients are dependent on exogenous insulin. The disease affects young patients **(juvenile-onset diabetes mellitus),** most commonly under 30 years of age, and there is a significant association with HLA-B8, -B15,

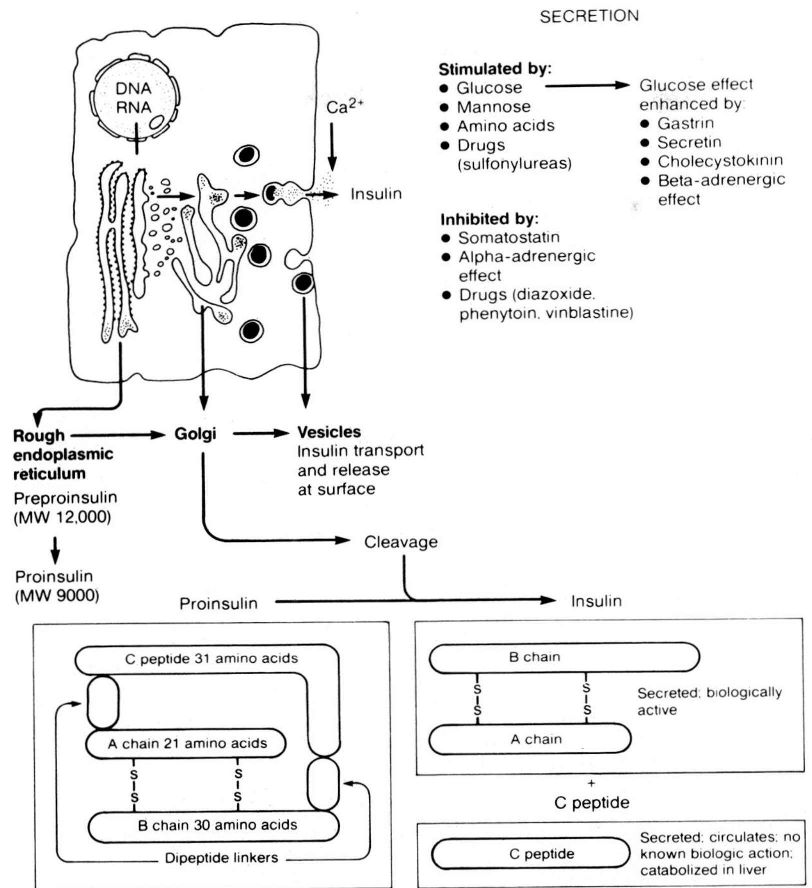

Figure 46-2. Insulin synthesis and secretion. The biochemical cleavage of proinsulin to insulin and C peptide that occurs in the Golgi zone is shown at the bottom.

-DR3, and -DR4. A genetic predisposition to type I diabetes is shown by the history of diabetes in about 20% of first-degree relatives—not as strong as in type II diabetes.

The cause of beta cell destruction in type I diabetes is unknown. A few cases have followed viral infections, most commonly with coxsackievirus B or mumps virus, and several viruses have been shown to cause beta cell damage when inoculated into mice. Despite these findings, the role of viruses in the etiology of human diabetes is thought to be minor.

Autoimmunity is believed to be the major mechanism involved. Islet cell autoantibodies are present in the serum of 90% of newly diagnosed cases. Such antibodies are directed against several cell components, including cytoplasmic and membrane antigens or against insulin itself (IgG and IgE antibodies). Sensitized T lymphocytes with activity against beta cells have also been demonstrated in some patients. Microscopic examination of the islets in patients with early type I diabetes shows the presence of a lymphocytic infiltrate in the islet ("insulitis"). One hypothesis is that a mild viral injury of beta cells induces an autoimmune reaction against the injured cells. HLA-linked immune response genes may explain the genetic susceptibility; HLA-B8, -B15, -DR3, and -DR4, in addition to their association with diabetes, also occur at increased frequency in Graves' disease, Addison's disease, and pernicious anemia, all of which are characterized by the presence of autoantibodies.

Toxins such as nitrophenylureas (in rat poisons) and cyanide from spoiled food have been implicated in rare cases.

B. Type II Diabetes Mellitus: The etiology of type II diabetes **(non-insulin-dependent diabetes mellitus, NIDDM)** is even less clearly understood (Fig 46–4). Two factors have been identified.

1. Impaired insulin release–Basal secretion of insulin is often normal, but the rapid release of insulin that follows a meal is greatly impaired, resulting in failure of normal handling of a carbohydrate load. The delayed phase of insulin secretion is also normal in the early stages but impaired in advanced disease. However, some level of insulin secretion is maintained in most patients, so that the abnormality of glucose metabolism is limited, and ketoacidosis is uncommon. In these pa-

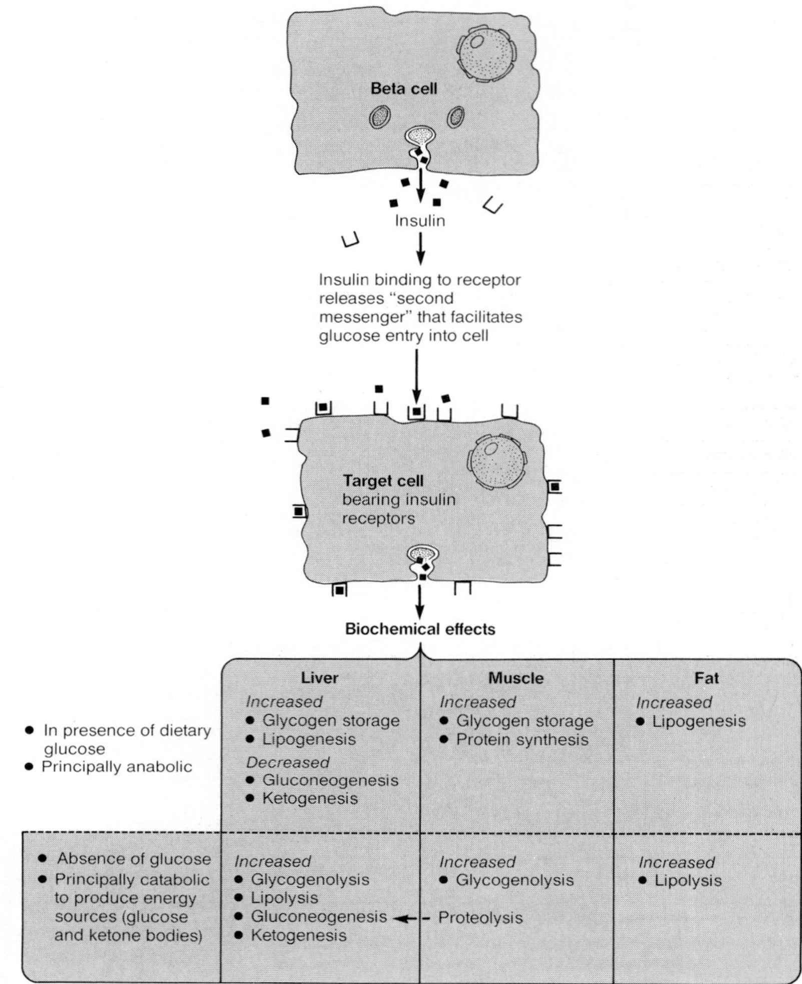

Figure 46-3. Mechanism of action of insulin on target cells and its principal biochemical actions. Note that the action of insulin on target cells is different in the presence and absence of adequate dietary glucose supply.

tients, insulin secretion can be stimulated by drugs such as sulfonylureas and exogenous insulin is therefore not essential in treatment. Most patients with type II diabetes first develop disease in adult life **(adult-onset diabetes)**.

It has been suggested that inheritance of a defective pattern of insulin secretion is responsible for the familial tendency of diabetes. The mechanism of inheritance is highly complex and probably involves multiple genes. The genetic factor is very strong in type II diabetes, with a history of diabetes present in about 50% of first-degree relatives.

2. Insulin resistance–A defect in the tissue response to insulin is believed to play a major role. This phenomenon is called "insulin resistance" and is caused by defective insulin receptors on the target cells.

Insulin resistance occurs in association with obesity and pregnancy. In normal individuals who become obese or pregnant, the beta cells secrete increased amounts of insulin to compensate. Patients who have a genetic susceptibility to diabetes cannot compensate because of their inherent defect in insulin secretion. Thus, type II diabetes is frequently precipitated by obesity and pregnancy.

In a few patients with extreme insulin resistance, antibodies against the receptors have been demonstrated in the plasma. These antibodies are mostly of the IgG class and may act in a manner analogous to the action of antiacetylcholine receptor antibodies in myasthenia gravis. Decreased numbers of insulin receptors, defective binding of insulin to receptors, and abnormalities in the series of cellular events that follow insulin binding have also been postulated as causes of insulin resistance.

Note that a different form of "insulin resistance" may occur following therapy with insulin and is due to the presence of antibodies against the bovine or porcine insulin preparation. This type of "insulin resistance" refers to the need for

Table 46–2. Classification of diabetes mellitus.

Primary diabetes mellitus (95%)
- Type I: Insulin-dependent diabetes mellitus (IDDM)
- Type II: Non-insulin-dependent diabetes mellitus (NIDDM)
- Impaired glucose tolerance: IGT ("latent diabetes")
- Gestational diabetes mellitus[1]

Secondary diabetes mellitus (5%)
- Destructive pancreatic disease
  - Chronic pancreatitis (Chapter 45)
  - Hemochromatosis (bronze diabetes; Chapter 43)
  - Total pancreatectomy
- Endocrine diseases (high levels of insulin-antagonistic hormones)
  - Acromegaly (growth hormone) (Chapter 57)
  - Cushing's syndrome (cortisol) (Chapter 60)
  - Hyperthyroidism (thyroxine) (Chapter 58)
  - Pheochromocytoma (catecholamines) (Chapter 60)
  - Glucagonoma (glucagon)
- Drug-induced diabetes (including diuretics such as thiazides, furosemide; propranolol; antidepressants; phenothiazines)
- Stress diabetes[1]
- Miscellaneous genetic syndromes with an increased incidence of diabetes
  - Down's syndrome (trisomy 21; mongolism)
  - Turner's syndrome (45,XO)
  - Friedreich's ataxia
  - Klinefelter's syndrome (47,XXY)
  - Glycogen storage disease type I
  - Laurence-Moon-Biedl syndrome[2]
  - Refsum's syndrome[3]

[1]Gestational and stress diabetes probably represent patients with IGT or with a genetic predisposition to diabetes who are decompensated by the physiologic changes of pregnancy or stress. The "diabetes" is often reversible, but such patients show a high incidence of diabetes in succeeding years.
[2]Retinitis pigmentosa, obesity, mental deficiency, skull defects with or without diabetes.
[3]Retinitis pigmentosa, polyneuropathy with or without diabetes.

increasing insulin dosage to maintain control of the diabetes in patients being treated with exogenous insulin.

Pathology

The pathologic changes in the pancreatic islets in diabetes mellitus are variable from one patient to another and are not specific for diabetes. In type I diabetes, there is frequently a lymphocytic infiltration of the islets in the early phase, followed by a decrease in the total number and size of the islets due to a progressive loss of beta cells.

The changes in type II diabetes are often minimal in the early stages. In advanced disease, there may be fibrosis and amyloid deposition in the islets; in diabetes, the amyloid appears to consist in part of precipitated insulin. Similar changes in the islets are sometimes present in elderly nondiabetic patients and are not considered diagnostic for diabetes.

Clinical Features

The classic symptoms of diabetes mellitus result from abnormal glucose metabolism. The lack of insulin activity results in failure of transfer of glucose from the plasma into the cells ("starvation in the midst of plenty"). The body responds as if it were in the fasting state, with stimulation of glycogenolysis, gluconeogenesis, and lipolysis producing ketone bodies (Fig 46–5).

The glucose absorbed during a meal is not metabolized at the normal rate and therefore accumulates in the blood **(hyperglycemia)** to be excreted in the urine **(glycosuria)**. Glucose in the urine causes osmotic diuresis, leading to increased urine production **(polyuria)**. The fluid loss and hyperglycemia increase the osmolarity of the plasma, stimulating the thirst center **(polydipsia)**. Stimulation of protein breakdown to provide

Table 46–3. Comparison of types of primary diabetes mellitus.

	Type I (Juvenile Onset)	Type II (Maturity [Adult] Onset)
Incidence	15%	85%
Insulin necessary in treatment	Always	Sometimes
Age (commonly; exceptions occur)	Under 30	Over 40
Association with obestiy	No	Yes
Genetic predisposition	Weak, polygenic	Strong, polygenic
Association with HLA system	Yes	No
Glucose intolerance	Severe	Mild
Ketoacidosis	Common	Rare
Beta cell numbers in the islets	Reduced	Variable
Serum insulin level	Reduced	Variable
Classic symptoms of polyuria, polydipsia, thirst, weight loss	Common	Rare
Basic cause	?Viral or immune destruction of beta cells	?Increased "resistance" to insulin

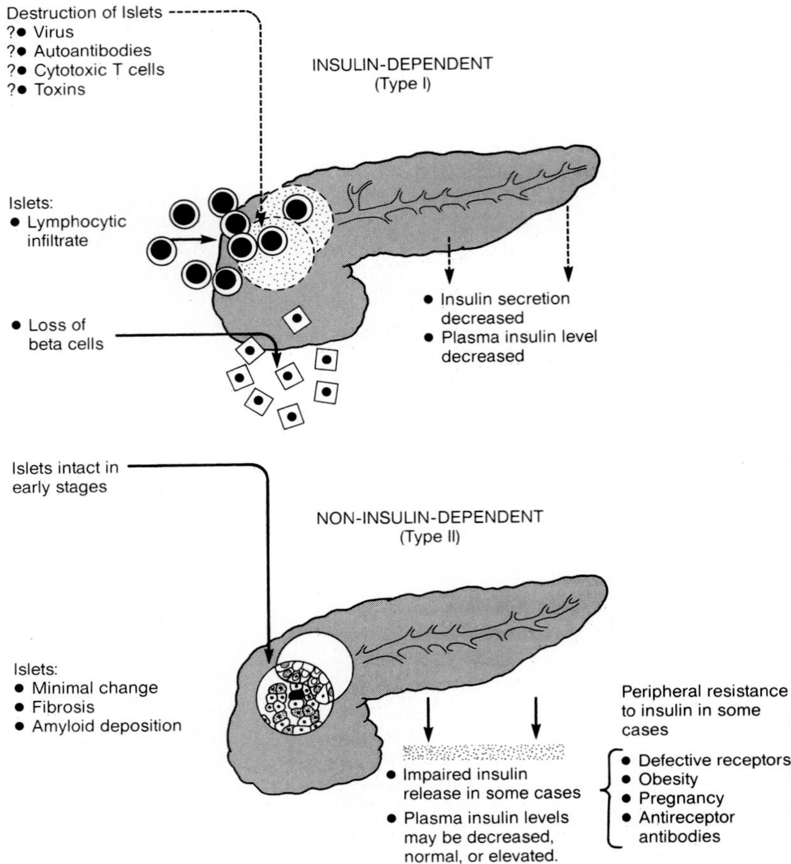

Figure 46-4. Etiology and pathogenesis of diabetes mellitus.

amino acids for gluconeogenesis results in **muscle wasting** and weight loss. These classic symptoms occur only in patients with severe insulin deficiency, most commonly in type I diabetes.

Many patients with type II diabetes do not have these symptoms and present with one of the complications of diabetes (see below).

Diagnosis

The diagnosis of diabetes is made by detecting abnormalities in glucose metabolism. In mild cases, the patient has a normal fasting plasma glucose level, the abnormality being restricted to deficient handling of a glucose load, as revealed by (1) an elevated postprandial plasma glucose concentration; (2) the presence of glucose in a postprandial sample of urine; and (3) an abnormal glucose tolerance test (Fig 46–6). The glucose tolerance test is the most sensitive method of diagnosis of diabetes mellitus. (***Note:*** There are numerous causes of glycosuria other than diabetes.)

In severe cases, there is fasting hyperglycemia and glycosuria.

All of the above tests provide information about the patient's glucose metabolism only at the time of the test. Estimation of **glycosylated hemoglobin** (HbA_{1c}) levels in blood is used as a guide to the degree of control over a long period. The level of HbA_{1c} is dependent on the serum glucose concentration and is increased in uncontrolled diabetes. HbA_{1c}, once formed, remains in the erythrocyte for the 120-day life span of the cell; HbA_{1c} levels thus provide an indication of blood glucose elevation in the previous 2–3 months. Normal HbA_{1c} is around 4% of total hemoglobin.

Acute Complications

A. Diabetic Ketoacidosis: Ketoacidosis occurs in severe diabetes, where insulin levels are greatly reduced. It is common in untreated type I diabetes but rare in type II diabetes, where insulin levels, although functionally inadequate, are still sufficient to prevent ketone body formation.

In the absence of insulin, lipolysis is stimulated (Fig 46–5), releasing free fatty acids that are oxidized in the liver cell to form acetylcoenzyme A. The entry of acetyl-CoA into the citric acid cycle is defective in diabetes. As a result, acetyl-CoA is converted in the liver to acetoacetate, β-hydroxybutyrate, and acetone (collectively called **ketone**

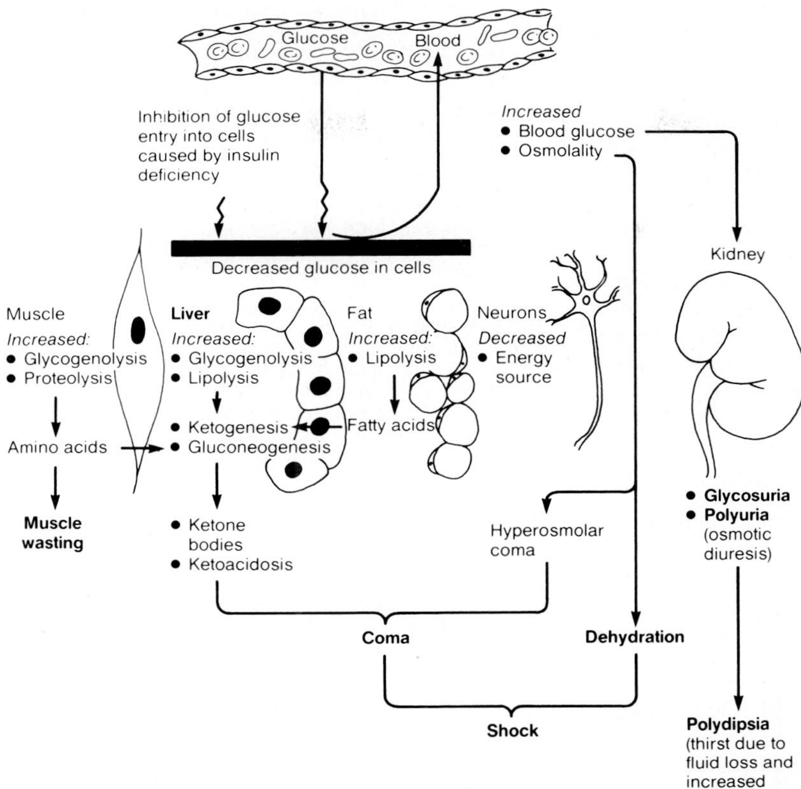

Figure 46-5. Abnormal metabolism and major symptomatology in diabetes mellitus.

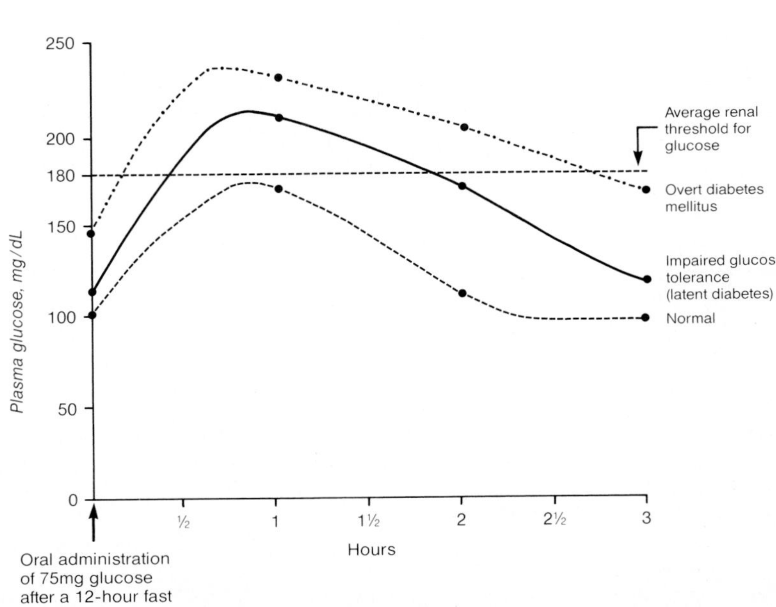

Figure 46-6. Response to an oral glucose load in normal and diabetic patients. (Normal fasting plasma glucose is 60–115 mg/dL.) Note the following points: (1) A normal glucose tolerance curve is defined as a fasting level < 115 mg/dL, 1 hour < 200 mg/dL, and 2 hours < 140 mg/dL. There is usually no glycosuria. (2) Impaired glucose tolerance is defined as a fasting level < 115 mg/dL, 1 hour > 200 mg/dL, 2 hours > 140 mg/dL. This was formerly called "latent diabetes." Five to 10 percent of these patients develop overt diabetes mellitus within 10 years. Because the other 90% of patients do not develop overt diabetes mellitus, the term "latent diabetes" has been dropped. (3) Overt diabetes mellitus is characterized by a fasting level > 115 mg/dL, 2 hours > 200 mg/dL. Many authorities hold that a value > 200 mg/dL at 2 hours is by itself sufficient for a diagnosis of diabetes mellitus.

bodies). The ketone bodies enter the blood (ketonemia, ketosis) and represent an important source of energy for skeletal muscle that cannot utilize glucose effectively in diabetes. They also spill over to be excreted in the urine (ketonuria).

Ketone bodies are moderately strong acids and cause a metabolic acidosis with decreased blood pH and low serum bicarbonate. Respiration is stimulated, washing out carbon dioxide and leading to a decrease in P_{CO_2}. An acid urine is excreted.

Clinically, patients present with altered consciousness as a result of general failure of energy production and acidosis. Coma occurs in severe cases. Marked volume depletion is usually present. The diagnosis is established by the presence of glycosuria, hyperglycemia, ketonemia, and ketonuria. Treatment requires aggresive fluid replacement, correction of electrolyte imbalance, and insulin therapy.

B. Hyperosmolar Nonketotic Coma: Patients who develop hyperosmolar coma are usually elderly, with severe uncontrolled diabetes. The disorder results from extremely high serum glucose levels that cause osmotic diuresis and marked fluid depletion, increasing plasma osmolarity. Hyperosmolar coma is treated with aggressive fluid replacement and insulin. It is associated with a high mortality rate.

C. Hypoglycemic Coma: Hypoglycemic coma is not a direct complication of diabetes but rather a complication of therapy. In treating diabetes it is essential to balance the insulin dose and the dietary intake of carbohydrate ("glucose dose"). A fall in blood glucose may follow overdosage of insulin but is seen more often when the usual daily schedule of insulin injections is given and one or more meals is missed or lost by vomiting (ie, when the "glucose dose" is reduced).

Chronic Complications (Table 46-4)

A. Diabetic Microangiopathy (Small-Vessel Disease): Microangiopathy is one of the most characteristic and most important pathologic changes in diabetes. It is characterized by diffuse thickening of the basement membranes of capillaries throughout the body. The kidney (Fig 46-7), retina, skin, and skeletal muscles are commonly involved. A similar change involves other basement membranes in renal tubules, placenta, and peripheral nerves. Basement membrane thickening in capillaries is associated with increased permeability to fluid and protein macromolecules.

The structure of the thick basement membrane in diabetics is abnormal. Increased amounts of collagen and laminin and decreased proteoglycans have been demonstrated. It has been suggested that prolonged elevation of serum glucose increases glycosylation of basement membrane proteins in a manner similar to glycosylation of hemoglobin. This would explain why strict control of diabetes decreases the incidence and severity of microangiopathy. It is widely accepted—though not proved—that control of diabetes decreases the risk of microangiopathy.

B. Large-Vessel Disease: Diabetes mellitus is a major risk factor for development of atherosclerotic vascular disease; myocardial infarction and cerebral arterial occlusion (stroke) represent the commonest causes of death in diabetics. The increased incidence of hyperlipidemia (both hypertriglyceridemia and hypercholesterolemia) in diabetes contributes to the development of atherosclerosis.

C. Neuropathy and Cataract: Neuropathy

Table 46-4. Chronic complications of diabetes mellitus by organ system.

Complication	Outcome
Kidney (see Chapter 48)	Renal failure
Glomerular microangiopathy	
Diffuse glomerulosclerosis	
Nodular glomerulosclerosis (Kimmelstiel-Wilson disease)	
Urinary infections	
Acute pyelonephritis	
Necrotizing papillitis	
Emphysematous pyelonephritis	
Glycogen nephrosis (Armanni-Ebstein lesion)	
Eye (see Chapter 33)	Visual failure
Retinopathy	
Nonproliferative retinopathy: capillary microaneurysms, retinal edema, exudates, and hemorrhages	
Proliferative retinopathy: proliferation of small vessels, hemorrhage, fibrosis, retinal detachment	
Cataracts	
Transient refractive errors due to osmotic changes in lens	
Glaucoma due to proliferation of vessels in the iris	
Infections	
Nervous system	
Cerebrovascular atherosclerotic disease: strokes, death	
Peripheral neuropathy: peripheral sensory and motor, cranial, autonomic	
Skin	
Infections: folliculitis leading to carbuncles	
Necrobiosis lipoidica diabeticorum: due to microangiopathy	
Xanthomata: secondary to hyperlipidemia	
Cardiovascular system	
Coronary atherosclerosis: myocardial infarction, death	
Peripheral atherosclerosis: limb ischemia, gangrene	
Reproductive system	
Increased fetal death rate[1] (placental disease, neonatal respiratory distress syndrome, infection)	
General	
Increased susceptibility to infection	
Delayed wound healing	

[1]Note that elevated maternal blood glucose levels produce elevated fetal blood glucose levels; the fetal pancreas often shows islet hyperplasia due to increased beta cells responding to the demand for more insulin.

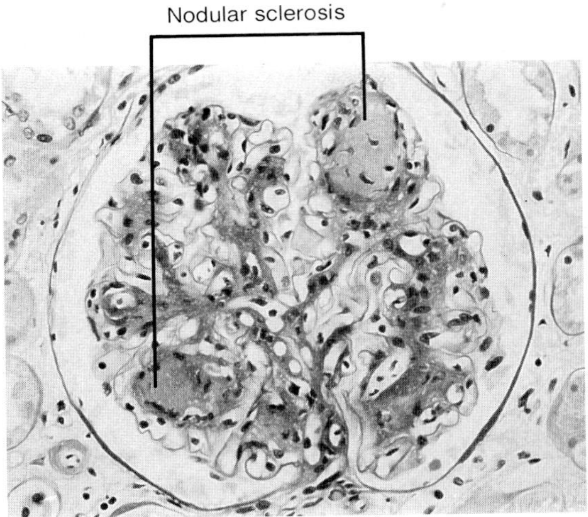

Figure 46-7. Diabetic nephropathy, showing nodular glomerulosclerosis (Kimmelstiel-Wilson disease).

and cataract in diabetic patients are believed to result from accumulation of sorbitol within nerve or lens tissue. The enzyme aldose reductase produces sorbitol in these tissues when glucose levels are high, and the accumulated sorbitol, which is osmotically active and nondiffusible, produces cellular swelling or death. It is postulated that nerve and lens tissue (and perhaps small vessels and kidney) may be particularly vulnerable to this effect since glucose can enter these cells even in low-insulin states—unlike other cells of the body, which require normal plasma levels of insulin for entry of glucose. Trials of drugs that inhibit aldose reductase are under way as a possible means of combating some of the chronic effects of diabetes.

D. Other Complications: Other complications include a general increased susceptibility to infection (Chapter 7) and impaired wound healing (Chapter 6).

Clinical Course

The average life expectancy of diabetics is reduced by 9 years for males and 7 years for females when compared with nondiabetics. The reduction is greatest when the onset of disease is at a young age.

Quality of life is seriously affected for all diabetics because of the many disabling complications. In addition, the requirement for strict dietary control and continuous drug treatment for many patients calls for a continuous emotional struggle.

Causes of death in diabetes (in order of frequency) are myocardial infarction, renal failure, cerebrovascular accidents, infections, ketoacidosis, hyperosmolar coma, and hypoglycemia.

Treatment

Type I diabetics require insulin treatment for life. Oral agents that act by stimulating the beta cells are not effective in these patients because of their beta cell-depleted state. Type II diabetics can be managed with measures to decrease "insulin resistance," such as decreasing body weight by diet, and by stimulation of the pancreatic beta cells with oral antidiabetic agents such as sulfonylureas. In many type II diabetics, insulin is also necessary for good control. An essential component of treatment is ensuring good control by repeated examinations of blood and urine for glucose. Serum HbA1c levels are useful for checking longer term control.

In animals, transplantation of pancreatic islets has resulted in a cure of experimental diabetes, but this method of treatment has not yet been applied successfully to humans.

HYPERFUNCTION OF THE PANCREATIC ISLETS

Excess secretion (Fig 46–8) of any one or several of the hormones of the islets of Langerhans may be caused by islet cell neoplasms or hyperplasia.

ISLET CELL NEOPLASMS

Adenomas derived from the islet cells are relatively common. In 10–15% of cases, multiple adenomas are present. Islet cell carcinomas occur, but less frequently.

Grossly, islet cell neoplasms are firm nodules that typically have a yellowish-brown color. They vary in size from microscopic (microadenomas) to large masses that may weigh several kilograms. They may or may not show encapsulation.

Microscopically, islet cell neoplasms are composed of uniform small cells arranged in nests and trabeculae separated by endothelium-lined vascular spaces. The islet cell origin of a pancreatic neoplasm can be established (1) by the presence of membrane-bound, electron-dense neurosecretory granules in the cytoplasm on electron microscopy; and (2) by positive staining for neuron-specific enolase, chromogranin, or specific hormones by immunoperoxidase techniques.

Differentiation of adenomas from carcinomas of islet cells is difficult by light microscopic examination. Invasion of the capsule and cytologic atypia are common in neoplasms that show benign behavior and cannot be used as evidence of malignant change. Conversely, islet cell carcinomas may be well circumscribed and have little cy-

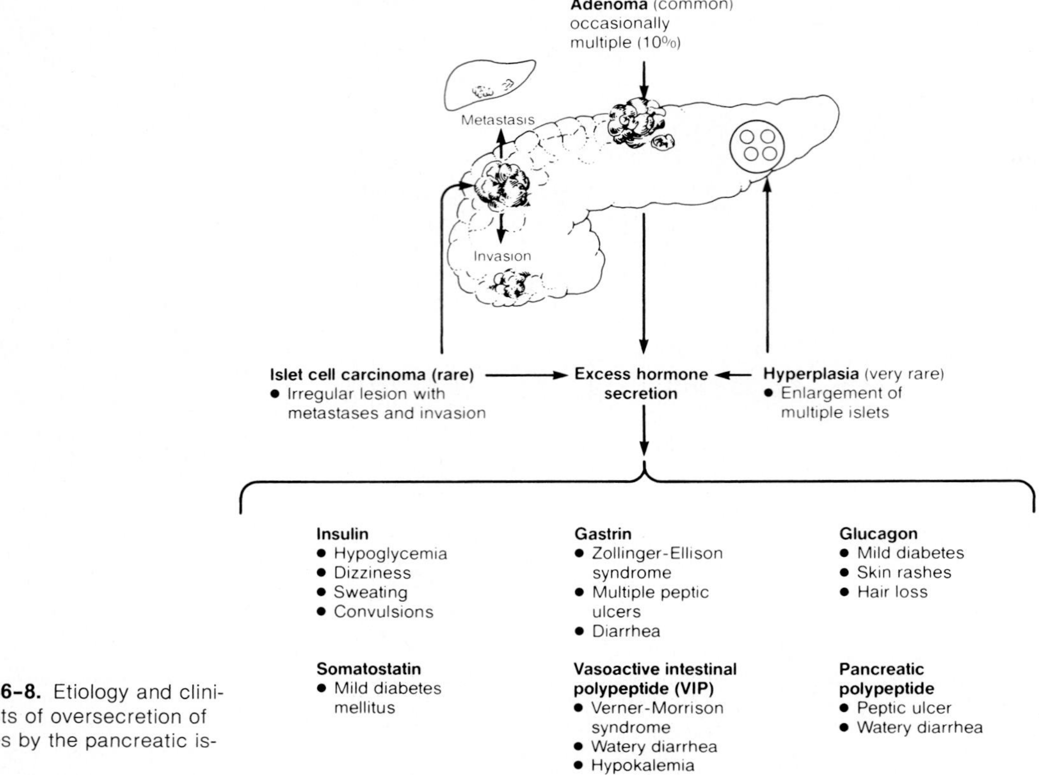

Figure 46–8. Etiology and clinical effects of oversecretion of hormones by the pancreatic islets.

tologic atypia. Features that favor a diagnosis of carcinoma are extensive invasion of the pancreatic stroma or peripancreatic tissue, venous involvement, and perineural invasion. The only definite evidence of malignancy is the presence of metastatic lesions.

Islet cell adenomas are cured by surgical excision; carcinomas tend to grow slowly but are difficult to control if surgery fails. Even in the presence of metastatic disease, patients may survive several years because of the slow growth rate of islet cell carcinoma.

Most islet cell neoplasms are composed of one cell type; less commonly, multiple cell types are involved. The diagnosis of the cell type is impossible by routine light microscopy and requires (1) electron microscopy, which demonstrates the characteristic granules of the different cells; (2) serum assay for the different pancreatic hormones; and (3) demonstration of hormone in the tumor cells by immunoperoxidase techniques. Some islet cell neoplasms do not produce sufficient hormone to be detectable in serum (''nonfunctioning islet cell neoplasms'').

ISLET CELL HYPERPLASIA

Diffuse hyperplasia of the islets is a rare cause of hypersecretion of pancreatic hormones, and there is some doubt about whether it is a real entity. Islet cell hyperplasia is characterized by the presence of islets in the size range 300–700 μm. Islets measuring less than 300 μm are normal; those above 700 μm are microadenomas. Microscopically, hyperplastic islets resemble normal islets; immunohistochemical studies sometimes show a dominance of one cell type.

In adults, the commonest situation in which hyperplastic islets are found is in the pancreas adjacent to an islet cell neoplasm. The finding of hyperplastic islets in a surgically removed pancreas should therefore lead to a careful search for an adenoma in the remaining pancreas. Marked islet cell hyperplasia (of insulin-producing beta cells) is also seen in fetuses born of diabetic mothers as a fetal response to the high glucose environment.

CLINICAL FEATURES OF PANCREATIC HORMONE EXCESS

The clinical features of hypersecretion of the islets depend on which hormone is secreted in excess and to what degree. In most cases, hypersecretion is restricted to one hormone; rarely, 2 or more hormones are involved.

Hyperinsulinism

The commonest clinical syndrome associated with hyperfunctioning islets is hyperinsulinism. Seventy percent of cases are caused by solitary beta cell adenomas (insulinomas); 10% by multiple adenomas; 10% by carcinomas; and 10% by islet cell hyperplasia.

Increased insulin secretion is characterized (1) by hypoglycemia, precipitated by fasting or exercise and causing dizziness, confusion, and excessive sweating which, if sustained, are followed by convulsions, coma, and death; (2) by prompt relief of symptoms after glucose administration; and (3) by a plasma glucose level under 40 mg/dL during an attack. The fasting plasma glucose is also decreased to less than half of normal. This symptom complex is known as Whipple's triad.

The diagnosis is established by the finding of an inappropriately high serum insulin level during a period of hypoglycemia.

Glucagon Excess

Glucagon stimulates glycogenolysis and gluconeogenesis, serving to maintain glucose levels between meals. Hyperfunction of alpha cells is rare and caused by an islet cell neoplasm (glucagonoma), 70% of which are carcinomas and 30% adenomas. Two-thirds of patients with carcinomas present with evidence of metastases, commonly in the liver.

Clinically, patients have mild diabetes mellitus, due to the insulin antagonistic action of glucagon, and a typical erythematous necrotizing migratory skin eruption. Alopecia, increased skin pigmentation, and glossitis are less common manifestations.

The diagnosis is made by finding an elevated serum glucagon level.

Gastrin Excess

Gastrin hypersecretion is second in frequency to hyperinsulinism among this group of diseases. It is usually caused by an islet cell neoplasm composed of G cells (gastrinoma), 70% of which are malignant. In 10% of cases, islet cell hyperplasia is present but no neoplasm is found in the pancreas. In 1% of cases, a microadenoma measuring about 1 mm in diameter is the cause. Gastrinomas rarely occur also in the duodenal and gastric wall.

Secretion of large amounts of gastrin leads to Zollinger-Ellison syndrome, characterized by continuous hypersecretion of gastric acid, causing a low pH of gastric juice. The resting acid secretion is greater than 60% of the maximum acid secretion in response to an injection of histamine or pentagastrin. Unrelenting, recurrent peptic ulcers occur in the stomach, duodenum, esophagus, and jejunum in 90% of patients. Severe diarrhea and hypokalemia—induced by the hyperacidity—are present in 30% of patients. Diarrhea may be associated with malabsorption of fat and steatorrhea due to inactivation of lipase by the low pH in the duodenum. Ten percent of patient with Zollinger-Ellison syndrome present with diarrhea and have no peptic ulcer disease. The gastric mucosal folds are commonly thickened.

The diagnosis of Zollinger-Ellison syndrome is made by demonstrating high serum gastrin levels. It can be distinguished from other causes of elevated serum gastrin by a paradoxic increase in gastrin levels in response to intravenous secretin and calcium injections.

Somatostatin Excess

D cell neoplasms of the pancreas (somatostatinomas) are very rare. Eighty percent are malignant. Clinically, mild diabetes mellitus resulting from impaired release of insulin is the most constant feature; diarrhea and gallstones also occur commonly.

Diagnosis by demonstration of an elevated serum level is difficult because of the short half-life of somatostatin.

Vasoactive Intestinal Polypeptide Excess

Excess secretion of vasoactive intestinal polypeptide (VIP) is rare and caused by a D_1 cell neoplasm of the islets (VIPoma). Clinically, the polypeptide stimulates intestinal secretion by an unknown mechanism, causing watery diarrhea with hypokalemia and alkalosis (WDHA syndrome; Verner-Morrison syndrome). The diagnosis is established by demonstrating elevated VIP levels in the serum and in an extract of the tumor.

Pancreatic Polypeptide Excess

Pancreatic polypeptide (PP)-producing neoplasms are extremely rare. They may be present in patients with no clinical symptoms. Some patients have watery diarrhea and hypokalemia; others have peptic ulcer disease.

Section XI.
The Urinary Tract & Male Reproductive System

The male reproductive system is discussed with the urinary system because they both come under the surgical subspecialty of urology. Nonsurgical diseases of the kidney come under the medical subspecialty of nephrology.

Urinary tract infections (Chapter 47) are very common, especially in women. Many glomerular diseases (Chapter 48) have an immunologic basis, and the reader will benefit by reviewing mechanisms of immunologic hypersenstitivity in Chapter 8. Chronic renal disease is associated with hypertension (see Chapter 20), anemia (see Chapter 24) and abnormalities in parathyroid gland function (see Chapter 59), and bone (see Chapter 67). Renal transplantation is routinely performed in most large medical centers for the management of chronic renal failure. This subject is not discussed in this section, and the reader should refer to Chapter 8.

Neoplasms of the kidney (Chapter 49) and urinary bladder (Chapter 50) are common. Prostate diseases, including benign prostatic hyperplasia and carcinoma (Chapter 51) are extremely common in elderly men. Testicular germ cell neoplasms, though not common, are of the greatest importance because they represent a group or neoplasms for which very successful chemotherapy is available.

47 The Kidney: I. Structure & Function; Tubulointerstitial Diseases

STRUCTURE OF THE KIDNEYS

The kidneys are located in the retroperitoneum and weigh 130–150 g each. The surface is smooth and invested in a capsule, which in turn is surrounded by perinephric fat and Gerota's fascia. The hilum of the kidney gives entrance to the renal artery and exit to the renal veins, lymphatics, and ureter.

The anatomic unit of the kidney is the nephron, which is composed of the glomerulus, proximal convoluted tubule, loop of Henle, distal convoluted tubule, and collecting tubule (Fig 47–1). Each kidney contains approximately 1 million nephrons.

The glomerulus (Figs 47–1 and 47–2) is the filtering mechanism of the kidney. It is composed of (1) an afferent and efferent arteriole; (2) intervening capillaries lined by endothelial cells (glomerular tuft); (3) the outer surface of the capillaries, which is covered by epithelial cells (podocytes), continuous with the epithelium of Bowman's space and the proximal tubule; (4) the mesangium, composed of mesangial cells and matrix; and (5) the basement membrane.

The renal tubules form the major part of the cortex (proximal and distal convoluted tubules) and medulla (collecting tubules and loops of Henle). A small amount of interstitial connective tissue separates the tubules in the normal kidney.

RENAL FUNCTION

Glomerular Filtration

Ultrafiltration of plasma occurs in the glomerular capillaries, driven by the hydrostatic pressure head in the arteriolar end of the capillary (Table 47–1). The normal glomerular capillary endothelium contains fenestrations that permit the passage of molecules up to a molecular weight of about 70,000 (Fig 47–2).

The glomerular filtration rate (GFR) is normally about 120 mL/min. It may be measured accurately by the clearance of exogenous inulin (inulin clearance test) or endogenous creatinine (creatinine clearance test).

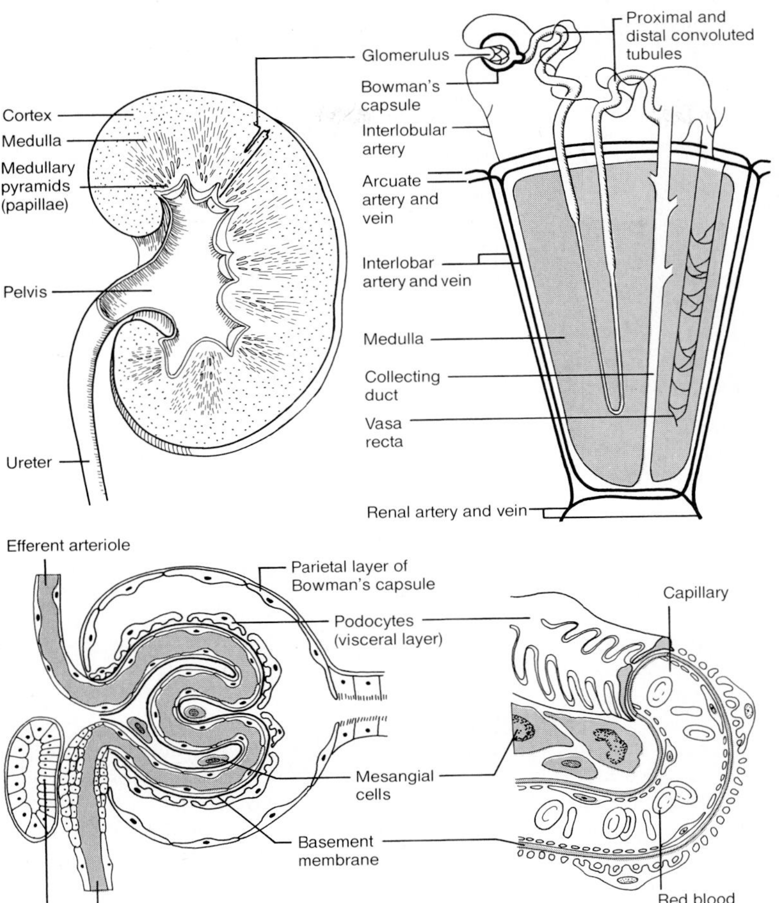

Figure 47–1. Structure of kidney, nephron, glomerulus, and glomerular capillary.

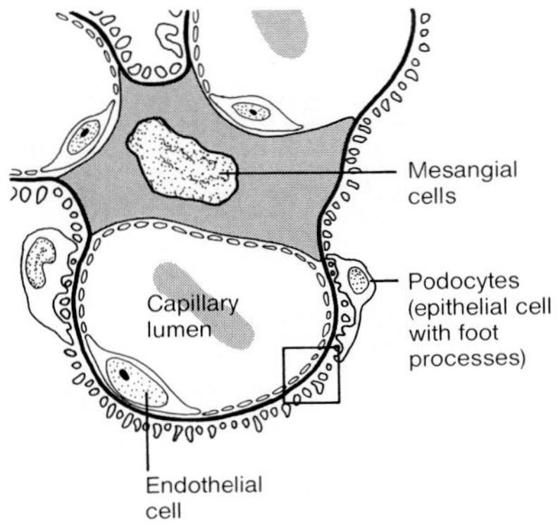

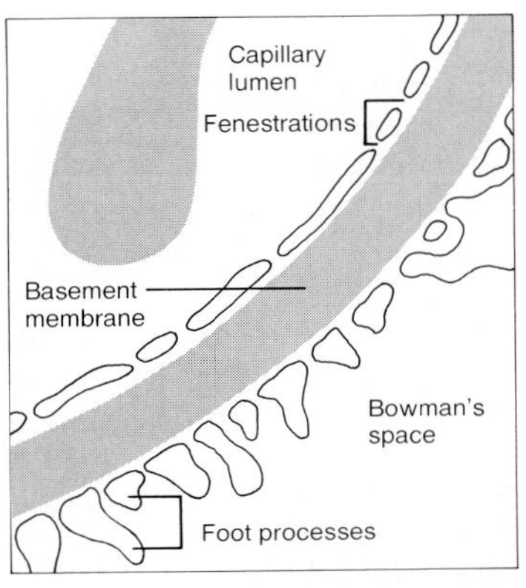

Figure 47–2. Detailed structure of glomerulus and glomerular filtration membrane composed of endothelial cell, basement membrane, and podocyte.

Table 47–1. Functional anatomy of the nephron.

Juxtaglomerular apparatus	Renin production
Glomerulus	Produces ultrafiltrate of plasma (glomerular filtration rate 120 mL/min)
Proximal convoluted tubule	Resorption of: Water (80%) Glucose (100%) K^+ (100%) Amino acids (100%)
Loop of Henle and vasa recta	Countercurrent exchange and multiplier mechanisms
Distal convoluted tubule and collecting duct	Resorption of: Water (antidiuretic hormone-controlled) Na^+ (in exchange for K^+ and H^+, controlled by aldosterone) Acidification

Tubular Reabsorption (Table 47–1)

Eighty percent of the glomerular ultrafiltrate volume is absorbed actively in the proximal tubule. Potassium, glucose, and amino acids are completely reabsorbed.

Approximately 30 mL/min of isotonic fluid is delivered to the loop of Henle. The loop of Henle passes down into the medulla and establishes a countercurrent exchange mechanism that causes a progressive increase in tonicity from the corticomedullary junction to the tip of the papillae. This mechanism is enhanced by the action of the vasa recta that accompany the loop of Henle (countercurrent multiplier system) (Fig 47–1). Establishment of the countercurrent exchange mechanism depends on active secretion of sodium into the interstitium by the ascending loop of Henle. There is otherwise little fluid or electrolyte exchange in the loop of Henle.

The following changes in the tubular fluid occur in the distal convoluted and collecting tubules:

(1) Water reabsorption occurs under the influence of antidiuretic hormone. Medullary hypertonicity produced by the countercurrent exchange and multiplier mechanisms is vital to the urine concentration mechanism. Of the 120 mL filtered at the glomerulus, only 1–2 mL normally passes through as urine.

(2) Sodium reabsorption occurs under the influence of aldosterone in exchange for potassium and hydrogen ions.

(3) Acidification of urine occurs. The total acid excreted per day by the kidney is only about 1% of that excreted by the lungs as CO_2. Nonetheless, failure of this mechanism will, after several days, result in metabolic acidosis.

Excreted urine contains precisely regulated quantities of sodium, potassium, water, chloride, bicarbonate, phosphate, and ammonium ions. Normal urine contains only a trace amount of protein, derived mainly from tubular secretion (Tamm-Horsfall protein) and no glucose or amino acids. It has a high concentration of excretory products, urea, uric acid, and creatinine.

CLINICAL MANIFESTATIONS OF RENAL DISEASE (Table 47–2)

Pain

The renal parenchyma contains no pain-sensitive nerve endings. Pain in renal disease is due to 2 mechanisms: Stretching of the renal fascia causes poorly localized pain in the flank, and severe muscular contraction of the ureters in conditions associated with ureteral obstruction produces ureteral colic. Ureteral colic is a severe, intermittent pain in the posterior renal angle that radiates around the flank to the pubic region.

Hematuria

Many renal diseases are characterized by the passage of blood in the urine (hematuria). There may or may not be pain. When bleeding is severe, hematuria is recognized by red discoloration of urine. When bleeding is slow, hematuria does not produce any visible change but can be diagnosed by the presence of erythrocytes in a sample of urinary sediment (microscopic hematuria). Hematuria has many causes (Table 47–3).

Proteinuria

Proteinuria is a common finding in many renal diseases, and testing for it is a useful screening test for renal disease. The trace amount of protein normally present in urine does not give a positive reaction with the usual screening tests. In a few individuals, orthostatic (postural) or exercise pro-

Table 47–2. Clinical manifestations of renal disease.

Pain, including ureteral colic
Enlargement of the kidney, including renal masses
Hematuria: the presence of red blood cells in the urine
Pyuria: the presence of neutrophils in the urine
Proteinuria: the presence of increased amounts of protein in the urine
Nephrotic syndrome: massive proteinuria (> 5 g/d), hypoproteinemia, and edema
Acute nephritic syndrome: oliguria (< 700 mL/d), hematuria, mild proteinuria, hypertension, and azotemia
Chronic renal failure
Hypertension

Table 47-3. Causes of hematuria.

	Additional Urinary Findings[1]
Renal diseases	
Acute and chronic glomerulonephritis Primary types, including Goodpasture's syndrome Secondary to systemic lupus erythematosus, polyarteritis nodosa, Henoch-Schönlein purpura	Red cell casts, granular casts,[2] leukocytes, protein
Acute and chronic pyelonephritis	Proteins, leukocytes, white cell and epithelial cell casts, organisms
Tumor	Protein, sometimes malignant cells
Calculi	Leukocytes
Trauma	None
Drug/chemical toxicity	Protein, casts
Papillary necrosis	Necrotic papillae occasionally
Polycystic disease	None
Diseases of bladder, ureters, urethra	
Cystitis	Leukocytes, organisms
Urethritis	Leukocytes, organisms
Tumor	Sometimes malignant cells
Calculi	Leukocytes
Trauma	None
Systemic disease causing bleeding from genitourinary tract	
Malignant hypertension	Protein
Systemic emboli as in bacterial endocarditis	Protein
Bleeding diathesis or anticoagulant therapy	None
Osler-Weber-Rendu disease	None
Hemoglobinopathies, hemolysis	Hemoglobinuria[3]
Exercise hematuria (after violent exercise)	None

[1]All hematurias by definition contain red cells, ranging from few (microscopic hematuria, detectable only by microscopic examination of urine) to many (grossly visible blood in urine).
[2]Hyaline casts indicate increased protein loss; white cell, epithelial cell, and granular casts indicate tubular or glomerular disease; they are formed in the damaged tubules.
[3]Red cells may be present in some hemoglobinopathies (eg, sickle cell disease). However, free hemoglobin will also cause red coloration of urine and give a positive result with the usual colorimetric and "dipstick" tests for hematuria. Microscopic examination for red cells is essential to differentiate hematuria from hemoglobinuria.

teinuria occurs following recumbency or vigorous physical activity; the condition has no clinical significance.

Urinary casts are formed when protein and other organic matter in the renal tubules solidifies. Casts are elongated cylindric structures with a diameter equal to that of the renal tubule. The presence of casts in urine is indicative of disease of the nephron. Casts may contain protein only (hyaline casts) or may include erythrocytes (red cell casts), leukocytes (white cell casts), and tubular cells (epithelial casts).

Nephrotic Syndrome

Nephrotic syndrome is characterized by massive proteinuria (over 5 g/24 h), hypoproteinemia, and edema (Table 47-4). Hypercholesterolemia is frequently also present. Nephrotic syndrome may result from any condition that causes increased glomerular capillary permeability to proteins (Table 47-5). The prognosis varies according to the underlying disease.

Acute Nephritic Syndrome ("Acute Nephritis")

Acute nephritic syndrome is a clinical syndrome characterized by decreased urinary volume (oliguria), hematuria, mild proteinuria, elevation of serum urea and creatinine (azotemia or uremia), hypertension, and mild edema. **Acute glomerular disease** associated with a decreased glomerular filtration is the major cause. Again, the prognosis depends upon the cause.

Acute Renal Failure

Acute renal failure is defined as marked diminution of urine output to less than 400 mL/d (oliguria; *anuria* would be complete absence of urine output). If persistent, it leads to elevation of serum creatinine and urea plus hypertension due to retention of sodium and water. Biopsy may be necessary to determine the cause (Table 47-6). In acute tubular necrosis, in some cases of glomerulonephritis, and in pre- and postrenal causes, the process is reversible and the patient may be ex-

Table 47-4. Major differential features of the principal clinical renal diseases.

	Urine Output	Proteinuria	Hematuria	Edema	Serum Albumin	Serum[1] Urea/ Creatinine	Blood Pressure	Other
Nephrotic syndrome	N or ↓	+++	− (Rarely +)	++	↓↓	N (until late)	N	↑ Serum cholesterol, casts
Acute nephritic syndrome (acute nephritis)	↓	+ to ++	+	+	N	↑	↑	Hyperkalemia
Acute renal failure	↓↓ or 0	+ to ++	±	±	N	↑↑	↑	Hyperkalemia, acidosis
Chronic renal failure	↑ (Cannot concentrate)	+ to ++	±	±	N	↑	↑	Isosthenuria
Acute pyelonephritis	N (Rarely ↓)	++	− (Rarely +)	−	N	N	N	White cells in urine (often purulent), frequency, dysuria, culture +

[1]Serum urea levels do not rise until 60% or more of the nephrons have lost function. Serum creatinine levels rise somewhat earlier than serum urea levels and are less subject to variation caused by overall hydration.

Table 47-5. Causes of nephrotic syndrome.

Primary renal disease
Minimal change glomerulonephritis (lipoid nephrosis)
Other forms of glomerulonephritis
Renal vein thrombosis
Nephrotoxins such as gold, bismuth, mercury
Systemic disorders with renal damage
Diabetes
Amyloidosis
Systemic lupus erythematosus
Allergic responses, poison ivy, insect stings, tumors
Infections, malaria, syphilis
Myeloma kidney
Goodpasture's syndrome, Henoch-Schönlein purpura, and other forms of secondary glomerulonephritis

pected to recover after treatment. Acute cortical necrosis and severe forms of glomerulonephritis are irreversible and often require long-term dialysis or renal transplantation.

Chronic Renal Failure

Chronic renal failure (chronic uremia) is characterized by a variety of abnormalities (Fig 47–3) resulting from a decrease in the total number of nephrons. The kidneys normally have a total of 2 million nephrons. Chronic renal failure appears only when the number of nephrons is reduced to about 25% of this number. Again, there are many causes (Table 47–7).

The manifestations of chronic renal failure are numerous and affect virtually every organ in the body.

A. Uremia and Azotemia: Failure of renal excretory function resulting in increased serum urea and creatinine occurs only when failure is advanced. A much more sensitive assessment of chronic renal failure is the **creatinine clearance test,** which is an estimate of the glomerular filtration rate. Decreased glomerular filtration is proportionate to the nephron loss. Serum urea and creatinine become elevated only when creatinine clearance decreases to about 30–40% of normal.

B. Inability to Concentrate Urine: This is one of the early clinical manifestations of chronic renal failure. It leads to polyuria (increased urine output), **nocturia** (excessive passage of urine at night), and **isosthenuria** (passage of a urine that varies little from a specific gravity of 1.010). Polyuria frequently causes dehydration.

C. Metabolic Acidosis: Failure of hydrogen ion excretion results in accumulation of acid in the blood (the body produces excess acid during cell metabolism), leading to metabolic acidosis.

D. Secondary Hyperparathyroidism and Renal Osteodystrophy: Failure of renal activation of vitamin D in chronic renal failure leads to defective intestinal absorption of calcium and hypocalcemia. The low plasma calcium causes compensatory parathyroid hyperplasia and increased parathyroid hormone secretion (secondary hyperparathyroidism). Abnormal calcium and phosphate metabolism leads to bone changes (renal osteodystrophy) and metastatic calcification. Renal osteodystrophy is a complex combination of osteomalacia and the effects of hyperparathyroidism (osteitis fibrosa cystica). Metastatic calcifica-

Table 47-6. Causes of oliguria or anuria.

Prerenal
Shock due to any cause: hypovolemia, renal vasoconstriction, and decreased renal blood flow
Postoperative oliguria (antidiuresis)
Dehydration (antidiuresis)
Renal
Acute glomerulonephritis
Acute tubular necrosis
Nephrotoxic
Drugs: aminoglycosides,[1] sulfonamides
X-ray contrast media[1]
Gold, mercury, arsenic
Industrial: carbon tetrachloride, ethylene glycol
Ischemic
Prolonged hypotension in shock
Includes trauma (crush syndrome),[2] incompatible transfusion,[2] burns,[2] eclampsia, hepatorenal syndrome
Transplant rejection
Acute cortical necrosis
Severe ischemia: Extreme shock, especially with infections, burns, and hemorrhage in pregnancy
Disseminated intravascular coagulation: Again, shock is usually present
Snakebite
Acute pyelonephritis when associated with papillary necrosis (rare)
Postrenal obstruction
To cause anuria, obstruction must involve both ureters, the bladder neck, or the urethra. Common causes include tumor, prostatic hyperplasia, calculus, and trauma (including abdominal surgery).

[1]Aminoglycosides (kanamycin, neomycin, etc) and x-ray contrast media are 2 of the most common causes in modern hospital practice.
[2]It has been argued that precipitation of hemoglobin, myoglobin, or fragmented red cell membranes in the tubules in these conditions may aggravate the effects of hypotension.

Table 47-7. Causes of chronic renal failure.[1]

Chronic glomerulonephritis: many causes	30%
Chronic pyelonephritis	15%
Obstructive nephropathy, hydronephrosis	10%
Hypertensive renal disease	10%
Polycystic disease	10%
Diabetic nephropathy	10%
Amyloidosis	5%
Multiple myeloma	rare
Nephrolithiasis, hypercalcemia	rare
Analgesic nephropathy, drugs, and chemicals	rare

[1]Note that many of these conditions occur together, eg, obstructive nephropathy, nephrolithiasis (stones), and pyelonephritis.

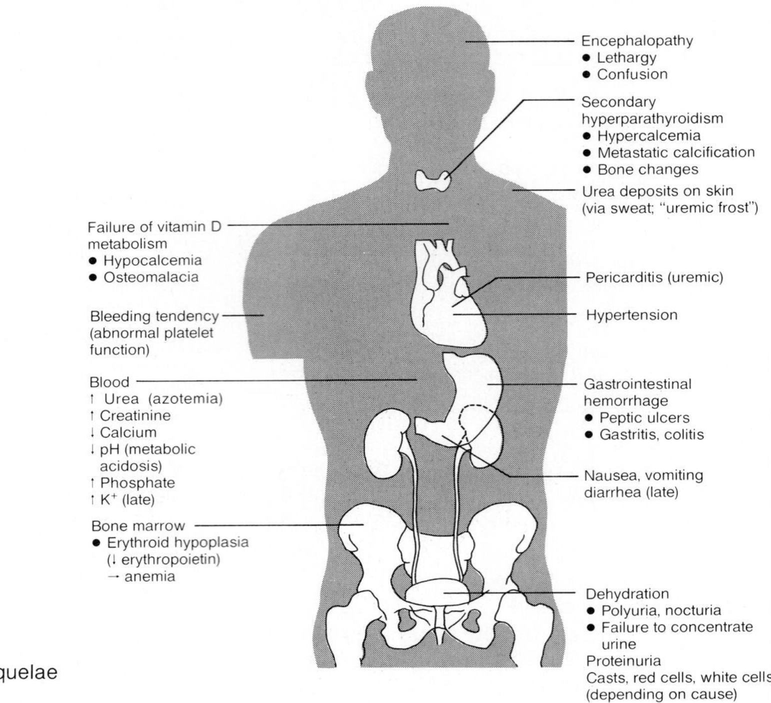

Figure 47-3. Clinical sequelae of chronic renal failure.

tion in the walls of small vessels may cause ischemic changes in affected tissues.

E. Hematologic Disorders: Decreased erythropoietin production by the kidney leads to normochromic normocytic **anemia**. Platelet function is abnormal, causing a **bleeding tendency**. Gastrointestinal hemorrhage is a common clinical manifestation of chronic uremia.

F. Cardiovascular Disorders: Chronic renal failure is frequently associated with **hypertension,** caused by sodium and water retention in the kidneys. In most cases, plasma renin levels are normal; in a few, they are elevated and contribute to the hypertension. Renal failure in an advanced stage may also cause acute fibrinous or hemorrhagic **pericarditis** by an unknown mechanism.

G. Encephalopathy: Chronic renal failure is often associated with abnormalities in cerebral function, causing disturbances in the level of consciousness. **Uremic encephalopathy** is presumed to be due to retention of unknown end products of protein metabolism.

Hypertension

Hypertension occurs in both acute and chronic renal failure and may be the presenting feature of renal disease; the principal mechanism is retention of sodium and water by the nephron. This may be the result of decreased glomerular filtration (a common cause in many renal diseases) or increased aldosterone levels (as in nephrotic syndrome). In a few patients with renal disease—most commonly renal artery stenosis—increased renin secretion contributes to hypertension.

METHODS OF EVALUATING RENAL STRUCTURE & FUNCTION

Physical Examination

The kidneys are difficult organs to palpate. When the kidney is enlarged (eg, in cystic disease, neoplasms), it can be palpated by bimanual examination.

Radiologic Examination

Many radiologic procedures are available for evaluation of renal structure: (1) Plain abdominal x-ray provides an estimate of renal size and shape. (2) Intravenous pyelography is an x-ray taken after intravenous administration of contrast dye which is excreted by the kidney. The pelvicaliceal system is outlined. Similar information may be obtained by retrograde injection of dye into the ureters at cystoscopy. (3) Ultrasonography and computerized tomography are sensitive methods of detecting cysts and neoplasms within the kidney. (4) Renal arteriography provides information regarding the vasculature of the kidney. It is useful in the diagnosis of renal artery stenosis and may also demonstrate the vascular pattern in mass lesions.

Examination of Urine

Routine urine examination should be part of every complete physical examination (Table 47–8). Most of the chemical tests and microscopic examination of the sediment can be easily performed by the physician in an office or ward laboratory. The availability of dipsticks has made urine testing relatively easy. Abnormalities detected by these means should be confirmed by formal testing in the pathology department.

Examination of Blood

Renal disease commonly results in abnormalities in serum levels of urea, creatinine, protein, and electrolytes (Table 47–4). Changes in red cell count, hemoglobin, and platelet function may occur in chronic renal failure.

Renal Biopsy

Percutaneous renal biopsy is a safe procedure that provides a cylindric core of renal tissue for histologic examination. Samples are also processed for electron microscopy and immunofluorescence. These studies have provided an objective method of diagnosis of renal diseases and have increased our understanding of many pathologic processes. Before biopsy is undertaken, it is necessary to demonstrate that both kidneys are present and that there is no bleeding abnormality.

CONGENITAL RENAL MALFORMATIONS

RENAL AGENESIS

Renal agenesis is failure of development of the renal anlage, resulting in a complete absence of the kidney. Renal agenesis may be bilateral or unilateral.

Bilateral renal agenesis is a rare anomaly resulting in death in utero or soon after delivery. Infants have renal failure associated with characteristic facial features, with wide-set eyes and prominent inner canthi; a broad, flattened nose; large and low-set ears; and a receding chin (Potter facies).

Unilateral renal agenesis is more common, occurring in 0.1% of the population. It is asymptomatic because the single kidney is capable of subserving normal renal function. The frequency of unilateral renal agenesis makes confirmation of the presence of 2 kidneys obligatory before nephrectomy or even biopsy is performed.

RENAL HYPOPLASIA

Renal hypoplasia is defined as a small kidney (< 50 g in an adult) with 5 or fewer calices (normal: 7–13) but otherwise normal in structure. The anomaly is rare and usually unilateral; renal failure occurs only when hypoplasia is extreme and bilateral.

ECTOPIC KIDNEY

Ectopic position of one or both kidneys is not unusual, the most common location being at the pelvic brim or in the pelvis. Renal ectopia is usually asymptomatic but may cause obstruction and infection if there is kinking of the ureter.

HORSESHOE KIDNEY

Horseshoe kidney is abnormal fusion of the 2 organs, with the lower poles being fused across the midline by a broad band of renal tissue. It occurs in 0.4% of individuals. The ureters pass anterior to the isthmus of the horseshoe kidney and may be narrowed. Most patients are asymptomatic; there is a higher incidence of urinary infection and renal calculi.

RENAL DYSGENESIS (Renal Dysplasia)

The term renal dysgenesis denotes maldevelopment of the renal anlage. (Note that the term "dysplasia" is used in an unusual manner and has nothing to do with cytologic abnormalities associated with neoplastic transformation. Renal dysgenesis is a better term.)

Renal dysgenesis may be total or segmental and may involve one or both kidneys (Table 47–9). Cysts are commonly present (see Chapter 15), and differentiation from some forms of cystic disease may be difficult. Depending upon the severity, renal failure may develop.

CYSTIC DISEASES OF THE KIDNEY

There are several different causes of multiple cysts within the kidney (Table 47–9). The cysts are fluid-filled spaces, usually formed by dilatation of

Table 47-8. Examination of urine.

	Method	Dipstick[1] Method Available	Conclusion/Comment
Physical evaluation			
Color			
Colorless	Inspection	–	Polyuria
Cloudy	Inspection	–	Phosphates, carbonates, urates, white blood cells, lipid
Dark	Inspection	–	Bilirubin, blood
Red, red/brown	Inspection	–	Blood, hemoglobin, porphyrins
Black	Inspection	–	Homogentisic acid, melanin
Various	Inspection	–	Drugs, food dyes
Odor			
Foul, ammoniacal	Smell	–	Probable infection with urea-splitting bacteria
Asparagus	Smell	–	Eating asparagus (some people)
Various unusual	Smell	–	Possible metabolic disorders such as phenylketonuria (mousy) or isovaleric acidemia (sweaty)
Volume (especially 24-hour)	Measure	–	Polyuria, oliguria; normal range is about 600–2000 mL for an adult. Nocturia: exceeds 400 mL at night
Specific gravity	Measure	+	Normal range 1.005–1.025; consistent value of 1.010 is isosthenuria and indicates inability to concentrate as in chronic renal failure
Taste[2] (sweet)	Tongue[2]	–	Diabetes mellitus (honey taste)
pH	Glass electrode/ pH meter	+	Dietary factors, renal tubular disorders, chronic renal failure, acidosis, alkalosis
Chemical evaluation			
Protein	Precipitation tests	+	Normally traces only; dipstick allows some quantitation; numerous causes, must exclude renal disease
Blood	Microscopy or orthotoluidine test	+	Chemical test may detect myo- and hemoglobinuria also; microscopy should always be used to confirm hematuria
Glucose	Copper reduction method	+	Strongly suspect diabetes; other causes rare
Bilirubin	Diazoreaction	+	Obstructive jaundice; liver disease
Ketones	Sodium nitroprusside	+	Starvation, diabetic ketotic coma
Urobilinogen	Erlich's aldehyde reaction (chloroform-soluble)	+	Increased in hemolytic or hepatocellular jaundice; absent in obstructive jaundice
Porphobilinogen	Erlich's aldehyde reaction (not chloroform soluble)	–	Detected by some urobilinogen dipsticks (eg, Ames), not others (eg, Chemstrip); positive in porphyrias; salicylates and other drugs may give positivity
Examination of sediment (microscopic evaluation)			
Red blood cells		–	Hematuria
Casts: red cell, white cell, granular, epithelial		–	Many renal diseases
White blood cells		–	Pyelonephritis, cystitis, other renal disease
Malignant cells	Cytologic examination	–	Cancer, especially bladder
Crystals		–	Often present; various types, little diagnostic value
Bacteriologic examination	Culture: fresh midstream clean-catch specimen	–	Specific organisms, pyelonephritis, cystitis, urethritis

[1]Multiple activity dipsticks (eg, Multistix-SG, Chemstrips) give an estimate of most or all of these. If critical to diagnosis, the results should be confirmed by formal laboratory assays; there are many causes of false-positive and -negative results which usually are indicated on the package labels.
[2]This test is currently unpopular but is of historical interest, distinguishing sweet polyuria (diabetes mellitus) from tasteless polyuria (diabetes insipidus).

Table 47-9. Cystic disease of the kidney.

Disease	Heredity	Age	Uni- or Bilateral	Gross Features	Microscopic Features	Associated Malformation or Disease
Dysgenesis						
Total renal dysgenesis	None	Usually infants	Bilateral or unilateral	Nonreniform "cluster of grapes"	Macrocysts, primitive mesenchyme; cartilage	Cardiovascular, gastrointestinal, central nervous system, and urinary tract abnormalities
Segmental dysgenesis	None	Any	Usually unilateral	Irregular cysts with scarring		
Polycystic renal disease						
Adult polycystic disease	Autosomal dominant	Adults; rarely children	Bilateral	Large, bosselated, reniform; cysts in cortex and medulla	Glomerular cysts and nondescript cysts anywhere along nephron	Gross cysts of liver, pancreas, lung; cerebral aneurysms
Infantile polycystic disease	Autosomal recessive	Infants, children	Bilateral	Large smooth kidney with radial fusiform cysts in cortex and medulla	Flat, cuboidal epithelium	Congenital hepatic fibrosis
Medullary cystic disease						
Medullary sponge kidney	None	Any age; usually adults	Unilateral or bilateral	Cysts at tip of papillae	Papillary cysts lined by flattened epithelium; medullary calcification	Renal stones
Uremic medullary cystic disease	Variable	Older children and adolescents	Bilateral	Small coarsely scarred kidneys with 1- to 20-mm cysts at corticomedullary junction	Flat epithelial lining of cysts; glomerular sclerosis with interstitial fibrosis and atrophy; patchy inflammatory infiltrate	None
Glomerulocystic disease	None	Newborns, infants, and children	Bilateral	Enlarged, reniform with 1- to 8-mm cysts throughout cortex	Glomerular and tubular cysts; collapsed tuft in glomerular cysts	None
Simple cyst	None	Adults; rarely children	Usually unilateral	Single cyst or few cysts usually in the cortex	Nondescript lining	None
Dialysis cystic disease	None	Adults on long-term dialysis	Bilateral	Multiple cysts throughout cortex	Flattened tubular epithelial lining	Increased incidence of renal adenocarcinoma

some part of the tubule that has lost its communication with the rest of the tubule. Most of the cysts are lined by flattened tubular epithelium.

ADULT POLYCYSTIC DISEASE

Adult polycystic disease is a relatively common inherited disorder affecting one of every 500 individuals and accounting for 5–10% of chronic dialysis patients and 5–10% of transplantation procedures for chronic renal failure. The pathogenesis is unknown.

Grossly, both kidneys are replaced by a mass of cysts involving both cortex and medulla (Fig 47–4). Microscopically the cysts are lined by renal tubular epithelium, both proximal and distal. Residual nephrons are progressively destroyed.

Patients with adult polycystic disease have increased frequency of cysts in the liver (about 30% of cases), pancreas, and spleen and, in 15% of cases, congenital (berry) aneurysms of cerebral arteries.

Clinically, patients present in adult life with hypertension, chronic renal failure, or hematuria. Acute infections occur with increased frequency.

The only available treatments are dialysis or transplantation.

INFANTILE POLYCYSTIC DISEASE

Infantile polycystic disease is a rare autosomal recessive disorder manifested as severe renal failure in infancy. The cut surface of the kidney shows innumerable radially oriented fusiform cysts lined by cuboidal epithelium. There is no normal renal parenchyma. Infantile polycystic disease is believed to result from failure of communication between the nephron and the pelvicaliceal system during development.

Many patients have associated bile duct dilatations (microhamartomas) as well as portal fibrosis (congenital hepatic fibrosis). In some patients, the liver changes dominate.

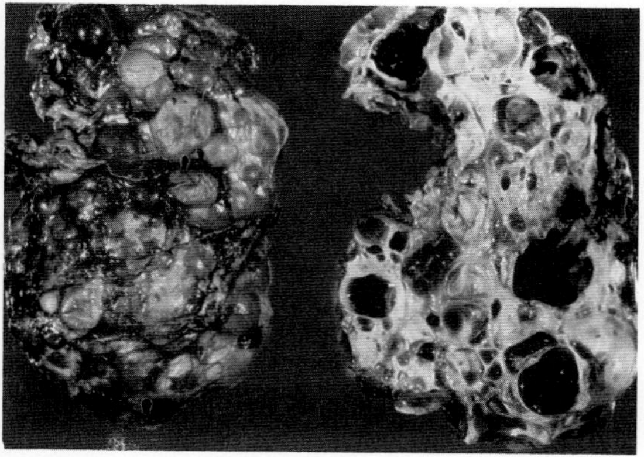

Figure 47–4. Adult polycystic disease of the kidneys. One kidney has been bisected to show both external (left) and internal (right) surfaces. Note multiple cysts with loss of renal substance.

MEDULLARY CYSTIC DISEASE

Medullary cystic disease affects the medulla selectively. Two separate conditions are recognized.

Medullary sponge kidney is relatively common, occurring in one or both kidneys of older patients (40–60 years). Small cysts are present in the renal papillae. The pathogenesis is unknown, and there are usually no symptoms. The frequency of urinary calculi is increased. Some patients have defective sodium reabsorption in the tubule.

Uremic medullary cystic disease is a rare disease of children and young adults characterized by the presence of multiple cysts in the medulla, cortical tubular atrophy, and interstitial fibrosis. The pathogenesis is unknown. Chronic renal failure progresses to death in 5–10 years.

GLOMERULOCYSTIC DISEASE

This rare lesion affects infants and young children. The entire cortex of both kidneys is replaced by small cysts (< 1 cm) composed microscopically of dilated Bowman spaces in glomeruli. The glomerular tuft is compressed. Glomerulocystic disease is associated with progressive renal failure.

SIMPLE RENAL CYSTS

Simple cortical cysts are present in over 50% of patients after age 50 years. They may be multiple and large. The pathogenesis is unknown, and they are of no clinical significance. Large cortical cysts may be difficult to differentiate clinically and radiologically from cystic renal adenocarcinoma.

DIALYSIS CYSTIC DISEASE

Multiple renal cysts occur in as many as 60% of patients receiving long-term hemodialysis for chronic renal failure. The cause of this cystic change is unknown. There is an increased incidence of renal adenocarcinoma arising in dialysis cystic disease.

TUBULOINTERSTITIAL DISEASE

Tubulointerstitial diseases are a group of renal disorders characterized by primary abnormalities in the renal tubules or interstitium. There are 4 principal causes: infectious, toxic, metabolic, and immunologic.

The morphologic changes in tubulointerstitial disease include the following.

(1) Acute tubular necrosis, which if widespread causes acute renal failure.

(2) Atrophy of tubules, with fibrosis of the interstitium, associated with nephron loss and chronic renal failure.

(3) Interstitial inflammation, either acute, with numerous neutrophils in the tubules and interstitium (acute interstitial nephritis); or chronic, with lymphocytes, plasma cells, macrophages, and fibroblasts (chronic interstitial nephritis).

(4) Tubular basement membrane thickening, as occurs in diabetes, amyloidosis, and transplant rejection.

(5) Deposition of abnormal substances such as calcium, amyloid, urate, myeloma proteins, and oxalate in the tubules and interstitium.

INFECTIOUS DISEASES

ACUTE PYELONEPHRITIS

Incidence

Acute pyelonephritis is extremely common—more so in females than in males (10:1). Acute pyelonephritis occurs at all ages, with highest frequency during early sexual activity and during pregnancy.

Etiology

Acute pyelonephritis is a bacterial infection, usually ascending from the lower urinary tract. Hematogenous infection of the kidney is uncommon. Factors important in etiology are as follows (Fig 47–5):

(1) A short urethra, as in females.

(2) Stasis of urine from any cause. The high incidence of urinary infections during pregnancy is believed to be the result of increased serum levels of progesterone, which decreases activity of the urinary tract smooth muscle, promoting stasis of urine.

(3) Structural abnormalities in the urinary tract that promote stasis of urine or establish a communication between the urinary tract and an infected site, such as fistulous tracts between the urinary tract and intestine, skin, or vagina.

(4) Vesicoureteral reflux of urine. Fifty percent

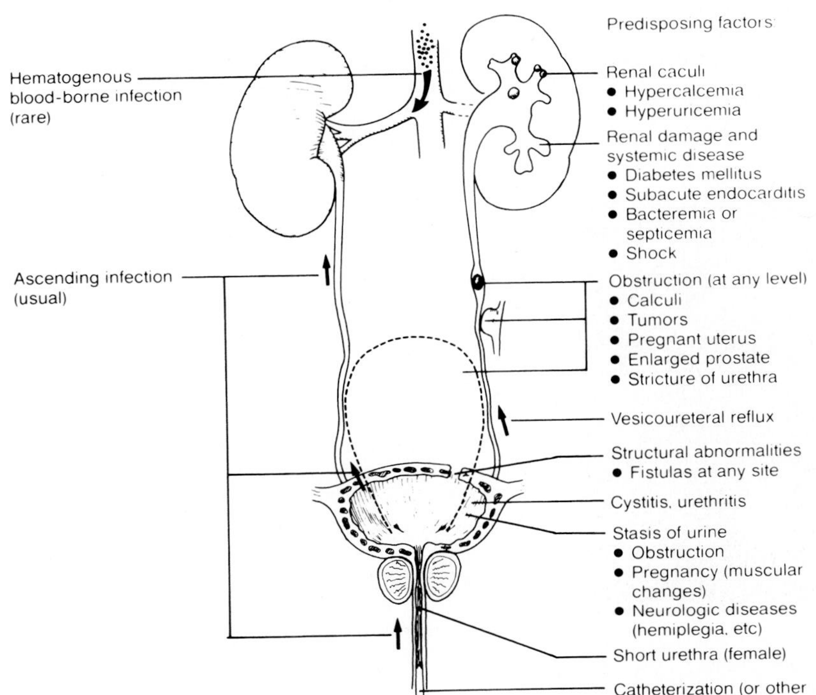

Figure 47–5. Etiologic factors associated with acute and chronic pyelonephritis.

of infants and young children with pyelonephritis show evidence of reflux, which is often familial and is due to an abnormality of the ureters entering the bladder wall.

(5) Catheterization of the bladder. Strict aseptic precautions must be taken, and even then an indwelling urinary catheter is almost invariably associated with infection.

(6) Diabetes mellitus.

Bacteriology

Seventy-five percent of cases of acute pyelonephritis are caused by *Escherichia coli.* When infections occur secondary to obstruction or catheterization, other organisms occur more often: *Klebsiella, Proteus, Streptococcus faecalis,* and *Pseudomonas aeruginosa.*

Postpubertal females have a significant incidence (5%) of asymptomatic bacteriuria (usually *E coli*), increasing to nearly 20% in pregnancy. The relationship of asymptomatic bacteriuria to acute pyelonephritis is not clearly established.

Pathology

Grossly, acute pyelonephritis may be unilateral or bilateral. The kidney is enlarged and shows areas of suppuration (abscesses) in the cortex with radial yellow streaks traversing the medulla (Fig 47–6). The renal pelvis is erythematous and frequently covered with exudate. Extension to the perinephric space to form a perinephric abscess is not uncommon.

Microscopically, there is an acute suppurative inflammation beginning in the renal tubules, which show infiltration by neutrophils and hyperemia (Fig 47–7). Liquefactive necrosis of the tubules (suppuration) follows. Involvement is characteristically patchy.

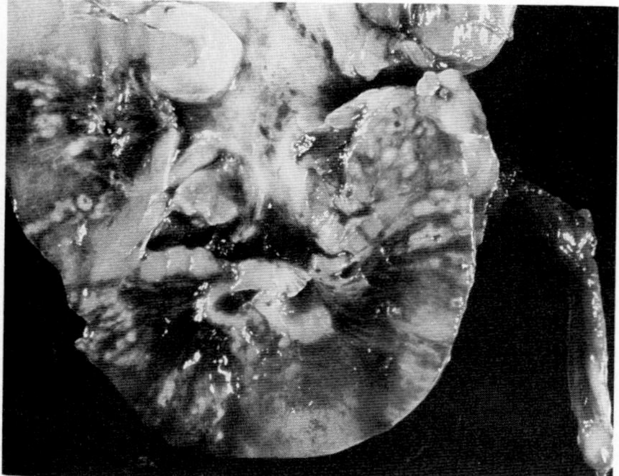

Figure 47–6. Acute pyelonephritis, showing diffuse hyperemia of the parenchyma and opened renal pelvis and multiple radially oriented suppurative streaks.

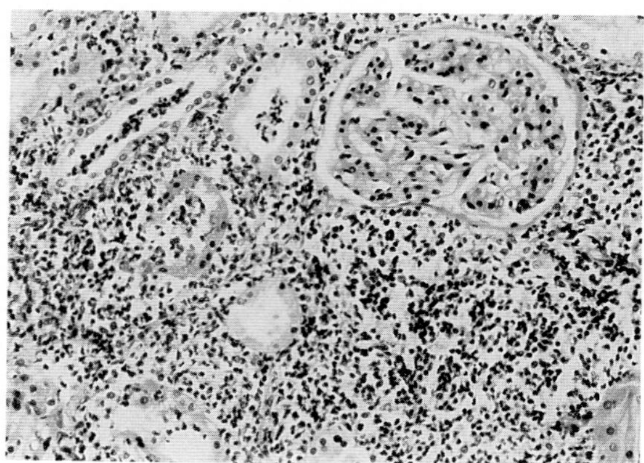

Figure 47–7. Acute pyelonephritis, showing replacement of renal tubules by acute inflammatory cells in the large part of the picture. An exudate with neutrophils is present in the lumens of some of the residual tubules.

Clinical Features

Onset is with high fever, chills, rigors, and flank pain. Dysuria and increased frequency are present in most cases.

The urine shows mild proteinuria, with neutrophils, white cell casts, and bacteria in the sediment (Table 47–4). The diagnosis is made by quantitative urine culture (colony count). A positive culture with over 100,000 organisms/mL is diagnostic. (Quantitative bacterial counts are necessary because although urine is normally sterile, it is almost always contaminated during collection, particularly in females. However, with a midstream "clean catch" specimen, colony cell counts above 100,000/mL usually indicate significant infection. Note that for these reasons urine should be cultured fresh—or stored at 4 °C if delay is unavoidable.)

Treatment & Prognosis

Treatment with antibiotics is effective. In an uncomplicated case, an antibiotic is selected that has activity against *E coli* (ampicillin or trimethoprim-sulfamethoxazole). When culture and antibiotic sensitivity results are available, the antibiotic may be changed accordingly.

The prognosis is excellent. Most patients recover completely, and there are no long-term sequelae from a single episode. Recurrent attacks are associated with increasing fibrosis and may lead to chronic pyelonephritis.

Complications

A. Gram-Negative Sepsis With Shock: Blood culture is frequently positive in patients with acute pyelonephritis. In a few cases, bacteremia is severe and causes gram-negative shock. The mortality rate is then high.

B. Renal Papillary Necrosis: Patients with diabetes mellitus who develop acute pyelonephritis tend to have more severe disease characterized by renal papillary necrosis (extreme inflammation of the papillae, which become necrotic and slough into the calyces).

C. Emphysematous Pyelonephritis: This disorder, characterized by anaerobic bacterial fermentation of glucose with gas formation in the renal parenchyma, occurs rarely in diabetic patients. Radiologic visualization of gas in the renal parenchyma is the basis for clinical diagnosis. Emphysematous pyelonephritis is a severe infection, often complicated by gram-negative shock and death. It is an indication for emergency nephrectomy.

CHRONIC PYELONEPHRITIS

Incidence & Etiology

Infectious pyelonephritis accounts for 15–20% of cases of chronic renal failure. Several different etiologic factors are recognized (Fig 47–5).

A. Chronic Obstructive Pyelonephritis: Chronic obstructive pyelonephritis is common and occurs at all ages in both sexes. Obstruction may be mechanical (eg, calculi, prostatic hyperplasia, tumors, congenital anomalies, retroperitoneal fibrosis) or paralytic (neurogenic [neuropathic] bladder). About 50% of patients give a history of a previous episode of acute pyelonephritis.

B. Chronic Pyelonephritis Associated With Vesico-ureteral Reflux: About 50% of children with vesicoureteral reflux develop chronic pyelonephritis; regurgitation of urine from the renal pelvis into the collecting tubules may be etiologically important. Early diagnosis of childhood vesicoureteral reflux (by voiding cystography) permits treatment to prevent chronic pyelonephritis.

C. Chronic "Nonobstructive" Pyelonephritis: Most cases previously classified as "nonobstructive" pyelonephritis have been found to have vesicoureteral reflux as their basis. A very small number of true nonobstructive cases occur, probably representing the end stage of a variety of noninfectious tubulointerstitial injuries.

Pathology (Fig 47–8)

Kidneys involved by chronic pyelonephritis usually show asymmetric involvement, with irregular scarring and contraction. Deformity of the pelvicaliceal system is common. Hydronephrosis and suppuration may be present in cases due to obstruction (chronic suppurative pyelonephritis).

Chronic pyelonephritis may be distinguished grossly from chronic glomerulonephritis by the asymmetry of renal involvement and the larger size of the cortical scars (pitted scarred kidney) in the former.

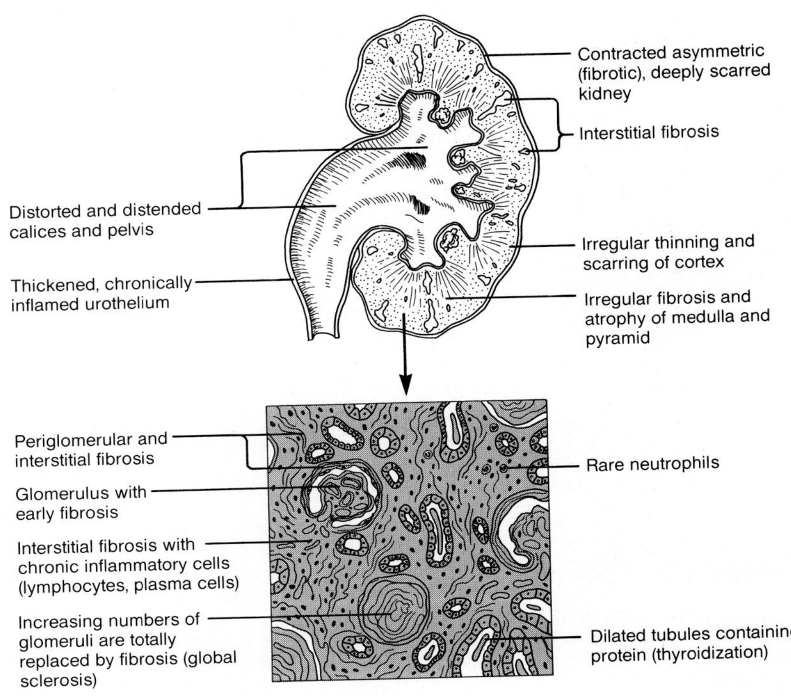

Figure 47–8. Pathologic features of chronic pyelonephritis.

Microscopically, there is marked patchy inflammation and fibrosis of the interstitium. The inflammatory cells are lymphocytes and plasma cells with scattered neutrophils. Periglomerular fibrosis later progresses to global sclerosis. Hypertrophy and dilatation of surviving tubules may be present (called thyroidization because superficially the numerous packed, dilated tubules resemble thyroid follicles). Immunofluorescence and electron microscopy do not show immune complex deposition in the glomeruli.

Cases in which lipid-laden foamy histiocytes are conspicuous are sometimes classified as **xanthogranulomatous pyelonephritis.** Xanthogranulomatous inflammation is associated with caliceal staghorn calculi. The inflammatory process frequently extends into the perinephric tissues and may involve adjacent organs (eg, colon, skin of the back, diaphragm, and pleura). Rarely, fistulas form between the renal pelvis and these organs.

Clinical Features

Chronic pyelonephritis usually manifests as hypertension or chronic renal failure. Pyuria (neutrophils in urine), mild proteinuria, and bacteriuria are present. In end-stage pyelonephritis, bacteriuria may be absent, and differentiation from chronic glomerulonephritis then becomes difficult.

RENAL TUBERCULOSIS

Renal tuberculosis is uncommon in the United States and Western Europe but still occurs frequently in parts of the world where tuberculosis is endemic.

The kidneys are initially infected in the primary pulmonary stage by hematogenous dissemination (see Chapter 34). The bacilli remain dormant and become reactivated much later. Renal tuberculosis is most common in patients 20–50 years of age. Approximately half of patients with renal tuberculosis have a normal chest x-ray, the original infection having long since healed.

The lesion usually begins in the corticomedullary region as a caseous granuloma (tuberculoma). Multiple granulomas are common. The kidney is grossly enlarged, and cut section shows several yellow crumbling foci. With progression, the granuloma opens into the pelvicaliceal system, leading to discharge of the caseous material in the urine and cavitation of the lesion. Microscopically, there is central caseous necrosis surrounded by epithelioid cells, lymphocytes, and fibroblasts. Marked fibrosis is usually present. Acid-fast bacilli can be demonstrated in most cases.

Clinically, patients have a combination of chronic inflammatory and urinary symptoms: low-grade fever, weight loss, hematuria, frequency, and mild lumbar pain. The urine shows numerous neutrophils. Ordinary urine culture is sterile (leading to the misnomer "sterile pyuria"); however, culture for mycobacteria is positive and diagnostic.

LEPTOSPIROSIS (Weil's Disease)

Leptospirosis is an uncommon infection caused by a spirochete of the genus *Leptospira,* most commonly *L icterohaemorrhagiae* (Table 47–10). Humans are infected by contact with infected rat urine, usually in occupations that necessitate working in open trenches, fields, or sewers, and recognition of this hazard is important in these groups.

Pathologically, there is focal renal tubular necrosis with interstitial infiltration by lymphocytes, histiocytes, and plasma cells. Leptospirae can be demonstrated in the tubules by silver stains.

Clinical onset is abrupt, with high fever, oliguria, proteinuria, and hematuria. Jaundice may occur as a result of liver involvement. Death may occur from acute renal failure. Meningitis, con-

Table 47-10. Leptospiral diseases.[1]

	Source: Urine of–	Clinical Findings[2]
L icterohaemorrhagiae	Rats, other rodents	Jaundice, nephritis, meningitis, petechiae
L canicola	Dogs	"Influenzalike"; meningitis
L bovis	Cattle	"Flulike"
L pomona	Swine, cattle	Meningitis
Other *Leptospira* species	Rodents, swine	Various fevers and flulike illnesses; Fort Bragg fever, etc

[1]Distribution is worldwide (some species are locally restricted), and infection of humans is usually by drinking or swimming in water contaminated by animal urine.
[2]Diagnosis: (a) Culture: Fletcher's or Stuart's media; (b) inoculation into young hamsters or guinea pigs; (c) microscopy: silver and Giemsa stains; (d) serology: rising titers of agglutinating antibody.

junctivitis, myositis, and myocarditis may also be present, with widespread petechial hemorrhages. The diagnosis is made by blood culture and demonstration of rising titers of specific agglutinating antibody.

If the patient recovers, the kidneys return to normal.

MALARIA

Plasmodium falciparum (malignant tertian) malaria (see Chapter 25) may cause (1) acute glomerulonephritis of immune complex type or (2) blackwater fever, so-called because of the passage of dark urine resulting from severe intravascular hemolysis and hemoglobinuria. Tubular damage may occur with acute renal failure.

Plasmodium malariae (quartan) malaria causes thickening of the basement membrane with deposition of immune complexes, leading to diffuse sclerosis of glomeruli, nephrotic syndrome, and chronic renal failure.

TOXIC TUBULOINTERSTITIAL DISEASE

RADIATION NEPHRITIS

Radiation nephritis occurs when the kidneys are in the field of radiation during treatment of malignant neoplasms. The dose required to produce radiation nephritis is about 23 Gy—lower in children or when radiation is given in combination with cytotoxic drugs.

Pathologically, the main changes are in the small arteries, which show fibrinoid necrosis. Tubular atrophy and interstitial fibrosis follow.

ANALGESIC NEPHROPATHY

Excessive use of analgesics is a relatively common cause of chronic renal disease in Australia and Europe but is rare in the United States. Analgesic nephropathy was first described following the use of analgesic "powders" containing phenacetin, aspirin, and caffeine. Phenacetin is believed to be the main offender.

Pathologically, analgesic nephropathy is characterized by necrosis of the apices of the renal papillae (renal papillary necrosis), which may be shed in the urine, causing ureteral colic (Fig 47–9). Interstitial medullary fibrosis and calcification may also occur. The mechanism of necrosis of renal papillae is unknown.

Clinically, there is hematuria, ureteral colic, hypertension, and progressive renal failure. The diagnosis may be suspected radiologically by the presence of calcification in the renal papillary region. In some cases, the shed necrotic renal papilla may be identified in a sample of urine.

DRUG-INDUCED NEPHROTOXICITY

Acute Interstitial Nephritis

Several drugs cause acute interstitial nephritis. Methicillin, other penicillin derivatives, sulfonamides, and various diuretics have been incriminated. Many cases show features of an immune hypersensitivity reaction. Immunofluorescence shows linear deposition of IgG, C3, and part of the methicillin molecule in the tubular basement membrane in methicillin-induced cases.

Pathologically, there is tubular degeneration and necrosis and marked inflammation of the interstitium with lymphocytes, plasma cells, and eosinophils.

Clinically, patients develop renal symptoms about 2 weeks after exposure to the drug. Fever, hematuria, proteinuria, skin rash, and eosinophilia are common. Acute renal failure develops

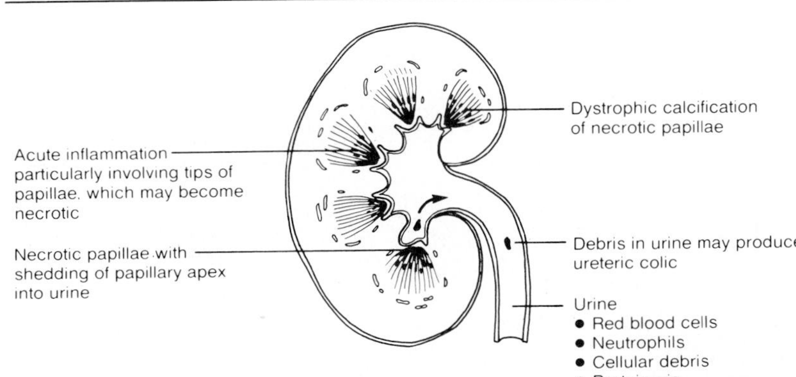

Figure 47–9. Analgesic nephropathy with renal papillary necrosis and calcification.

in 50% of cases. Recovery usually occurs when the drug is withdrawn.

Acute Renal Tubular Necrosis

Drug-induced acute renal tubular necrosis has been reported as a result of exposure to (1) aminoglycosides (gentamicin, kanamycin); (2) amphotericin B, an antifungal agent; (c) cephaloridine; and (4) methoxyflurane, an anesthetic agent.

Nephrotic Syndrome

Nephrotic syndrome may be caused by (1) mercurial compounds used as skin ointments and diuretics; (2) trimethadione, an antiepileptic drug; and (3) gold, used in the treatment of rheumatoid arthritis.

METAL TOXICITY

Mercury and lead poisoning result in renal damage. Mercurial compounds cause proximal convoluted tubule damage. Lead poisoning damages the entire tubule. The presence of intracytoplasmic and intranuclear eosinophilic inclusions in the cells is characteristic of lead poisoning. Both mercury and lead may cause acute or chronic renal failure.

"METABOLIC" TUBULOINTERSTITIAL DISEASES

GOUT (Urate Nephropathy)

Acute urate nephropathy occurs with very high serum uric acid levels; urate crystals deposited in the tubules cause obstruction. Chronic urate nephropathy occurs with protracted hyperuricemia, resulting in tubulointerstitial inflammation and fibrosis. Clinically, the manifestations are mild and progression slow.

HYPOKALEMIA

Hypokalemia causes tubular epithelial cell injury, leading to inability to concentrate urine, polyuria, loss of sodium in urine, and failure to excrete acid (renal tubular acidosis).

HYPERCALCEMIA

Acute hypercalcemia damages the distal convoluted tubular epithelium, resulting in failure to concentrate urine—manifested clinically as polyuria. With prolonged hypercalcemia, metastatic calcification occurs in the renal interstitium (nephrocalcinosis) and may lead to chronic renal failure.

Increased calcium excretion in the urine increases the risk of urinary calculi.

Table 47-11. Primary disorders of tubular function.

Disease	Defect	Comments
Renal tubular acidosis	Several forms; inability to absorb bicarbonate (proximal tubule) or excrete hydrogen ion (distal tubule)	Hyperchloremic metabolic acidosis with or without hypokalemia. Some forms inherited.
Vitamin D-resistant rickets	Inability to absorb phosphate	Hypophosphatemia, bone lesions of rickets in child and adult. X-linked dominant.
Nephrogenic diabetes insipidus	Tubular resistance to ADH;[1] excessive water loss	Presents in infants; inherited.
Cystinuria	Defective resorption of cystine (also lysine, arginine, and ornithine)	Recurrent renal (cystine) stones, infection.
Glycinuria	Defective resorption of glycine	Glycine stones.
Hartnup disease	Defective resorption of multiple amino acids, including phenylalanine, asparagine, and tyrosine	Skin rashes, ataxia.
Other aminoacidurias, including Fanconi's syndrome	Multiple tubular defects	Variable symptoms depending on amino acids lost; osteomalacia and mental retardation present in some cases.

[1]ADH = antidiuretic hormone.

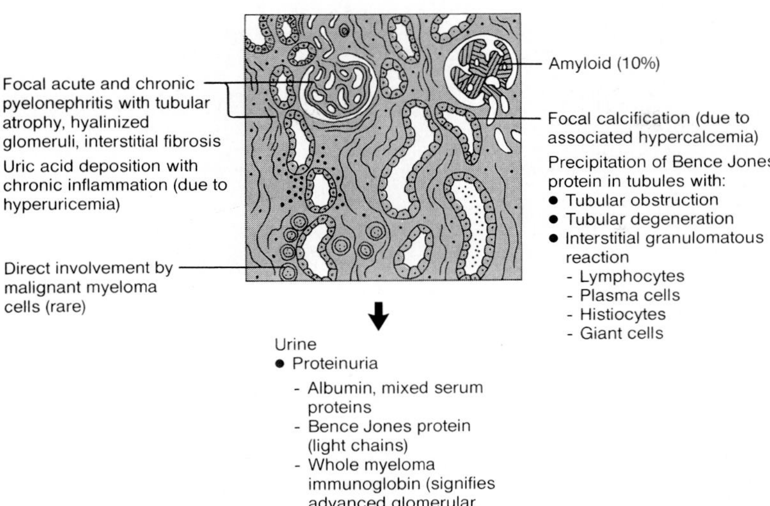

Figure 47-10. Pathologic features of the kidney in plasma cell myeloma.

MYELOMATOSIS ("Myeloma Kidney") (Fig 47-10)

Although not strictly a metabolic disease, plasma cell myeloma results in a renal interstitial disease caused by an interstitial granulomatous reaction to immunoglobulin light chains (Bence Jones proteins) in the renal tubules, interstitial calcification resulting from the accompanying hypercalcemia and vulnerability to infection. Renal interstitial involvement occurs commonly in myelomatosis, and renal failure is sometimes the cause of death in these patients. Bence Jones protein is deposited in the distal convoluted and collecting tubules as homogeneous eosinophilic casts surrounded by giant cells. Blockage of tubules results, causing renal dysfunction. Rarely, functional tubular failure, characterized by inability to absorb glucose, amino acids, and phosphate occurs (Fanconi's syndrome). Amyloidosis may also complicate myelomatosis. Patients with myelomatosis have an increased incidence of urinary calculi due to frequently elevated serum concentrations of calcium and uric acid.

DISORDERS OF TUBULAR FUNCTION

Tubular transport mechanisms are compromised in various tubulointerstitial diseases such as acute renal tubular necrosis. In addition, individual transport mechanisms may be impaired, leading to specific metabolic abnormalities (Table 47–11); these occur without associated morphologic changes.

IMMUNOLOGIC TUBULOINTERSTITIAL DISEASE

Immunologic mechanisms involving the renal tubules include transplant rejection (see Chapter 8) and some cases of drug-induced acute interstitial nephritis. The latter is discussed under drug-induced nephrotoxicity (see above).

48 The Kidney: II. Glomerular Diseases

This group of renal diseases is characterized by primary abnormalities of the glomerulus, both structural (inflammation, cellular proliferation, basement membrane thickening, fibrosis, epithelial cell changes) and functional (increased permeability causing proteinuria or hemorrhage of glomerular origin). Glomerular diseases may be acute or chronic.

The classification of glomerulonephritis is complicated and still evolving. As applied presently, the classification uses a combination of clinical (congenital or acquired; acute or chronic), morphologic (proliferative, membranous, minimal change), and immunologic criteria (Table 48–1).

Pathologic Changes

Glomerular diseases may be **focal,** showing abnormality in some but not all the glomeruli; or **diffuse,** where all glomeruli are affected. In **segmental** glomerular involvement, only a portion of each individual glomerulus is affected, in contrast to a **global** change, which involves entire glomeruli. Combinations of these terms are commonly used; eg, in focal segmental involvement the abnormality is present in some but not all glomeruli and the affected glomeruli are only partially involved.

Identification of exact morphologic changes in the glomerulus in renal biopsy specimens is important in the differential diagnosis of glomerular diseases (Fig 48–1). Some knowledge of these changes is necessary, because different glomerular diseases show varying combinations of these same basic features.

A. Proliferation of Cells in the Glomerulus: (Proliferative glomerulonephritis.) Any of the different cell types in the glomerulus may undergo proliferation in different diseases.

1. Mesangial cell proliferation is recognized by the presence of increased numbers of nuclei (in excess of 3) in the central part of a glomerular lobule. Mesangial cells are part of the phagocytic mechanism of the glomerulus.

2. Endothelial cell proliferation causes obliteration of the capillary lumen.

3. Epithelial cell proliferation, when extensive, leads to formation of a crescent-shaped mass of cellular or collagenized tissue that obliterates Bowman's space. Epithelial cell proliferation is believed to be stimulated by fibrin deposition in Bowman's space.

B. Infiltration of the Glomerulus by Inflammatory Cells: Infiltration with neutrophils, lymphocytes, and macrophages contributes to the appearance of glomerular hypercellularity that is present in many cases of acute proliferative glomerulonephritis. Acute inflammation is accompanied by fluid exudation and swelling of the glomerulus ("exudative glomerulonephritis").

C. Capillary Basement Membrane Thickening: Increased amounts of basement membrane material may be detected by light microscopy as a thickened capillary wall. The basement membrane can be specifically stained with silver stains and seen by electron microscopy. Basement membrane thickening is associated with deposition of immune complexes, immunoglobulins, and complement. Such deposition may be subepithelial, intramembranous, or subendothelial and is seen only by immunofluorescence and electron microscopy. Regardless of its cause, basement membrane thickening typically causes increased glomerular capillary permeability to proteins, leading to nephrotic syndrome.

D. Increased Mesangial Matrix Material: This pathologic picture is commonly due to deposition of immunoglobulins and complement in the

Table 48–1. Classification of glomerular diseases.

Congenital glomerulonephritis
Hereditary nephritis (includes Alport's syndrome)
Congenital nephrotic syndrome
Primary acquired glomerulonephritis (primary indicates that the renal involvement is the main manifestation of the disease)
Diffuse glomerulonephritis
Minimal change glomerulonephritis (glomerular epithelial cell disease)
Proliferative glomerulonephritis
Postinfectious (poststreptococcal) glomerulonephritis
Crescentic glomerulonephritis
Antiglomerular basement membrane disease (Goodpasture's syndrome)
Mesangial proliferative glomerulonephritis
Membranous glomerulonephritis
Membranoproliferative (mesangiocapillary) glomerulonephritis
Focal glomerulonephritis
Secondary acquired glomerulonephritis (secondary indicates that the renal involvement is part of a systemic disease such as systemic lupus erythematosus or progressive systemic sclerosis).
Chronic glomerulonephritis
Other glomerular diseases
Diabetic nephropathy
Amyloidosis

mesangium (positive staining on immunofluorescence and visible on electron microscopy).

E. Epithelial Foot Process Fusion: This feature can be seen only by electron microscopy. It is a nonspecific change that is believed to result whenever there is increased leakage of protein from the glomerular capillaries.

F. Fibrosis: Fibrosis (sclerosis) can affect part of the glomerulus (mesangium, Bowman's space) or may be global. Global sclerosis produces an obsolescent nonfunctioning glomerulus and is followed by atrophy and fibrosis of the corresponding nephron (tubules). It may follow any of the changes described above (Fig 48–1).

Pathogenesis of Glomerular Disease

Most forms of primary glomerular disease are caused by 2 principal immunologic mechanisms (Fig 48–2), sometimes acting in concert.

A. Immune Complex Disease (Type III Hypersensitivity): Immune complex disease is the most common cause of glomerular injury. Immune complexes are deposited on the glomerular filtration membrane or in the mesangium (Fig 48–2); complement fixation and inflammation follow.

Immune complex deposition may produce any or all of the pathologic features described above, one or the other predominating in different diseases (Table 48–2). Immunoglobulin and complement are demonstrable by immunofluorescence. The staining pattern on immunofluorescence is "lumpy-bumpy" (ie, irregular), corresponding to irregular deposition of the immune complexes. Immune complexes are visible with the electron microscope as electron-dense deposits.

B. Anti-Glomerular Basement Membrane Antibody (Type II Hypersensitivity): Deposition of anti-glomerular basement membrane antibodies on the basement membrane leads to complement fixation (Fig 48–2), with glomerular lesions that by light microscopy are identical to those seen in immune complex disease. Immunofluorescence, however, shows linear deposition of immunoglobulin and complement in the basement membrane.

Correlation between etiology, pathogenesis, pathologic change, and clinical outcome is poor (Table 48–2). **Hereditary defects** in basement membrane structure appear to be responsible for the renal changes in Alport's syndrome (dominant autosomal or X-linked pattern; associated with nerve deafness). Glomerular lesions of amyloidosis and diabetes are not caused by the mechanisms described above and will be discussed with those diseases later in this chapter.

MINIMAL CHANGE GLOMERULAR DISEASE (Epithelial Cell Disease)

Minimal change glomerular disease occurs most often in young children and is relatively rare in adults.

The cause and pathogenesis are unknown. A significant association between minimal change disease and allergic diseases suggests the possibility of a humoral immune mechanism.

Pathology

Light microscopy shows no abnormality (hence "minimal change"). Immunofluorescence shows absence of immunoglobulin or complement deposition. Electron microscopy shows fusion of the foot processes of the epithelial cells ("epithelial cell disease") (Fig 48–3; see also Fig 48–1). These changes disappear during remission.

Clinical Features

Minimal change disease is one of the most common causes of nephrotic syndrome, particularly in the young. The proteinuria is almost always **"highly selective,"** with loss of only low-molecular-weight proteins. "Selectivity" of proteinuria is assessed by the ratio of transferrin (low-MW) to IgG (high-MW) concentrations in urine. In highly selective proteinuria, the value is high; in nonselective proteinuria, it approaches 1. Hematuria, hypertension, and azotemia are absent.

Treatment & Prognosis

High-dosage corticosteroid therapy causes a dramatic decrease in proteinuria, with most pa-

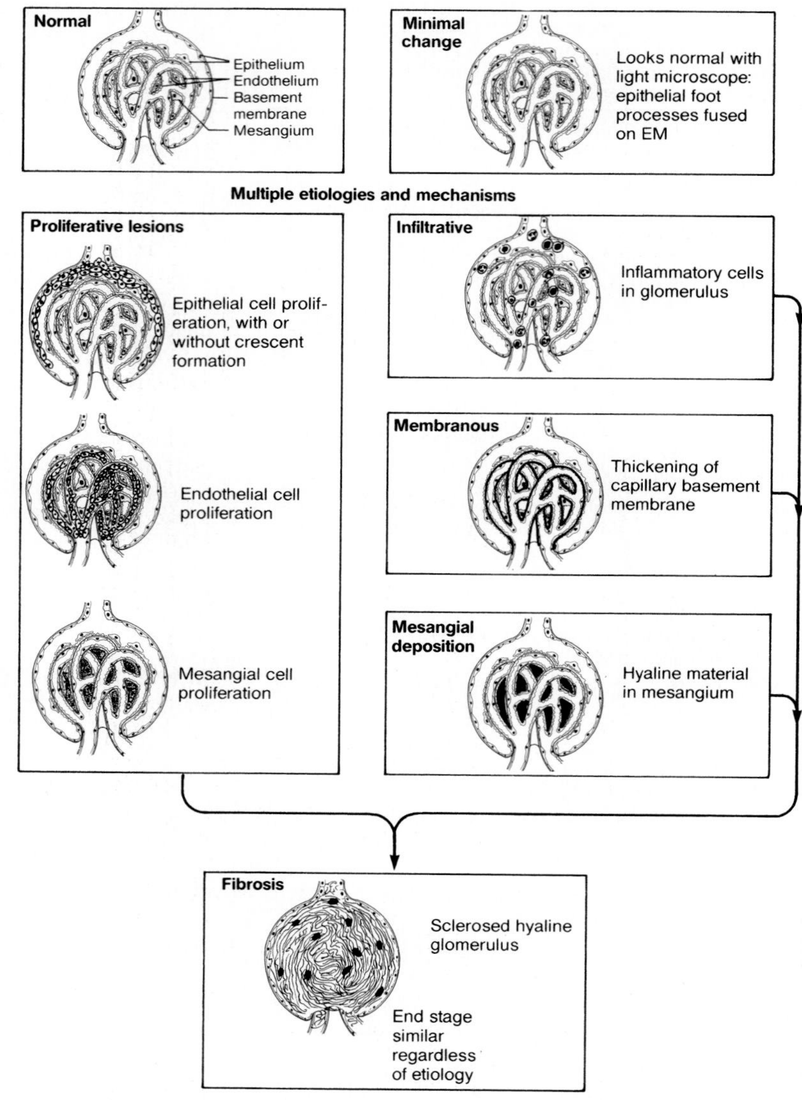

Figure 48–1. Basic pathologic changes that occur in glomerular diseases.

tients showing complete remission within 8 weeks. After withdrawal of steroids, about 50% of patients relapse intermittently for up to 10 years. Those who undergo relapses are steroid-sensitive; ie, each relapse responds well to steroid therapy.

Resistance to steroids or development of renal failure is rare and should prompt a search for some other diagnosis, usually focal glomerulosclerosis or membranoproliferative glomerulonephritis. The prognosis for life and renal function for patients with minimal change glomerular disease is almost the same as that of the general population.

POSTINFECTIOUS (POSTSTREPTOCOCCAL) GLOMERULONEPHRITIS (Acute Diffuse Proliferative Glomerulonephritis; Acute Exudative Nephritis)

Postinfectious glomerulonephritis is one of the most common renal diseases in childhood. It is less common in adults. Occurrence is worldwide, at times in epidemic distribution.

An infection precedes the glomerulonephritis by 1–3 weeks. In most cases, the infection is a group A beta-hemolytic streptococcal infection of the throat or skin. Not all streptococcal infections are associated with the risk of glomerulonephritis.

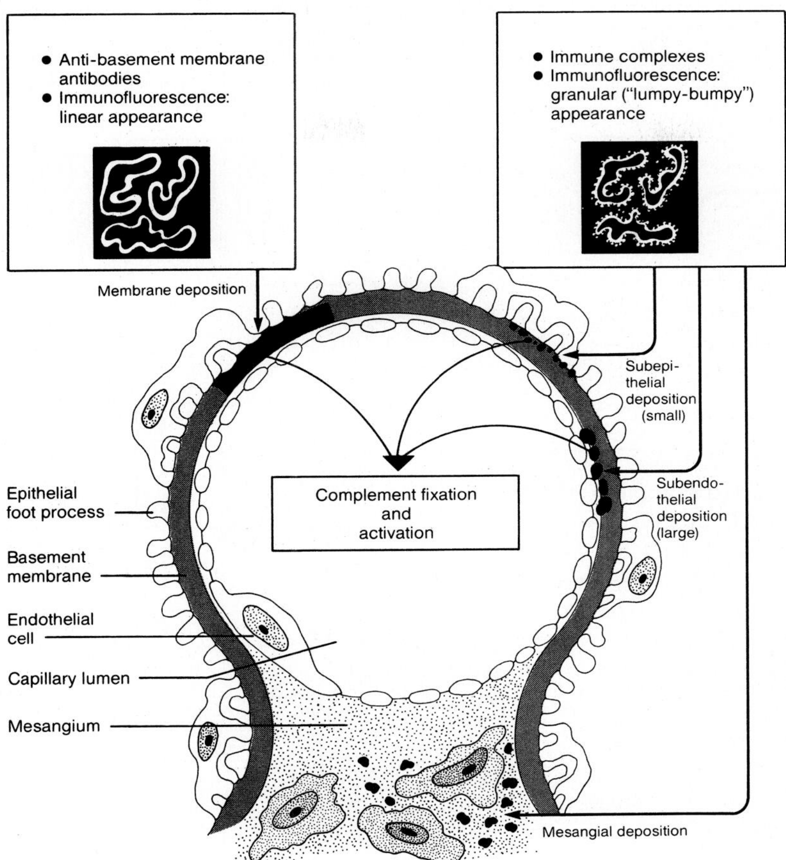

Figure 48-2. Basic types of glomerular injury resulting from (at left) the action of antiglomerular basement membrane antibody, and at right immune complex deposition. In both instances, complement activation results in damage. These 2 types of injury can be distinguished by their different staining patterns on immunofluorescence.

Certain streptococcal M types—especially types 12 and 49—are "nephritogenic."

Organisms other than beta-hemolytic streptococci may cause glomerulonephritis. Convincing data exist to incriminate *Staphylococcus aureus,* pneumococcus, meningococcus, and some viruses.

Immune complexes formed between antigens in the organism and host antibody are deposited in the glomerular filtration membrane, fix complement, and lead to inflammation.

Pathology

Grossly, the kidneys are slightly enlarged, with a smooth surface. In severe cases there are scattered petechial hemorrhages. Light microscopic examination shows diffuse glomerulonephritis. The glomeruli are enlarged, edematous, and hypercellular (Fig 48-4; see also Fig 48-1). The increased cellularity is due to proliferation of endothelial and mesangial cells plus infiltration with neutrophils and a few eosinophils. Epithelial proliferation producing crescents may be present in a few glomeruli. Rarely, crescent formation is extensive and results in rapidly progressive renal failure. Marked edema and endothelial swelling causes a narrowing of capillary lumens.

The immune complexes may be seen on light microscopy as characteristic "humps," particularly in trichrome-stained sections. These correspond to large, dome-shaped electron-dense deposits on the epithelial side of the basement membrane ("subepithelial humps") on electron microscopy (Fig 48-4). Deposits in other locations such as the mesangium and the subendothelial and intramembranous regions are frequently present.

Immunofluorescence shows a granular ("lumpy-bumpy") deposition of IgG and C3 along the glomerular basement membrane and in the mesangium (Fig 48-4).

Clinical Features

Most patients with postinfectious glomerulonephritis present with an abrupt onset of the acute nephritic syndrome, characterized by mild periorbital edema, hypertension, and elevated serum urea and creatinine. A few patients present with nephrotic syndrome.

Throat and skin cultures are usually negative because the streptococcal infection has usually re-

Table 48–2. Relationship of etiology, mechanisms, and clinical features of common glomerular diseases.

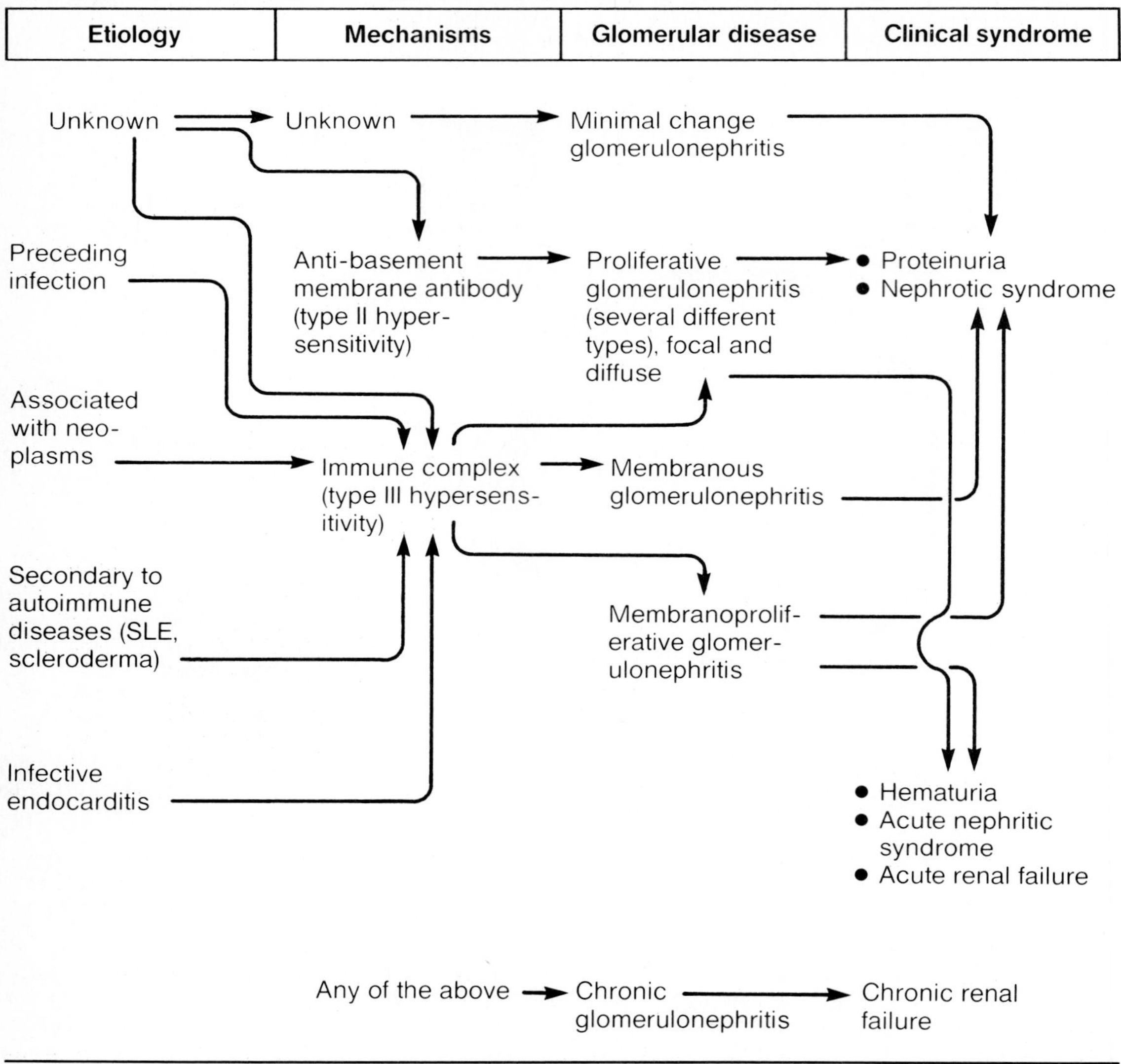

solved. Serum levels of antistreptococcal antibodies such as antistreptolysin O and antihyaluronidase are often elevated.

Treatment & Prognosis

Treatment is supportive. The short-term prognosis is excellent, most patients resuming normal renal function and blood pressure within a year. Abnormalities in urinary sediment may persist for several years. A small number of patients progress rapidly to renal failure within 1–2 years. These cases are associated with the presence of numerous epithelial crescents (**crescentic glomerulonephritis**—see below).

The long-term prognosis is controversial. Most studies indicate that children with postinfectious glomerulonephritis do not suffer progressive renal disease; however, a few studies report an increased incidence of chronic renal failure after initial resolution.

The prognosis is much worse (1) in adults, in whom chronic disease occurs in about half of cases; and (2) in patients who have an atypical clinical presentation.

CRESCENTIC GLOMERULONEPHRITIS (Proliferative Glomerulonephritis With Extensive Crescent Formation; Rapidly Progressive Glomerulonephritis; Subacute Glomerulonephritis)

Crescentic glomerulonephritis is a rare disease defined by the presence of epithelial crescents in

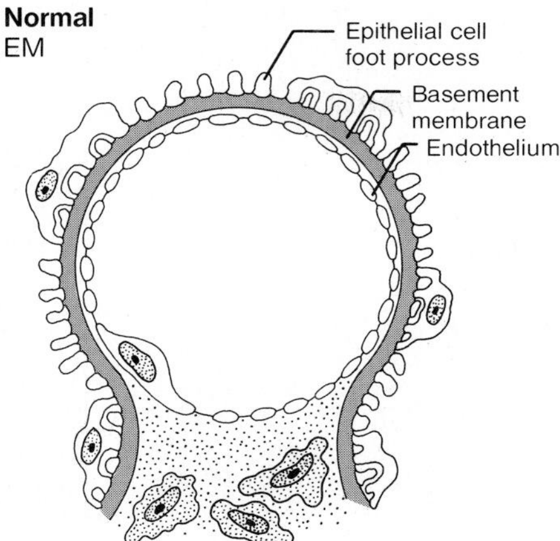

Minimal change glomerulonephritis
EM

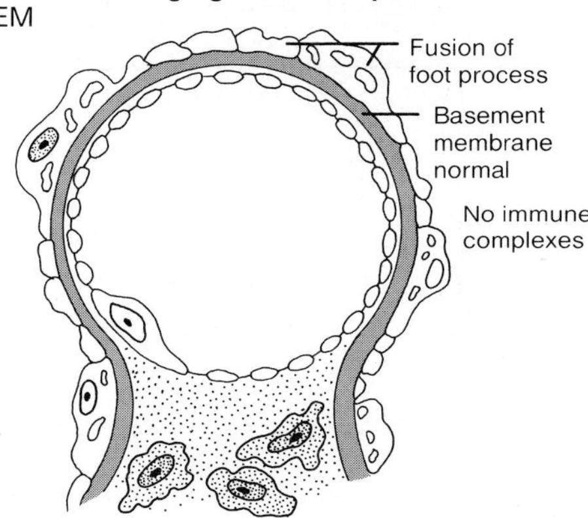

Immunofluorescence
- No immunoglobin or complement detectable
- Light microscopy looks normal

Figure 48-3. Minimal change glomerular disease. The only abnormality is fusion of epithelial foot processes, which is visible only by electron microscopy. Note that fusion of foot processes is not a specific abnormality.

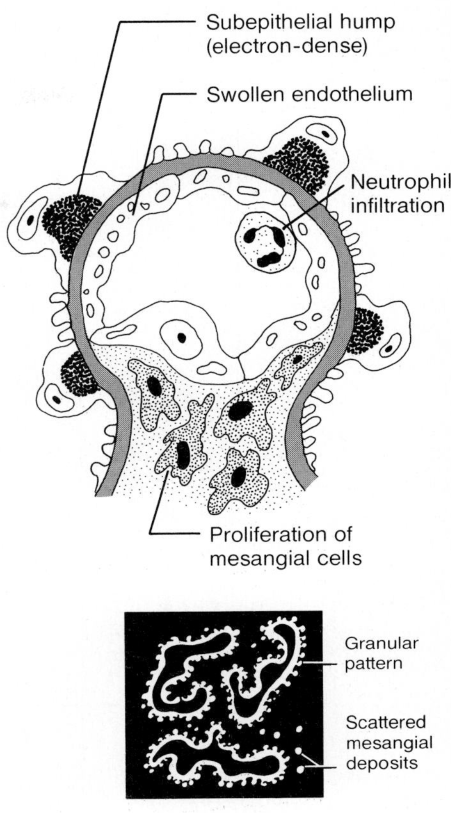

Figure 48-4. Poststreptococcal glomerulonephritis, characterized by the deposition of electron-dense immune complexes in the subepithelial and mesangial regions. Complement activation leads to proliferation of cells and inflammation.

more than 80% of the glomeruli. An epithelial crescent is a proliferation of epithelial cells in Bowman's space (Fig 48-5; see also Fig 48-1); it occurs in severe glomerular damage, frequently associated with visible necrosis. Crescents represent irreversible damage that always causes severe residual scarring of the affected glomerulus. Fibrin can be demonstrated in the crescent and is thought to induce its formation. Experimentally, anticoagulants prevent crescent formation.

In most cases of crescentic glomerulonephritis there is no known cause, and the causes are probably diverse. A few cases occur secondary to other diseases such as postinfectious glomerulonephritis and Goodpasture's syndrome (see below). In a few cases, anti-glomerular basement membrane antibodies are found in the serum.

Pathology

Eighty percent of glomeruli must show crescent formation for this diagnosis to be made, since scattered crescents are present in many glomerular diseases. Immunofluorescence studies show variable findings (Table 48-3). IgA and C3 may be present in some cases. Electron microscopy shows varying destructive changes in the glomeruli.

Treatment & Prognosis

Treatment is unsatisfactory, and the prognosis is very poor. A few cases of occurrence of the disease in transplanted kidneys have been reported.

Table 48–3. Differential features of glomerular disease.

Disease	Usual Clinical Findings	Proliferative	Membranous	Immunofluorescence				Electron Microscope	Diffuse/ Focal	Mechanism
				Pattern	Ig	Complement	Fibrin			
Minimal change glomerular disease (lipoid nephrosis)	Nephrotic syndrome	–	–	–	–	–	–	Foot process fusion	Diffuse	Unknown
Proliferative glomerulonephritis Poststreptococcal glomerulonephritis	Acute nephritic syndrome, nephrotic syndrome	+ Crescents (occasionally)	–	Granular	IgG	+	–	Subepithelial humps	Diffuse	Immune complex
Crescentic glomerulonephritis	Acute nephritic syndrome, rapidly progressive	+ Crescents	–	Granular or linear	IgG/ IgA	+	+	Variable deposits	Diffuse	Immune complex or basement membrane antibody
Anti-basement membrane disease (Goodpasture's syndrome)	Acute nephritic syndrome	+ Crescents	±	Linear	IgG	+	+	Thick basement membrane	Focal→ diffuse	Basement membrane antibody (also lung)
Mesangioproliferative glomerulonephritis IgG	Proteinuria, hematuria				IgG	+	–			
IgA (Buerger's disease)	Nephrotic syndrome, proteinuria, hematuria, acute nephritic syndrome	+ Mesangial	–	Mesangial	IgA	+	–	Mesangial deposits	Diffuse	Immune complex
IgA (Henoch-Schönlein purpura)	Nephrotic syndrome, proteinuria, hematuria, acute nephritic syndrome				IgA	+	+			
Membranous glomerulonephritis	Proteinuria, nephrotic syndrome, chronic renal failure	–	+	Granular	IgG	±	–	Subepithelial deposits, spikes, split basement membrane	Diffuse	Immune complex; probably formed in situ

Membranoproliferative glomerulonephritis (mesangiocapilary) I	Acute nephritic syndrome, nephrotic syndrome	+ Edothelial, mesangial	+	Granular	IgG	+	–	Subendothelial deposits, split basement membrane	Diffuse	Immune complex
II	Nephrotic syndrome, chronic renal failure			Granular	–	+	–	Thick basement membrane, dense deposits	Diffuse	Immune complex; probably alternative pathway
Focal glomerulonephritis	Proteinuria, nephrotic syndrome	+ Focal	±	Granular	IgM, IgA	+	+	Foot process fusion	Focal plus segmental	?Immune complex
Secondary glomerulonephritis, systemic lupus erythematosus, polyarteritis nodosa, etc	Variable	Variable +	Variable + (wireloops in systemic lupus erythematosus)	Granular	IgG	+	+	Variable	Diffuse/ focal	Immune complex
Chronic glomerulonephritis	Chronic renal failure	Any of above		Granular, linear: variable				Variable	Diffuse	Immune complex/antibasement membrane antibody
Diabetic nephropathy	Nephrotic syndrome, chronic renal failure	–	Focal sclerosis	None	–	–	–	Sclerosis	Diffuse/ focal	Unknown
Amyloidosis	Nephrotic syndrome, chronic renal failure	–	+	None	–	–	–	Fibrillar amyloid	Diffuse	Deposition of amyloid protein

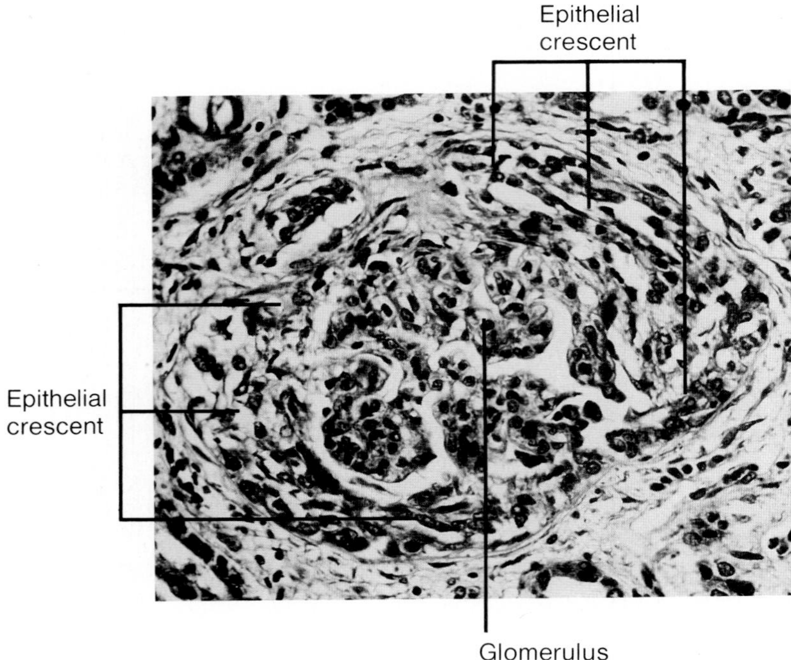

Figure 48-5. Glomerulus, showing an epithelial crescent.

ANTI-GLOMERULAR BASEMENT MEMBRANE DISEASE (Goodpasture's Syndrome; Proliferative Glomerulonephritis With Pulmonary Hemorrhage)

Goodpasture's syndrome is rare. It occurs in young adults, with males affected more frequently than females.

The serum contains anti-glomerular basement membrane antibodies of IgG type. These antibodies bind to both kidney and pulmonary alveolar basement membrane. Antibody binding to antigens on the glomerular basement membrane causes complement fixation (type II hypersensitivity) and a proliferative glomerulonephritis.

Pathology

Light microscopy initially shows a focal proliferative glomerulonephritis. In the later stages, diffuse glomerular involvement occurs. Proliferative changes are frequently associated with necrosis and epithelial crescent formation. Sclerosis becomes prominent in the late stages.

Immunofluorescence shows IgG and C3 deposition in a characteristic diffuse linear pattern along the basement membrane (Fig 48–2). C3 deposition is important for the diagnosis, linear IgG deposition alone being a nonspecific change in many conditions, notably diabetes mellitus. Similar linear C3 and IgG deposition is present in basement membranes in the lung in patients with Goodpasture's syndrome.

Electron microscopy shows diffuse and irregular thickening of the glomerular basement membrane. The electron microscopic findings are nonspecific.

In most patients, the lungs show extensive alveolar damage and intra-alveolar hemorrhages with hemosiderin-laden macrophages present in large numbers in the alveoli (Chapter 35).

Clinical Features

Goodpasture's syndrome commonly presents with proteinuria and hematuria followed by progressive renal failure. Patients with pulmonary involvement have recurrent hemoptysis, with dyspnea, cough, and bilateral pulmonary infiltrates on x-ray. Some patients have only lung or only kidney involvement.

Chronic loss of blood in the urine and lungs may cause severe iron deficiency anemia.

Treatment & Prognosis

Treatment of Goodpasture's syndrome is unsatisfactory, and the prognosis is poor. Most cases progress to renal failure within 1 year after diagnosis.

MESANGIAL PROLIFERATIVE GLOMERULONEPHRITIS

Proliferation of mesangial cells as the only abnormality in a renal biopsy specimen is a nonspecific finding. Mesangial proliferative glomerulonephritis is best classified according to the type of immunoglobulin present in the glomerulus.

1. WITH IgG IN MESANGIUM

IgG deposition is common and may occur as an isolated finding or in the healing phase of postinfectious glomerulonephritis. The pathogenesis is unknown in most cases.

Light microscopy shows increased numbers of mesangial cells in the glomeruli (more than the normal 3 nuclei per lobule; see Fig 48–1). The mesangial matrix material is increased. Immunofluorescence shows the presence of IgG and C3 in the mesangium. Electron microscopy shows the presence of mesangial electron-dense deposits in some cases.

2. WITH IgA IN MESANGIUM

IgA Nephropathy (Berger's Disease)

Berger's disease accounts for 2–5% of all cases of primary glomerulonephritis in the United States and England. The incidence is much higher (up to 20%) in France and Australia. Berger's disease is most common in the age group from 10 to 30 years and has a marked male predominance.

On light microscopy, there is mesangial hypercellularity and increased matrix material. Sclerosis is common with progressive disease. Immunofluorescence shows IgA deposits in the mesangium as confluent masses or discrete granules. C3 is frequently present. Electron microscopy shows mesangial hypercellularity, sclerosis, and electron-dense deposits.

Clinically, patients present with hematuria, often at the time of an upper respiratory infection. Hematuria is recurrent. Proteinuria and microscopic hematuria commonly persist. Though progression of the disease is very slow, the ultimate prognosis is not good. Most patients progress to chronic renal failure after a mean interval of 6 years.

Henoch-Schönlein Purpura

Henoch-Schönlein purpura is a rare disease, mainly affecting children. It is characterized clinically by a systemic vasculitis affecting skin, joints, intestine, and kidneys. Renal involvement is common and may cause hematuria, proteinuria, acute renal failure, or nephrotic syndrome.

Light microscopy shows mesangial hypercellularity and epithelial crescents. Immunofluorescence shows the presence of IgA deposition in the mesangium. Electron microscopy shows mesangial deposits and hypercellularity.

Henoch-Schönlein purpura is a progressive disorder. About 20% of patients develop chronic renal disease.

MEMBRANOUS NEPHROPATHY (Epimembranous Glomerulonephritis; Membranous Glomerulonephritis)

Membranous nephropathy is an important and common cause of nephrotic syndrome in adults (mean age 35 years). It is rare in children.

Membranous nephropathy is believed to result from accumulation of circulating immune complexes in the glomerular capillary. The reason why immune complex deposition does not produce complement-mediated inflammation and proliferative changes is unknown. Also unknown is the nature of the antigen involved.

Thus, most cases of membranous nephropathy are idiopathic. A few cases are associated with (1) systemic infections, including hepatitis B, malaria, schistosomiasis, syphilis, and leprosy; (2) drugs such as penicillamine and heroin; (3) toxic metals such as gold and mercury; (4) neoplasms, including carcinomas, malignant lymphomas, and Hodgkin's lymphoma; (5) collagen diseases such as systemic lupus erythematosus, progressive systemic sclerosis, and mixed connective tissue disease; and (6) miscellaneous conditions including renal vein thrombosis and sickle cell disease.

Pathology

Light and electron microscopy permit recognition of 3 stages of the disease (Fig 48–6; see also Fig 48–1):

(1) Stage I is characterized by the deposition of dome-shaped subepithelial electron-dense deposits. At this stage, the basement membrane is near normal, and a misdiagnosis of minimal change glomerulonephritis may be made on light microscopy. Protein leakage from the glomerulus leads to epithelial foot process fusion, but membranous nephropathy can be distinguished from minimal change disease by the presence of electron-dense immune complex deposits.

(2) Stage II is characterized by spikes of basement membrane material protruding outward toward the epithelial side between the deposits, which are now larger. These basement membrane spikes are seen on light microscopy with silver stains (deposits are not stained).

(3) In stage III, the spikes enlarge and fuse on the epithelial side of the deposits; on silver stains, the basement membrane now appears split, connected by the spikes (giving an appearance on sil-

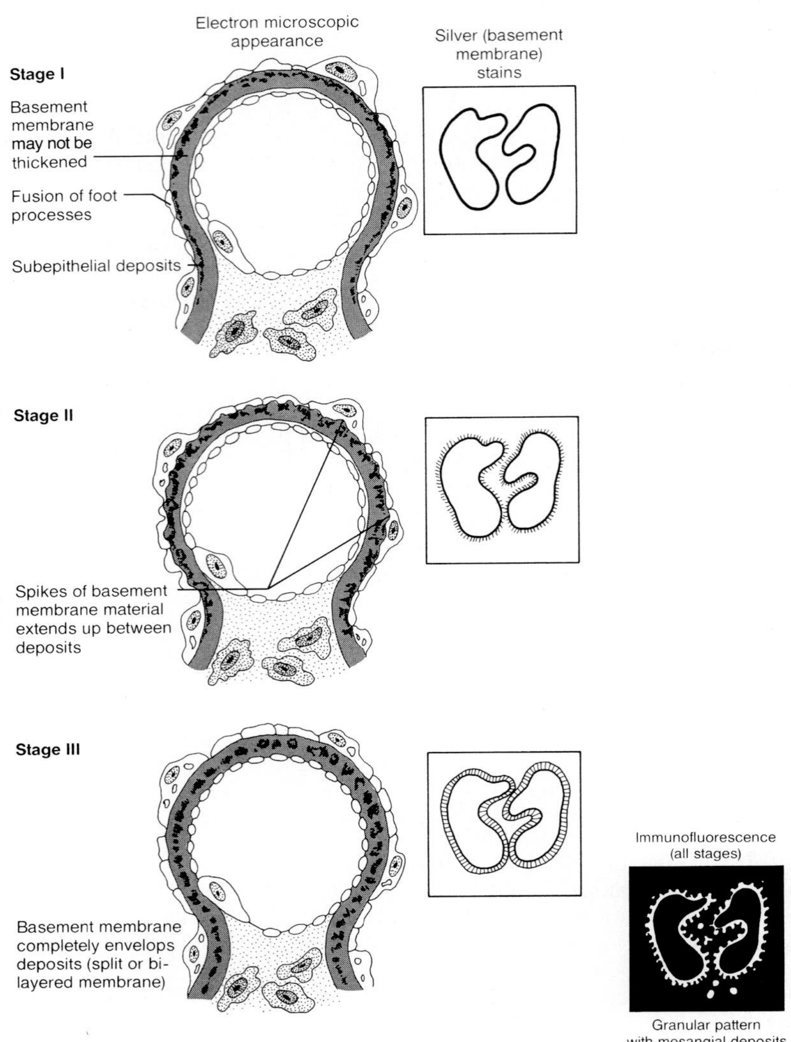

Figure 48-6. Membranous nephropathy. In stage I disease, light microscopy resembles minimal change disease but can be differentiated on electron microscopy and immunofluorescence because of the presence in membranous nephropathy of immune complexes. In later stages of the disease, protrusion of basement membrane material around the immune complexes produces spikes (stage II) and a bilayered appearance (stage III) when the basement membrane is stained with silver stains. Light microscopy shows thickened basement membrane in these later stages.

ver stain that has been likened to a chain with the unstained immune complex deposits appearing as bubbles or holes between the links of the chain). At this stage, basement membrane thickening can be detected on routine light microscopy (Fig 48–7).

There is no hypercellularity of the glomerulus in pure membranous nephropathy. With progression, increasing thickness of the basement membrane converts the glomerulus into a hyaline mass. The changes of idiopathic membranous nephropathy are identical to those of secondary disease.

Immunofluorescence shows granular deposits of IgG and C3 corresponding to the subepithelial deposits.

Clinically, patients with membranous nephropathy present with either the nephrotic syndrome or asymptomatic proteinuria. The proteinuria is nonselective. Even microscopic hematuria is absent in most cases.

Most patients have a slow progression to chronic renal failure. Recent evidence suggests that 70% of patients are alive at 10 years. The prognosis is better in females and much better in children.

MEMBRANOPROLIFERATIVE GLOMERULONEPHRITIS (Mesangiocapillary Glomerulonephritis; Hypocomplementemic Glomerulonephritis; Lobular Glomerulonephritis)

Membranoproliferative glomerulonephritis is characterized by the presence of a combination of

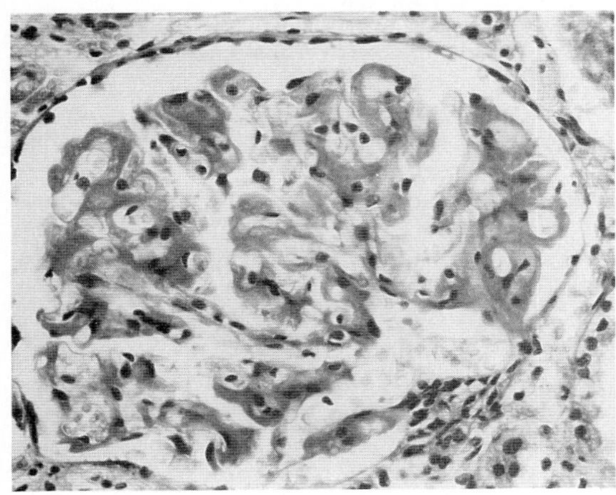

Figure 48–7. Membranous nephropathy, showing diffuse thickening of the glomerular basement membrane. Cellularity is normal.

thickening of the capillary wall and proliferation of mesangial cells. Two distinct patterns are recognized (Fig 48–8).

1. MEMBRANOPROLIFERATIVE GLOMERULONEPHRITIS TYPE I (With Subendothelial Deposits)

Type I membranoproliferative glomerulonephritis accounts for 65% of cases. It is characterized by deposition of subendothelial immune complexes in the glomerular capillary. Most cases have no known cause.

Light microscopy shows diffuse thickening of capillary walls and proliferation of mesangial cells. The basement membrane appears to be split (double-contour, or tram-track, appearance). Immunofluorescence shows granular deposition of IgG and C3 in the capillary wall. Electron microscopy shows the diagnostic subendothelial deposits.

Clinically, type I is a disease of children and young adults who present with nephrotic syndrome or a mixed nephrotic-nephritic pattern. Serum C3 levels are decreased in the majority of cases. Progression is variable, but the overall prognosis is poor.

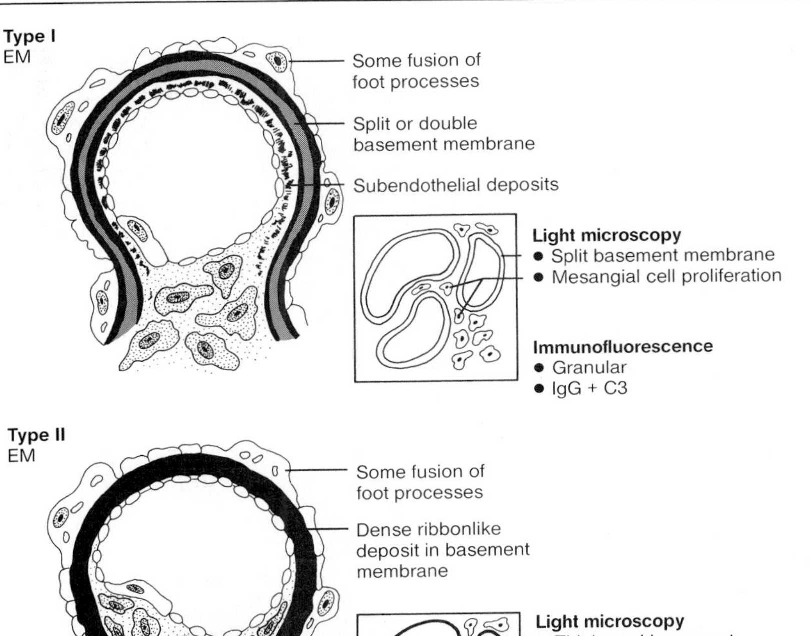

Figure 48–8. Membranoproliferative glomerulonephritis. Type I disease is characterized by subendothelial immune complexes, a split ("tram track") basement membrane, and deposition of IgG and C3. Type II is characterized by a densely thickened, ribbonlike basement membrane and the presence of C3 only on immunofluorescence.

2. MEMBRANOPROLIFERATIVE GLOMERULONEPHRITIS TYPE II ("Dense Deposit Disease")

Type II membranoproliferative glomerulonephritis accounts for the remaining 35% of cases. It is characterized by a dense intramembranous ribbonlike deposit on electron microscopy, leading to basement membrane thickening.

Light microscopy shows an eosinophilic, refractile, uniformly thickened basement membrane. Mesangial proliferation is less prominent than in type I. Immunofluorescence shows granular deposition of C3 in the capillary wall and mesangium. Immunoglobulins are not found.

Clinically, children and young adults tend to be affected most frequently. Presentation is identical to that of type I. Serum C3 levels are low, but C1q, C2, and C4 levels are normal, suggesting C3 activation by the alternative pathway. Many patients have a "C3 nephritogenic factor" in the serum—probably an immunoglobulin of the IgA class, which activates C3 by the alternative pathway. The prognosis is poor.

FOCAL GLOMERULOSCLEROSIS (Focal Sclerosing Glomerulonephritis; Segmental Hyalinosis)

Focal glomerulosclerosis is an uncommon disease that affects children and young adults predominantly. The cause is unknown. In a few patients, focal glomerulosclerosis is associated with intravenous heroin abuse, and a few cases have been described in patients with AIDS.

Pathology

Focal glomerulosclerosis is characterized by the presence of a focal segmental sclerotic area (pink hyaline material) in the peripheral part of the glomerulus, frequently near the hilum. The glomeruli affected first are in the juxtamedullary (deep cortical) region, and a superficial renal biopsy may easily miss the involved glomeruli, leading to a diagnosis of minimal change glomerulonephritis. (Many cases of "steroid-resistant" minimal change glomerulonephritis prove to be focal glomerulosclerosis.)

Immunofluorescence shows granular IgM, C3 and sometimes IgA, and fibrinogen deposition in the affected glomeruli. Electron microscopy shows an increase in the amount of mesangial matrix and collapse of the glomerular capillaries in areas of glomerulosclerosis. Epithelial cell foot processes are fused.

Clinical Features

Focal glomerulosclerosis is associated with nephrotic syndrome or asymptomatic proteinuria. The proteinuria is nonselective. Prognosis is poor, with slow progression to chronic renal failure. There is no response to corticosteroid therapy. A few patients have disease recurring in the allografts after renal transplantation.

SECONDARY ACQUIRED GLOMERULONEPHRITIS

Glomerulonephritis is a common manifestation of numerous collagen disorders and systemic vasculitides. These diseases are described elsewhere (Chapter 68), and only the renal manifestations are summarized here.

1. SYSTEMIC LUPUS ERYTHEMATOSUS (SLE)

Renal involvement (lupus nephritis) is the most common cause of death in SLE and the presenting feature in 5% of patients with SLE. Clinical manifestations include proteinuria, microscopic hematuria, nephrotic syndrome, acute nephritic syndrome, and renal failure. During the phase of active disease, serum complement levels are decreased.

Light microscopy shows a variety of changes (Table 48-4). Focal and diffuse proliferation of capillary endothelial cells is the most serious microscopic abnormality. Mesangial hypercellularity is commoner but less ominous. Diffuse or seg-

Table 48-4. World Health Organization categories of glomerular disease in systemic lupus erythematosus.

Class	Pathologic Change	% With Glomerulonephritis	Clinical Features
I	No change		Mild disease with microscopic hematuria or proteinuria; slow progression
II	Mesangial glomerulonephritis	10%	
III	Focal proliferative glomerulonephritis	30%	
IV	Diffuse proliferative glomerulonephritis	50%	Severe disease with rapid progression to renal failure
V	Diffuse membranous glomerulonephritis	10%	Nephrotic syndrome; slow progression to renal failure

mental basement membrane thickening produces the typical "wire loop" lesions (Fig 48–9) of SLE. Small, ill-defined basophilic bodies (hematoxyphil bodies) may rarely be found in areas of glomerular damage and are specific for SLE. Immunofluorescence shows lumpy IgG and C3 in the glomerular basement membrane and mesangium. Electron microscopy shows large immune complexes in the subendothelial, mesangial, and subepithelial regions. Wire loop lesions correspond with the presence of large subendothelial deposition of immune complexes and can be distinguished from membranous nephropathy of SLE in which there are subepithelial deposits.

The clinical features and prognosis depend on the histologic class of disease (Table 48–4). Eventually, most patients with SLE glomerular disease progress to chronic renal failure.

2. PROGRESSIVE SYSTEMIC SCLEROSIS (Scleroderma)

The kidneys are frequently involved in progressive systemic sclerosis, causing proteinuria that is sometimes severe enough to result in nephrotic syndrome, with progression to renal failure.

Light microscopy shows fibrinoid necrosis of the afferent arteriole and intimal fibrosis ("onion-skin" change) of the interlobular arteries. Glomeruli show fibrinoid necrosis and segmental basement membrane thickening ("wire loop" lesions) followed by sclerosis.

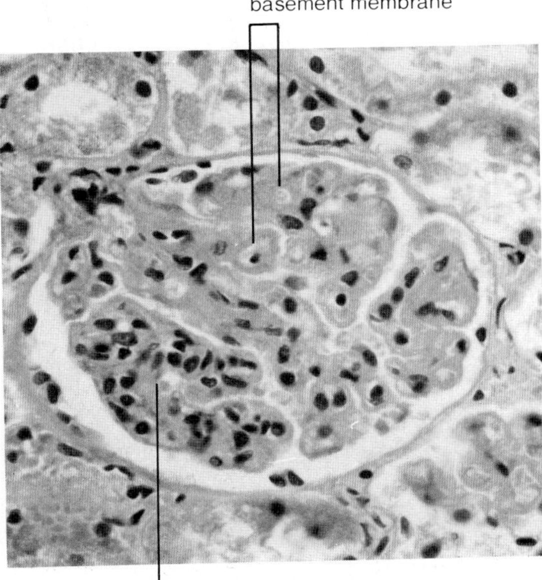

Figure 48–9. Systemic lupus erythematosus, showing focal mesangial cell proliferation and diffuse thickening of basement membrane.

Immunofluorescence shows granular deposits of IgM and C3 in the glomerular capillaries. Electron microscopy shows nonspecific changes.

3. MIXED CONNECTIVE TISSUE DISEASE (MCTD)

Renal involvement occurs in about 20–30% of cases of MCTD. Patients with renal disease have a very poor prognosis. Changes are mainly in glomeruli, which show a combination of proliferative and membranous glomerulonephritis.

4. POLYARTERITIS NODOSA

Renal involvement is present in 80% of cases of polyarteritis nodosa. Thirty percent of patients with polyarteritis nodosa die of renal failure.

Grossly, the kidneys are reduced in size and show evidence of infarction and multiple hemorrhages. Light microscopy shows fibrinoid necrosis, inflammation, thrombosis, aneurysm formation, and rupture of the segmental and arcuate arteries. The chronic lesions in the vessels are dominated by fibrosis of the wall and are not specific for polyarteritis.

Microscopically, glomeruli show fibrinoid necrosis and proliferative changes with crescents. Immunofluorescence shows immunoglobulin (mainly IgG) and fibrin in areas of fibrinoid necrosis. The increased incidence of serum positivity for hepatitis B surface antigen suggests that renal lesions are mediated by immune complexes formed with this antigen in some patients with polyarteritis.

Clinically, renal involvement is usually manifested as hematuria, proteinuria, and hypertension. Rapidly progressive renal failure is common.

5. WEGENER'S GRANULOMATOSIS

Renal involvement is one part of the classic triad of features of Wegener's granulomatosis—the others being upper respiratory tract and lung involvement. Renal disease occurs in 90% of cases and is characterized by proteinuria, hematuria, and rapidly progressive renal failure.

Light microscopy shows a necrotizing granulomatous arteritis involving small and medium-sized arteries. The glomeruli show a focal segmental proliferative glomerulonephritis. Fibrinoid necrosis, capillary thrombosis, and epithelial crescent formation are common. Immunofluorescence shows granular deposits of IgA, C3, and fibrin in the glomerular capillary wall, a pattern

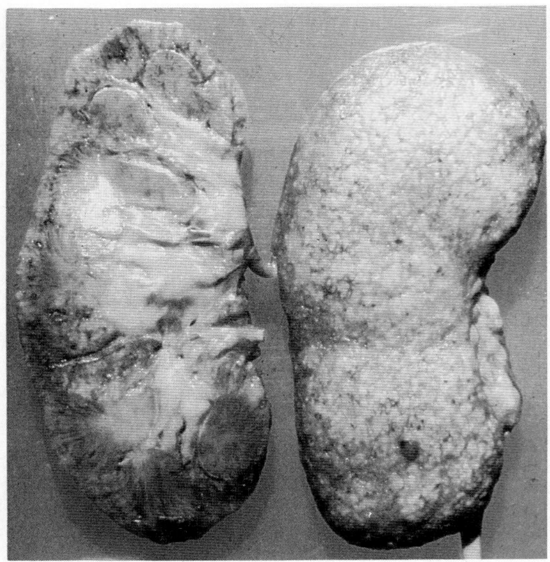

Figure 48-10. Chronic glomerulonephritis, showing a granular surface of the kidney. The cut surface shows a greatly thinned cortex and poor demarcation between cortex and medulla.

of staining that suggests mediation by immune complexes.

CHRONIC GLOMERULONEPHRITIS

Chronic glomerulonephritis is a common pathologic lesion in the kidney that probably represents the end stage of many diseases affecting glomeruli (Fig 48-1). Some patients give a past history suggestive of glomerular disease.

Grossly, the kidneys are greatly reduced in size, and the cortex shows a finely irregular surface ("granular contracted kidney"; Fig 48-10). The cortex is narrowed, corticomedullary demarcation is obscured, and the arteries stand out because of thickened walls.

Microscopically, the narrowed cortex shows a great decrease in number of nephrons. Glomeruli show diffuse sclerosis, many being converted to hyaline balls (Fig 48-11). There is atrophy of intervening tubules, and residual tubules often show dilatation and are filled with pink proteinaceous material ("thyroidization"). Interstitial fibrosis is present and may be severe.

Immunofluorescence and electron microscopy show variable changes. Less fibrotic glomeruli may show evidence of electron-dense deposits containing IgG, IgA, and C3. These are important in distinguishing chronic glomerulonephritis from other conditions such as hypertensive nephrosclerosis and chronic pyelonephritis that may result in sclerosis of glomeruli, granular contraction of the kidneys, and chronic renal failure. Immunoglobulin and complement deposition are not present in chronic pyelonephritis and hypertensive nephrosclerosis.

Clinically, patients show chronic renal failure and hypertension and frequently have microscopic hematuria, proteinuria, and sometimes nephrotic syndrome.

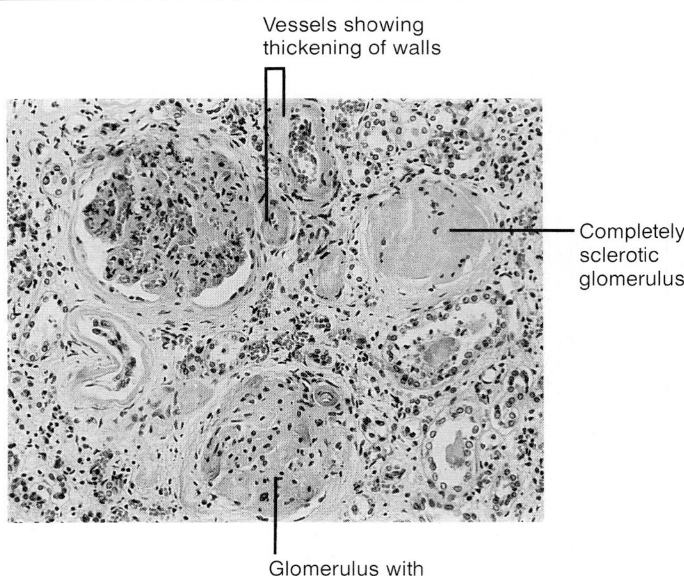

Figure 48-11. Chronic glomerulonephritis, showing 3 glomeruli with varying degrees of fibrosis.

DIABETIC NEPHROPATHY

Ten percent of patients with type II (adult-onset) diabetes mellitus die of chronic renal failure. The incidence of renal disease is still higher in type I (juvenile onset) diabetes. With the high frequency of diabetes in the population, diabetic nephropathy is one of the more common renal diseases.

Diabetic nephropathy is the result of diabetic microangiopathy (see Chapter 46) and is almost invariably associated with diabetic retinopathy. There is controversy about whether strict control of diabetes mellitus prevents the occurrence of nephropathy.

Pathology

Grossly, the kidney shows little abnormality in all but the most severe cases, when the organ may be contracted and show fine scarring. Light microscopy shows several changes (Fig 48–12; see also Chapter 46) the most common of which are focal and diffuse glomerulosclerosis. Electron microscopy of the focal nodular lesions shows them to be composed of increased mesangial matrix material. There are no discrete electron-dense deposits, and immunofluorescence is negative.

Exudative hyaline capsular "teardrop" lesions (not specific for diabetes).

Thickened capsule

Hyaline thickening of afferent and efferent arterioles (specific for diabetes).

Focal glomerulosclerosis (Kimmelstiel-Wilson lesions). (Specific for diabetes)

Diffuse glomerulosclerosis. Varying degrees to complete hyalinization of glomeruli (not specific for diabetes).

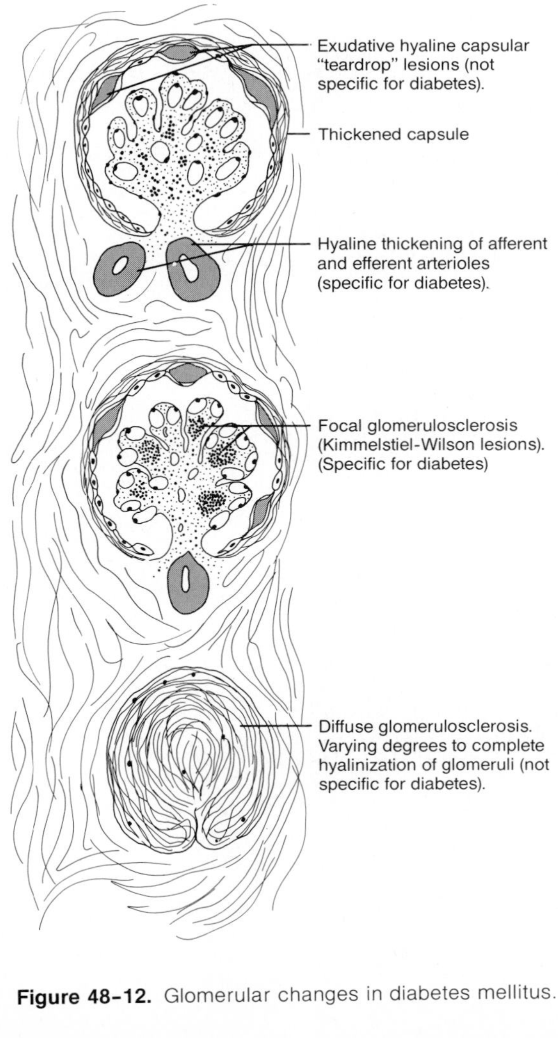

Figure 48–12. Glomerular changes in diabetes mellitus.

Clinical Features

Diabetic nephropathy presents with proteinuria, which may be sufficient to lead to nephrotic syndrome. Hypertension is commonly present. The renal lesion is progressive and causes progressive chronic renal failure.

RENAL AMLYLOIDOSIS (See Chapter 2.)

The kidneys are almost always affected in secondary amyloidosis and in about 30% of cases of primary amyloidosis.

Amyloid deposition occurs mainly in the glomerular capillaries, where it appears as a homogeneous thickening of the basement membrane. In severe cases, the entire glomerulus is converted into a ball of amyloid (Fig 48–13). Amyloidosis can be diagnosed by the presence of apple-green birefringence when Congo red-stained sections are examined under polarized light. Electron microscopy shows the diagnostic amyloid fibrillar material.

Clinically, deposition of amyloid increases the permeability of the glomerular capillary, resulting in proteinuria and the nephrotic syndrome. Amyloidosis is a progressive disease that usually results in chronic renal failure, a common cause of death in amyloidosis.

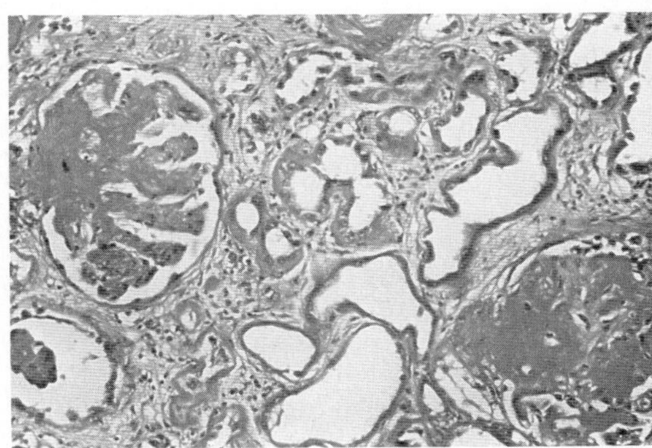

Figure 48–13. Renal amyloidosis, showing marked involvement of 2 glomeruli. Note also that the basement membrane of some tubules is thickened as a result of amyloid deposition.

GLOMERULAR INVOLVEMENT IN OTHER DISEASES

Many other diseases produce glomerular damage that may result in acute or chronic renal failure. Malignant hypertension is described elsewhere (see Chapter 20). Thrombotic thrombocytopenic purpura and hemolytic uremic syndrome produce coagulation in glomerular capillaries (see Chapter 27). Subacute infective endocarditis leads to microemboli and immune complex-mediated glomerulonephritis (see Chapter 22). Preeclampsia-eclampsia of pregnancy produces swelling of glomerular cells with glomerular ischemia (see Chapter 55).

The Kidney: III. Vascular Diseases; Neoplasms

49

RENAL VASCULAR DISEASES

HYPERTENSIVE RENAL DISEASE (Nephrosclerosis)

BENIGN NEPHROSCLEROSIS

Benign nephrosclerosis occurs in most patients with essential hypertension. Similar changes are seen at autopsy in nonhypertensive elderly patients, probably representing an aging change. There is bilateral symmetric reduction in the size of the kidneys. The renal surface has a fine, even granularity, and there is uniform thinning of the renal cortex (Table 49–1). Microscopically, there is hyaline thickening of the walls of small arteries and arterioles (luminal narrowing of these vessels causes chronic glomerular ischemia), global sclerosis of glomeruli, and atrophy of nephrons with interstitial fibrosis. Immunofluorescence and electron microscopy show no evidence of immune deposits.

The changes of benign nephrosclerosis are usually mild. Chronic renal failure occurs in less than 5% of cases.

MALIGNANT NEPHROSCLEROSIS

Malignant nephrosclerosis occurs with malignant hypertension (see Chapter 20). This complication occurs in about 5% of patients with hypertension.

The kidneys are normal in size or slightly enlarged and have a smooth surface with numerous small petechial hemorrhages (''fleabitten kidneys''). Microscopically, there is fibrinoid necrosis of arterioles and glomeruli (Fig 49–1). (Fibrinoid necrosis appears as pink granular material in which fibrin can be demonstrated by immunofluorescence.) Interlobar arteries show intimal cellular proliferation and laminated (onionskin) fibrosis. Luminal narrowing leads to ischemia.

Clinically, malignant nephrosclerosis is manifested by proteinuria and hematuria, rapidly followed by acute renal failure. Without treatment, 90% of patients die within 1 year. With modern antihypertensive therapy, over 60% of patients are alive 5 years after diagnosis.

RENAL ARTERY STENOSIS

Renal artery stenosis is uncommon but is an important disease in that it represents a potentially treatable form of hypertension. There are several causes.

(1) **Atherosclerosis** is the most common cause, particularly in older patients.

(2) **Fibromuscular dysplasia** of the renal artery is a rare condition of unknown cause, occurring in younger patients (20–40 years of age), particularly in women. It is characterized by unilateral or bilateral single or multiple constrictions of the renal arterial wall, caused by fibromuscular thickening of the media or, more rarely, the intima. Other arteries may be involved. Surgery is curative if the pathologic process is localized.

(3) **Posttransplantation stenosis** occurs in 10-

Table 49–1. Differential diagnosis of a granular, contracted kidney.

	Chronic Glomerulonephritis	Chronic Pyelonephritis	Benign Nephrosclerosis (Hypertension)
Renal involvement	Symmetric	Asymmetric	Symmetric
Granularity of surface	Fine	Coarse	Fine
Glomeruli	Global sclerosis	Periglomerular fibrosis	Global sclerosis
Interstitial inflammation	Mild or absent	Present	Mild or absent
Vascular changes	Present	Present	Present, marked
Ig, C3, immune complexes	Present	Absent	Absent
Bacterial culture	Negative	May be positive	Negative

20% of patients after renal transplantation, most commonly as a manifestation of rejection. Intimal thickening follows immunoglobulin deposition in donor vessel walls. Less commonly, the stenosis occurs at the site of anastomosis.

Pathology & Clinical Features

When a significant degree (> 75%) of narrowing of the renal artery is present, diffuse ischemia of the kidney occurs. Glomerular filtration pressure is decreased (Fig 49–2), resulting in increased renin secretion by the juxtaglomerular apparatus and leading to hypertension via aldosterone secretion and sodium retention. Renal artery stenosis is responsible for only about 2–3% of cases of hypertension overall, but it is important because it is surgically curable. Plasma renin levels are elevated. Differential renal vein renin assays show a significant difference between the stenotic side (high) and the normal side (normal).

Decreased glomerular filtration is associated with a slow transit time of fluid in the tubules, leading to increased reabsorption of water in the tubules. Intravenous pyelography shows a delay in excretion of dye on the affected side, but later films show an increased dye concentration. The diagnosis is made by renal arteriography.

Treatment & Prognosis

Transluminal dilatation of the stenotic segment with a balloon introduced via the arteriography catheter produces cure rates equivalent to those achieved by surgical resection of the stenosis. About 80–90% of patients so treated are cured. The prognosis depends on the duration of the disease. In long-standing stenoses, significant hypertensive changes in the opposite kidney prevent complete reversal of hypertension even when the stenosis is treated.

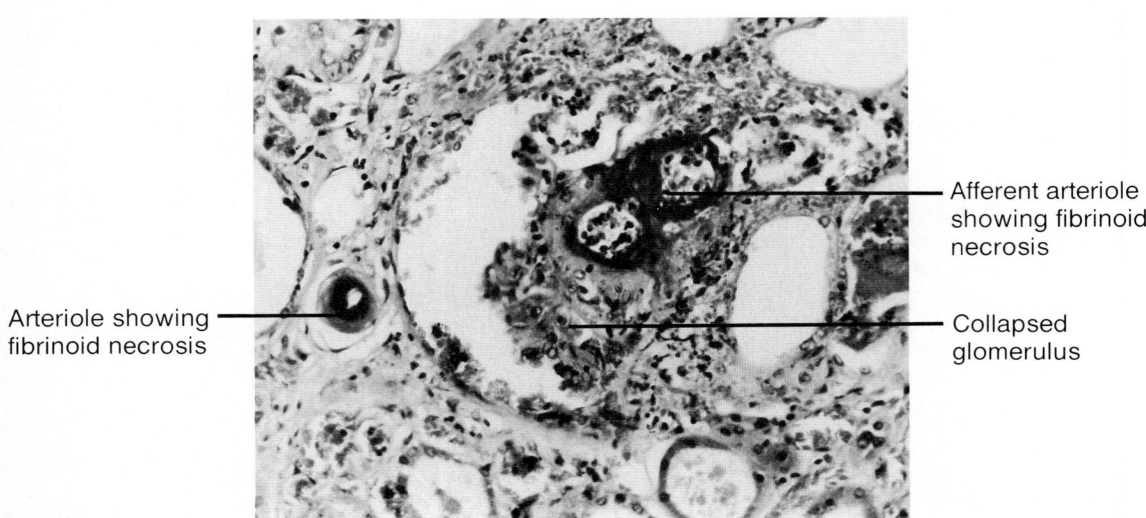

Figure 49–1. The kidney in malignant hypertension, showing fibrinoid necrosis of arterioles. The glomerulus is collapsed distal to the involved afferent arteriole.

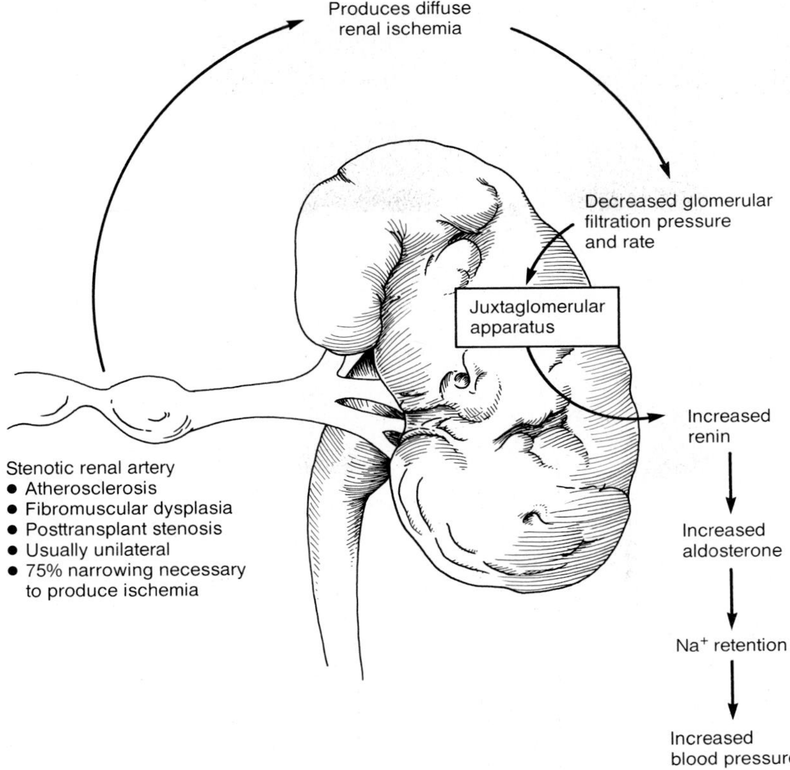

Figure 49–2. Renal artery stenosis—causes and pathogenesis of hypertension.

RENAL CHANGES IN SHOCK

The reduction in cardiac output in shock causes renal arteriolar constriction and a series of renal changes, as described below.

Prerenal Uremia ("Functional Renal Insufficiency")

Intense vasoconstriction serves to retain fluid and maintain blood pressure and as such is the appropriate physiologic response to hypotension in shock (Fig 49–3). Renal vasoconstriction leads to decreased glomerular filtration pressure, diminished glomerular filtration volume, and increased tubular reabsorption of water. The vasoconstriction also leads to increased secretion of renin, which causes sodium and water retention via the aldosterone mechanism. Oliguria results and may be severe enough (< 400 mL/d) to fall within the definition of acute renal failure. The urine is highly concentrated, with high levels of urea and creatinine, reflecting the fact that the tubules are still functioning normally. Serum urea levels rise.

No morphologic changes are seen in the kidney. Reversal of shock leads to return of normal renal function.

Ischemic Acute Renal Tubular Necrosis (ATN)

Acute tubular necrosis may occur following exposure to nephrotoxins (Chapter 47), as a manifestation of acute rejection in a transplanted kidney (Chapter 8), and in ischemic states. The commonest cause of acute tubular necrosis is severe shock, in which reflex vasoconstriction in the kidney is prolonged and severe enough to lead to necrosis of the renal tubular epithelium. In general, any cause of shock may induce ischemic necrosis of the tubules. In massive trauma (crush syndrome) and transfusion reactions, precipitation of myoglobin or hemoglobin or fragmented red cell membranes in the tubules aggravates the condition.

Microscopically, the tubules typically show patchy necrosis affecting both proximal and distal convoluted tubules. Disappearance of the brush border of proximal convoluted tubular epithelial cells is an early microscopic feature of acute tubular necrosis. Disruption of the tubular basement membrane occurs and distinguishes ischemic necrosis from "toxic" tubular necrosis, in which the

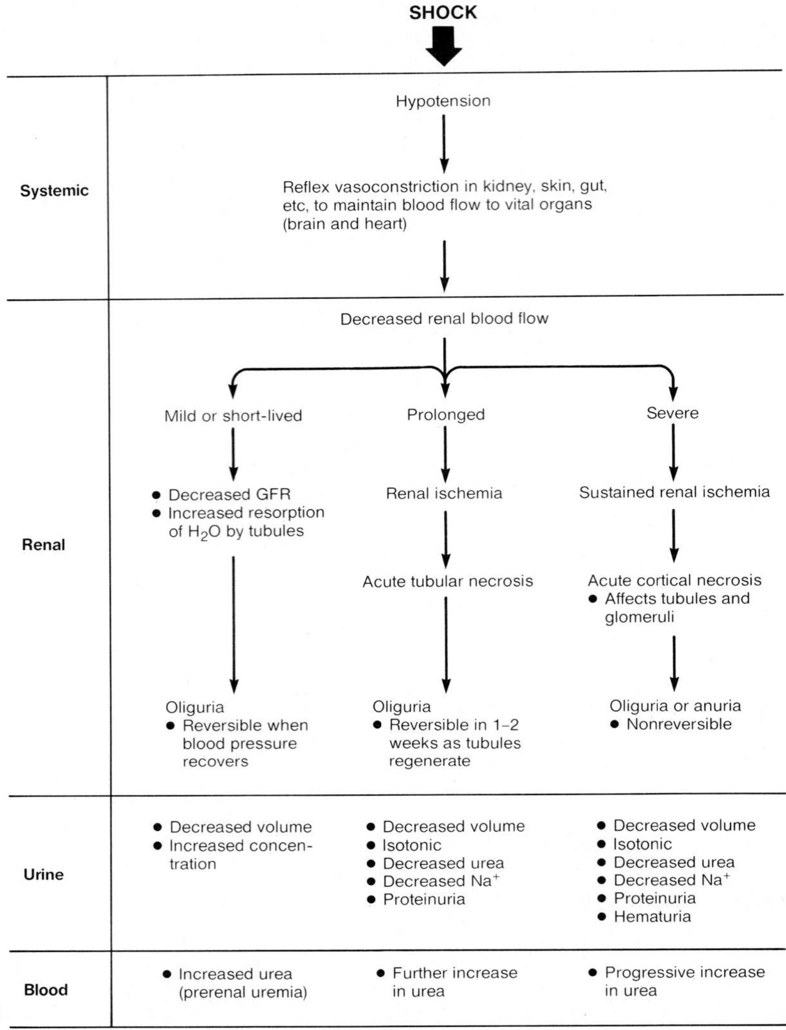

Figure 49–3. Renal changes in shock.

basement membrane is intact. Eosinophilic hyaline casts are present in the distal convoluted and collecting tubules. If the patient survives, evidence of tubular epithelial regeneration is seen in the second week.

Clinically, acute tubular necrosis is characterized by acute renal failure, with oliguria and azotemia. As tubular necrosis develops, urine volume remains low but osmolality approaches that of glomerular ultrafiltrate (specific gravity 1.010, ie, isosthenuria), indicating failure of tubular function. Failure of the tubules to concentrate urine and handle urea and electrolytes permits differentiation of tubular necrosis from the prerenal uremic state (Fig 49–3). The urine contains red cells and tubular epithelial casts.

The **oliguric phase** of tubular necrosis usually lasts 10–14 days. In patients who recover, this is followed by the **diuretic phase,** in which urine output increases—still without tubular reabsorption. In this diuretic phase, where there is unregulated loss of an increasing volume of isotonic urine, there is a risk of fluid and electrolyte imbalance. Tubular function is restored only 2–3 weeks after the occurrence of tubular necrosis, representing the time necessary for complete cell regeneration. Mild urinary abnormalities may persist for 2–3 months.

Renal Cortical Necrosis

Renal cortical necrosis is rare, being caused by severe, prolonged shock (hypotension). It is characterized by necrosis of the entire renal cortex, including the glomeruli. It is irreversible. In the acute phase the cortex is yellow and of normal thickness, but it shrinks rapidly and may undergo calcification.

Clinically, renal cortical necrosis presents in a

similar manner to tubular necrosis except that the oliguric phase is profound and prolonged and the diuretic phase does not appear. The glomeruli do not regenerate, and function cannot be restored.

Renal cortical necrosis has a very high mortality rate unless hemodialysis or transplantation is undertaken. A few patients who have a sufficient number of viable glomeruli recover some renal function after a prolonged period of hemodialysis.

RENAL INFARCTION

Renal infarction is an uncommon condition with several causes. **Arterial occlusion by embolism** is the most common cause. Emboli usually originate in the heart in infective endocarditis, myocardial infarction, mitral stenosis, or atrial fibrillation. Rarely, cholesterol emboli from aortic atherosclerotic plaques are responsible.

Arterial occlusion by thrombosis is usually secondary to atherosclerosis. More rarely, thrombosis of smaller intrarenal arteries in polyarteritis nodosa, progressive systemic sclerosis, or malignant hypertension may result in infarction.

Renal vein occlusion by thrombosis or neoplasms may rarely cause ischemia to the degree that hemorrhagic infarction occurs.

Pathologic & Clinical Features

Grossly, arterial infarcts are pale and wedge-shaped, with the occluded vessels at the apex of the wedge (see Chapter 9). Venous infarcts are hemorrhagic and often involve large areas, frequently the entire kidney. Microscopically, the infarcted area shows coagulative necrosis. A narrow zone of cortex supplied by capsular arteries is frequently spared. The infarct heals by progressive enzymatic liquefaction, macrophage phagocytosis of debris, and scar formation over a period of a few weeks. The ultimate result is a depressed cortical scar.

Clinically, infarction produces sudden-onset flank pain followed by hematuria. Unless infarction is bilateral and extensive, there is no impairment of renal function.

NEOPLASMS OF THE KIDNEYS (Table 49–2)

BENIGN NEOPLASMS

RENAL CORTICAL ADENOMA

Renal cortical adenoma is a common incidental finding at autopsy, appearing as a well-circumscribed, round, yellowish nodule in the cortex, composed of cytologically benign cells arranged in a papillary or solid pattern.

When found during life—usually incidentally during radiologic examination of the abdomen—differentiation from early carcinoma is difficult or impossible. A diameter in excess of 3 cm, the presence of necrosis or hemorrhage, or cytologic features of cancer indicate renal carcinoma. When a small renal cortical tumor is found incidentally, either at surgery or during computerized tomography, it should be resected if possible.

RENAL ONCOCYTOMA ("Proximal Tubular Adenoma")

Renal oncocytoma is a special kind of cortical adenoma believed to be derived from proximal tubular cells. Unlike other adenomas, an oncocytoma may reach a large size but remain benign. Distinction from carcinoma is difficult.

The gross appearance is distinctive. Oncocytomas have a uniform mahogany brown color without necrosis or hemorrhage, though frequently there is a central scarred area. Histologically, oncocytomas are composed of a uniform population of large cells having small round nuclei and abundant pink, granular cytoplasm.

ANGIOMYOLIPOMA

Renal angiomyolipoma is an uncommon but important renal tumor. It may be solitary or multiple and bilateral. In the latter event, it is often part of the syndrome of tuberous sclerosis (Chapter 62).

Renal angiomyolipoma is best regarded as a renal hamartoma, but it may produce a large mass that clinically resembles carcinoma (Fig 49–4). Its content of fat gives it a characteristic appearance on computerized tomography, permitting accurate radiologic diagnosis preoperatively. Histologically, it is composed of a variable admixture of mature adipose tissue, proliferating smooth muscle cells, and abnormal blood vessels. The ves-

Table 49-2. Renal neoplasms.

	Frequency	Gross Features	Microscopic Features	Clinical Features	Comments
Benign					
Renal cortical adenoma	Common	< 3 cm; firm circumscribed yellowish nodule in cortex	Cytologically benign cells; papillary or solid pattern	Asymptomatic; usually an incidental autopsy finding	When found during life, difficult to differentiate from a small renal adenocarcinoma
Renal oncocytoma	Rare	May be large; circumscribed, mahogany brown, uniform; central scar	Uniform large cells with small, regular nuclei and abundant granular cytoplasm	Mass, slowly growing; hematuria	Difficult to differentiate from oncocytic renal carcinoma
Angiomyolipoma	Uncommon	May be large; solitary or multiple; circumscribed yellow mass; may be bilateral	3 components: mature fat cells, abnormal blood vessels, and smooth muscle cell proliferation	Mass, hematuria; CT scan shows fat density	Associated with tuberous sclerosis
Juxtaglomerular apparatus tumor	Very rare	Small, solid cortical mass	Small, round, uniform cells arranged in nests and sheets	Hypertension due to increased renin secretion by tumor	Rare cause of secondary hypertension in a young patient
Congenital mesoblastic nephroma	Rare	May be large; circumscribed, firm, pale mass; whorled surface	Benign fibroblastic spindle cell proliferation	Mass during neonatal period	Occurs in first 3 months of life
Medullary fibroma	Common	< 1 cm/ firm, circumscribed mass in medulla	Benign fibroblastic spindle cell proliferation	Asymptomatic; incidental finding at autopsy	Of little clinical significance
Malignant					
Renal adenocarcinoma	Common	Usually large; variegated appearance; pseudoencapsulated, may invade renal vein	Clear cells of varying cytologic malignancy; solid, papillary, cystic, oncocytic variants	Mass; hematuria, metastatic disease	1–2% of all cancers in adults
Nephroblastoma (Wilms's tumor)	Common in children	Large; firm, solid mass; frequently replaces kidney	Primitive small spindle cells; tubular differentiation; mesenchymal elements	Mass in childhood; abdominal enlargement	25–30% of cancers in children under age 10 years
Transitional cell neoplasms of renal pelvis	Common	Papillary mass in renal pelvis; may invade kidney	Papillary urothelial neoplasms of varying grades	Hematuria; mass; malignant cells in urine	Multiple tumors may be present
Primary sarcomas	Very rare	Large masses; usually in capsule and perinephric fat	Depends on type of sarcoma; liposarcoma, leiomyosarcoma, and fibrosarcoma most common	Mass	
Primary renal malignant lymphoma	Very rare	Large mass; solid and fleshy	Commonly aggressive large cell and immunoblastic lymphomas	Mass; hilar nodes commonly involved	Renal involvement in systemic lymphoma is more common

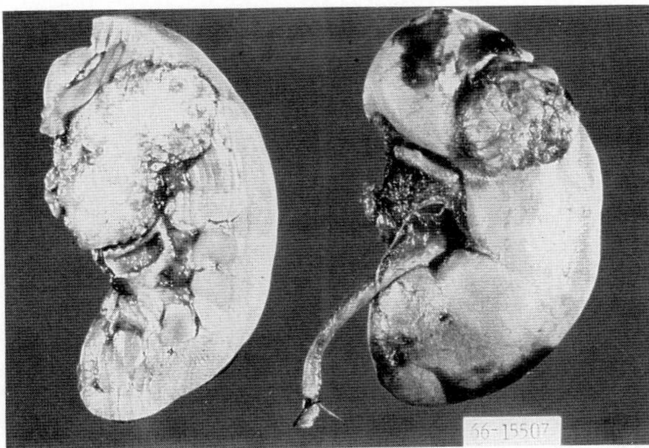

Figure 49–4. Renal angiomyolipoma presenting as a mass in the upper pole of the kidney (left) that protrudes on the surface (right).

sels have a typical appearance with irregularly proliferative medial smooth muscle and an eccentric lumen. The smooth muscle cells often show considerable cytologic pleomorphism, which may lead to a misdiagnosis of sarcoma.

Renal angiomyolipoma is a benign lesion. Rarely, similar hamartomas are present in the lymph nodes in the renal hilum; these do not constitute metastases.

MALIGNANT NEOPLASMS (Tables 49–2 and 49–3)

RENAL ADENOCARCINOMA (Hypernephroma; Grawitz's Tumor)

Renal adenocarcinoma is the most common malignant neoplasm of the kidney and accounts for 1–2% of all cancers in adults. It occurs most frequently in the sixth decade but is not rare in younger patients. It is believed to be derived from proximal tubular epithelial cells. No strong etiologic factors have been identified; patients with von Hippel-Lindau syndrome and dialysis cystic disease of the kidney have an increased incidence of renal adenocarcinoma.

Pathology

Grossly, renal adenocarcinoma varies in size from small to massive. Commonly solid (Fig 49–5), it may contain cystic areas or may be predominantly cystic (Fig 49–6). The cut surface is variegated, with yellow-orange areas mottled with hemorrhagic (red-black) and fibrous (gray) areas (Fig 49–5). Calcification is common. The yellow color of the neoplasm is caused by the high lipid content of the neoplastic cells.

Renal adenocarcinomas may infiltrate locally through the capsule of the kidney and rarely through the fascia around the perinephric fat to infiltrate surrounding organs (Fig 49–7). Invasion into renal vein is common; occasionally, tumor extends along the lumen of the inferior vena cava—rarely, all the way into the right atrium.

Microscopically, renal adenocarcinomas are composed of a mixture of clear cells and pink granular oncocytic cells. In well-differentiated neoplasms, the cells are arranged in glandular papillary and tubular formations separated by a highly vascular stroma. The cells in well-differentiated (grade I) carcinomas are large, with small nuclei and abundant clear cytoplasm rich in lipid and glycogen (clear cell carcinoma; Fig 49–8). There is little cytologic atypia. In less well differentiated neoplasms, the cells become more pleomorphic, with nuclear enlargement and atypia, the appearance of large nucleoli, and may be arranged in irregular sheets. Necrosis, cystic change, calcification, and hemorrhage are commonly present.

A histologic grading system ranging from grade I (well-differentiated) to grade IV (anaplastic) has been shown to correlate with prognosis. The nuclear size and appearance form the main basis for histologic grading.

Table 49–3. Malignant renal neoplasms: Risk factors.

	Renal Adenocarcinoma	Transitional Carcinoma of Renal Pelvis	Nephroblastoma
Age	50+	50+	0–10 years
Sex	M > F	M > F	M = F
Frequency	90% of adult renal cancers	10% of adult renal cancers	99% of childhood renal cancers
Genetic factors	Rare familial cases	None	Deletion of part of chromosome 11 in some cases
Associated conditions	Von Hippel-Lindau syndrome (rare); dialysis cystic disease	Other urothelial neoplasms	Aniridia
Identified etiologic factors	Thorotrast (rare); smoking (slight effect)	Smoking (marked influence), calculi, aniline dyes	None

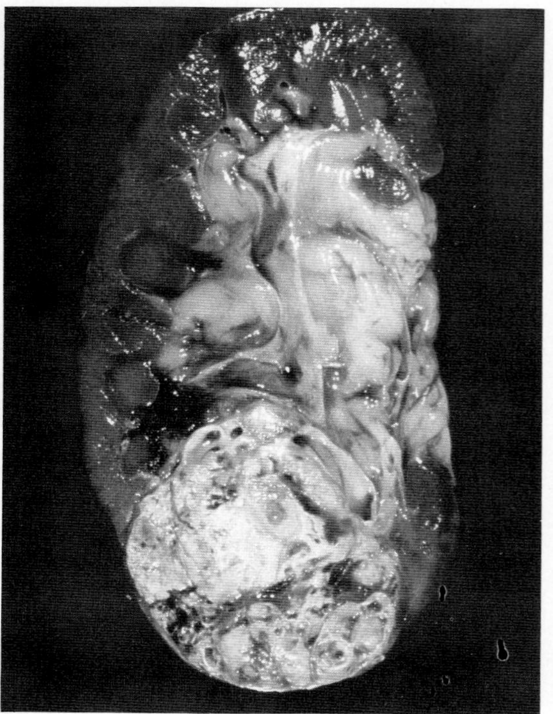

Figure 49-5. Renal adenocarcinoma. Typical appearance, showing a solid mass with a variegated cut surface. The tumor is confined to the kidney in this example.

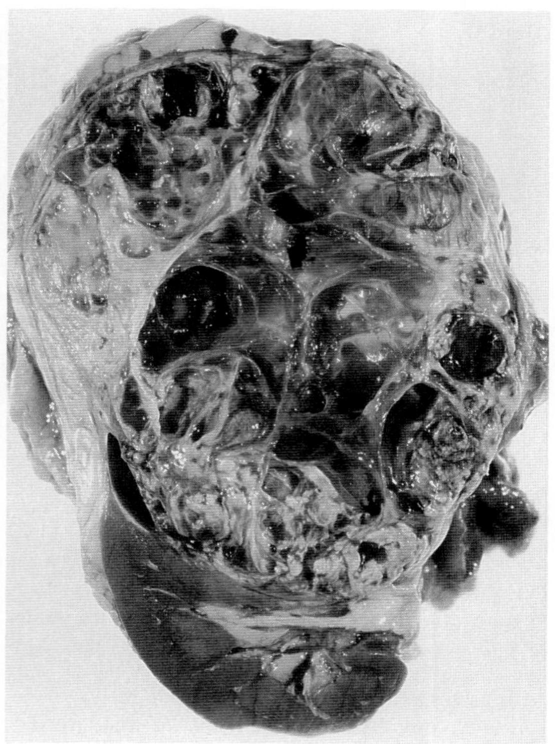

Figure 49-6. Renal adenocarcinoma, predominantly cystic. Solid foci are seen at the bottom and on the left side of the mass.

Clinical Features

The usual presentation is with hematuria (Table 49-4). A renal mass may be palpable when the tumor reaches a large size. Metastases occur early and may be the reason for clinical presentation when they occur with relatively small asymptomatic tumors. Common metastatic sites are lungs, bone, liver, brain, and skin.

Extension of the neoplasm into the renal vein on the left side may obstruct the testicular vein, which drains into it, causing a scrotal varicocele. Extension into the renal vein may also very rarely cause venous infarction of the kidney. Extension into the inferior vena cava may occlude it, leading to edema in the lower extremities.

A few renal adenocarcinomas secrete hormones, including (1) parathyroid hormone-like substances that cause hypercalcemia, low serum phosphate, and a clinical syndrome resembling primary hyperparathyroidism; (2) erythropoietin, causing polycythemia; and (3) other hormones such as prolactin (causing galactorrhea), renin (hypertension), prostaglandins, and gonadotropins.

The diagnosis is made by intravenous pyelography, CT scan, or angiography, which show the presence of a renal mass. These radiologic studies are important in identifying the extent of invasion, such as involvement of a renal vein or inferior vena cava, which may require special handling at surgery.

Treatment & Prognosis

Treatment of renal adenocarcinoma is surgical removal, which is very successful in clinical stage 1 carcinomas. The prognosis correlates well with clinical stage (Table 49-5). Histologic grade is a relatively minor prognostic indicator.

Table 49-4. Clinical presentation of renal adenocarcinoma.

Hematuria	70%
Flank mass	50%
Flank pain	50%
Fever	5%
Metastatic disease	5%
Left scrotal varicocele Inferior vena caval obstruction Polycythemia (erythropoietin production) Hypercalcemia (parathyroid hormone-like molecule) Hypertension (renin production) Cushing's syndrome (adrenocorticotropic hormone-like molecule) Galactorrhea (prolactin production)	Rare

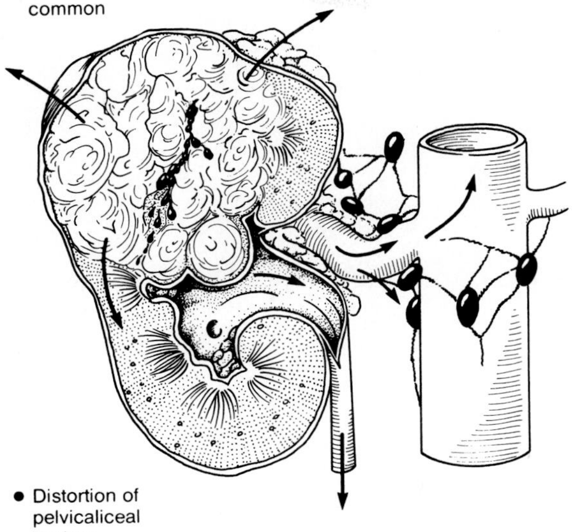

Tumor
• Enlarging mass often appears encapsulated
• Necrosis and hemorrhage are common
• Distortion of pelvicaliceal system
SPREAD
Direct
• Through capsule into perinephric fat
• Renal pelvis
• Rarely to adjacent organs
Hematogenous
• Lung, bone, brain, skin are common sites
Contiguous venous spread
• Renal vein
• Inferior vena cava as solid tumor mass
• To right atrium
Lymphatic
• Renal hilar nodes
• Para-aortic nodes
• Cervical nodes (rare)
Urine
• Red blood cells
• Occasional malignant cells
• Proteinuria

Figure 49-7. Pathologic features and spread of renal carcinoma.

Renal adenocarcinoma is unpredictable in its biologic behavior. It has been known in rare cases to regress spontaneously, and it is not uncommon for metastases to regress, at least temporarily, after removal of the primary neoplasm. Renal adenocarcinoma may also remain dormant for long periods, and cases have been recorded in which a metastatic lesion has occurred up to 50 years after treatment of the primary tumor.

NEPHROBLASTOMA (Wilms's tumor)

Nephroblastoma constitutes about 25–30% of cancers in childhood, being second in frequency to leukemia and lymphoma as a cause of cancer in childhood. Most cases occur between 1 and 7 years of age. Adult nephroblastoma occurs rarely.

The cause is unknown. Nephroblastoma is be-

Muscle wall of renal vein
Tumor thrombus in renal vein
Endothelial lining of renal vein

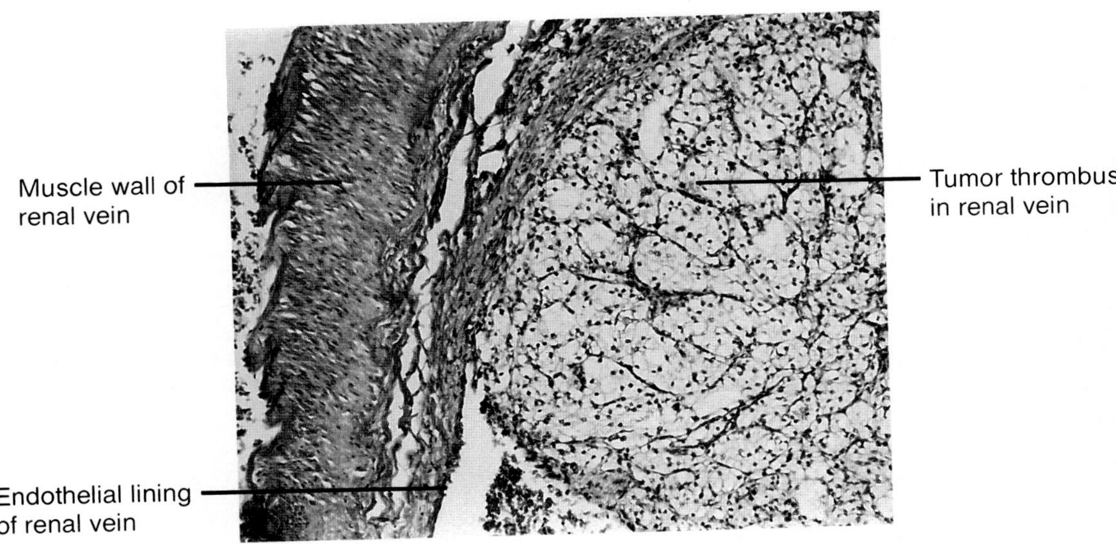

Figure 49-8. Renal adenocarcinoma, clear cell type, showing tumor in the renal vein at the hilum.

Table 49-5. Renal adenocarcinoma: Staging.

Stage	Criteria	5-Year Survival Rate[1]
I	Confined to kidney; no capsular invasion	70%
II	Invades perinephric fat	30%
III	Involvement of renal vein[2] or regional nodes	< 10%
IV	Extension beyond perinephric fat (Gerota's fascia) or distant metastases	< 5%

[1]Five-year survival rate following aggressive surgery, radio- and chemo-therapy where appropriate.
[2]Recent evidence suggests that survival rates in patients with renal vein involvement, including cases where the tumor thrombus extends into the inferior vena cava, are much higher than 10% if patients are treated with radical surgery. Reevaluation of renal vein involvement as a criterion for stage III disease is necessary.

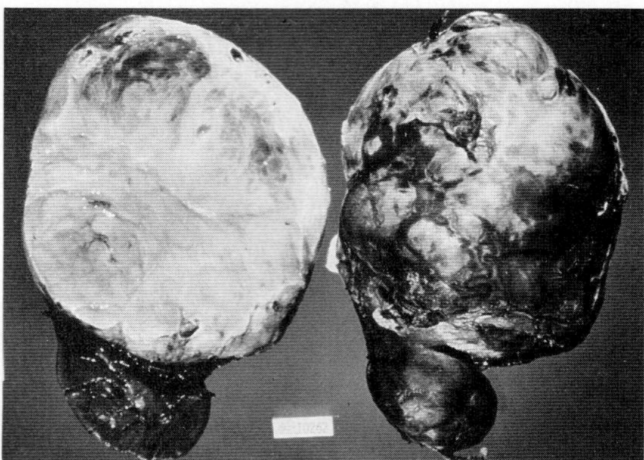

Figure 49-9. Nephroblastoma (Wilms's tumor). The cut surface (left) has a fleshy homogeneous appearance with focal hemorrhage. The kidney is greatly enlarged.

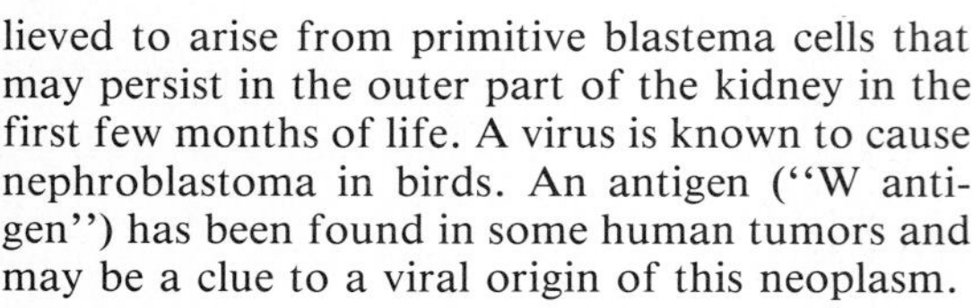

lieved to arise from primitive blastema cells that may persist in the outer part of the kidney in the first few months of life. A virus is known to cause nephroblastoma in birds. An antigen (''W antigen'') has been found in some human tumors and may be a clue to a viral origin of this neoplasm.

Genetic Features

All bilateral and approximately one-third of unilateral nephroblastomas are hereditary, with an apparent dominant mode of transmission and 60% penetrance. However, molecular studies suggest that homozygous recessive genes are responsible, both of which must have undergone mutation for the neoplasm to develop. According to this theory, in the hereditary form of the disease one recessive gene would be inherited in the mutant form (creating a predisposition to the disease); the second gene (allele) would then undergo an acquired mutation (leading to development of the neoplasm); this would mimic dominant inheritance with incomplete penetrance. In the acquired form, both genes would have to undergo acquired mutations. (See retinoblastoma, Chapter 33, for an analogous situation.)

Some patients with nephroblastoma have a distinctive chromosomal abnormality—deletion of part of the short arm of chromosome 11 (see page 293). This may be accompanied by aniridia.

Pathology

Grossly, nephroblastoma is commonly a large, firm tumor that is usually soft but may undergo cystic change (Fig 49–9). Bilateral nephroblastoma occurs in about 8% of cases. Microscopically, the most primitive nephroblastomas resembles renal blastema, which is the primitive mesodermal tissue of the embryonic renal anlage and is composed of small, somewhat spindle-shaped cells with hyperchromatic nuclei and scant cytoplasm. Undifferentiated neoplasms may display anaplasia, necrosis, and a high mitotic rate. Differentiation may occur into epithelial tubular structures, primitive glomerular structures (Fig 49–10), and a variety of mesenchymal tissues such as cartilage, smooth muscle, striated muscle, and bone. Rarely, tumors of childhood resembling Wilms's tumor are composed of cells showing primitive skeletal muscle differentiation (rhabdoid sarcoma) or clear cells (clear cell sarcoma). These histologic subtypes have a more aggressive behavior than the usual Wilms tumor.

According to the degree of differentiation, 3 histologic grades are recognized. Grade I (differentiated) neoplasms have the best prognosis. Grade III (anaplastic) neoplasms have the worst prognosis.

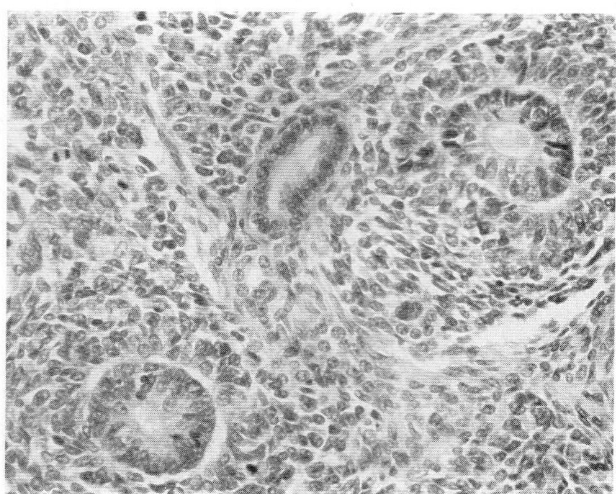

Figure 49–10. Nephroblastoma, showing primitive oval cells resembling renal blastema with focal differentiation into tubules.

Clinical Features & Treatment

Most patients with nephroblastoma present with a large abdominal mass that is usually felt by a parent. Nephroblastoma is staged clinically according to the size of tumor, the presence of tumor on either side of the midline, and distant spread. Treatment combines surgery, radiation, and chemotherapy. The prognosis has improved dramatically with introduction of more effective chemotherapeutic agents (dactinomycin, vincristine) in the last decade. Currently, the 5-year survival rate exceeds 50% even when metastases are present. For tumors confined to the kidney and resected surgically, the 5-year survival rate exceeds 80%.

UROTHELIAL NEOPLASMS OF THE RENAL PELVIS

These may present as renal masses (Fig 49–11) and are considered in the next chapter.

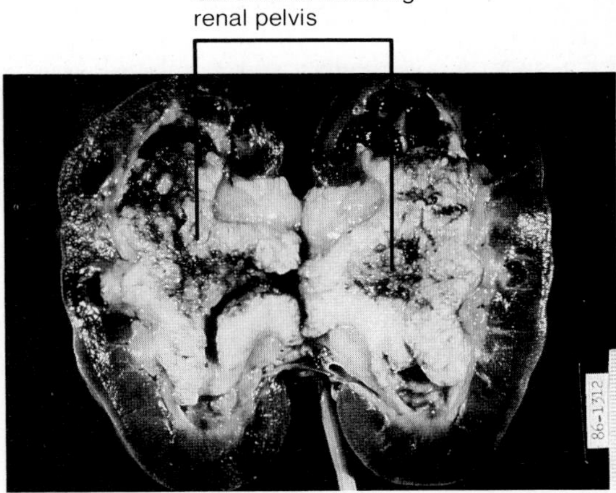

Figure 49–11. Transitional cell carcinoma of the renal pelvis. The tumor has involved a large part of the renal pelvis.

50 The Ureters, Urinary Bladder, & Urethra

THE RENAL PELVIS & URETERS

The ureters are narrow urothelium-lined muscular structures that transport urine from the renal pelvis to the bladder. Diseases of the ureter are manifested essentially as obstruction of the urinary passage, causing dilatation proximal to the obstruction (hydroureter) and renal pelvis (hydronephrosis) (Fig 50–1).

Acute obstruction of the ureter may result in hyperactivity of ureteral muscle and severe spasmodic pain called ureteral colic. Ureteral colic originates in the flank and radiates down and around to the suprapubic region. With chronic ureteral obstruction, there is no pain.

CONGENITAL ANOMALIES

ANATOMIC ANOMALIES

Anatomic anomalies of the urinary tract occur in about 2% of autopsies as incidental findings. They include abnormalities in position and number of ureters (eg, double and bifid ureter). Severe abnormalities may be associated with ureteral obstruction in the neonate.

URETEROCELE

A ureterocele is a thin-walled cystic swelling of the lowermost part of the ureter in its course through the bladder muscle. The cyst usually protrudes into the bladder lumen. Ureterocele is believed to be the result of congenital stenosis of the ureteral orifice in the bladder wall.

Ureterocele is common both in children and in young adults and is bilateral in 10% of cases. It tends to be more common in females. Other congenital anomalies of the urinary tract are often present as well.

Ureteroceles are frequently asymptomatic but may be associated with ureteral obstruction, hydroureter, and hydronephrosis.

MEGAURETER (Megaloureter)

Megaureter is a rare anomaly characterized by marked dilatation of the ureter associated with increased thickness of the muscle wall. The ureteral lumen is patent. It is believed to be caused by an abnormal arrangement of the muscle in the lower

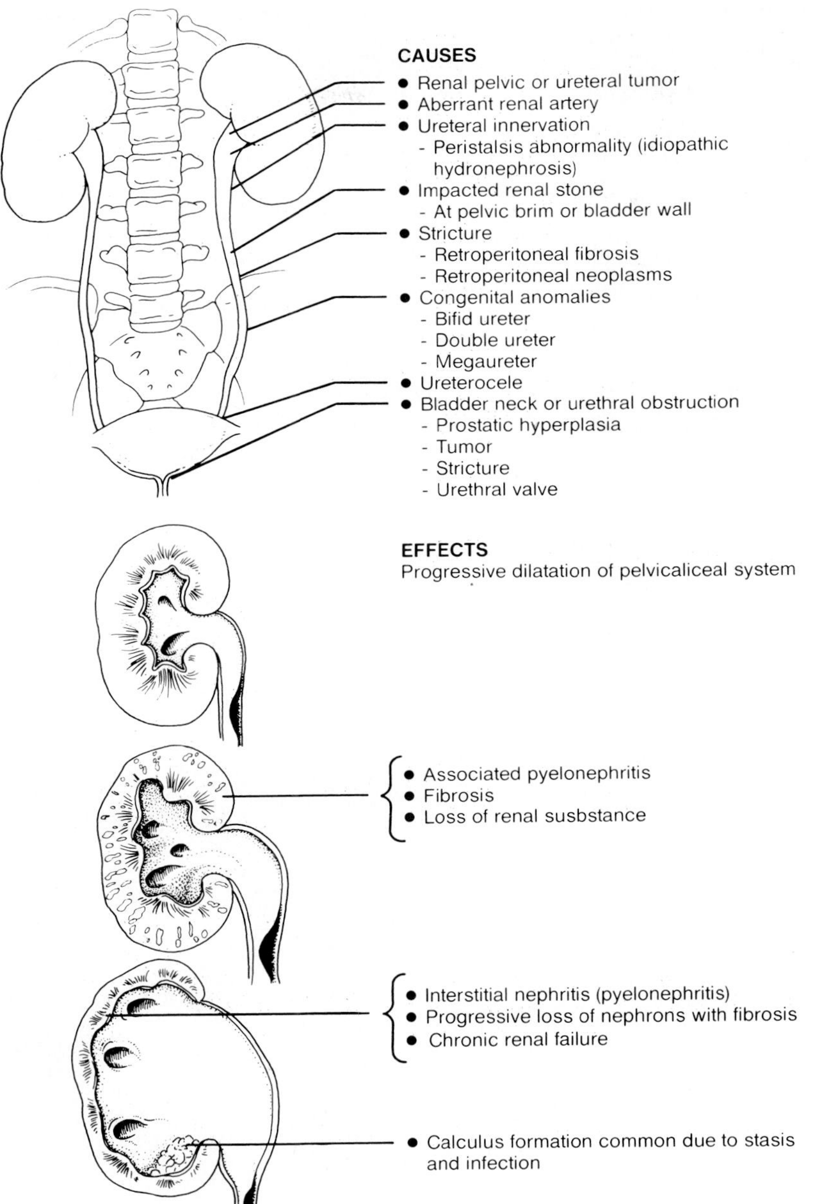

Figure 50–1. Causes and effects of hydronephrosis.

ureter, which results in abnormal peristalsis and functional obstruction.

IDIOPATHIC HYDRONEPHROSIS

Idiopathic hydronephrosis involves functional obstruction at the ureteropelvic junction, leading to massive hydronephrosis (Fig 50–2). The lumen is patent. In a few cases, an abnormal renal artery draped around the ureteropelvic junction has been incriminated in causing obstruction. In other cases, there is no physical obstruction, and it has been suggested that congenital abnormalities in innervation or arrangement of muscle fibers result in failure of peristalsis at the ureteropelvic junction. Surgical removal of the junction zone followed by restoration of anatomic continuity is curative. In many cases, however, prolonged hydronephrosis has produced considerable atrophy of the kidney before the diagnosis is made.

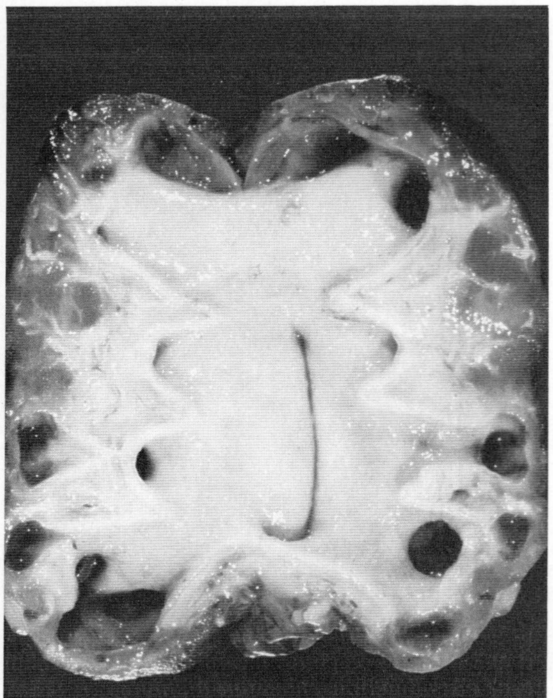

Figure 50-2. Idiopathic hydronephrosis, showing marked dilatation of renal pelvis and caliceal system. The kidney has been sectioned longitudinally in the plane of the dilated renal pelvis.

URINARY TRACT CALCULI (Urolithiasis)

Urolithiasis is a common clinical problem, occurring in about 0.5–2% of the general population (accounts for one of every 1000 hospital admissions in the United States). Urinary calculi may form in any part of the urinary tract, but the vast majority form in the renal pelvis (renal calculi) or bladder.

Etiology & Classification (Table 50-1)

Seventy percent of patients with urinary calculi have calcium oxalate calculi. In most of these patients, there is no biochemical abnormality to account for the calculi. Hypercalciuria or hyperoxaluria is present in a minority of patients. Calcium oxalate calculi are small, hard calculi with jagged edges that damage the ureteric mucosa as they pass down. Phosphate calculi account for 15% of urinary calculi and tend to be associated with urinary infections caused by urea-splitting organisms such as *Proteus* that produce ammonia and make the urine alkaline. Alkalinity of the urine is necessary for formation of phosphate calculi. These tend to be solitary, large, and soft and may fill the pelvicaliceal system (staghorn calculus; Fig 50-3). Uric acid calculi (10%) are important because they are radiolucent and therefore not seen on plain abdominal x-rays.

Clinical Features (Fig 50-4) & Diagnosis

Calculi typically present with acute ureteral obstruction, ureteral colic, and hematuria due to mucosal trauma. Small stones are successfully pushed down the ureter by peristalsis into the bladder and then passed out with urine.

Urinary tract obstruction occurs when a stone becomes impacted in the ureter. Hydronephrosis, urinary stasis, urinary tract infection, and acute pyelonephritis commonly follow.

Diagnosis of ureteral calculi is made by plain x-ray (radiopaque calculi) or intravenous or retrograde pyelography (radiolucent stones). Ninety percent of urinary calculi are radiopaque (Table 50-1). Serum and urinary studies are necessary to identify a predisposing cause (hypercalcemia, hyperoxaluria, cystinuria, gout, urinary infection). It should be noted that the presence of crystals in the urine does not correlate with the presence of urinary calculi.

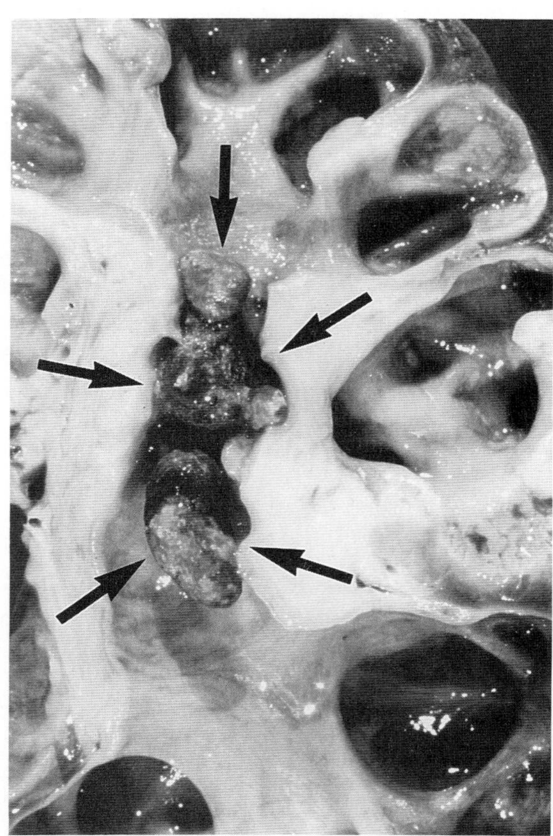

Figure 50-3. Staghorn calculus in the renal pelvis.

Table 50-1. Urinary tract calculi.

Type	Frequency	Predisposing Factors	Urine pH	Morphology
Calcium oxalate	70%	Hypercalcemia: Primary hyperparathyroidism Metastatic neoplasms in bone Idiopathic hypercalciuria Hyperoxaluria: Inherited Intestinal diseases (Crohn's ileitis, ileoileal bypass) High dietary intake of green vegetables, decaffeinated coffee High vitamin C intake Ethylene glycol poisoning	Any pH	Hard, small (< 5 mm), multiple stones; may be smooth, round, or jagged; radiopaque
Phosphate calculi (mixture of calcium phosphate and magnesium ammonium phosphate)	15%	Urinary infections by urea-splitting bacteria, commonly *Proteus* spp.	Alkaline	Soft, gray-white; often large and solitary, filling the pelvicaliceal system ("staghorn calculus"); radiopaque
Uric acid (urates)	10%	Most cases occur in patients with normal serum uric acid levels Gout; frequency has decreased after allopurinol therapy	Acidic	Yellow-brown; small, hard, smooth; often multiple; radiolucent—not visible on plain x-ray
Cystine and xanthine stones	Rare	Cystinuria, xanthinuria	Any pH	Yellowish; soft, waxy, small; smooth, round, multiple; cystine stones are slightly radiopaque; xanthine stones are radiolucent

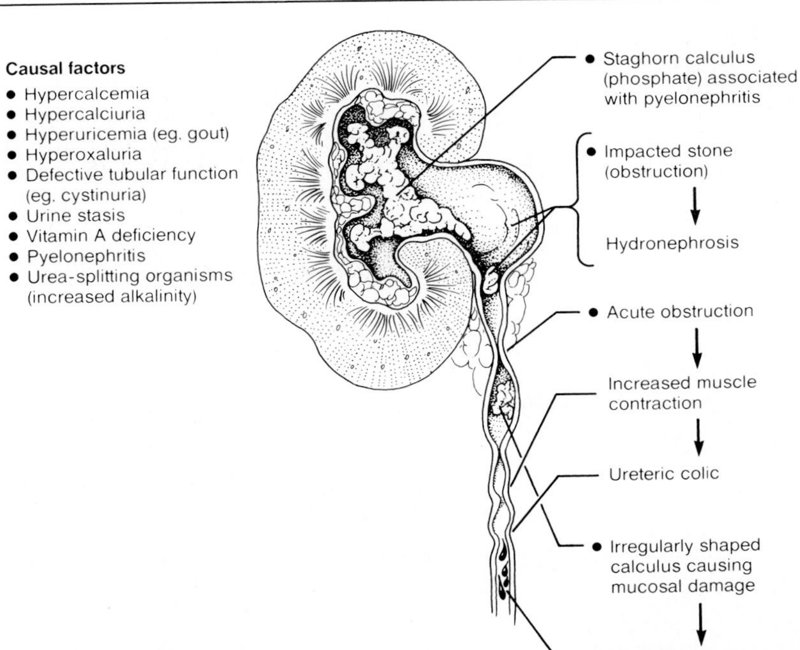

Figure 50-4. Causes and clinical effects of ureteric calculi.

Treatment

Treatment of ureteral calculi consists of observation of the stone as it passes down the ureter, combined with alleviation of pain. With large and impacted calculi, surgery to remove the calculi is indicated. Recently, a nonsurgical technique of fracturing stones with a machine called a lithotriptor that generates ultrasonic waves has proved effective.

FIBROUS STRICTURE OF THE URETERS

A variety of nonneoplastic conditions cause fibrosis and narrowing of the ureters.

(1) Chronic nonspecific ureteritis. This disorder of unknown cause is characterized by chronic inflammation, fibrosis, and cystic dilatation of epithelial nests in the submucosa (ureteritis cystica). Although usually an incidental finding, fibrosis may rarely be sufficient to cause ureteral obstruction.

(2) Tuberculosis of the ureter, usually secondary to renal tuberculosis, may be associated with fibrosis and strictures.

(3) Injury to the ureter may sometimes occur in extensive pelvic operations for gynecologic cancer and may be followed by fibrosis and strictures.

(4) Radiation often causes fibrous thickening of the ureteral wall and may cause obstruction.

(5) Retroperitoneal fibrosis. Retroperitoneal fibrosis is a form of idiopathic fibromatosis that involves the retroperitoneum, producing distortion and medial displacement of both ureters, a finding of diagnostic importance on radiologic studies. Microscopically, there is a cellular infiltrative fibroblastic proliferation in the retroperitoneum that surrounds and constricts the ureters, resulting in hydronephrosis, which may be bilateral.

(6) Endometriosis of the ureteral wall associated with cyclic hemorrhage and fibrosis is a rare cause of ureteral stricture in women.

UROTHELIAL NEOPLASMS

Primary urothelial neoplasms occur fairly frequently in the renal pelvis but are rare in the ureters. They have features identical with those of urothelial neoplasms of the bladder (see below).

Involvement of the ureters by retroperitoneal neoplasms, both primary and metastatic, is more common. Metastatic neoplasms involve the ureters in one of 2 ways: (1) by involving the retroperitoneal lymph nodes and extending outward to involve the ureters—most commonly in carcinomas of the urinary bladder or uterine cervix, testicular germ cell neoplasms, and malignant lymphomas; or (2) by direct metastasis to the ureteral wall, producing malignant strictures—seen rarely with carcinoma of the breast.

THE URINARY BLADDER

STRUCTURE & FUNCTION

The urinary bladder acts as a reservoir for urine, this function being dependent on the internal muscular sphincter at the bladder neck. Bladder filling results in a sensory input that leads to socially acceptable voluntary urination. Normal bladder emptying requires higher impulses from the brain, spinal cord, and pelvic autonomic nerves. Muscular contraction of the wall with relaxation of the internal sphincter causes complete evacuation. Interference with innervation of the bladder—as in spina bifida, spinal cord neoplasms, spinal trauma (paraplegia), or multiple sclerosis—leads to various forms of bladder dysfunction, resulting in urinary incontinence, infection, stone formation, and hydronephrosis.

The bladder, like the renal pelvis, ureters, and urethra, is lined by urothelium, which is a stratified transitional epithelium up to 6 layers of cells in thickness.

CONGENITAL ANOMALIES

ANATOMIC ABNORMALITIES

Anatomic abnormalities such as duplication—complete or incomplete—and congenital fistulas caused by abnormal development of the cloaca and urogenital sinus are rare.

URACHAL ABNORMALITIES

The urachus is the canal that connects the fetal bladder with the allantois. After delivery, it becomes obliterated or remains as a fibrous cord, the median umbilical ligament. Persistence of the entire urachus causes a vesicoumbilical fistula; persistence of parts of the urachus predisposes to infection, sinuses, and fistula formation. Urachal cysts and neoplasms occur rarely.

EXSTROPHY OF THE BLADDER (Ectopia Vesicae)

Exstrophy of the bladder is a rare congenital anomaly associated with failure of development of the anterior wall of the bladder and the overlying abdominal wall, including the pubic symphysis. The bladder is open to the skin surface as a large defect (complete exstrophy). Lesser defects also occur.

The exposed bladder is red and granular at birth and is covered by transitional epithelium. Repeated infections cause epithelial metaplasia of the squamous or intestinal type. Isolated defects can be corrected surgically. Exstrophy is often associated with numerous other congenital anomalies.

A higher incidence of cancer (usually adenocarcinoma) is reported in exstrophic bladders.

INFLAMMATORY LESIONS

ACUTE CYSTITIS

Etiology

A. Acute Bacterial Cystitis: Acute bacterial cystitis is a common ascending infection caused by coliform bacteria, commonly *Escherichia coli, Proteus* species, and *Streptococcus faecalis.* It occurs more commonly in females and is etiologically related to sexual intercourse, pregnancy, and instrumentation (Fig 50–5). In older individuals, chronic retention of urine in patients with prostatic hyperplasia is the major predisposing factor. The etiologic agent can be cultured from urine, which also contains protein, red cells, and neutrophils (casts are present only if the kidney is also involved). Many cases of acute cystitis are associated with acute pyelonephritis.

B. Acute Radiation Cystitis: Radiation cystitis occurs in cases where the bladder is included in the field of pelvic irradiation for malignant neoplasms.

C. Drugs Effects: Drugs used in the treatment of cancer (eg, cyclophosphamide) cause acute hemorrhagic cystitis with marked atypia of the lining transitional epithelium that may be mistaken for cancer on cytologic examination of urine.

Pathology

Acute cystitis is characterized by hyperemia of the mucosa with neutrophilic infiltration of the lamina propria. The term **"encrusted cystitis"** is used for nonspecific cystitis in which alkalinity of the urine causes precipitation of crystalline phosphates on the bladder mucosa; phosphate precipitation occurs in infections by organisms such as *Proteus* that split urea to form ammonia. **Bullous cystitis** is a variant of acute cystitis in which large fluid-filled spaces form in the submucosa.

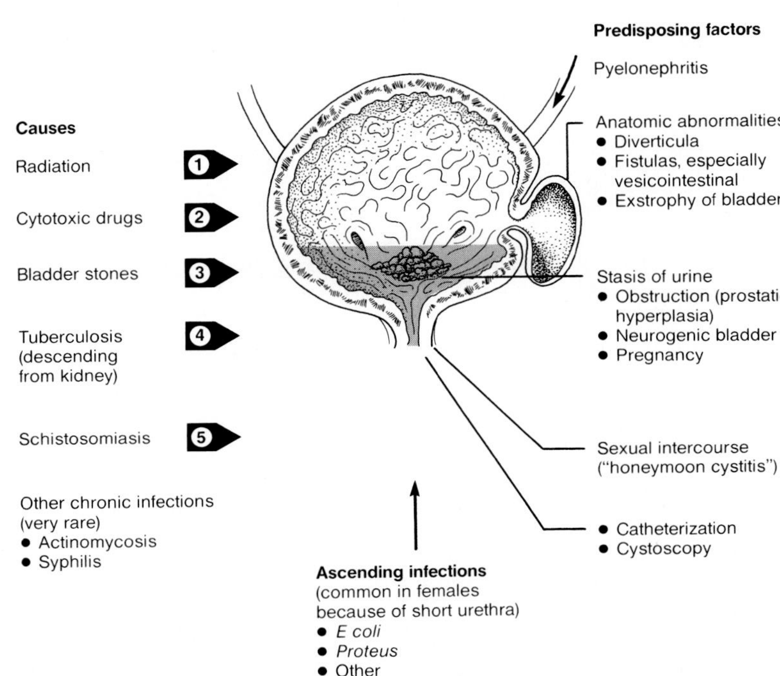

Figure 50–5. Causes and predisposing factors of bladder infections. Most cases are due to ascending infections caused by enteric bacteria such as *E coli* and *Proeus* species. Rare specific causes of cystitis are enumerated at left.

Clinical Features

Acute cystitis is characterized by fever, low abdominal pain, frequency of micturition, and dysuria. Frequency is the result of trigonal irritation, which stimulates the sensory arc of the micturition reflex.

Diagnosis & Treatment

Diagnosis is established by quantitative culture (colony count) of a midstream urine specimen. Specific treatment depends on the results of culture and sensitivity tests. While waiting for culture results, treatment should be started with an antibiotic effective against the common agents (ampicillin, trimethoprim-sulfamethoxazole). The prognosis is excellent.

TUBERCULOSIS

Vesical tuberculosis occurs in 70% of patients with renal tuberculosis and is a common presenting symptom in patients with urinary tract tuberculosis. The ureters and epididymis may also be involved.

The trigone is affected first, the early lesions appearing as small submucosal granulomas. Extensive caseous granulomas may cause nodules and ulceration, while the associated fibrosis may cause retraction of the ureteral orifice into the wall of the bladder ("golf-hole ureter") with vesicoureteral reflux. Diffuse involvement of the bladder is associated with marked fibrous contraction of the bladder ("thimble bladder"). At this stage, urinary frequency is extremely severe.

Clinically, there is frequency, pain, dysuria, and pyuria. Low-grade fever and weight loss may be present. Cultures for mycobacteria are diagnostic.

SCHISTOSOMIASIS

The perivesical venous plexus is the favored habitat of *Schistosoma haematobium,* a species that is common in Egypt and the Middle East. The ova pass through the bladder wall to enter the lumen and are excreted in urine. Finding typical ova in the urine is diagnostic.

In their passage through the wall, the ova cause marked inflammation, with abscesses and granulomas in which there are large numbers of eosinophils. Vesical schistosomiasis is associated clinically with fever, frequency, dysuria, and hematuria. Cystoscopic examination shows scarring and small nodules in the bladder mucosa. Marked fibrosis occurs in the chronic stage.

The bladder epithelium frequently shows squamous metaplasia. There is a greatly increased risk of squamous carcinoma.

CHRONIC NONSPECIFIC CYSTITIS

Chronic nonspecific cystitis is characterized by epithelial hyperplasia and infiltration of the bladder mucosa with lymphocytes and plasma cells. Cystic dilatation of epithelial nests in the submucosa (Brunn's nests) may produce multiple epithelium-lined cysts in the mucosa **(cystitis cystica)**. Glandular metaplasia may occur **(cystitis glandularis)**. These forms of epithelial change have little clinical significance. The cause is not known. One form of chronic nonspecific cystitis characterized by ulceration of the mucosa with submucosal fibrosis, vasculitis, and infiltration by eosinophils is called **Hunner's interstitial cystitis.**

A histologically distinct type of chronic inflammation occurs in patients with chronic bladder dysfunction and trauma, especially those with neurologic disease. This is characterized by a peculiar metaplasia of the urothelium called nephrogenic metaplasia. In some cases, this metaplastic epithelium becomes polypoid (nephrogenic "adenoma").

MALAKOPLAKIA

Malakoplakia is a peculiar chronic inflammation characterized by yellowish plaques, nodules, or polyps in the bladder mucosa. The lesions are composed microscopically of dense collections of macrophages with abundant granular cytoplasm. Within the cytoplasm are round, laminated concretions—called Michaelis-Gutman bodies—that stain positively with PAS (periodic acid-Schiff stain) as well as calcium and iron stains. The macrophages also contain partially digested bacterial remnants, leading to the theory that malakoplakia is caused by defective removal of phagocytosed bacteria by macrophages.

Malakoplakia is most commonly found in the bladder; other sites include the renal pelvis, ureter, prostate, epididymis, colon, and lungs.

MISCELLANEOUS DISEASES

BLADDER DIVERTICULA

Bladder diverticula may be congenital or acquired and may occur in childhood or in the elderly. Most acquired diverticula result from bladder neck obstruction, the most common cause of which is prostatic hyperplasia. Bladder neck obstruction results in muscular hypertrophy and increased intraluminal pressures leading to "pulsion" diverticula.

The most common location of diverticula is near the ureteral orifice. The presence of a bladder diverticulum results in stasis of urine and susceptibility to infection and formation of bladder calculi. There is also an increased incidence of urothelial neoplasms in diverticula, probably due to increased contact time between the mucosa and urinary carcinogens.

BLADDER FISTULAS

Bladder fistulas may communicate with the skin, intestine, or female reproductive organs. Such fistulas may be **(1) congenital,** eg, urachal vesicoumbilical fistula or, rarely, vesicovaginal fistula; **(2) traumatic**—mainly obstetric trauma, which may be complicated by vesicovaginal fistula; **(3) inflammatory,** as in diverticulitis of the colon, salpingitis, and Crohn's disease—diverticulitis is the most common cause of vesicointestinal fistula; or **(4) neoplastic,** particularly carcinoma of the cervix, colon, and bladder.

The clinical effects of bladder fistulas depend on the organs involved. Vesicovaginal fistula produces constant dribbling of urine through the vagina. Vesicointestinal fistula causes passage of feces (fecaluria) and gas (pneumaturia) with urine. All fistulas predispose to vesical infection.

BLADDER CALCULI

Calculi may form in the bladder (primary) or descend from the kidney (secondary). They have the same composition and causes as renal calculi.

AMYLOIDOSIS OF THE BLADDER

Amyloidosis is rarely localized in the bladder and presents as hematuria. Amyloid deposition may appear as a mucosal plaque or nodule or may involve the bladder more diffusely, causing irregular thickening of the mucosa and wall. Hemorrhage caused by rupture of amyloid-affected vessels is common.

NEOPLASMS OF THE BLADDER

UROTHELIAL NEOPLASMS

Bladder cancer is fairly common, being responsible for about 2% of cancer deaths in the United States and Europe. It has a marked geographic variation. In Japan, the incidence is extremely low, while in Egypt it accounts for 40% of cancers (because of the high incidence of schistosomiasis).

Etiology

Bladder cancer has been related to several chemical carcinogens such as aniline dyes containing benzidine and 2α-naphthylamine, which were responsible for bladder cancer in workers in the dye, rubber, and insulating cable industries. The latent period may be many years.

Artificial sweeteners such as saccharin and cyclamate cause bladder cancer in experimental animals. Although there is still some concern about their carcinogenic potential, there is no evidence that they cause cancer in humans.

Probably the most important etiologic factor in the genesis of human bladder cancer in the United States is cigarette smoking. The relationship between bladder cancer and smoking has been established by statistical methods. The mechanism by which smoking causes bladder cancer is unknown. In Egypt, schistosomiasis is important, producing squamous metaplasia, dysplasia, and squamous carcinoma.

Pathology

A. Overt Urothelial Neoplasms: Urothelial neoplasms may occur anywhere in the bladder mucosa. The most common locations are near the trigone or in a diverticulum. Large tumors may involve a large area of the mucosal surface and cause obstruction of the ureteral orifices (Fig 50–6).

The better-differentiated urothelial neoplasms commonly project into the lumen and have a delicate papillary appearance. In contrast, poorly differentiated neoplasms are solid ulcerative lesions that frequently show evidence of infiltration of the bladder wall.

Microscopically, most are transitional cell carcinomas. Squamous or glandular differentiation commonly occurs in transitional cell carcinomas.

The international (World Health Organization) histologic grading system for urothelial neoplasms recognizes 4 histologic grades.

1. Transitional cell papilloma is a well-differentiated papillary neoplasm that has less than 6 layers of cytologically normal transitional cells lining the papillary fronds. This tumor is rare and benign but tends to be multifocal, often recurring after surgery.

2. Grade I transitional cell carcinoma shows well-formed papillary structures lined by an epithelium that is cytologically normal but thicker than 6 layers.

3. Grade II transitional cell carcinoma has papillary and solid areas. The cells show mild to moderate cytologic atypia and have a greater degree of pleomorphism (Fig 50–7).

4. Grade III transitional cell carcinoma has a predominantly solid growth pattern with or without a papillary structure and shows cytologic anaplasia and a high mitotic rate. It may be difficult to recognize its transitional cell nature. Some authorities recognize a **grade IV carcinoma,** which represents a more anaplastic variant of grade III with evidence of cell necrosis.

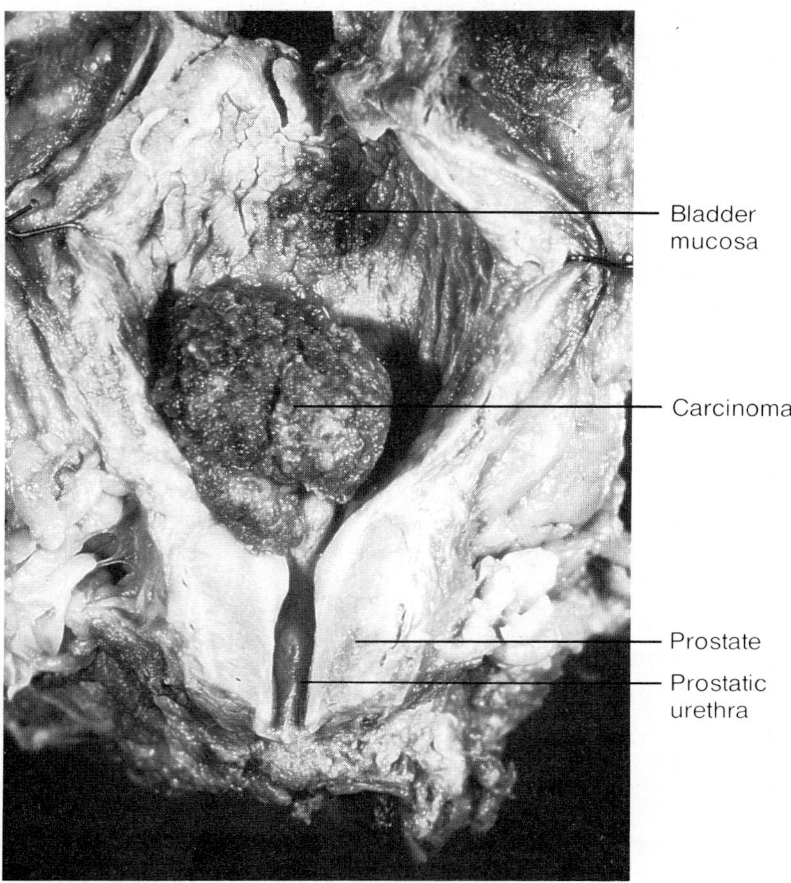

Figure 50–6. Bladder carcinoma, showing a large neoplasm almost filling the lower half of the bladder.

The critical distinction in terms of behavior and treatment is between grade I or II (well-differentiated) and grade III or IV (poorly differentiated) carcinomas. Grade III carcinomas are frequently associated with carcinoma in situ of the adjacent mucosa (see below).

Infiltration of the tumor must be assessed independently of histologic grade. Infiltration of the smooth muscle wall or blood vessels has adverse prognostic significance.

B. Dysplasia and Carcinoma in Situ: In high-grade bladder carcinomas, the urothelium is believed to progress through dysplasia to carcinoma in situ before it invades the basement membrane. Carcinoma in situ usually occurs in men over 40 years of age and causes no symptoms or gross changes in the bladder mucosa. Random bladder biopsy or cytologic examination of urine is necessary for diagnosis. Microscopically, the epithelium shows disturbed maturation and cytologic abnormalities such as an increased nuclear:cytoplasmic ratio, disturbed chromatin pattern, and hyperchromasia. Cytologic examination of urine shows malignant transitional cells.

Carcinoma in situ is frequently multifocal and may extend into the urethra and ureters. The prognosis is bad, with many patients developing high-grade invasive carcinoma.

Clinical Features

Painless hematuria is the commonest presenting symptom of bladder carcinoma. Involvement of the trigone may cause frequency and dysuria. Involvement of the ureteral orifice may lead to hydronephrosis and infection. Rarely, invasion of adjacent organs (Fig 50–8) (colon, usually) leads to fistulous tracts. Dysplasia and carcinoma in situ are asymptomatic.

The diagnosis is made by cystoscopy and biopsy.

Clinical Staging

Clinical staging depends on the degree of invasion by the neoplasm and the presence of lymph node and distant metastases (Table 50–2).

Treatment & Prognosis

The mainstay of treatment of bladder cancer is surgery. Radical cystectomy is indicated for poorly differentiated carcinomas and well-

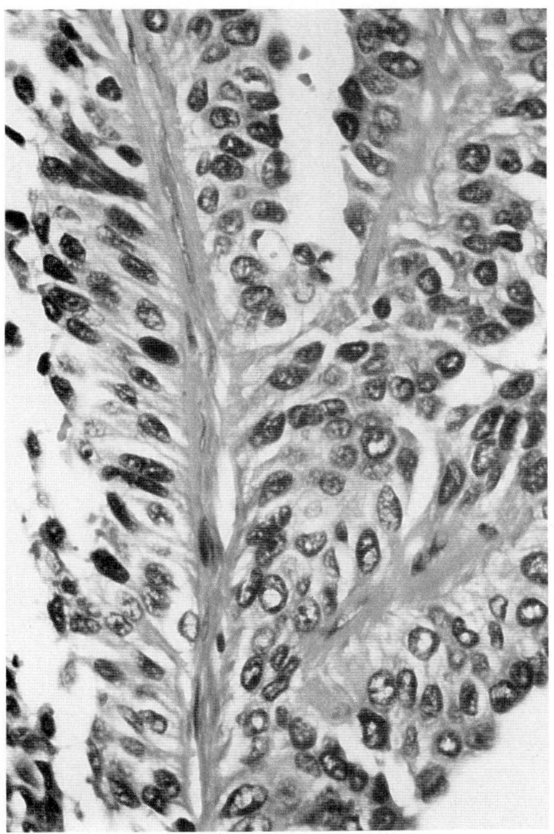

Figure 50-7. Transitional cell carcinoma of the bladder, showing papillary fronds lined by atypical transitional epithelium.

Table 50-2. Staging of transitional cell carcinoma of the bladder.[1]

Stage 0	PIS	Carcinoma in situ
	Pa	Papillary neoplasm without invasion
Stage A	P1	Invasion of lamina propria
Stage B1	P2	Invasion of superficial half of the muscle wall
Stage B2	P3a	Invasion of deep half of the muscle wall
Stage C	P3b	Invasion through bladder wall into perivesical fat
Stage D1	P4a	Invasion of prostate, vagina, or uterus
	P4b	Tumor fixed to pelvic or abdominal wall
	N1-3	Pelvic nodes involved
Stage D2	M1	Distant metastases
	N4	Involvement of lymph nodes above the aortic bifurcation

[1]These designations are based on the TNM staging system which is being used more frequently. In this system, P = characteristics of the primary tumor based on pathologic examination; N = node status; M = metastatic status.

differentiated carcinomas in which there is muscle invasion. Local resection or partial cystectomy suffices for better-differentiated noninvasive neoplasms.

The prognosis depends both on clinical stage and histologic grade. With appropriate surgical resection, 50–80% of patients with stage II neoplasms survive 5 years. With local extension outside the bladder, the 5-year survival rate drops to 20–30%. The better differentiated the neoplasm (lower grade), the better the prognosis.

OTHER EPITHELIAL NEOPLASMS

Pure Squamous Carcinoma

Pure squamous carcinoma is rare except where schistosomiasis is endemic, in which case it represents the commonest type.

Well-differentiated keratinizing squamous carcinoma tends to form large, bulky exophytic masses that protrude into the lumen. They tend to remain confined to the bladder until a late stage and have a better prognosis than transitional carcinomas of similar size.

Pure Adenocarcinoma of the Bladder

Adenocarcinoma is rare but may arise (1) in urachal epithelial remnants in the dome of the bladder; (2) in bladder mucosa that has undergone glandular metaplasia; and (3) in cystitis glandularis.

NONEPITHELIAL NEOPLASMS

Paraganglioma (Pheochromocytoma)

Paragangliomas of the urinary bladder are rare and originate in paraganglionic structures in the bladder wall. They resemble pheochromocytomas of the adrenal gland. Most are nonfunctioning. Functioning paragangliomas secrete bursts of catecholamines during urination, causing palpitations and hypertension.

Mesenchymal Neoplasms

Mesenchymal neoplasms are rare. Smooth muscle tumors (leiomyoma and leiomyosarcoma) are the most common of these; embryonal rhabdomyosarcoma occurs in young children.

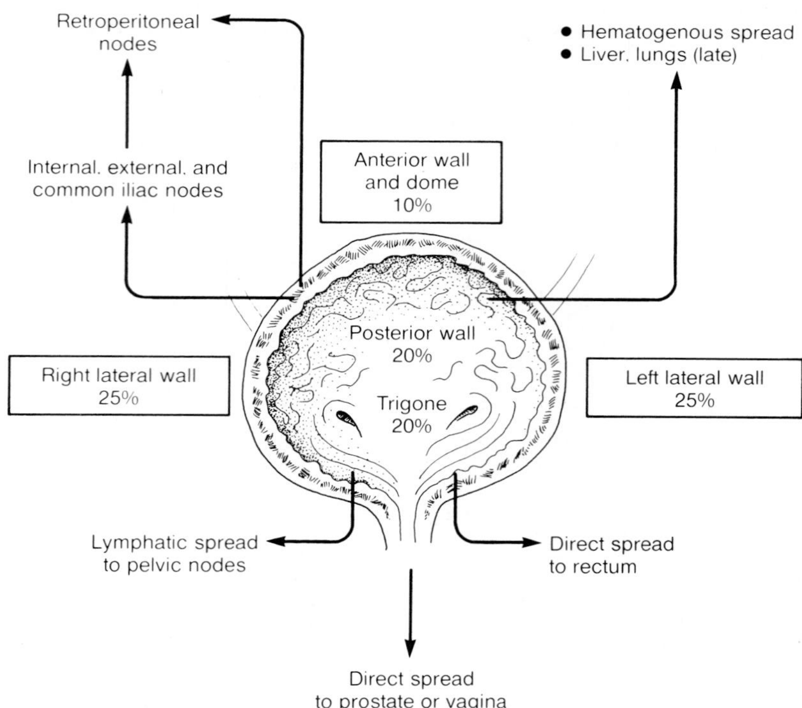

Figure 50–8. Mode of dissemination of urothelial neoplasms of the bladder. The percentages refer to the distribution of cancers in different parts of the bladder.

THE URETHRA

CONGENITAL ANOMALIES

POSTERIOR URETHRAL VALVE

Posterior urethral valve is a congenital anomaly that occurs mainly in males. It is characterized by the presence of folds of mucous membrane in the posterior urethra that cause partial valvular obstruction to the passage of urine, leading to infection and hydronephrosis in childhood.

ECTOPIC URETERS

Ectopic ureters opening into the urethra are rare. Continuous dribbling of urine results.

URETHRAL INFECTIONS (Urethritis)

Most infections of the urethra are sexually transmitted. Gonorrhea and nonspecific urethritis, which is probably caused by chlamydiae, are the most common. These infections are discussed in Chapter 54.

Urethral strictures may follow chronic infections and urethral trauma. When severe, urinary flow is obstructed.

URETHRAL NEOPLASMS

URETHRAL CARUNCLE

A caruncle is a common lesion of the urethra, occurring mainly in older women. It usually presents as a small (< 2 cm) nodular, red, friable mass situated at the external urethral orifice. It frequently becomes ulcerated and bleeds.

Microscopically, a urethral caruncle is composed of inflamed, highly vascular granulation tissue. The cause is uncertain, but it is more apt to be a reactive change than a neoplasm.

Surgical excision is curative.

CARCINOMA OF THE URETHRA

Urethral carcinoma is extremely rare. The most common form is transitional cell carcinoma of the prostatic urethra in males. Lower urethral carcinomas are highly malignant, frequently squamous carcinomas or adenocarcinomas. These have a very poor prognosis, with a 5-year survival rate close to zero.

The Testis, Prostate, & Penis

51

EMBRYOLOGY

The reproductive system develops from the urogenital ridge in the posterior coelomic cavity of the early embryo. The early gonad is identical in both sexes.

In the absence of a Y chromosome (in the female), the gonads develop into ovaries and the müllerian ducts into the internal female reproductive organs—uterine (fallopian) tubes, uterus, and vagina (Fig 51–1).

In the presence of a Y chromosome (male), the gonads develop into testes. The müllerian ducts regress under the influence of a factor produced by the testis (müllerian duct regression factor). The wolffian ducts, in the presence of testicular androgenic hormones, develop to form the internal male reproductive organs—vasa deferentia, seminal vesicles, and ejaculatory ducts (Fig 51–1).

THE TESTIS & EPIDIDYMIS

STRUCTURE & FUNCTION

The testes are small before puberty, enlarging to reach adult size at about age 10 years. The prepubertal testis is composed of seminiferous tubules lined by inactive cuboidal germ cells and Sertoli cells; a lumen develops in the tubules at about 4 years. Considerable proliferation occurs at puberty, causing enlargement of the seminiferous tubules and the onset of spermatogenesis.

The normal adult testis is composed of **seminiferous tubules,** which show active spermatogenesis, with spermatocytes, spermatids and spermatozoa; and the **interstitial cells of Leydig,** which lie between the tubules and are the source of testosterone. The seminiferous tubules are lined by a delicate basement membrane, and there is little interstitial connective tissue.

The functions of the adult testis are (1) production of spermatozoa, which are then transported via the epididymis and vas deferens to the seminal vesicle, where they are stored; and (2) secretion of androgens, mainly testosterone, which are responsible for development and maintenance of male secondary sexual characteristics.

MANIFESTATIONS OF TESTICULAR DISEASE

Infertility

Either the male, the female, or both partners may be responsible for infertility, which is defined

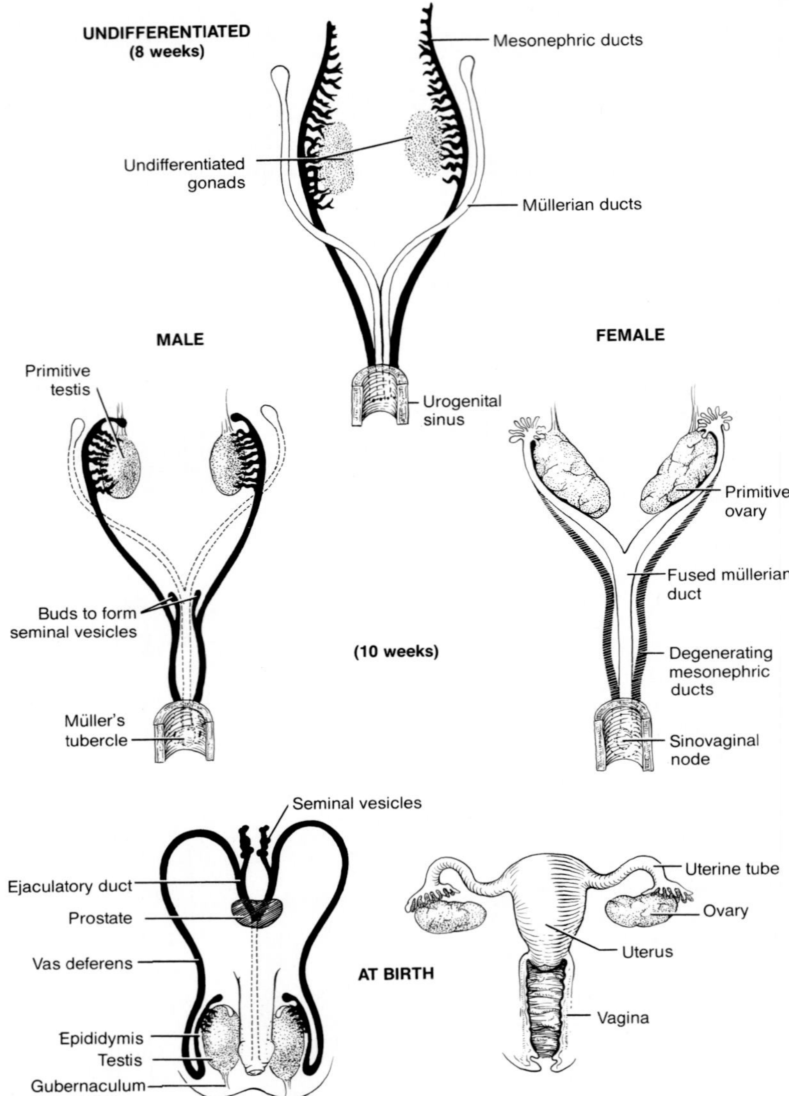

Figure 51–1. Differentiation of the embryonic genital system into the definitive male and female reproductive systems.

as the failure to conceive after 1 year of regular coitus without contraception. Male infertility, usually recognized by absence of spermatozoa (azoospermia) or decreased numbers of spermatozoa in semen (oligozoospermia), may result from one of 3 categories of disease:

A. Pretesticular Causes: These consist of endocrine disorders—most commonly hypopituitarism—in which failure of production of gonadotropins leads to testicular failure. These diseases are recognized by decreased pituitary gonadotropin levels in serum.

B. Posttesticular Causes: The most common mechanism is obstruction to the outflow of spermatozoa. Bilateral obstruction results in azoospermia. Obstructive infertility is responsible for up to 50% of cases of infertility and may be corrected surgically. The diagnosis is established by vasograms, in which dye is introduced into the duct system for radiographic visualization; and by testicular biopsy, which shows normal spermatogenesis.

C. Testicular Causes: Most of these conditions are untreatable and include any disorder associated with testicular atrophy (Table 51–1) plus either of the following specific abnormalities identifiable on testicular biopsies: (1) germ cell aplasia, in which there is a total absence of spermatocytes and the seminiferous tubules are lined entirely by Sertoli cells (also called "Sertoli cell only" syndrome); and (2) spermatocytic maturation arrest.

Testicular Masses or Enlargement

The presence of masses or enlargement of the testis represents the most common symptom of

Table 51-1. Causes of atrophy of the testes.

Cryptorchidism
Klinefelter's syndrome
Obstruction to outflow of semen
Administration of estrogens, most commonly in the treatment of prostatic carcinoma
Hypopituitarism
Aging
Malnutrition and cachexia
Inflammatory diseases such as mumps orchitis
Radiation
Alcoholic cirrhosis

testicular disease. In general, acute inflammatory lesions are painful; chronic inflammatory lesions and neoplasms are usually painless. Scrotal swelling (Fig 51-2) should be carefully examined for evidence of an enlarged testis, and any patient with a testicular mass should be considered to have a neoplasm until proved otherwise.

Abnormal Production of Hormones

Hormones from functioning testicular stromal tumors may produce precocious puberty in the child (androgens) or gynecomastia (estrogens).

ASSESSMENT OF TESTICULAR FUNCTION

Physical examination should be supplemented when necessary by ultrasonography and computerized tomography in the evaluation of testicular mass lesions. Testicular biopsy is useful in the diagnosis of mass lesions and in determining whether the cause of azoospermia is testicular or posttesticular. Serum levels of gonadotropins and androgens may be abnormal in testicular failure secondary to hypopituitarism and in functioning testicular neoplasms.

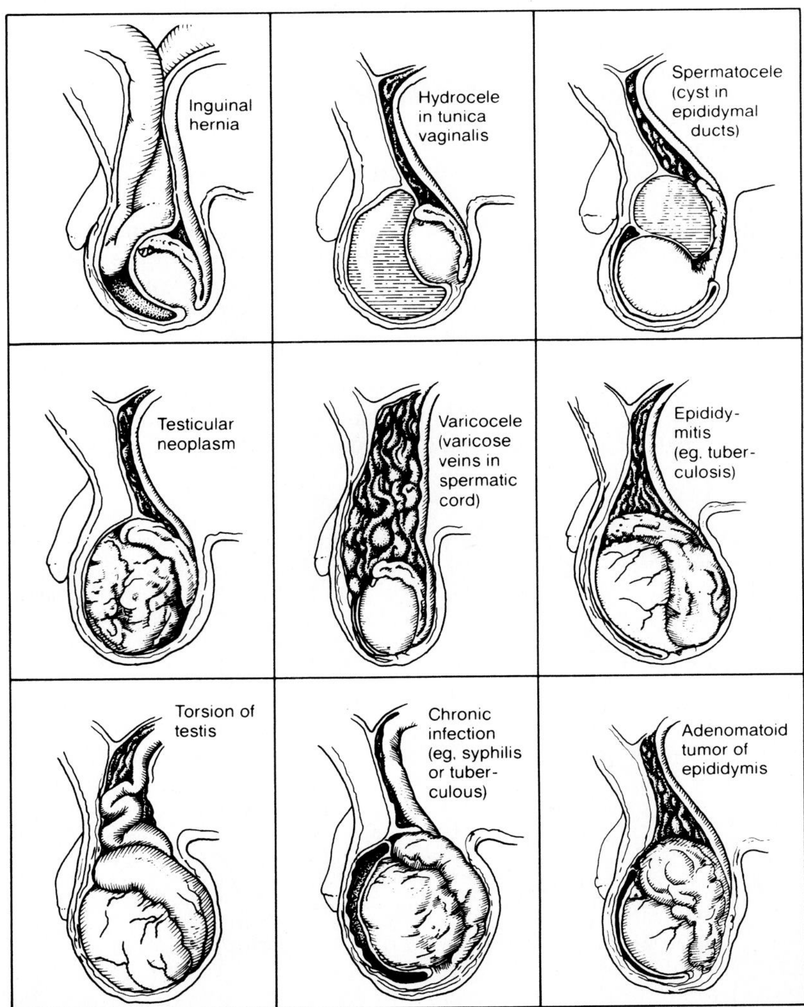

Figure 51-2. Principal causes of scrotal swelling, including testicular mass lesions.

A normal semen specimen has a volume of 3–4 mL, a sperm count of 30 × 10^6/mL, and 80% morphologically normal and motile spermatozoa.

CONGENITAL TESTICULAR ANOMALIES

Absence of one or both testes and **fusion** of testes are very rare anomalies. **Klinefelter's syndrome** (testicular dysgenesis) results in failure of normal testicular development at puberty (Chapter 15).

Abnormalities of Testicular Descent (Undescended Testis; Ectopic Testis; Cryptorchidism)

Normal descent of the testis through the inguinal canal into the scrotum occurs in the last trimester of pregnancy. The mechanism and factors that stimulate descent are uncertain.

Arrest of testicular descent is common, occurring in 3% of full-term male infants; in most of these cases, complete descent occurs in the first year of life. A testis that remains arrested at an extrascrotal location along the normal path of migration is called an undescended testis (Fig 51–3).

Rarely, the testis comes to be located outside its normal descent route (ectopic testis; Fig 51–3).

An extrascrotal testis appears normal until about puberty, and placement in the scrotum before age 6–8 years assures normal function. After puberty, a misplaced testis becomes atrophic. Failure of spermatogenesis is believed to be due to the higher temperature of an extrascrotal testis, the normally lower scrotal temperatures being necessary for normal spermatogenesis.

Individuals with undescended testes have a greatly increased risk of developing malignant germ cell neoplasms if the maldescent is not corrected. A slightly increased risk of testicular cancer persists after the testis is replaced in the scrotum. In patients with one undescended testis, the normal testis also has a slightly increased risk of developing testicular cancer.

TESTICULAR ATROPHY

Atrophy of the seminiferous tubules is common, usually symptomless, and occurs secondary to many diseases (Table 51–1). The testes are smaller than normal. Microscopically, the seminiferous tubules show decreased diameter, increased thickness of the basement membrane, marked decrease in germ cells, and absent spermatogenesis. In complete atrophy, the tubules either contain only Sertoli cells or become completely occluded by fibrosis. The interstitium shows fibrosis. Leydig cells are usually present in normal numbers (Fig 51–4).

INFLAMMATORY LESIONS OF THE TESTIS & EPIDIDYMIS

ACUTE EPIDIDYMO-ORCHITIS

Acute epididymo-orchitis is a common infection caused by bacteria that reach the epididymis from the urethra. *Escherichia coli* and the gonococcus are common culprits. Organisms reach the epididymis via the vas deferens secondary to reflux of infected urine from the prostatic urethra, or via the lymphatics of the spermatic cord. Acute pyogenic inflammation of the epididymis ensues, commonly extending into the testis (Fig 51–5).

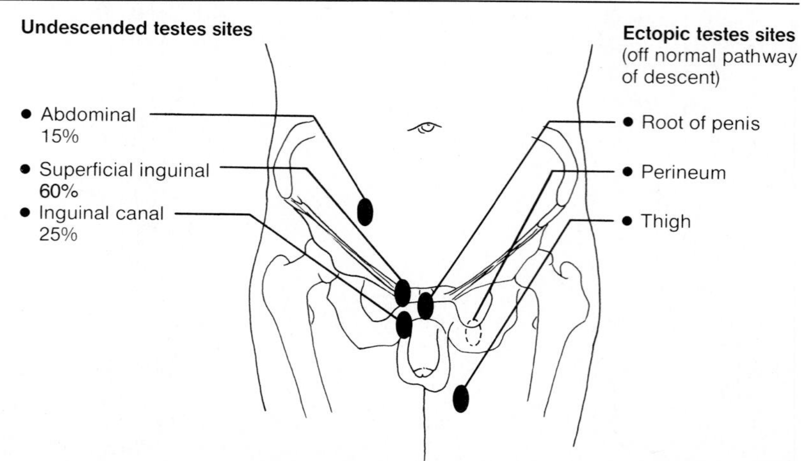

Figure 51–3. Sites at which undescended and ectopic testes are commonly found.

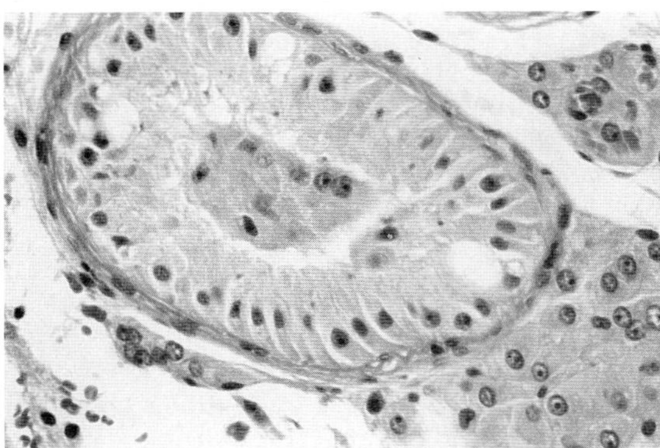

Figure 51-4. Cryptorchid testis, showing marked atrophy of the seminiferous tubules, which are lined by Sertoli cells only, with absent germ cells. The interstitium contains Leydig cells.

Clinically, patients present with acute onset of fever, pain, and tenderness and redness of the scrotum extending along the spermatic cord. Resolution occurs rapidly with specific antibiotic therapy.

Complications include (1) fibrosis leading to obstruction of the epididymis, resulting in sterility only in those cases where both sides are affected; (2) vascular compromise, leading rarely to infarction of the testis; and (3) abscess formation in the scrotum.

TUBERCULOUS EPIDIDYMO-ORCHITIS

Tuberculosis of the epididymis is common wherever there is a high incidence of tuberculosis. Eighty percent of patients have demonstrable (though often subclinical) lesions in the urinary tract. Tubercle bacilli gain access to the epididymis from the urethra.

Pathologically, there is a chronic granulomatous inflammation with caseous necrosis and fibrosis, leading to thickening of the epididymis. The inflammatory reaction frequently spreads to involve the testis (Fig 51-5).

Clinically, patients present with enlargement of the scrotum. Pain is usually not a major complaint. Caseous material may ulcerate and drain through the skin of the scrotum, usually the posterior aspect. The diagnosis is made by culture or by demonstration of acid-fast bacilli in caseous granulomas on tissue sections.

MUMPS ORCHITIS

Orchitis occurs in 10-20% of cases of mumps in postpubertal males. It usually causes mild acute inflammation with testicular pain and mild swelling that resolves rapidly. In a small number of cases, severe inflammation results in testicular atrophy and sterility.

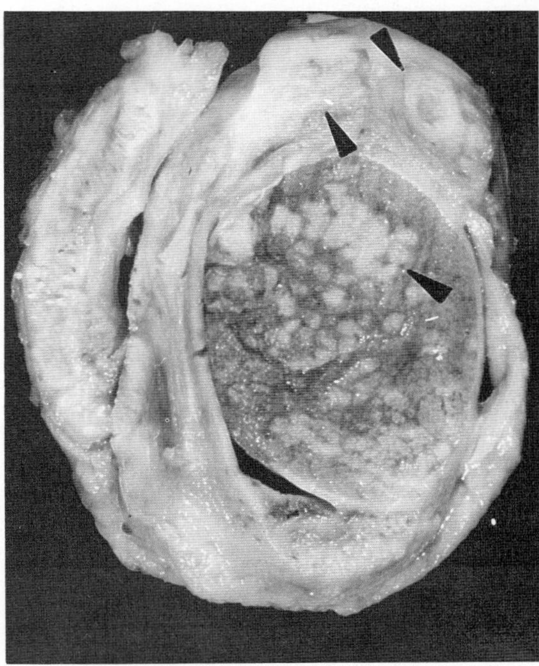

Figure 51-5. Tuberculous epididymo-orchitis, showing caseating granulomas in the testis and epididymis (arrows).

SYPHILIS

Syphilis affects the testis in the tertiary (late) stage and is characterized by formation of a rubbery firm mass of necrotizing chronic granulomatous inflammation known as a gumma. It is rare today because of better treatment of early syphilis. Syphilis is discussed in Chapter 54.

IDIOPATHIC GRANULOMATOUS ORCHITIS

This uncommon inflammatory lesion of the testis is of unknown cause; some patients have autoantibodies to testicular antigens, leading to the hypothesis that it is an autoimmune disease.

Grossly, the testis is enlarged, with a smooth capsule. On cut section, the normal structure of the testis is replaced by a firm, grayish-white multinodular lesion. Microscopically, there is destruction of seminiferous tubules and the presence of multiple epithelioid granulomas with giant cells. Caseation does not occur.

Patients are usually postpubertal and present with moderately painful enlargement of the testis; clinically, this disorder is frequently mistaken for a neoplasm.

SPERM GRANULOMA

A sperm granuloma is a fairly common lesion that occurs in the testis and epididymis when there is leakage of spermatozoa into the interstitium. A common cause is a slipped vasectomy ligature.

Extravasation of spermatozoa leads to a granulomatous response with progressive fibrosis. The diagnosis is made by identification of spermatozoa within the inflammatory lesion.

FOURNIER'S SCROTAL GANGRENE

This rare disease of adults is characterized by necrotizing cellulitis and fasciitis of the scrotum, caused usually by anaerobic bacteria. Acute inflammation with marked edema progresses rapidly to vascular thrombosis and gangrene of the scrotal skin, which then ulcerates and sloughs, leaving the testes exposed. The mortality rate is high unless treatment is started expeditiously.

HYDROCELE

A hydrocele is a collection of fluid within the potential space between the 2 layers of the tunica vaginalis (Fig 51–2). The usual causes are trauma, infection, or tumor of the underlying testis. Congenital hydroceles also occur but are rare. Hydrocele fluid is usually clear and straw-colored; if it contains much blood, the term "hematocele" may be appropriate.

TESTICULAR TORSION

Torsion of the testis is a common condition caused by twisting of the spermatic cord, leading to vascular obstruction. Abnormalities of the testis or its ligaments are predisposing factors. Torsion occurs commonly in incompletely descended testes.

Pathologically, there is edema, hemorrhage, and finally venous infarction of the testis. Clinically, the torsion causes sudden onset of severe pain with marked swelling of the scrotum (Fig 51–2). The testis is intensely tender. Orchiectomy is required in cases that have progressed to necrosis of testicular tissue.

TESTICULAR NEOPLASMS

Testicular neoplasms are classified on a histogenetic basis. There are 2 main groups: germ cell neoplasms and stromal neoplasms (Table 51–2).

Table 51–2. Classification of testicular neoplasms.

Tumor Type	Frequency	Age	Gross
Germ cell tumors			
Seminoma	30%	30–50	Solid, yellowish-white, firm.
Embryonal carcinoma[1]	20%	15–30	Solid, fleshy, soft, friable, hemorrhagic.
Teratoma[1]	10%	10–30	Cystic, solid areas, cartilage.
Yolk sac (entodermal sinus) carcinoma	Rare	10–30	Solid, fleshy, soft, friable.
Choriocarcinoma[1]	Rare	10–30	Solid, hemorrhagic.
Mixed germ cell neoplasms[1]	35%	10–50	Variable, usually have a cystic teratomatous component.
Gonadal stromal tumors			
Undifferentiated	1%	Any age	Usually small round circumscribed nodule
Leydig cell	1%	Any age	Usually small round circumscribed nodule
Sertoli (granulosa-theca) cell	1%	Any age	Usually small round circumscribed nodule
Mixed stromal	Rare	Any age	Usually small round circumscribed nodule
Mixed germ cell and stromal	Rare	10–50	Variable
Lymphoma	2%	60–80	Solid nodules
Metastasis and other	Rare	Any age, usually elderly	Solid nodules

[1]Note that the British Testicular Tumor Panel classifies these neoplasms as varieties of teratoma: embryonal carcinoma = malignant teratoma undifferentiated; teratoma = teratoma differentiated (mature); mixed germ cell neoplasms = malignant teratoma intermediate; choriocarcinoma = malignant teratoma trophoblastic.

GERM CELL NEOPLASMS

Germ cell neoplasms account for over 95% of testicular tumors. They occur with an incidence of 2 per 100,000 males. In the age group from 15 to 34 years, they cause 10–12% of cancer deaths. They are more common in whites than blacks.

Etiology

The etiology of testicular germ cell neoplasms is unknown. Extrascrotal testes have an increased incidence of neoplasia (especially seminomas); 5% of testes in the abdominal cavity and 1% of testes in the inguinal canal develop cancer. The risk—approximately 30 times normal—is sufficient to warrant prophylactic orchiectomy if an undescended testis is discovered in an adult. When undescended testis is detected early in life and surgically placed in the scrotum, the risk of germ cell neoplasia is only slightly increased.

The taking of diethylstilbestrol (DES) by the mother during pregnancy is associated with an increased incidence of testicular cancer in male offspring. There is no familial predisposition.

Classification

Germ cell tumors are presumed to arise in a primitive germ cell in the seminiferous tubules. They are classified according to their differentiation (Fig 51–6; Table 51–2). Germ cell neoplasms that show minimal differentiation and are composed of primitive germ cells are called embryonal carcinomas. Those that show recognizable differentiation are called seminomas (seminiferous dif-

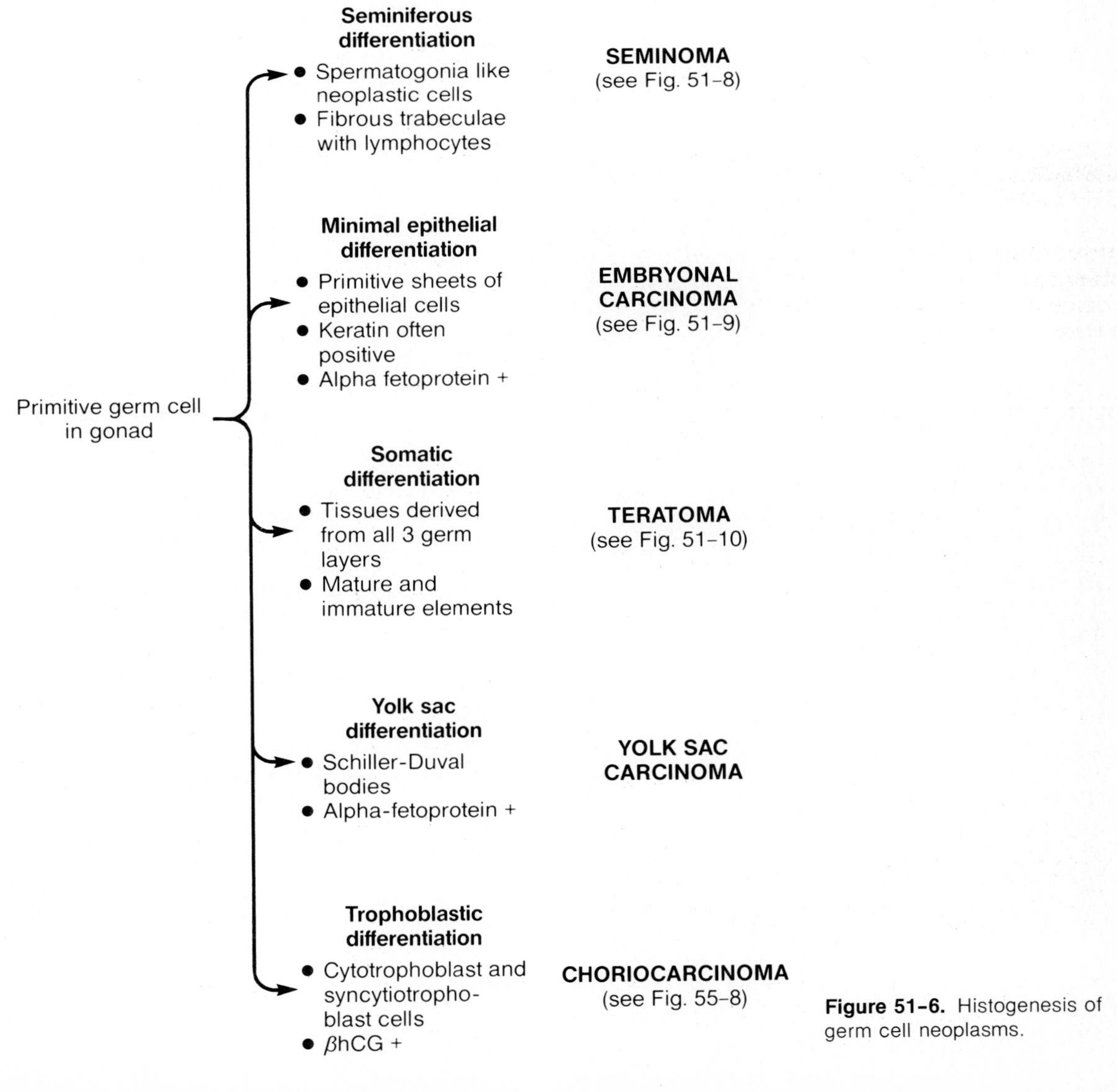

Figure 51–6. Histogenesis of germ cell neoplasms.

ferentiation), teratomas (somatic differentiation), choriocarcinomas (trophoblastic differentiation), or yolk sac carcinomas (yolk sac differentiation). Neoplasms composed of a single element account for 60%; the remainder are mixed tumors.

This has been accepted as the international classification by the World Health Organization and is the one used in the United States. Other classifications exist (see footnote 1 in Table 51–2).

From a clinical standpoint, it is important to differentiate between seminoma and nonseminomatous germ cell neoplasms because the 2 groups may be treated differently.

Pathology

A. Gross Appearance: (Fig 51–7.) All germ cell neoplasms appear as masses causing destruction of testicular substance. In small neoplasms, there may be residual testicular tissue, partially infiltrated by tumor. Seminomas and teratomas are often better circumscribed than other types. Some gross differences exist between the different types of tumor (Table 51–2).

B. Microscopic Appearance:

1. Seminoma–"Classic seminoma" is characterized by nests of uniform large round cells that have distinct cell membranes, centrally placed nuclei, prominent nucleoli, and clear cytoplasm containing abundant glycogen; these cells resemble the primary spermatocytes in the seminiferous tubule. The nests of cells are separated by fibrous trabeculae infiltrated by numerous lymphocytes (Fig 51–8). Granulomatous inflammation with giant cells and necrosis is present in about 50% of cases and may dominate the histologic picture. There is some evidence that the presence of a lymphocytic or granulomatous infiltrate (?immune response) indicates a better prognosis.

Two additional variants of seminoma are recognized: **(1) Spermatocytic seminoma** accounts for about 5% of cases, occurs in older individuals, and is characterized by maturation of the tumor cells, which resemble secondary spermatocytes. It does not metastasize. **(2) Anaplastic seminoma** is more pleomorphic and has a higher mitotic rate (> 3 per high-power field). It tends to present at a more advanced stage of disease, but stage for stage it has a prognosis similar to that of classic seminoma.

2. Embryonal carcinoma–Embryonal carcinoma is characterized by highly malignant primitive-appearing undifferentiated cells showing frequent mitoses and necrosis. The cells may be arranged in solid sheets or may show glandular and papillary patterns (Fig 51–9).

3. Teratoma–Teratoma is characterized by somatic differentiation. By definition, all 3 germ

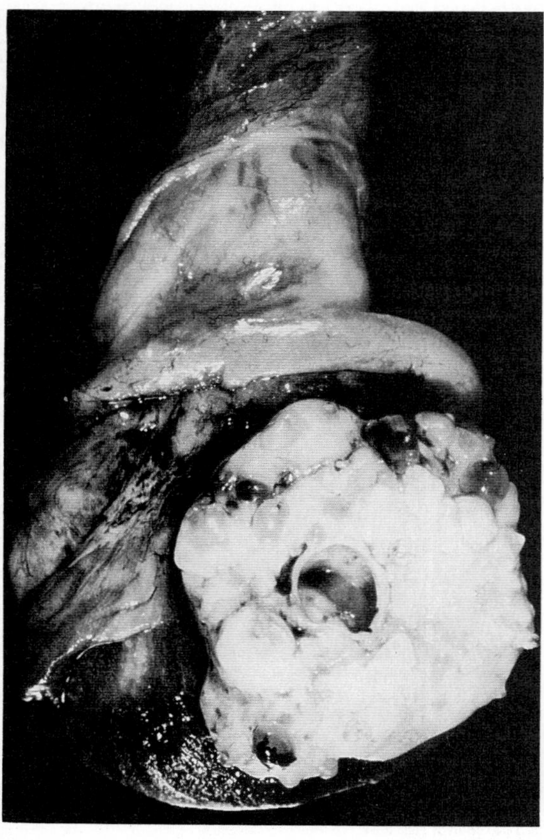

Figure 51–7. Mixed germ cell tumor of the testis. Note the cystic area in the center, which is characteristic of teratoma.

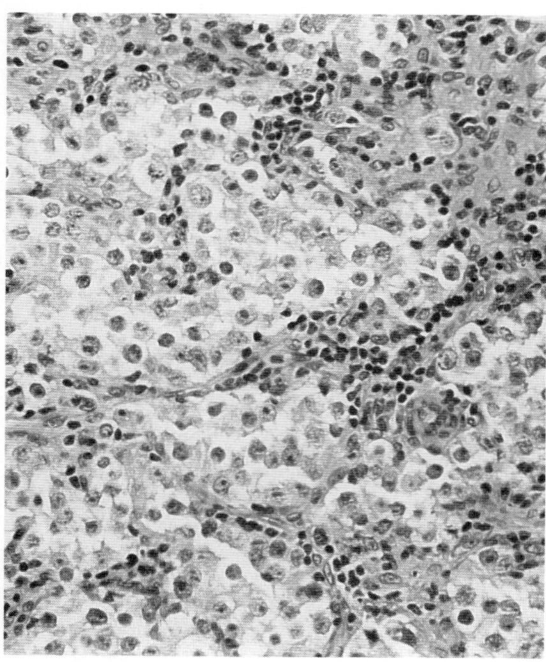

Figure 51–8. Seminoma of the testis, showing nests of large round cells resembling spermatogonia separated by fibrous trabeculae infiltrated by lymphocytes.

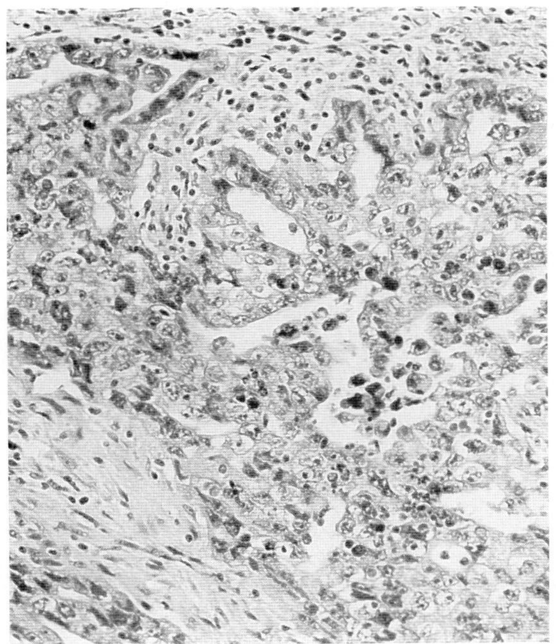

Figure 51-9. Embryonal carcinoma of testis, showing solid masses of primitive epithelial cells forming irregular glandlike spaces.

layers are represented. When mature somatic structures such as skin and nerves (ectoderm), gut and respiratory epithelium (entoderm), and cartilage, bone, and muscle (mesoderm) are present, the term mature teratoma is used (Fig 51-10). When immature somatic structures like neuroblastic tissue and undifferentiated mesenchymal cells are present, the neoplasm is called an immature teratoma. All testicular teratomas in adults are biologically malignant; in contrast, in children under age 12 years, teratomas behave as benign neoplasms.

4. Yolk sac carcinoma-This tumor is characterized by differentiation toward yolk sac-like structures. Tumor cells assume a delicate reticular (lacelike) pattern or a papillary pattern in which structures that resemble glomeruli (glomeruloid or Schiller-Duval bodies) are present. Pink hyaline globules are often present in the cytoplasm of the cells of yolk sac carcinoma; these globules frequently stain positively for alpha-fetoprotein.

5. Choriocarcinoma-The presence of cytotrophoblastic and syncytiotrophoblastic giant cells, arranged in a manner resembling their relationship in chorionic villi, is characteristic. There is almost always extensive hemorrhage. The syncytiotrophoblastic cells secrete human chorionic gonadotropin (hCG) and stain positively for βHCG.

It must be emphasized that the presence of syncytiotrophoblastic giant cells alone does not permit a diagnosis of choriocarcinoma. Such cells are not uncommonly found scattered in all of the other germ cell neoplasms.

Tumor Markers

βHCG and alpha-fetoprotein (AFP) are ex-

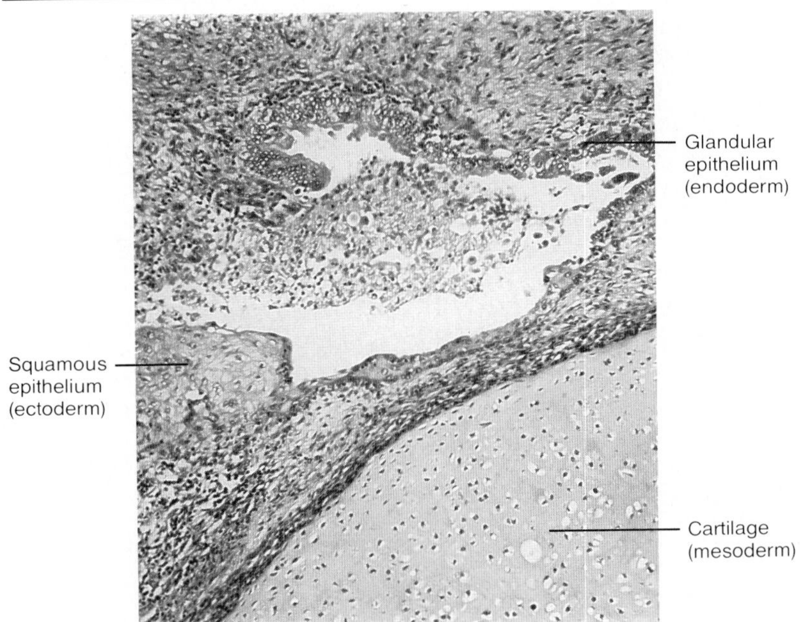

Figure 51-10. Teratoma of testis, showing elements of all 3 germ layers.

tremely important tumor markers in germ cell neoplasms. High levels of βHCG are present in the serum in patients with choriocarcinoma. Mildly elevated serum βHCG levels occur in patients with other germ cell neoplasms containing a subpopulation of syncytiotrophoblastic giant cells. Alpha-fetoprotein levels in serum are markedly elevated in patients with yolk sac carcinoma and embryonal carcinoma. The absence of elevated βHCG and AFP in the serum indicates the absence of choriocarcinoma and yolk sac carcinoma. It should be noted that other neoplasms are associated with elevation of βHCG (eg, rare cases of lung carcinoma) and AFP (eg, 90% of hepatocellular carcinomas) (see Chapter 19).

These 2 tumor markers are also very useful in monitoring the treatment of patients with germ cell neoplasms. Elevation of βHCG or AFP in serum is a very sensitive indicator of the presence of that particular tumor type in the body. With removal of the tumor, either by surgery or by chemotherapy, the levels of these tumor markers drop; subsequent elevation indicates recurrence.

Biologic Behavior

All germ cell neoplasms of the testis should be considered malignant. The only exception is teratoma in children, which behaves as a benign neoplasm.

The metastatic potential is very high for these neoplasms. They spread by lymphatics to the retroperitoneal and para-aortic lymph nodes and via the bloodstream to the lungs and liver (Fig 51–11).

Clinical Presentation

Germ cell neoplasms usually present as a painless mass in the testis, often associated with a hydrocele.

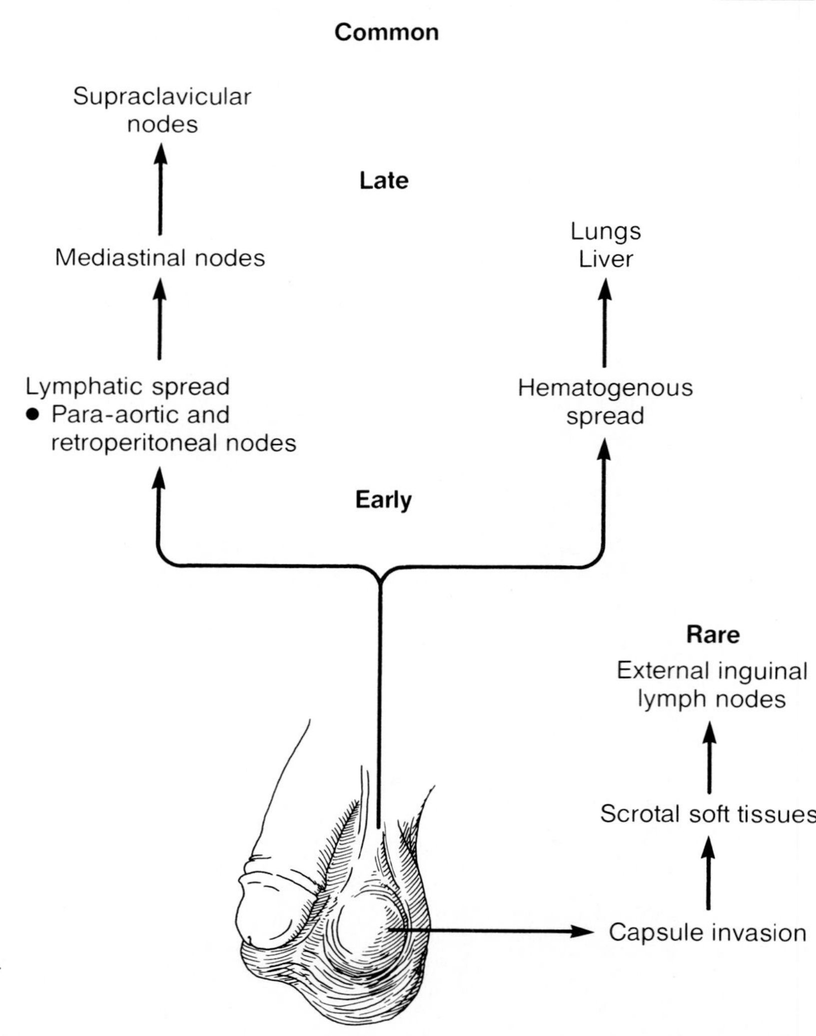

Figure 51–11. Pathways of metastasis of testicular germ cell neoplasms.

Not uncommonly, the first manifestation of the neoplasm is at a metastatic site (retroperitoneum, lung). Germ cell tumors have a tendency to remain small at the primary site while metastases may become large (eg, in the retroperitoneum).

Treatment

Seminomas are extremely radiosensitive. All germ cell neoplasms are highly sensitive to modern combined chemotherapy. The use of orchiectomy and surgical removal of metastases from the lungs and retroperitoneum combined with aggressive chemotherapy has greatly improved the prognosis. While 90% of patients with testicular germ cell neoplasms died of their disease 20 years ago, the survival rate is now close to 90%, representing one of the most remarkable successes of cancer treatment (Table 51–3).

GONADAL STROMAL NEOPLASMS (Table 51–2)

Interstitial (Leydig) cell tumors constitute about 1% of testicular neoplasms and occur mainly in children and young adults. They often produce androgens, causing precocious puberty in children. More rarely, they secrete estrogens.

These neoplasms vary from 0.5 cm to over 10 cm in diameter and are usually well-circumscribed and yellowish-brown. Microscopically, there are sheets of large cells resembling interstitial cells. In 50% of cases, typical rod-shaped crystalloids of Reinke occur. Cytologic atypia may be present but is not necessarily an indicator of malignancy. Immunoperoxidase stains for steroid hormones are positive in the tumor cells.

The biologic behavior of these tumors is usually benign, but about 10% are malignant. Prediction of malignant behavior is not possible by histologic examination.

Sertoli cell tumors (sometimes called androblastomas) are rare. They typically contain structures resembling seminiferous tubules with Sertoli cells. Production of estrogens may induce gynecomastia. Most are benign.

MALIGNANT LYMPHOMA

Primary malignant lymphoma of the testis occurs most often in patients over 60 years of age and represents the commonest neoplasm of the testis in this age group. It accounts for 2% of all testicular neoplasms. B-immunoblastic sarcoma is the most common histologic type.

ADENOMATOID TUMOR

Adenomatoid tumor is a benign neoplasm that usually arises in the epididymis, probably from mesothelial cells in the tunica vaginalis. Immunoperoxidase stains for keratin are positive. A similar tumor occurs also in the pelvic cavity in females, commonly on the external surface of the uterus and uterine tubes.

Adenomatoid tumors appear as small circumscribed firm nodules with a homogeneous grayish-white cut surface. Microscopically, they are composed of glandlike or slitlike spaces (hence "adenomatoid") lined by flat to cuboidal mesothelial cells in a stroma composed of fibroblasts, smooth muscle cells, and collagen.

THE PROSTATE

STRUCTURE & FUNCTION

The prostate gland weighs about 20 g and encircles the upper (prostatic) urethra (Fig 51–12). It is composed of 2 lateral lobes, a median lobe, and one anterior and one posterior lobe. The ejaculatory ducts pass through the gland to open into the prostatic urethra. Histologically, the prostate is a compound tubuloalveolar gland with a stroma composed of smooth muscle.

Prostatic secretion is the major volume compo-

Table 51–3. Prognostic factors in testicular germ cell tumors.

Good Prognosis	Poor Prognosis[1]
Confined to testis	Invasion of upper spermatic cord or spread outside testis
Absence of metastases	Distant metastases
Presence of dense lymphocytic infiltrate (in seminoma)	Histologic diagnosis of choriocarcinoma, immature teratoma, embryonal carcinoma, and yolk sac carcinoma
Histologic diagnosis of teratoma in a child and spermatocytic seminoma	Incomplete response to chemotherapy; recurrence after chemotherapy[1]
Good response to chemotherapy[1]	

[1]Five-year survival rates for nonseminomatous germ cell neoplasms that were about 10% 20 years ago are about 90% today. The main prognostic factor today is the response to chemotherapy, which has superseded all other factors.

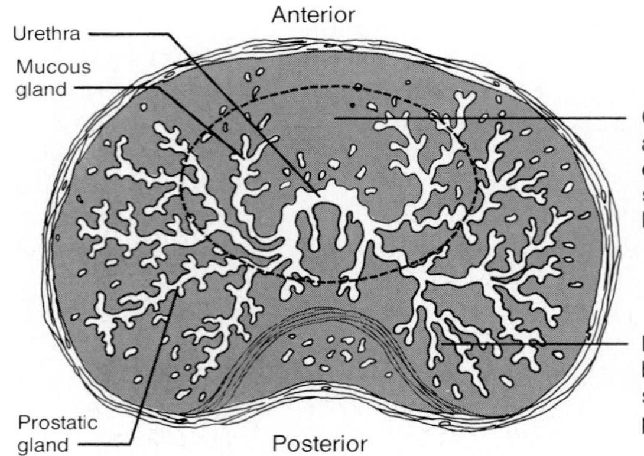

Figure 51-12. Structure of the prostate as seen in a transverse section through the gland.

nent of seminal fluid. It is rich in acid phosphatase.

Anatomically, the prostate is closely related to the rectum, and rectal examination permits digital palpation of its posterior aspect. Needle biopsy is also possible through the rectal wall. Both fine-needle aspiration and core-needle biopsy can be performed, providing specimens for cytologic and histologic examination, respectively.

MANIFESTATIONS OF PROSTATIC DISEASE

Obstruction of Urinary Outflow

Enlargement of the prostate from any cause may cause acute retention of urine, with acute painful dilatation of the bladder; or chronic retention of urine, characterized by incomplete emptying of the bladder, frequency, and a poor stream (decreased urinary flow). The bladder is dilated, and its wall undergoes hypertrophy. There is an increased incidence of infection of the stagnant bladder urine. Chronic renal failure may occur as a result of hydroureter and hydronephrosis.

Pain

Inflammatory lesions of the prostate cause perineal pain, aggravated by urination or by palpation of the prostate at rectal examination.

Hematuria

Hematuria may occur in benign prostatic hyperplasia, especially when there is infarction of a nodule. Hematuria is a late manifestation of prostatic cancer because that tumor most frequently arises in the peripheral zone of the gland.

INFLAMMATION OF THE PROSTATE

ACUTE PROSTATITIS

Acute prostatitis is a common disease caused by gram-negative coliform bacteria, most commonly *Escherichia coli.* Gonococcal prostatitis is also common. Prostatitis is a frequent complication of lower urinary tract surgery.

Acute inflammation—sometimes with suppuration—involves the gland focally or diffusely. Clinically, acute prostatitis is manifested as pain associated with urination or ejaculation. Marked tenderness is present over the enlarged prostate on rectal examination.

CHRONIC PROSTATITIS

Chronic prostatitis is common. While bacterial infection is frequently present, in many cases the cause is uncertain (''abacterial prostatitis'').

The gland is irregularly enlarged, firm, and infiltrated by numerous lymphocytes, plasma cells, macrophages, and neutrophils. Extravasation of secretions may provoke a foreign body type of granulomatous reaction (granulomatous prostatitis).

The symptoms of chronic prostatitis are vague. On examination, the gland feels irregular and firm, arousing a suspicion of cancer.

TUBERCULOSIS OF THE PROSTATE

Tuberculous prostatitis is rare and always secondary to a focus of tuberculosis elsewhere in the urinary tract; the epididymis is also usually involved.

NODULAR HYPERPLASIA OF THE PROSTATE (Benign Prostatic Hyperplasia; BPH)

When defined as an increase in the weight of the prostate, BPH is present in 50% of men between 40 and 60 years of age and 95% of men over 70. In most of these individuals, the condition is symptomless; however, clinically significant BPH is present in about 5–10% of men over 60 years of age. A small proportion of these individuals have symptoms severe enough to require surgery.

Etiology

The cause of prostatic hyperplasia is unknown. Changes in hormonal status are believed to be important; declining levels of androgens relative to estrogen levels are believed to stimulate glandular and stromal hyperplasia.

Pathology

A. Gross Findings: The periurethral part of the gland is most commonly involved (Fig 51–12). Overall, the gland is enlarged, often reaching massive size, and has a firm, rubbery consistency. Small nodules are present throughout the gland, usually 0.5–1 cm in diameter but sometimes much larger. Some of the larger nodules show cystic change. The urethra appears slitlike and compressed.

B. Microscopic Findings: The nodules are composed of a variable mixture of hyperplastic glandular elements and hyperplastic stromal muscle. The glands are larger than normal and lined by tall epithelium that is frequently thrown into papillary projections (Fig 51–13). Infarction of a nodule is common and may be associated with acute swelling that may precipitate acute pain and urinary retention. When infarction of a periurethral nodule occurs, the patient may develop hematuria.

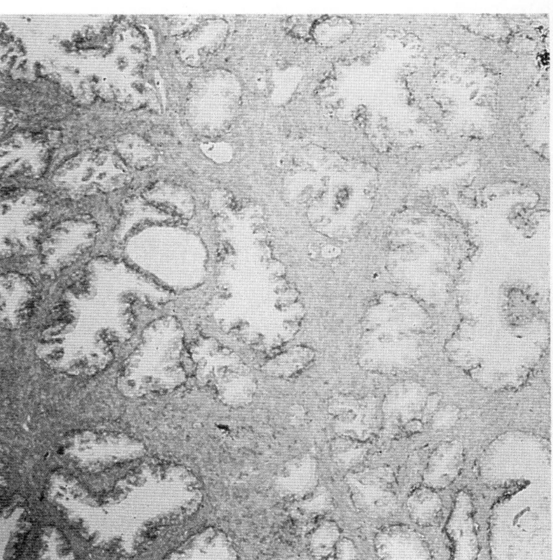

Figure 51–13. Benign prostatic hyperplasia, showing regular proliferation of glands. The epithelium shows hyperplasia characterized by papillary ingrowth. Note the separation of glands by stroma.

Clinical Features

Obstruction to urinary outflow is responsible for the major symptoms. The patient commonly has difficulty initiating urination, and the decreased flow causes a poor urinary stream. Incomplete emptying of the bladder leads to chronic retention of urine and frequency. Bladder neck obstruction is caused by urethral compression and enlargement of the periurethal median lobe, which protrudes into the bladder and acts as a ball valve.

Complications include (1) chronic retention of urine, hypertrophy of bladder musculature, and the development of bladder diverticula; (2) acute retention of urine, often due to swelling of the prostate caused by infarction; (3) hematuria, also the result of infarction; (4) urinary infection, because of urinary stasis; and (5) bilateral hydronephrosis and chronic renal failure.

Treatment of prostatic hyperplasia is surgical removal of the obstructing part of the glands, either by transurethral resection or open prostatectomy. The condition is not premalignant.

NEOPLASMS OF THE PROSTATE

CARCINOMA OF THE PROSTATE

Carcinoma of the prostate is a common incidental finding at autopsy, being present in 15–20% of men over 50 years and over 70% of men at 90 years. Tumors not manifested clinically during life are called occult cancers. The incidence of clinically evident carcinoma is about 30 per 100,000 in the United States (about 75,000 cases per year). Prostatic cancer is most common in American blacks, fairly common in whites, and uncommon in Orientals.

There is no difference in the histologic appearances of occult as compared with clinically evident prostatic cancer.

Etiology

The etiology of prostatic carcinoma is unknown. A study of the geographic distribution provides some insight. The low incidence in Japanese men increase to approach that of American whites when they emigrate to the United States, suggesting an important role for environmental factors.

Androgens are involved in the growth of prostatic carcinoma if not their causation. Most prostatic carcinomas arise in the subcapsular peripheral region of the posterior lobe of the prostate, a region of the gland that is most sensitive to changes in androgen levels. The fall in androgen levels in later life is associated with involutionary changes in the outer part of the gland, and it is in this region affected by these regressive changes that cancer arises.

The growth of prostatic carcinoma is androgen-dependent. Some degree of androgen dependency is shown by all prostatic carcinomas, permitting control of prostatic cancer by removing androgens. Bilateral orchiectomy or administration of estrogens causes regression of tumor, albeit temporarily.

Nodular hyperplasia of the prostate is not associated with an increased incidence of carcinoma.

Pathology

Prostatic carcinoma appears grossly as a hard, irregular, ill-defined gray or grayish-yellow area on cut section. Nearly all cancers occur in the outer part of the gland—about 75% in the posterior part. The size of the neoplasm varies from microscopic to massive.

Histologically, prostatic carcinomas are adenocarcinomas arising in the glandular epithelium. The cancer may be well-differentiated, forming small or large glands (Fig 51–14A); or poorly differentiated, extensively invading the stroma. Several different histologic grading systems have been suggested, because there is fairly good correlation between histologic grade and prognosis. The most widely used and the one that correlates best with survival is Gleason's system which uses 2 numbers representing the 2 predominant patterns in the tumor. The best- and worst-differentiated patterns, according to this system, are 1,1 (pure grade 1 lesions) and 5,5 (pure grade 5 lesions), respectively; a grade 2,4 carcinoma would show a mixture of moderately and poorly differentiated areas.

Since prostatic cancers occur in the outer part of the gland, urethral involvement occurs relatively late in the course of the disease. Urethral obstruction and hematuria occur only with large tumors.

Perineural invasion (Fig 51–14B) is a common feature of prostatic adenocarcinoma and is useful in making the histologic diagnosis of carcinoma in difficult cases. Its presence has no prognostic significance.

Spread

Local extension through the prostatic capsule into pelvic fat occurs early. Local structures such as the seminal vesicles, the base of the bladder, and the ureters are commonly involved. The rectum is rarely invaded, probably because of the presence of the rectovesical fascia.

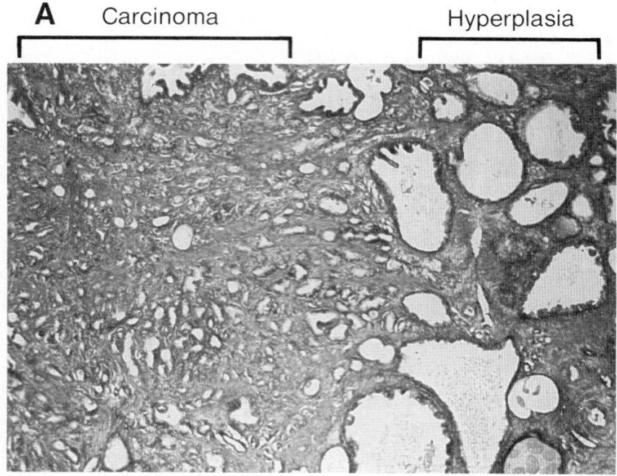

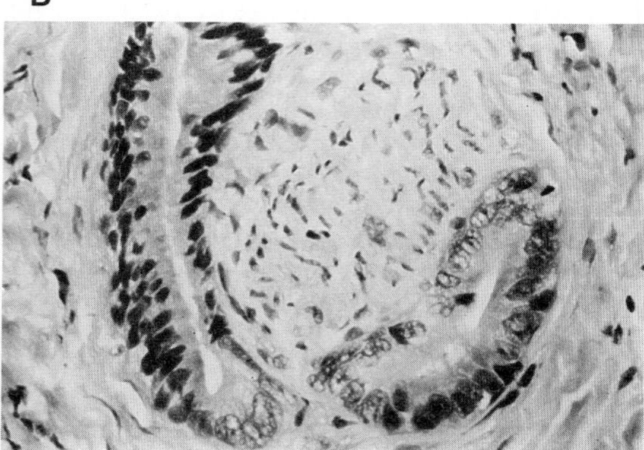

Figure 51–14. A: Prostatic carcinoma, low magnification, showing disorganized mass of small carcinomatous glands contrasting with the more regular glands of benign hyperplasia. **B:** High magnification, showing perineural invasion.

Lymphatic spread to the regional lymph nodes (iliac, periaortic, inguinal; Fig 51–15) is common. Hematogenous spread to the lumbosacral spine occurs early, via communications that exist between the prostatic and vertebral venous plexuses (Fig 51–16). Systemic hematogenous spread occurs late in the course of prostatic cancer and is more common in high-grade lesions.

Pathologic Staging

The clinicopathologic stage, which depends on the size of the tumor and the extent of spread (Table 51–4), has a much greater prognostic impact than any other factor, including histologic grading.

Clinical Features

Urinary symptoms such as altered flow, hematuria, and frequency occur late because of the usual peripheral posterior location of the tumor.

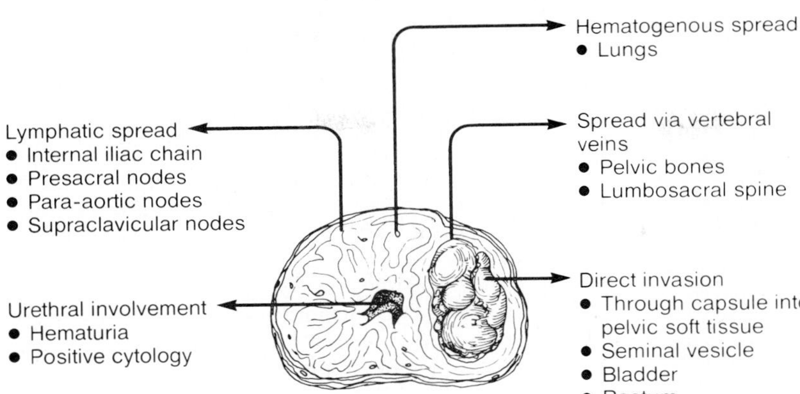

Figure 51-15. Spread of prostatic carcinoma.

The diagnosis can often be made by digital palpation of the gland at rectal examination. The cancerous area can be felt as a hard, irregular nodule. Back pain due to vertebral metastases is a common presenting feature. Skeletal metastases of prostatic cancer are associated with increased osteoblastic activity, leading to sclerotic lesions.

Prostatic cancer cells produce acid phosphatase. Serum prostatic acid phosphatase becomes elevated when the tumor infiltrates outside the capsule and is therefore not of great help in the diagnosis of early stage A or B carcinoma; it is a good confirmatory test in stage C and D carcinoma. An antigen derived from prostatic cancer cells—prostate epithelial antigen—may also be found in increased amounts in the blood; its detection is a useful diagnostic test.

Needle biopsy of a suspicious area provides tissue for histologic diagnosis. Recently, fine-needle aspiration cytology—a much less painful procedure than needle biopsy—has proved very effective in diagnosis of prostatic cancer. In cases where doubt exists about whether an adenocarcinoma is of prostatic origin, as with a metastatic lesion, immunohistochemical staining for prostatic acid phosphatase or prostate epithelial antigen reliably establishes prostatic origin (Fig 51–17).

Figure 51-16. Metastatic prostatic adenocarcinoma in bone. The marrow space between bony trabeculae is completely filled with malignant gland-forming epithelial cells.

Prognosis

The prognosis depends on the clinicopathologic stage and to a lesser extent on histologic grade. With early disease (stage B), 80% of patients survive 5 years and 60% survive 10 years following aggressive surgery with adjuvant radiotherapy and chemotherapy. Unfortunately, less than 20% of patients are diagnosed at this early stage. With advanced disease (stage D), the prognosis is poor, only 20% surviving 5 years.

OTHER PROSTATIC NEOPLASMS

Neoplasms other than prostatic adenocarcinoma are rare. Embryonal rhabdomyosarcoma (a malignant tumor of immature muscle cells) is worthy of mention since it is the most common prostatic neoplasm in childhood. It is highly malignant.

Table 51-4. Staging of prostate carcinoma.

Stage A: Occult or latent carcinoma Found by the pathologist in a prostatectomy specimen from a patient in whom carcinoma was not suspected prior to surgery. Latent carcinoma is subdivided into stages A1 and A2 depending on extent.
Stage B: Clinically suspected carcinoma Confined within the prostatic capsule: stage B1, a tumor less than 1.5 cm in diameter, involving only one lobe; stage B2, a larger tumor or involvement of more than one lobe.
Stage C: Extracapsular extension
Stage D: Distant metastases

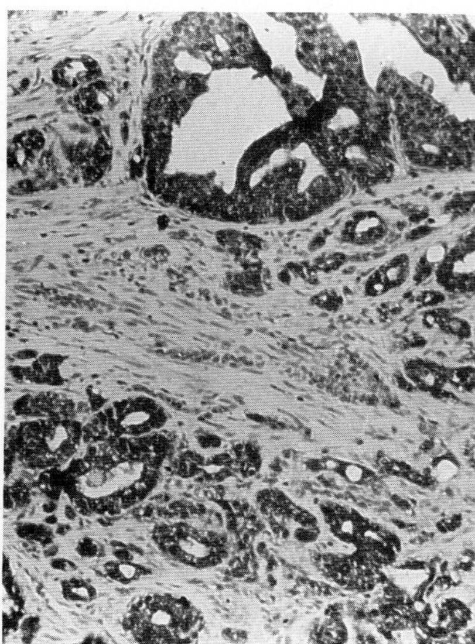

Figure 51-17. Adenocarcinoma of prostate stained by immunoperoxidase technique for acid phosphatase. The dark positive staining of the cells confirms the prostatic origin of the carcinoma.

THE PENIS

CONGENITAL PENILE ANOMALIES

The commonest congenital anomalies relate to the position of the urethral opening on the penis.

In **hypospadias,** the opening is situated on the ventral aspect of the penis at a variable distance from the tip. Minor degrees of hypospadias are common. In the most extreme form of hypospadias, the urethra opens at the root of the penis, resembling the clitoris and urethra in the female (ambiguous genitalia; Chapter 15).

Epispadias (uncommon) is opening of the urethra on the dorsal aspect of the penis. It is rare.

Phimosis is a frequent disorder that may be congenital or may be acquired by trauma or recurrent infection. It is characterized by an excessively small preputial orifice that prevents retraction over the glans and in extreme cases obstructs urinary outflow.

INFECTIONS

Urethritis and the sexually transmitted diseases are discussed in Chapter 54.

PENILE NEOPLASMS

CONDYLOMA ACUMINATUM

Condyloma acuminatum is a common benign neoplasm caused by human papilloma virus, which is transmitted sexually. Penile condylomas occur commonly on the coronal sulcus of the glans or the inner surface of the prepuce. They vary in size from 1 mm to several centimeters and appear grossly as wartlike or raspberrylike masses; they are frequently multiple.

Penile condylomas have histologic features of benign papillomas of squamous epithelium. Vacuolization of the cytoplasm ("koilocytosis") is common and characteristic. The larger lesions—also called giant condylomas of Buschke and Lowenstein—are difficult to distinguish from well-differentiated verrucous type of squamous carcinoma.

PENILE CARCINOMA IN SITU (Bowen's Disease; Erythroplasia of Queyrat)

Penile carcinoma in situ appears clinically as a red plaque on the glans or prepuce. There is a high risk of subsequent invasive carcinoma.

CARCINOMA OF THE PENIS

Carcinoma of the penis is uncommon in the United States, representing less than 1% of cancers in males. The incidence is low in the circumcised male. Penile carcinoma is almost nonexistent in Jews, in whom circumcision is performed at birth, and is seen very infrequently in Moslems, in whom circumcision is performed in the early teens.

Penile carcinoma is common in Oriental races, accounting for as much as 10% of male cancers in some Asian countries. It occurs in the age group from 40 to 70 years.

Pathology & Clinical Features

The common sites for carcinoma of the penis are the glans and inner surface of the prepuce. The lesion is detected at an early stage, when the prepuce is retractable; detection may be delayed in patients with phimosis. The early lesion is commonly an area of epithelial thickening (leukoplakia) followed by formation of an elevated white papule. Ulceration follows, producing the characteristic indurated, painless ulcer with raised, everted edges (Fig 51–18). Less commonly, carcinoma appears as a papillomatous or warty growth.

Microscopically, penile carcinoma is a squa-

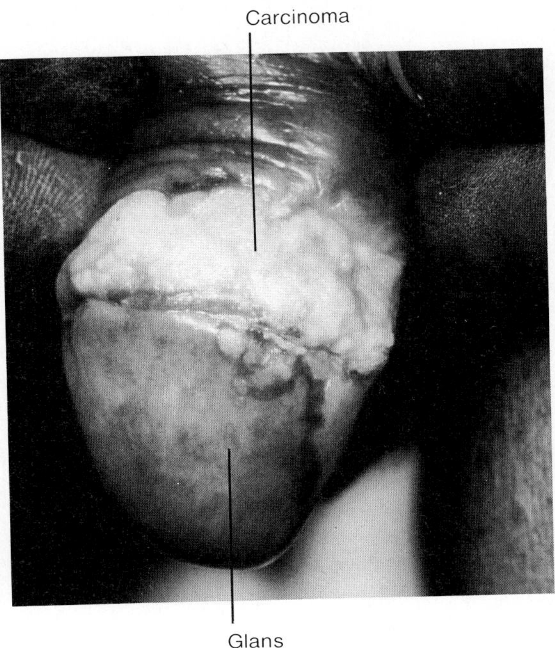

Figure 51–18. Carcinoma of the penis, showing an ulcerated mass at the base of the glans penis.

mous carcinoma of variable differentiation. The degree of differentiation is not important from a prognostic standpoint. Penile carcinoma with a wartlike appearance and minimal cytologic abnormality is called verrucous carcinoma.

Behavior & Treatment

Penile carcinoma usually shows slow infiltrative growth locally, with invasion of the corpora cavernosa occurring early. At the time of presentation, about 25–30% of patients have regional (inguinal) lymph node involvement. Distant metastases occur only at a late stage.

With adequate surgical removal of the primary, which frequently entails penectomy and excision of regional inguinal lymph nodes, the overall 5-year survival approaches 50%. Radiation therapy is useful in controlling recurrent disease.

THE SCROTUM

Scrotal disease is common secondary to underlying disorders of the testis or epididymis (eg, tuberculous epididymo-orchitis). In addition, the scrotum may be involved by skin diseases (Chapter 61), most commonly epidermal cysts, which frequently calcify. Necrotizing fasciitis of the scrotum (Fournier's gangrene) has been described earlier in this chapter. The scrotum may rarely be the site of squamous carcinoma; historically, the scrotum was the first known site of a carcinogen-induced tumor (soot in chimney sweeps—Percivall Pott, 1714–1788; Chapter 18).

Section XII. The Female Reproductive System

Gynecology and obstetrics (Chapters 52, 53, and 55) represents a large proportion of medical practice, and many large medical centers have hospitals dedicated entirely to this area.

Many infections of the female reproductive system are sexually transmitted (Chapter 54). We decided to include sexually transmitted infections in this section, although they equally affect males. AIDS, which is probably the most serious sexually transmitted infection at the present time, is discussed in Chapter 7.

Neoplasms are important diseases of the female reproductive system. The recognition of epithelial dysplasia of the cervix by cervical smears was the beginning of the use of cytology in the detection of cancer (see Chapter 16). Cancer of the breast (Chapter 56), cervix and endometrium (Chapter 53), and ovaries (Chapter 52) are all common; it is estimated that 1 out of approximately every 11 women in the USA will develop breast cancer during her lifetime. Early detection of carcinoma of the cervix by cervical smears and breast cancer by mammography represent two major cancer screening programs in the USA.

52 The Ovaries & Uterine Tubes

THE OVARIES

EMBRYOLOGIC DEVELOPMENT OF THE FEMALE REPRODUCTIVE SYSTEM

The internal reproductive system of the female develops from the paired müllerian ducts of the embryo (see Fig 51–1). The ducts remain paired in their cephalad part as the uterine (fallopian) tubes but fuse caudad to form the uterus and the upper part of the vagina. The lower vagina develops from the embryonic urogenital sinus.

The primitive gonad of the female develops into the ovaries, which descend into the pelvis and remain covered by coelomic epithelium (germinal epithelium). The peritoneal opening of the uterine tube comes to lie in close apposition to the ovary on either side.

Congenital anomalies are commonly the result of incomplete fusion of the paired müllerian ducts (Fig 52–1); these congenital anomalies are important because they may cause subfertility or recurrent abortion. Rarely, the ovaries are abnormally situated or underdeveloped; the best-known example is Turner's syndrome (see Chapter 15), in which only streaks of ovarian tissue composed of stroma without primordial germ cells are present.

PHYSIOLOGY OF THE MENSTRUAL CYCLE

In prepubertal females, the ovaries are small and composed of stroma and primordial germ cells; the normal female ovary at birth has the full complement of germ cells required for the entire reproductive life of the individual. The uterus too is small before puberty and is lined by inactive thin endometrium.

The onset of menstruation **(menarche)** signifies onset of **puberty** in the female. The age at which menarche occurs varies between 10 and 14 years of age and is dictated by pituitary secretion of follicle-stimulating hormone (FSH), which in turn is controlled by the hypothalamus via gonadotropin-releasing hormones (Fig 52–2). Hypothalamic initiation of secretion of releasing hormones is influenced by a variety of higher psychosocial stimuli. After its initial stimulation by the hypothalamus, FSH secretion is controlled primarily by feedback from ovarian hormones, and cyclic menstruation begins (Fig 52–2).

Repeated cycles of menstruation, sometimes interrupted by pregnancy, continue to the **menopause** (cessation of menstruation), which marks the end of reproductive life in the female. Menopause appears to be caused by primary failure of the ovary, which fails to respond to FSH stimulation. It is characterized by (1) failure of ovulation, (2) marked decrease in estrogen and absence of progesterone secretion by the ovary, (3) atrophy of the endometrium, and (4) marked increase of pituitary FSH secretion (due to decreased negative feedback by estrogen). Elevated FSH is responsi-

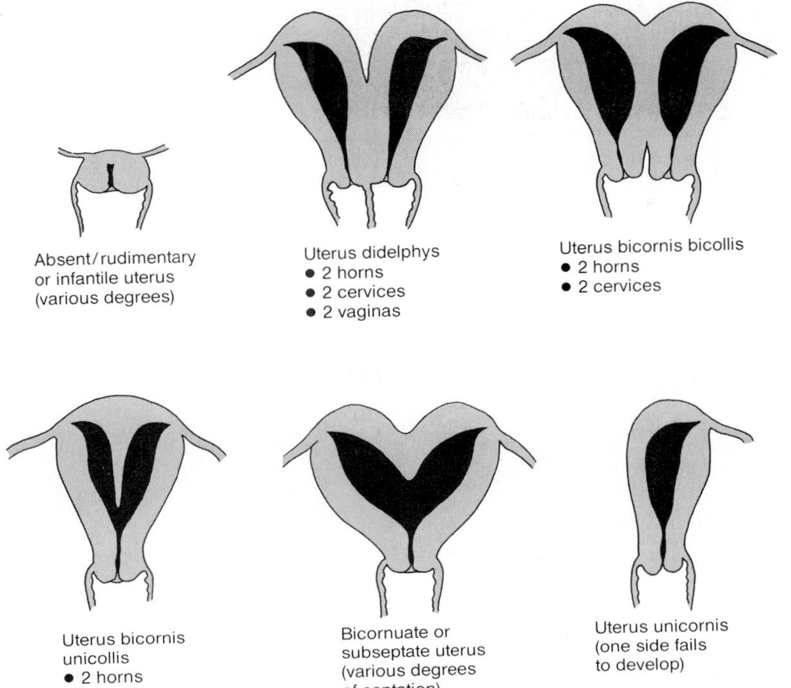

Figure 52-1. Congenital anomalies of the uterus.

ble for many of the symptoms of menopause such as hot flushes.

FERTILIZATION

Fertilization of the ovum usually occurs in the uterine tube. The early zygotic divisions occur in the tube as the fertilized ovum migrates to the uterus. Normal **implantation** occurs in the fundus of the uterus.

The fertilized ovum differentiates into the **embryo,** which develops into the fetus; and the **trophoblast,** which forms the placenta. Trophoblastic cells secrete human chorionic gonadotropin (hCG), which maintains and promotes further development of the corpus luteum. The corpus luteum of pregnancy continues progesterone secretion and prevents shedding of the endometrium, which becomes thicker, hypersecretory, and completely decidualized.

STRUCTURE OF THE OVARIES

The ovaries are paired ovoid structures weighing 5–8 g each situated in the retrouterine space in relation to the lateral part of the uterine tube on each side. Each ovary is covered by **germinal epithelium** except where it is attached to the broad ligament of the uterus, at which point the germinal epithelium covering the ovary is continuous with the peritoneum (both are derived from the embryonic coelom).

The bulk of the ovary consists of dense mesenchymal ovarian stromal cells plus **germinal follicles** and, after puberty, **corpora lutea** at various stages of maturation (Fig 52–3). The exact appearance of the ovary depends on the age of the patient and the phase of the menstrual cycle. If the patient is closer to menarche, there are more primordial follicles; if she is closer to menopause, there are more regressed, hyalinized corpora lutea **(corpora albicantia)**. Scattered embryonic epithelial remnants and hilar cells are often present; hilar cells possess abundant lipid-filled cytoplasm and are believed analogous to the testicular interstitial cells of Leydig.

MANIFESTATIONS OF OVARIAN DISEASE

Failure of ovarian function may be manifested as **infertility,** caused by failure of ovulation; and by **menstrual irregularities** due to abnormal patterns of secretion of ovarian hormones.

Mass lesions also occur but are usually asymptomatic until they become very large. Ovarian masses may be palpated at an early stage by vaginal examination and visualized by ultrasonography and computerized tomography. Very large ovarian masses may cause pelvic discomfort.

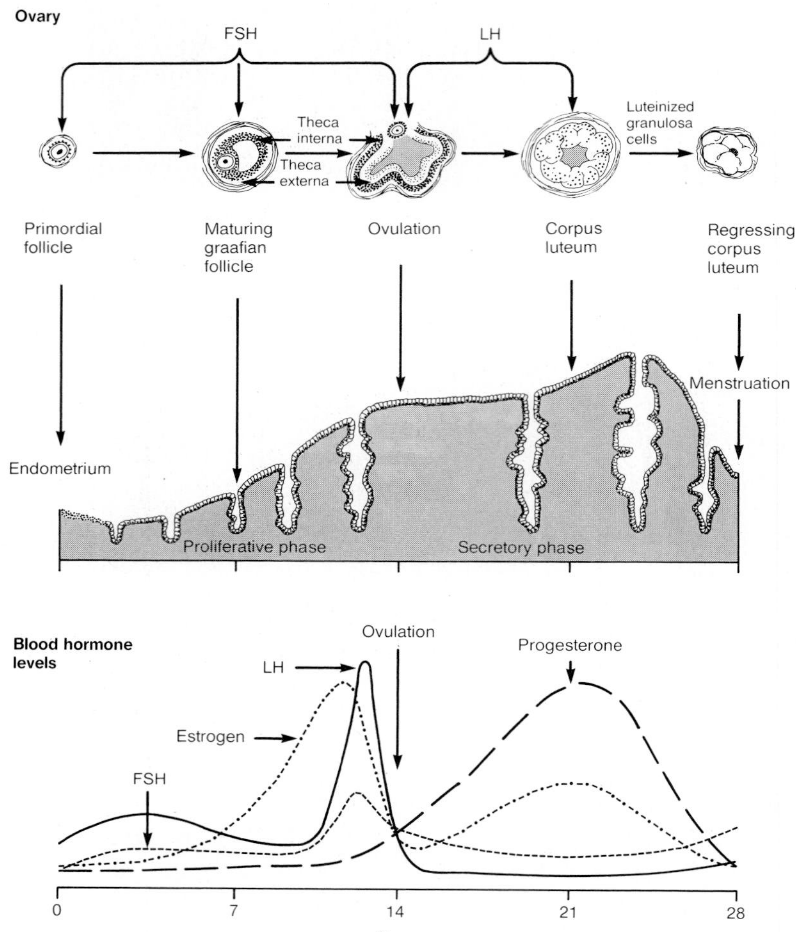

Figure 52-2. Changes in the ovary, endometrium, and blood hormone levels during the menstrual cycle.

NONNEOPLASTIC OVARIAN CYSTS & TUMORS

Physiologically normal structures in the ovary such as follicles and corpora lutea may occasionally become sufficiently enlarged or cystic (Table 52–1) to present as an ovarian mass that may be difficult to distinguish from a neoplastic lesion.

1. FOLLICULAR CYST

Follicular cysts are extremely common variations of developing or atretic graafian follicles. They contain serum fluid, rarely exceed 1–5 cm in diameter, and are lined by flattened layers of granulosa cells. Follicular cysts are of no clinical significance, disappearing spontaneously in 1–2 months.

2. POLYCYSTIC OVARY SYNDROME

Polycystic ovary syndrome is characterized by (1) bilaterally enlarged ovaries; (2) multiple follicular cysts in the outer, subcapsular region; (3) absence of corpora lutea (resulting from failure of ovulation); and (4) hyperplastic ovarian stroma with thickening of the capsule (Fig 52–4).

It is associated clinically with (1) amenorrhea, infertility, and virilism (Stein-Leventhal syndrome); (2) excess androgen secretion (usually androstenedione); (3) normal or elevated estrogen levels, which may cause endometrial hyperplasia and abnormal uterine bleeding (menorrhagia); and (4) an increased incidence of endometrial carcinoma.

The cause of polycystic disease is probably abnormal secretion of pituitary gonadotropins; the normal luteinizing hormone (LH) surge that causes ovulation is lacking, and continuous FSH and LH stimulation leads to the development of multiple follicular cysts. Treatment with clomiphene, which stimulates ovulation, is effective;

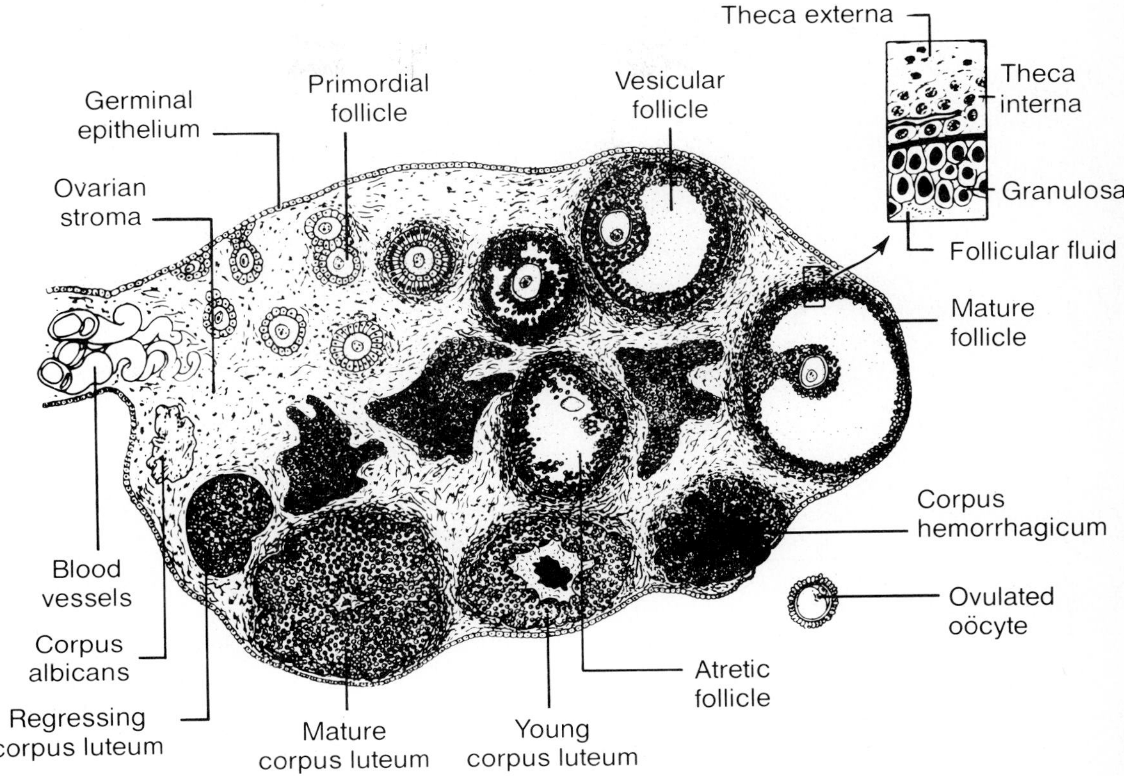

Figure 52–3. Diagram of mammalian ovary, showing the sequential development of a follicle and the formation of the corpus luteum. An atretic follicle is shown in the center, and the structure of the mature follicle is detailed at the upper right. Normally, all of these stages are not present together.

surgical wedge resection of the ovary, which was standard treatment in the past, is now rarely needed.

3. LUTEINIZED FOLLICULAR CYSTS (Theca Lutein Cysts)

Multiple luteinized follicular cysts occur in patients with abnormally elevated secretion of chorionic gonadotropins, as occurs in the trophoblastic neoplasms hydatidiform mole and choriocarcinoma. hCG stimulates luteinization of granulosa and theca interna cells in normal and atretic follicles, forming cystic structures that resemble corpus luteum cysts. (They are not true corpus luteum cysts since they occur in follicles where ovulation has not taken place.)

Table 52–1. Ovarian cysts.

Follicular cysts	Derived from regressing follicles; no clinical significance; disappear spontaneously
Multiple follicular cysts (polycystic ovary syndrome)	Associated with virilism and infertility (Stein-Leventhal syndrome)
Luteinized follicular cysts (theca lutein cysts)	Result of elevated hCG levels; associated with hydatidiform mole
Corpus luteal cysts	Derived from corpus luteum of pregnancy; produce estrogens and occasionally androgens; disappear spontaneously
Endometriotic cysts	Blood-containing (chocolate) cysts in endometriosis
Neoplastic cysts	Many neoplasms have cystic component, especially cystadenomas and teratomas (dermoid cysts; see Table 52–2)

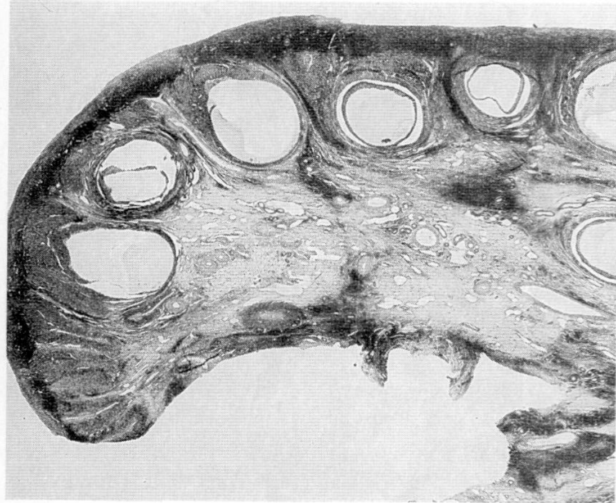

Figure 52-4. Polycystic ovary syndrome (Stein-Leventhal syndrome), showing multiple follicular cysts, thickened capsule, and absence of corpora lutea.

4. VARIATIONS RELATING TO THE CORPUS LUTEUM

Rarely, a corpus luteum may be large enough to be palpable—particularly when it becomes hemorrhagic **(corpus luteum hematoma)** or cystic **(luteal cyst)**.

Luteoma of pregnancy is an extreme form of luteal hyperplasia that produces a nodular mass in the ovary in the last trimester. It may reach a large size and may be bilateral. Luteomas are commonly encountered during cesarean sections and should not be mistaken for neoplasms. Grossly, they are a solid yellowish-brown masses composed, microscopically, of sheets of large luteinized cells with abundant eosinophilic cytoplasm. Rarely, luteomas produce androgens and cause virilization. They involute spontaneously within a few weeks after delivery.

5. ENDOMETRIOTIC CYSTS

The ovary is the commonest site for extrauterine endometriosis (see Chapter 53). Ovarian endometriosis is characterized by the appearance of multiple hemorrhagic cysts ("chocolate cysts") characterized microscopically by a lining of endometrial epithelium and stroma.

NEOPLASMS OF THE OVARIES

Neoplasms of the ovary are relatively common; 75–80% are benign. Malignant ovarian neoplasms account for about 5% of all cancers in women (the fifth most common cancer in American women). Benign neoplasms occur in a younger age group (20–40 years) than malignant ones (40–60 years), but there is considerable overlap.

Classification

Ovarian neoplasms are classified according to their histogenesis (Fig 52–5) in a scheme that shows some parallels with the classification of testicular neoplasms (Table 52–2; compare Table 51–2) except for the absence of neoplasms derived from coelomic epithelium in the latter.

Clinical Features (Fig 52–6)

Ovarian neoplasms are often found incidentally during pelvic examination, radiography, or abdominal surgery. Large neoplasms may produce a sensation of "heaviness" or discomfort in the lower abdomen. Pressure on the bladder may cause frequency of micturition. Malignant neoplasms often remain silent until they have metastasized.

Hormone-secreting ovarian neoplasms present with manifestations of hormone excess. Estrogen-secreting granulosa-theca cell tumors cause endo-

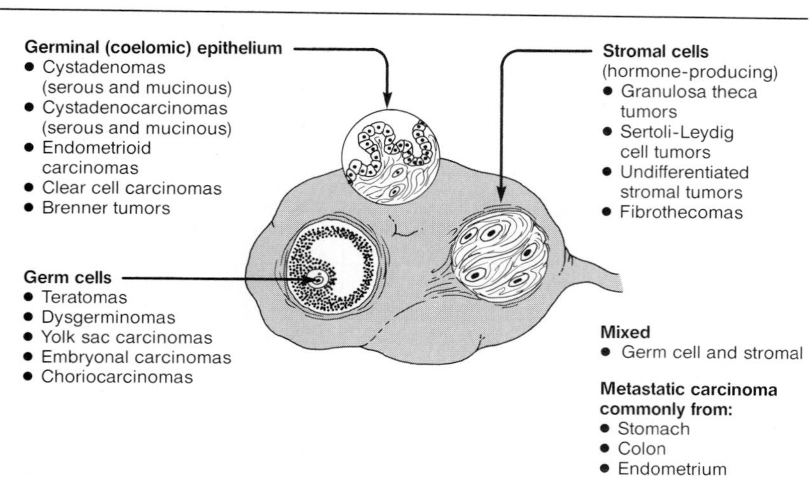

Figure 52-5. Histogenesis of ovarian neoplasms.

Table 52-2. Classification of ovarian neoplasms.

Tumor Type	Frequency[1] (%)	Age[2] (Years)	Gross
Tumors of coelomic (germinal) epithelium	**75**		
Serous tumors Benign serous cystadenoma Borderline serous tumor Serous cystadenocarcinoma	40	15–50	Solid or cystic, may be large; often bilateral
Mucinous tumors Benign mucinous cystadenoma Borderline mucinous tumor Mucinous cystadenocarcinoma	20	15–50	Large solid or cystic
Endometrioid tumors Borderline type (rare) Carcinoma	5	30–70	Large solid or cystic
Clear cell carcinoma	2	50–70	Usually unilateral, solid or cystic
Brenner tumors Benign Borderline (rare) Malignant (very rare)	2	30–70	Usually small and solid; small cystic areas
Undifferentiated carcinoma	5–10	30–70	Bilateral, necrotic, hemorrhagic
Germ cell tumors	**20**		
Teratoma Benign ("dermoid cyst") Immature (rare)	15	1–80 > 20 < 20	Frequently cystic; may be large, occasionally bilateral
Dysgerminoma	5	1–80	Solid, occasionally bilateral
Yolk sac carcinoma	Rare	1–30	Solid with necrosis
Embryonal carcinoma	Very rare	—	Solid with necrosis; associated with teratoma
Choriocarcinoma[3]	Very rare	—	Associated with teratoma
Gonadal stromal tumors	**5**	1–80	
Granulosa-theca cell	2	Especially 50+	Solid, often hemorrhagic; hormonal effects
Undifferentiated	Rare	Especially 50+	Aggressive, often bilateral
Fibrothecoma	3	Especially 50+	Solid with or without ascites
Sertoli-Leydig cell	Rare	10–30	Solid, with necrosis
Mixed germ cell and stromal (gonadoblastoma)	**Rare**		Occurs in dysgenetic ovaries in patients with chromosomal abnormalities
Metastatic neoplasms	**Common**	Usually 40+	Often bilateral

[1]Frequencies are approximate percentages of all primary ovarian tumors; the text also gives figures as a percentage of malignant tumors only.
[2]Represents the usual age range; occasional tumors will occur outside the range given.
[3]Choriocarcinoma also occurs in the ovary secondary to gestational choriocarcinoma.

metrial hyperplasia and adenocarcinoma, leading to abnormal uterine bleeding. Androgen-secreting tumors cause virilization. Very rarely, thyroid tissue or neuroendocrine (carcinoid) elements in an ovarian teratoma lead to hyperthyroidism and carcinoid syndrome, respectively.

Spread
(Fig 52–6)

Malignant ovarian neoplasms tend to spread locally in the peritoneal cavity, leading to ascites. Cytologic examination of aspirated peritoneal fluid may offer a diagnosis in such cases. In many of these cases, metastases in the omentum cannot be seen grossly, and random omental biopsies should be taken at the time of excision of the ovarian cancer. In other cases, omental deposits appear as extensive flat, solid masses (likened to pancakes). Lymphatic spread, to iliac and para-aortic lymph nodes, and bloodstream spread, most commonly to the lungs, occurs in the high-grade malignant neoplasms.

Treatment

Surgical removal represents the primary mode of therapy for treatment of ovarian neoplasms. With benign and most borderline neoplasms, surgery is curative. For malignant neoplasms, radia-

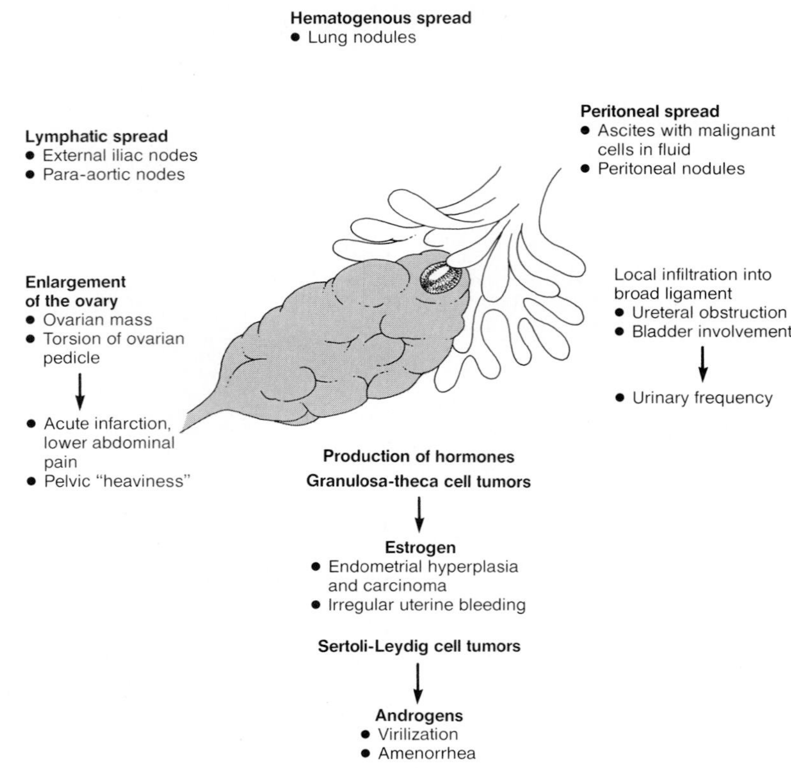

Figure 52-6. Pathologic and clinical effects of malignant ovarian neoplasms.

tion therapy and chemotherapy are used in conjunction with surgery.

1. COELOMIC (GERMINAL) EPITHELIAL NEOPLASMS

Neoplasms derived from the surface coelomic epithelium are the commonest group of ovarian neoplasms. They may differentiate into a variety of different cell types that recapitulate the differentiating potential of müllerian epithelium (Table 52–3). Within these groups, 3 biologic types of tumor may be recognized based on histologic criteria (Table 52–3 and Fig 52–7).

Serous Tumors

Serous tumors are the commonest ovarian neoplasms, accounting for approximately 40% of primary ovarian neoplasms and 20% of primary cancers. They occur in the age group from 15 to 50 years. Benign neoplasms tend to occur in younger

Table 52-3. Nomenclature of ovarian neoplasms of coelomic epithelial origin.[1]

Cell Differentiation	Benign	Borderline[2]	Malignant
Tubal (serous tumors)	Serous cystadenoma (100%)	Borderline tumor (95%)	Cystadenocarcinoma (20%)
Endocervical (mucinous tumors)	Mucinous cystadenoma (100%)	Borderline tumor (95%)	Cystadenocarcinoma (45%)
Endometrial	?Endometriosis[3]	Very rare	Endometrioid carcinoma (50%)
Uncertain			Clear cell carcinoma (40%)
Urothelial	Brenner tumor	Proliferating Brenner tumor (rare)	Malignant Brenner tumor (very rare)
Undifferentiated	...	...	Undifferentiated carcinoma (10%)

[1]Figures in parentheses are 5-year survival rates. Note that 10-year survival rates are generally lower, because late recurrence of tumor is not uncommon in ovarian neoplasms. Survival figures are not available for the very rare tumor types.
[2]Borderline tumors are also called tumors of low malignant potential.
[3]The origin of endometrial tissue in endometriosis is uncertain, whether by displacement from the uterus or by differentiation of the ovarian coelomic epithelium.

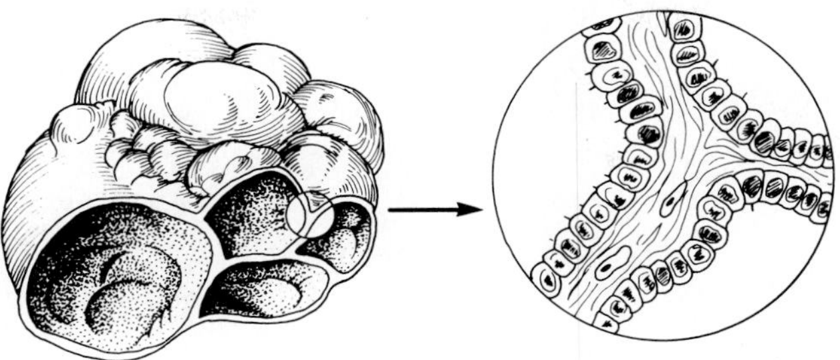

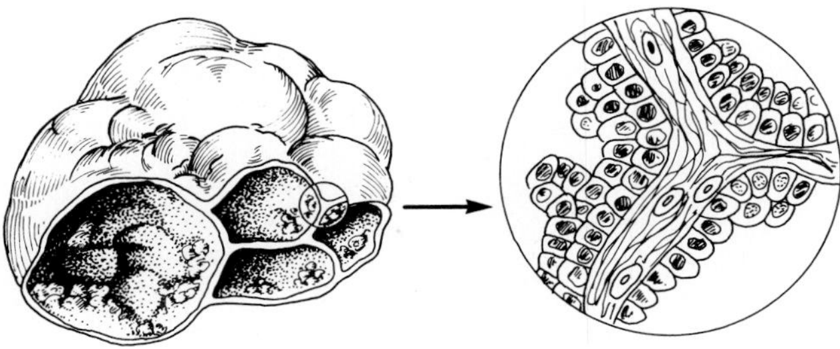

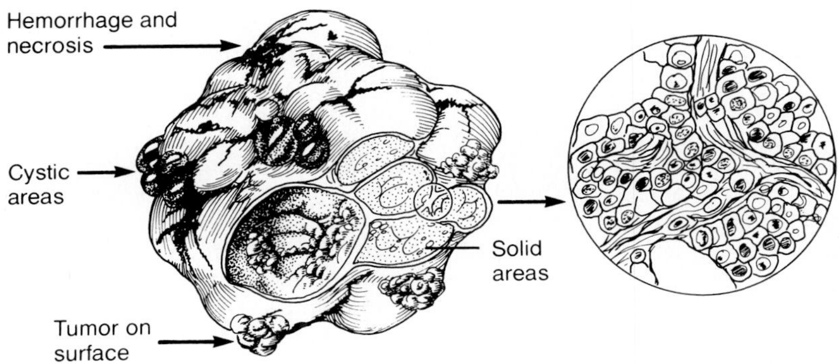

Figure 52–7. Serous tumors of the ovary, showing criteria used for differentiating benign, borderline, and malignant counterparts of these tumors.

women than malignant ones. Serous tumors are frequently bilateral; 25% of benign, 50% of borderline, and 70% of malignant serous tumors are bilateral.

Based on the microscopic appearance, 3 different biologic types are recognized (Fig 52–7).

A. Benign Serous Cystadenoma: Benign serous tumors vary in size from small cysts in the ovary (germinal inclusion cysts; serous cystomas) to large multilocular cystic neoplasms reaching a size of over 40 cm. They have a smooth external surface and a smooth or papillary internal lining (Fig 52–8) of cuboidal or flattened epithelium. Taller columnar cells—sometimes ciliated—resembling uterine tubes may be seen.

A variant of serous cystadenoma containing, in addition, a mass of proliferating fibrous connective tissue between the cystic spaces is known as **serous cystadenofibroma.**

Benign serous tumors do not infiltrate the capsule or metastasize. Surgical removal is curative.

B. Borderline Serous Tumor: Borderline serous tumors (also called serous tumors of low malignant potential) are distinguished from benign

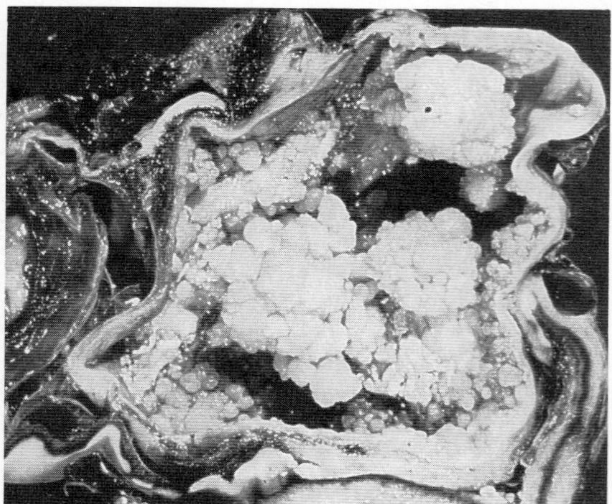

Figure 52-8. Cystic serous tumor of the ovary showing internal surface of the cyst. Note the multiple nodular and papillary projections. Microscopic examination is necessary to classify this as benign, borderline, or malignant.

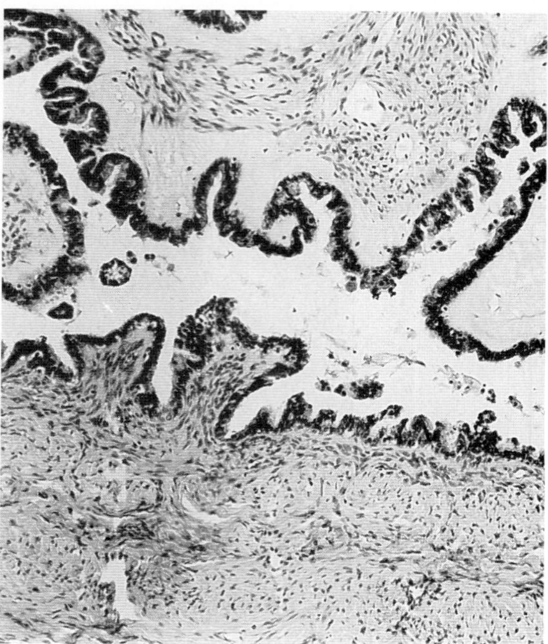

Figure 52-9. Borderline serous tumor of the ovary, showing complex papillary architecture and stratification of lining epithelial cells. There is no stromal invasion.

serous cystadenomas in having more exuberant papillary ingrowths and a complex histologic pattern. The neoplastic cells lining the papillae are taller than those lining benign neoplasms, with stratification (up to 3 cell layers) and mild cytologic atypia (Figs 52–7 and 52–9). Calcification in the form of round, laminated psammoma bodies is commonly present.

Borderline tumors are distinguished from serous cystadenocarcinoma by the lack of infiltration of the stroma or capsule of the neoplasm. Carcinomas also have a greater degree of cell stratification and cytologic atypia (see below).

Borderline serous tumors behave in a low-grade malignant manner, metastasizing to the peritoneal cavity and rarely to the lungs. They have a good prognosis (5-year survival rate of 95%) even in the presence of peritoneal metastases.

C. Serous Cystadenocarcinoma: Serous cystadenocarcinomas show irregular solid and cystic areas. The outer surface may be irregular due to infiltrating tumor (Fig 52–7). Microscopically, the cyst epithelial lining has a highly complex papillary pattern with cell stratification (more than 3 cell layers), marked cytologic atypia, and stromal or capsular invasion (Fig 52–7). Calcification in the form of round, laminated psammoma bodies is commonly present.

High-grade serous cystadenocarcinoma loses its papillary appearance and becomes indistinguishable from undifferentiated carcinoma.

Serous cystadenocarcinoma is a highly malignant neoplasm, infiltrating and metastasizing early in its course. Spread locally to the peritoneum and omentum occurs early. Lymph node involvement also occurs early, with metastases in pelvic and para-aortic lymph nodes. Distant metastases occur late, with lung and liver being the main sites. The 5-year survival rate is about 20%.

Mucinous Tumors

Mucinous tumors account for 20% of ovarian neoplasms. They occur most often in the age group from 15 to 50 years. Most are benign. Mucinous cystadenocarcinoma accounts for less than 5% of ovarian cancers. Mucinous tumors are less frequently bilateral than serous tumors (20% bilaterality for borderline and malignant mucinous tumors).

Based on their histologic features, 3 types of mucinous tumors are recognized.

A. Benign Mucinous Cystadenoma: Mucinous cystadenoma tends to be larger than serous cystadenoma and typically is a cystic multiloculated neoplasm filled with thick mucoid fluid (Fig 52–10). The inner lining is smooth and is composed of uniform tall columnar cells with flattened basal nuclei, and the apical part of the cell is distended with mucin (Fig 52–11). The lining epithelium resembles that of the endocervix.

Surgical removal is curative.

B. Borderline Mucinous Tumor: Borderline tumors are distinguished from benign tumors by the presence of complex papillary projections, stratification less than 3 layers thick, and mild cytologic atypia of the epithelial lining; and from carcinoma by the lesser degree of stratification and cytologic atypia and the absence of stromal and capsular invasion.

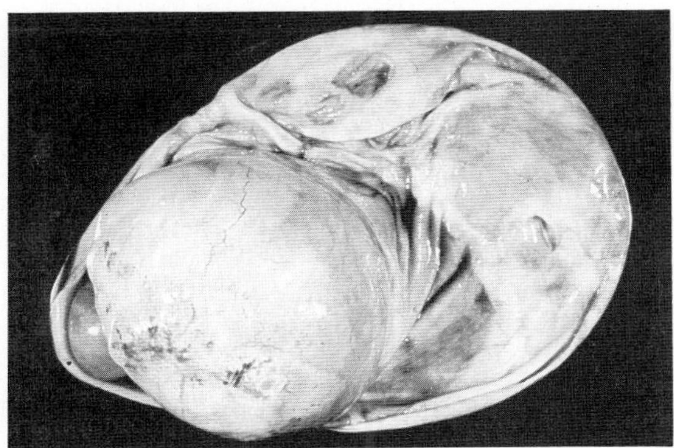

Figure 52-10. Multilocular mucinous cystadenoma of the ovary. Note smooth internal surface.

Borderline mucinous tumors grow slowly and may spread to the peritoneum, producing multiple mucoid masses with extensive adhesions (pseudomyxoma peritonei). Distant metastases are rare. The 5-year survival rate is around 90%, but the overall long-term prognosis is poor when there is extensive peritoneal disease.

C. Mucinous Cystadenocarcinoma: Mucinous cystadenocarcinoma can be recognized by the presence of solid areas and evidence of invasion. Microscopically, there is marked cytologic anaplasia and extensive infiltration. This highly malignant neoplasm infiltrates locally and metastasizes to the peritoneal cavity, lymph nodes, and distant organs in a manner similar to serous cystadenocarcinoma. Prognosis is poor.

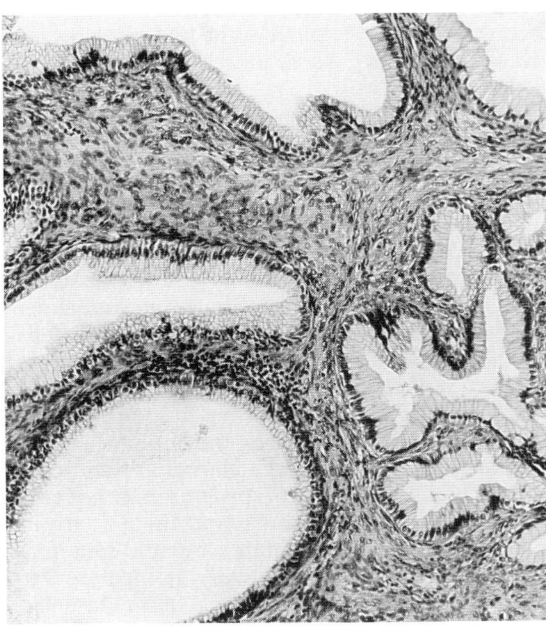

Figure 52-11. Mucinous cystadenoma. The lining cells are tall columnar cells with basally situated nuclei. The epithelium is flat, and there is no stratification of cells.

Endometrioid Carcinoma

Endometrioid carcinoma accounts for 15% of malignant ovarian neoplasms. It is defined by its microscopic resemblance to endometrial carcinoma. Associated endometriosis is found in about 25% of cases, and in some cases concurrent endometrial carcinoma is present, raising the question whether the ovarian neoplasm is metastatic or a second independent primary. Origin of some endometrioid carcinomas from endometriosis has been demonstrated, but the frequency with which this occurs is probably very low; in most cases, the tumor is believed to represent endometrioid differentiation of a neoplasm derived from the coelomic epithelium.

Endometrioid carcinomas grossly appear as solid and cystic masses that frequently show areas of hemorrhage and necrosis. Microscopically, the cells resemble endometrial carcinoma (Fig 52-12). Squamous metaplasia is seen in 50% of cases.

Endometrioid carcinoma has the best prognosis among ovarian carcinomas, with a 5-year survival rate of 50%. Borderline endometrioid tumors have been described but are very rare.

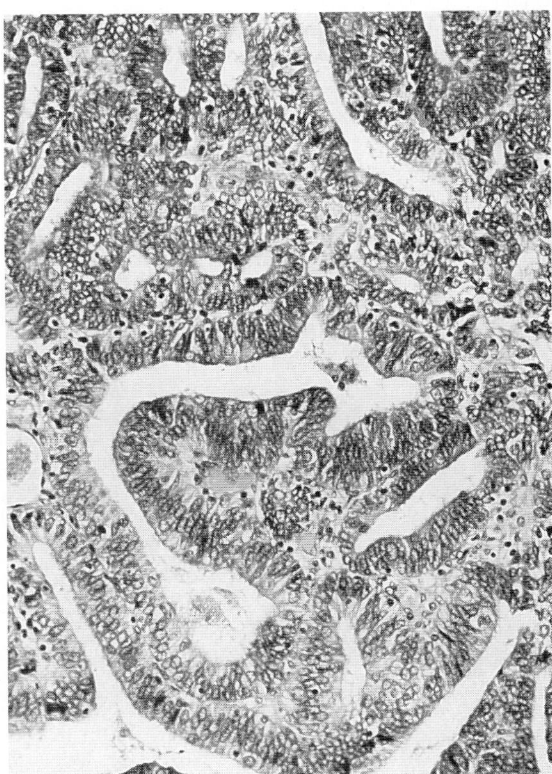

Figure 52-12. Endometrioid carcinoma, showing glandular spaces lined by tall, stratified carcinoma cells resembling the pattern of endometrial carcinoma.

Clear Cell Carcinoma

Clear cell carcinoma of the ovary was originally called mesonephric carcinoma because of a presumed origin from mesonephric rests. This theory has been discredited, and this rare type of ovarian cancer is now regarded as originating from the coelomic epithelium. Clear cell carcinoma accounts for 5% of malignant primary neoplasms of the ovary and is characterized histologically by large cells with clear cytoplasm arranged in solid glandular, tubular, or papillary patterns (Fig 52–13). Clear cell carcinoma has a prognosis similar to that of endometrioid carcinoma.

Brenner Tumor

Brenner tumor is uncommon, accounting for 2% of ovarian neoplasms. It occurs at all ages but is most frequently encountered as an incidental finding in older patients.

Grossly, it is a solid, firm white neoplasm that varies from 1 to 30 cm in size. Small cysts containing mucinous material are common. Microscopically, Brenner tumors are characterized by a cellular fibroblastic stroma in which there are epithelial islands composed of uniform, cytologically benign cells that resemble transitional epithelium.

Brenner tumors are usually benign. Rare Brenner tumors show evidence of proliferation of the transitional epithelium; these "proliferating" Brenner tumors are analogous to borderline tumors. Malignant Brenner tumors are very rare and resemble transitional cell carcinoma.

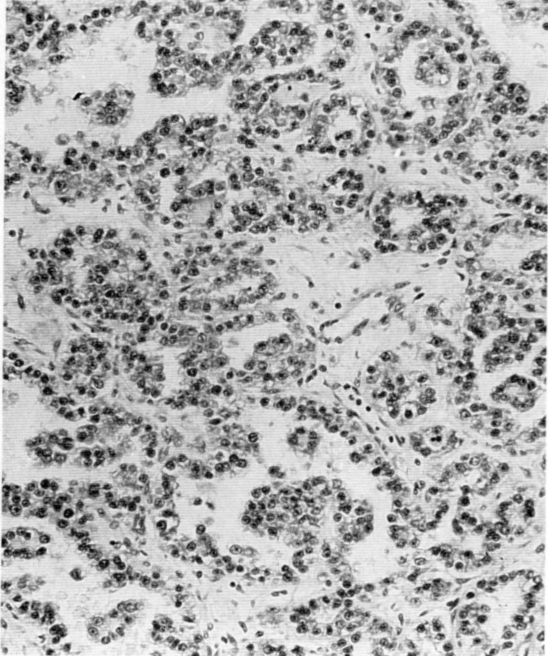

Figure 52–13. Clear cell carcinoma, showing glands with papillary infoldings lined by hobnail epithelium.

Undifferentiated Carcinoma

The term undifferentiated carcinoma is used for an epithelial neoplasm of the ovary that does not show any kind of differentiation. Such tumors are composed of solid masses of cells with necrosis, hemorrhage, and a high mitotic rate. They have the poorest prognosis, with a 5-year survival rate of less than 10%.

2. GERM CELL NEOPLASMS

Germ cell tumors of the ovary are similar in derivation to their counterparts in the testis, but there are some striking differences. Mature teratoma of the ovary is biologically benign at all ages—not true of teratomas of the testis—and are responsible for 80% of all germ cell tumors of the ovary. Dysgerminoma (which is histologically identical to seminoma in the testis) and yolk sac carcinoma are similar to their testicular counterparts. Immature teratoma of the ovary occurs mainly in the age group under 20 years and is a highly malignant neoplasm, whereas teratomas of the testis in young boys have a benign biologic behavior. Embryonal carcinoma and choriocarcinoma are extremely rare in the ovary.

Benign Cystic Teratoma (Dermoid Cyst)

Benign cystic teratoma is a common neoplasm of the ovary, accounting for about 15% of ovarian neoplasms. It is bilateral in 10% of cases and occurs in all age groups, most commonly over 20 years.

Benign teratoma appears grossly as a cyst containing thick sebaceous material and hair (which is why it is sometimes called dermoid cyst). The internal lining is mostly smooth but frequently has a knoblike nodular protrusion in one area (the "umbo"), in which cartilage, bone, and well-formed teeth may be present (Fig 52–14A). Microscopically, skin elements dominate, including dermal appendages such as hair follicles and sebaceous glands. In most cases, however, structures of entodermal (respiratory and gastrointestinal epithelia) and mesodermal (muscle, fat, cartilage) origin are present, satisfying the definition of teratoma (Fig 52–14B). Glial elements are also commonly present. Rare ovarian teratomas are composed almost entirely of thyroid tissue ("struma ovarii") or tissue resembling carcinoid tumor.

Cystic teratomas of the ovary are benign. Very rarely, malignant transformation occurs in one of the elements of a benign teratoma, most commonly the squamous epithelium, giving rise to squamous carcinoma.

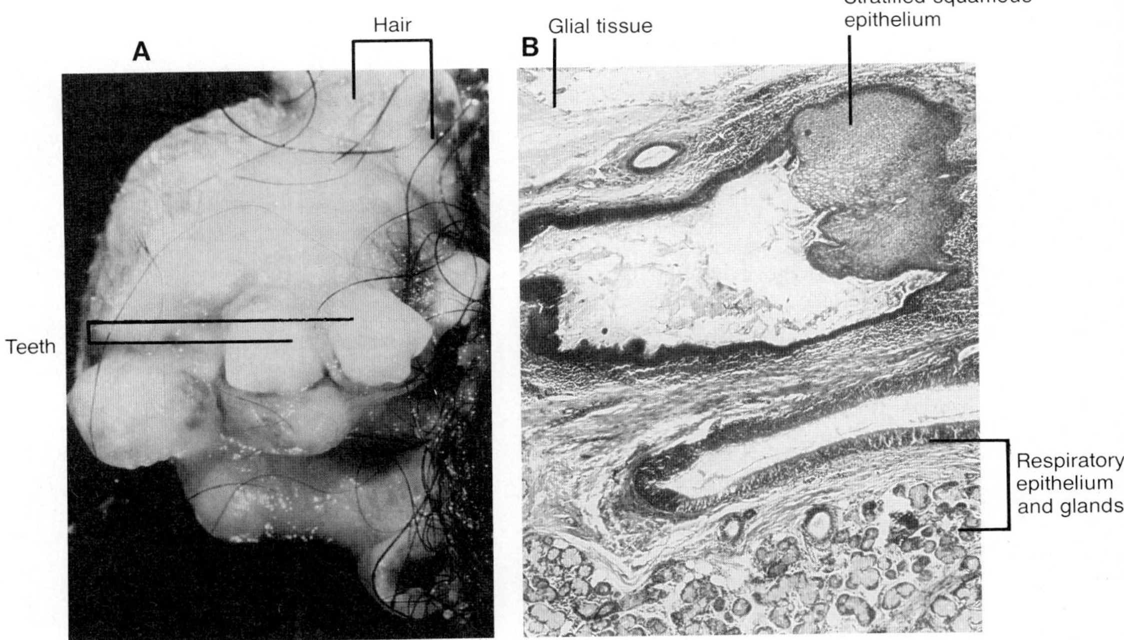

Figure 52–14. A: A portion of a benign cystic teratoma (dermoid cyst) containing teeth and hair. **B:** Microscopic features of cystic teratoma, showing stratified squamous epithelium, pseudostratified columnar epithelium with adjacent peribronchial glands, and glial tissue.

Immature Teratoma (Malignant Teratoma)

Immature teratoma is a rare malignant variant of teratoma that occurs mainly in patients under 25 years of age.

Grossly, immature teratomas are usually solid neoplasms with minimal cystic change. Microscopically, they are composed of immature (poorly differentiated) elements derived from all 3 germ layers. Primitive neuroectodermal (neuroblastic) elements are especially common. Immature teratoma is graded histologically according to the amount of primitive neuroectodermal tissue it contains; tumors with large areas of neuroblast are the highest grade (grade 3) and have the worst prognosis.

Dysgerminoma

Dysgerminoma is the ovarian counterpart of seminoma of the testis. It accounts for about 2% of ovarian cancers. Dysgerminomas commonly occur in the age group from 10 to 30 years.

Grossly, dysgerminomas are usually solid, rarely (5–10%) bilateral, and range in size from very small to enormous. They have a firm, homogeneous yellowish-white cut surface. Microscopically, nests of round germ cells are separated by fibrous trabeculae infiltrated by lymphocytes—an appearance identical to that of testicular seminoma (Fig 52–15). Necrosis and granulomatous inflammation are common.

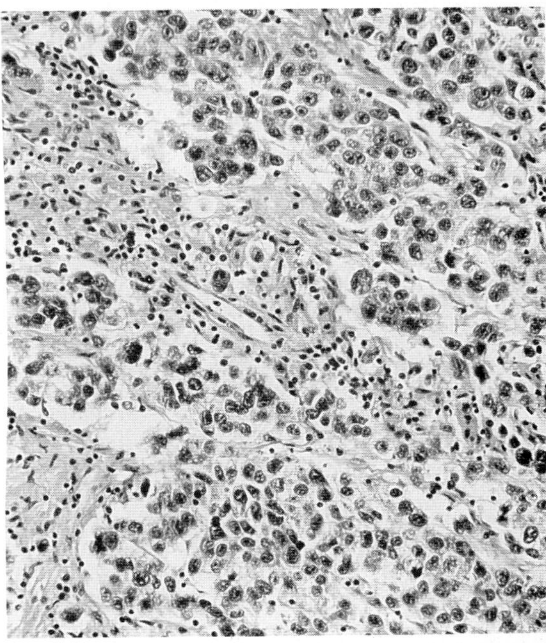

Figure 52–15. Dysgerminoma, showing nests of round germ cells separated by fibrous trabeculae infiltrated by lymphocytes.

Though potentially malignant, small dysgerminomas confined to the ovary are usually cured by simple resection. The overall prognosis is good, with a 5-year survival rate of 80%.

Yolk Sac Tumor (Entodermal Sinus Tumor)

Yolk sac tumors are rare, accounting for 1% of ovarian cancers. They occur mainly in females under 20 years of age and are solid neoplasms with areas of necrosis and hemorrhage. Histologically, yolk sac tumors are composed of a lacelike arrangement of primitive cells in which are found structures resembling immature glomeruli (glomeruloid or Schiller-Duval bodies). Yolk sac tumors of the ovary are identical with their testicular counterpart. They are highly malignant neoplasms with a bad prognosis. Alpha-fetoprotein can be detected in the cytoplasm as well as in the serum. Serum alpha-fetoprotein assay provides a mechanism for following therapy.

3. GONADAL STROMAL NEOPLASMS

Gonadal stromal neoplasms account for 5% of ovarian neoplasms. They are composed of variable mixtures of granulosa cells, theca cells, stromal fibroblasts, and cells resembling testicular Sertoli cells and Leydig cells. While most neoplasms can be categorized into the types described below, some of them defy accurate classification. The term "ovarian stromal neoplasm of unknown biologic potential" is used for such tumors.

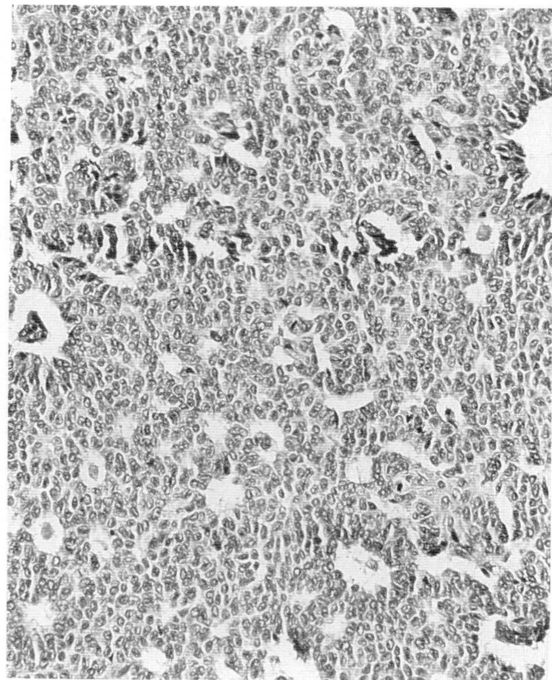

Figure 52-16. Granulosa cell tumor, showing solid sheetlike arrangement of granulosa cells with multiple spaces representing Call-Exner bodies.

Granulosa-Theca Cell Tumors

Granulosa-theca cell tumors are derived from the follicular epithelium of the primordial follicles and account for 2% of ovarian neoplasms. They may occur at any age but are most frequently seen in postmenopausal women. About 5% are bilateral.

Grossly, granulosa-theca cell tumors are solid yellowish fleshy masses that frequently show extensive hemorrhage and cystic change. Microscopically, they are composed of a variable mixture of granulosa and theca cells (Fig 52–16). The granulosa cells appear as small, uniform cells arranged in solid masses with a follicular or trabecular pattern; the formation of small spaces filled with eosinophilic fluid, recapitulating the normal structure of the graafian follicle (Call-Exner bodies), is characteristic. The more elongated theca cells tend to surround the granulosa cell masses.

Granulosa-theca cell tumors typically secrete estrogens, which produce hyperplasia of the endometrium and predispose to endometrial adenocarcinoma. Abnormal uterine bleeding is the most common mode of presentation.

The biologic behavior of these tumors cannot be predicted on the basis of their histologic features. About 25% behave in a locally aggressive manner. Distant metastases occur in about 10–15% of cases. The 5-year survival rate for patients with granulosa-theca cell tumors is 85%.

Undifferentiated Stromal Cell Tumors

Like the corresponding tumors of the testes, these tumors are best recognized by immunohistochemical demonstration of steroid hormones in the tumor cells. Tumor cells are large and anaplastic. The prognosis is poor.

Fibroma (Fibrothecoma)

Ovarian fibromas are benign neoplasms that arise in the ovarian mesenchymal stroma. They account for 3% of ovarian neoplasms and occasionally (5%) are bilateral. Fibromas are most often seen in postmenopausal women.

Grossly, fibromas form encapsulated white masses, usually less than 20 cm in diameter. Tumors that have a significant theca cell component are yellow. Microscopically, they are composed of fibroblasts and interspersed theca cells. Approximately 20% are associated with marked ascites, and a small proportion also show pleural effusions (Meigs's syndrome).

Sertoli-Leydig Cell Tumor (Androblastoma; Arrhenoblastoma)

Sertoli-Leydig cell tumors are rare. They occur at all ages, most commonly in the 10- to 30-year age group. Less than 5% are bilateral.

Grossly, they are solid grayish-white neoplasms with areas of hemorrhage, necrosis, and cystic degeneration. Histologically, they are composed of large cells with abundant eosinophilic cytoplasm arranged in nests or tubules.

Sertoli-Leydig cell tumors commonly produce androgens and cause virilization. Rarely, they secrete estrogens. They resemble the corresponding testicular tumors. Most have a benign biologic behavior; the 5-year survival rate is 90%. Malignant behavior is associated with the less well differentiated neoplasms.

4. GONADOBLASTOMA

Gonadoblastoma is a rare ovarian neoplasm composed of a mixture of stromal cells (usually Sertoli-Leydig cells) and germ cells (usually dysgerminoma). Extensive calcification is a common feature. Gonadoblastoma occurs almost exclusively in dysgenetic ovaries in patients with sex chromosome abnormalities (usually in streak ovaries of phenotypic females who have a Y chromosome in their karyotype, eg, XX/XY mosaics). The biologic behavior of gonadoblastoma depends on the amount of germ cell neoplasm: The more there is, the more malignant the tumor is.

5. METASTATIC NEOPLASMS

The ovary is a common site for metastases, particularly in carcinoma of the endometrium, breast, stomach, and colon. Metastatic carcinoma causes solid enlargement of one or both ovaries, which may reach a large size. In some cases, differentiation from primary ovarian carcinoma can be difficult, particularly in undifferentiated carcinoma and metastatic colon and endometrial carcinoma, which resemble endometrioid carcinoma of the ovary.

Krukenberg's tumor consists of bilateral involvement of the ovaries by a desmoplastic signet ring cell carcinoma of gastric origin (Fig 52–17); some authorities extend the term to denote any metastatic adenocarcinoma of the ovary.

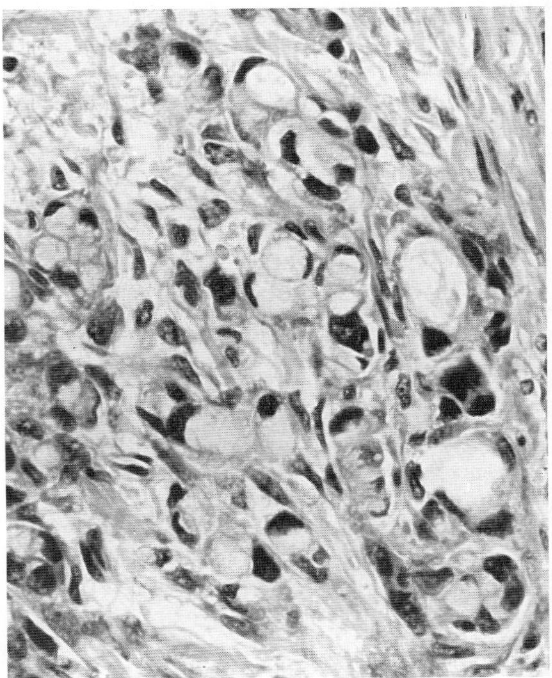

Figure 52–17. Signet ring cell carcinoma of the stomach metastatic to the ovary (Krukenberg tumor).

THE UTERINE (FALLOPIAN) TUBES

INFLAMMATORY LESIONS

ACUTE SALPINGITIS

Acute inflammation of the uterine tubes—which is also called **pelvic inflammatory disease (PID)**—is most commonly the result of gonococcal infection. In the past, acute streptococcal salpingitis was a frequent complication of abortion or childbirth.

Acute salpingitis is characterized by hyperemia and edema of the tube. The external surface is covered by a fibrinopurulent exudate, and the lumen contains pus. One or both tubes may be affected. Microscopically, all the typical features of acute inflammation are present. Suppuration occurs frequently, producing an abscess that involves the tube and ovary (tubo-ovarian abscess).

Patients with acute salpingitis present clinically with fever and lower abdominal pain. Treatment with appropriate antibiotics is effective.

CHRONIC SALPINGITIS

Chronic salpingitis follows recurrent attacks of acute inflammation. Incomplete resolution causes luminal adhesions and progressive fibrosis. **Salpingitis isthmica nodosa** is a disorder characterized by nodular thickening of the isthmus of the tube in which internal adhesions divide the lumen into multiple small channels.

Complete luminal obliteration may also occur, resulting in dilatation of the distal ampullary part of the tube, which is filled with serous fluid (hydrosalpinx). Subsequent infection produces a dilated pus-filled tube (pyosalpinx); culture commonly yields a polybacterial flora with many anaerobic bacteria.

Clinically, chronic salpingitis is characterized by recurrent lower abdominal pain. Luminal narrowing prevents normal migration of the ovum and spermatozoa, causing infertility. In some cases, a fertilized ovum becomes arrested in the narrowed tube, leading to tubal ectopic pregnancy (see Chapter 55).

TUBERCULOUS SALPINGITIS

The uterine tube is a relatively common site for tuberculosis. The gross appearance differs little from that of nonspecific chronic salpingitis. The diagnosis is made by microscopic examination, which shows caseating granulomas with acid-fast bacilli.

NEOPLASMS OF THE UTERINE TUBES

Neoplasms of the uterine tube are rare. The commonest benign neoplasm is adenomatoid tumor, which arises in the mesothelial covering of the tube and is identical to its counterpart in the epididymis (Chapter 51).

Carcinoma of the uterine tube is very rare. It resembles papillary serous cystadenocarcinoma of the ovary.

The Uterus, Vagina, & Vulva 53

THE UTERUS (BODY & ENDOMETRIUM)

STRUCTURE & FUNCTION

The uterus is a pear-shaped muscular organ situated in the pelvis between the bladder anteriorly and the rectum posteriorly. It is partially covered by the peritoneum of the pelvic floor. The cavity of the uterus communicates with the uterine tubes on either side and the vagina below.

The uterus is customarily divided into the **body** and the **cervix** (Fig 53–1). The body is lined by the endometrium, whose thickness varies at different ages and stages of the menstrual cycle. The endometrium is composed of endometrial glands and mesenchymal stromal cells, both of which are very sensitive to the action of female sex hormones. At the internal os, the endometrium becomes continuous with the endocervical canal, which is lined by columnar epithelium and contains mucous glands. The epithelium changes again at the junction of the endocervix and ectocervix, where it becomes stratified squamous epithelium.

The wall of the uterus is composed of smooth muscle (myometrium).

THE NORMAL ENDOMETRIAL CYCLE

The normal endometrium shows cyclic changes caused by corresponding changes in ovarian hormone production. Histologic examination of the endometrium in a biopsy or curettage specimen permits evaluation of the phase of the endometrial cycle (Fig 53–2). Along with the patient's menstrual history, this can provide important information about possible causes of abnormal uterine bleeding.

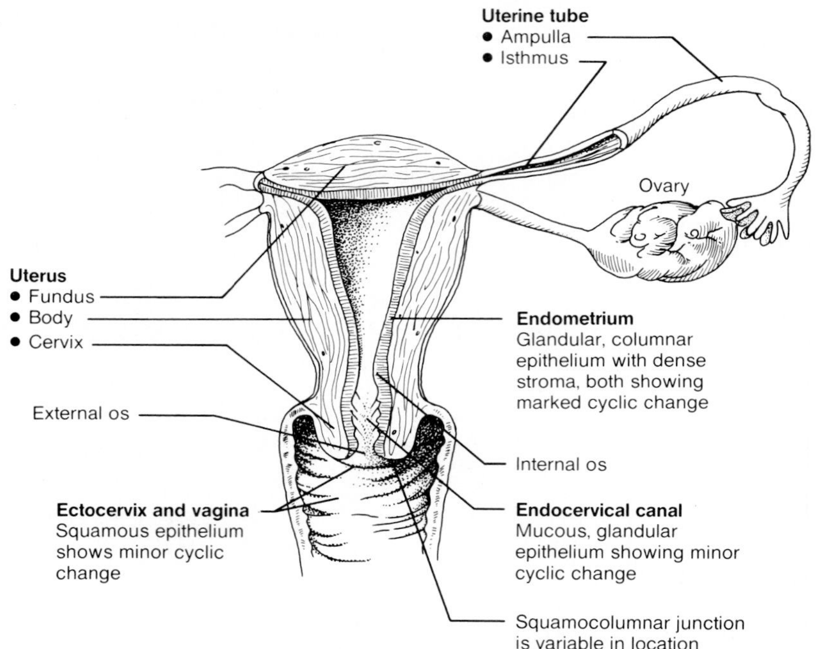

Figure 53-1. Anatomic landmarks of the uterus and adjacent organs.

The endometrial cycle is divided into a preovulatory proliferative phase that is the result of estrogenic stimulation (Fig 53-2) and a postovulatory secretory phase that is directed by progesterone secretion by the corpus luteum. Day 1 of the cycle is the onset of menstruation.

In the **proliferative phase,** there is a rebuilding of the shed endometrium from the basal layer, and mitotic figures are present in both glandular and stromal cells. The endometrium thickens, and the glands start becoming tortuous. The **secretory phase** begins after ovulation with luteal progesterone secretion. The first histologic evidence that the endometrium is in the secretory phase is seen 2–4 days after ovulation, when subnuclear secretory vacuoles appear in the glands. Later, the cell secretions move to the apex of the cell, the nuclei moving back to the base. Stromal edema appears on about the seventh postovulatory day. The glands become progressively more tortuous and

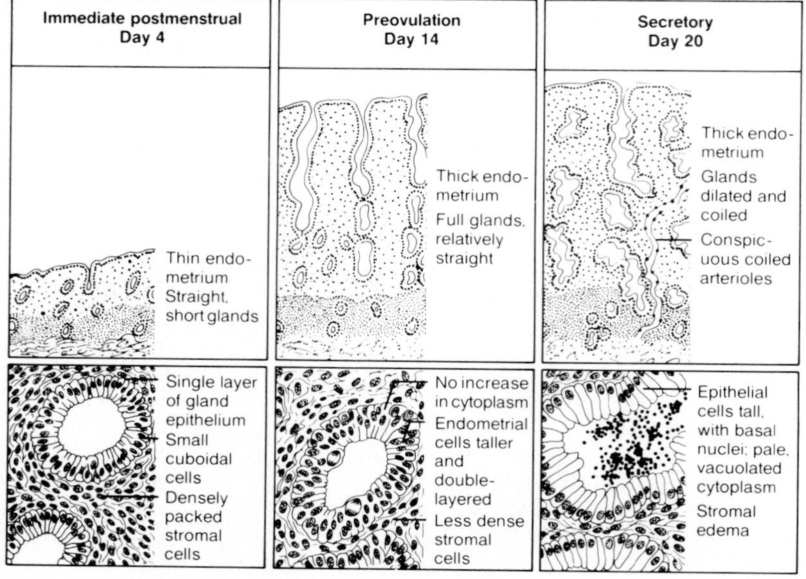

Figure 53-2. Endometrial changes during the menstrual cycle.

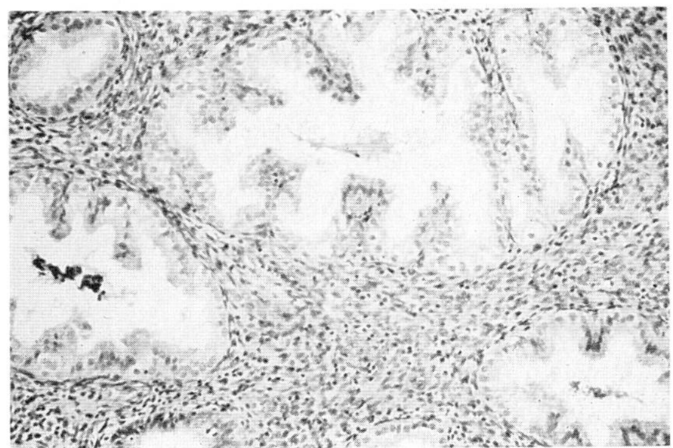

Figure 53-3. Secretory endometrium, showing dilated tortuous endometrial glands lined by a single layer of cells.

typically serrated in the later part of the cycle (Fig 53-3). Spiral arterioles become prominent on the ninth day after ovulation. Beginning on about the ninth day after ovulation, the stromal cells become larger, with increase in the amount and glycogen content of the cytoplasm (predecidual change). In the absence of fertilization, neutrophils appear in the stroma on about day 13 after ovulation, accompanied by increasing hemorrhage and focal necrosis of the glands **(premenstrual phase)**. In the secretory phase of the cycle, endometrial histology permits fairly accurate (within 2 days) assessment of the date of the cycle in relation to ovulation (Table 53-1).

Menstruation is the result of a sudden decrease in estrogen and progesterone due to degeneration of the corpus luteum. Spiral arterioles collapse, causing ischemic degeneration of the endometrium. The menstrual endometrium shows breakdown of glands, hemorrhage, and infiltration with neutrophil leukocytes. The entire endometrium superficial to the basal layer sheds during menstruation, the whole process taking 3-5 days.

MANIFESTATIONS OF UTERINE DISEASE

Abnormal Uterine Bleeding

Abnormalities in uterine bleeding represent the commonest clinical manifestation of uterine disease. Abnormal uterine bleeding may represent an increased amount of regular bleeding **(menorrhagia)** or irregular noncyclic bleeding **(epimenorrhea)**. In some instances, an organic cause can be identified. In others, bleeding is the result of abnormal hormonal stimulation (dysfunctional uterine bleeding).

Table 53-1. Features observed in normal endometrium at different stages of the endometrial cycle that are useful in ascribing a "date" to the endometrium.

Date[1]	Changes[2]
Proliferative phase	
1st-4th day	Menstruation; neutrophils, necrosis, and a mixture of late secretory and early proliferative glands
4th-7th day (early proliferative)	Thin regenerating surface epithelium; straight, short glands; compact stroma; few mitotic figures in epithelium and stroma
8th-10th day (mid proliferative)	Columnar surface epithelium; long glands; numerous mitotic figures in epithelium and stroma; moderately dense stroma
11th-14th day (late proliferative)	Long glands showing stratification of nuclei with numerous mitoses; dense stroma with numerous mitotic figures
Secretory phase	
14th-15th day	No microscopic changes from late proliferative endometrium
16th-17th day	Subnuclear vacuoles appear in the epithelium, which loses its nuclear stratification; mitotic activity in epithelium and stroma disappears
18th-20th day	Subnuclear vacuoles shrink, and the nuclei of the orderly row of epithelial cells in the glands move toward the base; intraluminal eosinophilic secretions appear; glands tortuous
21st-22nd day	Stromal edema appears; gland tortuosity increased with serrated lumens
23rd day	Spiral arterioles become prominent
24th-25th day	Stromal cells show predecidual changes with an increase in cytoplasm
26th-28th day (premenstrual)	Neutrophils appear; increasing necrosis and hemorrhage of the endometrium

[1]The date is given with day 1 being the onset of menstruation. Note that the date of ovulation is assumed to be day 14 of the cycle. Because the date of ovulation varies considerably, it is probably more accurate to date the secretory phase changes as days after ovulation rather than day of the cycle; eg, the 18th to 20th days in this table will become the 4th to 6th days after ovulation.

[2]Note that the changes in the proliferative phase do not permit accurate dating; however, in the secretory phase it is possible to date a given endometrium within 2 days of its actual date.

Pain Associated With Menstruation

Menstruation is commonly associated with a dull ache or with cramping pain. Severe pain during menstruation is called **dysmenorrhea**. Primary dysmenorrhea appears with the onset of menstruation at menarche, and there is usually no organic basis for the pain, which is believed to be due to abnormal activity of the nerves and muscle of the uterine cervix. Secondary dysmenorrhea begins later in life and is often associated with underlying organic disease (eg, endometriosis).

Infertility & Spontaneous Abortion

Uterine abnormalities such as congenital anatomic anomalies, neoplasms, and endometrial disease interfere with implantation and development of the embryo, causing spontaneous abortion or infertility.

Uterine Masses

Neoplasms of the uterus often cause uterine enlargement. However, because of the location of the uterus, such masses must reach a large size before they produce clinical symptoms.

METHODS OF EVALUATING THE UTERUS

Physical Examination

Vaginal examination permits direct palpation of the cervix and assessment of the uterine body for changes in position and in size and for the presence of masses. Ultrasonography and computerized tomography are effective tools for visualizing the uterus.

Cervical (Pap) Smears (Table 53-2)

Routine smears taken with a spatula from the surface epithelium of the cervix provide material for cytologic evaluation of the phase of the cycle, the presence of certain infections, and dysplasia or neoplasia. Samples are also taken for cytologic evaluation of the endocervix.

Colposcopy & Biopsy of Cervix & Endometrium

The cervix can be directly visualized and biopsied by colposcopy. Biopsy of the endocervical canal and endometrium can be performed by passage of an instrument through the endocervical canal. Biopsies must be evaluated in conjunction with a complete history, including the patient's menstrual status.

Table 53-2. Papanicolaou ("Pap") smear of cervix.

Involves cytologic evaluation of exfoliated cells stained by the Papanicolaou method.

A cervical smear is taken by lightly sweeping the surface of the cervix with a spatula (Ayre's spatula) through a vaginal speculum or at colposcopy. The spatula covers the ectocervix, squamocolumnar junction, and lower endocervix. An endocervical smear is usually obtained additionally with a cotton swab.

A Pap smear report may include the following:

Degree of estrogen effect (stage of cycle, or postmenopausal). The evaluation of hormonal status by Pap smear is not accurate.

Presence of any infectious agent (eg, *Trichomonas, Chlamydia, Candida,* evidence of papillomavirus cytomegalovirus, or herpesvirus).

A description of the cervical epithelial cells:

This may use the following grading system:

Class I	Normal
Class II	Slightly abnormal or inflammatory change
Class III	Marked abnormality, uncertain significance
Class IV	Dysplasia (mild, moderate, severe, carcinoma in situ)
Class V	Squamous carcinoma or adenocarcinoma

A class II result requires a repeat smear. A class III, IV, or V report requires formal cervical biopsy to confirm diagnosis histologically.

More commonly, the Pap smear report describes the cytologic changes observed without using a grading system (eg, inflammatory atypia, repair, dysplasia, squamous carcinoma).

ABNORMAL ENDOMETRIAL CYCLES (Fig 53-4)

Exogenous Progestational Hormone Effect

Exogenous administration either of progesterone or of a combined progesterone-estrogen oral contraceptive is followed by abnormal development of the endometrium. The stroma becomes relatively more abundant and shows predecidual change and edema, but the endometrial glands remain small and show minimal secretory activity due to lack of priming by estrogen (Fig 53-4A).

Unopposed Estrogen Effect (Fig 53-4B)

Prolonged estrogen stimulation of the endometrium, unopposed by progesterone, occurs as a result of exogenous estrogen administration or the action of estrogen-secreting neoplasms, most commonly granulosa cell tumor of the ovary and, more rarely, adrenal cortical neoplasms. In **anovulatory cycles,** failure of ovulation results in persistence of the graafian follicle, continued estrogen production, and failure of corpus luteum

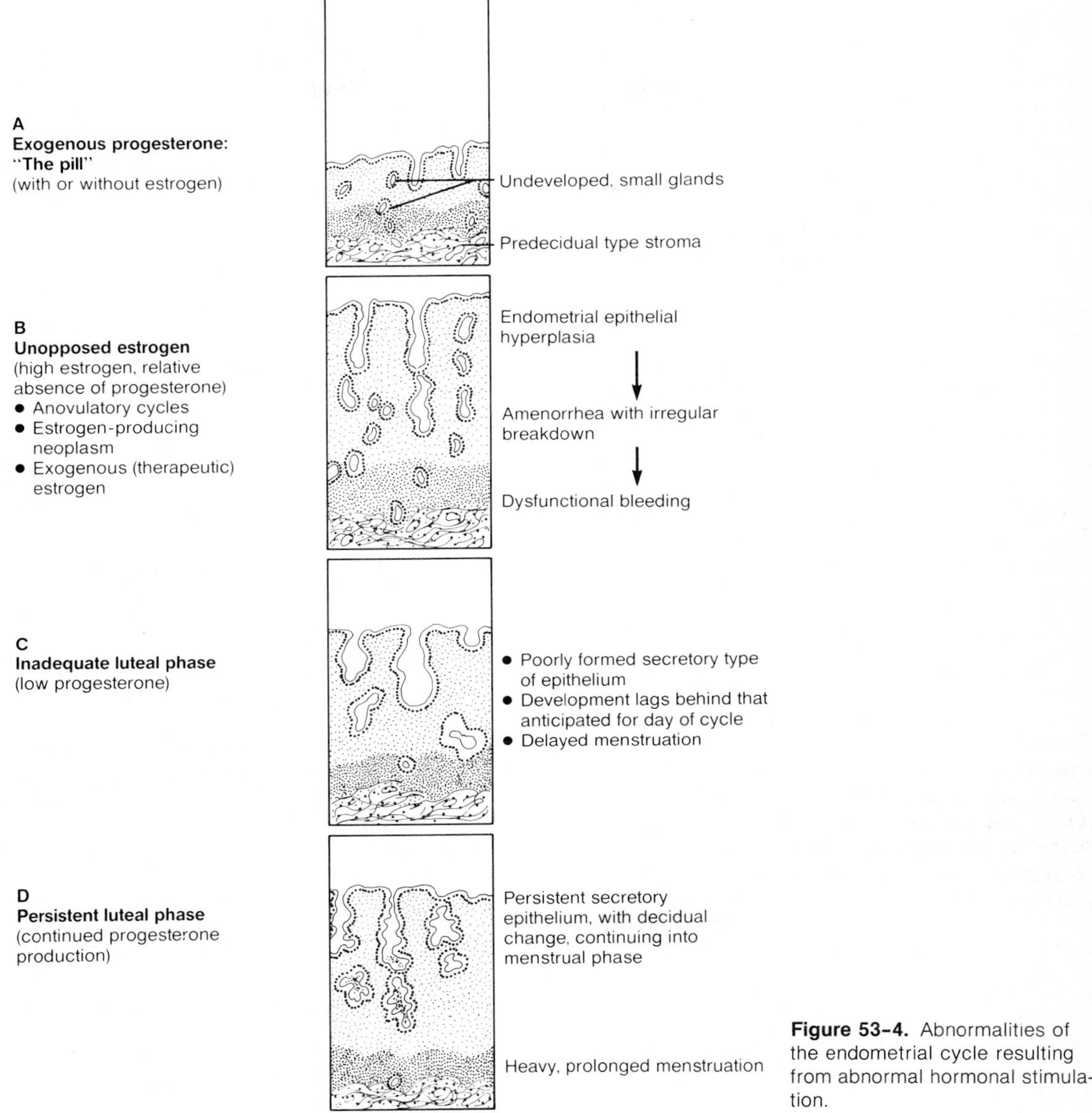

Figure 53–4. Abnormalities of the endometrial cycle resulting from abnormal hormonal stimulation.

formation. Anovulatory cycles occur irregularly at the extremes of reproductive life (postmenarcheal and premenopausal) and in polycystic ovary (Stein-Leventhal) syndrome.

The result of unopposed estrogen effect is prolongation of the proliferative phase of the endometrial cycle. With low-level stimulation, the endometrium remains in the proliferative phase but breaks down in an irregular manner to produce **dysfunctional uterine bleeding**. In these cases, endometrial biopsy during the bleeding phase shows proliferative phase endometrium and lack of secretory activity.

With more intense estrogen stimulation, various degrees of **endometrial hyperplasia** occur: (1) In mild endometrial hyperplasia, there are increased numbers of cystically dilated glands of varying sizes ("Swiss cheese" appearance). The epithelium is commonly stratified and shows increased mitotic activity. The stromal cells also are increased in number, appearing dense with numerous mitoses. (2) Moderate endometrial hyperplasia shows a more marked increase in the number of glands, with extreme proliferation of epithelial cells, which are stratified and frequently thrown into papillary folds. Mitotic figures are numerous. The stroma also is hyperplastic and shows numerous mitoses. (3) Severe endometrial hyperplasia is distinguished by the presence of cytologic atypia, which in its most severe form is sometimes severe enough to warrant the designation of carcinoma in situ of the endometrium (Fig 53-5).

The above terminology is currently coming into vogue, replacing the traditional terms cystic or adenomatous hyperplasia (mild to moderate hyperplasia) and atypical adenomatous hyperplasia (severe hyperplasia).

The most important aspect of unopposed estrogen stimulation is that it predisposes to endometrial adenocarcinoma. The risk of carcinoma varies from less than 1% for mild hyperplasia to 15% for severe atypical hyperplasia.

Clinically, prolonged estrogenic excess produces prolonged periods of **amenorrhea** followed by bleeding which is usually heavier than normal. If hyperplasia develops, the endometrium becomes unstable, and irregular breakdown bleeding occurs. Unopposed estrogen effect is the most common cause of excessive uterine bleeding.

Treatment consists of administering **progestogens,** which reverse all of the changes including severe hyperplasia.

Inadequate Luteal Phase

Inadequate function of the corpus luteum leads to low progesterone output and a poorly developed secretory endometrium, which tends to break down irregularly, resulting in abnormal uterine bleeding late in the cycle (Fig 53-4C). Endometrial biopsy shows poorly formed secretory endometrium, which does not correspond to the date of the cycle. (The phase of histologic development of the endometrium lags 4 or more days behind that predicted by the menstrual history.) The diagnosis is based on clinical and histologic criteria and the results of hormonal studies (low serum progesterone, FSH, and LH levels).

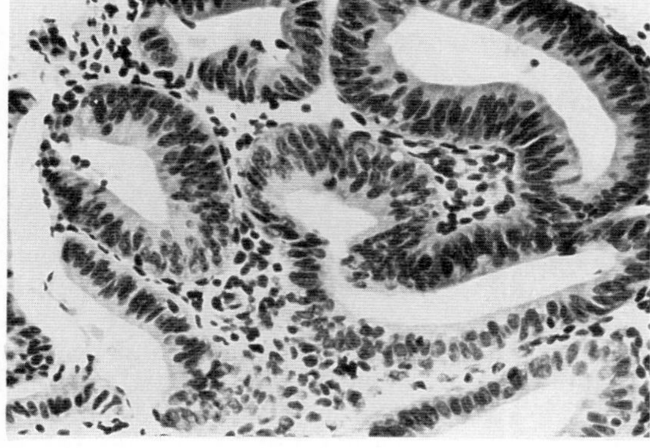

Figure 53-5. Severe endometrial hyperplasia, showing crowded endometrial glands lined by stratified, cytologically atypical cells.

Persistent Luteal Phase; Irregular Shedding of Menstrual Endometrium

At the end of the normal cycle, the corpus luteum abruptly discontinues progesterone secretion, leading to shedding of the menstrual endometrium, which is usually complete in 4 days. Rarely, the corpus luteum maintains low levels of progesterone secretion, causing protracted and irregular shedding of the menstrual endometrium.

Clinically, the patient has regular periods, but menstrual bleeding is excessive and prolonged, frequently lasting 10-14 days. The diagnosis is made by the finding of persistent secretory endometrium after the fifth day of menstruation.

ENDOMETRIOSIS

Endometriosis is the occurrence of endometrial tissue at a site other than the lining of the uterine cavity (Fig 53-6). The "ectopic" endometrial tissue is usually composed of both epithelial and stromal cells and responds to ovarian hormones somewhat like the uterine endometrium.

Pathology

There appear to be 2 types of endometriosis with different pathogenetic mechanisms.

A. Adenomyosis (Endometriosis Interna): Adenomyosis is defined as the presence of endometrial glands and stroma abnormally situated deep in the myometrium (at a depth of more than 3 mm—one low-power field—from the base of the endometrium) (Fig 53-6).

Adenomyosis is common in older women (over 40 years of age) and is documented in about 10% of uteri at autopsy. In about half of cases, adenomyosis is restricted to the inner third of the myometrium. In the remainder, it extends more deeply, not infrequently reaching the serosa.

Two distinct forms are recognized: (1) Diffuse adenomyosis, involving much or all of the uterus; and (2) focal adenomyosis, forming a nodular mass that resembles a leiomyoma (sometimes called an adenomyoma).

Adenomyosis responds cyclically to ovarian hormones, leading to hemorrhage with hemosiderin deposition at sites of disease.

B. Extrauterine Endometriosis (Endometriosis Externa): Endometriosis occurring outside the uterus is pathogenetically unrelated to adenomyosis. In order of decreasing frequency, endometriosis externa is found in (1) an ovary; (2) the wall of a uterine tube; (3) parametrial soft tissue; (4) the serosa of the intestine, most commonly the sigmoid colon and appendix; (5) the umbilicus; (6) the urinary tract; (7) the skin at the site of laparotomy scars, usually after surgery on the uterus and most commonly after cesarian sec-

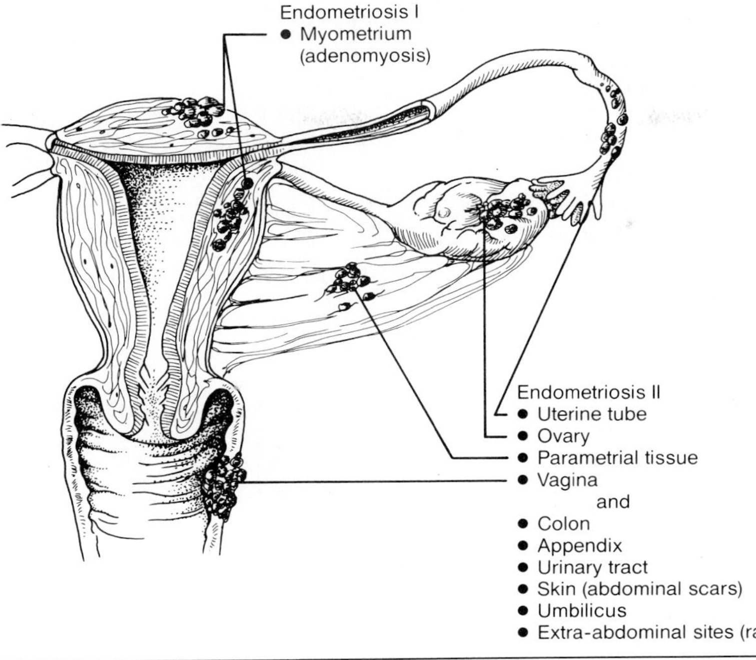

Figure 53–6. Endometriosis, showing sites of involvement.

tion; and (8) extra-abdominal sites such as the lungs, pleura, and bones.

Pathologically, foci of endometriosis appear as cysts that contain areas of new and old hemorrhage **("chocolate cysts")**, due to cyclic bleeding that occurs during menstruation. Microscopically, foci are characterized by the presence of endometrial glands surrounded by stroma (Fig 53–7). Evidence of hemorrhage, hemosiderin deposition, and fibrosis are common. Endometriosis of the uterine tube is a common cause of infertility because of luminal obliteration by fibrosis.

Pathogenesis

A. Adenomyosis: Adenomyosis (endometriosis interna) is believed to be the result of abnormal downgrowth of the endometrium into the myometrium, with entrapment of foci of endometrium deep in the uterine muscle.

B. Endometriosis Externa: Two main theories have been advanced. The first is that endometriosis results from metaplasia (differentiation) of the coelomic epithelium into endometrial tissue. A theory more favored in current opinion is that endometriosis results from transport of fragments of normal menstrual endometrium from the uterus, through the uterine tubes, and into the peritoneal cavity.

Both theories are consistent with the observation that the main concentration of endometriosis is in the pelvic peritoneum. In favor of the second theory are the following observations: (1) menstrual endometrium has been shown in animals to be viable after it is shed into the peritoneal cavity; (2) retrograde flow of menstrual blood through the uterine tubes has been shown to occur during menstruation; and (3) experimental introduction of menstrual flow into the peritoneal cavity in animals has led to endometriosis, often after a considerable latent period.

Clinical Features

Clinically, patients with endometriosis are in the reproductive phase of life; endometriotic foci regress after menopause when the hormone levels decrease. Endometriosis may be asymptomatic.

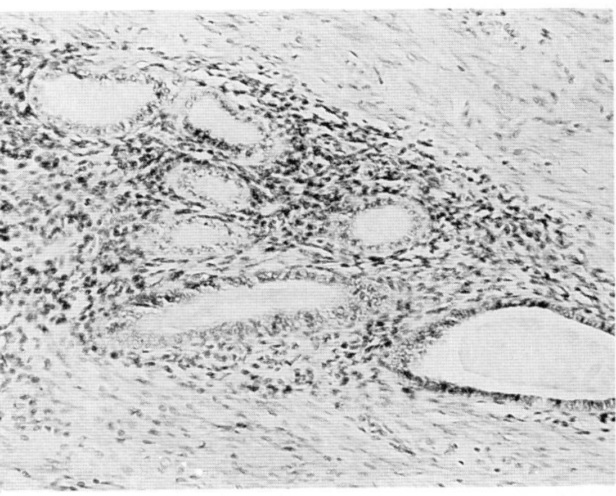

Figure 53–7. Endometriosis, showing endometrial glands surrounded by stroma. This was from a nodule on the serosal aspect of the sigmoid colon.

The commonest symptoms of adenomyosis are dysmenorrhea, menorrhagia, and infertility. With extrauterine endometriosis, cyclic bleeding may be visible—as in endometriosis involving the umbilicus, surgical scars, urinary tract (cyclic hematuria), or colon (rectal bleeding)—or occult, producing cyclic abdominal pain.

Repeated episodes of bleeding result in fibrosis, which may cause peritoneal adhesions and intestinal obstruction. Endometriosis of the uterine tubes results in infertility and an increased risk of tubal pregnancy.

Pregnancy causes decidualization of endometriotic foci, leading to their involution in many cases. Regression also follows oral progesterone therapy.

INFLAMMATORY LESIONS OF THE ENDOMETRIUM

1. ACUTE ENDOMETRITIS

Acute endometritis occurs (1) as a postpartum or postabortion infection, where the usual organisms are streptococci; and (2) as an ascending gonococcal infection. In the past, prior to sterile delivery procedures and antibiotic therapy, acute endometritis was a major cause of morbidity ("puerperal sepsis") and death.* The diagnosis is suggested by fever 2–4 days after delivery, with offensive lochia (uterine discharge).

Acute inflammation may also result when there is obstruction to the outflow of the uterus at the cervical os, either by neoplasm or fibrosis. This leads to accumulation of blood in the endometrial cavity (hematometron), which may be followed by infection and the accumulation of pus (pyometron).

2. CHRONIC NONSPECIFIC ENDOMETRITIS

Chronic endometritis is common in patients harboring foreign material in the uterine cavity, specifically an intra-uterine contraceptive device or retained products of conception. Less often, it is associated with chronic salpingitis. Bacteriologic studies rarely produce a positive culture.

Chronic endometritis interferes with the cyclic development of the endometrium. The endometrial glands remain small throughout the cycle, while the stromal reaction is often heightened, producing an unstable endometrium in which the glands and stroma are out of phase. Irregular uterine bleeding results. The diagnosis depends on the finding of plasma cells in the endometrium. Plasma cells are normally not found in the endometrium (unlike lymphocytes and neutrophils).

*In the 1840s, the recorded maternal mortality rate at childbirth in the General Hospital in Vienna was 10–30%, mainly from puerperal sepsis. Semmelweiss succeeded in lowering the rate to 1–2% by the simple expedient of hand washing by obstetricians and midwives.

3. TUBERCULOUS ENDOMETRITIS

Tuberculosis of the endometrium is rare even in regions where tuberculosis is endemic. It is usually associated with tuberculous salpingitis and may cause irregular uterine bleeding and infertility. The diagnosis is usually made by finding caseating epithelioid cell granulomas in an endometrial biopsy. It can be confirmed by culture.

NEOPLASMS OF THE ENDOMETRIUM

1. ENDOMETRIAL POLYPS

Endometrial polyps are common, particularly around menopause. They vary in size from 0.5 to 3 cm and are covered by endometrial epithelium. Microscopically, these polyps are composed of endometrial glands—which may or may not show cyclic changes—and a fibrovascular stroma.

Clinically, endometrial polyps may be asymptomatic or may cause excessive uterine bleeding. They probably represent disproportionate reactive responses of parts of the endometrium to estrogen rather than true neoplasms. Very rarely, they undergo carcinomatous transformation.

2. ENDOMETRIAL CARCINOMA

Endometrial adenocarcinoma is common, accounting for about 10% of cancers in women, and the incidence is increasing in many countries. Ninety percent of cases occur in postmenopausal women, the most common age being 55–65 years. The epidemiology of carcinoma of the endometrium is very different from that of carcinoma of the cervix (Table 53–3).

Etiology

Prolonged unopposed estrogen stimulation of the endometrium is believed to be the major etiologic factor. Endometrial hyperplasia precedes cancer in most cases.

Endometrial carcinoma is associated with obesity, diabetes mellitus, and hypertension (so-called **corpus cancer syndrome**). The mechanism of this association is unknown. Pregnancy appears to have a protective effect in endometrial carcinoma,

Table 53-3. Carcinoma of the uterus and cervix.

	Carcinoma of Body (Corpus)	Carcinoma of Cervix
Incidence in USA	39,000/year	16,000/year
Deaths	4000/year	8000/year
Site	Body of uterus	Cervix
Age	50 plus	40 plus
Etiologic factors	Nulliparity, obesity, hypertension, diabetes	Multiparity, human papilloma virus, herpes simplex virus; multiple sexual partners
5-year survival rate (overall)	80%	60%
Histology	Adenocarcinoma (occasionally with squamous metaplasia)	Squamous carcinoma (except endocervical carcinoma which is adenocarcinoma)

probably by opposing estrogenic stimulation; there is a decreased incidence in multiparous as compared with nulliparous women.

Pathology

Most endometrial carcinomas present as polypoid fungating masses in the endometrial cavity (Fig 53–8). The uterus is often asymmetrically enlarged. Invasion into the myometrium occurs early.

Microscopically, endometrial carcinoma is an **adenocarcinoma** (Fig 53–9), and most are well-differentiated, with irregular glands lined by malignant columnar epithelial cells. Papillary variants also occur. Endometrial carcinomas are graded according to their degree of histologic differentiation. Well-differentiated carcinomas are grade 1. The presence of large solid areas (grade 2) and poor differentiation (grade 3) implies a worse prognosis.

Areas of squamous differentiation are common, and if this feature is prominent the neoplasm is called an **adenoacanthoma**. When the squamous areas are poorly differentiated and show cytologic features of malignancy, the term **adenosquamous carcinoma** is used.

The pathologic stage of the neoplasm, determined by the degree of spread (Fig 53–10), is the most important prognostic factor.

Clinical Features

Abnormal uterine bleeding is the earliest symptom. At the usual age at which endometrial cancer occurs, it is **postmenopausal bleeding**. Physical examination may be normal or may disclose enlargement of the uterus. Examination of a cervical smear may be diagnostic but is not reliable unless special techniques are used to obtain material from the endometrium. Endometrial biopsy or curettage is usually diagnostic.

Prognosis

The prognosis of patients with endometrial carcinoma depends mainly on the stage of disease.

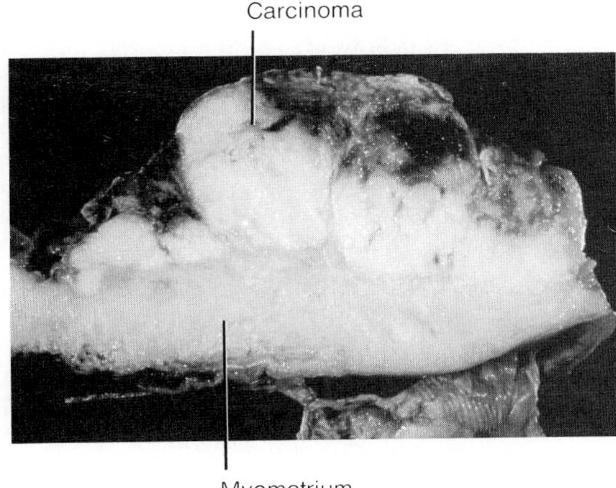

Figure 53-8. Endometrial carcinoma, showing a bulky mass projecting into the uterine cavity. There is invasion of the inner third of the myometrium.

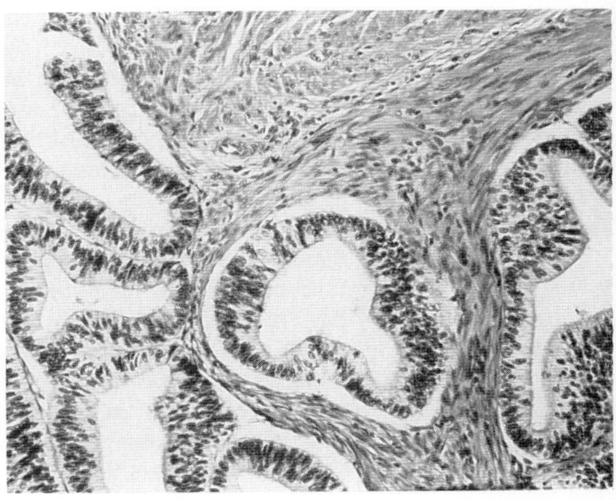

Figure 53-9. Microscopic section from previous figure showing a well differentiated endometrial carcinoma infiltrating the myometrium.

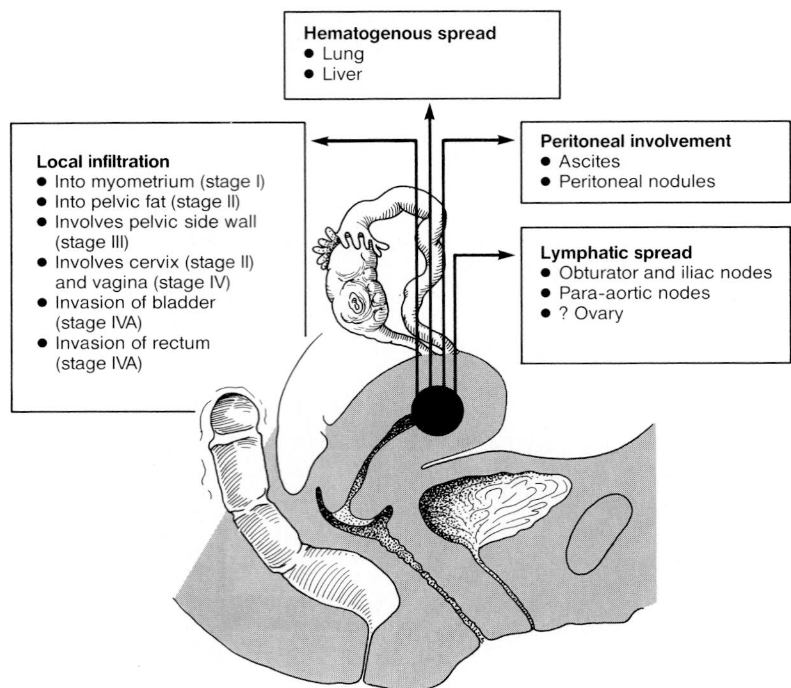

Figure 53-10. Spread of endometrial carcinoma. The clinical stages corresponding to the degree of spread are shown in the figure.

With treatment, 90% of patients with stage I disease, 40% with stage II, and 10–20% with more advanced disease will survive 5 years. The histologic grade of the neoplasm is of secondary importance; the overall 5-year survival rate is 70% in grade 1 and 20% in grade 3 carcinomas.

3. MIXED MESODERMAL TUMOR (Malignant Mixed Müllerian Tumor)

Mixed mesodermal tumor is a rare neoplasm that usually occurs in women over age 55. It is believed to originate from residual müllerian mesodermal cells in the endometrium. Grossly, these tumors appear as bulky, fleshy masses that commonly fill the uterine cavity. They often show extensive necrosis and hemorrhage.

Microscopically, mixed mesodermal tumors are composed of a malignant epithelial component (usually an adenocarcinoma) and a malignant mesenchymal component (usually leiomyosarcoma; occasionally rhabdomyosarcoma, chondrosarcoma, or osteosarcoma). The mesenchymal elements are often poorly differentiated, with a high mitotic rate (Fig 53–11). Extensive necrosis and hemorrhage are commonly present.

Mixed mesodermal tumors of the uterus present with uterine bleeding, which is usually postmenopausal. They are highly malignant neoplasms that tend to metastasize early. The overall 5 year-survival rate is about 20%.

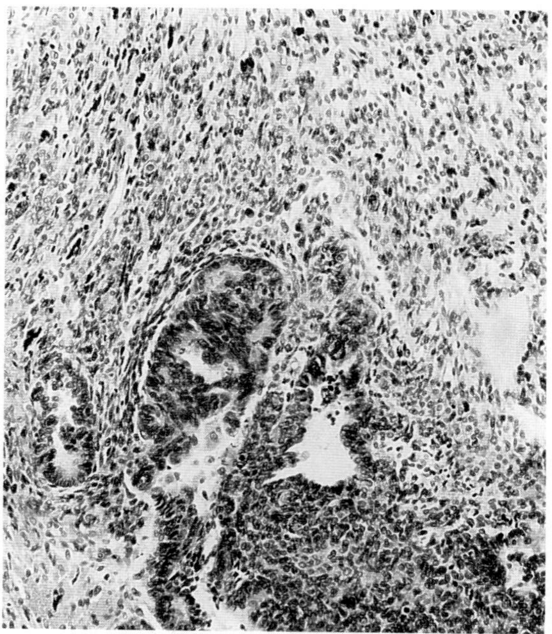

Figure 53-11. Mixed mesodermal tumor. Both stromal and epithelial elements are malignant.

4. ENDOMETRIAL STROMAL NEOPLASMS

Several different types of endometrial stromal neoplasms have been described. All are rare.

(1) Benign stromal nodule is a focal collection of stromal cells that appears as a circumscribed nodule. The cells resemble normal endometrial stromal cells and have a very low mitotic rate.

(2) Endolymphatic stromal myosis (low grade stromal sarcoma) consists of collections of well-differentiated stromal cells lying between myometrial bundles or penetrating lymphatic spaces. This disorder behaves like a low-grade malignant neoplasm, with a tendency to spread outside the uterus. It almost never metastasizes, but local recurrence is common.

(3) Stromal sarcoma, high grade, is a malignant proliferation of stromal cells characterized by cytologic atypia and a high mitotic rate (over 10 mitoses per 10 high-power fields). It usually produces a bulky, infiltrating, friable mass. Hemotogenous metastases occur early. The disorder occurs in older women, and postmenopausal bleeding is the common method presentation. The prognosis is poor.

NEOPLASMS OF THE MYOMETRIUM

1. LEIOMYOMA ("Fibroid")

Leiomyoma is a benign neoplasm of uterine smooth muscle. It is one of the most common neoplasms in females, being found in one of every 4 women in the reproductive years. Leiomyomas are responsible for 30% of gynecologic admissions to hospitals.

Leiomyomas are most common between 20 and 40 years of age and tend to stop growing actively or to regress after menopause. Growth appears to be dependent on estrogens and may be rapid during pregnancy.

Leiomyomas may be solitary or multiple and may be located anywhere in the uterine smooth muscle (Fig 53–12). They often reach large size. Grossly, leiomyomas are circumscribed (Fig 53–13), firm, grayish-white masses with a characteristic whorled appearance on cut section. Histologically, they are composed of a uniform proliferation of spindle-shaped smooth muscle cells (Fig 53–14). Cytologic atypia is sometimes present, particularly in areas of hyalinization, but mitotic

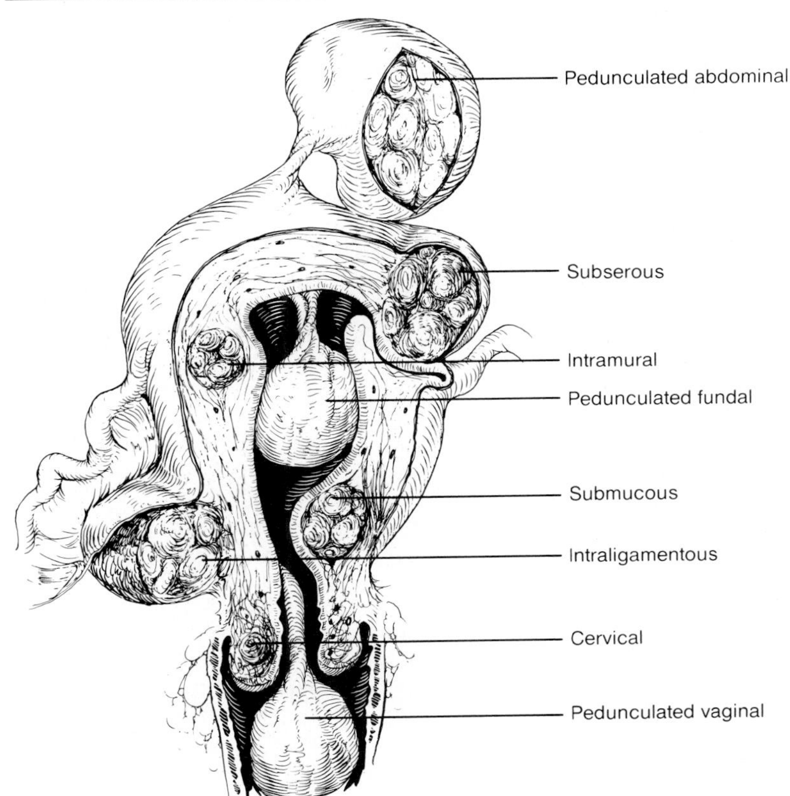

Figure 53–12. Leiomyomas of the uterus, showing different locations where these neoplasms are found in the uterus.

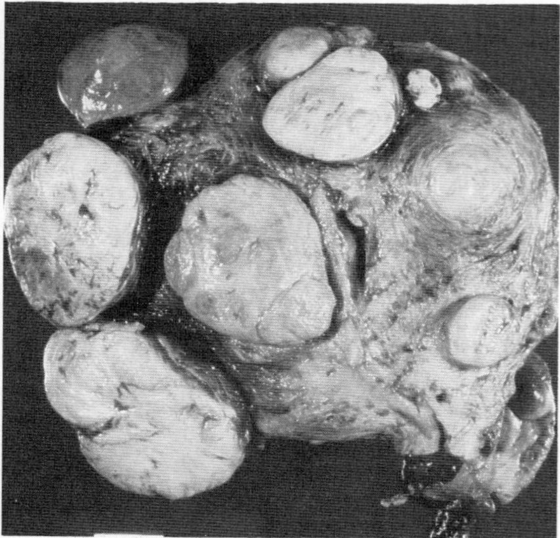

Figure 53-13. Uterine leiomyomas, showing multiple well-circumscribed nodules of varying size with the typical whorled appearance on cut surface.

figures are scarce. Collagen is present in varying amounts (hence "fibroid").

Degenerative changes occur frequently: (1) Red degeneration (necrobiosis) is typically seen during pregnancy, when the neoplasm undergoes necrosis and develops a beefy-red color. This change is associated with acute abdominal pain. (2) Cystic degeneration is common and usually does not cause symptoms. (3) Hyalinization, with broad bands of collagen appearing in the tumor, may be associated with marked cytologic atypia ("bizarre leiomyoma") but is still benign, the cytologic atypia probably representing a degenerative phenomenon. (4) Calcification may rarely be so extensive that the tumor appears as a radiopaque mass on plain x-ray. (5) Leiomyomas very rarely undergo malignant change.

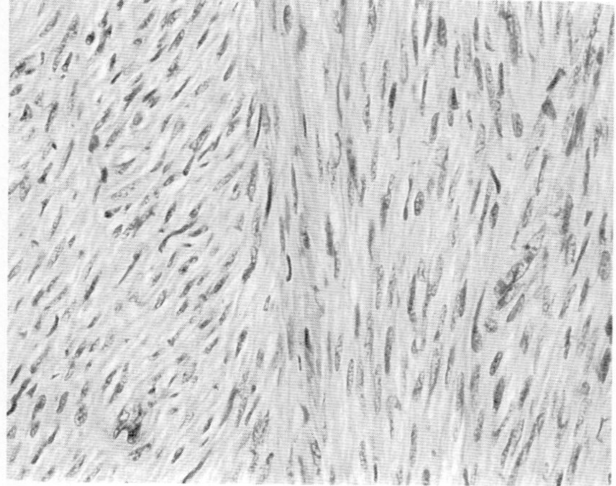

Figure 53-14. Uterine leiomyoma, showing interlacing fascicles of cytologically uniform smooth muscle cells.

Leiomyomas are a common cause of excessive uterine bleeding (menorrhagia) and an important cause of infertility. However, most patients are asymptomatic.

2. LEIOMYOSARCOMA

Leiomyosarcoma is a rare uterine neoplasm, accounting for 3% of uterine malignant neoplasms. It is nonetheless the most common uterine sarcoma. It arises from smooth muscle of the myometrium, usually de novo rather than from a preexisting leiomyoma.

Leiomyosarcomas appear as bulky, fleshy masses that show hemorrhage and necrosis. Marked cytologic pleomorphism and atypia are usually present. The most important diagnostic criterion is a high mitotic rate (over 10 mitoses per 10 high-power fields).

Leiomyosarcoma is most common in older women, presenting as postmenopausal bleeding or a uterine mass. Local recurrence and hematogenous metastases are frequent. The 5-year survival rate is about 40%.

THE UTERINE CERVIX

STRUCTURE & FUNCTION

The uterine cervix is the part of the uterus that lies distal to the internal os. It is composed of the endocervix, which extends from the internal to the external os and contains the endocervical canal. The endocervical canal is lined by columnar epithelium and has complex mucous glands. At the external os or close to it, the columnar epithelium of the endocervix gives way to the squamous epithelium of the ectocervix. The ectocervix has no glands, and its epithelium becomes continuous with that of the vagina at the vaginal vault and fornices.

The cervix secretes mucus, whose quality changes during the menstrual cycle and is dependent on hormonal status. The quality of the mucus influences penetration of the cervix by the spermatozoon. The cervix also plays an important role in retaining the developing embryo in the uterus during pregnancy and in the first stage of labor, when it dilates and finally is effaced, permitting exit of the fetus into the birth canal.

INFLAMMATORY CERVICAL LESIONS

1. ACUTE CERVICITIS

Acute cervicitis is a common condition characterized by erythema, swelling, neutrophilic infiltration, and focal epithelial ulceration. The endocervix is more frequently involved than the ectocervix.

Acute cervicitis is usually a sexually transmitted infection, commonly with gonococci, *Trichomonas vaginalis,* and herpes simplex (see Chapter 54). Non-sexually transmitted agents such as *Escherichia coli* and staphylococci may also be isolated from acutely inflamed cervices, but their role is not clear. Acute cervicitis also follows the trauma of childbirth and surgical instrumentation.

Clinically, there is a purulent vaginal discharge and pain. The severity of symptoms does not correlate well with the degree of inflammation.

2. CHRONIC CERVICITIS

Moderate numbers of lymphocytes, plasma cells, and histiocytes are present in the cervix in all females. Chronic cervicitis is therefore difficult to define pathologically. The presence of detectable cervical abnormalities such as granularity and thickening along with increased numbers of chronic inflammatory cells in a biopsy specimen is considered to warrant a diagnosis of chronic cervicitis.

Chronic cervicitis is most commonly seen at the external os and endocervical canal. It may be associated with fibrous stenosis of gland ducts, leading to retention (nabothian) cysts. When lymphoid follicles are present on microscopic examination, the term follicular cervicitis is sometimes used.

Clinically, chronic cervicitis is often an incidental finding. However, it may produce a vaginal discharge, and in a few cases associated fibrosis of the endocervical canal may cause stenosis, leading to infertility.

NONNEOPLASTIC CERVICAL PROLIFERATIONS

1. SQUAMOUS METAPLASIA

Squamous metaplasia of the endocervical epithelium is common, probably representing a response to irritation.

2. MICROGLANDULAR HYPERPLASIA

Microglandular hyperplasia is an unusual proliferation of endocervical glands that has been associated with the use of oral contraceptive agents. It presents grossly as a polypoid lesion that protrudes into the endocervical canal. Microscopically, it is characterized by an abnormal mass of endocervical glands lined by a flattened cuboidal epithelium.

3. ENDOCERVICAL POLYP

Polyps are common lesions of the endocervical canal, usually occurring at about the time of menopause. When large, a polyp may protrude out of the external os. Microscopically, endocervical polyps contain hyperplastic endocervical glands and a highly vascular stroma and may show marked chronic inflammation. The surface epithelium of a polyp commonly shows squamous metaplasia. Endocervical polyps are benign, with no increased incidence of neoplasia.

Rarely, decidualization of the cervical stroma in pregnancy may produce polypoid lesions clinically resembling neoplasm. These are called decidual polyps.

NEOPLASMS OF THE CERVIX

1. CONDYLOMA ACUMINATUM

Condyloma acuminatum is a common lesion of the cervix caused by the human papilloma virus, which is transmitted by sexual contact. It occurs in 2 forms: (1) as a wartlike papillomatous lesion that resembles condylomata in other sites; and (2) as elevated flat areas in the epithelium with no papillomatous growth. Flat condylomas, which are commonly caused by types 16 and 18 human papilloma virus, are frequently associated with epithelial dysplasia.

Condyloma acuminatum is characterized by hyperplasia of the squamous epithelium with marked cytoplasmic vacuolation (koilocytosis) and nuclear chromatin condensation. Nuclear atypia is often present. Immunoperoxidase studies using antibodies against human papilloma virus are positive (Fig 53–15). A large number of different types of papilloma virus have been identified in condylomas; some of these, particularly types 16, 18, 31, and 33, are also associated with cervical squamous carcinoma, suggesting that some condylomas carry an increased risk of carcinoma.

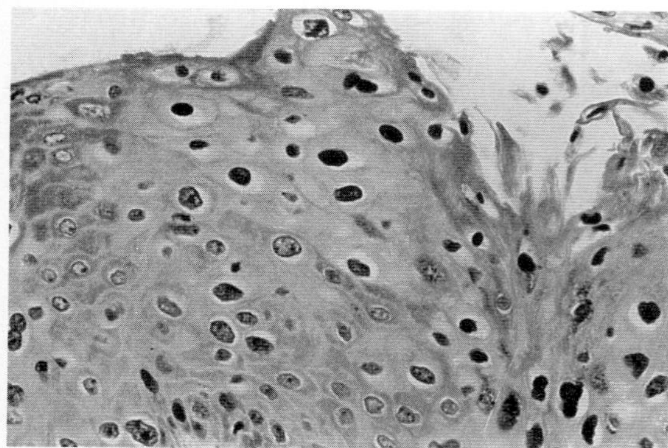

Figure 53–15. Flat condyloma acuminatum of the cervix, showing marked vacuolation of the cytoplasm and nuclear pyknosis (koilocytosis). This slide has been stained by the immunoperoxidase technique for papilloma virus and shows positive nuclear staining in many of the cells.

2. SQUAMOUS CARCINOMA

Cervical squamous carcinoma is common, causing 8000 deaths annually in the United States. It ranks sixth as a cause of cancer death in women. The incidence of cervical carcinoma has been falling, partly due to early detection of premalignant epithelial dysplasia by routine cytologic screening of cervical smears ("Pap smears"); many cases are detected and treated in the preinvasive stage.

In contrast to carcinoma, dysplasia of the cervical epithelium remains common and appears to be occurring in younger women.

Etiology

Considerable evidence suggests that carcinoma of the cervix is caused by a sexually transmitted carcinogenic agent, probably viral (Table 53–3). The risk of developing carcinoma increases with early onset of sexual activity, frequency of coitus, and greater number of sexual partners. It is common in multiparous women who have married early and in prostitutes but vanishingly rare in nuns. In general, cervical carcinoma tends to affect the lower socioeconomic stratum of society.

Cervical carcinoma is uncommon in Jewish and Moslem women, leading to a theory that male circumcision reduces the incidence of cervical cancer in women. It has been shown recently that there is a 3-fold increase in the incidence of cervical cancer among the sexual partners of men who have been married before to women with carcinoma of the cervix.

Two viruses are suspected of having an etiologic role in cancer of the cervix:

(1) Herpes simplex virus type 2 (HSV-2). HSV-2 antibodies are present in a high percentage of patients with cervical carcinoma when compared with controls. Though entire viral particles have not been demonstrated in the cells of cervical carcinoma, HSV-2 viral DNA, messenger RNA, and viral proteins have been found in some cases. The incidence of cervical carcinoma in patients infected with HSV-2 virus is, however, low, indicating that carcinogenic potential of the virus is not great.

(2) Human papilloma virus—particularly serologic types 16 and 18, which cause atypical flat condyloma acuminatum—has been found in both squamous carcinoma and dysplastic lesions of the cervix. This is presently considered to be an important etiologic agent. Recent studies show that the presence of human papilloma virus, as demonstrated by immunologic or molecular techniques in cervical smears or vaginal fluid, is associated with a 20-fold increase in the risk for cervical carcinoma (see also Chapter 18).

Dysplasia of the Cervix (Fig 53–16)

Most cervical carcinomas arise in a stratified squamous epithelium that shows precancerous change (dysplasia; see Chapter 16). Dysplasia commonly involves the region of the squamocolumnar junction and the endocervical canal that has undergone squamous metaplasia. Dysplasia is recognized by the presence of cytologic abnormalities in a cervical (Pap) smear (Table 53–2) and confirmed by cervical biopsy (Fig 53–17). The cytologic changes include increased nuclear size, increased nuclear:cytoplasmic ratio, hyperchromatism, abnormal chromatin distribution, and nuclear membrane abnormalities. The extent of these changes permits classification (in order of increasing severity) as mild, moderate, or severe dysplasia and carcinoma in situ (Fig 53–16). These cytologic changes on a Pap smear correlate accurately with the degree of abnormal maturation of the epithelium in a subsequent cervical biopsy specimen. In carcinoma in situ, biopsy reveals that maturation is totally lacking, and most of the cytologic changes of carcinoma are present except invasion through the basement membrane.

Dysplasias are reversible lesions, but the more severe the degree of dysplasia the less the tendency to reverse. Twenty-five percent of patients with carcinoma in situ develop invasive carcinoma within 5 years if left untreated. The time span for progression of dysplasia is variable. The median time for carcinoma to develop is 7 years for mild dysplasia and 1 year for severe dysplasia. This observation has led to the recommendation that routine cervical Pap smears should be performed in all women at least once every 3 years after 2 initial examinations 1 year apart have proved negative.

The term **cervical intraepithelial neoplasia (CIN)** is currently in vogue and has the same denotation as dysplasia. CIN I is equivalent to minimal dysplasia, CIN II to moderate dysplasia, and CIN III includes severe dysplasia and carcinoma

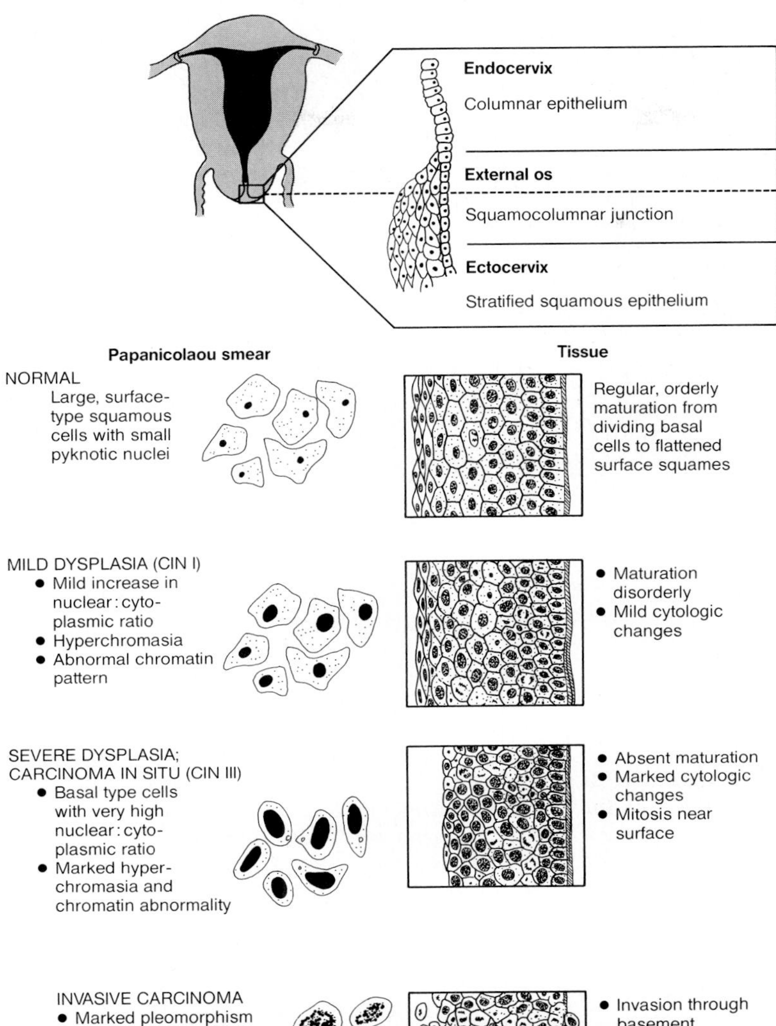

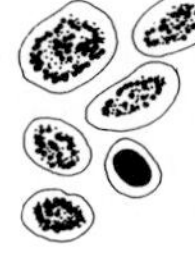
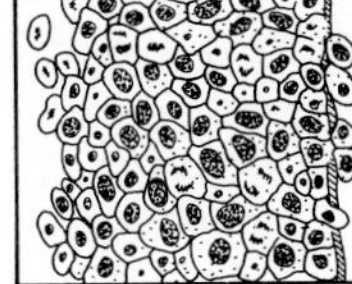

Figure 53–16. Squamous epithelial dysplasia and carcinoma of the cervix, showing criteria used to grade dysplasia. Dysplasia commonly occurs at the squamocolumnar junction.

in situ. This terminology, of course, raises basic questions about the exact definition of neoplasia versus dysplasia (see Chapter 16).

Dysplasia affects cervical surface epithelium as well as extending down into endocervical glands (gland duct involvement). The significance of gland duct involvement is the same as that of dysplasia of the surface epithelium.

Dysplasia and carcinoma in situ produce no symptoms. Changes in the mucosa on inspection are minimal, but some lesions may be recognized by means of the magnified image provided at colposcopy (eg, abnormal vascular pattern, thickening, and white coloration). Colposcopy and biopsy should be performed in all patients in whom dysplasia of any grade is found on routine cervical cytologic examination (see Table 53–2). The Schiller test, which consists of painting the cervix with aqueous iodine, is helpful in locating areas of dysplasia, since dysplastic epithelium lacks glycogen and will appear as a pale area whereas normal epithelium stains dark brown with iodine.

The treatment of dysplasia is local and conservative. Cryosurgery, electrocoagulation, laser coagulation, and conization—removal of a cone of cervical tissue, including the entire squamocolumnar junction—are all effective.

Microinvasive Carcinoma (Stage IA)

Microinvasive carcinoma of the cervix is defined as cervical carcinoma in which the total

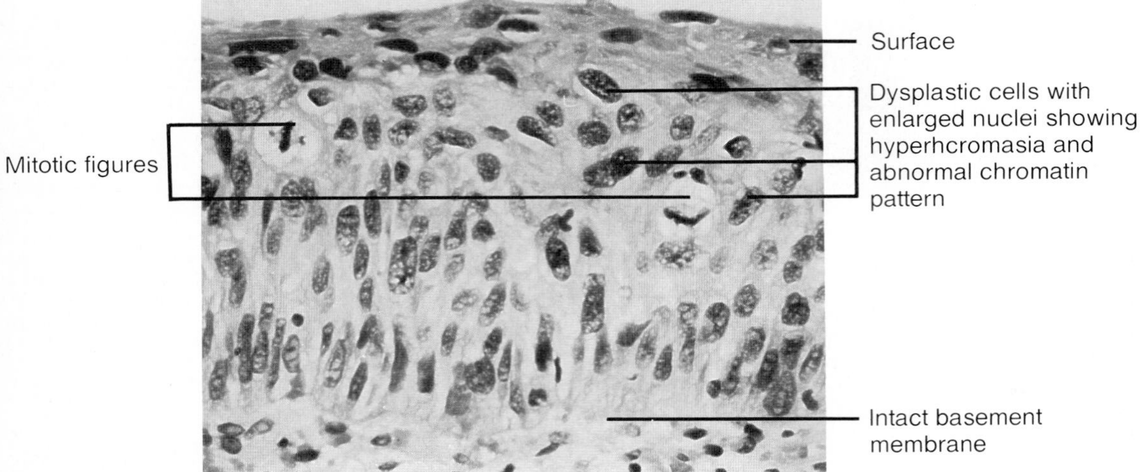

Figure 53-17. Moderate to severe dysplasia of the cervical squamous epithelium, showing disordered maturation, increased nuclear:cytoplasmic ratio, hyperchromasia, chromatin clumping, and mitotic figures in the upper part of the epithelium.

depth of invasion is less than 3 mm from the basement membrane (Table 53-4). Microinvasive carcinoma so defined is rarely associated with metastases, and local surgical excision is curative. It should be recognized that the submucosa of the cervix within this 3-mm zone below the basement membrane does contain lymphatics and blood vessels, and metastases are a theoretic possibility. Nonetheless, the rarity of metastases is a statistical fact.

Table 53-4. Clinical staging of cervical carcinoma.[1,2]

Stage 0:	Carcinoma in situ (100%)
Stage IA:	Microinvasive carcinoma; invasion to a depth less than 3 mm from the basement membrane (> 95%)
Stage IB:	Invasive carcinoma, infiltrating to a depth greater than 3 mm but confined to the cervix (90%)
Stage II:	Extension of tumor beyond the cervix to involve the endometrium, vagina (but not the lower third), or paracervical soft tissue (but has not extended to the pelvic side wall) (75%)
Stage III:	Extension to the pelvic side wall or involvement of the lower third of the vagina or the presence of hydronephrosis from ureteral involvement (35%)
Stage IV:	Extension beyond the pelvis or clinical involvement of bladder or rectal mucosa (10%)

[1]Adapted from American Joint Committee for Cancer Staging and End-Results Reporting; Task Force on Gynecologic Sites: Staging System for Cancer at Gynecologic Sites, 1979.
[2]Figures in parentheses represent 5-year survival rates for the stage.

Invasive Squamous Carcinoma (Stage IB & More Extensive)

Invasive carcinoma is defined as carcinoma infiltrating to a depth of greater than 3 mm from the basement membrane. It occurs most frequently in the age group from 30 to 50 years.

Invasive carcinoma may present grossly as an exophytic, fungating, necrotic mass (Fig 53-18), the most common appearance; as a malignant ulcer; or as a diffusely infiltrative lesion with only minimal surface ulceration or nodularity (uncommon). Microscopically, there are 3 different types: (1) large cell, nonkeratinizing squamous carcinoma—the most common type, with the best prognosis; (2) keratinizing squamous carcinoma—next most common, with an intermediate prognosis; and (3) small cell carcinoma—rare, with a poor prognosis.

Invasive cervical carcinoma is manifested as abnormal uterine bleeding (commonly irregular and excessive menstrual bleeding or postmenopausal bleeding) or vaginal discharge. Obstruction of the cervical canal may cause blood to accumulate in the uterine cavity and result in infection (pyometron). Colposcopy permits direct visualization and biopsy to make a definitive histologic diagnosis. Cervical carcinoma is staged according to the degree of spread (Table 53-4).

Treatment is a combination of surgery and radiation therapy, depending on the extent of disease. The prognosis depends primarily on the clinical stage of the disease. The histologic type is a lesser prognostic factor.

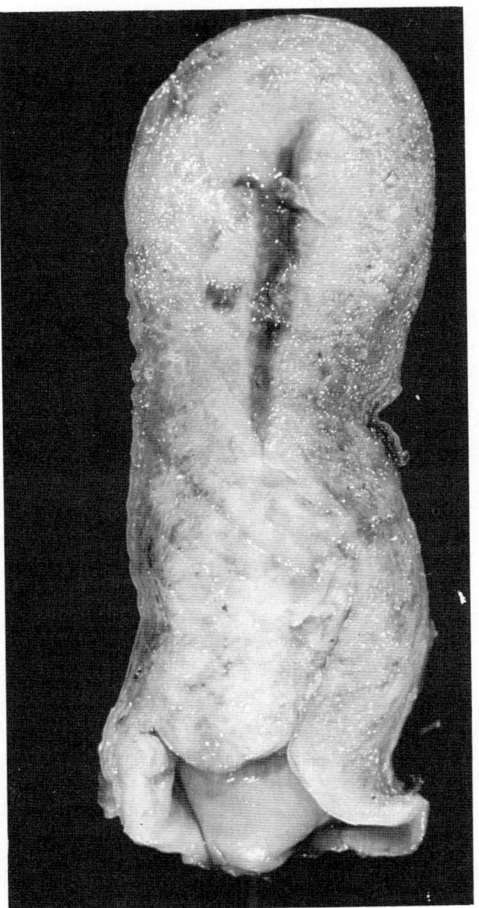

Figure 53–18. Squamous carcinoma of the cervix involving the squamocolumnar junction and most of the endocervical canal. The tumor is mainly to the left of the displaced endocervical canal in this figure.

3. ENDOCERVICAL ADENOCARCINOMA

Endocervical adenocarcinoma accounts for 10–15% of cervical cancers. It arises in the endocervical glands, presenting as a mass in the endocervical canal. It frequently obstructs the endocervical canal, predisposing to pyometron.

Microscopically, endocervical adenocarcinoma is usually a well-differentiated lesion, often with a papillary appearance. It may show squamous differentiation (adenoacanthoma, adenosquamous carcinoma). The prognosis is less favorable than that of squamous carcinoma. Adenosquamous carcinoma behaves in a highly malignant fashion.

THE VAGINA

The vagina is a muscular tube lined by nonkeratinizing stratified squamous epithelium. Its upper part is derived from the müllerian duct, its lower part from the urogenital sinus. The vagina normally contains no glands but exudes fluid throughout the epithelium. The vaginal epithelium undergoes cyclic changes during the menstrual cycle, mainly relating to the glycogen content of the superficial cells. Examination of a vaginal scraping was used in the past as a means of evaluating hormonal status, but this technique has been discarded. The vagina is effectively evaluated by direct examination using a speculum, which also permits taking of biopsies from abnormal areas.

INFLAMMATORY VAGINAL LESIONS (Fig 53–19)

1. ACUTE VAGINITIS (Non-Sexually Transmitted)

Before puberty, pyogenic bacterial infection of the vagina may occur. After puberty, the vaginal mucosa is protected by the low pH produced by the commensal Döderlein bacillus *(Lactobacillus acidophilus),* and vaginitis is relatively rare during the reproductive years.

Non-sexually transmitted vaginitis may be caused by *Gardnerella (Haemophilus) vaginalis, Trichomonas vaginalis,* and *Candida albicans.* Atrophic vaginitis is a specific form of acute inflammation that occurs in postmenopausal women when the vaginal mucosa undergoes extreme atrophy as a result of estrogen withdrawal. The atrophic mucosa is susceptible to secondary infection.

Vaginitis presents clinically with vaginal discomfort and discharge. The diagnosis may be established by examination of a smear and culture.

TUMORS (MASS LESIONS) OF THE VAGINA

1. GARTNER'S DUCT CYST

Gartner's duct cysts are derived from vestigial remnants of the mesonephric ducts. They occur in the anterolateral wall of the vagina and are lined by cuboidal or columnar epithelium.

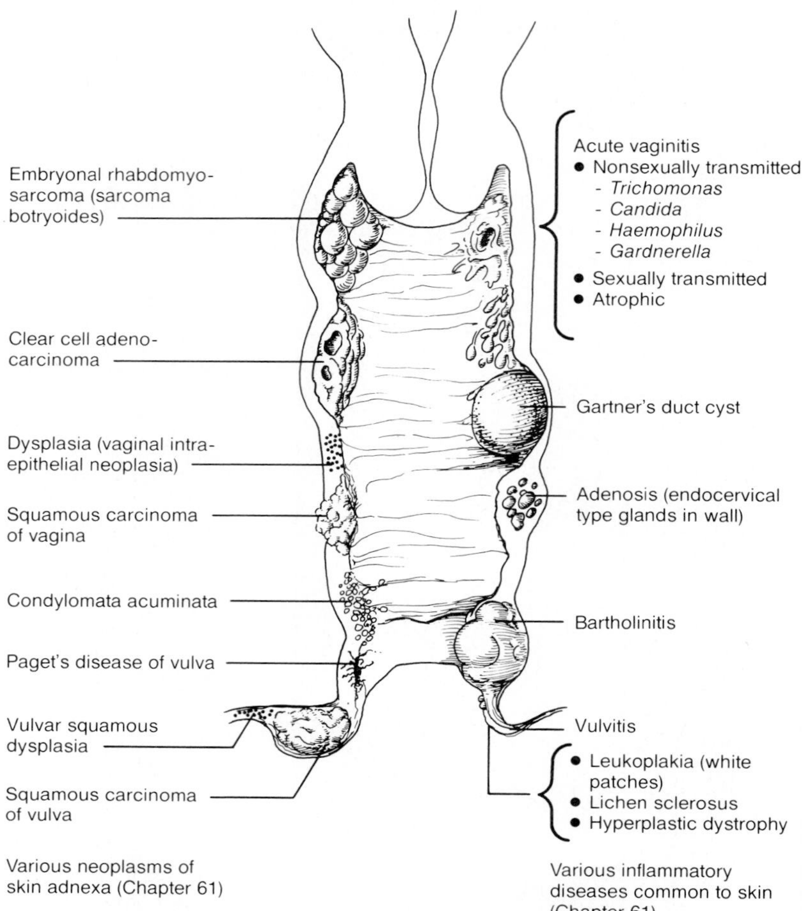

Figure 53-19. Principal diseases of the vagina and vulva.

2. VAGINAL ADENOSIS

Vaginal adenosis is the occurrence of endocervical type glands in the vaginal wall in women. The incidence is uncertain, but its frequency is greatly increased in women whose mothers received diethylstilbestrol (DES) during pregnancy. It is postulated that DES inhibits transformation of the müllerian epithelium of the embryonic vagina into adult squamous epithelium.

In most cases, there is no visible lesion, and the condition is of little significance clinically except for its yet uncertain relationship to clear cell adenocarcinoma of the vagina (see below). If vaginal adenosis is the precursor lesion for clear cell adenocarcinoma, the risk is small.

3. SQUAMOUS CARCINOMA

Squamous carcinoma is the most common vaginal neoplasm. It is rare and accounts for only 1–2% of cancers in the female genital tract.

Grossly, vaginal carcinoma presents as a polypoid, fungating, exophytic mass or as an ulcerative, infiltrative tumor. Microscopically, it has the typical appearance of a squamous carcinoma, with keratinization and formation of epithelial pearls. Not uncommonly, the tumor is poorly differentiated. The adjacent epithelium commonly shows dysplasia.

Local extension beyond the vagina occurs early. Lymphatic spread varies with the location: tumors in the upper two-thirds drain mainly to pelvic nodes; tumors in the lower third, mainly to inguinal nodes. Vaginal carcinoma is staged according to its degree of spread (Table 53–5).

Treatment is by a combination of surgery and radiation therapy. The overall prognosis is poor, with a 5-year survival rate of 30–40%. The prognosis varies with the clinical stage, and the overall low survival rate indicates that many cancers are detected at a late stage.

4. CLEAR CELL ADENOCARCINOMA

Clear cell adenocarcinoma of the vagina is rare, accounting for about 0.1–0.2% of cancers in the female genital tract. It occurs in young females,

Table 53-5. Clinical staging of vaginal carcinoma.

Stage 0:	Carcinoma in situ (intraepithelial neoplasia)
Stage I:	Carcinoma limited to vaginal wall
Stage II:	Involvement of subvaginal tissues without extension to the pelvic side walls
Stage III:	Extension to one or both pelvic side walls
Stage IV:	Involvement of mucosa of bladder or rectum (stage IVA) or extension beyond the true pelvis (stage IVB)

usually between 10 and 35 years of age, and has a definite association with exposure of the mother to diethylstilbestrol (DES) during pregnancy. Clear cell adenocarcinoma was not reported until about 15 years ago, whereupon its incidence increased; this increase is probably related to the use of DES to prevent first-trimester abortion in the early 1950s. About 500,000 fetuses were exposed to DES before this practice was discontinued; thus, there may be a further rise in the incidence of this type of carcinoma. As noted above, the relationship of clear cell carcinoma to vaginal adenosis is controversial, but both are associated with DES exposure.

Clear cell carcinoma most often appears as a polypoid mass. Microscopically, it is composed of clear cells arranged in a tubuloglandular pattern. The neoplastic cells have a "hobnail" appearance.

Treatment with surgery and radiation is effective in the short term. Data relating to long-term survival are not yet available.

5. EMBRYONAL RHABDOMYOSARCOMA (Sarcoma Botryoides)

Embryonal rhabdomyosarcoma is the commonest sarcoma of the vagina. It occurs in the first 5 years of life and appears as a large, lobulated tumor mass (Gk *botryoides* "like a bunch of grapes") that frequently protrudes at the vaginal orifice. Microscopically, it is an anaplastic embryonal rhabdomyosarcoma. It behaves as a highly malignant neoplasm with early hematogenous dissemination.

THE VULVA

The vulva is composed of the labia majora, labia minora, vestibule, and clitoris. The vagina and urethra open into the vulva, as do several different glands, the largest being the paired Bartholin's glands, which are mucus-secreting glands that open at the vaginal introitus. Skene's glands are situated around the urethral opening.

INFLAMMATORY VULVAL LESIONS

Inflammatory lesions of the vulva are similar to those occurring in the skin. Furuncles are common, and erysipelas and severe necrotizing vulvitis have been reported. All of the sexually transmitted diseases may produce lesions in the vulva (Chapter 54).

Acute inflammation of Bartholin's gland, frequently leading to abscess formation, is a common lesion. *Staphylococcus aureus, Streptococcus pyogenes, Neisseria gonorrhoeae,* and *Escherichia coli* are the common organisms. Acute bartholinitis presents as a painful, tender, erythematous swelling in the inferior part of the labium majus. Treatment with surgical drainage and appropriate antibiotics is effective.

VULVAL DYSTROPHIES

The vulval dystrophies are manifested by opaque white plaques (leukoplakia) on the mucosal surface of the vulva. Leukoplakia may be due to a variety of different conditions, including vulval dystrophies, chronic dermatitis, psoriasis, and carcinoma in situ.

There are 2 main types of vulval dystrophy: lichen sclerosus and hyperplastic dystrophy. In about 30% of cases, both types are present.

1. LICHEN SCLEROSUS (Kraurosis Vulvae)

Lichen sclerosus is a chronic, progressive disease usually occurring in postmenopausal women. Its cause is unknown. It is characterized by scaly and pruritic white plaques. Sclerosis and shrinkage of the dermis causes the vulva to be smooth, glazed, and parchmentlike.

Microscopically, lichen sclerosus is characterized by thinning of the epidermis, with a relatively prominent stratum corneum, flattened rete pegs, and some basal layer degeneration. Dense hyaline collagen is present in the upper dermis. The condition was formerly called lichen sclerosus et atrophicus, but true atrophy is not present.

Lichen sclerosus is not premalignant.

2. HYPERPLASTIC DYSTROPHY

Hyperplastic dystrophy is a common lesion occurring mainly in postmenopausal women. It appears clinically as leukoplakia. Microscopically, there is

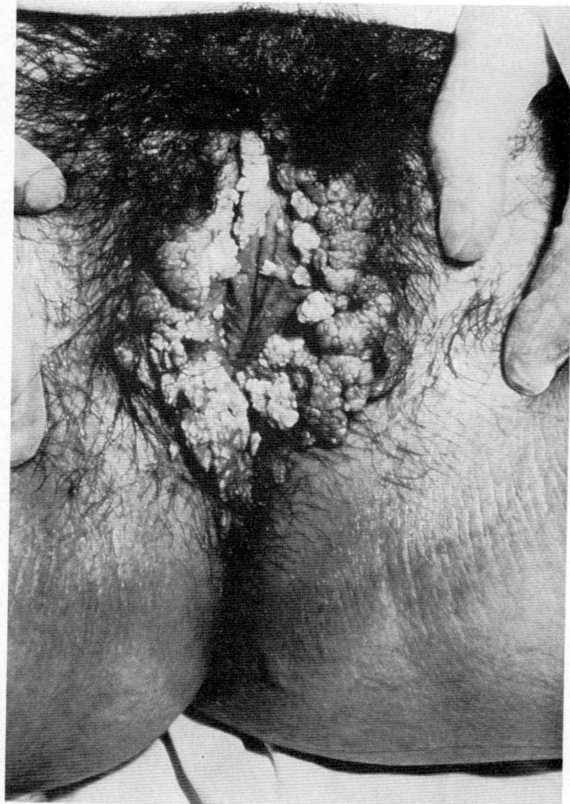

Figure 53-20. Condylomata acuminata of the vulva.

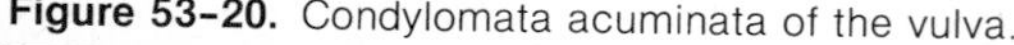

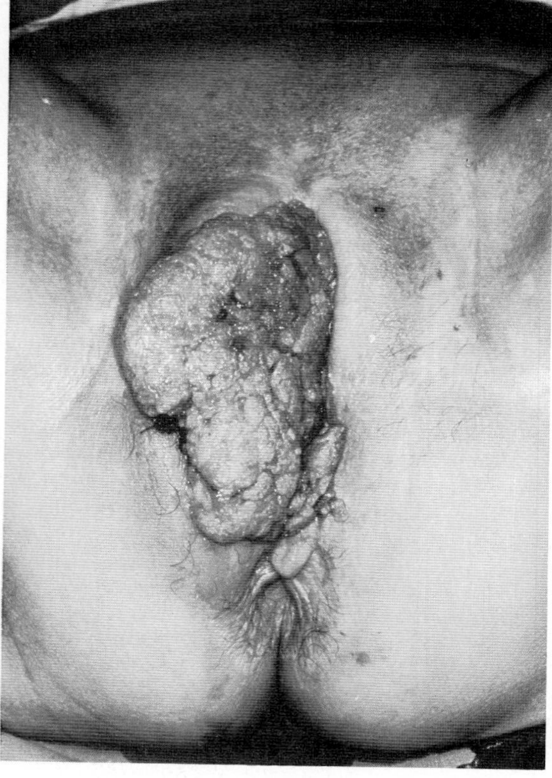

Figure 53-21. Large, exophytic squamous carcinoma of the vulva.

hyperplasia of the epidermis, with hyperkeratosis and chronic dermal inflammation. In some cases, maturation is normal; in others, cytologic dysplasia occurs. The more severe forms of dysplasia are equivalent to carcinoma in situ of the vulva. Hyperplastic dystrophy is a premalignant lesion, the risk being proportionate to the degree of dysplasia.

NEOPLASMS OF THE VULVA

Condyloma acuminatum is a benign verrucous lesion caused by the sexually transmitted papilloma virus (Figure 53–20). It is common in the vulva and is identical to its counterpart on the penis.

Adnexal skin tumors occur commonly in the vulva. The most common of these is hidradenoma papilliferum, which is a benign papillary neoplasm derived from the apocrine glands of the vulva. It presents as a labial nodule, frequently with ulceration.

Melanocytic lesions of all types occur in the vulva. Most frequently, these are benign compound nevi. Vulval malignant melanoma is rare.

1. SQUAMOUS CARCINOMA IN SITU (Bowen's Disease)

Squamous carcinoma in situ of the vulva occurs as the extreme form of dysplasia in hyperplastic dystrophy. In such cases, it presents clinically as leukoplakia. In some cases, carcinoma in situ occurs without preceding vulval dystrophy and then appears as a slightly elevated, red-brown plaque on the vulva. It may be associated with carcinoma in situ in the cervix and vagina, suggesting a common etiologic agent.

Carcinoma in situ is characterized by absence of normal maturation of the squamous epithelium, cells which have a high nuclear:cytoplasmic ratio, abnormal chromatin distribution in the nucleus, and numerous mitotic figures. Invasion of the basement membrane is absent.

Carcinoma in situ of the vulva carries a high risk of development of squamous carcinoma, but the latent period may vary from 1 to 10 years. Patients with carcinoma in situ of the vulva should have the entire lesion excised surgically.

2. INVASIVE SQUAMOUS CARCINOMA

Though it is the commonest malignant neoplasm of the vulva, squamous carcinoma accounts for only 4% of female genital tract cancers. It usually occurs in women over 60 years of age. The cause is unknown, but an association with cervical carcinoma suggests that a common etiologic agent, probably human papilloma virus infection, may be involved.

Grossly, the early lesion is an indurated plaque, progressing to a firm nodule that ulcerates (Fig 53–21). It may involve any part of the vulva, the most common site being the anterior two-thirds of the labia majora. Microscopically, squamous carcinoma of the vulva is usually well-differentiated. The degree of differentiation correlates poorly with prognosis.

Lymphatic spread to inguinal and pelvic nodes occurs early, with bilateral involvement being common. About 60% of patients have involved nodes at the time of diagnosis. Hematogenous dissemination occurs in advanced disease. The clinical stage of the disease (Table 53–6) correlates well with prognosis. Cases with negative lymph nodes (stage II) have a 70% 5-year survival rate, in contrast with a 40% rate in those with lymph node involvement. Patients with early, small lesions (stage I) treated by radical vulvectomy have an 80% 5-year survival rate. Chemotherapy and radiotherapy are useful when used in conjunction with surgery and for temporary control of advanced lesions.

Table 53–6. Clinical staging of vulvar carcinoma.[1]

Stage 0:	Carcinoma in situ (100%)
Stage I:	Lesion less than 2 cm in diameter and confined to vulva, with no suspicious groin nodes (80%)
Stage II:	Lesion greater than 2 cm in diameter and confined to vulva, with no suspicious groin nodes (70%)
Stage III:	Lesion of any size with extension beyond vulva to involve urethra, vagina, perineum, and anus without suspicious groin nodes, *or* lesion confined to vulva with suspicious or positive groin nodes (40%)
Stage IV:	Extension beyond vulva with positive groin nodes, *or* involvement of mucosa of rectum, bladder, or upper urethra, *or* distant metastases (20%)

[1]Figures in parentheses represent 5-year survival rates for the stage.

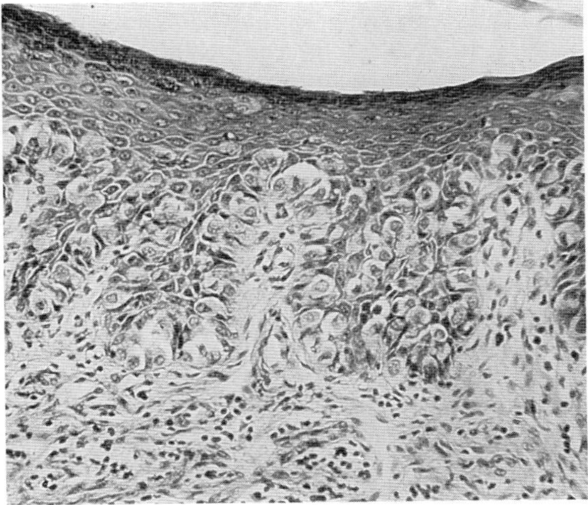

Figure 53–22. Paget's disease of the vulva with adenocarcinoma cells in the basal zone of the squamous epithelium.

3. VERRUCOUS CARCINOMA

Verrucous carcinoma is a variant of well-differentiated squamous carcinoma, characterized by a polypoid growth pattern with little infiltrative tendency. Distinction from condyloma acuminatum may be difficult. Verrucous carcinomas tend to remain localized and are cured by wide excision. They are, however, resistant to radiation therapy—indeed, radiation has been reported to induce aggressive behavior associated with increased anaplasia histologically. For this reason, it is important to distinguish verrucous carcinoma from the more common well-differentiated squamous carcinoma.

4. EXTRAMAMMARY PAGET'S DISEASE

The vulva is the most common site for extramammary Paget's disease. It is, however, a rare lesion when compared to Paget's disease of the breast. Paget's disease presents as an eczemalike red, crusted lesion in the labia majora, usually in elderly women.

Microscopically, large anaplastic tumor cells are present singly or in small groups in the epidermis (Fig 53–22). The tumor cells contain mucin, evidence of their glandular origin. Thirty percent of cases have an associated underlying carcinoma in vulval glands.

The prognosis of extramammary Paget's disease is poor if it is associated with an underlying invasive cancer.

54 Sexually Transmitted Infections

- Gonorrhea
- Syphilis
  - Primary Syphilis
  - Secondary Syphilis
  - Tertiary or Late Syphilis
  - Congenital Syphilis
- Herpes Genitalis
- Chancroid
- Chlamydial Urethritis and Cervicitis
- Lymphogranuloma Venereum
- Granuloma Inguinale

A large variety of infectious agents are transmitted by sexual contact (Table 54–1). Diseases transmitted mainly by sexual contact were traditionally classified as venereal diseases (after Venus, the Roman goddess of beauty and love) but are now conventionally called sexually transmitted diseases. They are considered separately because they present special problems relating to transmission and prevention.

The sexual revolution of the past 3 decades has been associated with an increase in the incidence of sexually transmitted diseases, many of which now represent major public health problems. New sexually transmitted diseases—most importantly AIDS—have also emerged.

The diseases traditionally regarded as venereal or sexually transmitted infections are gonorrhea, syphilis, herpes genitalis, chancroid, chlamydial urethritis and cervicitis, lymphogranuloma venereum, and granuloma inguinale. More recently, AIDS, hepatitis B, and human papilloma virus infection have been included in this category. In this chapter, only the traditional sexually transmitted diseases are discussed.

GONORRHEA

Gonorrhea is one of the most common sexually transmitted diseases, with a reported incidence of over 300 per 100,000 population in the United States. It is estimated that approximately 1% of the population (ie, 2–3 million persons) in the United States have had gonorrhea. Since large numbers of cases may go unreported, 1% is probably an underestimate.

Pathology

Gonorrhea is caused by the gram-negative diplococcus, *Neisseria gonorrhoeae.* The organism infects chiefly the urethra in the male, producing acute urethritis. In the female, the cervix is the main site of infection.

Infection occurs also at other sites in the genital tract. In men, the prostate, seminal vesicles, and epididymides are commonly involved, causing suppurative acute inflammation followed by fibrosis and sometimes sterility. In women, the urethra, Bartholin's and Skene's glands, and the uterine tubes are commonly involved. Salpingitis (pelvic inflammatory disease) leads to fibrosis of the uterine tube, causing infertility and an increased risk of ectopic pregnancy.

With varied sexual practices, gonococcal pharyngitis and anal gonorrhea may occur; gonococcal proctitis is frequent in male homosexuals.

Entry of gonococci into the pelvic peritoneum in the female via the uterine tubes may cause peritonitis. Entry of gonococci into the bloodstream may cause (1) bacteremia, with fever and a skin rash; (2) gonococcal endocarditis, which tends to affect both the right- and left-sided valves of the heart; and (3) gonococcal arthritis, frequently monarticular, affecting large joints, most commonly the knee joint.

In addition, gonococcal infection may be transmitted to the fetus during delivery through the birth canal, producing neonatal ophthalmitis, the end result of which is often blindness. Prophylactic instillation of 1% silver nitrate solution into the conjunctiva prevents this complication and is mandatory in obstetric practice in the United States.

Clinical Features & Diagnosis

In men, the common presentation is with dysuria and purulent urethral discharge. In women, cervicitis may produce a vaginal discharge. Systemic symptoms are usually absent. In both sexes, gonorrhea may be asymptomatic, constituting a source of apparently healthy carriers. The risk of infection during a single act of intercourse with an infected partner is estimated to be 10–20%.

The diagnosis of gonorrhea is made by direct smear of the urethral or vaginal discharge. Gram staining reveals gram-negative diplococci both ex-

Table 54–1. Major sexually transmitted diseases.

Disease	Additional Features	Organism
Gonorrhea	Urethritis, cervicitis, pelvic inflammatory disease, prostatitis, epididymitis, arthritis	*Neisseria gonorrhoeae*
Syphilis		*Treponema pallidium*
Primary syphilis	Chancre	
Secondary syphilis	Fever, lymph node enlargement, skin rashes, mucosal patches and ulcers, condyloma latum	
Tertiary syphilis	Gumma, tabes dorsalis, general paresis (dementia paralytica), aortitis	
Congenital syphilis	See text	
Herpes genitalis	Penile, vulvular, or cervical ulcers	Herpes simplex type 2
Chancroid	Soft chancres, lymphadenopathy	*Haemophilus ducreyi*
Chlamydial urethritis/cervicitis	Conjunctivitis, Reiter's syndrome, pelvic inflammatory disease	*Chlamydia trachomatis* (D–K)
Lymphogranuloma venereum	Ulcers, lymphadenopathy, rectal strictures	*C trachomatis* (L1–L3)
Granuloma inguinale	Ulcerating nodules, lymphadenopathy	*Calymmatobacterium donovani*
Trichomonas vaginitis	Vaginitis	*Trichomonas vaginalis*
Acquired immune deficiency syndrome (AIDS)	Opportunistic infections, Kaposi's sarcoma, lymphoma	Human immunodeficiency virus (see Chapter 7)
Condyloma acuminatum	Cervical cancer	Human papilloma virus
Viral B hepatitis	(See Chapter 42)	Hepatitis B virus

tracellularly and inside neutrophils. The diagnosis should be confirmed by culture, which requires special media and a high CO_2 environment. Commercial media such as Transgrow are effective in culturing gonococci. Culture is essential because Neisseria species other than gonococci may be present as commensals in the vagina.

The gonococcus is sensitive to penicillin in most cases. The recent emergence of penicillin-resistant *N gonorrhoeae* represents one of the major problems of management. Penicillin resistance is due to β-lactamase (penicillinase) production; the β-lactamase gene is plasmid-associated and is transferable to other gonococci by conjugation. Spectinomycin and trimethoprim-sulfamethoxazole are alternative antimicrobial agents.

SYPHILIS

Syphilis is caused by *Treponema pallidum,* a spirochete. While the incidence of syphilis has increased, the incidence of late syphilis has declined because of effective antibiotic treatment of early disease. The incidence of syphilis is difficult to estimate because of underreporting. It is probable that there are about 1 million active cases of syphilis in the United States. The common age for contracting syphilis is shifting from the mid 20s to the teen years. There has been a recent increase in the incidence of syphilis among individuals that are at high risk for developing AIDS (male homosexuals, intravenous drug users).

Routine testing of transfused blood and pregnant women for syphilis has resulted in a dramatic decline of transfusion syphilis and congenital syphilis.

Pathology & Clinical Features

Syphilis is best considered in terms of its early (primary and secondary) and late (tertiary) manifestations (Fig 54–1). Features of late syphilis occur 4 or more years from the date of infection.

Treatment

Early syphilis responds to penicillin. Tertiary manifestations of syphilis do not respond to antibiotic therapy and represent a chronic progressive disease that frequently causes considerable morbidity and ultimately death.

1. PRIMARY SYPHILIS

T pallidum is a delicate organism, rapidly killed by drying or temperature change. Transmission requires intimate sexual contact, because mucous membranes are the optimal sites of infection. *T pallidum* can penetrate intact mucous membranes and abraded skin. It cannot penetrate intact skin.

The incubation period after infection is 9–90 days. During this time, treponemes multiply lo-

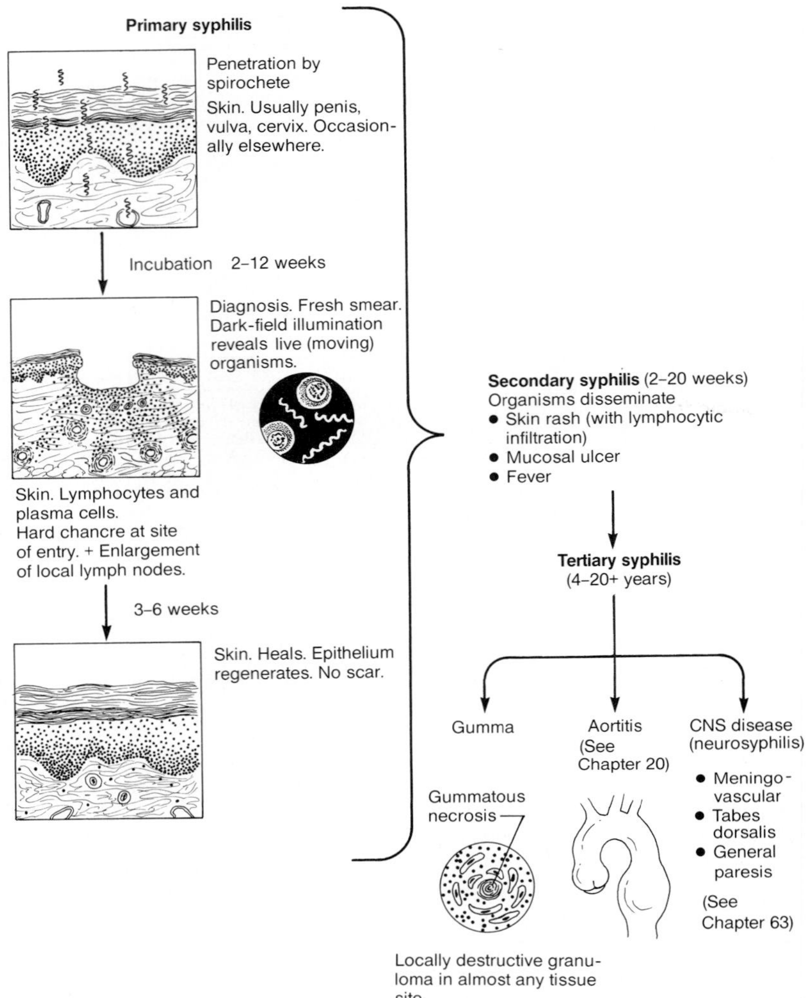

Figure 54–1. Course and pathologic features of syphilis.

cally and spread to lymph nodes and blood. The first visible lesion is termed the **primary chancre.** The chancre appears at the site of initial invasion—usually the penis (glans or shaft) in the male and the vulva in the female. Other sites include the cervix, scrotum, anus, rectum, and oral cavity.

The primary chancre is a painless, punched-out ulcer with an indurated base (hard chancre) consisting of chronic inflammatory tissue. Its surface exudes a serous fluid containing large numbers of treponemes. Painless enlargement of the inguinal lymph nodes may be present, but there are no systemic symptoms and the patient feels well.

The diagnosis of syphilis is best made at this stage by identifying spirochetes in the serous exudate from the chancre by dark-field microscopy. Serologic tests for syphilis may be negative in the early primary stage (Tables 54–2 and 54–3), and the organism cannot be cultured.

The primary chancre heals spontaneously in 3–6 weeks.

2. SECONDARY SYPHILIS

Secondary syphilis usually follows the primary stage after 2–20 weeks but may begin before the primary chancre heals. It is characterized by fever, generalized lymph node enlargement, and a red maculopapular skin rash. Orogenital mucosal lesions are common and include mucous membrane patches, irregular (''snail track'') ulcers in the mouth, and plaquelike lesions in the perineum (condylomata lata). Hepatitis, meningitis, nephritis (immune complex type), and osteochondritis may also occur.

Microscopically, these lesions are characterized by a nonspecific chronic inflammatory response with numerous plasma cells. Spirochetes are present in large numbers and can be demonstrated in tissue sections with Dieterle's silver stain.

Diagnosis is by demonstration of the living organism in smears made from lesions and examined by dark-field microscopy, silver stains of

Table 54–2. Serologic tests for syphilis.

Nonspecific reagin[1] tests
WR (Wassermann reaction: complement fixation test)
VDRL (Venereal Disease Research Laboratory: flocculation test)
RPR (rapid plasma reagin: flocculation test)

Become positive in late primary or early secondary syphilis, frequently revert to negative in tertiary syphilis.

Biologic false-positives occur in malaria, leprosy, infectious mononucleosis, collagen diseases.

Value as useful screening tests; if positive, should be followed by a specific confirmatory test. VDRL is most widely used; the antigen is a controlled complex of cardiolipin, cholesterol, and lecithin.

Specific confirmatory tests[2]
Treponema pallidum immobilization test (TPI)
Fluorescent treponemal absorption test (FTA-ABS)
Microhemagglutination test for treponemal antibodies (MHA-TP)

Become positive in primary and secondary syphilis, usually remain positive in tertiary syphilis.

Biologic false-positives rare; include other treponemal diseases, bejel, yaws, and pinta, which occur in the tropics and Central America but are rare in the USA and Europe.

Value as a confirmatory test in serum or cerebrospinal fluid. FTA-ABS is widely used but is technically difficult; many laboratories have adopted the MHA-TP. Both use killed treponemes grown in rabbit. The TPI uses live treponemes and is largely obsolete.

[1]The term "reagin" as used in syphilis serology has no connection with the IgE reagins of type I hypersensitivity. Syphilitic reagin is a mixture of IgG and IgM antibodies against a nontreponemal lipid antigen that is released from the tissues in syphilis and some other diseases.
[2]All test for specific antibody to *Treponema pallidum.*

tissue section from a lesion such as a condyloma latum, or positive serologic tests (Tables 54–2 and 54–3).

3. TERTIARY OR LATE SYPHILIS

Manifestations of late syphilis appear any time after 4 years following primary infection. Even without treatment, only 30% of cases of early syphilis ever develop tertiary syphilis. Primary and secondary stages may have been so subtle (subclinical) that patients with tertiary syphilis frequently give no history of symptoms.

Tertiary syphilis takes one of 3 forms (Fig 54–1).

Gumma

A gumma is a localized destructive granuloma. It may occur anywhere but is more common in the liver, bones, oral cavity, and testes. Grossly, it produces a large mass that may be mistaken for a neoplasm. Microscopically, a gumma is composed of a central area of gummatous ("rubbery") necrosis, surrounded by epithelioid cells, lymphocytes, numerous plasma cells, and fibrosis.

Spirochetes cannot usually be demonstrated in gummas. Type IV immunologic hypersensitivity is probably involved in the pathogenesis of the granuloma.

Syphilitic Aortitis

Involvement of the aorta is common in tertiary syphilis, leading to the development of aneurysms in the ascending thoracic aorta, aortic valve incompetence, and myocardial ischemia secondary to coronary ostial narrowing due to aortic fibrosis (Chapter 20).

Neurosyphilis

Neurosyphilis may be manifested as chronic meningovascular inflammation, tabes dorsalis, or general paresis (Chapter 63).

Diagnosis is by a combination of clinical, pathologic (biopsy), and serologic findings (Tables 54–2

Table 54–3. Syphilis serology.[1]

	Percent Serum Positivity by Stage of Disease			Neurosyphilis	
Test	Primary	Secondary	Late Tertiary	Serum	CSF
VDRL (reagin)	70%	99%	<5%	50%	60%
FTA-ABS	85%	100%	98%	95%	80%[2]

[1]Congenital syphilis is difficult to diagnose because maternal IgG antibodies cross the placenta; the fetus will give positive serology whether infected or not. An IgM FTA-ABS test, measuring only fetal IgM, has been developed; however, its use is not fully accepted.
[2]FTA-ABS test should not be used alone because it yields up to 5% of technical false-positives in cerebrospinal fluid.

and 54–3). Organisms are not demonstrable except in general paresis, where silver stains may reveal organisms in the brain.

4. CONGENITAL SYPHILIS

Transplacental infection of the fetus occurs in the second and third trimesters of pregnancy if the mother has untreated early (first 4 years) syphilis. Routine serologic testing and treatment of women in early pregnancy prevents congenital syphilis, which now occurs only when there is deficient prenatal care.

Intrauterine infection causes disease of varying degree.

(1) Abortion and intrauterine death of the fetus.

(2) Neonatal or infantile congenital syphilis (Fig 54–2), with lesions containing numerous spirochetes and resembling those of early syphilis in the adult, ie, desquamative skin rashes and ulcerating patches on mucous membranes. Osteochondritis and perichondritis have severe effects on growing bone and cartilage—especially the nose, causing nasal bridge collapse (“saddle nose”), and tibia (“sabre shins”). Liver involvement leads to hepatic fibrosis and pulmonary involvement to fibrosis and inflammation of the lungs (“pneumonia alba”).

(3) Late childhood congenital syphilis, characterized by interstitial keratitis, leading to blindness; nerve deafness, due to meningovascular inflammation; abnormalities in permanent teeth—Hutchinson’s teeth, Moon’s molars; and abnormalities in bones and cartilage, including saddle nose and sabre shins.

Gummas and neurosyphilis may occur in all forms of congenital syphilis; syphilitic aortitis is extremely uncommon.

The diagnosis of congenital syphilis is based on clinical manifestations, dark-field microscopy, and serologic tests (Table 54–3).

HERPES GENITALIS

Infection with herpes simplex virus type 2 is currently at the epidemic level (at least 500,000 cases per year in the USA for a total of more than 5 million infected). Rarely, type 1 virus, which usually infects the oral cavity and eye, is associated with genital infection.

Herpes simplex virus causes painful shallow ulcers on the penis, vulva, and cervix (Fig 54–3). The ulcers heal spontaneously, but the virus remains latent in lumbar and sacral ganglia and may cause lifelong recurrent infections. Several therapeutic agents are under trial, but none control relapses.

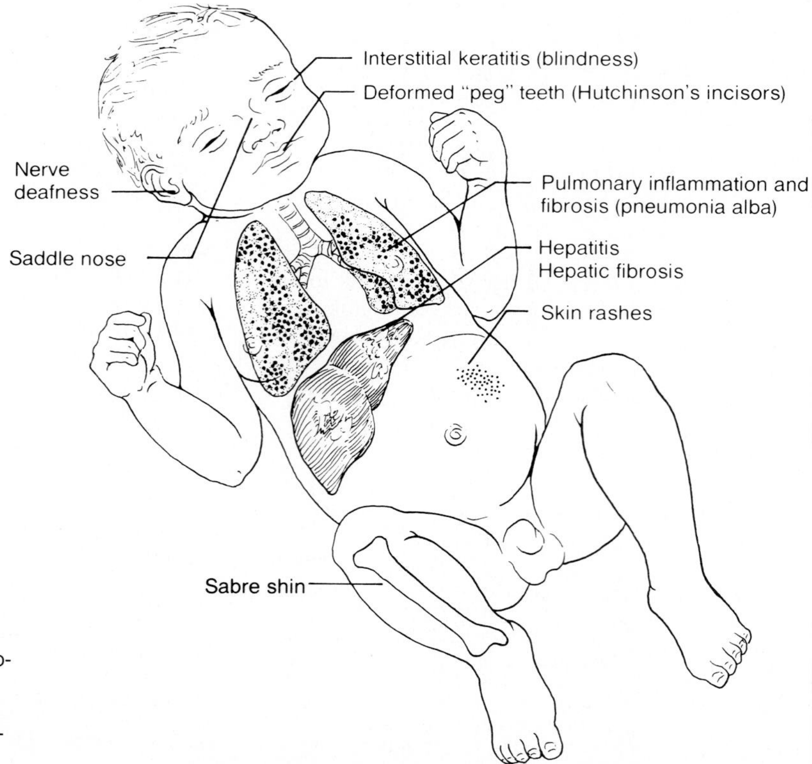

Figure 54–2. Clinical and pathologic features of congenital syphilis. Saddle nose and saber shins are aspects of osteochondritis.

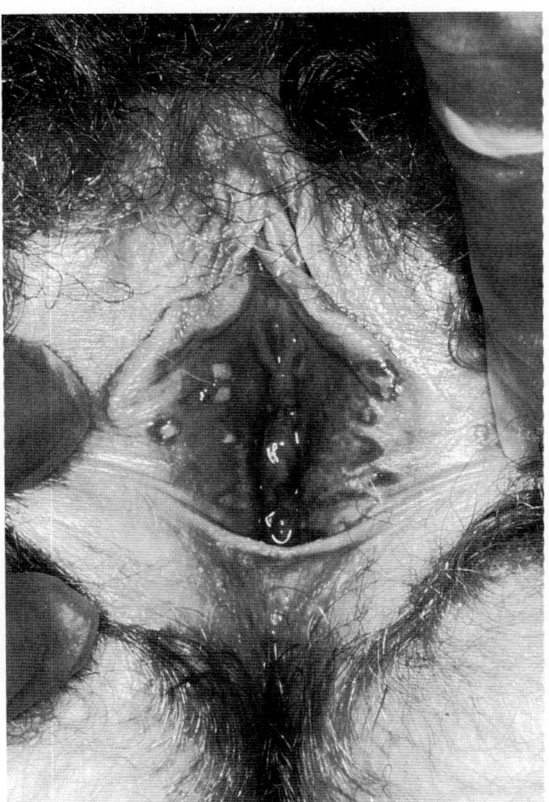

Figure 54–3. Herpes simplex infection of the vulva, showing multiple shallow ulcers.

The main danger of herpes genitalis is in a pregnant woman who has active infection at the time of delivery. The fetus has a high risk of becoming infected during passage down the infected birth canal, leading to disseminated neonatal herpes simplex infection or herpes encephalitis, either of which are frequently fatal. Detection of active herpes genitalis during pregnancy is an absolute indication for cesarean section. More rarely, the virus infects the amniotic cavity and causes fetal infection in utero.

A relationship of herpes simplex virus to carcinoma of the cervix has been suggested but not proved (Chapter 53).

CHANCROID

Chancroid is an uncommon sexually transmitted disease caused by *Haemophilus ducreyi,* a gram-negative bacillus. It is characterized clinically by the development of one or more painful, shallow, necrotic ulcers (soft chancres) at the site of inoculation on the external genitalia. Regional lymph nodes are enlarged and tender and show suppurative acute inflammation. Systemic symptoms are mild.

The diagnosis is established by culture from either an ulcer or a lymph node aspirate. Ducrey's skin test against killed *H ducreyi* antigen remains positive for life, but immunity is short-lived. Treatment with antibiotics (tetracycline, trimethoprim-sulfamethoxazole) is effective.

CHLAMYDIAL URETHRITIS & CERVICITIS

Chlamydia trachomatis serotypes D–K are increasingly being recognized as a cause of sexually transmitted disease. In some studies, chlamydial infection ranks as the commonest sexually transmitted disease in the United States. It causes urethritis and cervicitis that clinically resembles gonorrhea. In male homosexuals, chlamydial proctitis is common. Because routine bacterial cultures are negative, this infection is sometimes called nonspecific or nongonococcal urethritis. The same organism may also cause concurrent conjunctivitis, particularly in neonates. Reiter's syndrome—conjunctivitis, arthritis, skin lesions, and urethritis—may complicate chlamydial infection in adults.

The diagnosis may be made by culturing the organism in living cell culture media or by demonstration of typical intracytoplasmic inclusions in smears from lesions (Fig 54–4).

Chlamydial infections respond to treatment with tetracyclines.

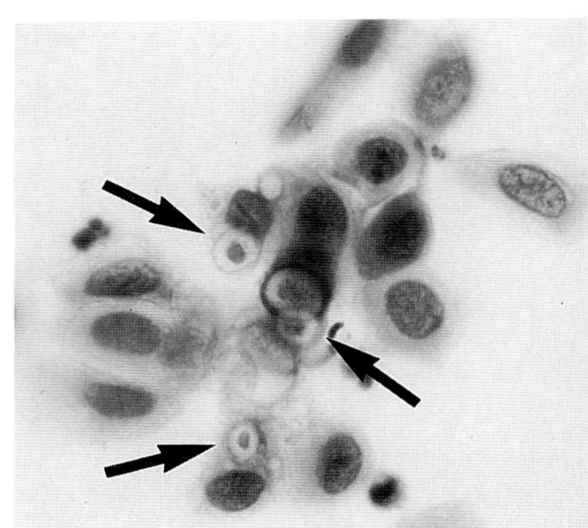

Figure 54–4. Cervical smear in a patient with chlamydial infection, showing intracytoplasmic inclusions (arrows) in infected cells.

LYMPHOGRANULOMA VENEREUM

Lymphogranuloma venereum (LGV) is an uncommon sexually transmitted disease caused by *Chlamydia trachomatis* L1–L3 (LGV serotype). The acute phase of the illness is characterized by an ulcerative lesion at the site of entry. Enlarged, tender, fluctuant regional lymph nodes develop 1–2 weeks later.

The histologic appearance of the nodes is distinctive, with large stellate granulomas containing central suppuration. Chlamydial inclusions are rarely demonstrated. Chronic LGV is characterized by extensive fibrosis, which extends around the pelvic organs up into pelvic soft tissues. The fibrosis may cause rectal strictures and extensive lymphatic obstruction, leading to chronic lymphedema (''elephantiasis'') of the vulva and penis.

The diagnosis is made by a combination of clinical, histologic, and serologic findings. The Frei test is a skin test for LGV that uses antigen extracted from LGV lesions. A more accurate complement fixation test is available.

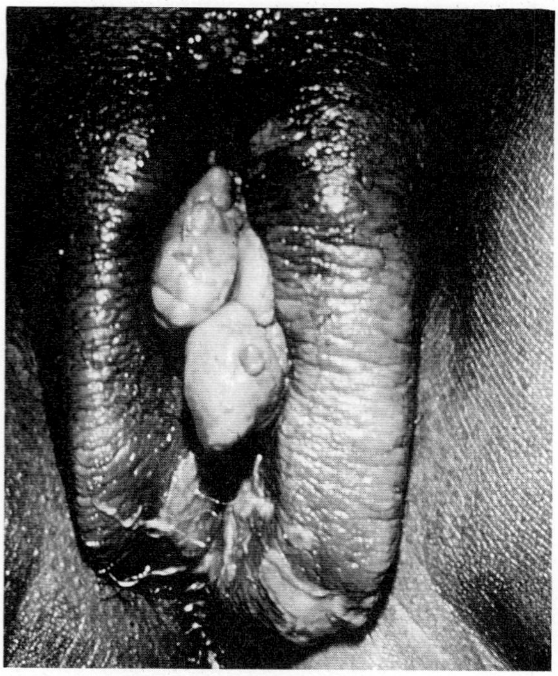

Figure 54–5. Granuloma inguinale, showing nodular lesion in the vulva. Biopsy is necessary to exclude neoplasm, and culture is necessary for specific diagnosis.

GRANULOMA INGUINALE

Granuloma inguinale is a rare sexually transmitted disease caused by *Calymmatobacterium donovani* (formerly Donovan's bacillus), a small gram-negative coccobacillus related to the klebsiellae.

The lesion at the site of inoculation begins as a papule that slowly enlarges, ulcerates, and spreads, resulting in a nodular mass with extensive scarring and regional lymph node involvement (Fig 54–5). Intracellular organisms may be identified with some difficulty in the involved lymph nodes using Giemsa's stain or silver stains.

The diagnosis is based on the clinical presentation and may be confirmed by demonstrating Donovan bodies in smears or biopsies of the lesions. Culture is possible but difficult.

Treatment with antibiotics (eg, tetracycline, erythromycin) is effective.

Diseases of Pregnancy; Trophoblastic Neoplasms

55

The ovum is fertilized by the sperm in the ampullary portion of the uterine tube, whence it passes into the uterine cavity prior to implantation.

The ovum divides rapidly, differentiating into (1) the embryo, which develops over the next 40 weeks into the full-term fetus; and (2) the trophoblast, which invades the progestational endometrium to form the placenta. The developing fetus becomes enclosed in an amniotic cavity that contains amniotic fluid. The amniotic cavity is lined by amnion and chorion (fetal membranes). The amnion also covers the fetal surface of the placenta and umbilical cord. The chorion is accentuated at one pole of the uterus to form the placenta, which is usually located in the fundus of the uterus. The fetus is connected to the placenta by the umbilical cord.

At term—usually around the 40th week after the last menstrual period—uterine contractions of labor begin and the fetus, placenta, and membranes are delivered per vaginam.

ECTOPIC PREGNANCY

An ectopic pregnancy is one in which implantation of the fertilized ovum occurs at a site other than the uterine cavity (Fig 55–1).

TUBAL PREGNANCY

Tubal pregnancies are common, representing about 0.3–0.5% of all pregnancies. The incidence is believed to be increasing, possibly as a consequence of the general increase in the incidence of pelvic inflammatory disease, which causes tubal narrowing and adhesions that interfere with passage of the fertilized ovum. Endometriosis involving the uterine tube is also associated with an increased risk of tubal pregnancy. In many cases of tubal pregnancy, however, no etiologic factor is identified.

Pathology

In spite of the abnormal implantation site, the ovum develops normally in the first few weeks, forming a placenta, an embryo, and an amniotic sac. Later development is greatly impeded by the lack of space, poor vascular supply, and limited placental size.

Rupture of the tube containing the pregnancy frequently occurs 2–6 weeks after fertilization, causing massive, potentially fatal intraperitoneal hemorrhage (Fig 55–2). This may occur so early in the course of the pregnancy that the patient may not have missed a menstrual period. The embryo may still be alive (in which case the pregnancy test for serum or urinary hCG will still be positive). In most cases, the released embryo dies soon after tubal rupture. When rupture of a tubal pregnancy releases a live embryo into the peritoneal cavity, it can move to a secondary implantation site on the peritoneal surface (secondary abdominal pregnancy). Very rarely, such a pregnancy progresses to term, though of course normal delivery cannot occur.

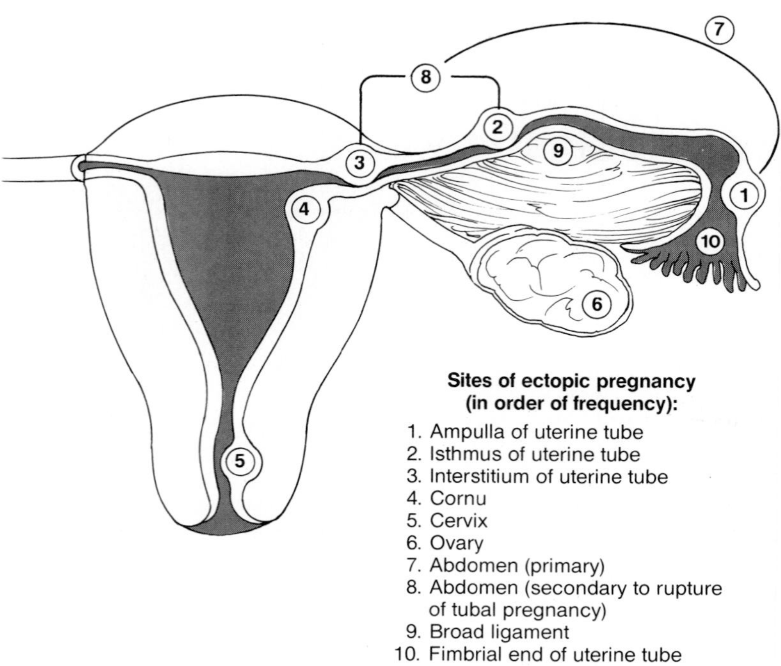

Figure 55-1. Sites in which ectopic pregnancies may occur.

If the tubal pregnancy does not rupture, death of the embryo occurs at about 10 weeks, with one of several consequences: (1) absorption of the products of conception; (2) calcification of the fetus to form a lithopedion (Gk *lithos* "stone," *paidion* "child"); or (3) extrusion of the dead fetus into the peritoneum through the fimbrial end of the tube—again associated with severe intraperitoneal hemorrhage.

Clinical Features

Patients with tubal pregnancy present with evidence of early pregnancy such as a missed menstrual period, vomiting of pregnancy, or a positive pregnancy test. This is associated with an absence of appropriate uterine enlargement and the presence of a tender mass in the adnexa, representing the expanded uterine tube.

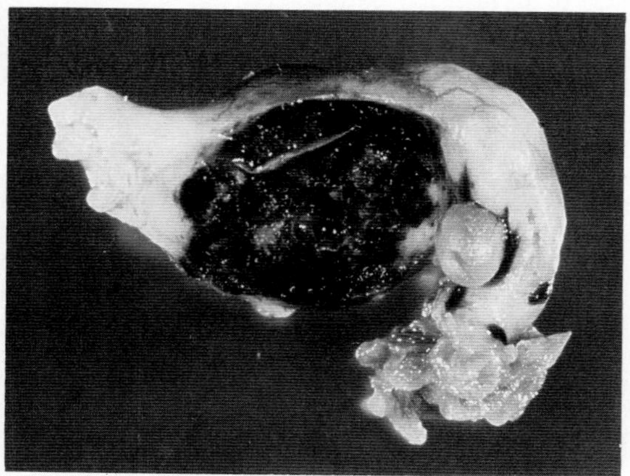

Figure 55-2. Tubal pregnancy, showing hemorrhagic mass in the ampulla of the uterine tube. No products of conception are seen in this photograph, but they were identified on microscopic examination.

Rupture of a tubal pregnancy produces severe abdominal pain and intraperitoneal bleeding, often rapid and severe. The presence of blood in the peritoneal cavity can be confirmed by aspiration or laparoscopy. Many patients are in a state of hypovolemic shock at the time of presentation.

Death of the fetus in a tubal pregnancy results in rapid decline in the serum level of chorionic gonadotropin, leading to a negative pregnancy test. Decline in hCG levels causes the corpus luteum to degenerate. This leads to decreased estrogen and progesterone levels, which causes the endometrium to break down. Uterine bleeding results.

The diagnosis of tubal pregnancy is established by clinical examination. The absence of chorionic villi in endometrial curettings from a woman who appears to be pregnant requires exclusion of the presence of tubal pregnancy. Endometrial curettage is performed in a patient who shows evidence of pregnancy only when there is persistent severe vaginal bleeding. In such patients, the differential diagnosis includes spontaneous abortion and ectopic pregnancy.

Treatment

The diagnosis and treatment of tubal pregnancy is urgent. Traditionally, the treatment of choice has been to remove the uterine tube on the affected side (salpingectomy). Recently, attempts have been made to save the tube (salpingostomy), particularly if bilateral tubal disease is present, in order to preserve maximum fertility. In such patients, there is a high risk of recurrence of tubal pregnancy.

SPONTANEOUS ABORTION

The developing pregnancy is called an **embryo** for the first 8 weeks and a **fetus** thereafter. Most of the major organs have formed at 12 weeks (at which time the fetal crown-rump length is 7–10 cm and the genitalia are recognizably male or female). In most countries, the fetus is considered viable at 20 weeks, though as a practical matter the proportion of fetuses that survive after delivery at 20–28 weeks is small.

Delivery of the embryo or fetus before 20 weeks is termed **abortion;** after 20 weeks and up to term at 40 weeks, **premature delivery**. Spontaneous abortion is common, and the causes are many (Table 55–1). It has been estimated that 25% of fertilized ova abort—many so early that the pregnancy is never recognized and others during the eighth to twelfth weeks. Spontaneous abortion is characterized clinically (1) by vaginal bleeding, which may be rapid and severe, leading to hypovolemia and shock; or (2) by lower abdominal pain due to uterine contraction. Pregnancy tests become negative. It is not uncommon for products of conception to be retained in the uterus (incomplete abortion; Fig 55-3). This may cause continued irregular bleeding over the next several weeks. For this reason, most patients with spontaneous abortion require surgical evacuation of the uterus (dilatation and curettage).

Table 55-1. Causes of spontaneous abortion.

Ovular/fetal
Failure to implant
Lethal chromosomal defects
Hydatidiform mole
Maternal/uterine
Uterine abnormalities, eg, leiomyoma, septate uterus
Ectopic pregnancy
Incompetent cervix
Endocrine abnormalities: failure of the corpus luteum, diabetes, hypertension, hyperthyroidism, hypothyroidism
Various systemic diseases, including renal failure, hypertension, malnutrition, severe anemia
Infections: toxoplasmosis, rubella, *Chlamydia,* cytomegalovirus, herpes simplex virus, syphilis, brucellosis
Drugs and chemicals: lead poisoning, thalidomide, anticoagulants
Chemotherapy for cancer in the mother
Physical agents
Severe maternal trauma and shock
Irradiation
Electric shock: lightning

PLACENTAL ABNORMALITIES

PLACENTA PREVIA

The fertilized ovum normally implants in the fundus, and the placenta forms in that location.

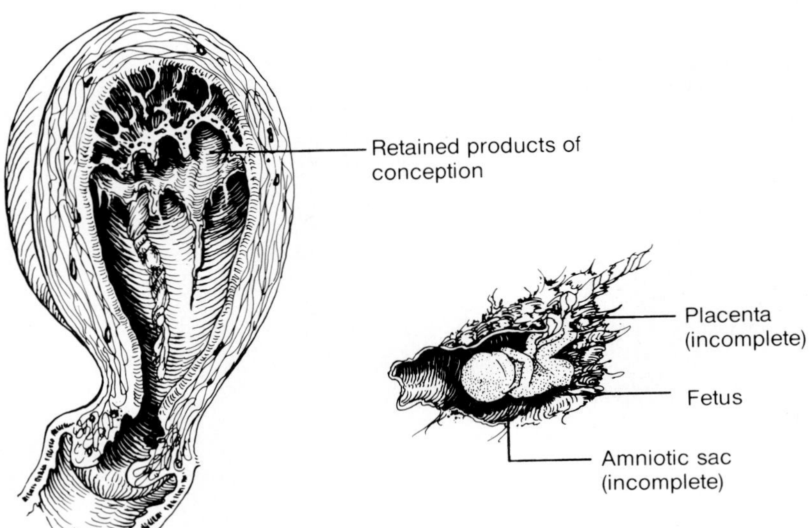

Figure 55-3. Incomplete abortion, showing retained products of conception in the uterus after evacuation of the fetus and part of the fetal membranes and placenta.

Abnormally low implantation may lead to formation of the placenta in the lower uterine segment. When the placenta is formed over the internal os (Fig 55-4A), it is called placenta previa.

Placenta previa causes problems only in late pregnancy, chiefly at the onset of labor. Uterine contractions in the first stage of labor cause effacement, stretching, and dilatation of the cervix, leading to premature separation of the placenta previa, which results in bleeding, often severe, at the onset of labor **(antepartum hemorrhage)**.

The availability of ultrasonography for placental localization permits early detection of placenta previa. Treatment is elective cesarian section before the onset of labor.

ABRUPTIO PLACENTAE

Abruptio placentae is premature separation of a normally situated placenta after 20 weeks of gestation, leading to antepartum hemorrhage due to rupture of vessels between the myometrium and separated placenta. In 20% of cases, blood is retained in the placental bed (Fig 55-4B) as **concealed hemorrhage,** and extensive loss may result in shock and disseminated intravascular coagulation (Chapter 9). In the remainder, severe bleeding occurs vaginally due to opening of the retroplacental hematoma into the cervical os (Fig 55-4C) **(revealed hemorrhage)**. In both instances, fetal death and premature labor are likely.

PLACENTA ACCRETA

The normal placental villi are separated from the myometrium by a plate of decidual tissue (modified endometrial stroma). This decidual plate is the plane of normal separation of the placenta in the third stage of labor after the fetus has been delivered. Placental separation and expulsion (as afterbirth) must occur to permit sustained contraction of the uterine muscle at the end of la-

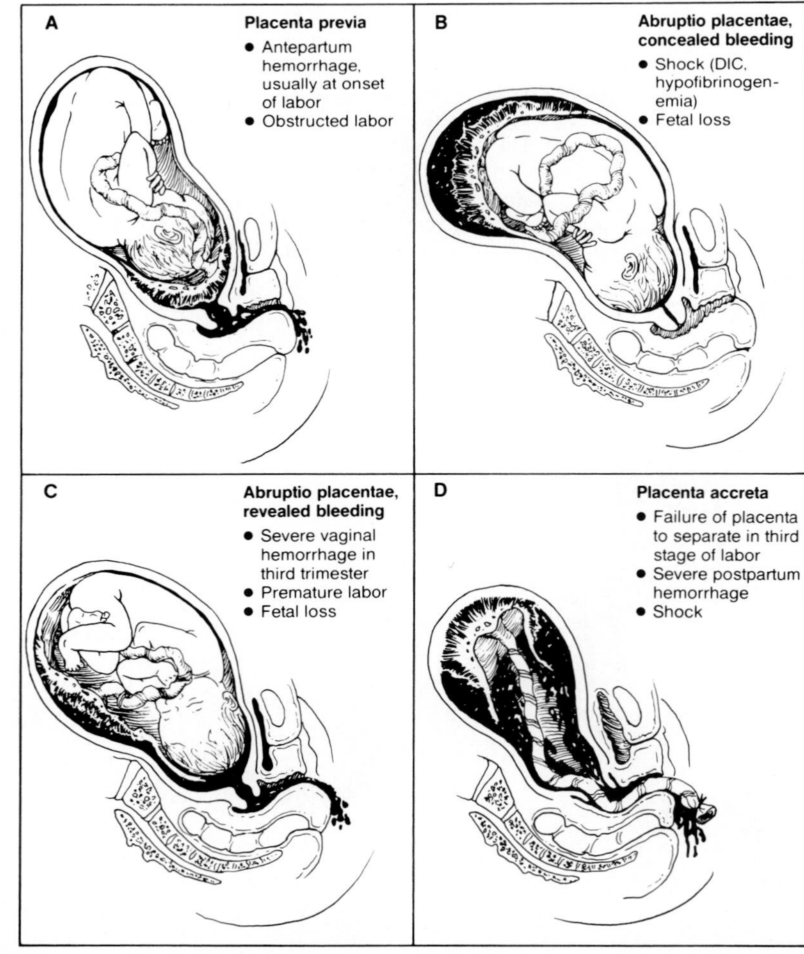

Figure 55-4. Abnormalities of the placenta.

bor, the principal mechanism whereby bleeding from the raw placental site is controlled (Fig 55–4D).

Placenta accreta is absence of a plane of separation between the placental villi and myometrium. The placenta fails to separate in labor, leading to severe postpartum hemorrhage. Placenta *increta* is a further stage of this abnormality in which the villi actually penetrate the myometrium. Placenta *percreta* is the most severe degree, with penetration of villi through the full thickness of the myometrium to reach the serosa.

In this group of placental abnormalities, hysterectomy is frequently necessary to arrest bleeding.

PLACENTAL INFARCTS

True placental infarcts occur in maternal hypertension and preeclampsia-eclampsia but are otherwise rare because of the rich placental blood supply. The term "infarct" is often misapplied to other nodular lesions in the placenta, including local areas of fibrin deposition, hemorrhage, or cystic degeneration.

PLACENTAL INFECTION

Placental infection may be classified into 2 types, as follows:

(1) Infection of the fetal membranes (chorioamnionitis), which represents ascending infection from the vagina and cervix. *Escherichia coli*, *β*-hemolytic streptococci, and anaerobes are the usual organisms. Rupture of the membranes not followed by delivery of the fetus within 24–48 hours almost always leads to chorioamnionitis.

(2) Maternal hematogenous infections involving the placenta, which include syphilis, tuberculosis, cytomegalovirus infection, toxoplasmosis, listeriosis, rubella, and herpes simplex. These organisms cause focal abscesses, granulomas, and necrosis of the placenta; rarely, the organism can be identified in the inflamed villi.

AMNIOTIC FLUID EMBOLISM

Amniotic fluid and debris may gain entry to uterine veins at the time of placental separation in labor and travel in the maternal circulation as emboli. Though amniotic fluid embolism is rare, it accounts for a significant percentage of maternal deaths in developed countries, where maternal mortality rates are very low. Predisposing factors include premature placental separation and a dead fetus.

Amniotic debris, which consists mainly of fetal squames, may be found in the lungs. The identification of squamous epithelial cells in pulmonary capillaries at autopsy is a reliable method of diagnosis (see Chapter 9). The amniotic fluid contains thromboplastic substances that cause disseminated intravascular coagulation, which is responsible for the main clinical manifestations.

RUPTURE OF THE UTERUS

A normal uterus in normal labor "never" ruptures. Factors that predispose to rupture during labor include fibroids, placenta increta or percreta, the presence of a fibrous scar from a previous cesarian section, prolonged labor due to malposition (eg, breech presentation), instrumentation (forceps), and extensive uterine stimulants (oxytocin, prostaglandins, ergot infusions). Rupture not associated with labor may be associated with choriocarcinoma, invasive hydatidiform mole, or endometrial carcinoma.

PREECLAMPSIA-ECLAMPSIA

The term eclampsia (Gk *eklampo* "shine, flash forth") was initially applied to fits occurring in pregnancy, which were commonly accompanied by visual symptoms of flashing lights. The condition has been recognized for over 2000 years, and a prodromal condition, thought to be due to a toxin, was described—thus the term preeclamptic toxemia (PET). Today, while the cause is still unclear, it is universally accepted that blood-borne toxins are not involved, and the term preeclampsia is used.

Preeclampsia is a syndrome consisting of 3 principal signs: hypertension, proteinuria (albuminuria), and generalized edema. The term gestational edema with proteinuria and hypertension (GEPH) is sometimes used for preeclampsia. The condition is distinct from pregnancy occurring in a patient with preexisting hypertension.

Incidence

Preeclampsia complicates about 5% of pregnancies in the United States, and 10% of patients with preeclampsia develop seizure symptoms (eclampsia). Presentation is usually in the third trimester.

Predisposing factors include (1) primigravida status—two-thirds of cases of preeclampsia occur in first pregnancies; (2) multiple pregnancies and hydramnios (excess amniotic fluid); (3) preexisting diabetes or hypertension; (4) hydatidiform mole; and (5) malnutrition and familial factors.

Etiology

The cause of preeclampsia-eclampsia is unknown. Theories include (1) placental ischemia; (2) immunologic reaction against placental vessels; (3) deficient production of prostaglandin E by the placenta, resulting in increased sensitivity to the hypertensive effects of renin and angiotensin, and (4) DIC, which certainly occurs in established eclampsia due to substances with thromboplastic activity released by the placenta. DIC is probably a complication rather than an etiologic factor in preeclampsia-eclampsia.

Pathology

The placenta shows degeneration, hyaline deposition, calcification, and congestion (premature aging). The maternal decidua shows hemorrhage and necrosis with thrombosis of spiral arteries. Placental infarcts may occur.

In eclampsia, the maternal kidneys show swelling of glomerular endothelial cells, mesangial proliferation, and marked narrowing of glomerular capillary lumens. Significant cortical ischemia with renal cortical necrosis may follow. The liver typically shows periportal necrosis and congestion in severe cases. Endothelial thickening, hemorrhages, and edema also occur in other tissues, including the brain, heart, lungs, and pituitary.

Clinical Findings

Edema is common in pregnancy and does not of itself warrant a diagnosis of preeclampsia. Hypertension is the most critical feature, together with proteinuria, which usually is last to appear. Fetal growth may be less than expected because of placental insufficiency (small-for-gestational age fetus).

Eclampsia is preceded by increasing hypertension. Individual twitchings of muscles are followed by generalized clonic contractions. Eclampsia may occur before or during labor and carries a high mortality rate.

Treatment

Treatment of preeclampsia is aimed at reducing the blood pressure and preventing eclampsia. Diet and sedatives are used widely, and antihypertensive drugs in severe cases. Induction of labor or cesarian section when the fetus is judged sufficiently mature is dramatically effective.

TROPHOBLASTIC NEOPLASMS

HYDATIDIFORM MOLE (Molar Pregnancy)

The incidence of hydatidiform mole varies greatly in different parts of the world. It occurs in one in every 2000 pregnancies in the United States but has a much higher frequency (1:150) in India and the Far Eastern countries.

Etiology

There is controversy about the cause of hydatidiform mole. The currently favored theory is that it represents a benign neoplasm of trophoblastic tissue. An older theory was that hydatidiform mole was the result of a blighted (damaged) ovum, with the trophoblastic villi continuing to proliferate and function, absorbing fluid and becoming cystic. Edematous (hydropic) villi are widely associated with blighted or degenerated ova, but probably as an entity distinct from hydatidiform mole.

A fetus and fetal membranes are almost never present in molar pregnancy. Those rare cases in which a dead fetus is also present are sometimes called partial moles.

Cytogenetic studies of hydatidiform moles have shown that most have an XX karyotype. Studies also show that both X chromosomes are derived from spermatozoa, suggesting that an abnormal zygote that has lost the female X chromosome is the stimulus for trophoblastic proliferation into a mole.

Pathology

The uterus is usually enlarged. The uterine cavity is filled with a mass of grapelike structures—thin-walled, translucent, cystic, and grayish-white. This represents the hydatidiform mole. The weight of this evacuated mass is usually in excess of 200 g. In most cases, no normal fetal parts are identified.

Microscopically, the cysts are composed of dilated chorionic villi, the interior being filled with an avascular, loose myxoid stroma. Trophoblastic proliferation produces sheets of cytotrophoblastic and syncytiotrophoblastic cells (Fig 55–5). Cytologic atypia may be present.

Hydatidiform mole is associated with greatly elevated levels of chorionic gonadotropin. The high gonadotropin level causes multiple bilateral theca lutein cysts in the ovary in about 30% of cases (see Chapter 52). These regress after removal of the mole.

Clinical Features

The initial features are those of early preg-

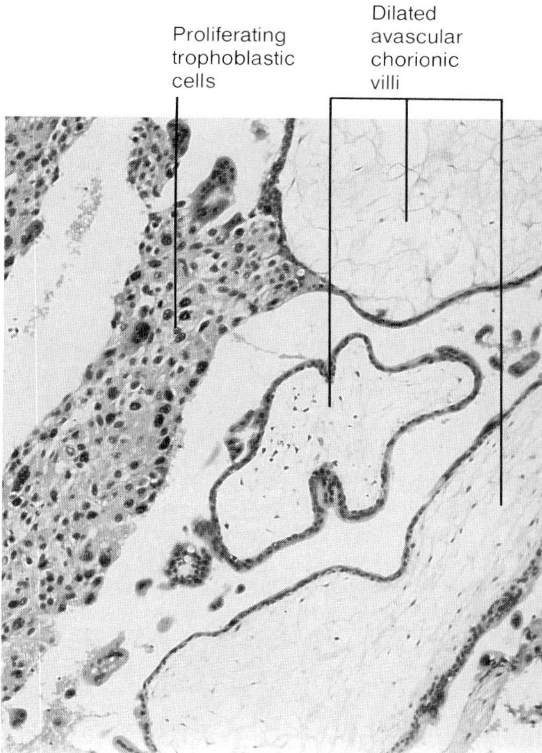

Figure 55–5. Hydatidiform mole, showing dilated, avascular chorionic villi lined by proliferative trophoblastic tissue.

nancy, including amenorrhea, vomiting of pregnancy—often severe—and a positive pregnancy test. Uterine enlargement is usually greater than in the case of normal pregnancy. Vaginal bleeding usually begins in the third to fourth month. Passage of grapelike clusters admixed with blood may also be observed. Ultrasound examination is usually diagnostic, showing the enlarged, multicystic placenta and the absence of a fetus. Diagnosis is confirmed by the greatly elevated levels of βHCG in the serum.

Hydatidiform mole is treated surgically, with evacuation of the mole from the uterine cavity by curettage. This is curative in the great majority of cases. After evacuation, the serum βHCG level falls rapidly to normal; failure to do so indicates residual mole.

Complications

About 2.5% of molar pregnancies lead to subsequent choriocarcinoma. The presence of marked cytologic atypia in a hydatidiform mole shows some correlation with later development of choriocarcinoma, though not to the extent that would permit reliable prediction. The most precise method of detecting cancer after molar pregnancy is by follow-up determination of serum βHCG; following return to normal after evacuation of the mole, a later elevation of βHCG raises a suspicion of choriocarcinoma.

CHORIOADENOMA DESTRUENS (Invasive Mole)

Chorioadenoma destruens is a hydatidiform mole that shows extensive penetration of the villi and trophoblast into the myometrium. Some extension into superficial myometrium is usually present in hydatidiform mole. In invasive mole, extension often reaches the serosal surface.

Invasive mole is associated with necrosis and hemorrhage in the myometrium (Fig 55–6), and uterine rupture may occur. Villi may embolize to distant sites—commonly the lungs—but regress spontaneously. Invasive mole is associated with persistent elevation of βHCG levels after evacuation of the uterine cavity. Without treatment, the mortality rate from hemorrhage or uterine rupture is about 10%. Treatment with chemotherapy is effective.

GESTATIONAL CHORIOCARCINOMA

Gestational choriocarcinoma of the uterus is rare, complicating about one in 40,000 pregnancies. About half follow a hydatidiform mole; others occur after abortion (25%), normal pregnancy (23%), or ectopic pregnancy (2%).

Choriocarcinoma, like hydatidiform mole, has a relatively high incidence in some parts of Asia and Africa. It may be considered as the malignant counterpart of hydatidiform mole, both being neoplasms of the trophoblastic epithelium. Histologically, gestational choriocarcinoma arising from a pregnancy is identical to ovarian (or testicular) choriocarcinoma having a germ cell origin.

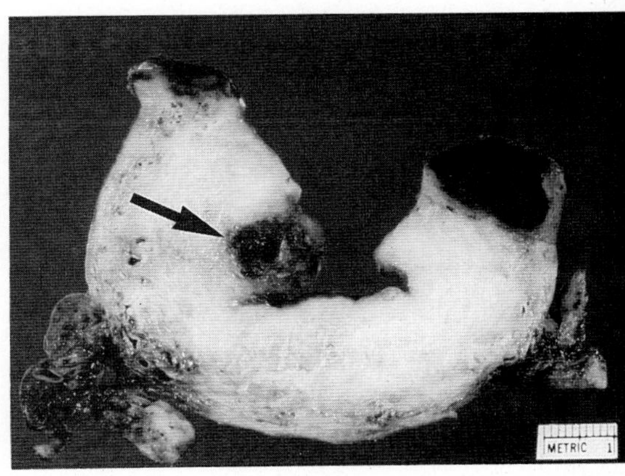

Figure 55–6. Invasive mole (chorioadenoma destruens), showing hemorrhagic mass invading the myometrium (arrow).

Pathology

Choriocarcinoma presents grossly as a friable hemorrhagic mass in the uterine cavity. It infiltrates the myometrium extensively, and vascular invasion occurs early, with widespread metastases in lungs, brain, liver, and bone marrow. Microscopically, choriocarcinoma is composed of cytologically malignant sheets of cytotrophoblastic and syncytiotrophoblastic cells associated with necrosis and hemorrhage (Fig 55–7). Formed chorionic villi are absent. βHCG can often be demonstrated in the tumor cells.

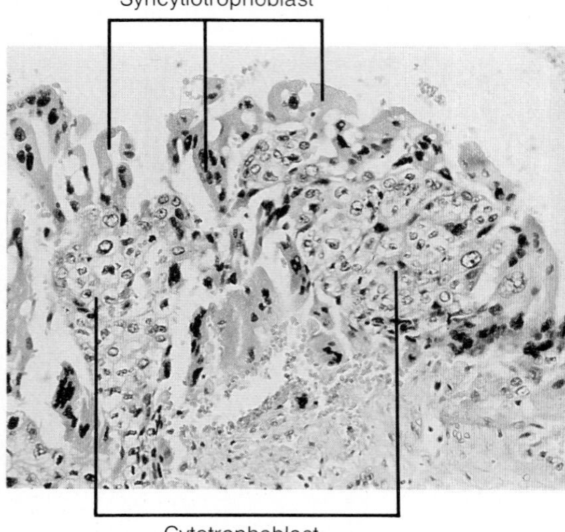

Figure 55–7. Choriocarcinoma, showing proliferating cytotrophoblast and syncytiotrophoblast cells.

Clinical Features & Treatment

Patients with choriocarcinoma present with abnormal uterine bleeding, commonly occurring within a few months after normal pregnancy, abortion, or hydatidiform mole. Many patients have metastatic lesions at the time of diagnosis.

Serum βHCG is markedly elevated. The diagnosis is made by histologic examination of a biopsy specimen, which shows malignant trophoblastic cells. Many tumors (most commonly lung carcinomas) other than choriocarcinoma secrete βHCG, though at lower levels.

The prognosis of choriocarcinoma was hopeless less than 20 years ago. With aggressive combined chemotherapy using methotrexate and dactinomycin, the 5-year survival rate has improved to over 50% even in patients with widespread metastases at presentation. Serum βHCG levels are extremely useful in monitoring treatment. Elevated βHCG levels in serum indicate persistence of viable trophoblastic tissue and the need for further chemotherapy.

PLACENTAL SITE TROPHOBLASTIC TUMOR (PSTT)

This is a rare lesion characterized by the diffuse proliferation in the uterus of sheets of intermediate trophoblastic cells resembling cytotrophoblast, most commonly after abortion or normal pregnancy. No chorionic villi or fetal parts are identified. The proliferating cells may show considerable cytologic abnormalities, which results in a resemblance of this lesion to choriocarcinoma. The neoplastic cells contain human placental lactogen, demonstrable by immunoperoxidase techniques. Unlike choriocarcinoma, PSTT shows only a slight elevation of βHCG and no syncytiotrophoblastic cells. The biologic behavior of PSTT is usually benign. Most cases are cured by curettage. A few cases have demonstrated a more aggressive biologic behavior, and rare cases with metastases have been reported.

The Breast

56

I. THE FEMALE BREAST

STRUCTURE & FUNCTION

Embryologic Development

The breast develops from the epidermal milk line, an embryonic ridge of tissue between the upper and lower limb buds. The ridges normally atrophy except in the thoracic region, where 2 thickenings develop into the nipples. Cords of cells grow downward from the nipple, developing lumens to form the ducts of the breast. This degree of development occurs in both sexes during fetal life.

Pubertal Development

At puberty, under the influence of female sex hormones, the female breast develops further. Outpouchings arise from the terminal ducts that branch extensively into the lobules of the breast. The adult female breast is composed of 5–10 segments, each draining at the nipple by a separate lactiferous duct (Fig 56–1).

In the nonpregnant breast, the parenchyma represents only about 10% of the volume. Much of the breast enlargement that occurs at puberty is due to an increase in the amount of fibroadipose stroma, which is also directed by the female sex hormones. Histologically, the normal nonpregnant breast is composed of breast lobule units, comprised of approximately 10–20 acini around a terminal ductule. Lobular units are separated from one another by abundant fibroadipose stroma.

The breast responds cyclically to menstruation. During the preovulatory phase, estrogen causes the glands and ducts to undergo mild dilatation and hypertrophy. During the postovulatory phase, progesterone causes stromal proliferation and edema. These changes may result in mild enlargement of the breast toward the end of the cycle.

Changes in Pregnancy

During pregnancy, there is marked hyperplasia of the glands that displace the fibroadipose stroma of the breast (Fig 56–2). Enlargement of the breast occurs in the third trimester and becomes prominent during lactation. Secretion begins in the third trimester of pregnancy. The lactating breast is composed of closely packed dilated glands with little intervening stroma.

After lactation, the glands atrophy to a level that approaches the prepregnant state. After menopause, glands, ducts, and adipose tissues atrophy further (see Chapter 16), causing progressive shrinkage in breast size.

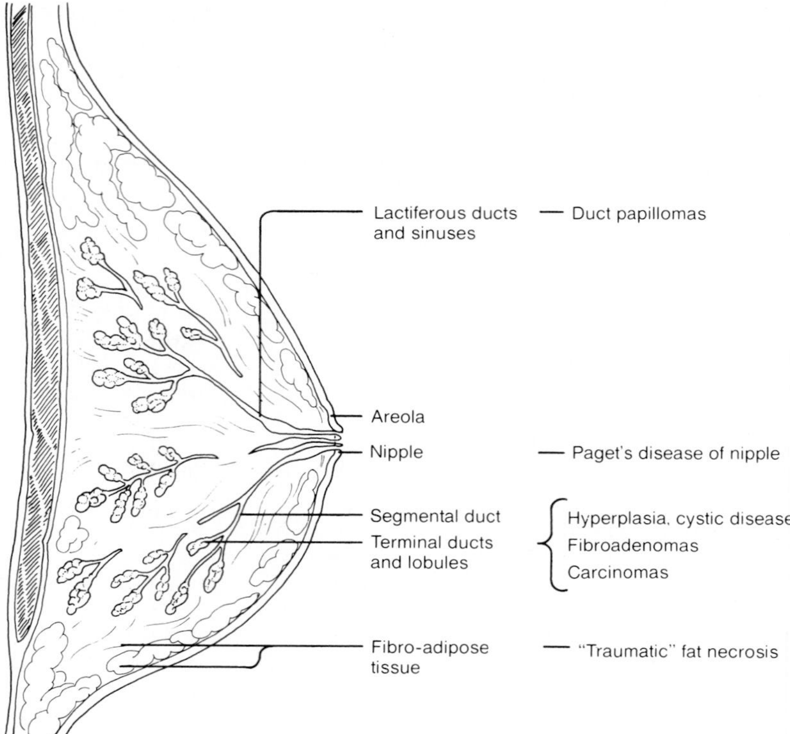

Figure 56-1. Structure of the breast and sites in which common pathologic lesions originate.

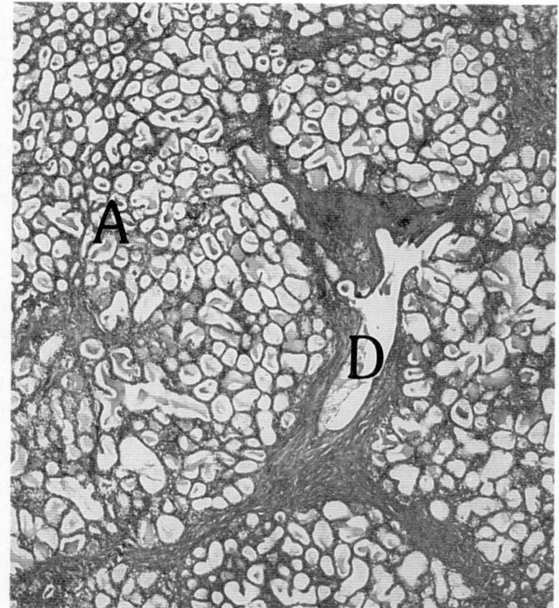

Figure 56-2. Lactating breast, showing extreme hyperplasia of the acini **(A),** which have replaced the normal interlobular adipose tissue. Many acini show secretion in the lumen. D = ductule.

MANIFESTATIONS OF BREAST DISEASE

Breast Mass

A mass in the breast is the earliest manifestation of breast carcinoma and therefore the most important symptom of breast disease. Any mass in the breast must be evaluated for its cancer potential. This is particularly important (1) if the patient is over 30 years of age, (2) if the mass is of recent onset, (3) if the mass has increased in size recently, (4) if the mass is solitary, or (5) if the mass is solid. A mass that disappears when its fluid content is aspirated is probably a simple cyst. However, if the mass does not completely disappear on aspiration, it is still suspect and should be biopsied.

Nipple Discharge

Discharge from the nipple is a common symptom of a variety of breast diseases. A discharge of milk occurs in pregnancy and lactation and rarely at other times (galactorrhea). Nonhemorrhagic nipple discharge is a common symptom in breasts showing fibrocystic change. Bloody discharge occurs in fibrocystic change and intraductal neoplasms, most commonly intraductal papilloma and carcinoma.

Skin Changes

Skin changes may be present overlying an advanced cancer of the breast. Infiltration of the skin may cause tethering and dimpling of the skin over the mass, followed by ulceration. Extensive involvement of dermal lymphatics results in lymphedema and other changes of inflammation such as erythema and pain ("inflammatory carcinoma"). Lymphedema produces skin thickening and a pitted appearance that is known as "peau d'orange" from its resemblance to orange peel.

Acute inflammatory signs may also be present overlying a breast abscess. Paget's disease of the nipple is an eczemalike appearance of the nipple and surrounding skin caused by intraepidermal spread of cancer cells.

Pain

Diffuse mild pain in the breast occurs commonly during the premenstrual phase in many women. A painful mass usually denotes an inflammatory lesion but may occur in advanced inflammatory carcinoma. Pain is rare in early breast carcinoma, but its presence in relation to a breast mass should not prevent the mass from being evaluated for carcinoma.

METHODS OF EVALUATING BREAST DISEASE

Physical Examination

Physical examination of a breast mass is useful in differentiating carcinoma from other causes only in advanced disease. Fixation of the mass to skin or to the chest wall, ulceration of skin, nipple retraction and lymphedema are late signs of breast carcinoma.

Mammography

A mammogram is a soft tissue radiograph of the breast that is of value in identifying the presence of breast carcinoma before it reaches a clinically palpable stage. Mammography is extremely useful as a screening procedure for monitoring patients at high risk for breast carcinoma (see below) and as a means of detecting a clinically occult primary tumor in a patient who has presented with a lesion metastatic from breast cancer.

Biopsy

Microscopic examination of a sample of tissue is the definitive means of evaluation of a breast mass. Tissue may be obtained in any of 3 ways: **(1) Fine needle aspiration** provides a sample for cytologic examination. This method is effective and very accurate in recognizing the presence of carcinoma. **(2) Core needle biopsy** provides a core of tissue for histologic examination. **(3) Incisional or excisional open biopsy** recovers part or all of the mass for histologic examination. Histologic examination is more accurate than cytologic examination, since the latter method bases diagnosis upon examination of isolated cells while histologic examination permits assessment of both the cells and the architecture in tissue sections.

Nipple aspiration is an experimental approach in which cells obtained from the breast ducts by suction aspiration of the nipple are examined cytologically.

CONGENITAL BREAST ANOMALIES

Supernumerary Breast (Polymastia, Polymazia) & Supernumerary Nipples (Polythelia)

Accessory breast tissue may occur anywhere along the milk line, most commonly in the axilla and more rarely at the caudal end of the line, presenting as a mass in the vulva. Accessory breast tissue usually does not have a nipple but is subject to the same changes with menstruation, pregnancy, and lactation as normal breast.

Accessory nipples are common and more varied in distribution, being seen fairly frequently on the chest, axillas, and abdominal wall.

Absence of the Breast (Amastia, Amazia)

Absence of the breast is extremely rare; breasts may, however, remain rudimentary in ovarian dysgenesis (eg, Turner's syndrome).

INFLAMMATORY BREAST LESIONS

ACUTE MASTITIS & BREAST ABSCESS

Acute inflammation of the breast, often with abscess formation, occurs commonly in the postpartum period at the onset of lactation (puerperal mastitis). Cracks in the nipple provide the portal of entry of bacteria (Fig 56–3A). Stasis of milk in cystically dilated ducts predisposes to infection.

Staphylococcus aureus is the most common infecting agent. Acute mastitis causes redness, swelling, pain, and tenderness in the affected area

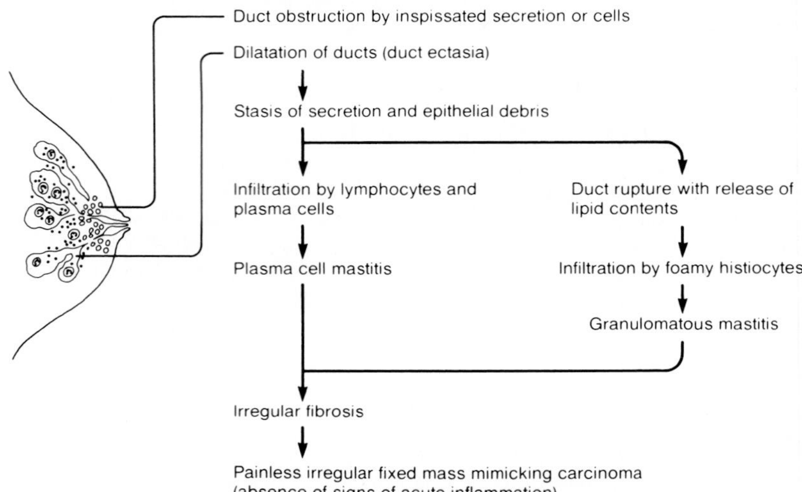

Figure 56–3. Etiology and pathologic features of acute and chronic mastitis.

of the breast. Abscess formation occurs rapidly, requiring drainage of pus.

CHRONIC MASTITIS

Chronic inflammation of the breast is uncommon. It usually occurs in perimenopausal women as a result of obstruction of the lactiferous ducts by inspissated luminal secretions. Obstruction leads to dilatation of the ducts (mammary duct ectasia) and periductal chronic inflammation (Fig 56–3B). In most cases, the inflammatory cells are predominantly plasma cells, and the term **plasma cell mastitis** is used.

In other instances, rupture of small ductules releases secretions into the periductal stroma and evokes a cellular reaction characterized by accumulation of numerous foamy histiocytes (lipid phagocytosis). Foreign body type giant cells appear along with fibrosis. This entity is called **granulomatous mastitis.**

Grossly, both plasma cell mastitis and granulomatous mastitis produce irregular fibrosis with induration of the involved area of the breast. This may cause nipple retraction and produce a clinical appearance that closely mimics breast carcinoma.

FAT NECROSIS

Fat necrosis is an uncommon yet important disease in the breast. The cause is unknown. Physical trauma was believed to be the main factor—leading to the term traumatic fat necrosis—but is now thought to play a minor role. Ischemia resulting from stretching and narrowing of arteries in pendulous breasts may be a factor.

In the early stage, fat necrosis is characterized by collection of neutrophils and histiocytes around the necrotic fat cells. Later, the necrotic tissue is replaced by granulation tissue and collagen, with numerous foamy histiocytes. Calcification may occur. Grossly, fat necrosis appears as an ill-defined grayish-white nodular lesion. Localized scarring results in a palpable mass that is firm and irregular, clinically resembling cancer. This resemblance may be heightened by the presence of skin retraction over the mass. Histologic examination is essential to differentiate it from carcinoma.

FIBROCYSTIC CHANGES
(Fibrocystic Disease; Cystic Mastopathy)

Fibrocystic "disease" of the breast has recently become a controversial issue. For a long time it was considered to be a very common lesion of the female breast affecting about 10% of women. In recent autopsy studies, many of the same changes have been found in up to 50% of women who had no symptoms of breast disease during life, suggesting that they may be physiologic variations rather than disease. The changes occur after puberty, reach a maximum during the late reproductive period, and persist into the postmenopausal period.

Some of the histologic changes of fibrocystic "disease" are associated with an increased risk of breast carcinoma. It is important, therefore, not to use the diagnosis of fibrocystic "disease" indiscriminately. It has been recommended that the diagnosis be discarded altogether in favor of the term "fibrocystic changes" followed by a description of the histologic features observed in the individual case (Table 56–1).

Etiology

Fibrocystic changes in the breast are believed to result from response of the breast to cyclic changes in levels of female sex hormones, mainly estrogens. No constant endocrine abnormality has been identified. Oral contraceptives do not increase the incidence of fibrocystic changes.

Table 56–1. Relative risk for invasive breast carcinoma based on pathologic examination of breast tissue with fibrocystic changes.[1]

No increased risk
Adenosis, sclerosing or florid
Apocrine metaplasia
Cysts, macro- or micro- (or both)
Duct ectasia
Fibrosis
Hyperplasia, mild
Mastitis (inflammation)
Slightly increased risk (1½–2 times[2])
Hyperplasia, moderate or florid, solid or papillary
Moderately increased risk (4–5 times[2])
Atypical hyperplasia (borderline lesion)
Ductal
Lobular

[1]Modified from Consensus Meeting: Is "fibrocystic disease" of the breast precancerous? October 3–5, 1985, New York. *Arch Pathol Lab Med* 1986;**110:**171.
[2]Risk is expressed as the risk compared with the general female population.

Pathology (Table 56–1 and Fig 56–4)

A. Changes Not Associated With Increased Risk of Breast Carcinoma:

1. Fibrosis–An increase in stromal fibrous tissue is common; when fibrosis predominates, the term fibrous mastopathy is used. Ill-defined masses may result; these are rubbery in consistency.

2. Cyst formation–Cysts occur commonly, probably as result of duct obstruction. They vary in size from small (microcysts) to several centimeters in diameter, the latter forming palpable

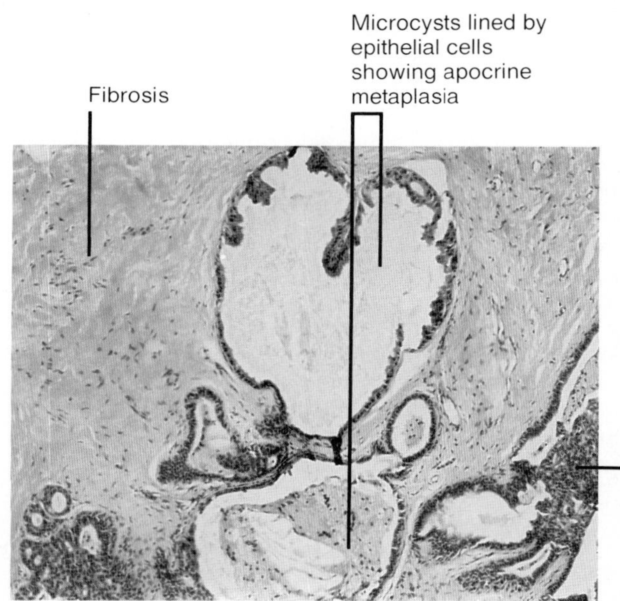

Figure 56–4. Fibrocystic change, showing fibrosis, formation of microcysts, apocrine metaplasia, and focal ductal epithelial hyperplasia.

masses. The cysts are lined by flattened or apocrine epithelium and contain a glairy, turbid fluid. On gross examination, many have a bluish color and for that reason are sometimes called blue-domed cysts. Needle aspiration of cysts causes them to collapse.

3. Inflammation-Chronic inflammation, with lymphocyte and plasma cell infiltration, is commonly present. ("Chronic cystic mastitis" was once an alternative term for fibrocystic changes.) Rupture of cysts may evoke a histiocytic response resembling granulomatous mastitis.

4. Mild ductal or lobular hyperplasia-Mild hyperplasia of lobules (adenosis) or epithelium within ducts is very common. Hyperplasia may be accompanied by sclerosis (fibrosis), leading to marked distortion of the normal lobular pattern and making histologic distinction from carcinoma difficult. The terms sclerosing adenosis and microglandular adenosis are used for this histologic appearance.

5. Apocrine metaplasia-Metaplasia of the ductal epithelium to an apocrine type (large cells with abundant pink cytoplasm and decapitation type secretion) is very common.

B. Changes Associated With Increased Risk of Carcinoma:

1. Atypical lobular hyperplasia-Marked proliferation of lobular epithelium is considered to carry a 4- to 5-fold increased risk of carcinoma. The proliferating cells distend the lobule and show cytologic atypia but do not satisfy the histologic criteria of lobular carcinoma in situ (see below). The histologic differentiation from lobular carcinoma in situ may sometimes be difficult.

2. Ductal hyperplasia without atypia-(Also called ductal hyperplasia of the usual type, "papillomatosis," and "epitheliosis.") Moderate to severe hyperplasia of the ductal epithelium without features of intraductal carcinoma carries a $1\frac{1}{2}$- to 2-fold increased risk of carcinoma. This type of ductal hyperplasia is characterized by proliferation of small oval cells with overlapping nuclei, poorly demarcated cell outlines, and absence of necrosis and cribriform spaces.

3. Atypical ductal hyperplasia-Marked atypical proliferation of ductal epithelium, causing stratification and often filling the lumen of the distended duct, is associated with a 4- to 5-fold increased risk of cancer. The risk of cancer associated with atypical ductal hyperplasia doubles if the patient has a family history of breast cancer. The term "borderline lesion" is sometimes used for this process.

The histologic differentiation of atypical ductal hyperplasia from intraductal carcinoma may sometimes be difficult (see below).

Clinical Features

Patients with fibrocystic changes may present with pain, nipple discharge, and an irregular "lumpy" consistency of the breast. Bilateral involvement is common. On occasion, there may be breast masses that mimic carcinoma. Needle aspiration may yield fluid from a cyst, resulting in disappearance of the mass. In many cases, however, biopsy is necessary to rule out carcinoma.

NEOPLASMS OF THE BREAST

BENIGN NEOPLASMS

FIBROADENOMA OF THE BREAST

Fibroadenoma is a common benign breast neoplasm that occurs at all ages, with the highest incidence in young women. It presents as a discrete, firm, freely movable nodule in the breast. Multiple fibroadenomas occur in 10% of cases. Grossly, fibroadenomas are encapsulated, firm, and uniformly grayish-white. Fibroadenomas are usually 1–5 cm in diameter but may be larger ("giant fibroadenoma").

Histologic examination reveals proliferation of both glandular and stromal elements. The relative amount of each component varies from case to case. When the glandular component dominates, the term "tubular adenoma" or "pericanalicular fibroadenoma" is used; when the stroma dominates, the term "intracanalicular fibroadenoma" is used (Fig 56–5). These histologic variants have no significance.

LACTATING ADENOMA

A lactating adenoma is probably a fibroadenoma in which lactational changes have supervened. Lactating adenomas may be associated with rapid increase in size, raising a suspicion of carcinoma. Biopsy is advisable.

DUCTAL PAPILLOMA

Ductal papillomas are benign neoplasms, commonly originating in a major lactiferous duct near the nipple (Fig 56–6). They present with a bloody nipple discharge. Most ductal papillomas are small—about 1 cm in diameter; the larger tumors are palpable as a subareolar mass.

Grossly, the tumor is seen as a papillary mass projecting into the lumen of a large duct (Fig 56–6). Histologically, there are numerous delicate papillae composed of a fibrovascular core, covered by a layer of epithelial and myoepithelial cells.

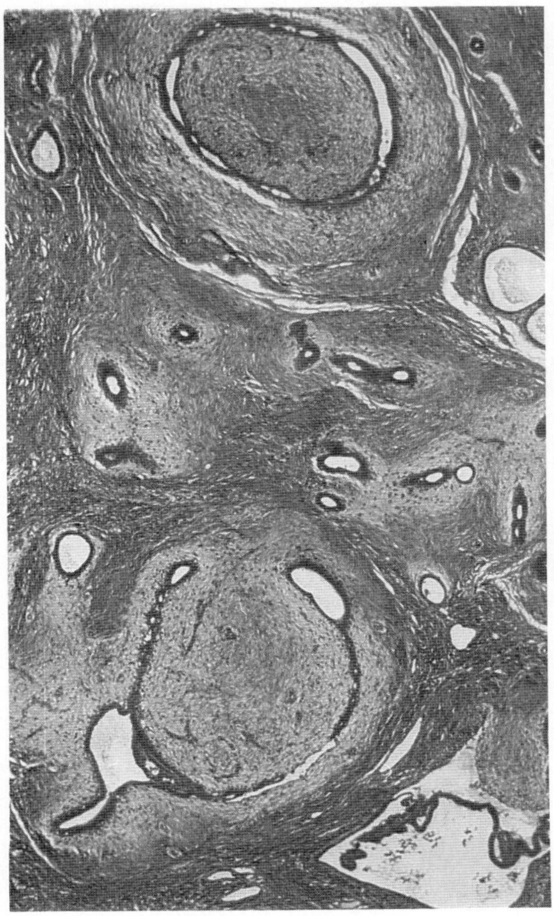

Figure 56-5. Fibroadenoma, showing the typical relationship of glands and stroma.

Rarely, papillomas are histologically very complex, and distinction from papillary carcinoma may be difficult.

GRANULAR CELL TUMOR

Granular cell tumor (previously called granular cell myoblastoma) is a rare benign neoplasm of the breast. It is probably derived from neural Schwann cells. It presents clinically and on gross pathologic examination as a hard infiltrative mass that resembles breast cancer. Microscopic examination, which shows large cells with small nuclei and abundant granular cytoplasm, is essential to make the diagnosis.

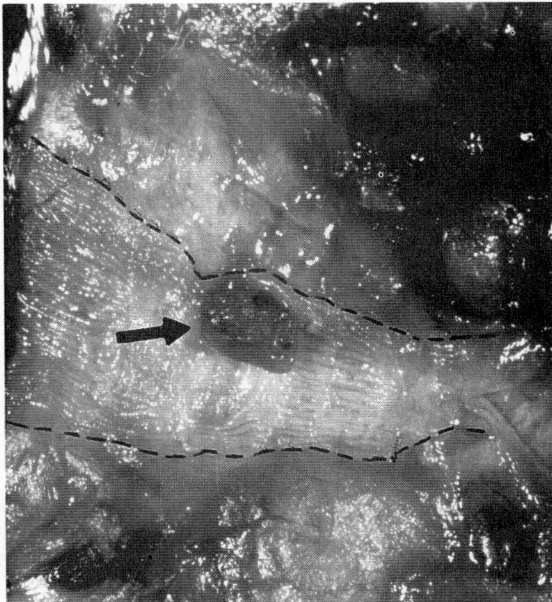

Figure 56-6. Intraductal papilloma. The lactiferous duct has been opened longitudinally (outline of duct marked by dotted lines) to show the small tumor within the duct (arrow). The patient presented with a bloody discharge from the nipple.

MALIGNANT NEOPLASMS

CARCINOMA OF THE BREAST

There are more than 100,000 new cases of breast cancer every year in the United States and 35,000 deaths, and it has been estimated that one of every 10 women in the United States will develop breast carcinoma during her lifetime. Until 1983, breast cancer was the leading cause of cancer death among females; it is now second to lung cancer because of the increase in the number of women developing lung cancer.

There is a marked geographic variation in the incidence of breast cancer. It is especially common in North America and Western Europe but rare in Japan, where the incidence is about 20% that in the United States.

Breast carcinoma is rare before 25 years of age and uncommon before 30 years, but the incidence increases sharply after 30 years, with a mean and median age of 60 years.

Risk Factors (Table 56-2)

Statistically, the risk of breast cancer is increased in nulliparous women (nuns have a high incidence), in women who have early menarche and late menopause, and in those who have their

Table 56-2. Breast cancer: Risk factors.

Sex	Female
Race	Caucasians, Jews
Age	30+ years, median 60 years
Family history	Mother or sister with breast cancer (5-fold), especially if bilateral or premenopausal
Medical history	Previous breast cancer
	Fibrocystic changes with atypical ductal or lobular hyperplasia (4- to 5-fold)
Menstrual history	Early menarche (< 12 years)
	Late menopause (> 50 years)
Pregnancy history	Nulliparous
	Late age at first pregnancy
	Absence of breast feeding

first pregnancy after age 30. Breast feeding appears to have a protective effect. Evidence linking oral contraceptives to breast carcinoma is scant; a few studies suggest a very slightly increased incidence in women who use oral contraceptives.

The presence of atypical lobular and ductal hyperplasia in a breast biopsy increases the risk 4- to 5-fold. A family history (limited to first-degree relatives—ie, mother, sister, daughter) of breast carcinoma increases the risk 5-fold. The first-degree relatives of a woman who develops bilateral breast cancer before menopause are at greatly increased risk. The increased risks resulting from atypical hyperplasia and family history are additive (ie, the presence of both increases the risk 8- to 10-fold).

The occurrence of carcinoma in one breast increases the risk of carcinoma in the other breast about 6-fold.

Etiology

The cause of breast carcinoma is unknown but is probably multifactorial. The following factors have been proposed.

A. Genetic Factors: Genetic factors are suggested by the strong familial tendency. There is no inheritance pattern, suggesting that the familial incidence is due either due to the action of multiple genes or to similar environmental factors acting on members of the same family. A "marker chromosome" (1q+) has been reported, and increased expression of an oncogene *(HER2/NEU)* has been detected in some cases. The presence of *NEU* oncogene in breast cancer cells correlates with a poor prognosis.

B. Hormones: Hormones are widely believed to play a role in the etiology of breast cancer. Estrogen has been the most extensively studied hormone, because of the epidemiologic evidence that prolonged estrogen exposure (early menarche, late menopause, nulliparity, and delayed pregnancy) increases the risk of breast cancer. A weaker case can be made for prolactin as a possible cause.

While the role of hormones in the induction of breast carcinoma is uncertain, there is no doubt that some breast cancers are hormone dependent. Hormone dependency is related to the presence of estrogen, progesterone, and other steroid hormone receptors on the surface of breast carcinoma cells. In neoplasms that possess such receptors, hormone (antiestrogen) therapy dramatically slows the growth of the tumor.

C. Viruses: Viruses are also suspected of causing breast carcinoma. The Bittner milk factor is a virus (mouse mammary tumor virus; see Chapter 18) that causes breast carcinoma in mice; it is transmitted via breast milk. The virus has also been found in the genome of these mice, being transmitted vertically and leading to genetic strains of mice with a high incidence of breast carcinoma. Antigens similar to those present in mouse mammary tumor virus are present in some cases of human breast carcinoma, but their significance is not clear.

Pathology

Based upon histologic criteria, several different types of breast carcinoma are recognized, subclassified according to origin (lobular versus ductal) or invasiveness (in situ versus infiltrating) (Table 56–3).

A. In Situ (Noninvasive) Carcinoma:

1. Lobular carcinoma in situ (LCIS)-(Fig 56–7.) LCIS is a neoplastic proliferation of lobular epithelial cells that fill and distend at least one complete lobular unit, obliterating their lumens. The basement membrane is intact; there is no risk of disseminated disease as long as the tumor remains in situ. LCIS tends to be multifocal and bilateral.

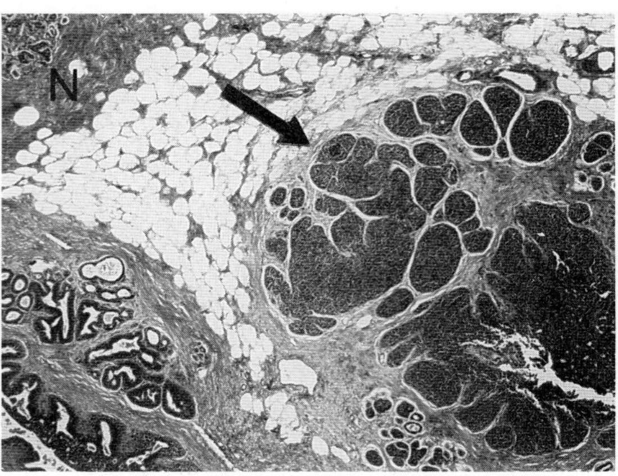

Figure 56-7. Lobular carcinoma in situ. The involved lobule (arrow) shows complete filling and distention of all constituent acini by small round cells. Compare with normal breast lobule at top left (labeled N).

Table 56-3. Pathologic types of breast carcinoma.

Lobular carcinoma (10%)
Lobular carcinoma in situ (LCIS)
Does not produce a mass; often discovered incidentally in breast biopsies
Multifocal, bilateral in 70%
Long in situ phase
High risk (10–12 fold) of breast carcinoma (either infiltrating ductal or lobular) in both ipsilateral and contralateral breast
Invasive lobular carcinoma
Approximately 10% of infiltrating breast carcinoma
Differentiated from infiltrating ductal carcinoma by histologic features only
More frequently bilateral than infiltrating ductal carcinoma
More frequently estrogen receptor-positive than ductal carcinoma
Prognosis similar to that of infiltrating ductal carcinoma
Ductal carcinoma (85%)
Ductal carcinoma in situ (DCIS)
Produces a breast mass or is detected by mammography
Short in situ phase
Multifocal, bilateral in about 20%
Type of carcinoma most often associated with Paget's disease of the nipple
Infiltrating ductal carcinoma (lacking other specific features)
Diagnosis made by histologic features; invasion present
Histologic variants of breast carcinoma
With a better prognosis than regular infiltrating ductal carcinoma
Medullary carcinoma
Tubular carcinoma
Mucinous (colloid) carcinoma
Papillary carcinoma
With a worse prognosis than regular infiltrating ductal carcinoma
Inflammatory carcinoma (dermal lymphatic carcinomatosis)
Others (5%)
Paget's disease of the nipple
Unclassifiable and anaplastic types
Mixed lobular and ductal carcinoma

LCIS does not produce a palpable lesion and is not apparent on mammography. It is usually an incidental pathologic finding in a patient who has had breast tissue removed for some other reason.

The presence of LCIS increases the risk of future development of breast carcinoma 10- to 12-fold. Both breasts are at risk, the ipsilateral slightly more so than the contralateral breast. Infiltrating carcinoma associated with LCIS may be either ductal or lobular.

The management of a patient with LCIS is highly controversial, and recommended treatment ranges from careful follow-up to bilateral simple mastectomy. LCIS without invasion is cured by simple mastectomy, which also removes any increased risk of breast carcinoma.

2. Ductal carcinoma in situ (DCIS)–(Fig 56–8.) Intraductal carcinoma is a neoplastic proliferation

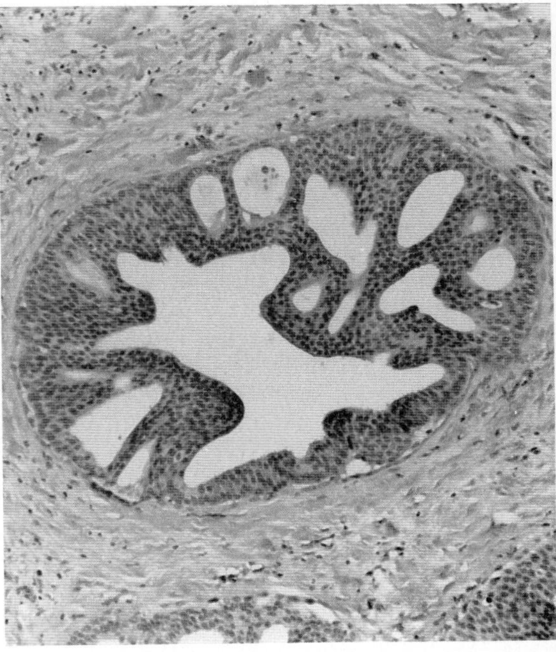

Figure 56-8. Intraductal carcinoma, cribriform type, showing the duct to be distended by a uniform population of cells. The basement membrane is intact.

of ductal epithelial cells confined within the basement membrane. Pure DCIS does not metastasize. However, DCIS is commonly associated with infiltrating ductal carcinoma elsewhere in the breast. DCIS is frequently multifocal, and is bilateral in 15–20% of cases.

Grossly, DCIS may produce a hard mass composed of thickened cordlike structures from which necrotic material can sometimes be expressed. Calcification is a common feature; DCIS is detectable by mammography. In some cases, however, DCIS is neither palpable nor visualized by mammography and can be diagnosed only on microscopic examination of a breast biopsy.

Histologically, the involved ducts are distended by malignant cells that may be arranged in cribriform, papillary, or solid patterns. The cells are large and uniform, with well-defined cell membranes and nonoverlapping, round nuclei. Central necrosis is a common feature ("comedo" carcinoma).

DCIS is treated similarly to infiltrating ductal carcinoma, though recent reports indicate that more limited resection than mastectomy may suffice for tumors of small size (< 2.5 cm).

B. Infiltrating (Invasive) Carcinoma:

1. Invasive ductal carcinoma–Invasive ductal carcinoma is the most common type of breast cancer, comprising more than 80% of all cases. Grossly, it forms a gritty, rock-hard, grayish-white infiltrative mass (Fig 56–9). Yellowish-white

A

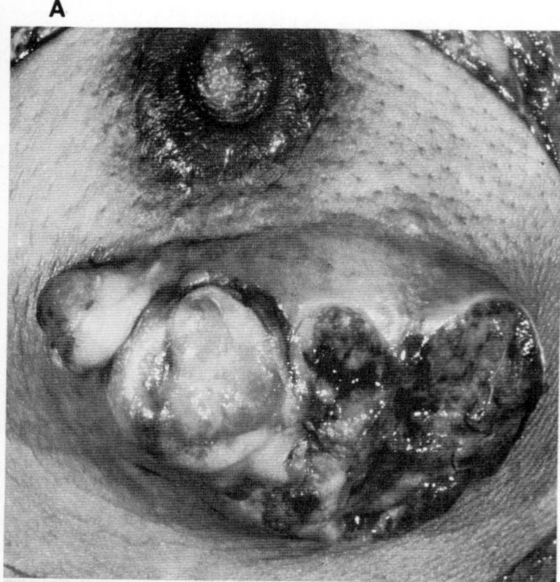

B

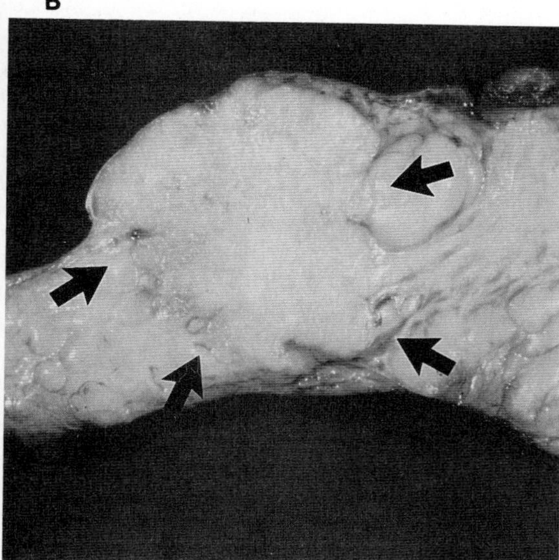

Figure 56-9. Invasive carcinoma of the breast. **A:** Surface view, showing the carcinoma ulcerating through the skin. **B:** Cut surface of the same breast, showing a large infiltrative mass extending from the skin almost to the deep surface (arrows).

chalk streaks are characteristic and correspond to a peculiar deposition of elastic tissue (elastosis) around ducts in the area of involvement. Fibrosis may be extensive (desmoplasia), producing a hard (scirrhous) type of cancer.

Microscopically, highly pleomorphic ductal epithelial cells infiltrate the fibrous stroma. Lymphatic invasion is common.

2. **Infiltrating lobular carcinomas-**Infiltrating lobular carcinomas constitute 5–10% of all breast carcinomas. They are similar to infiltrating ductal carcinomas except for (1) a different histologic pattern of infiltration, with a tendency to form single rows of cells (''Indian filing''; Fig 56-10) and concentric arrangement of cells around ducts (''targetoid appearance''); (2) a higher incidence of bilaterality; and (3) a greater frequency of estrogen receptor positivity.

3. **Morphologic variants of breast carcinoma-**Variant forms of breast carcinoma have been recognized (Table 56-3). Some of them—like medullary carcinoma, mucinous (colloid) carcinoma, and tubular carcinoma—are important to recognize because they have a better prognosis than the usual infiltrating ductal carcinoma. Medullary carcinomas tend to be large, soft, and very well circumscribed and consist of sheets of large polygonal cells associated with a marked lymphocytic infiltrate (which may contribute to the good prognosis). Mucinous carcinomas form gelatinous lakes of mucoid material in which cancer cells are suspended. Tubular carcinoma is composed of small, irregular infiltrative cancerous glands.

Clinical Features of Infiltrating Breast Carcinoma (Table 56-4)

Most patients present with a painless mass. Any breast mass should be regarded as a carcinoma until proved otherwise. Initially, the mass may be small and movable, but typically it enlarges, sometimes rapidly, and in the later stages it becomes fixed to the chest wall and skin. Skin and nipple retraction and ulceration are late features with an unfavorable prognosis. A few patients present with a bloody nipple discharge. Carcinoma may present in pregnancy, when diagnosis is often delayed because of the overall breast enlargement and nodularity.

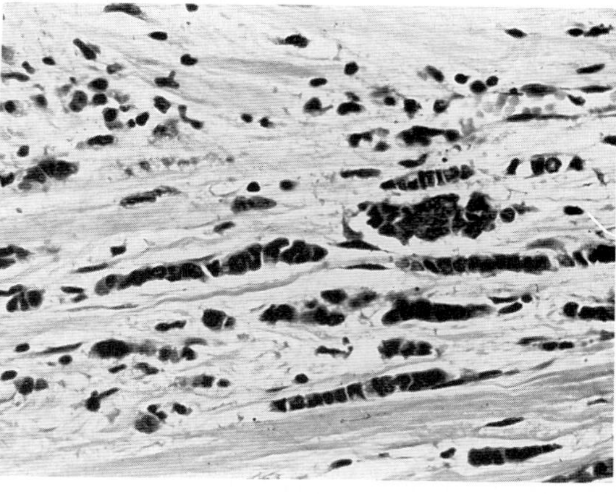

Figure 56-10. Infiltrating lobular carcinoma of the breast, showing tumor cells arranged in single rows (Indian file appearance) and fibrosis.

Table 56-4. Clinical presentation of breast cancer.

	Percentage of All Cases[1]
Breast mass, painless	66
Breast mass, painful	11
Nipple discharge	9
Nipple retraction or crusting	5
Local edema and inflammation	4
Metastatic disease in lymph nodes, bone, brain, lung, pleura	5

[1]The percentage of asymptomatic patients detected by mammography screening is proportionate to the number of women screened. Annual mammograms are recommended for women at increased risk, including all women over 40 years of age.

Early detection of breast carcinoma is very important, because the smaller the lesion is, the greater the likelihood of cure. Self-examination of the breast is strongly recommended at monthly intervals for all women. At present, the majority of breast cancers are discovered by self-examination. Mammography is capable of showing breast cancer at a stage before it is palpable. Small masses or speckled areas of calcification are visible, and biopsy is directed by a needle placed into the suspicious areas under radiologic guidance. Mammography is an effective screening technique that is currently recommended for high-risk groups such as patients with a family history, or a previous breast biopsy showing atypical hyperplasia, or a previous history of breast carcinoma. It is also recommended annually for all women over the age of 40 years.

A small number of breast carcinomas have a distinctive clinical presentation.

A. Paget's Disease of the Nipple: Paget's disease presents clinically as an eczematous change in the nipple and surrounding skin. It is characterized microscopically by the presence of carcinoma cells in the epidermis (Fig 56–11; and see also Chapter 53, the section on extramammary Paget's disease). These cells are believed to spread within the epidermis. The cells are large, with abundant cytoplasm that stains positively for mucin and resembles the cells of ductal carcinoma of the breast. In most cases, the underlying breast shows the presence of a ductal carcinoma.

Patients with Paget's disease have the prognosis of the underlying breast carcinoma. When Paget's disease occurs in a patient without a palpable mass or in one with only intraductal carcinoma, it is an early manifestation of cancer, and the prognosis is good.

B. Inflammatory Breast Carcinoma: This rare form of breast carcinoma is characterized by the presence of swelling producing the typical peau-d'orange appearance of the overlying skin, redness, pain, and tenderness of the breast. The underlying breast shows diffuse induration, frequently without a definite breast mass. This clinical picture resembles that of acute inflammation of the breast. Inflammatory carcinoma is the result of extensive involvement of the dermal lymphatics by carcinoma (dermal lymphatic carcinomatosis) (Fig 56–12). It has a very bad prognosis, with few patients surviving 5 years.

Mode of Spread

Direct spread occurs along the ductal system at an early stage, often before invasion has occurred. Such intraepithelial spread may result in involvement of multiple ducts and lobules ("cancerization of lobules"). Extension to the nipple in this manner results in Paget's disease. Local invasion may also occur into the breast stroma and then into overlying skin and underlying pectoralis major. The latter has a poor prognosis.

Lymphatic spread follows predictable routes according to the site of the primary lesion (Fig 56–13). The axillary lymph nodes are the primary node group affected. The nodes along the internal mammary artery may be involved in carcinomas located in the medial half of the breast. Spread beyond the axillary nodes into supraclavicular and cervical nodes is evidence of advanced disease. Local dermal lymphatic obstruction, most commonly due to extensive axillary node involvement, causes edema of the skin (peau d'orange).

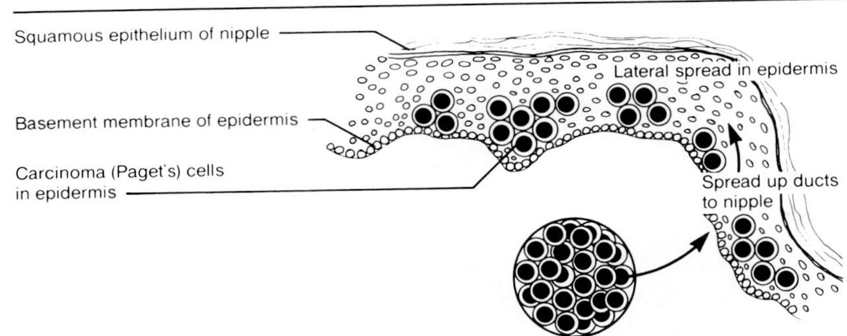

Figure 56–11. Paget's disease of the nipple.

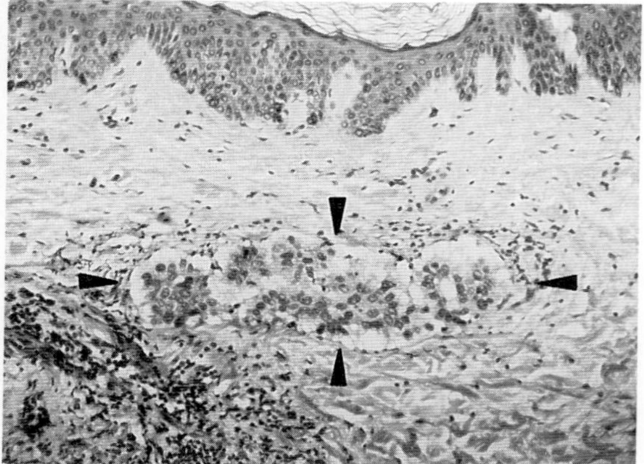

Figure 56-12. Inflammatory breast carcinoma, showing dermal lymphatic containing carcinoma cells (arrows).

Bloodstream spread with metastatic deposits in bone, liver, and lungs occurs in the later stages in almost all cases not cured by initial treatment. Entry of cancer cells into the bloodstream probably occurs early in the course of invasive breast carcinoma, but most of these cells are either killed by the immune system or remain dormant in distant organs. The mechanisms underlying dormancy of metastatic cancer cells and the reasons for their later activation to cause clinically detectable tumor masses are unknown. Dormancy and activation of cancer cells are necessary to explain the occurrence of metastases many years after treatment of the primary.

Spread via the pleural or peritoneal cavity occurs when the pleura or peritoneum is secondarily involved by the breast cancer.

Diagnosis

Histologic examination of a biopsy of the mass is the definitive diagnostic method. Excisional, incisional, or needle biopsies may be performed. Immediate diagnosis of a biopsy specimen by frozen section examination has a high degree of accuracy in experienced hands.

A complete pathologic diagnosis of breast carcinoma should provide the following information: (1) the histologic type of carcinoma; (2) the size of the tumor; (3) the stage of disease (Table 56–5); and (4) the estrogen and progesterone receptor status.

Receptor status is currently established by bioassay, for which a specimen from the tumor must be removed by the pathologist immediately after excision for freezing. Delay in preservation greatly interferes with the results of receptor assay. Immunohistochemical techniques being developed for receptor determination may facilitate management in the future.

Cytologic diagnosis utilizing a specimen obtained by fine-needle aspiration is increasing in popularity because it is rapid and cost-effective. Cytologic diagnosis is capable only of identifying carcinoma cells. Definitive diagnosis of the histo-

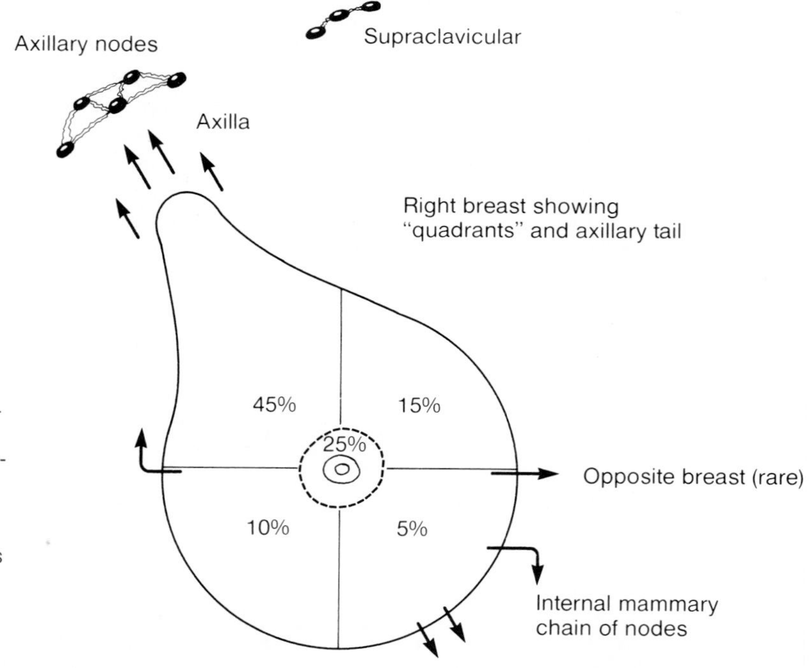

Figure 56-13. Pathways of lymphatic spread of breast cancer. The percentages refer to the frequency of breast cancer by location within the breast. All breast cancers spread primarily to axillary lymph nodes. Cancers in the inner quadrants have a higher incidence of internal mammary chain involvement than those in the outer quadrants.

Table 56-5. Clinicopathologic staging of breast cancer.[1]

Stage	Tumor Size and Metastasis	5-Year Survival Rate
I	Tumor < 5 cm diameter; no involved nodes, no distant metastases	85%
II	Tumor < 5 cm diameter; involved axillary nodes, no distant metastases	66%
III	Tumor > 5 cm diameter, or any size with attachment to skin or chest wall; no distant metastases	41%
IV	Distant metastases (includes lymph nodes outside axilla)	10%

[1]Several slightly different staging systems exist; all are based on similar principles.

logic type of the carcinoma still requires histologic examination of tissue sections.

Treatment

A. Surgery: Surgery has been the mainstay of treatment of breast cancer for the past several decades. The standard treatment was radical mastectomy, which involves removal of the breast with the pectoral muscles and axillary contents. The realization that this type of surgery may be too extensive led to new approaches. Currently, most surgeons perform a modified radical mastectomy in which the pectoral muscle is not removed. This provides a much better cosmetic effect. It has been demonstrated that a breast carcinoma under 4 cm in size has equivalent survival rates when treated with either modified radical mastectomy or complete lump excision plus axillary dissection followed by radiotherapy. A trend therefore exists to perform lesser degrees of surgery for the treatment of breast carcinoma.

B. Radiotherapy: Breast carcinoma is a moderately radiosensitive tumor. Radiotherapy is very useful as an adjunct to surgery, particularly when it is necessary to control locally recurrent disease in the chest wall.

C. Chemotherapy: Chemotherapy has improved the short-term prognosis in breast carcinoma but is not curative. The rationale for chemotherapy after successful surgical treatment (adjuvant chemotherapy) is that it removes microscopic foci of neoplastic cells in distant sites, thus complementing the role of surgery. Adjuvant chemotherapy has not increased overall cure rates in breast cancer.

D. Hormonal Therapy: Hormonal manipulation—usually antiestrogen therapy—is most effective in patients with estrogen or progesterone receptor-positive carcinomas. (Sixty to 80% of such patients respond; only 10% of receptor-negative patients respond.) Removal of estrogens may be achieved surgically (removal of ovaries and adrenal glands) or by antiestrogenic drugs such as tamoxifen. Antiprogesterone agents have recently become available and are under trial.

Prognosis

Infiltrating carcinoma of the breast has a 5-year survival rate of about 70%. About 20% of patients who survive 5 years will develop late recurrences. Recurrences of breast carcinoma have been recorded as late as 25 years after the primary tumor was successfully treated. The most important factors affecting prognosis are the following:

A. The Clinicopathologic Stage: Several staging systems are in use for breast carcinoma; that given in Table 56–5 is widely used. Stage I is a mass less than 5 cm that is localized to the breast. Stage II is a similar mass with involved axillary lymph nodes. Stage III is a larger mass or one that has infiltrated locally outside the breast, irrespective of axillary nodal status. Stage IV represents the presence of disease outside the breast and axilla, irrespective of any other factor.

B. The Histologic Type: (Table 56–3.) The prognosis for any patient must be individualized according to the histologic type and the stage of the disease. The 5-year survival rates of patients with breast carcinoma may then vary from almost nil for a patient with inflammatory breast carcinoma to almost 100% for one with a small stage I medullary carcinoma.

C. The presence of *NEU* oncogene, especially when large numbers (more than 20 copies per cell) are present, indicates a poor prognosis. This has been shown to be a powerful prognostic factor.

D. Absence of steroid hormone receptors indicates a poor prognosis quite apart from the lack of response to hormonal therapy that is associated with absence of receptors.

CYSTOSARCOMA PHYLLODES (Phyllodes Tumor)

Cystosarcoma phyllodes is (in 80–90% of cases) a low-grade malignant neoplasm that is locally infiltrative, with a tendency to recur locally after simple excision. In 10–20% of cases, the tumor behaves like a high-grade neoplasm, metastasizing to distant sites, mainly the lungs.

Cystosarcoma phyllodes typically forms a large mass, commonly over 5 cm in diameter. Grossly, it is a fleshy tumor with poorly circumscribed margins and areas of cystic degeneration. Histologically, it is composed—like a fibroadenoma—of epithelial and stromal components. The epithelial component resembles that of fibroadenoma. The stroma is much more cellular than that of fibroadenomas and frequently shows cytologic atypia. The presence of increased mitotic activity in the stroma (> 3 mitotic figures per 10 high-power fields) and stromal overgrowth at the expense of the epithelial component are useful criteria to predict metastatic potential in cystosarcomas.

Because of its infiltrative behavior, cystosarcoma phyllodes must be removed with a surrounding margin of breast tissue. With large tumors, simple mastectomy may be necessary. Tumors that metastasize usually cause death, since chemotherapy and radiotherapy are not very effective.

OTHER MALIGNANT NEOPLASMS OF THE BREAST

Primary malignant neoplasms other than carcinomas and cystosarcoma phyllodes occur very rarely in the breast. They include angiosarcoma, acute myeloblastic leukemia (granulocytic sarcoma), malignant lymphomas, and sarcomas derived from stromal cells. Metastases to the breast from cancers in other organs are rare.

II. DISEASES OF THE MALE BREAST

GYNECOMASTIA

Enlargement of the male breast may be unilateral or bilateral; it usually presents as a nodule or plaque of firm tissue under the nipple and may be painful.

Gynecomastia is uncommon; most cases are idiopathic (without any identifiable cause). In a few cases, a cause can be identified: (1) testicular atrophy or destruction, as in Klinefelter's syndrome, cirrhosis of the liver, and lepromatous leprosy; (2) conditions associated with increased estrogen levels, such as an estrogen-secreting tumor of the testis or adrenal; (3) increased gonadotropin levels, as in choriocarcinoma of the testis; (4) increased prolactin levels, as in diseases of the hypothalamopituitary axis, where breast enlargement may be accompanied by galactorrhea; and (5) drugs, most commonly digoxin.

Histologically, gynecomastia is characterized by proliferation of the ducts of the breast, which become surrounded by proliferating edematous stroma. A moderate degree of epithelial hyperplasia is common. Lobular units are absent in most cases.

Gynecomastia is a benign condition and carries no increased risk of malignancy.

CARCINOMA OF THE MALE BREAST

Carcinoma of the male breast is extremely rare. It presents with a painless breast mass. Histologic features are identical to those of infiltrating ductal carcinomas in the female. In spite of the small bulk of the breast in men, the diagnosis of male breast carcinoma is usually delayed; 50% of patients have axillary lymph node metastases at the time of diagnosis. As a result, male breast cancer has a worse overall prognosis than female breast cancer.

Section XIII. The Endocrine System

Diseases of the endocrine glands are relatively uncommon. Multinodular goiter is common in parts of the world where iodine deficiency is common, but has decreased in the USA with the use of iodized salt. Endocrine diseases are frequently characterized by over- or undersecretion of hormones. Hormone production by nonendocrine neoplasms such as lung cancer represents one of the so-called paraneoplastic manifestations of neoplasia (see Chapter 19).

This section discusses the main endocrine glands, which include the pituitary, thyroid, parathyroid, and adrenal glands. Other organs in the body such as the pancreas (islets of Langerhans; Chapter 46), ovaries (granulosa cells and luteal cells; Chapter 52), testes (interstitial cells of Leydig), gastrointestinal tract (eg, pyloric antral G cells), and placenta (chorionic gonadotropin; Chapter 55) have endocrine components which are discussed in those chapters.

The pituitary secretes tropic hormones that control the function of the thyroid (thyrotropin, or thyroid-stimulating hormone [TSH]), the cortisol-producing zones of the adrenal cortex (adrenocorticotropin, or adrenocorticotropic hormone, [ACTH]), and gonads (gonadotropins, follicle-stimulating hormone [FSH], and luteinizing hormone [LH]). The pituitary in turn is controlled by releasing hormones secreted by the hypothalamus.

All endocrine glands have elaborate control mechanisms that regulate secretion strictly according to body needs. In many cases, this involves feedback inhibition whereby elevated serum levels of the product stimulated by the hormone causes inhibition of hormone secretion by the gland.

Hormones usually bind to receptors on target cells in the body. The receptors may be located in the cell membrane (catecholamines, polypeptide hormones), or the nucleus (thyroid hormones and estrogen). The combination of the hormone with the receptor leads to a series of changes in the cell that results in the metabolic action of the hormone. In the case of catecholamines and polypeptide hormones, there is activation of adenylate cyclase that stimulates intracellular production of cAMP. cAMP acts as an internal messenger, effecting the specific biochemical change dictated by the hormone on the target cell. Other hormones such as corticosteroids and thyroid hormone cause increased mRNA synthesis, leading to protein (enzyme) synthesis.

Endocrine diseases are frequently characterized by abnormal patterns of hormone secretion: excessive secretion, diminished secretion, and abnormal or inappropriate secretion.

Excessive secretion of hormones may be due to the presence of increased numbers of cells of the type that normally secrete the hormone. This may occur as **primary hyperfunction,** due to hyperplastic or neoplastic proliferation of the cells; or **secondary hyperfunction,** due to increased stimulation by increased levels of tropic hormones or decreased feedback inhibition. Excessive secretion may also be due to production of hormones by cells that do not normally secrete the hormone, resulting in what have come to be called **ectopic hormone syndromes**.

Decreased secretion of hormones may be due to decreased numbers of hormone-secreting cells, which may in turn be due to **primary hypofunction,** from congenital absence or hypoplasia or destruction of the gland by trauma, infection, ischemia, immunologic mechanisms, or neoplasms; or **secondary hypofunction,** from absence of stimulation by the tropic hormones on which the cells are dependent. Secondary hypofunction is characterized by atrophy of the hormone-secreting cells. Diminished secretion may also be due to **deficiency of enzymes** required to synthesize the hormone. Decreased hormone activity may be caused by a **defect in the target organ receptors,** usually congenital. Receptor defects result in failure of hormone action, which has the same clinical effect as hormone lack. Because serum hormone levels are normal in such patients, the prefix *pseudo-* is attached to these hypofunctional states, eg, pseudohypoparathyroidism (see Chapter 59).

Secretion of abnormal hormones by endocrine glands is usually due to enzyme deficiency, eg, in congenital adrenal hyperplasia (see Chapter 60).

The Pituitary Gland

57

- Structure and Function
- Hypersecretion of Anterior Pituitary Hormones; Pituitary Adenoma
- Hyposecretion of Pituitary Hormones
- Diseases of the Posterior Pituitary
  - Diabetes Insipidus
  - Excessive Secretion of Antidiuretic Hormone

STRUCTURE & FUNCTION

The pituitary (hypophysis) is a small gland (350–900 mg) located in the sella turcica, a bony compartment in the base of the skull. It is composed of an anterior lobe (adenohypophysis), which comprises about 75% of the gland; a posterior lobe (neurohypophysis), which comprises about 25% of the gland; and a vestigial intermediate lobe (Fig 57–1).

Histologically, the anterior pituitary is composed of small round cells in nests and cords separated by a rich vascular network. The cells have variably staining cytoplasm on routine sections and were at one time called acidophils, basophils, and chromophobes. They are now classified according to the specific hormones they produce (Table 57–1), as identified by immunohistochemical methods. About 15–20% of the cells in the anterior pituitary are nonreactive to immunohistochemical tests and are classified as nonsecretory cells.

The posterior lobe is composed of a mass of nerve fibers with supporting glial cells. These unmyelinated nerves are the axons of hypothalamic neurons. As shown by electron microscopy, they contain membrane-bound secretory granules (composed either of antidiuretic hormone [ADH] or of oxytocin). ADH and oxytocin are complexed with specific binding proteins (neurophysins).

The anterior and posterior lobes of the pituitary are under hypothalamic control. Control is direct in the case of the posterior lobe; neurons in the hypothalamic nuclei secrete ADH and oxytocin, which pass down the axons in the pituitary stalk for storage and are released into the blood by the posterior pituitary. Hypothalamic control of the anterior pituitary is effected by releasing and inhibiting hormones produced in the hypothalamus and carried to the anterior lobe via the portal venous system (Table 57–2 and Fig 57–1).

HYPERSECRETION OF ANTERIOR PITUITARY HORMONES; PITUITARY ADENOMA

Nearly all cases of anterior pituitary hypersecretion are due to primary hyperfunction caused by benign neoplasms of a single cell type (pituitary adenoma). Hyperplasia of pituitary cells and pituitary carcinoma are extremely rare.

Pituitary adenomas are uncommon, constituting about 10% of primary intracranial neoplasms. They occur at all ages but are most common in the age group from 20 to 50 years. They occur in men slightly more frequently than in women.

About 30% are nonfunctional, causing destruction of the normal gland and presenting with general or selective hypopituitarism. About 30% secrete prolactin, 25% growth hormone, and 10% ACTH. The remainder secrete thyrotropin or gonadotropins.

Occasionally, pituitary adenoma occurs as part of the multiple endocrine adenoma syndrome (MEA, Werner's syndrome; see Chapter 60).

Pathology

Grossly, pituitary adenomas vary greatly in size from microscopic to very large. Microadenomas (diameter < 1 cm) are commonly found in autopsy glands, but their significance is unclear. ACTH- and prolactin-secreting adenomas tend to be small at the time of presentation, whereas nonfunctioning and growth hormone-secreting adenomas tend to reach a large size before they are discovered. Larger tumors expand the sella turcica and compress surrounding structures, especially the optic chiasm (Table 57–3).

Pituitary adenomas are circumscribed and often have a thin fibrous capsule. In a few cases—particularly when the adenoma recurs after sur-

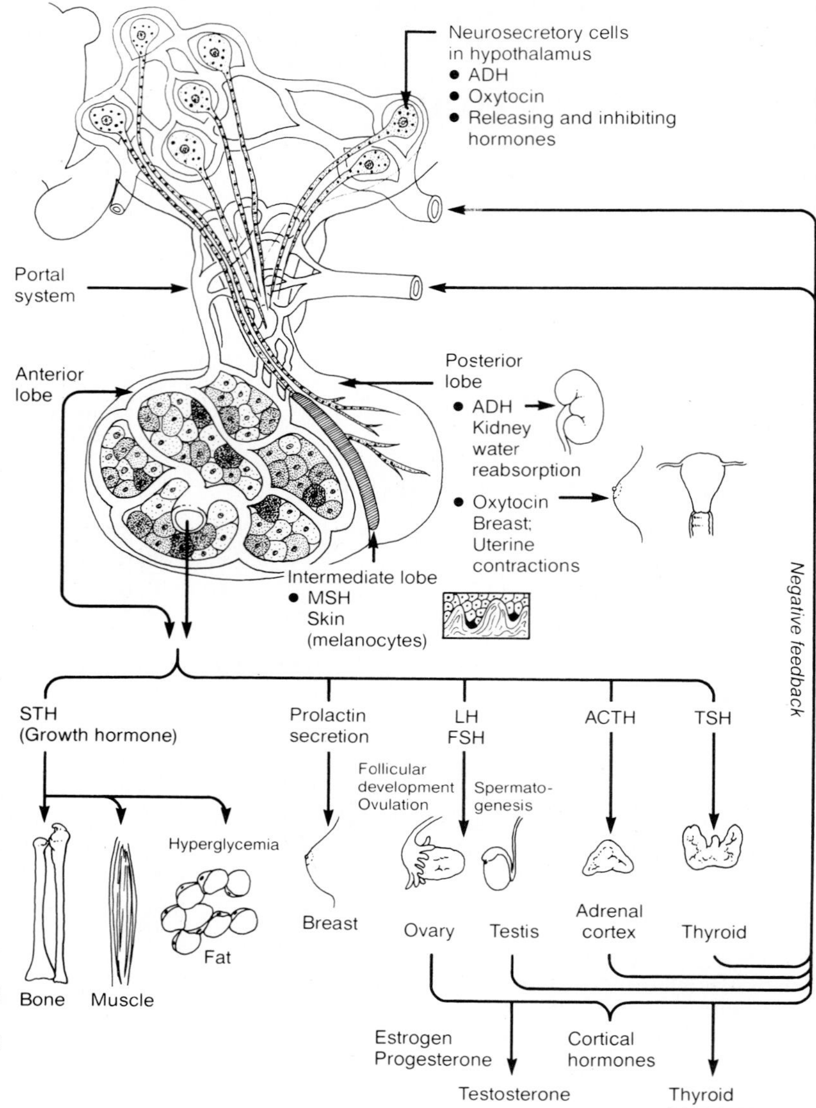

Figure 57–1. Principal hormones of the pituitary and hypothalamus. Hypothalamic neurosecretory cells secreting ADH and oxytocin have direct axonal connections with the posterior pituitary. Hypothalamic cells secreting releasing and inhibiting hormones that control pituicytes in the anterior lobe exert their controlling influence via the portal venous system in the pituitary stalk. STH = somatotropic hormone; LH = luteinizing hormone; FSH = follicle-stimulating hormone; ACTH = adrenocorticotropic hormone (corticotropin); TSH = thyroid-stimulating hormone (thyrotropin); ADH = antidiuretic hormone.

gical removal—the neoplasm is locally infiltrative. Such locally aggressive adenomas are called invasive adenomas; the diagnosis of carcinoma is made only when distant metastases are documented.

On cut section, pituitary adenomas are fleshy, gray to red masses that frequently show cystic degeneration, hemorrhage, and necrosis due to ischemia. Rarely, infarction of the entire tumor may occur.

Microscopically, the cells in a pituitary adenoma are mostly of one morphologic type and are arranged in nests and trabeculae separated by sinusoidal blood vessels. The cells are uniform, resembling normal pituitary cells in most cases. However, in a few tumors, particularly recurrent cases, there is cytologic pleomorphism and increased mitotic activity. These cytologic features correlate with locally aggressive behavior but are not sufficient to make a diagnosis of carcinoma.

The characterization of cell type requires either immunohistochemical (Table 57–4) or electron microscopic study (differences in granule types). The classification of pituitary adenomas into basophilic (ACTH, TSH), acidophilic (GH, prolactin), and chromophobic (nonfunctioning) is inexact and should be discarded. Chromophobe adenomas can be shown immunohistochemically to produce hormones in many cases.

Clinical Features

The clinical features of pituitary adenoma may be divided into effects resulting from local growth of the neoplasm and those resulting from hor-

Table 57–1. Cell types and hormones of the pituitary.

Cell Type	Quantity	Hormone	Action
Anterior pituitary Somatotroph	40–50%	Growth hormone (somatotropin)	Growth of all body tissues; antagonist to insulin
Lactotroph	15–20%	Prolactin	Proliferation of breast and initiation of milk secretion
Corticotroph[1]	15–20%	Corticotropin (ACTH)	Stimulation of adrenocortical steroid synthesis and secretion
		Beta-lipotropic hormone	. . .
		Beta-endorphin	Endogenous opiate
		Alpha-melanocyte stimulating hormone	Dispersion of melanin in skin
Thyrotroph	5%	Thyrotropin (TSH)	Stimulation of thyroid hormone synthesis and secretion
Gonadotroph[2]	5%	Follicle-stimulating hormone (FSH)	Preovulatory growth of graafian follicle and estrogen secretion; with LH, induces ovulation
		Luteinizing hormone (LH)	With FSH, induces ovulation, formation of corpus luteum, and progesterone secretion
Nonsecretory (null) cells	15–20%	None	. . .
Posterior pituitary Hypothalamic nuclei		Antidiuretic hormone (ADH)	Water resorption in distal nephron; arteriolar constriction
		Oxytocin	Contraction of smooth muscle of uterus, breast ducts

[1]Beta-lipotropic hormone, beta-endorphin, and alpha-melanocyte stimulating hormone are peptides that are split off during corticotropin synthesis.
[2]The same cell probably secretes both FSH and LH. Note that in the male, LH is identical to the interstitial cell-stimulating hormone (ICSH), which stimulates the testicular Leydig cells to secrete androgens.

Table 57–2. Control mechanisms for pituitary hormones.

Hormone	Control
Antidiuretic hormone (ADH)	Serum osmolality
Oxytocin	Neural
Growth hormone	Serum glucose; hypothalamic GHRH,[1] GHIH[1]
Prolactin	Hypothalamic PRH,[1] PIH[1]
Thyrotropin	Serum thyroxine; hypothalamic TRH[1]
Gonadotropins	Serum estrogen, progesterone, testosterone; hypothalamic GRH[1] (LHRH[1] and FRH[1])
Corticotropin	Serum cortisol; hypothalamic CRH[1]

GHRH = growth hormone-releasing hormone
GHIH = growth hormone-inhibiting hormone (somatostatin)
PRH = prolactin-releasing hormone
PIH = prolactin-inhibiting hormone
TRH = thyrotropin-releasing hormone
CRH = corticotropin-releasing homone
GRH = gonadotropin-releasing hormone
LHRH = leutinizing hormone-releasing hormone
FRH = FSH-releasing hormone
FSH = follicle-stimulating hormone
[1]These releasing and inhibiting hormones (factors) are produced by cells in the hypothalamus and transmitted to the anterior pituitary by a portal system (see Fig 57–1).

mone secretion (Table 57–3). The former depend on the size of the neoplasm and its invasive capability; the latter depend on the type of hormone secreted.

A. Local Effects: Enlargement of the sella turcica can be detected by radiologic examination and is one of the earliest manifestations of pituitary neoplasm. As the neoplasm expands into the suprasellar cistern, it impinges on the large blood vessels (causing dull headache) and the central inferior part of the optic chiasm (leading to visual field defects, typically superior quadrantic bitemporal hemianopia). Large neoplasms compress the more peripheral part of the chiasm, the hypothalamus, and sometimes the third ventricle, resulting in hydrocephalus.

Infiltrative neoplasms may open into the paranasal sinuses (with a high risk of meningitis) or the cavernous sinus (producing thrombosis with orbital edema and congestion).

B. Systemic Effects Due to Hormone Excess:

1. Hyperprolactinemia–The commonest hormone produced by a pituitary adenoma is prolactin. In women, prolactin causes amenorrhea, infertility, and galactorrhea (milk secretion in the absence of pregnancy). In men, it causes decreased libido, impotence, and galactorrhea.

Table 57-3. Pituitary adenoma: Clinical effects.

Mass Effects	Excessive Hormone Secretion (Only Manifestation in Small Adenomas)
Large adenomas Usually nonfunctioning or growth-hormone producing ↓ Destruction of normal pituitary cells → hypopituitarism, diabetes insipidus Expansion of sella turcica → visible on x-ray Suprasellar extension through diaphragma sella ↓ Compression of optic chiasm or nerves → visual field defects Compression of hypothalamus → diabetes insipidus Interference with outflow of CSF from 3rd ventricle → raised intracranial pressure → hydrocephalus Compression of vessels → headache Cranial nerve compression (rare) May invade brain ("invasive adenoma"), paranasal sinuses, cavernous sinus	Absent in 30% of cases 30% Prolactin → galactorrhea 25% Growth hormone → gigantism (child) → acromegaly (adult) 10% Corticotropin → Cushing's syndrome 5% Thyrotropin, gonadotropins

These clinical features may be mimicked by other conditions, including hypothalamic diseases in which there is decreased production of prolactin inhibiting factor, and may occur as a toxic response to drugs that block dopaminergic transmission (eg, methyldopa and reserpine) and hence produce hyperprolactinemia. Since prolactin-secreting tumors are commonly microadenomas, the differential diagnosis may be very difficult.

2. Growth hormone (somatotropin) excess- Increased growth hormone levels cause increased growth of nearly every tissue in the body. The clinical effect depends on the age of the patient. In children, there is excessive uniform bone growth at the epiphyses, resulting in a massive but proportionate increase in height (gigantism). In adults, in whom adenomas occur much more commonly, the fused epiphyses do not permit increased height, but there is generalized enlargement of bones, most visible in the hands (spade-like hands), jaw, and skull (acromegaly: Gk *acros* "extreme" + *megale* "great").* Tissues other than bone are also affected. Increased size of cartilages leads to enlargement of the nose and ears. Joint abnormalities occur, particularly in the vertebral column, causing osteoarthritis. Increased size of soft tissues produces coarsening of facial features and enlargement of all the viscera, notably the heart, liver, kidneys, adrenals, thyroid, and pancreas.

Table 57-4. Classification of pituitary adenomas based on immunohistochemical tests.

Type of Adenoma	Frequency
Lactotroph adenoma	30%
Somatotroph adenoma	25%
Corticotroph adenoma	10%
Thyrotroph adenoma	Rare
Gonadotroph adenoma	Rare
Mixed cell adenoma[1]	Rare
Oncocytoma[2]	Rare
Null cell (nonsecretory) adenoma[3]	30%

[1]Mixed cell adenoma is most commonly composed of a mixture of lactotrophs and somatotrophs.
[2]An oncocytoma is composed of nonsecretory cells that have abundant eosinophilic cytoplasm containing numerous mitochondria.
[3]Absence of staining for all hormones.

Many patients with acromegaly have evidence of decreased secretion of other pituitary hormones, because of compression atrophy of the residual normal pituitary cells. Impotence (in the male), amenorrhea (in the female), and infertility (both sexes) result.

Growth hormone also antagonizes the action of insulin and results in secondary diabetes mellitus. Ten percent of patients with acromegaly have overt diabetes; over 40% have abnormalities in the glucose tolerance test.

The diagnosis is established by a finding of elevated serum levels of growth hormone that cannot be suppressed by glucose administration.

3. Corticotropin (ACTH) excess- Increased production of corticotropin (ACTH) by a pituitary adenoma stimulates hyperplasia of the zona fasciculata of the adrenal cortex, causing exces-

*Many dogs appear to have been bred for pituitary disease: Bulldogs are acromegalic; Irish Wolfhounds have pituitary gigantism; and many "miniatures" are pituitary dwarfs.

sive secretion of cortisol (Cushing's syndrome). The high serum cortisol levels fail to depress ACTH secretion by the partially autonomous adenoma (lack of feedback inhibition). Increased skin pigmentation is variously attributed to increased production of MSH or to the melanogenic effect of high ACTH levels.

High serum levels of both cortisol and ACTH strongly suggest a diagnosis of pituitary adenoma. However, identical findings may be seen in other neoplasms that secrete ACTH (eg, ectopic ACTH in lung carcinoma), and the diagnosis then depends on demonstrating the pituitary adenoma by radiographic studies. Since most ACTH-secreting adenomas are very small, this may be difficult. Indeed, before it was realized that most cases of adrenal hyperplasia and Cushing's syndrome were due to pituitary microadenomas, it was customary to treat these patients by bilateral adrenalectomy. The sudden reduction in serum cortisol that followed adrenalectomy removed any residual partial feedback inhibition of the tumor and led to rapid proliferation of pituitary adenoma cells, with very high ACTH levels and skin pigmentation (Nelson's syndrome).

4. Thyrotropin (TSH) and gonadotropin excess–These disorders are very rare.

Treatment & Prognosis

The treatment of pituitary adenoma is surgical removal. The tumor can be approached from below through the nasopharynx (transsphenoidal approach) or from above through a craniotomy. Surgery is curative in most cases. The adenoma recurs in a small percentage of cases and may show locally aggressive behavior. Metastasis (ie, carcinoma) is very rare.

HYPOSECRETION OF PITUITARY HORMONES

Hypopituitarism in adults (Simmonds' disease) is rare. The commonest cause in the past was ischemic necrosis of a gland that had undergone hyperplasia during pregnancy (Sheehan's syndrome) (Table 57–5). This was due to shock, usually precipitated by postpartum hemorrhage. With improved obstetric care, it is now very uncommon in developed countries.

Nonfunctioning neoplasms involving the sella now represent the commonest cause of hypopituitarism in developed countries. Such tumors include nonfunctioning pituitary adenoma and craniopharyngioma (see Chapter 65). Pituitary dwarfism occurs if hypopituitarism develops early in life, due either to tumor or to other causes.

Table 57–5. Causes of hypopituitarism.

Ischemic necrosis of the pituitary
Postpartum necrosis (Sheehan's syndrome)
Head injury
Vascular disease, commonly associated with diabetes mellitus
Neoplasms involving the sella turcica
Nonfunctioning adenoma
Craniopharyngioma
Suprasellar chordoma
Histiocytosis X (eosinophilic granuloma; Hand-Schüller-Christian disease)
Intrasellar cysts
Chronic inflammatory lesions
Tuberculosis, syphilis, sarcoidosis
Infiltrative diseases
Amyloidosis
Hemochromatosis
Mucopolysaccharidoses
Congenital pituitary dwarfism
Lorain type: normal proportions and intelligence but delayed sexual development
Fröhlich type: obese with stunted growth, mental retardation, and abnormal sexual development

Pathology

Over 90% of the gland must be destroyed before clinical evidence of hypopituitarism is manifested. The pathologic changes depend on the cause. In cases due to ischemic necrosis, the initial area of coagulative necrosis is replaced by scar tissue.

Clinical Features

The clinical effects of hypopituitarism depend on whether the patient is a child or an adult.

Hypopituitarism in children results in a proportionate failure of growth due to absence of growth hormone (pituitary dwarfism). These children have normal intelligence and remain childlike, failing to develop sexually (Lorain type of dwarfism). This is different from the Fröhlich type, characterized by obesity, mental retardation, and abnormal sexual development, due probably to associated hypothalamic dysfunction.

In adults, hypopituitarism is characterized mainly by the effects of gonadotropin deficiency. In the female, there is amenorrhea and infertility; in the male, infertility and impotence. Thyrotropin and corticotropin deficiency may result in atrophy of the thyroid and adrenal cortex. However, decreased secretion of thyroxine and cortisol is rarely severe enough to cause clinical manifestations. Isolated growth hormone deficiency produces little abnormality in the adult.

Treatment

Treatment of hypopituitarism is by replacement of all the deficient hormones. When a neoplasm is responsible, surgical removal of the mass is necessary.

DISEASES OF THE POSTERIOR PITUITARY

DIABETES INSIPIDUS

Diabetes insipidus is caused by failure of the hypothalamus and posterior pituitary to secrete antidiuretic hormone (ADH). Deficient water reabsorption in the renal collecting tubule then leads to the excretion of an increased amount of urine (polyuria) of very low specific gravity. Serum osmolality is increased, inducing thirst and polydipsia (excessive water intake). The superficial resemblance of the clinical features (polyuria, polydipsia) to diabetes mellitus, combined with the absence of a sweet ("insipid") taste of the urine led to the term diabetes insipidus.

Diabetes insipidus may be caused by any condition that interferes with the hypothalamopituitary axis: (1) hypothalamic or pituitary neoplasms or (2) disruption of the pituitary stalk by trauma, meningeal disease (metastatic carcinoma, sarcoidosis, tuberculous meningitis), or bone disease (Hand-Schüller-Christian disease).

Diagnosis is based on the clinical features with confirmation by the water deprivation test. Deprivation of water fails to increase urine concentration in patients with diabetes insipidus.

EXCESSIVE SECRETION OF ANTIDIURETIC HORMONE

Inappropriate excessive secretion of ADH (SIADH; Schwartz-Bartter syndrome) by the posterior pituitary is a common phenomenon seen in a large variety of clinical conditions, including (1) pulmonary disorders, eg, tuberculosis and pneumonia; (2) cerebral neoplasms and trauma; (3) drugs, eg, vincristine and chlorpropamide; (4) cirrhosis of the liver; and (5) adrenal and thyroid insufficiency.

ADH may also be produced by several different malignant neoplasms, most commonly small cell undifferentiated (oat cell) carcinoma of the lung and pancreatic carcinoma (ectopic ADH syndrome).

High levels of ADH cause water to be retained in the renal collecting tubule; concentrated urine is excreted, leading to decreased serum osmolality (< 275 mosm/kg) and hyponatremia. The clinical manifestations are those of hyponatremia and include weakness, lethargy, confusion, convulsions, and coma.

The Thyroid Gland

58

STRUCTURE & FUNCTION

Embryology

The thyroid gland develops from a tubular invagination of the embryonic pharynx (the thyroglossal duct), which migrates downward into the neck and there develops into the thyroid gland.

Thyroid gland ectopia results when there is arrest of this downward migration. The most extreme form is the very rare lingual thyroid, at the root of the tongue. More frequently, ectopic thyroid tissue in the midline of the neck along the path of descent is present in addition to the normal gland. Rarely, migration may proceed too far, resulting in a gland located in the superior mediastinum.

Epithelial remnants of the thyroglossal duct may persist in the midline of the neck and may produce cysts, lined by either squamous or respiratory epithelium with thyroid tissue in the wall **(thyroglossal duct cyst)**. Thyroglossal duct cysts are commonly found between the hyoid bone and the isthmus of the thyroid gland. They present in late childhood or early adult life. Infection and abscess formation may occur.

Structure

The adult thyroid weighs 20–25 g and is composed of 2 lateral lobes joined across the midline by an isthmus. A pyramidal lobe of varying size extends upward from the isthmus and represents the point of attachment of the thyroglossal duct. The pyramidal lobe cannot be palpated in a normal gland. The thyroid is firm, reddish-brown, and smooth. It is surrounded by a fibrous capsule that blends with the deep cervical fascia.

Histologically, the thyroid is composed of closely packed follicles separated by a rich vascular supply and little intervening stroma. The follicles are lined by cuboidal epithelial cells and contain colloid, a proteinaceous material composed mainly of thyroglobulin and stored thyroid hormones.

Dispersed between the thyroid follicles are the parafollicular or C cells, which secrete **calcitonin**.

Synthesis of Thyroid Hormone

The rate of synthesis of thyroid hormone is controlled by the level of pituitary thyrotropin (TSH) in the blood (Fig 58–1). Thyrotropin regulates all the steps in the synthesis of thyroid hormone. The effect of TSH on the rate of iodide trapping by the thyroid is believed to be the principal factor determining the rate of hormone secretion by the gland. TSH also induces an increase in the number and size of thyroid follicular cells.

After trapping, the iodide is oxidized to iodine in the thyroid cell and is incorporated into tyrosine molecules to form monoiodotyrosine (MIT) and diiodotyrosine (DIT) (Fig 58–1), which are linked with the thyroglobulin molecule in the colloid. These are then coupled enzymatically to form thyroxine (T_4) and triiodothyronine (T_3). T_4 is the major hormone secreted by the thyroid, the T_4:T_3 ratio being about 10:1.

Peripheral Metabolism of Thyroid Hormone

T_4 and T_3 are transported in the plasma bound to the plasma proteins thyroxine-binding globulin (TBG) and thyroxine-binding prealbumin (TBPA).

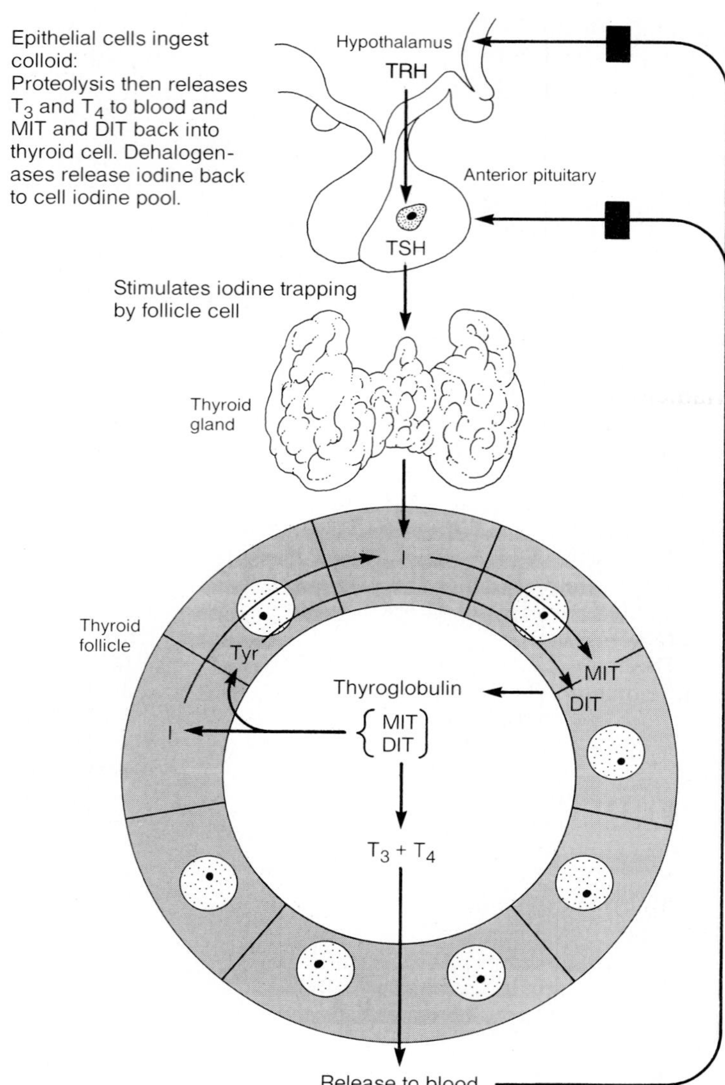

Figure 58-1. Thyroid hormone production and its control. TRH = thyrotropin-releasing hormone; TSH = thyroid-stimulating hormone; MIT = monoiodotyrosine; DIT = diiodotyrosine.

Eighty percent of T_4 in the plasma is bound to TBG. Protein-bound hormone, which represents over 99% of the total plasma thyroid hormones, is inactive but is in equilibrium with the biologically active free hormone. The plasma total T_4:T_3 ratio is about 40:1 because of greater affinity of the binding proteins to T_4 and slower metabolism of T_4.

The metabolic effects of thyroid hormone result from binding of free hormone to target cell receptors. Combination of thyroid hormone with receptors increases cellular mRNA synthesis, which is believed to be the mechanism by which thyroid hormone exerts its effects.

T_4 is converted in the peripheral tissues to T_3, which is the much more potent hormone. While T_4 has independent capability, the main physiologic effects of thyroid hormones are probably mediated by T_3.

Functions of Thyroid Hormone

Thyroid hormone influences basic energy metabolism of the target cell, increasing protein synthesis as well as oxidative phosphorylation in the mitochondria. The net result is an increase in cell metabolism, with enhanced turnover of carbohydrates and lipids plus calcium mobilization in bone. Thyroxine also appears to modulate the number or activity of β-adrenergic receptors at the cell membrane, thus potentiating adrenergic effects.

ASSESSMENT OF THYROID STRUCTURE

Clinical Examination

When enlarged, the thyroid becomes easily palpable. Its close fascial attachment to the larynx causes the thyroid to move upward with the larynx during swallowing, a maneuver that permits clinical identification of a neck mass as being in the thyroid.

Radiologic Examination

Radioisotopic scans, utilizing radioactive ^{125}I, are widely used for detection of thyroid neoplasms, which appear as areas of low uptake of iodine as compared with the normal gland ("filling defects"; "cold nodules"). Ultrasonography is useful in differentiating cystic from solid thyroid nodules.

Thyroid Biopsy

Fine-needle aspiration biopsy of the thyroid has become very popular in evaluation of thyroid nodules. A 21-gauge needle is inserted directly into the nodule. The material aspirated is smeared on a slide for cytologic examination.

ASSESSMENT OF THYROID FUNCTION

Total Serum T_4 & T_3

Total serum T_4 and T_3 can be determined by radioimmunoassay, which measures both protein-bound and free hormone. The value of this assay is limited, because only the free hormone is active biologically, and total serum T_4 and T_3 levels are influenced by changes in levels of thyroid-binding globulins (reduced in liver and kidney disease and in certain congenital diseases; elevated in pregnancy and by oral contraceptives).

T_3 Resin Uptake

T_3 resin uptake provides a measure of thyroid-binding protein (TBG). The test is useful because it can be combined with total serum T_4 and T_3 in a mathematical calculation that gives a reliable estimate of the free T_4 and free T_3 levels in serum (called the free thyroxine and T_3 index). TBG, free T_4, and free T_3 may also be measured directly.

Serum Thyrotropin (TSH)

Estimation of serum thyrotropin (TSH) is the most sensitive test in the diagnosis of primary hypothyroidism. Reduction of pituitary feedback inhibition in primary hypothyroidism (ie, low T_3 and T_4 levels) results in elevated levels of TSH.

DISORDERS OF THYROID SECRETION

Thyroid disorders present clinically as abnormalities of thyroid function or as enlargement of the thyroid gland (goiter). The discussion below of the major causes of hyperthyroidism and hypothyroidism will be followed by details of the principal disease processes.

EXCESSIVE SECRETION OF THYROID HORMONE (Hyperthyroidism; Thyrotoxicosis)

Etiology

Over 95% of cases of hyperthyroidism are caused by Graves' disease, an autoimmune thyroid disease in which autoantibodies stimulate the cells to produce excess hormone.

Rare causes of hyperthyroidism other than Graves' disease can be listed as follows: (1) toxicity in a multinodular goiter; (2) functioning follicular adenoma or, rarely, carcinoma; (3) thyrotropin-secreting pituitary adenoma (sometimes called "secondary" hyperthyroidism); (4) germ cell tumors such as choriocarcinoma (which may rarely produce a TSH-like substance) or teratoma (which may contain functioning thyroid tissue); (5) thyroiditis, of both subacute and Hashimoto type, either of which may be associated with transient hyperthyroidism in the early phase; and (6) hypothalamic disease with production of excess TRH (thyrotropin-releasing hormone).

Pathology

Pathologic changes in the thyroid depend on the cause (see individual diseases, below).

Clinical Features (Table 58-1)

Hyperthyroidism results in a general increase in cellular metabolism of target cells, which is responsible for many of the clinical features: (1) Nervousness, anxiety, insomnia, and fine tremors. (2) Weight loss despite a good appetite. Thyroid hormone increases basal metabolic rate. (3) Heat intolerance and increased sweating. (4) Palpita-

Table 58-1. Contrasting features in disorders of thyroid function.

	Hyperthyroid	Hypothyroid
Laboratory Free thyroxine index	↑	↓
T_4 and T_3 levels	↑[1]	↓
TSH[2] levels	↓[3]	↑[3]
Physiologic mechanisms Cellular metabolism and protein synthesis	↑	↓
Potentiation of ß-adrenergic effects	↑	↓
Insulin antagonism	↑	↓
Clinical effects Basal metabolic rate	↑	↓
Goiter	Usually present	May be present
Body weight	↓	N or ↑
Activity	Hyperactive, insomniac	Lethargic, somnolent
Reflexes	Brisk	Slow
Cardiovascular	Tachycardia, arrhythmias	Bradycardia
Gastrointestinal	Mild diarrhea	Constipation
Hair	Fine	Coarse, brittle; hair loss
Myxedema[4]	Circumscribed patches, mainly pretibial	Generalized, especially extremities and face
Temperature tolerance	Heat-intolerant	Cold-intolerant
Other	Exophthalmos (in Graves' disease)	Mental and growth retardation (in childhood cretinism); anemia, hypercholesterolemia

[1]Occasionally only T_3 is elevated.
[2]TSH = thyroid-stimulating hormone.
[3]Reflects changes in biofeedback in primary thyroid disease; in hyperthyroidism caused by pituitary disease, the TSH level will be increased; if hypothyroidism is due to pituitary failure, TSH will be decreased.
[4]The term myxedema refers to accumulation of mucopolysaccharides in the dermis. Although myxedema occurs in both hyper- and hypothyroidism, the distribution and pathogenesis are different.

tions, tachycardia, cardiac arrhythmias, and cardiac failure, which may occur as a result of the effect of thyroxine on myocardial cells. Atrial fibrillation is common. (5) Amenorrhea and infertility. (6) Muscle weakness, particularly involving the limb girdles (proximal myopathy). (7) Osteoporosis with bone pain.

Laboratory Diagnosis (Tables 58-1 and 58-2)

Elevated total serum T_4 and T_3 are not very reliable indices of thyroid hyperfunction because of variations in levels of binding proteins; increased T_3 is more valuable than T_4, since T_3 is less affected by these variations. Free thyroxine index is elevated in hyperthyroidism and is currently the best diagnostic test. In about 10% of cases, T_4 secretion is within normal limits, the hyperthyroidism being the result of elevated T_3 levels (so-called T_3 toxicosis).

All conditions associated with hyperthyroidism are characterized by increased thyroid hormone levels in the blood and the clinical effects of hyperthyroidism. Graves' disease is distinguished from other causes of hyperthyroidism by the additional presence of eye changes and serum thyroid-stimulating autoantibodies (see below). Serum TSH levels are decreased in all cases of hyperthyroidism except in those rare cases where the hyperthyroidism is secondary to a thyrotroph adenoma of the pituitary.

DECREASED SECRETION OF THYROID HORMONE (Hypothyroidism)

Decreased secretion of thyroid hormones results in cretinism if deficiency is present from birth and myxedema if it develops in an adult (Table 58-1).

Hypothyroidism may be broadly classified as primary, due to decrease in thyroid hormone resulting from a disease process in the thyroid gland (common); or secondary, resulting from failure of pituitary TSH secretion (rare).

The diagnosis of hypothyroidism may be confirmed in the laboratory by decreased levels of T_4 (not very reliable) and a decreased free thyroxine index (reliable). The T_3 level is of little value, since

Table 58-2. Differential features in thyroid disease.

	Thyroid Gland	Thyroid Hormones[1]	Thyroid-Stimulating Hormone	Autoantibodies
Hyperthyroidism **Primary** Graves' disease	Diffuse enlargement	Elevated	Decreased	Thyroid-stimulating Ig; exophthalmos-producing factor
Toxic nodular goiter	Multinodular goiter	Elevated	Decreased	None
Toxic adenoma	Solitary nodule	Elevated	Decreased	None
Subacute thyroiditis	Tender enlargement	Elevated	Normal	None
Secondary Pituitary thyrotropic adenoma	Diffuse enlargement	Elevated	Elevated	None
Hypothyroidism **Primary** Thyroid agenesis	Absent	Absent	Elevated	None
Enzyme deficiency	Diffuse enlargement	Decreased	Elevated	None
Iodine deficiency	Diffuse/nodular goiter	Decreased	Elevated	None
Hashimoto's thyroiditis	Diffuse enlargement	Decreased	Elevated	Antithyroglobulin, anti-microsomal, anticolloid
Secondary Pituitary failure	Atrophy	Decreased	Decreased	None

[1]Thyroid hormone levels may be assessed by total T_4, total T_3, and free T_4 index. In most thyroid diseases, all 3 are elevated; free T_4 index is more reliable than total T_4 and total T_3 levels. In a few cases of hyperthyroidism, T_4 levels are normal and only T_3 is elevated ("T_3 toxicosis").

it only falls in extreme hypothyroidism. The most sensitive diagnostic test in primary hypothyroidism is elevation of serum thyrotropin (TSH) concentration. This test is also useful in the differentiation of primary (increased serum TSH) and secondary (decreased serum TSH) hypothyroidism.

1. CRETINISM

Etiology

Cretinism is an uncommon disease of childhood, but diagnosis is important because thyroxine administration soon after birth can in many cases prevent severe consequences.

The causes can be listed as follows:

(1) Failure of development of the thyroid (thyroid agenesis).

(2) Failure of hormone synthesis due to severe iodine deficiency in the diet of both the mother during pregnancy and the baby after birth. This condition is now rare in countries in which table salt is iodized but still occurs in some mountainous Third World countries (endemic cretinism).

(3) Failure of hormone synthesis due to the presence of dietary substances (goitrogens) that block hormone synthesis. Thiocyanate in the cassava plant eaten in Central Africa is the best known of these substances. Goitrogens represent a very rare cause of endemic cretinism.

(4) Failure of hormone synthesis due to autosomal recessive enzyme deficiency (sporadic cretinism). Many enzyme deficiencies have been identified, causing failure of iodide trapping, organification of iodide, coupling, and dehalogenation of MIT and DIT.

Pathology

The appearance of the thyroid depends on the cause. In cretinism due to thyroid agenesis, the gland is absent. In cretinism caused by failure of thyroid hormone synthesis, the gland undergoes enlargement and hyperplasia owing to increased secretion of pituitary thyrotropin resulting from decreased feedback inhibition (goitrous cretinism).

Clinical Features

Babies with cretinism show lethargy, somnolence, hypothermia, feeding problems, and persistent neonatal jaundice. A hoarse cry, hypotonia of muscles, large protruding tongue, and umbilical hernia are common features. If the diagnosis is not made at birth, there is growth retardation (failure to thrive, delayed bone growth) and irreversible mental retardation. Replacement of thyroid hormones after diagnosis of cretinism in the perinatal period prevents mental retardation to a large extent.

2. MYXEDEMA

Etiology

Causes of hypothyroidism in the adult include the following:

A. Hashimoto's Autoimmune Thyroiditis: This disorder is responsible for most cases and is discussed below.

B. Pituitary Failure: Secondary hypothyroidism due to pituitary failure is uncommon but may be recognized by the markedly decreased thyrotropin level in the blood.

C. Iatrogenic Hypothyroidism: Hypothyroidism may result from administration of antithyroid drugs or ablation of the gland by surgery (total thyroidectomy) or radiation.

D. Dietary Causes: Failure of thyroid hormone synthesis due to extreme dietary iodine deficiency very rarely results in hypothyroidism. In patients with iodine deficiency, decreased hormone production is usually compensated for by hyperplasia of the thyroid via the thyrotropin feedback mechanism, the enlarged gland maintaining adequate hormone secretion. Certain dietary factors appear to induce similar effects by interfering with iodine metabolism (goitrogens).

Pathology

The changes in the thyroid depend on the cause of hypothyroidism (see Hashimoto's thyroiditis and multinodular goiter, below).

Clinical Features (Table 58-1)

Decreased levels of thyroid hormones cause a decreased rate of metabolism in all target cells, with the following results: (1) Lethargy, cold intolerance, weight gain, and constipation. (2) Loss of hair all over the body, but typically in the scalp and eyebrows. (3) Neurologic manifestations, including psychomotor retardation and slow thought processes and bodily movements. In many patients, overt psychotic features appear ("myxedema madness"). A useful physical finding is a prolonged relaxation phase in the deep tendon reflexes. (4) Anemia, usually normochromic normocytic, due to decreased erythropoiesis. (5) Pleural and pericardial effusions. (6) Increased serum cholesterol and atherosclerosis.

The term **myxedema** is used for adult hypothyroidism because of the deposition of increased amounts of mucopolysaccharides in connective tissues. It is not known why this occurs. Mucopolysaccharides are deposited (1) in the skin, producing a peculiar kind of diffuse nonpitting doughy swelling; (2) in the larynx, causing hoarseness, an almost constant feature in severe hypothyroidism; and (3) in the heart, involving the interstitium between myocardial fibers and causing cardiac enlargement. Myocardial fiber degeneration also occurs. Hypothyroid patients may present with heart failure owing to the combined effect of this change and myocardial ischemia due to the associated atherosclerotic coronary artery disease. In treating hypothyroid patients with thyroid hormone replacement, care must be taken to ensure that the cardiac stimulation caused by administered thyroid hormone does not precipitate failure in the myxedematous heart.

DISEASES OF THE THYROID

IMMUNOLOGIC DISEASES OF THE THYROID

1. GRAVES' DISEASE

Graves' disease is responsible for the great majority of cases of hyperthyroidism. It is a relatively common disease affecting females 4–5 times more commonly than males. It has its highest incidence in the 15- to 40-year age group. There is a familial tendency and an association with the histocompatibility antigen HLA-DR3. Patients with Graves' disease frequently suffer from other autoimmune diseases such as pernicious anemia.

Etiology (Fig 58-2)

Graves' disease is an autoimmune disease characterized by the presence in serum of thyroid-stimulating immunoglobulins (TSI), which are autoantibodies of the IgG class. These include (1) long-acting thyroid stimulator (LATS), (2) human thyroid stimulator (HTS), and (3) LATS protector (LATS-P). Another group of antibodies that stimulate the growth of thyroid epithelial cells has been described.

The thyroid-stimulating immunoglobulins are directed against antigens on the thyroid cell membrane. The combination of antibody with TSH receptors mimics the action of TSH on the thyroid cell, stimulating many enzyme reactions in hormonogenesis and resulting in increased hormone secretion (stimulatory type II hypersensitivity; see Chapter 8).

The precipitating cause is unknown. Serum levels of antibodies do not correlate precisely with severity of disease.

Since the stimulating antibodies are IgG, they cross the placenta in pregnancy and stimulate the fetal thyroid, causing neonatal hyperthyroidism; this condition spontaneously reverses after delivery as the maternal antibodies disappear from the baby's blood, providing good evidence that the antibodies are responsible for the disease.

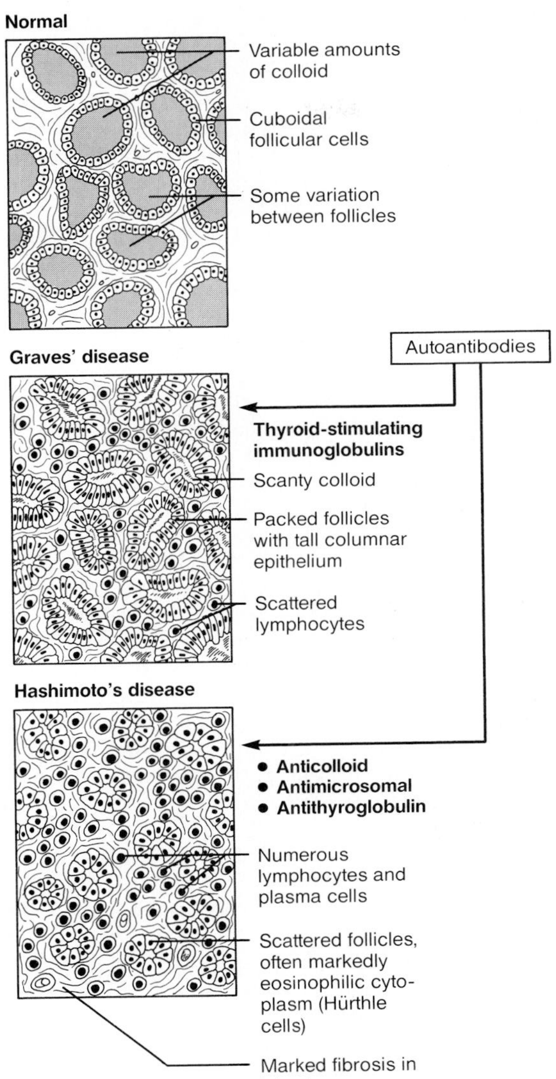

Figure 58-2. Immunologic diseases of the thyroid. Thyroid-stimulating antibodies in Graves' disease directly stimulate follicular epithelial cells, which undergo hyperplasia and secrete excessive hormone. In Hashimoto's disease, the precise role played by the different autoantibodies in causing thyroid epithelial cell destruction is uncertain.

Pathology

The thyroid gland is diffusely and symmetrically enlarged and extremely vascular. Microscopically, thyroid follicular epithelial cells are increased in size and number. The follicles are closely packed and lined by tall columnar epithelium which is frequently thrown into papillary infoldings (Fig 58-3). Colloid is scanty, and its periphery is scalloped because of rapid thyroglobulin proteolysis. Lymphocytic infiltration of the interstitium is common, and lymphoid follicles with germinal centers may be present. Treatment with antithyroid drugs causes regression of these hyperplastic changes.

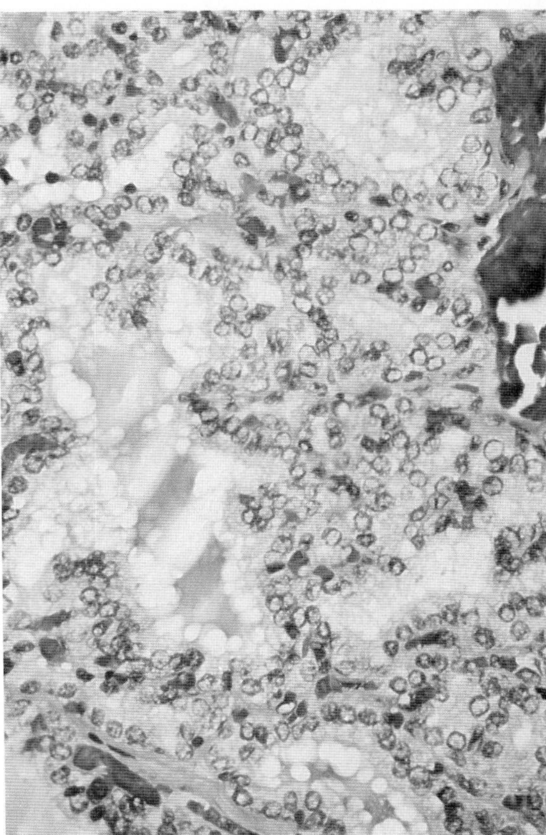

Figure 58-3. Graves' disease, showing small follicles with scanty colloid and enlarged lining epithelial cells.

Clinical Features & Diagnosis (Tables 58-1 and 58-2)

The thyroid gland is diffusely enlarged and appears as a mass in the neck. A bruit resulting from the greatly increased blood flow is often present over the gland.

Eye changes are present in most patients with Graves' disease. These include exophthalmos (see below), a staring gaze due to decreased blinking, and impaired eye muscle function; eye changes help to distinguish Graves' disease from other causes of hyperthyroidism.

Laboratory evidence of hyperthyroidism—most reliably elevation of free thyroxine index—is present. Ten percent of patients show normal T_4 but elevated levels of free T_3 (T_3 toxicosis).

Thyroid scan shows increased uptake of radioiodine but is rarely needed for diagnosis. Most patients have thyroid stimulating immunoglobulins (TSI) in their blood, and this is of diagnostic value.

Associated Conditions

The following conditions may be associated with Graves' disease but are not always present.

A. Exophthalmos: Exophthalmos—protrusion of the eyeballs—occurs in 70% of patients with Graves' disease. Its presence is unrelated to the severity of Graves' disease, and it may rarely occur in the absence of hyperthyroidism. Exophthalmos is related to the presence in serum of an autoantibody known as exophthalmos-producing factor (EPF) that is independent of other autoantibodies. Lymphocytic infiltration of the orbital soft tissues with edema fluid and mucopolysaccharides produces the exophthalmos. When severe, there is risk of ocular infections and blindness.

B. Pretibial Myxedema: Pretibial myxedema occurs in 5% of patients and is due to localized accumulation of mucopolysaccharide, forming circumscribed patches in the pretibial skin. It is of diagnostic value, since it almost never occurs in the absence of Graves' disease. It causes no symptoms other than itching.

Treatment

Graves' diseases may be treated with antithyroid drugs, by ablation, or by counteracting the peripheral effects of thyroxine, many of which are the result of β-adrenergic potentiation.

A. Antithyroid Drugs: Drugs such as propylthiouracil, which block the synthesis of thyroid hormones, are effective in controlling the symptoms of Graves' disease. They are usually given an initial trial in the hope that the disease process will remit spontaneously.

B. Thyroid Ablation: The thyroid gland may be ablated, either by surgical removal (subtotal thyroidectomy) or by therapeutic doses of radioactive iodine, which selectively destroys the thyroid gland. Treatment with radioiodine is preferred in older individuals; in younger patients, the increased risk of developing hypothyroidism or even thyroid carcinoma after radioiodine therapy restricts its use.

C. Propranolol: Some of the more troublesome effects of thyrotoxicosis relate to the potentiation of catecholamines by thyroxine. Propranolol may be effective in controlling these effects.

Treatment of Complications

Treatment of Graves' disease has no effect on the exophthalmos, which pursues its course independently. In most cases, the eye changes remit spontaneously. In severe cases, immunosuppressive therapy with corticosteroids and even surgical decompression of the orbit may be required to prevent blindness.

2. HASHIMOTO'S AUTOIMMUNE THYROIDITIS

Hashimoto's thyroiditis is responsible for most cases of primary hypothyroidism. The entity that was previously called idiopathic primary myxedema is now believed to represent the end stage of Hashimoto's thyroiditis.

Hashimoto's thyroiditis affects middle-aged individuals—females 10 times more frequently than males.

Etiology (Fig 58-2)

Hashimoto's disease is believed to be the result of an autoimmune response against the thyroid. Neither the cause for development of autoimmunity nor the exact mechanism by which the thyroid is destroyed is known.

Most patients with Hashimoto's disease have in their serum several different IgG autoantibodies with specificity against thyroid antigens: (1) antithyroglobulin antibody, which may be detected by the immunofluorescent technique; (2) antimicrosomal antibody, detected by the complement fixation test; and (3) a third antibody directed against a component of colloid other than thyroglobulin. Serum levels of these antibodies do not correlate with severity of disease, and their exact relationship to thyroid cell destruction is uncertain. They are, however, of diagnostic value.

It has been suggested that T cell-mediated hypersensitivity may be involved in Hashimoto's disease, but no good test exists to establish this.

Pathology

In the early stages, the thyroid is enlarged diffusely. The gland is firm and rubbery, with a coarsely nodular ("bosselated") appearance. As the disease progresses, the gland becomes smaller; the end result is a markedly atrophic fibrosed thyroid.

Microscopically, there is evidence of destruction of the thyroid follicles associated with severe lymphocytic infiltration of the gland (Fig 58–4). Large lymphoid follicles with germinal centers are commonly present. Surviving follicular epithelial cells are commonly transformed into large cells with abundant pink cytoplasm known as Hürthle cells. Progressive fibrosis occurs.

The histologic changes are diagnostic of Hashimoto's disease only if the clinical background is consistent. Similar changes, usually of lesser degree and usually without the presence of Hürthle cells, occur commonly without Hashimoto's disease and are referred to as nonspecific lymphocytic thyroiditis.

Clinical Features

Most patients with Hashimoto's thyroiditis

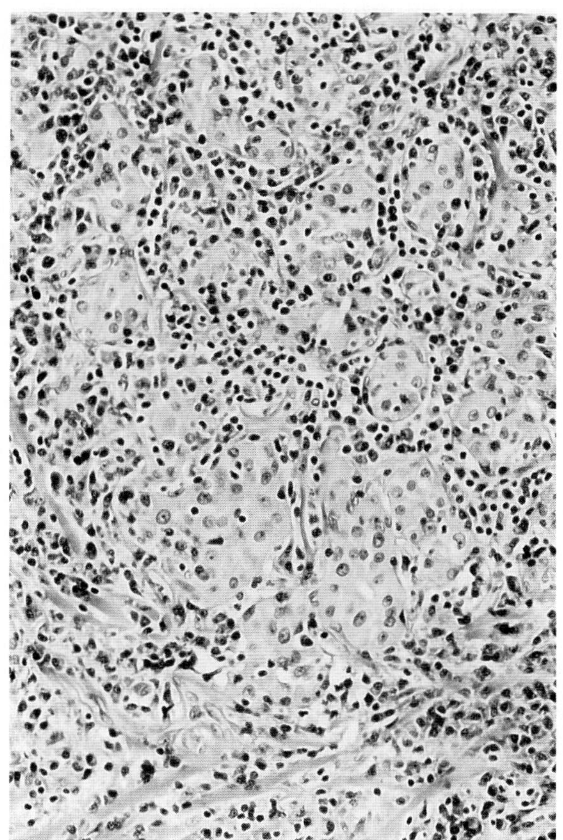

Figure 58–4. Hashimoto's autoimmune thyroiditis, showing marked lymphocytic infiltration and loss of thyroid follicles. Residual thyroid follicular epithelial cells are enlarged and have abundant cytoplasm (Hurthle cells).

present with gradual enlargement of the thyroid that may raise a suspicion of neoplasm.

Thyroid function at the time of presentation is variable. Patients are commonly either euthyroid (normal hormone levels) or mildly hypothyroid. Rarely, there is mild hyperthyroidism in the early phase. In most cases, the disease progresses with increasing degrees of hypothyroidism.

Thyroid autoantibodies can be detected in the serum of almost all patients. High titers of these antibodies are diagnostic of Hashimoto's disease. Moderate titers may be present in patients with Graves' disease, multinodular goiter, and thyroid neoplasms, and low levels are seen in 50% or more of elderly males and 90% of elderly females.

Treatment of Complications

Without treatment, Hashimoto's disease progresses to primary hypothyroidism. Thyroid replacement therapy is effective in maintaining the euthyroid state.

About 5% of patients with long-standing Hashimoto's disease develop malignant neoplasms of the thyroid, either papillary carcinoma or malignant B cell lymphoma.

INFLAMMATORY THYROID DISEASES

1. SUBACUTE THYROIDITIS

Subacute thyroiditis—also called granulomatous thyroiditis and DeQuervain's thyroiditis—is an uncommon inflammatory condition of the thyroid. It affects both sexes and all ages.

A viral origin is considered most likely. Thyroid inflammation frequently follows upper respiratory infection. Viruses that have been implicated include adenoviruses, mumps virus, echovirus, influenza virus, Epstein-Barr virus, and—most consistently—coxsackieviruses. However, neither culture nor electron microscopy has demonstrated the virus in affected thyroid.

Autoimmunity has also been suggested as a possible mechanism but is considered an unlikely one since antithyroid antibodies are present only transiently in a few patients. Subacute thyroiditis has no relationship to either Graves' disease or Hashimoto's thyroiditis.

Pathology

The thyroid is diffusely enlarged, firm, and often adherent to surrounding structures. Microscopically, there is extensive destruction and fibrosis of thyroid follicles with aggregates of macrophages and giant cells around fragments of colloid.

Clinical Features

There is acute onset of painful enlargement of the thyroid, often associated with fever, malaise, and muscle aches. Most patients are euthyroid but in a few cases there is a transient hyperthyroidism, due probably to the sudden release of hormone from the damaged gland.

The disease is self-limited and does not lead to hypothyroidism.

2. RIEDEL'S THYROIDITIS

Riedel's thyroiditis is a rare chronic disorder occurring in older patients, with women being affected more frequently than men.

Thyroid autoantibodies are usually not present. Riedel's thyroiditis is sometimes associated with similar fibrosing lesions in the retroperitoneum and mediastinum, suggesting that it may be a systemic disorder involving fibroblasts.

Pathology

The gland is usually mildly enlarged and replaced wholly or in part by stony hard, grayish-white fibrous tissue ("woody" or "ligneous" thyroiditis), which extends beyond the capsule.

Microscopically, there is atrophy of thyroid follicles, which are replaced by dense scarlike collagen. Scattered lymphocytes and plasma cells are present.

Clinical Features

Clinically and at surgery, Riedel's thyroiditis resembles a malignant neoplasm of the thyroid. It presents with painless rock-hard enlargement of the thyroid. The fibrosis may constrict the trachea, producing dyspnea and stridor; the esophagus, causing dysphagia; or the recurrent laryngeal nerve, causing hoarseness. Patients are usually euthyroid.

Treatment is difficult. In most cases the disorder causes slowly increasing fibrosis of the neck structures.

DIFFUSE NONTOXIC & MULTINODULAR GOITER

Diffuse nontoxic and multinodular goiter represent the culmination of mild deficiency of thyroid hormone production, followed by feedback increase of TSH secretion by the pituitary, which results in thyroid hyperplasia. Hyperplasia of the gland corrects the hormone deficiency and maintains the euthyroid state at the expense of thyroid enlargement. There is therefore a fine balance between thyroid hormone output, TSH secretion, and thyroid enlargement. (Note that "goiter" means enlargement of the thyroid gland due to any cause.)

Etiology

The basic cause of diffuse nontoxic and multinodular goiter is failure of normal thyroid hormone synthesis.

A. Endemic Goiter: Endemic goiter is the result of chronic dietary deficiency of iodine. It occurs mainly in inland mountainous regions of the world such as the Alps, Andes, and Himalayas and inland regions of Asia and Africa away from coastal waters. In these populations, up to 5% of individuals may have thyroid enlargement, sometimes massive. Endemic goiter is not common in coastal communities because of the high iodine content of seawater and seafood. Endemic goiter is more common in women, because of increased iodine requirements in pregnancy and lactation.

The incidence of endemic goiter decreased greatly in countries such as the United States and Western Europe after iodization of common table salt was instituted.

Much less commonly, goitrogens are responsible for endemic goiter. Goitrogens are dietary factors that block thyroid hormone synthesis. They are found in plants such as cabbage and cassava and have been identified as a cause of goiter in South America, Netherlands, and Greece.

B. Sporadic Goiter: Sporadic goiter may occur anywhere and is usually due to increased physiologic demand for thyroxine at puberty or during pregnancy (also called physiologic goiter). Less commonly, sporadic goiter may result from mild deficiency of enzymes involved in thyroid hormone synthesis. Abnormalities relating to synthesis of thyroid-binding globulin may cause goiter because excess TBG in plasma decreases delivery of free hormone to the periphery. In some patients, no cause can be identified.

Pathology

Changes in the thyroid gland progress through diffuse enlargement (diffuse nontoxic goiter) to multinodular goiter (Fig 58–5). Nodularity is the result of alternating periods of hyperplasia during times of iodine deficiency and involution, when dietary iodine levels increase.

In the early stages, diffuse hyperplasia is induced by excess TSH stimulation (in response to a reduced hormone output by the gland). Small follicles lined by tall columnar cells resemble the microscopic changes of Graves' disease. (The term diffuse nontoxic goiter is used for this stage because the patient is clinically euthyroid.) Involution follows, due probably to transient phases of adequate iodine intake (the thyroid hormone output rises, TSH falls). The follicles become distended with colloid, and the lining epithelial cells become flattened or cuboidal. These changes are not uniform, and there may be a mixture of colloid-filled large follicles and small hyperplastic follicles. At this stage, the thyroid is enlarged, and its cut surface appears gelatinous and glistening

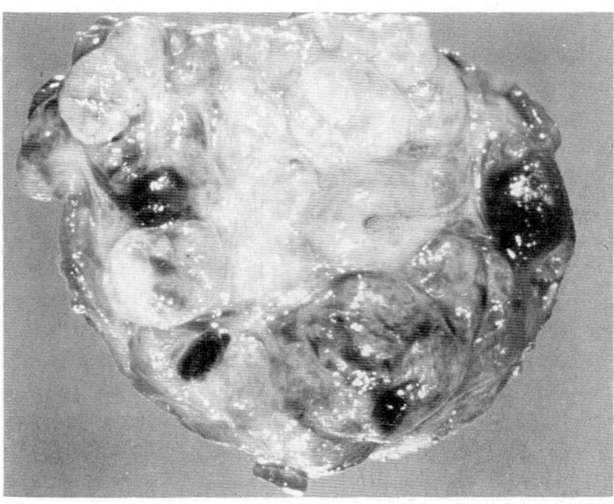

Figure 58–5. Multinodular goiter, showing part of a massively enlarged gland containing multiple nodules of varying size, some showing hemorrhage.

owing to its colloid content (also called diffuse colloid goiter).

Repeated episodes of hyperplasia and involution over a long period result in a markedly enlarged multinodular goiter. In endemic areas, it is not uncommon to see goiters hanging to the chest. Multinodular goiter is characterized by nodules composed of colloid-filled enlarged follicles, areas of hyperplasia in which small follicles are lined by active epithelium, fibrosis, areas of hemorrhage, cystic degeneration, fibrosis, and calcification.

Clinical Features

Patients present with painless diffuse enlargement of the thyroid. As the disease progresses, the thyroid becomes larger and more nodular. Patients are euthyroid as a rule. The most common reason for surgical treatment is that the mass is cosmetically unacceptable. In a few patients, the presence of a dominant nodule may mimic a neoplastic process.

Abnormal thyroid hormone production may rarely occur in multinodular goiter. Hyperthyroidism is commoner than hypothyroidism and is due to the development of autonomous hyperplastic nodules in the gland (toxic nodular goiter). Hypothyroidism results when thyroid hyperplasia cannot compensate for severe deficiency of hormone synthesis.

The risk of development of carcinoma in a multinodular goiter is small.

Treatment

In the earliest stage, providing iodine or thyroxine will remove the TSH stimulus and result in cessation of the hyperplastic process. In the later stages, where gland enlargement has resulted in a large neck mass, surgery is the treatment of choice.

THYROID NEOPLASMS (Fig 58-6)

SOLITARY THYROID NODULE

The solitary thyroid nodule is a common clinical problem that deserves special consideration before a discussion of thyroid neoplasia is undertaken.

In studies on autopsy material, it is found that 4–12% of all patients have small thyroid nodules; clinical studies have shown that careful palpation of the thyroid reveals the presence of thyroid nodules in 4–7% of cases. Having detected a nodule clinically, the question is what to do about it.

A solitary thyroid nodule is malignant in less than 5% of cases. About 30% of solitary nodules are benign follicular neoplasms (adenomas). The remainder represent nonneoplastic lesions such as Hashimoto's thyroiditis, early nodular goiter (colloid nodule), subacute thyroiditis, or normal thyroid. The physician's task is to identify those nodules that have a high likelihood of being carcinoma.

Fine-needle aspiration is probably the best method of evaluating a solitary thyroid nodule and is quite accurate in identifying papillary and anaplastic carcinomas of the thyroid. It is less accurate in distinguishing follicular carcinoma from follicular adenoma or a cellular portion of nodular goiter.

Thyroid scan is less reliable than fine-needle aspiration. Thyroid neoplasms, including carcinoma, usually take up iodine less avidly than the surrounding normal thyroid ("cold nodule"). However, some thyroid neoplasms take up radioiodine and appear as "hot" nodules, and many other types of nodules—including those of nodular goiter and Hashimoto's thyroiditis—are cold; about 20% of cold nodules turn out to be carcinomas.

FOLLICULAR ADENOMA

Follicular adenoma of the thyroid is the commonest neoplasm of the thyroid, accounting for about 30% of all cases of solitary thyroid nodules. It may occur at any age; females are affected 4 times as frequently as males.

Pathology

Grossly, thyroid adenomas present as a solitary, firm gray or red nodule up to 5 cm in diameter (Fig 58-7); hemorrhage, fibrosis, calcification, and cystic degeneration may be present.

Microscopically, follicular adenomas are usually composed of follicles of varying size (microfollicular adenoma; macrofollicular adenoma). Less often, solid cords of thyroid epithelial cells form only rudimentary follicular structures (embryonal adenoma). Other adenomas are composed of cells with abundant pink granular cytoplasm (Hürthle cell adenoma). The cytologic features of adenomas are usually uniform; a few adenomas, however, show cellular pleomorphism and atypia (atypical adenoma).

Follicular adenomas are surrounded by a complete fibrous capsule of varying thickness, and the normal thyroid parenchyma around the adenoma is compressed (Fig 58-8). The capsule is intact, and there is no vascular invasion. Absence of capsule and vascular invasion are the criteria used to differentiate follicular adenoma from follicular carcinoma.

Clinical Features, Diagnosis, & Treatment

Patients are usually euthyroid. Thyroid scan shows the presence of a circumscribed cold nod-

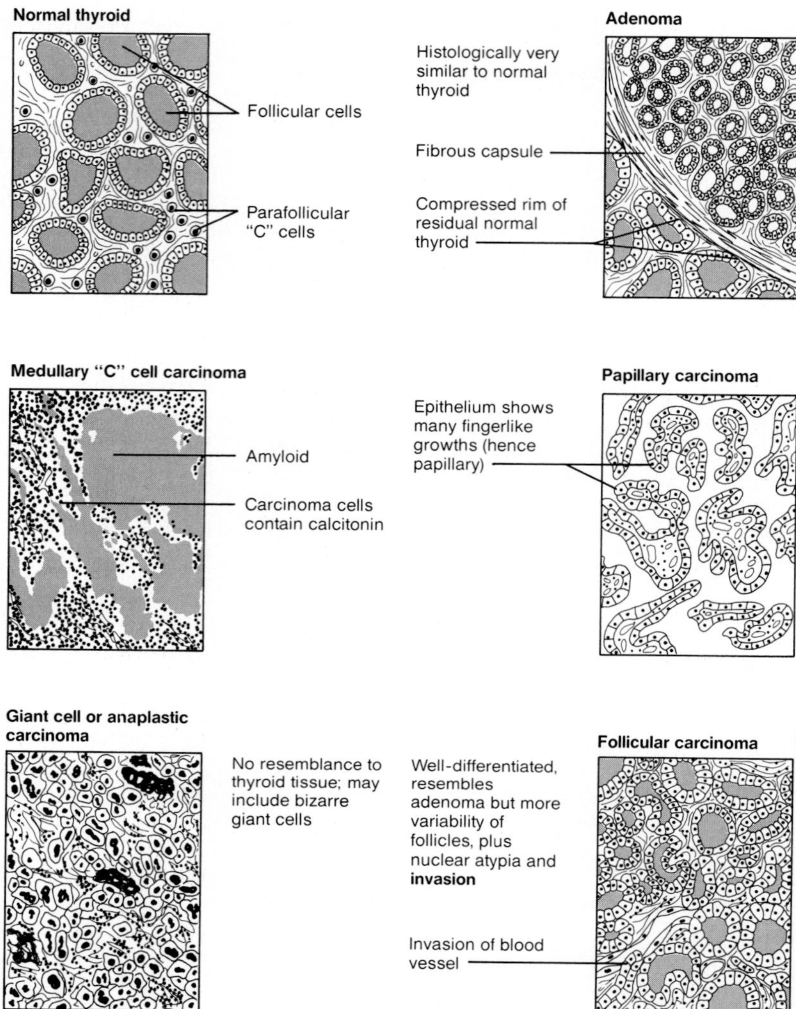

Figure 58-6. Common thyroid neoplasms, showing basic pathologic features.

ule. Fine-needle aspiration usually shows a cellular smear with many microfollicles. Rare "toxic" adenomas produce sufficient hormone to cause hyperthyroidism.

In the initial phases, an adenoma may be dependent for its continued growth on TSH and can theoretically be treated by suppression of TSH (with exogenous thyroid hormone). Later, such tumors become autonomous and are difficult to control. Furthermore, there are no laboratory tests that permit absolute differentiation of an adenoma from a thyroid carcinoma short of surgical removal and complete pathologic evaluation. For these reasons, thyroid adenomas are excised surgically.

CARCINOMA OF THE THYROID

Thyroid cancer is uncommon, with an incidence in the United States of about 25–30 cases per million population. It is responsible for about 2000 deaths per year, or 0.5% of all cancer deaths in the United States. Thyroid cancer affects females about 3 times as frequently as males.

The incidence has increased greatly in the last 50 years, probably as a result of increased exposure to radiation. Radiation-induced thyroid carcinoma is most commonly of the papillary or follicular type.

Two types of radiation are known to cause thyroid cancer:

A. Therapeutic Radiation: External neck radiation was used in the 1950s for treatment of thymic enlargement, which was believed incorrectly to cause respiratory distress in infants. About 5% of all infants so treated developed thyroid cancer 15–40 years later.

B. Nuclear Mishaps: Radioactive isotopes of iodine are selectively taken up by the thyroid and lead to thyroid cancer—again, 15–40 years after exposure. The population exposed to the Hiro-

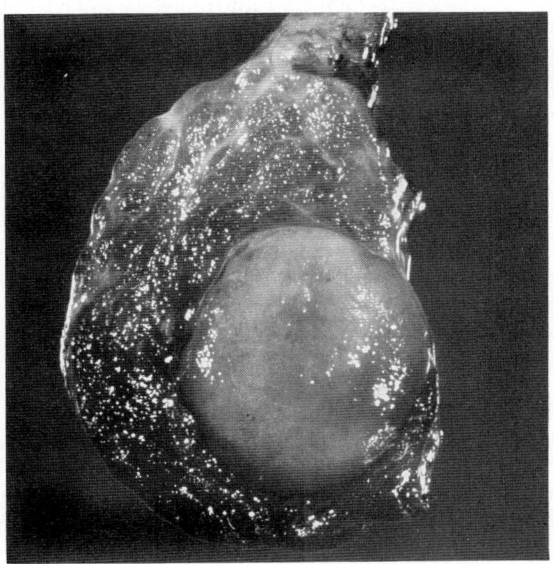

Figure 58-7. Follicular adenoma, showing a well-encapsulated solitary nodule in the thyroid. Microscopic evaluation is necessary to rule out carcinoma.

shima and Nagasaki atomic bombs—and the Marshall Islanders who were exposed to nuclear test explosions in the South Pacific—had an incidence of thyroid cancer of 5–10%. More recently, the nuclear power accident at Chernobyl in the Soviet Union has put a large population at risk.

Pathology

Thyroid carcinoma is classified on the basis of its microscopic appearance into 4 types (Fig 58–6 and Table 58–3). Three of these—papillary, follicular, and anaplastic—are derived from thyroid follicular epithelium. Medullary carcinoma is distinct and arises from calcitonin-secreting C cells. Mixed papillary and follicular carcinomas also occur but behave exactly like pure papillary carcinoma.

A. Papillary Carcinoma: Papillary carcinoma is the most common type (Table 58–3). It affects females 3 times more commonly than males; younger individuals in the age range 15–35 years are predominantly affected.

Grossly, papillary carcinomas range from microscopic lesions to large masses over 10 cm in diameter. They are usually infiltrative lesions, but a small number appear as circumscribed nodules.

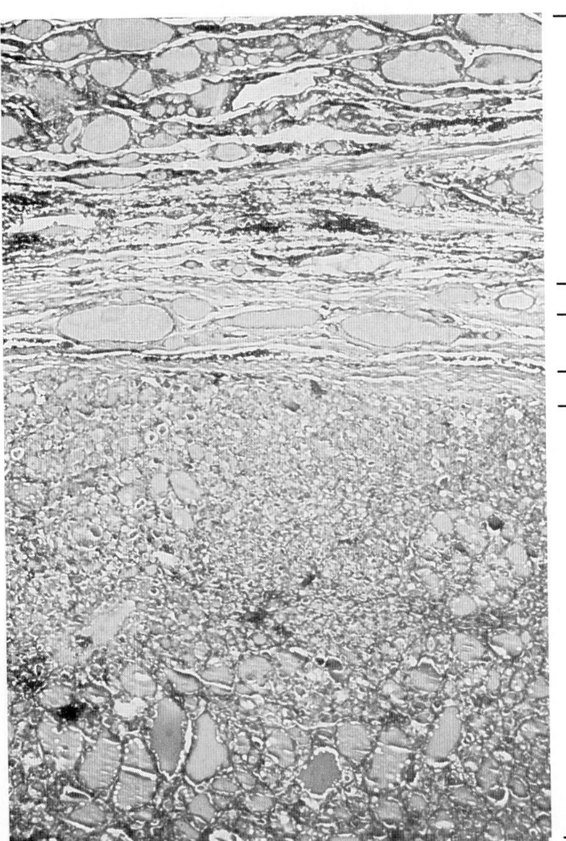

Figure 58-8. Follicular adenoma, showing microfollicular structure of the neoplasm, a thin fibrous capsule, and compressed normal thyroid.

Table 58-3. Differential features of thyroid carcinomas.

Neoplasm	Cell of Origin	Frequency[1]	Age/Sex Incidence	Local Features	Lymphatic Metastasis	Blood-Borne Metastasis	5-Year Survival Rate	Tumor Markers
Papillary carcinoma	Follicular epithelial cell	70%	F > M = 3:1 15–35 yrs	Infiltrative masses; multifocal and bilateral; lymph nodes often +	+ + +	Late/ uncommon	90%	Thyroglobulin
Follicular carcinoma	Follicular epithelial cell	20%	F > M all ages; > 30 yrs	May be grossly infiltrative or "encapsulated" angioinvasive	+	+ + +	65%	Thyroglobulin
Anaplastic carcinoma	Follicular epithelial cell	5%	F > M; > 50 yrs	Massively infiltrating locally	+ + +	+ + +	0%	None
Medullary carcinoma	Parafollicular or "C" cell	5%	F = M; 30–60 yrs	Slowly growing mass; infiltrative	+	+	50%	Calcitonin

[1]Percentages relate to frequency among thyroid carcinomas.

Microscopically, they are characterized by (1) an arrangement of cells in papillary structures (Fig 58–9); (2) clear nuclei—resembling the eyes of the cartoon character Orphan Annie—which are virtually diagnostic of papillary carcinoma even though they represent an artefact produced by formalin fixation; (3) intranuclear inclusions caused by cytoplasmic invaginations into the nucleus; and (4) psammoma bodies, which are round, laminated, calcified bodies that are present in about 40% of papillary carcinomas.

Papillary carcinomas grow very slowly. They commonly spread by local invasion, and most have invaded the thyroid capsule at the time of presentation. Lymphatic spread produces additional intraglandular foci of papillary carcinoma; in over 60% of cases, foci of tumor are present in the opposite lobe. Cervical lymph node metastases—once mistakenly thought to be nodules of congenitally "aberrant" thyroid—are present in 40% of cases of papillary carcinoma at the time of presentation. Bloodstream dissemination is rare in papillary carcinoma.

B. Follicular Carcinoma: Follicular carcinomas comprise 20% of thyroid carcinomas. Again, females are affected more commonly than males. All ages are vulnerable, but the disease is more common in middle age.

Grossly, follicular carcinoma may be indistinguishable from adenoma ("encapsulated" follicular carcinoma) or it may form a large infiltrative mass. Microscopically, follicular carcinomas are composed of follicles of varying size lined by thyroid epithelial cells that resemble normal thyroid cells. Rarely, cells have clear cytoplasm (clear-cell variant) or are composed of Hürthle cells (Hürthle cell carcinoma). Solid areas composed of cells showing cytologic atypia, pleomorphism, and increased mitotic activity are common. The diagnosis of carcinoma depends on the presence of invasion of the capsule or vascular structures (Fig 58–10).

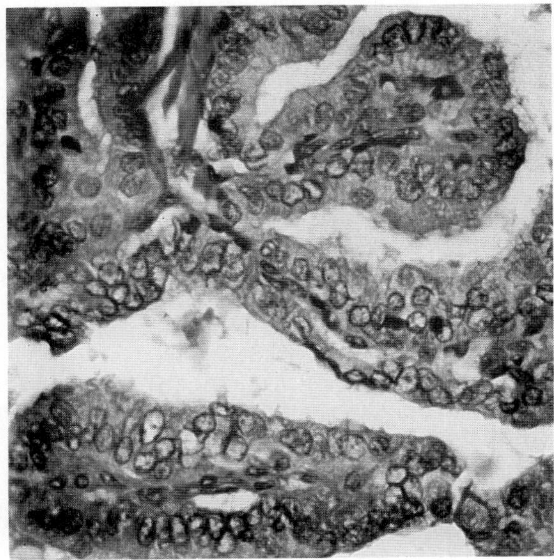

Figure 58–9. Papillary carcinoma, showing typical papillary structures composed of a fibrovascular core and lined by enlarged epithelial cells. Note that many of the cells have enlarged, clear nuclei.

Follicular carcinoma is a slowly growing neoplasm that may, however, spread via the bloodstream at an early stage, producing metastases in bone and lungs. Lymphatic metastasis to cervical nodes also occurs but to a lesser extent than in papillary carcinoma.

C. Anaplastic Carcinoma: Anaplastic carcinoma is rare, comprising 5% of thyroid carcinomas. It occurs most commonly in patients over the age of 50 years.

Grossly, anaplastic carcinoma appears as a massive infiltrative lesion. It is hard, gritty, and grayish-white and frequently shows areas of necrosis and hemorrhage. Microscopically, it is composed of highly malignant-appearing spindle or giant cells, showing extreme pleomorphism and frequent mitotic figures.

Anaplastic carcinomas are highly malignant, rapidly growing neoplasms that disseminate extensively. Death usually occurs within a year after diagnosis and is mainly due to local invasion of neck structures.

D. Medullary Carcinoma: Medullary carcinoma is uncommon, accounting for about 5% of thyroid carcinomas. It is derived from the calcitonin-secreting parafollicular cells (C cells) of the thyroid. Ninety percent of medullary carcinomas occur as sporadic lesions; 10% are familial and may form part of the multiple endocrine neoplasia (MEN type II) syndrome (concurrence of medullary carcinoma of the thyroid, pheochromocytoma of the adrenal, and parathyroid adenoma; see Chapter 60). The familial form may be distinguished from the sporadic type by the occurrence of C cell hyperplasia in the residual noncancerous thyroid in the former.

Grossly, medullary carcinoma forms a hard, grayish-white infiltrative mass. Microscopically, it is composed of small spindle-shaped and polygonal cells arranged in nests, cords, and sheets (Fig 58–11). The stroma contains amyloid in most cases; the amyloid consists of calcitonin fragments (Chapter 2). Electron microscopy shows the presence of membrane-bound dense-core neurosecretory granules in the neoplastic cells and fibrillar amyloid material in the stroma.

Medullary carcinomas have a slow but progressive growth pattern. Local invasion of neck structures is common. Both lymphatic and bloodstream metastasis occurs.

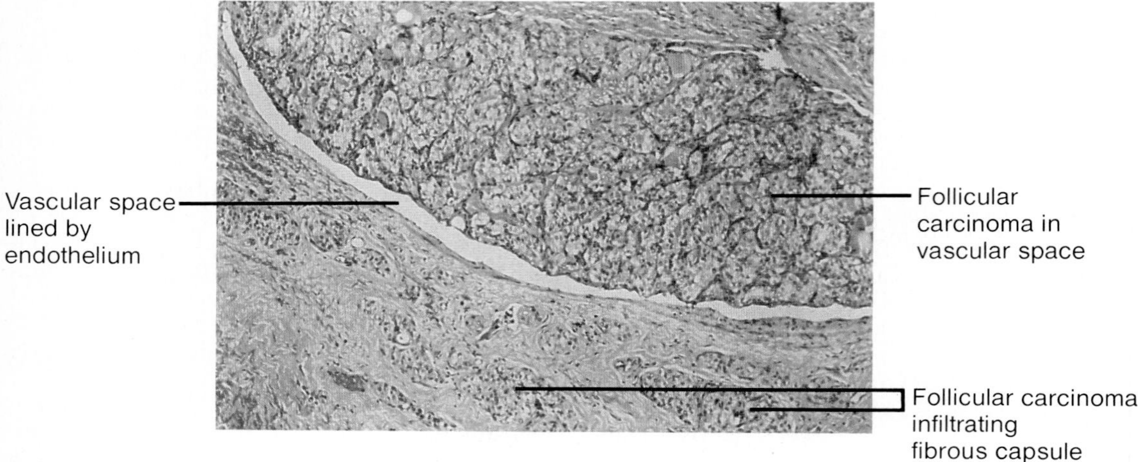

Figure 58-10. Follicular carcinoma, showing large vessel in the capsule of the neoplasm filled with tumor. Note also the irregular infiltration of the fibrous capsule by tumor.

Clinical Features (Fig 58-12)

Thyroid carcinomas commonly present with a painless solitary nodule in the thyroid. Thyroid scan commonly shows a lack of uptake (cold nodule). Fine-needle aspiration may be diagnostic of papillary carcinoma, medullary carcinoma, and anaplastic carcinoma, but the distinction of follicular carcinoma from follicular adenoma is not possible in most cases.

Patients with thyroid carcinoma are euthyroid as a rule. Very rarely, well-differentiated carcinomas secrete hormones and cause hyperthyroidism.

Important modes of presentation of thyroid carcinoma are with local invasion of neck structures or distant metastases. In the case of papillary carcinoma, this is commonly in a cervical lymph node. In follicular carcinoma, the first manifestation of disease may be due to a metastasis in bone or lung.

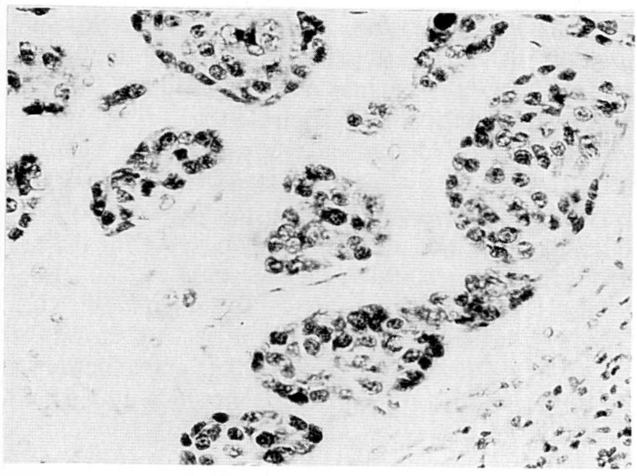

Figure 58-11. Medullary carcinoma of the thyroid. This is a section stained by immunoperoxidase for calcitonin, showing positive cytoplasmic staining in nests of neoplastic cells. The normal tissue comprising the stroma of the tumor is completely unstained.

Tumor Markers

Medullary carcinoma of the thyroid secretes calcitonin, which can be detected in the blood (by radioimmunoassay) and is useful in diagnosis and following response to treatment. Rarely, calcitonin production is sufficient to induce hypocalcemia. Identification of a thyroid carcinoma as medullary in type is facilitated by staining sections for calcitonin using immunoperoxidase methods (Fig 58-11).

Well-differentiated thyroid carcinomas (papillary and follicular types) form thyroglobulin, which can be demonstrated in tumor cells in histologic sections by immunoperoxidase techniques—useful in identifying a neoplasm as a thyroid carcinoma (Fig 58-13). However, not all thyroid carcinomas are positive. Small amounts of thyroglobulin, released by the tumor cells into the blood, can be detected by ultrasensitive assays for thyroglobulin. Thyroglobulin is also found in the blood after any form of damage to the thyroid.

Anaplastic carcinomas do not commonly stain for thyroglobulin and have no tumor markers in the blood.

Treatment & Prognosis

Surgery—either total thyroidectomy or thyroid lobectomy—is the primary mode of treatment for well-differentiated thyroid carcinoma and medullary carcinoma.

Well-differentiated papillary and follicular carcinomas are dependent on thyrotropin for growth. Suppression of TSH secretion by admin-

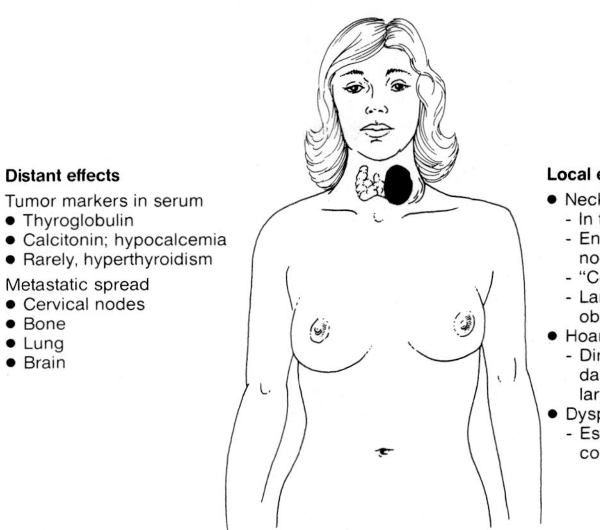

Figure 58-12. Clinical effects of thyroid carcinoma.

istration of thyroxine is effective in slowing neoplastic growth temporarily.

Well-differentiated papillary and follicular carcinomas also take up iodine. Administration of therapeutic doses of radioactive iodine provides an effective means of specifically radiating the tumor cells. It is important to stimulate tumor cells to maximum activity (with TSH) before administration of radioiodine.

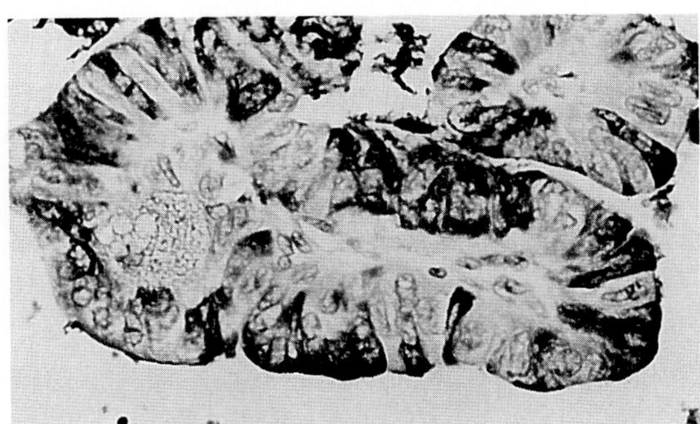

Figure 58-13. Papillary carcinoma of the thyroid stained for thyroglobulin by the immunoperoxidase technique, showing dark staining of the cytoplasm of most of the cells. Positive staining for thyroglobulin establishes the carcinoma as being of thyroid epithelial origin.

External radiation is useful for temporary control only but is the only feasible therapy for anaplastic carcinoma.

The prognosis of papillary carcinoma is good, with a 5-year survival rate of 90% and a 20-year survival rate of 85%. Even when metastases are present, patients survive for long periods after surgical excision. Follicular carcinoma has a 5-year survival rate of about 65% and a 20-year survival rate of 30%. The presence of distant blood-borne metastases is a bad prognostic sign. Medullary carcinoma has a 5-year survival rate of 50%. Anaplastic carcinoma is a highly malignant neoplasm, and most patients die within a year after diagnosis; the 5-year survival rate is almost nil.

MALIGNANT LYMPHOMA

Primary malignant lymphoma of the thyroid is extremely rare. It occurs mainly in elderly persons, particularly as a complication of Hashimoto's thyroiditis. The commonest type of malignant lymphoma is B-immunoblastic lymphoma.

59 The Parathyroid Glands

STRUCTURE & FUNCTION (Fig 59-1)

Normally, there are 4 parathyroid glands, situated in 2 pairs one above the other on the posterior aspect of the thyroid gland. In about 10% of individuals, the number exceeds 4, and rarely there are less. The inferior pair of parathyroids, which arise in the same branchial arch that gives rise to the thymus, may rarely descend into the mediastinum.

Grossly, each parathyroid gland is an encapsulated ovoid structure with a distinctive yellowish-brown color. Its maximal diameter is 5 mm and its weight is 35–40 mg.

Microscopically, the normal parathyroid contains 3 types of cells: chief cells, water-clear cells, and oxyphil cells. All 3 are believed to produce hormone, and their relative numbers are of little significance. Variable amounts of adipose tissue are interspersed between parenchymal cells; the amount of adipose tissue increases with age. Cells of the normal parathyroid gland contain cytoplasmic lipid granules that are absent in cells of hyperplastic and neoplastic parathyroid glands.

The parathyroid glands secrete parathyroid hormone (PTH), an 84-amino-acid polypeptide (MW 9500), which is synthesized on the parathyroid cell ribosome as a 115-amino-acid precursor, preproPTH. PTH is split off from preproPTH in the Golgi zone and secreted directly into the blood. In the blood and peripheral tissues, PTH undergoes final cleavage into N-terminal and C-terminal fragments. The N-terminal fragment is the active component, with a very short half-life; it is removed from the plasma by attachment to PTH receptors of target cell membranes, renal excretion, and degradation. The C-terminal fragment is inactive, with a molecular weight of 7000 and a long half-life. It is removed from plasma exclusively by renal excretion. Serum assays for PTH using radioimmunoassay measure chiefly the inactive C-terminal fragment. Newer assays are now available that measure the N-terminal and C-terminal fragments individually. N-terminal PTH assay has the most accurate correlation with the rate of PTH secretion by the gland.

PTH regulates the concentration of ionic calcium in plasma. Its main target cells are the renal tubular epithelial cells and osteoclasts in bone. PTH increases reabsorption of calcium in the distal tubules and decreases reabsorption of phosphate in the proximal tubule. It also stimulates renal activation of vitamin D, which in turn increases intestinal absorption of calcium. PTH increases bone resorption (releasing calcium and phosphate) by stimulating osteoclastic activity. This function of PTH requires the synergistic action of active vitamin D. It also increases collagenase activity in bone, causing breakdown of the bony matrix.

The overall effect of PTH is an increase in total and ionized plasma calcium and a decrease in plasma inorganic phosphate.

The action of PTH is dependent on combination with cell membrane receptors to cause activation of intracellular adenylate cyclase. The result is increased synthesis of cAMP, which mediates the physiologic actions of PTH.

The rate of PTH synthesis and secretion are controlled by the serum ionized calcium level (feedback regulation).

EXCESS PTH SECRETION (Hyperparathyroidism)

Hyperparathyroidism is defined as elevated serum PTH due to increased secretion. Primary hyperparathyroidism results from an intrinsic abnormality of the parathyroid gland. Secondary hyperparathyroidism is excessive secretion of PTH by a normal parathyroid gland in response to a lowered serum ionized calcium level.

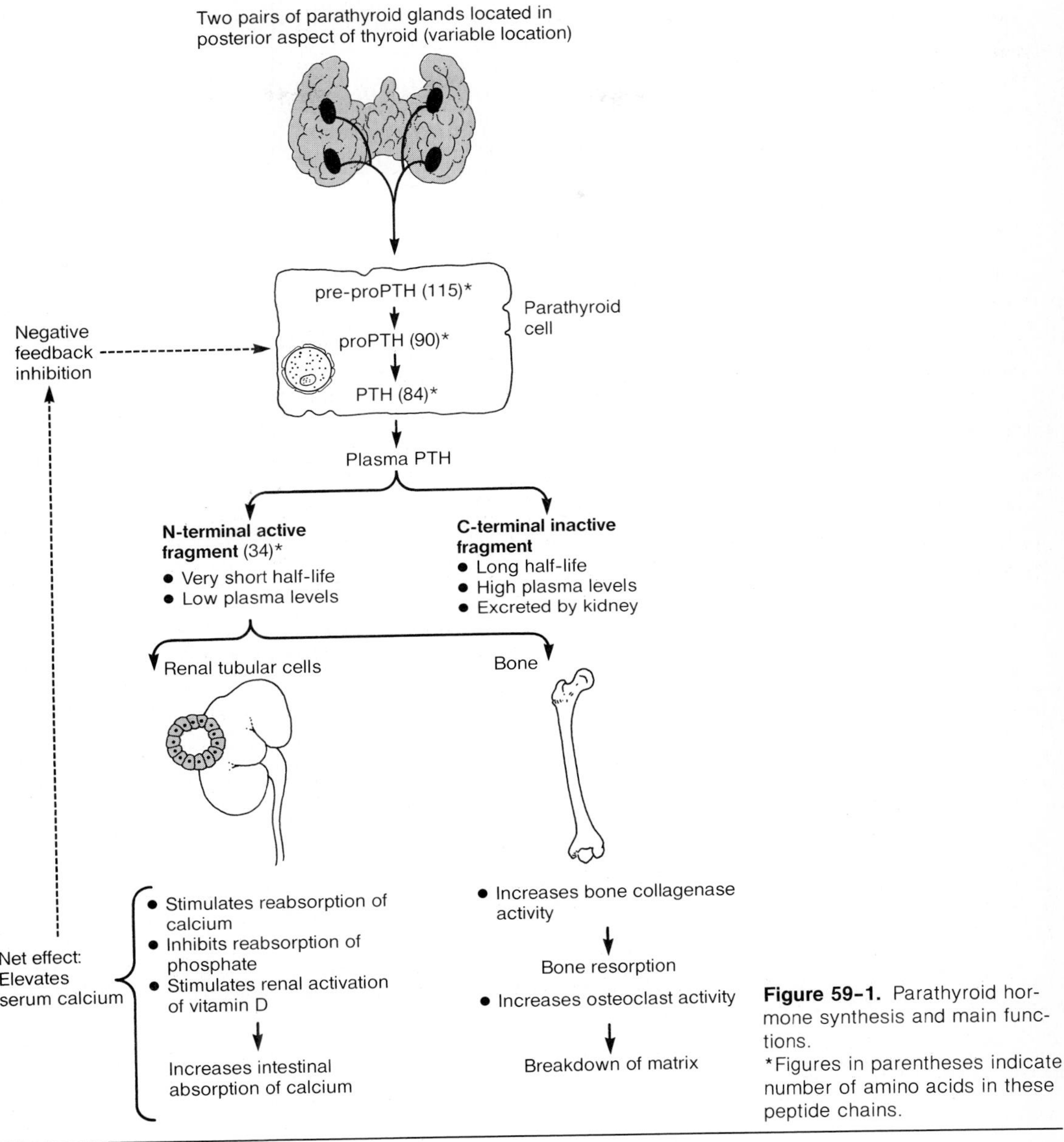

Figure 59–1. Parathyroid hormone synthesis and main functions.
*Figures in parentheses indicate number of amino acids in these peptide chains.

Primary hyperparathyroidism is most commonly due to a solitary adenoma involving one gland; less often, diffuse hyperplasia of all 4 glands occurs (Table 59–1). In about 10% of cases, the gross findings at surgery are atypical, with 2 or 3 slightly enlarged glands being found (Fig 59–2). These represent either irregular parathyroid hyperplasia or multiple adenomas.

Secondary hyperparathyroidism is a compensatory hyperplasia of all 4 glands aimed at correcting a lowered serum calcium. In most cases, serum calcium levels are corrected toward normal but are not elevated. Rarely, overcorrection occurs, and serum calcium levels exceed normal; the patient may then develop symptoms of hypercalcemia (so-called tertiary hyperparathyroidism).

Ectopic PTH Syndromes. PTH or PTH-like polypeptides may also be secreted by a variety of malignant neoplasms, producing a syndrome that is very similar to primary hyperparathyroidism. Squamous carcinomas of the lung, anocarcinomas of the kidney and endometrium, and bladder carcinoma are the common sources of ectopic PTH.

Pathology (Fig 59–2)

A. Parathyroid Adenoma: Parathyroid adenoma is a benign solitary neoplasm that involves

Table 59-1. Causes of hyperparathyroidism.

Primary hyperparathyroidism	
Single adenoma	80–90%
Multiple adenomas	1–4%
Diffuse hyperplasia	3–15%
Carcinoma	1–4%
Secondary hyperparathyroidism	
Chronic renal failure	
Malabsorption syndrome	
Vitamin D deficiency	
Medullary carcinoma of the thyroid	
Ectopic parathyroid hormone (PTH) syndromes[1]	
Squamous carcinoma of lung	
Renal adenocarcinoma	
Others	

[1]Most malignant neoplasms secrete a hormone that activates PTH receptors on target cells but does not cross-react with immunologic testing reagents used in PTH assays. These patients have high urinary cAMP levels (indicating activation of cells) and low (suppressed) plasma PTH levels associated with marked hypercalcemia.

one gland only; very rarely, multiple adenomas are present.

Grossly, parathyroid adenomas are usually small (commonly 1–2 cm in diameter and weighing 1–3 g) and may be difficult to locate at surgery. However, once located, they are well-encapsulated masses that are easily removed.

Microscopically, parathyroid adenomas are composed of a mixed population of chief, water-clear, and oxyphil cells, arranged in sheets, trabeculae, or glandular structures. The cells are usually small and uniform; rarely, there may be cytologic pleomorphism. Mitotic activity is very rare. There is no correlation between predominant cell type and hormone levels.

Parathyroid adenoma is differentiated from a normal gland by its increased size, the absence of fat in the mass, and the presence of a compressed rim of normal parathyroid tissue around the adenoma. In many parathyroid adenomas, there is no compressed rim of normal gland. In patients with a solitary adenoma, the other 3 parathyroid glands are normal in size and microscopic appearance.

B. Parathyroid Hyperplasia:

1. Primary hyperplasia–Primary hyperplasia of the parathyroid is hyperplasia of all 4 glands in

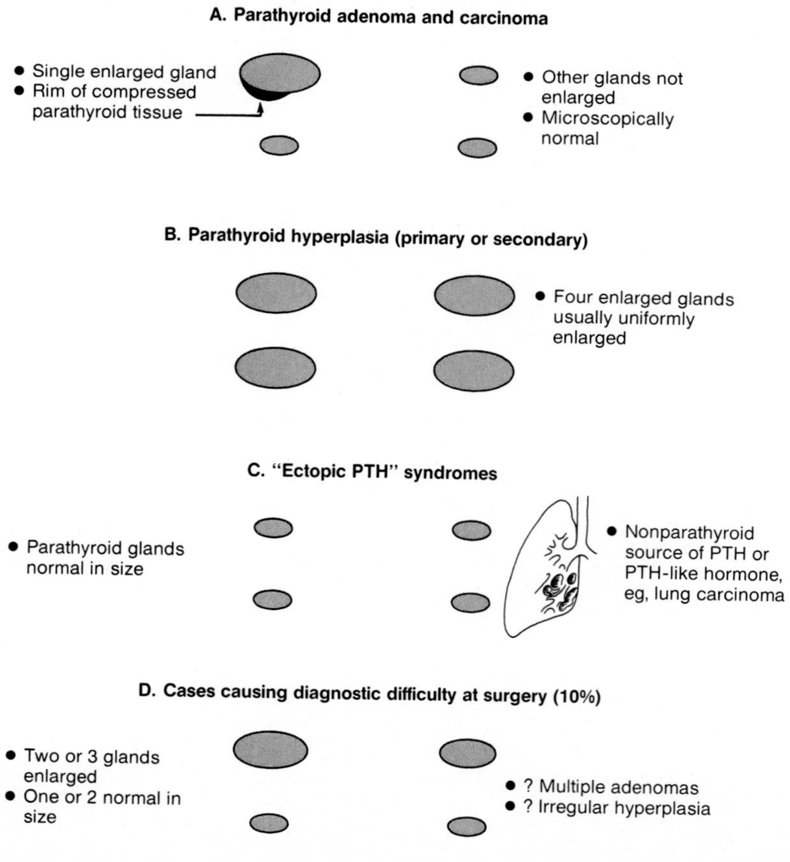

Figure 59-2. Operative findings in hyperparathyroidism. In cases that are atypical, where 2 or 3 glands are enlarged **(D),** the diagnosis is facilitated by biopsy of a normal-appearing gland. In adenoma, this will a histologically normal gland; in hyperplasia, it will be histologically abnormal.

the absence of a known inciting cause. Hyperplasia usually affects all glands equally; rarely, one or 2 glands are disproportionately enlarged. The most accurate method of diagnosis of hyperplasia is to demonstrate increased weight of all 4 glands above 40 mg each. Gland weight can be assessed at surgery by estimating the volume by measurement and multiplying the result by the specific gravity of 1.06.

Microscopically, parathyroid hyperplasia is characterized by proliferation of all 3 cell types at the expense of the intraglandular fat. The nature of the cells in hyperplasia is identical to that of an adenoma. Microscopic examination of a single enlarged gland does not permit differentiation of parathyroid adenoma from hyperplasia except in cases where a rim of compressed normal gland is present in an adenoma. Differentiation of hyperplasia from adenoma requires biopsy of a second parathyroid gland; in hyperplasia, the second gland is microscopically abnormal, whereas in adenoma the second gland is normal. Normality of the second gland is best established by demonstrating the presence of cytoplasmic lipid. Lipid is absent in hyperplastic and neoplastic parathyroid cells.

2. Secondary hyperplasia–The pathologic findings in secondary parathyroid hyperplasia are identical to those of primary hyperplasia.

C. Parathyroid Carcinoma: Carcinoma of the parathyroid is very rare. Patients with parathyroid carcinoma tend to have higher serum calcium and PTH levels. Carcinoma differs pathologically from adenoma in the following respects: (1) carcinoma tends to infiltrate outside the capsule, so that it is difficult to remove at surgery; (2) there is a high mitotic rate; and (3) broad bands of collagen frequently are present in the substance of a carcinoma. The pathologic differentiation of parathyroid carcinoma from adenoma is difficult.

Parathyroid carcinoma tends to recur locally after excision. However, metastasis to regional lymph nodes or distant sites is the only proof of malignancy.

Clinical Features & Diagnosis (Figs 59-3 and 59-4)

A. Primary Hyperparathyroidism: Primary hyperparathyroidism is characterized by elevated serum PTH, elevated serum calcium, and decreased serum phosphate (Table 59-2 and Fig 59-3). The degree of elevation of serum calcium is

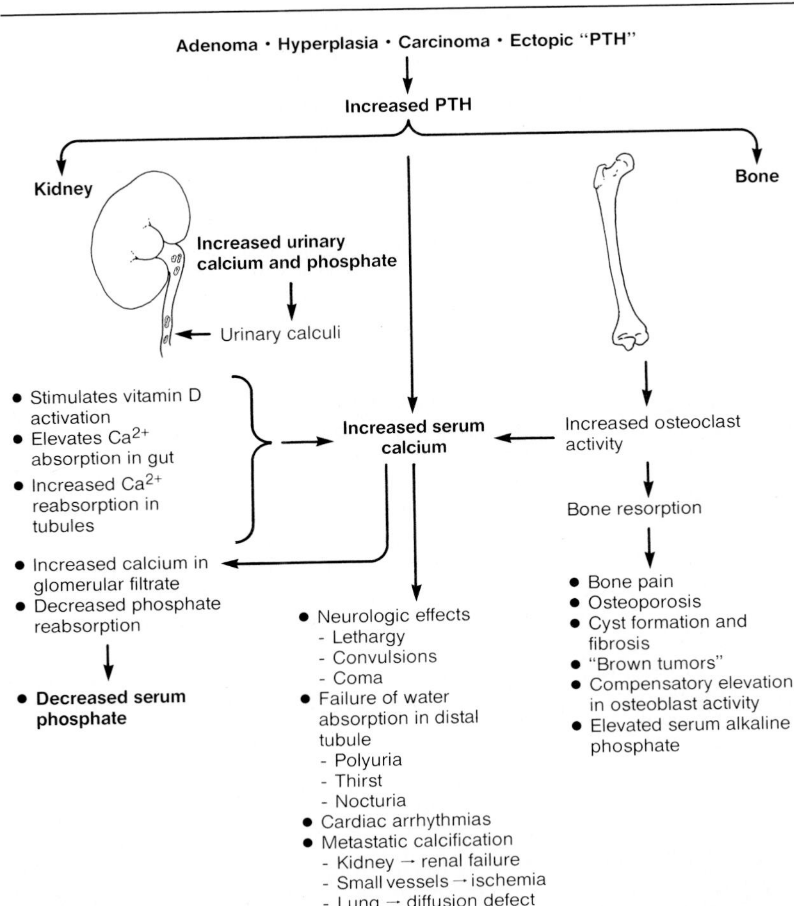

Figure 59-3. Clinicopathologic changes in primary hyperparathyroidism.

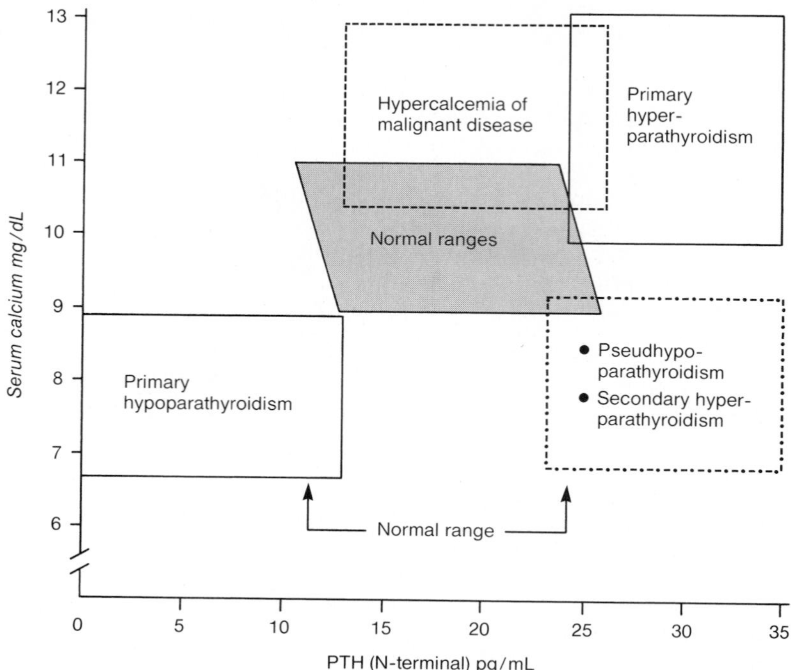

Figure 59-4. Changes in serum calcium and parathyroid hormone levels in parathyroid diseases.

usually not great, being in the 11–12 mg/dL range (normal, 9–11 mg/dL). However, when serum calcium and PTH levels are considered together, the PTH level is seen to be inappropriately increased. In rare patients with parathyroid carcinoma, serum calcium levels may be very high (15–20 mg/dL). One diagnostic pitfall is that there is reduced clearance of the inactive C-terminal fragment of PTH in patients with renal failure, causing falsely elevated total serum PTH. Determination of N-terminal PTH is therefore recommended for assessment of parathyroid function in patients with renal failure.

1. Urinary calculi–Urine calcium is increased owing to increased filtration of calcium, despite the fact that calcium reabsorption in the distal tubule is also increased. Phosphate excretion in urine is increased by direct PTH action. The result is an increased incidence of urinary calculi composed of calcium phosphate; 25% of patients with primary hyperparathyroidism present with renal calculi.

2. Metastatic calcification–Calcification occurs as a result of elevated serum levels of ionized calcium. Calcium is deposited in the renal interstitium (nephrocalcinosis), causing renal failure, and in the walls of small blood vessels throughout the body. When extensive, this may result in widespread ischemic changes.

Increased calcium levels also interfere with cellular function (1) in the distal convoluted tubule, resulting in inability to concentrate urine and causing polyuria, nocturia, and thirst; (2) in the nervous system, causing disturbances in levels of consciousness, convulsions, and coma; and (3) in the heart, producing arrhythmias and electrocardiographic abnormalities.

3. Bone changes–Bone changes are characteristic and may be the presenting feature. Increased bone resorption leads to osteoporosis, fibrosis of the intertrabecular zone, and cyst formation (osteitis fibrosa cystica). Compensatory osteoblastic proliferation causes elevation of serum alkaline phosphatase. "Brown tumors"—solid masses of osteoclastic giant cells, fibroblasts, and collagen—resemble giant cell tumor of bone in histologic appearance, but they are nonneoplastic. The brown color is due to hemorrhage and hemosiderin deposition.

B. Secondary Hyperparathyroidism: Secondary hyperparathyroidism usually is accompanied by normal or slightly decreased serum calcium with high PTH (Fig 59–4) and low serum phosphate levels. Bone changes caused by high PTH concentrations are similar to those seen in primary hyperparathyroidism. A few patients have high serum calcium levels and are liable to develop all the renal, vascular, and neurologic complications that are caused by hypercalcemia.

Treatment

Treatment of severe hypercalcemia is a medical emergency; death may occur from neurologic or cardiac dysfunction. Hydration with saline solution is usually adequate to control life-threatening hypercalcemia. Diuretics may also be used to in-

Table 59-2. Pathologic abnormalities in diseases associated with abnormal calcium and phosphorus metabolism.

	Size of Parathyroid Glands	Serum Ca	Serum Phosphate	Serum PTH	Alkaline Phosphatase	Urine Ca	Urine cAMP[1]	Comments
Primary Hyperparathyroidism Adenoma	Only 1 enlarged	↑	↓	↑	↑	↑	↑	Bone lesions and urinary calculi, peptic ulcer, metastatic calcification
Hyperplasia	All 4 large	↑	↓	↑	↑	↑	↑	Bone lesions and urinary calculi, peptic ulcer, metastatic calcification
Ectopic parathyroid hormone (PTH)	All 4 normal	↑↑	↓	↑[2]	N(↑)	↑	↑	Bone lesions, calculi rare; underlying malignant neoplasm
Secondary Hyperparathyroidism	All 4 large	N, ↑ or ↓	N(↓↑)	↑	N(↑)	N↑↓	↑	Features of underlying disease[3]
Other causes of hypercalcemia Lytic metastases to bone, including myeloma	All 4 normal	↑	↑	↓	↑	↑	↓	Caused by (a) bone lysis, (b) production of vitamin D-like molecule by tumor, (c) production of osteoclast-activating factor (myeloma).
Sarcoidosis	All 4 normal	↑	↑	↓	N(↑)	↑	↓	Systemic granulomas: hypersensitivity to vitamin D with high 1,25-$(OH)_2D_3$levels[4]
Vitamin D intoxication	All 4 normal	↑	↑	↓	N	↑	↓	Elevated 25(OH)D levels
Milk-alkali syndrome	All 4 normal	↑	↑	↓	N	↑	↓	Associated with alkalosis
Familial hypercalcemia with hypocalciuria	All 4 slightly enlarged	↑	↓	↑	N	↓	↑	Autosomal dominant
Hypoparathyroidism Idiopathic	All 4 normal	↓	↑	↓	N	N↓	↓	Metastatic calcification
Pseudo-	All 4 normal	↓	↑	N↑	N	N↓	↓	Albright's dystrophy

[1]Urine cAMP is increased when there is excessive renal cell stimulation by PTH or PTH-like hormones that combine with cell membrane PTH receptors.
[2]In some cases PTH-like hormone is not detected by PTH assays; PTH levels may then be decreased.
[3]Findings vary with underlying causal disease (see Table 59-1).
[4]Vitamin D is converted in the liver to 25(OH)D (hydroxycholecalciferol), which is further changed to biologically active 1,25-$(OH)_2D_3$ (dihydroxycholecalciferol) in the kidney; this latter step appears to be accelerated in sarcoidosis.

crease calcium excretion. High doses of glucocorticoids are useful in treating hypercalcemia resulting from vitamin D intoxication, sarcoidosis, and lytic metastatic bone tumors. Mithramycin inhibits bone resorption, but this toxic drug should only be used in the short term.

The definitive treatment of symptomatic hyperparathyroidism is surgery. If one gland is found to be enlarged and the others normal, the diagnosis of parathyroid adenoma may be made and the involved gland excised. Frozen section is required to confirm that tissue identified as parathyroid grossly actually does represent parathyroid tissue. If more than one gland is enlarged, a diagnosis of parathyroid hyperplasia is made, and $3\frac{1}{2}$ glands are removed. Parathyroid tissue may be preserved by snap freezing in liquid nitrogen so that it can be reimplanted in case hypoparathyroidism develops after surgery.

If a diagnosis of adenoma or hyperplasia cannot be made or if all 4 glands cannot be found in the neck, a search must be made for ectopic parathyroid tissue. Ectopic sites in which parathyroid glands are found include the mediastinum and within the capsule of the thyroid gland.

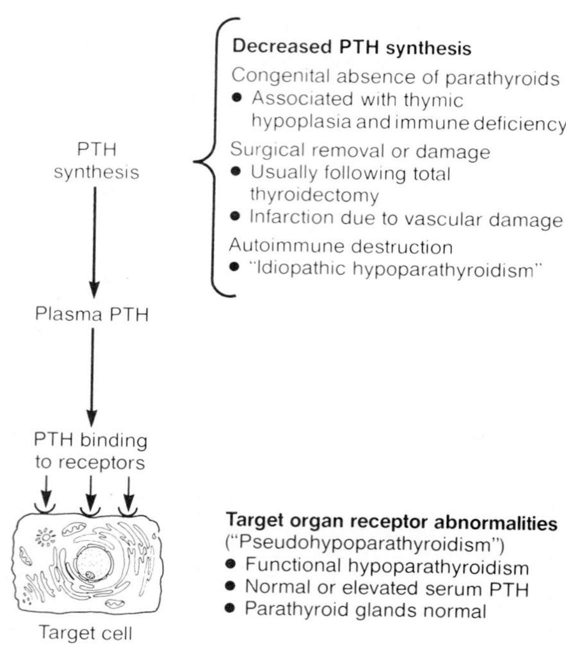

Figure 59–5. Etiology of hypoparathyroidism.

DECREASED PTH SECRETION (Hypoparathyroidism)

Etiology & Pathology (Fig 59–5)

A. Hypoparathyroidism Complicating Neck Surgery: Accidental removal of parathyroid glands during neck surgery is the commonest cause of hypoparathyroidism. Two to 10 percent of patients undergoing total thyroidectomy develop hypoparathyroidism after surgery.

It is not uncommon to have transient hypocalcemia after thyroidectomy even when the parathyroids have not been removed; this is believed to be due to transient parathyroid edema or ischemia. Permanent hypoparathyroidism may result from infarction of the glands caused by interference with their arterial supply during surgery.

B. Idiopathic Hypoparathyroidism: Idiopathic hypoparathyroidism is a rare disease with slight female predominance. It is believed to be the result of autoimmune destruction of the parathyroid cells. Parathyroid-specific autoantibodies are demonstrable in about 40% of patients, and there is an association with other autoimmune diseases such as pernicious anemia, Addison's disease, and Hashimoto's thyroiditis. Microscopically, there is atrophy of parathyroid cells, lymphocytic infiltration, and fibrosis.

C. Congenital Absence of Parathyroids: Absence of parathyroids most commonly occurs when there is a generalized failure of development of the third and fourth branchial arches. It is then associated with thymic agenesis and marked deficiency of cellular immunity (DiGeorge's syndrome; see Chapter 7). Patients with congenital absence of parathyroids present with hypocalcemia and convulsions soon after birth.

D. Pseudohypoparathyroidism: This term denotes a group of rare inherited disorders characterized by lack of end-organ response to PTH and in some instances due to abnormal PTH receptors. The term *pseudo*hypoparathyroidism is used because there is evidence of clinical hypoparathyroidism but serum PTH levels are normal. Examples of both autosomal and X-linked inheritance have been reported.

Pseudohypoparathyroidism is commonly associated with Albright's osteodystrophy, characterized by short stature, short neck, abnormally developed metacarpal and metatarsal bones, and subcutaneous ossification. These features provide clues to diagnosis. Rarely, these skeletal abnormalities are present in a patient who has no evidence of clinical hypoparathyroidism (sometimes called **pseudopseudohypoparathyroidism**).

Clinical Features & Diagnosis

Hypoparathyroidism is characterized by decreased serum levels of ionized calcium (Table 59–2 and Fig 59–4). This causes increased irritability of nerves, leading to numbness and tingling of the hands, feet, and lips and tetany. Tetany is manifested clinically as muscular spasms that first affect the hands and feet (carpopedal spasms). Laryngeal spasm may occur, leading to respiratory obstruction. Muscular contraction is easily stimulated by such maneuvers as (1) inflating a blood pressure cuff (to above systolic pressure for at least 3 minutes) to produce transient ischemia, which precipitates carpal spasms (Trousseau's sign); and (2) tapping the facial nerve at its exit at the stylomastoid foramen, which precipitates facial twitching (Chvostek's sign). With severe hypocalcemia, particularly in children, there are generalized convulsions.

Serum phosphate is increased because of defective renal excretion of phosphate when PTH is deficient. High phosphate levels are associated with deposition of calcium phosphate in tissues (metastatic calcification). Increased bone density, calcification of the basal ganglia, and mineral deposition in the lens to form cataracts may be seen in patients with hypoparathyroidism.

Treatment

Treatment of hypoparathyroidism consists of correction of the major metabolic abnormality, ie, hypocalcemia. This is most easily achieved by the administration of vitamin D analogues and by ensuring adequate intake of calcium in the diet. When serum calcium has reached normal levels, the dosage of vitamin D is adjusted to maintain it at these levels.

60 The Adrenal Cortex & Medulla

I. THE ADRENAL CORTEX

STRUCTURE & FUNCTION

The paired adrenal glands are situated in the retroperitoneum above the kidneys. They are variably shaped and irregularly folded, flattened structures whose cut surface reveals an outer yellow cortex and an inner gray medulla. The normal adrenals have an aggregate weight of about 6 g (the upper limit is 8 g).

The adrenal cortex is derived from the mesoderm of the urogenital ridge and has an origin independent of the adrenal medulla, which is derived from the neural crest.

The cortex is composed of the zona glomerulosa beneath the capsule (10–15%), the zona fasciculata (80%), and the zona reticularis (5–10%). The clinical effects of adrenal disease are quite predictable depending upon which part of the adrenal is hyper- or hypofunctioning (Fig 60–1). The zona glomerulosa secretes aldosterone and is controlled mainly by the renin-angiotensin mechanism, being independent of the pituitary. The zona fasciculata and reticularis secrete cortisol and androgenic hormones and are under the regulatory control of the pituitary via corticotropin (ACTH). ACTH secretion by the pituitary is under the control of (1) hypothalamic corticotropin-releasing factor (Chapter 57) and (2) the feedback inhibitory effect of serum cortisol.

Adrenocortical hormones are synthesized from cholesterol (Fig 60–2) by a series of enzyme-directed reactions.

CONGENITAL ADRENAL HYPERPLASIA

Congenital adrenal hyperplasia (adrenogenital syndrome) is a group of uncommon diseases that result from inherited deficiency of one of the several enzymes in the cortisol synthetic pathway (Fig 60–2). Decreased secretion of the end product (cortisol) stimulates, via the feedback mechanism, pituitary ACTH secretion, which in turn stimulates the zona fasciculata and reticularis to undergo bilateral hyperplasia and to secrete excessive amounts of precursor hormones. The clinical effects depend on the enzyme that is deficient and upon the products that accumulate prior to the block induced by the deficiency.

(1) Complete 21-hydroxylase deficiency (30%) is a severe disease manifested in early childhood by failure of cortisol and aldosterone secretion (Fig 60–3). There is marked sodium loss in urine, leading to severe hypotension (sometimes called salt-losing congenital adrenal hyperplasia). Increased androgen synthesis from the 17-hydroxyprogesterone that accumulates results in virilism in females.

(2) Partial 21-hydroxylase deficiency (60%) is the commonest of the group. 21-Hydroxylase levels are adequate to maintain normal aldosterone secretion under the renin-angiotensin stimulus, so

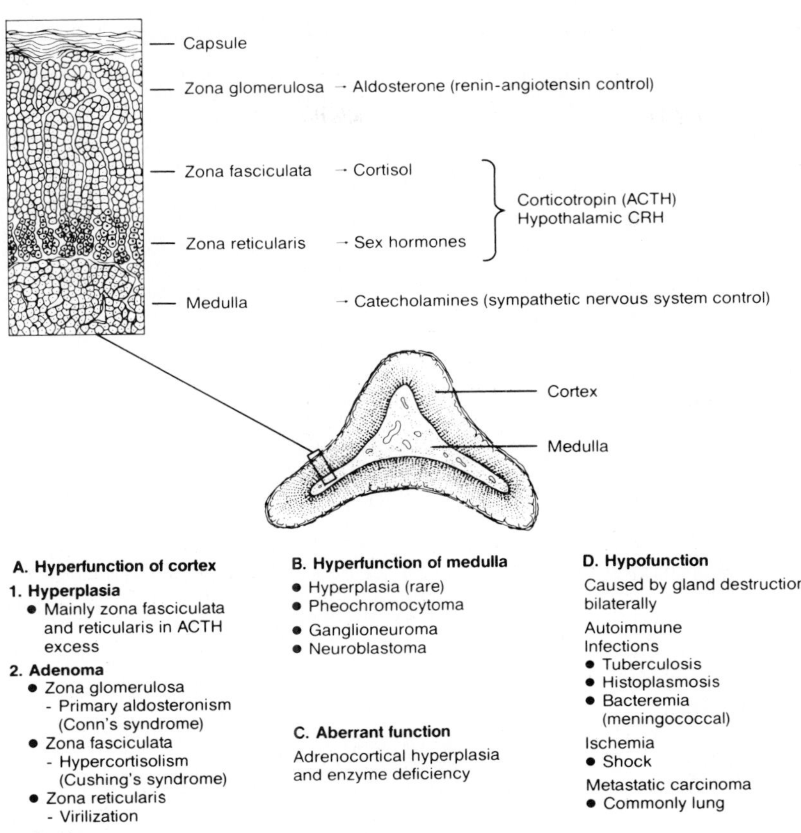

Figure 60–1. Principal diseases of the adrenal glands.

that there is no sodium loss. Cortisol levels are also normal, the tendency to hypocortisolism having been compensated by adrenal hyperplasia via increased pituitary ACTH levels.

The main effects of partial 21-hydroxylase deficiency are (1) adrenal hyperplasia; (2) high serum ACTH levels; and (3) increased secretion of androgens by the overstimulated zona reticularis, producing virilism in the female and precocious puberty in the male. Detection of elevated serum levels of 17-hydroxyprogesterone and androgens permit diagnosis.

(3) 11-Hydroxylase deficiency (5%) is rare. It causes the hypertensive form of congenital adrenal hyperplasia. The enzyme deficiency leads to accumulation of 11-deoxycortisol and deoxycorticosterone, both of which are strong mineralocorticoids that cause sodium retention in the kidneys and hypertension. Virilization due to androgen excess is also present as a result of increased ACTH stimulation of the zone reticularis.

(4) Other enzyme deficiencies, including desmolase deficiency, 17-hydroxylase deficiency, and 3β-dehydrogenase deficiency, are all extremely rare.

EXCESS SECRETION OF ADRENOCORTICAL HORMONES

EXCESS CORTISOL SECRETION (Cushing's Syndrome)

Cushing's syndrome is a relatively common clinical abnormality of the adrenal gland, usually affecting middle-aged individuals, women more often than men. It can be caused by several different disease processes (Table 60–1).

Pathology

A. Adrenocortical Adenoma: Grossly, adrenocortical adenomas appear as well-circumscribed nodular masses that are usually small (< 5 cm in greatest diameter and 5–50 g in weight; Fig 60–4). They usually have a bright yellow color and may show areas of cystic degeneration, fibrosis, and hemorrhage. The contralateral adrenal usually is atrophic.

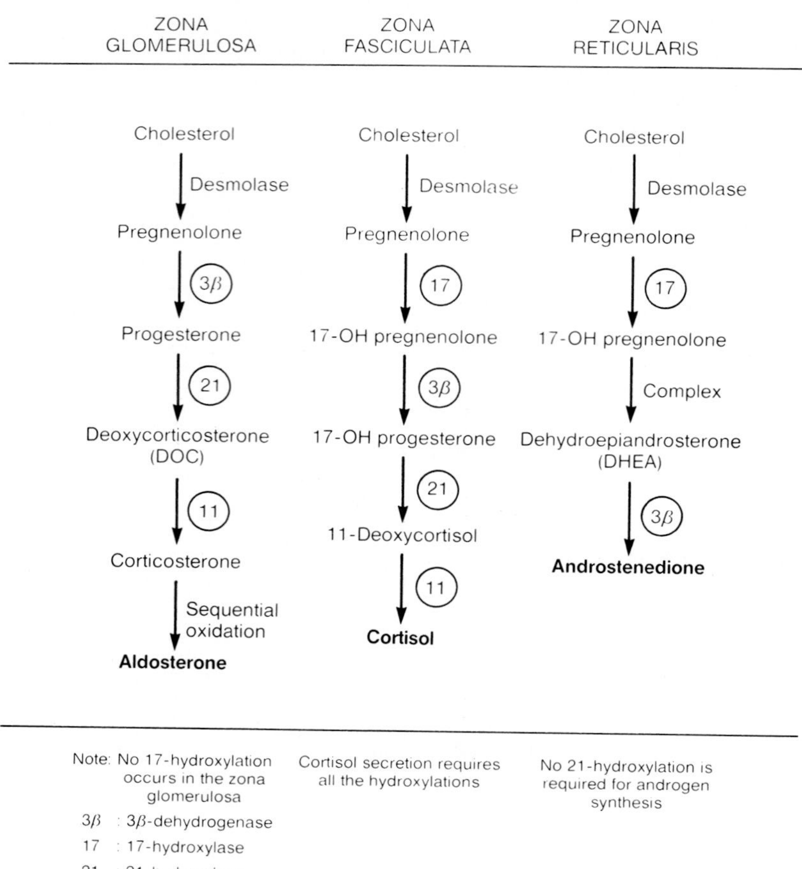

Figure 60–2. Simplified pathways of steroid synthesis in the different zones of the adrenal cortex. Note the differences in the types of enzyme necessary and the different order of enzymic reactions in the different zones.

Microscopically, adenomas are composed of uniform large cells arranged in nests and trabeculae. The cells have abundant lipid-filled cytoplasm and small uniform nuclei. Nuclear enlargement and pleomorphism are not uncommon, but mitotic figures are rare. They may show different functional attributes depending upon the precise "zone" of origin (Fig 60–1).

Not all adrenocortical adenomas produce hormones. Nonfunctioning adrenocortical adenomas are present in about 5% of all autopsies and are being increasingly detected as an incidental finding when abdominal CT scans are performed for other reasons. The diagnosis of functioning adrenocortical adenoma is best made by careful chemical assays for hormones in the serum before the adenoma is removed. Pathologic features of nonfunctioning adenomas and those that secrete different hormones are similar and do not allow diagnosis of specific hormone-secreting adenomas.

B. Adrenocortical Carcinoma: Adrenocortical carcinomas usually appear as large (> 6 cm and > 50 g), poorly circumscribed masses that commonly show infiltration of the kidney and perinephric fat. Gross involvement of the adrenal and renal vein by the neoplasm may occur.

Microscopically, adrenal carcinomas are composed of large, pleomorphic cells arranged in diffuse sheets. Mitotic figures are frequent and abnormal. Areas of necrosis, capsular invasion, and vascular invasion are common. The microscopic features permit accurate differentiation of adenoma and carcinoma.

Adrenal carcinoma behaves as a highly malignant neoplasm, metastasizing both to lymph nodes and via the bloodstream. Not all produce excess hormones; like adenomas, the pathologic features of nonfunctioning carcinomas are similar to those that secrete hormones.

C. Bilateral Adrenal Hyperplasia: Once thought to be a primary disorder of the adrenal, bilateral adrenal hyperplasia is now believed to be almost invariably secondary to increased ACTH production, whether from a pituitary adenoma or a malignant nonpituitary neoplasm (usually small-cell undifferentiated carcinoma of lung). Both adrenal glands are enlarged to greater than their aggregate upper weight limit of 8 g. Careful weigh-

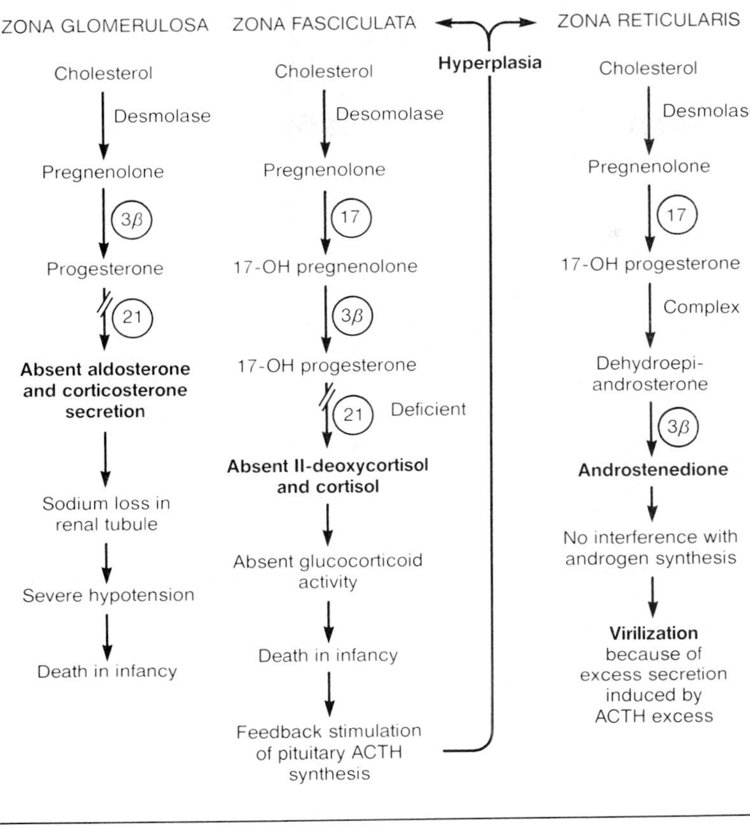

Figure 60–3. Pattern of abnormal steroid synthesis in a patient with complete 21-hydroxylase deficiency. Patients with complete 21-hydroxylase deficiency die in early life as a result of failure of synthesis of both mineralocorticoids and glucocorticoids. Note that partial 21-hydroxylase deficiency which is compatible with longer survival is more common.

ing of the adrenal removed at surgery or autopsy after all periadrenal connective tissue has been dissected away is the most reliable means of making a diagnosis of adrenal hyperplasia. The enlarged glands may be nodular or diffuse. Microscopically, the zona fasciculata and reticularis are greatly widened.

D. Iatrogenic Hypercortisolism: In cases where hypercortisolism is the result of exogenous glucocorticoid administration, both adrenal cortices show diffuse atrophy due to inhibition of pi-

Table 60–1. Etiology of excess cortisol secretion.

Iatrogenic
Glucocorticoid administered in high doses in the treatment of nonendocrine diseases
Noniatrogenic
Functioning adrenocortical neoplasms (25%)
Adenoma (20%)
Carcinoma (5%)
Bilateral adrenal hyperplasia (75%)
ACTH-secreting pituitary adenoma (60%)
ACTH-secreting nonpituitary neoplasms (ectopic ACTH syndrome; 15%)

ACTH = adrenocorticotropic hormone.

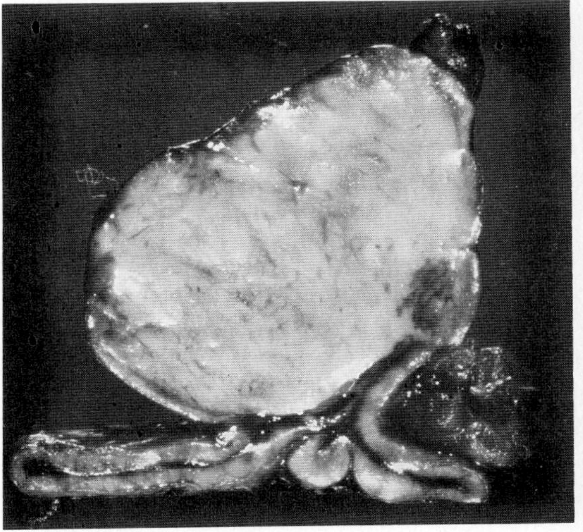

Figure 60–4. Cross section of adrenal, showing an adrenocortical adenoma in a patient with primary aldosteronism. The gross and microscopic features do not permit differentiation of aldosterone- and cortisol-secreting adenomas in most cases.

tuitary ACTH secretion by the exogenous steroids.

Clinical Features

Cortisol excess causes an extensive array of metabolic abnormalities (Fig 60–5):

(1) Redistribution of body fat from the extremities to the trunk results in moon facies and truncal obesity with thin extremities. Hypercholesterolemia and aggravated atherosclerosis also occur.

(2) The antagonistic effect of cortisol on the action of insulin produces diabetes mellitus.

(3) Protein catabolism is increased. Gluconeogenesis is stimulated by cortisol, leading to muscle wasting. Growth retardation occurs in children. Other consequences of increased protein catabolism include thinning of the skin with development of striae, easy bruising, and delayed wound healing. Decrease in the amount of the protein matrix of bone leads to osteoporosis.

(4) Cortisol has a significant mineralocorticoid action that results in retention of sodium in the distal renal tubule at the expense of potassium and hydrogen. Hypertension and hypokalemic alkalosis may occur as a result.

(5) Cortisol has an inhibitory effect on lymphocyte, macrophage, and neutrophil function, resulting in increased susceptibility to infections.

(6) Cortisol in excess has an effect on brain cells, and patients with Cushing's syndrome frequently have psychiatric symptoms such as euphoria, mania, and psychosis (steroid encephalopathy).

(7) Some degree of androgen excess coexists with cortisol excess in many patients, leading to hirsutism, acne, infertility, and menstrual disturbances in females.

Diagnosis (Table 60–2)

The first step in the diagnosis is to establish the presence of excess cortisol secretion. Plasma levels of cortisol and its metabolites, the 17-hydroxycorticosteroids, are high. The 24-hour urinary free cortisol level also is elevated. The diurnal rhythm of cortisol secretion is lost. Normally, cortisol secretion is maximal in the morning and reaches a nadir at night. One of the first abnormalities is the finding of a high cortisol level in a midnight sample. Once it has been established that a given patient has hypercortisolism, it is necessary to determine the cause (Table 60–2).

Treatment

Functioning adrenal neoplasms and pituitary neoplasms that produce ACTH are surgically re-

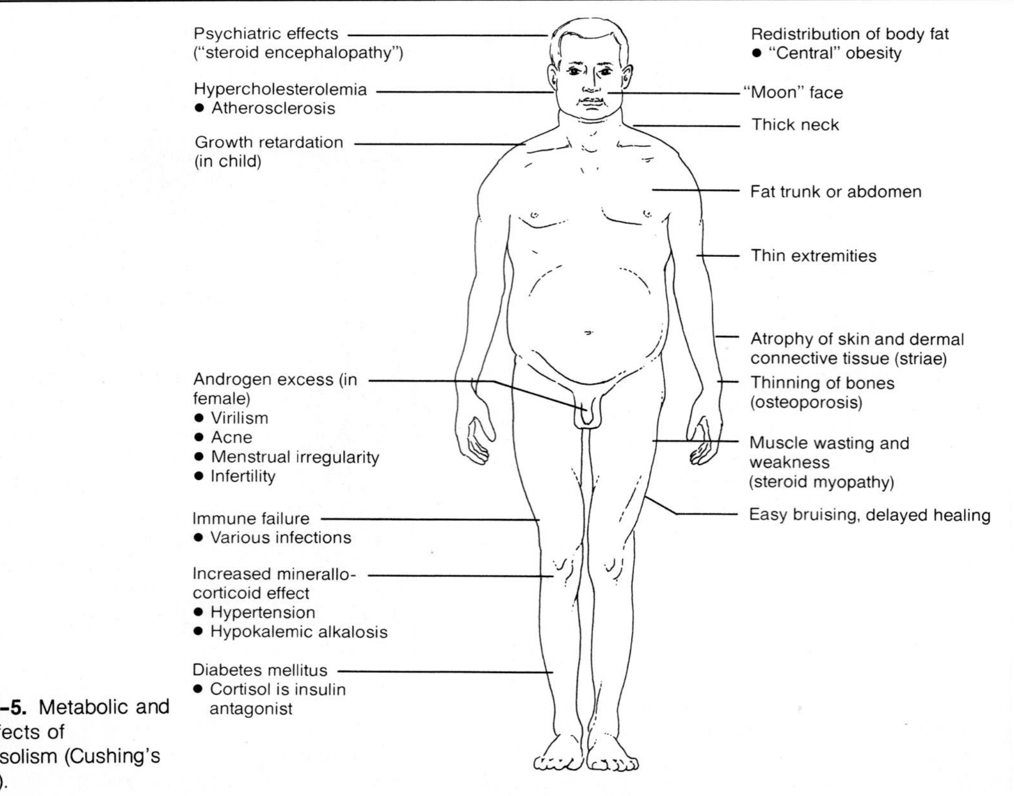

Figure 60–5. Metabolic and clinical effects of hypercortisolism (Cushing's syndrome).

Table 60–2. Laboratory diagnosis of Cushing's syndrome.

Step A: Establishment of presence of hypercortisolism
Plasma cortisol: elevated
Loss of normal diurnal variation: high plasma level in a midnight sample when cortisol levels are normally very low

Urinary 24-hour free cortisol level is elevated: a very good screening test

Low-dose 2-day dexamethasone suppression:
Suppresses plasma cortisol in all but patients with Cushing's syndrome[1]

Step B: Differential diagnosis of Cushing's syndrome

	Plasma ACTH[2]	Suppression With High-Dose Dexamethasone[1]	CT Scan Findings
Pituitary-induced adrenal hyperplasia	Elevated	Yes	Pituitary adenoma (may be small); bilateral adrenal hyperplasia
Adrenal adenoma	Low	No	Adrenal neoplasm: small
Adrenal carcinoma	Low	No	Adrenal neoplasm: large
Ectopic ACTH[2] production	Very high	No	Bilateral adrenal hyperplasia; normal pituitary; some other malignant neoplasm

[1]Dexamethasone is a synthetic glucocorticoid that suppresses ACTH secretion. At low doses suppression is not adequate to decrease excess cortisol secretion in any patient with Cushing's syndrome. At high doses it suppresses excessive ACTH secretion by pituitary adenomas.
[2]ACTH = adrenocorticotropic hormone.

moved. In the ectopic ACTH syndrome, therapy is aimed at the tumor responsible, eg, chemotherapy for small-cell carcinoma of the lung.

EXCESS ALDOSTERONE SECRETION

Incidence & Etiology

A. Primary Hyperaldosteronism (Conn's Syndrome): This disorder is rare and is most commonly the result of an aldosterone-secreting adrenocortical adenoma. Less commonly, it may result from bilateral hyperplasia of the zona glomerulosa. Adrenal carcinomas only very rarely secrete aldosterone. In a few cases of hyperaldosteronism, no definite abnormality is detected in the gland.

B. Secondary Hyperaldosteronism: Secondary hyperaldosteronism is common. It is caused by a high renin output from the juxtaglomerular cells of the kidney in response to (1) renal ischemia, such as occurs in renal artery stenosis and malignant hypertension; (2) reduced effective plasma volume, as occurs in cardiac failure and hypoproteinemic states; or (3) juxtaglomerular cell hyperplasia (Bartter's syndrome) or neoplasia.

Pathology

Most cases of primary aldosteronism are associated with adrenocortical adenoma indistinguishable from an adenoma that produces cortisol except that it tends to be smaller (usually < 2 cm in diameter).

The adrenals appear grossly normal in patients with secondary hyperaldosteronism; microscopic demonstration of hyperplasia of the zona glomerulosa is difficult and subjective.

Clinical Features

Aldosterone causes sodium retention in the distal renal tubule in exchange for potassium and hydrogen ions, resulting in hypertension and hypokalemic alkalosis. Hypertension is the usual presenting feature. Less than 1% of patients with hypertension have primary hyperaldosteronism, but this cause is important to identify since it represents a surgically curable cause. Hypokalemic symptoms may occasionally dominate and include muscle weakness, fatigue, paralyses, and paresthesias. Alkalosis may cause a decrease in serum ionized calcium, leading to tetany.

Secondary hyperaldosteronism occurs as a complication of a variety of diseases whose clinical manifestations usually dominate the clinical picture. In this situation, increased aldosterone secretion is a normal compensatory phenomenon and produces few symptoms except that it does cause sodium retention, thereby contributing to the genesis of edema in these conditions. Hypokalemic alkalosis and its effects may also be present.

It is of interest that edema is rare in patients with primary hyperaldosteronism even though there is marked sodium and water retention. This paradox has given rise to the postulated existence of a renal mechanism ("third factor") that limits the amount of sodium retained in the body.

Diagnosis

The diagnosis of primary hyperaldosteronism must be suspected in any hypertensive patient who has hypokalemia without an apparent cause or who develops profound hypokalemia when treated with diuretics.

The diagnosis of primary hyperaldosteronism may be made by the presence of elevated serum aldosterone levels associated with low serum renin levels. Salt-loading tests and furosemide stimulation tests are being less widely used as serum aldosterone and renin assays become more readily available. Renin and aldosterone levels are elevated in secondary hyperaldosteronism.

Differentiation of aldosterone adenoma and bilateral hyperplasia of the zona glomerulosa requires (1) demonstration of changes in serum aldosterone level in the supine and upright positions (no change in adenoma; increased in upright position in hyperplasia); and (2) serum 18-hydroxycorticosteroid level ($>$ 100 units in adenoma, $<$ 100 units in hyperplasia).

Preoperative localization of the adrenal adenoma responsible for primary hyperaldosteronism is achieved (1) by computerized tomography, which is successful in demonstrating adrenal adenoma in about 95% of cases; (2) by measurement of adrenal vein aldosterone concentrations, which are elevated on the side of the adenoma; and (3) by iodocholesterol scan. Iodocholesterol (tagged with radioiodine) is taken up by the zona glomerulosa and delineates an adenoma (unilateral) and hyperplasia (bilateral).

Treatment

Primary hyperaldosteronism is best treated by surgical removal of the adrenal gland that contains the adenoma. Aldosterone antagonist drugs (eg, spironolactone) are useful in the management of patients with secondary hyperaldosteronism.

EXCESS SEX HORMONE SECRETION

Excessive secretion of androgenic hormones by the adrenals is very rare. It may be due to adrenocortical neoplasms (particularly carcinomas) or congenital adrenal hyperplasia (adrenogenital syndrome) or may occur as an associated phenomenon in patients with Cushing's syndrome.

Excessive estrogen secretion occurs very rarely with adrenocortical carcinomas.

DECREASED SECRETION OF ADRENOCORTICAL HORMONES (Addison's Disease)

Incidence & Etiology

Decreased secretion of adrenocortical hormones is uncommon.

Acute insufficiency may follow destruction of the adrenal glands in severe bacteremias, most commonly meningococcal bacteremia (Waterhouse-Friderichsen syndrome). Clinically, this is a fulminant illness characterized by high fever, bacteremia, hemorrhagic skin rash, and shock, which progresses rapidly to death in most cases. Disseminated intravascular coagulation is believed to be responsible for petechial hemorrhages throughout the body, including the adrenals.

Acute adrenocortical insufficiency ("addisonian crisis") is most commonly seen today as an iatrogenic disease in patients being treated with synthetic glucocorticoids (eg, prednisone) in high doses. These drugs suppress pituitary ACTH and result in atrophy of the adrenal cortex, destroying the patient's ability to secrete cortisol normally. If such a patient has a sudden increased demand for cortisol (as during stress or an infection) or if the exogenous steroids are withdrawn rapidly, acute adrenocortical insufficiency may occur.

Chronic insufficiency of adrenocortical hormone synthesis occurs in a variety of conditions associated with chronic destruction of the adrenal glands (Fig 60–1).

(1) Autoimmune destruction of the adrenal gland. 50% of these patients have antiadrenal antibodies in their serum, and there is an association with other autoimmune diseases such as Hashimoto's thyroiditis and pernicious anemia. Autoimmune Addison's disease is now the commonest cause of chronic adrenal insufficiency.

(2) Infections, such as tuberculosis and histoplasmosis.

(3) Metastatic carcinoma, particularly lung carcinoma, which has a predilection for producing adrenal metastases.

(4) Metabolic diseases such as hemochromatosis and amyloidosis, which in rare instances involve the adrenal glands and produce adrenal insufficiency.

(5) Congenital adrenal hyperplasia, particularly that due to complete 21-hydroxylase deficiency.

(6) Deficient ACTH secretion in conditions of hypopituitarism (see Chapter 57).

Pathology

When the adrenals are the site of a disease (tuberculosis, fungal infection, metastatic carcinoma, hemochromatosis, amyloidosis, etc), the gland shows the specific morphologic features associated with those disorders.

In autoimmune Addison's disease, the adrenals are markedly atrophic, with an aggregate weight less than 4 g. There is loss of normal architecture and lipid depletion of cells, resulting in a brown color. Microscopically, the cortex is greatly narrowed, with a diffuse lymphocytic infiltrate and fibrosis.

Clinical Features

The dominant clinical features of Addison's disease are caused by decreased mineralocorticoid activity. There is increased sodium excretion in the renal tubules with retention of potassium and hydrogen ions. Loss of sodium results in hyponatremia and contraction of plasma volume, leading to hypotension. Serum chloride is decreased, and there is a hyperkalemic acidosis. Hyperkalemia may cause muscular weakness and electrocardiographic abnormalities.

A decreased cortisol level in plasma does not cause immediate symptoms. However, such patients are unable to respond to stresses such as infections, surgery, and trauma, which precipitate life-threatening circulatory collapse (addisonian crisis).

A compensatory increase in pituitary ACTH secretion occurs in all cases of adrenal insufficiency (except when caused by hypopituitarism). Plasma ACTH levels are increased. This causes increased skin pigmentation because of the melanocyte-stimulating property of ACTH.

II. THE ADRENAL MEDULLA

STRUCTURE & FUNCTION

The adrenal medulla is derived from the neural crest and is therefore closely related to the sympathetic ganglia and paraganglia. Paraganglia are a group of small organs located in the paravertebral region from the base of the skull to the parasacral region. Paraganglia have also been described at the aortic bifurcation (organ of Zuckerkandl) and in the wall of the urinary bladder.

The medulla comprises about 10% of the adrenal weight. It is present only in the head and body regions of the adrenal, being absent in the tail. Microscopically, it is composed of large cells arranged in nests and trabeculae, separated by a rich vascular stroma. The cells of the adrenal medulla are richly innervated and form part of the sympathetic nervous system. Adrenal medullary secretion is controlled by the activity of the sympathetic nerves.

The adrenal medulla secretes the catecholamines norepinephrine (noradrenaline) and epinephrine (adrenaline). The adrenal medulla differs from extra-adrenal paraganglia in having the enzyme phenylethanolamine N-methyltransferase, which converts norepinephrine to epinephrine; the adrenal medulla secretes chiefly epinephrine.

ASSESSMENT OF MEDULLARY STRUCTURE & FUNCTION

Clinical Examination

Signs and symptoms of excess catecholamine production may be present (see below).

Radiologic Examination

Computerized tomography can show lesions in the adrenal in the 1- to 2-cm range but cannot differentiate between cortical and medullary lesions. Contrast studies, including intravenous pyelography and renal angiography, should not be used in patients suspected of having an adrenal medullary lesion, since they may induce a sudden release of catecholamines and precipitate a potentially fatal hypertensive crisis.

A more specific method of evaluating the adrenal medulla involves the intravenous administration of a radiolabeled guanine compound (metaiodobenzylguanidine; MIBG) that is taken up selectively by paraganglionic cells. An abnormal "hot" spot correlates with the presence of a functioning paraganglionic or adrenal medullary neoplasm.

Serum & Urinary Enzyme Assays

Several tests are used for the assessment of adrenal medullary secretion:

(1) Urinary metanephrine and vanillylmandelic acid (VMA) levels are good screening tests.

(2) Catecholamines can be assayed directly both in serum and in urine, but levels fluctuate greatly and unpredictably during a single day. A timed 24-hour urine collection provides a better estimate than a random plasma level.

(3) The ratio between epinephrine and norepinephrine in serum provides an indication of the source of the catecholamines. Adrenal medullary secretion contains considerable amounts of epinephrine as well as norepinephrine, whereas extra-adrenal secretion contains mainly norepinephrine.

Adrenal Vein Hormone Assays

Catheterization of the adrenal vein to obtain samples for assays has largely been supplanted by the improved radiologic methods mentioned above.

DISEASES OF THE ADRENAL MEDULLA

Neoplasms constitute the only common disease process to affect the adrenal medulla (Table 60–3). Very rarely, adrenal medullary hyperplasia occurs as part of the multiple endocrine neoplasia syndrome (MEN type II).

PHEOCHROMOCYTOMA

Pheochromocytomas are catecholamine-producing neoplasms of the adrenal medulla or extra-adrenal paraganglia. The term paraganglioma is commonly used for these tumors when they occur outside the adrenal.

Pheochromocytoma is an uncommon neoplasm. It usually occurs sporadically, but occasional patients give a positive family history for the following diseases: (1) Familial occurrence of pheochromocytoma, with an autosomal dominant pattern of inheritance is very rare. (2) Generalized neurofibromatosis (von Recklinghausen's disease) is associated with an increased incidence of pheochromocytoma. (3) Multiple endocrine neoplasia types IIa and IIb (see below) should raise the possibility of bilateral pheochromocytoma, since these patients have bilateral neoplasms in about 50% of cases.

Pathology

Pheochromocytoma is sometimes called "the 10% tumor" for the following reasons: (1) Its commonest location is in the adrenal medulla, but 10% of pheochromocytomas occur in extra-adrenal paraganglia—most often intra-abdominal, occasionally in the mediastinum, neck, or wall of the urinary bladder. Carotid body tumors, formerly termed chemodectomas, are now considered to be paragangliomas and may secrete catecholamines. (2) Ten percent of patients with pheochromocytoma have multiple tumors, most commonly involving both adrenal glands but also the extra-adrenal paraganglia. (3) Most pheochromocytomas behave as benign neoplasms, but 10% are malignant, with local invasion and metastasis.

Pheochromocytomas vary in size from very small (1 cm) to massive tumors, are well circumscribed, and frequently show areas of hemorrhage and necrosis (Fig 60–6). Fixation in a chromium salt fixative (such as Zenker's solution) imparts a brown color to the tumor—hence the older term chromaffin paraganglioma.

Microscopically, the tumor consists of large cells arranged in sheets and nests separated by a rich vascular stroma. Pleomorphism is common, but mitoses are rare. Invasion of capsule and vessels is common even in those neoplasms that behave in a benign fashion.

Electron microscopy shows the presence of membrane-bound, dense-core neurosecretory granules in the cytoplasm. Immunologic studies show the presence of markers for neuroendocrine cells such as neuron-specific enolase and chromogranin. Catecholamines can be demonstrated in the tumor if a sample is assayed.

The biologic behavior of a pheochromocytoma cannot be predicted by microscopic examination. The diagnosis of malignant pheochromocytoma is made only when metastasis is demonstrated. Distinction must also be made between true metasta-

Table 60–3. Primary neoplasms of the adrenal medulla.

	Pheochromocytoma	Ganglioneuroma	Neuroblastoma[1]
Age	Adults	Adults/children	Children
Biologic behavior	90% benign; 10% malignant	Benign	Highly malignant
Secretion	High levels of catecholamines	Slight increase in catecholamines	Slight increase in catecholamines
Clinical presentation	Hypertension, sweating, palpitations	Abdominal mass	Abdominal mass, metastases
Macroscopic features	Mass, often hemorrhagic	Solid, firm mass	Mass, often necrotic
Microscopic features	Nests of large cells, vascular	Ganglion cells and neural tissue	Primitive small neuroblasts
Immunohistochemical markers	Chromogranin, NSE[2]	S100 protein	NSE[2]

[1]Neuroblastomas may spontaneously show evidence of maturation characterized by the appearance of multinucleated ganglion cells. The end result of maturation resembles a benign ganglioneuroma and has a benign biologic behavior.
[2]NSE = neuron-specific enolase.

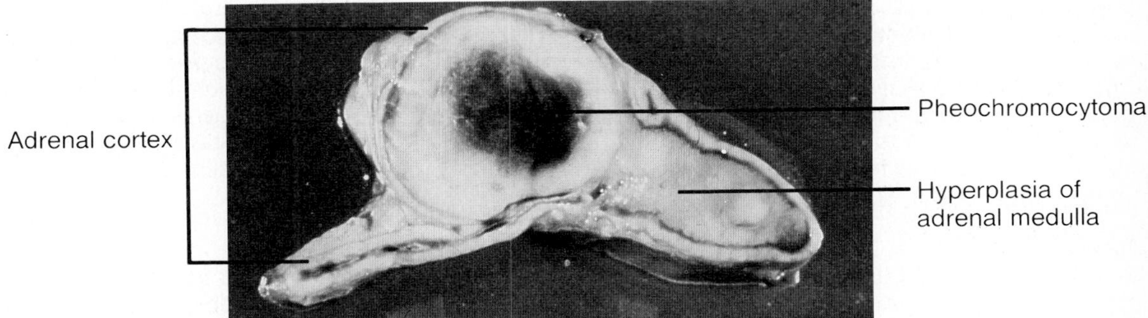

Figure 60-6. Cross section of adrenal, showing a pheochromocytoma associated with hyperplasia of the medulla in a patient with multiple endocrine neoplasia type IIa. (He also had a medullary carcinoma of the thyroid and a large pheochromocytoma in the opposite adrenal.)

ses and multiple primary paragangliomas, which occur rarely and are usually benign. A diagnosis of metastatic pheochromocytoma is made only when a pheochromocytoma occurs in a site where paraganglia are not found (eg, lung, bone, liver, brain).

Clinical Features

The clinical manifestations of pheochromocytoma are due to increased catecholamine secretion.

Hypertension is the commonest presenting feature. Blood pressure elevation is the result of peripheral vasoconstriction and increased cardiac output caused by the alpha and beta effects of catecholamines. Hypertension is commonly persistent but may be paroxysmal, with return of the blood pressure to normal between paroxysms. Paroxysmal hypertension is caused by sudden release of hormone from the neoplasm and may be precipitated by bending, increased abdominal pressure (as during physical examination), meals, and—in those rare cases where the tumor is located in the urinary bladder wall—by micturition. During a hypertensive crisis, the systolic pressure can rise to 300 mm Hg.

Hypertension, particularly when episodic, is accompanied by other manifestations of catecholamine excess such as palpitations, tachycardia, feelings of anxiety, and excessive sweating. Impaired glucose tolerance (diabetes mellitus) is common, being the result of the insulin-antagonistic action of catecholamines.

Untreated, patients with pheochromocytomas die of cardiac failure or cerebral hemorrhage during a hypertensive crisis.

Diagnosis

Patients with hypertension—particularly if they are under 40 years of age—must be evaluated for the possibility of pheochromocytoma. The best screening tests are urinary metanephrine and vanillylmandelic acid (breakdown products of catecholamines), one or both of which is elevated in almost all cases. The diagnosis may be confirmed by urinary and serum catecholamine assays.

When the diagnosis of pheochromocytoma has been made, the neoplasm or neoplasms should be localized radiologically prior to surgical removal.

Treatment

Surgical removal of the tumor is the treatment of choice but is a complex procedure that requires sympathetic blockade, expert anesthesiologic support, and meticulous fluid balance. Removal of the neoplasm may cause a sudden drop in blood pressure; if some fall in blood pressure does not occur, the possibility of a second pheochromocytoma must be suspected.

NEUROBLASTOMA

Neuroblastoma is a malignant neoplasm composed of primitive neural crest cells. It occurs chiefly in very young children; the median age is 2 years, and 80% of cases occur under the age of 5 years. Neuroblastoma is rare past puberty.

The adrenal medulla is by far the most common site, followed by neural crest derivatives in the retroperitoneum. Extra-abdominal neuroblastomas may occur in the posterior mediastinum, pelvis, head, neck, and cerebral hemispheres. A specific form of the neoplasm—olfactory neuroblastoma—occurs in the nasal cavity in older individuals.

Neuroblastoma is the third most common malignant neoplasm in childhood, following leukemia-lymphoma and nephroblastoma. Most cases are sporadic. Very rarely, neuroblastoma occurs in families.

Genetic Abnormalities

Three distinctive cytogenetic features have been

described: (1) Most cases of neuroblastoma show a near-terminal deletion of part of the short arm of chromosome 1 (partial monosomy 1), a finding that is of diagnostic value. (2) Chromosome 2 frequently shows a dense homogeneously stained region (HSR). (3) Multiple double-minute (DM) chromatin bodies may be observed apart from the chromosomes (Fig 60–7).

Both HSR and DM chromatin bodies are believed to represent amplification sites of an oncogene N-*MYC* (N-*MYC* is a recently described relative of C-*MYC*, part of a growing "*MYC*" family of oncogenes). N-*MYC* amplification is most often present in advanced disease (stages III and IV), and demonstration of N-*MYC* amplification is thus considered a poor prognostic factor.

Pathology

Grossly, neuroblastomas tend to be very large infiltrative tumors. They are soft and friable and often show extensive hemorrhage and necrosis.

Microscopically, the neoplastic cells are small and round, with large round nuclei and scanty cytoplasm. They are arranged in diffuse sheets with very little intervening stroma. The cells often bear nerve fibrils that appear as delicate pink filamentous structures. The formation of "rosettes"—groups of cells arranged in a ring around a central mass of pink neural filaments—is characteristic (Fig 60–8).

Electron microscopy shows neurosecretory granules in the cytoplasm. Immunohistochemical studies show positivity for neuron-specific enolase. These findings permit differentiation of neuroblastoma from malignant lymphomas and other primitive mesenchymal neoplasms such as embryonal rhabdomyosarcoma, which can present similar gross and microscopic appearances.

Maturation, signified by differentiation of primitive cells into large multinucleated ganglion cells, is not uncommon in neuroblastoma. When ganglionic differentiation is present, the tumor is called a ganglioneuroblastoma or differentiating neuroblastoma, and the prognosis is better than for an undifferentiated neuroblastoma. In a few cases of neuroblastoma with metastases, complete ganglion cell differentiation has been described, producing ganglioneuromas that then behave in benign fashion.

Clinical Features

Most patients with neuroblastoma present with an enlarging mass in the abdomen. Seventy-five percent of patients have increased catecholamine secretion, which can be identified by increased urinary levels of metanephrine and vanillylmandelic acid. Clinical evidence of catecholamine excess is, however, rare.

Hematogenous dissemination occurs very early. Patients fall into 3 fairly distinct patterns based on the pattern of metastasis: (1) extensive skull metastases, involving particularly the orbit and producing exophthalmos (Hutchinson type); (2) extensive liver metastases (Pepper type); and (3) extensive bone marrow involvement. It is not uncommon for patients with neuroblastoma to present with a metastatic lesion.

Treatment & Prognosis

Treatment of neuroblastoma is with combined surgery, chemotherapy, and radiation. Surgery is necessary to provide tissue for diagnosis and reduce tumor bulk. The increased effectiveness of chemotherapy has greatly improved the survival statistics.

The prognosis of a patient with neuroblastoma depends on the age at presentation—the younger the patient, the better the prognosis—and the clinical stage of the disease. Histologic evidence of ganglionic differentiation is a good prognostic sign. Amplification of N-*MYC* oncogene in the cancer cells is a bad prognostic sign.

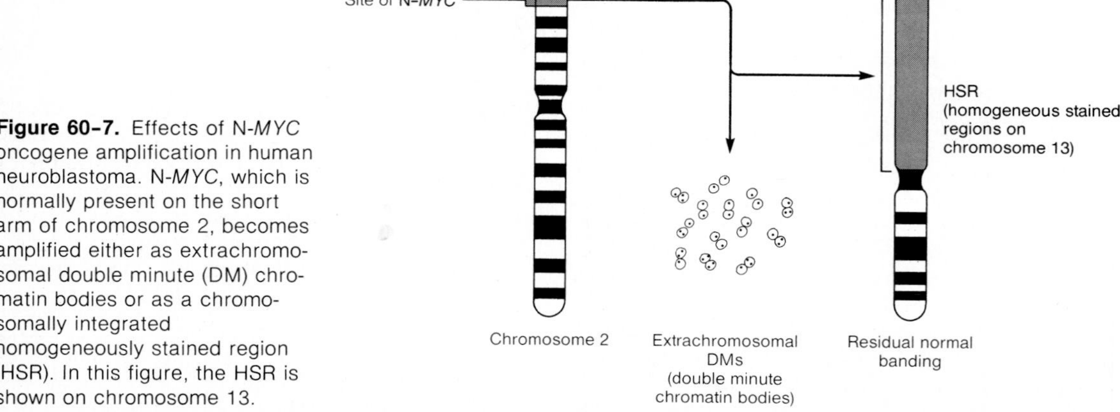

Figure 60–7. Effects of N-*MYC* oncogene amplification in human neuroblastoma. N-*MYC*, which is normally present on the short arm of chromosome 2, becomes amplified either as extrachromosomal double minute (DM) chromatin bodies or as a chromosomally integrated homogeneously stained region (HSR). In this figure, the HSR is shown on chromosome 13.

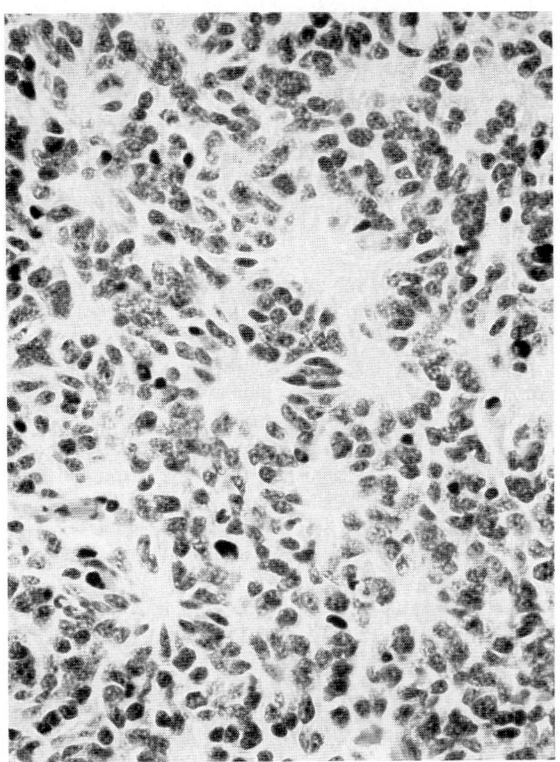

Figure 60–8. Neuroblastoma, showing primitive neuroblasts forming rosettes.

Neuroblastomas are staged as follows according to the degree of spread of tumor:

Stage I: Tumor confined to the organ of origin.

Stage II: Local spread, confined to one side.

Stage III: Local spread across the midline, with involved regional lymph nodes.

Stage IV: Distant metastasis.

Surgery plays a greater role in stage I disease; radiation therapy is useful in stage II and stage III disease; and chemotherapy is useful at all stages but has improved the prognosis most dramatically in the later stages.

III. MULTIPLE ENDOCRINE NEOPLASIA SYNDROMES

The multiple endocrine neoplasia (MEN) or multiple endocrine adenomatosis (MEA) syndromes are characterized by the familial occurrence of multiple endocrine neoplasms. They are rare and are inherited as an autosomal dominant trait with variable penetrance.

Three types of MEN syndromes are recognized:

(1) MEN (MEA) type I. MEN type I consists of pituitary adenoma, parathyroid hyperplasia or adenoma, and pancreatic islet cell neoplasms, including gastrinoma. Peptic ulcers also occur in these patients, probably related to gastrin production (Zollinger-Ellison syndrome). Adrenocortical adenomas rarely occur.

(2) MEN type IIa (Sipple syndrome). MEN type IIa consists of medullary carcinoma and parafollicular cell hyperplasia of the thyroid and adrenal medullary hyperplasia or pheochromocytoma (Fig

Table 60–4. "APUDomas" (neuroendocrine tumors).

Site	Tumor	Secretory Products[1]
Anterior pituitary	Pituitary adenoma	GH, ACTH, prolactin, FSH, LH, TSH
Bronchus	Carcinoid, small cell undifferentiated carcinoma	5HT, ACTH, ADH, parathormone
Gastrointestinal tract	Carcinoid	5HT, VIP, gastrin
Pancreas	Islet cell adenoma and carcinoma	Insulin, glucagon, VIP, PP, somatostatin, 5HT, ACTH, bombesin
Thyroid	Medullary carcinoma	Calcitonin
Parathyroid	Adenoma, carcinoma	Parathormone
Adrenal medulla and autonomic ganglia	Pheochromocytoma, neuroblastoma	Catecholamines
Paraganglia, glomus jugulare, carotid body	Paraganglioma, glomus tumor, chemodectoma	Catecholamines
Skin	Merkel cell tumor	Calcitonin, parathormone

[1]GH = growth hormone; ACTH = adrenocorticotropic hormone; FSH = follicle-stimulating hormone; LH = luteinizing hormone; TSH = thyroid-stimulating hormone; 5HT = 5-hydroxytryptamine; ADH = antidiuretic hormone; VIP = vasoactive intestinal polypeptide; PP = pancreatic polypeptide.

60–6). Parathyroid hyperplasia or adenoma may also be present. These patients do not have pancreatic islet cell neoplasms and have no increased incidence of peptic ulcer.

(3) MEN type IIb. A subgroup of MEN type II has been identified in which patients have mucocutaneous (tongue, eyelids, bronchus, intestine) neuromas in addition to the thyroid and adrenal neoplasms. This is sometimes also called MEN type III.

THE APUD (NEUROENDOCRINE CELL) SYSTEM

The occurrence of multiple neoplasms involving several endocrine glands as a consequence of the inheritance of a single abnormal gene suggests that these cells are related in some way. The term APUD or neuroendocrine cell system has been applied to these interrelated cells. These cells are distributed throughout the body in virtually all organs. They have certain characteristics in common:

(1) They are believed to be derived embryologically from neuroectodermal cells of the neural crest. This common origin has recently been disputed, particularly for bronchial and intestinal APUD cells, which are believed to take origin from a primitive entodermal cell that can differentiate into both epithelial and neuroendocrine cells.

(2) They have the ability to take up amine precursors such as tryptophan and possess an enzyme that decarboxylates these into amines. Hence the acronym APUD, for amine precursor uptake and decarboxylation.

(3) The cells secrete physiologically active amines (serotonin, catecholamines) or polypeptide hormones.

(4) The cells contain membrane-bound dense-core neurosecretory granules in their cytoplasm, as seen by electron microscopy.

(5) When stained with immunoperoxidase techniques they stain positively for neuroendocrine markers such as neuron-specific enolase and chromogranin as well as for individual specific products (biogenic amines and polypeptide hormones; see Table 60–4).

APUDomas are neoplasms derived from APUD cells and retain the features that characterize these cells (Table 60–4). More recently, the term "neuroendocrine tumor" has been used in preference to APUDoma. Neuroendocrine tumors are classified by the cell of origin or the principal cell product.

Section XIV. The Skin

Chapter 61: Diseases of the Skin

Dermatologic pathology is presented in this section in a very simplified manner. We stress skin neoplasms, including carcinomas and malignant melanoma, and common skin infections. Only those dermatologic diseases that have characteristic clinicopathologic bases and which are encountered commonly are discussed.

61 Diseases of the Skin

STRUCTURE OF THE SKIN (Fig 61-1)

Epidermis

The epidermis is composed of stratified squamous epithelium in which several cell types can be identified.

A. Keratinocytes: Keratinocytes are subdivided according to degree of differentiation into **(1) basal cells,** which are the germinative cells (epidermal stem cells); **(2) prickle or spinous cells** (stratum spinosum), characterized by the presence of keratin and desmosomes and names for the desmosomal intercellular attachments, which appear as spines or prickles connecting cells; **(3) granular cells** (stratum granulosum), containing numerous large basophilic keratohyalin granules in the cytoplasm; and **(4) cornified cells** (stratum corneum)—flat, anucleate cells that form the most superficial layer of the epidermis. The stratum corneum is continuously shed at the surface and varies greatly in thickness—greatest in the soles and palms.

The normal rate of maturation from a basal cell to a surface cornified cell is 2 weeks. The cell remains in the stratum corneum another 2 weeks before it is shed.

B. Melanocytes: Melanocytes are epidermal cells derived from the embryologic neural crest. They produce melanin and are situated singly in the basal layer, appearing as larger clear cells. The dopa reaction, which is positive in the presence of enzymes of the tyrosine-melanin pathway is a histochemical means of identifying melanocytes. Melanocytes have dendritic processes that ramify in the epidermis and transfer melanin to keratinocytes.

Melanocytes can be identified electron microscopically by the presence of **melanosomes,** which are membrane-bound ellipsoidal structures containing concentric internal lamellae. Positive staining for **S100 protein** and melanosomal antigen are useful immunohistochemical markers for melanocytes.

The number of melanocytes in the skin is relatively constant. Skin pigmentation is dependent on the rate of synthesis of melanin, which is governed by (1) racial factors, being greater in dark-skinned races; (2) ultraviolet radiation, which increases melanin synthesis; and (3) hormones—melanocyte-stimulating hormone and adrenocorticotropin increase melanin pigmentation.

C. Langerhans Cells: Langerhans cells are clear dendritic cells situated among the cells of the stratum spinosum. They are believed to be antigen-processing cells related to the interdigitating reticulum cells of lymph nodes. They are S100 protein-positive on immunohistochemical studies. On electron microscopy, they lack melanosomes but contain a characteristic organelle known as a Birbeck granule.

D. Merkel Cells: Merkel cells are neuroendocrine cells that are present in the basal layer of the epidermis. They cannot be recognized in routine histologic sections but can be identified in electron micrographs by the presence of cytoplasmic neurosecretory granules.

Basement Membrane

The basement membrane is not seen on routine sections but appears as a homogeneous band in sections stained with periodic acid-Schiff (PAS) stain. It is composed of collagen and mucopoly-

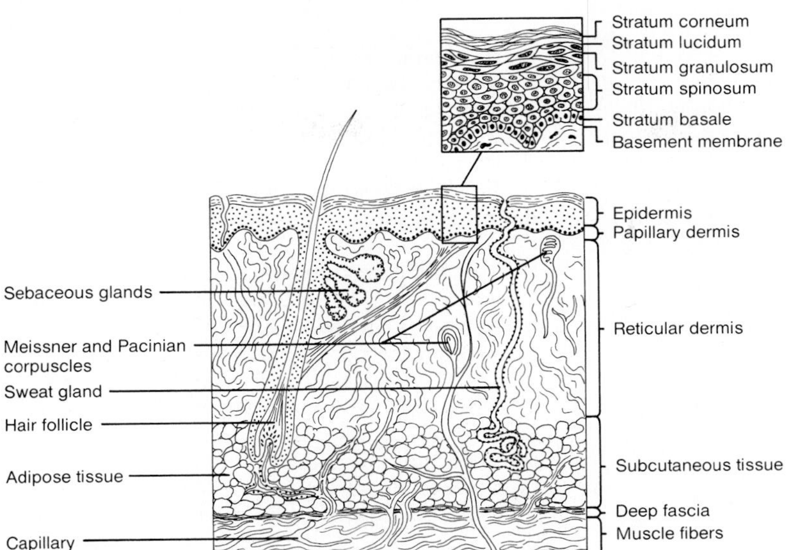

Figure 61-1. Structure of the skin.

saccharides, to which basal cells are bound by attachment plaques (modified desmosomes) and anchoring filaments.

The Dermis

The dermis is a layer of connective tissue 1–4 mm thick subjacent to the epidermis. It is composed of mucopolysaccharide ground substance, fibrillar proteins (reticulin, collagen, and elastin), and cells (fibroblasts, macrophages, mast cells, and a few lymphocytes). The dermis contains blood vessels, lymphatics, and nerves.

Epidermal Appendages

Epidermal appendages include modified keratinaceous structures such as nails and hair and adnexal glands of the epidermis and hair follicles, including sebaceous glands, sweat (eccrine) glands, and apocrine glands. Apocrine glands are found mainly in the axillas and anogenital region.

FUNCTIONS OF THE SKIN

The epidermis is impermeable to water and electrolytes, permitting maintenance of an essentially aqueous medium (body cells and tissue fluids) in a relatively dry atmospheric environment.

The skin is a major organ of temperature regulation. Cutaneous vasoconstriction decreases and vasodilatation increases heat loss. Sweating also permits heat loss as a function of evaporation. Both cutaneous blood flow and sweating are regulated by the sympathetic nervous system.

The skin also serves to protect the internal organs from the action of toxic chemicals and radiation. The epidermis is impervious to all but corrosive chemicals, while melanin pigment in the epidermis absorbs damaging ultraviolet radiation.

The skin is an effective physical barrier to the entry of infectious agents, with the stratum corneum presenting an inhospitable environment for most microorganisms. The chemical effect of sweat and sebum and the presence of commensal bacteria also help to defend against infection by virulent organisms. The barrier effect of the skin is lost if it is chronically wet or if its continuity is destroyed by trauma.

MANIFESTATIONS OF SKIN DISEASE

The skin responds to injury in a limited number of ways.

General Responses

Acute inflammation may involve the epidermis and the dermis. Redness, heat, and swelling are readily apparent in the skin, and pain and tenderness are usually marked because of the rich nerve supply. Accumulation of fluid in the epidermis between the keratinocytes is called **spongiosis**. Extreme spongiosis leads to a vesicle (a localized fluid collection). Dermal swelling causes elevation of the epidermis (wheal formation).

Severe injuries to the skin lead to necrosis. Epidermal necrosis leads to ulceration. Dermal necrosis produces a variety of different clinical appearances depending on the structures involved and the extent of necrosis.

The changes of chronic inflammation in the skin are less obvious but include thickening of the epidermis (acanthosis), thickening of the stratum corneum (hyperkeratosis), and dermal fibrosis.

Specific Responses

In addition to general responses to injury, the skin shows a variety of specific changes (Table 61–1); these responses in varying combinations produce the histologic changes seen in the different skin diseases.

INFECTIONS OF THE SKIN

BACTERIAL INFECTIONS (Fig 61-2)

Impetigo

Impetigo is a superficial epidermal infection caused by *Staphylococcus aureus.* Streptococci may also be present, probably as secondary invaders. Impetigo most commonly occurs in children—particularly on the face, whence it may spread by scratching. Transmission is by direct contact; impetigo is highly contagious.

Grossly, impetigo begins as a pustule (a blister filled with pus) that ruptures to form the typical thick, yellow, translucent crust. Microscopically, the blister is in the superficial part of the epidermis. Eradication of the infection with antibiotics leads to rapid healing without scarring.

Neonatal impetigo is an extremely serious specific variant in infants caused by strains of staphylococci that produce an epidermolytic toxin. Bullae (large blisters) extend and enlarge, resulting in denudation of large areas of the superficial epidermis ("scalded skin syndrome").

Hair Follicle Infections

"Folliculitis" is extremely common, occurring in any part of the body where there is hair—often the face and upper trunk. *Staphylococcus aureus* is the usual pathogen and produces typical acute inflammation with pain, swelling, and erythema. Suppuration leads to an abscess, or furuncle (the common boil or pimple). A boil in relation to an eyelash is called a sty, or hordeolum.

A **carbuncle** is a much more serious infection that begins as a folliculitis but spreads deep and laterally to form a large inflammatory mass with multiple areas of suppuration. Carbuncles are especially common in diabetics and may lead to bacteremia.

Acne Vulgaris

While not primarily an infection, the lesions of acne vulgaris frequently become infected by low-grade pathogens. The lesion of acne vulgaris is the comedo (blackhead or whitehead), which consists of a pilosebaceous structure plugged with keratin and lipids. The retained keratin and sebaceous secretions are degraded by anaerobic bacteria such as *Propionibacterium acnes,* leading to acute inflammation that may—especially if secondary infection occurs—evolve into an abscess very similar to a furuncle.

Table 61-1. Skin responses to injury.

Response	Terminology	Clinical Appearance
Hyperplasia of keratinocytes → thickening of the epidermis	Acanthosis	Diffuse thickening or localized elevated plaque (papule)
Increased rate of maturation of keratinocyte → thickening of stratum corneum	Hyperkeratosis	Silvery surface scales
Increased rate of maturation of keratinocytes with premature shedding → nucleated cells in stratum corneum	Parakeratosis	None
Abnormal keratinization	Dyskeratosis	None
Epidermal atrophy → thin epidermis	Atrophy	Thinning of skin
Degeneration of basal layer	. . .	Subepidermal vesicle[1]
Separation of epidermal cells	Acantholysis	Intraepidermal vesicle[1]
Epidermal edema	Spongiosis	Intraepidermal vesicle[1]
Dysplasia of keratinocytes	Dysplasia	Papule[2]
Inflammatory cells in epidermis	Exocytosis	None
Epidermal abscess formation	Pustule	Pus-filled vesicle[1]
Dermal inflammation, edema	. . .	Macule;[2] wheal
Dermal hemorrhage	. . .	Petechiae, purpura

[1]Vesicles appear clinically as blisters, or bullae (see Table 61-3).
[2]Macule = a change in the skin that is flat and level with the skin surface; papule = an elevated, flat lesion.

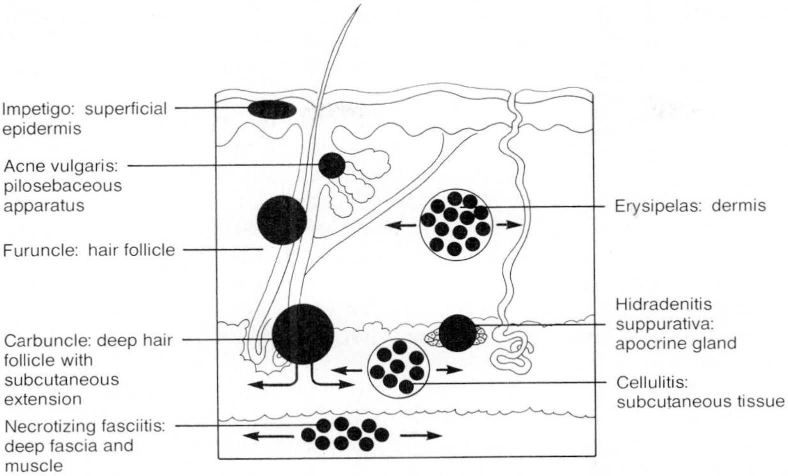

Figure 61-2. Bacterial infections of the skin. Solid areas represent suppuration and abscess formation. Dotted areas represent spreading acute inflammation, with the arrows showing the plane of spread of the infection and inflammatory reaction.

Acne affects most adolescents at about the age of puberty. Its cause is uncertain. Elevated sex hormone levels at puberty may influence the quality of sebaceous secretions, and certain foodstuffs appear to exacerbate the condition in some individuals, suggesting an allergic phenomenon. Poor hygiene plays an uncertain role in initiation of the comedo (the blackhead is oxidized lipid, not dirt) but predisposes to secondary infection.

Hidradenitis Suppurativa

Staphylococcal infection of apocrine glands may lead to acute suppurative inflammation with abscess formation. The axillas and anogenital regions are the usual sites. The process may become chronic, with increasing fibrous scarring and recurrent abscesses.

Erysipelas

Erysipelas is an acute spreading inflammation of the skin, commonly of the face or scalp. It is usually caused by streptococci. The involved skin is red, hot, swollen, and thickened. The dermis shows hyperemia and neutrophil infiltration. Local abscess formation is not a feature. Patients have systemic signs of acute inflammation, with high fever.

Cellulitis

Rapidly spreading acute inflammation of subcutaneous tissue occurs as a complication of wound infection. The usual infecting organism is *Streptococcus pyogenes*. The inflamed area is red, hot, and swollen. Bacteremia is frequent, and the patient is febrile.

Two severe forms of necrotizing cellulitis caused by anaerobic bacteria are Ludwig's angina, affecting the floor of the mouth and neck; and Fournier's gangrene of the scrotum.

Necrotizing Fasciitis

Necrotizing fasciitis is an uncommon spreading infection of the deep subcutaneous tissue, deep fascia, and underlying skeletal muscle, most commonly affecting the extremities and abdominal wall. It is usually caused by anaerobic bacteria. It is characterized by extensive necrosis of muscle, fascia, and overlying skin. The presence of skin hemorrhage, necrosis, and large bullous lesions filled with blood-stained fluid is characteristic. The lesion tends to spread rapidly and requires emergent and aggressive surgical debridement.

A specific type of necrotizing fasciitis is caused by *Vibrio vulnificus,* which is a frequent contaminant of fish in coastal waters. A history of ingestion of raw oysters contaminated with the vibrio is present in 90% of cases. Ingestion of the vibrio results in bacteremia in patients with chronic liver disease, who comprise the main susceptible group. Necrotizing fasciitis follows bacteremia and spreads rapidly to a fatal outcome. Early recognition of the agent permits antibiotic treatment, which is very effective.

Anthrax

Anthrax is a rare infection caused by *Bacillus anthracis,* a spore-bearing gram-positive bacillus found mainly in and around farm animals. Anthrax has a strong occupational relationship to industries dealing with animal products and hides (farming, textile and leather industries). About 95% of cases are cutaneous as a result of skin inoculation; 5% are pulmonary, resulting from inhalation of spores.

Anthrax is characterized by severe necrotizing hemorrhagic acute inflammation of the skin due to the virulence of the organism and its tendency to produce vasculitis.

Clinically, anthrax produces a "malignant pustule"—a large hemorrhagic blister that ruptures and leaves an ulcer with a black crust. The surrounding skin is markedly inflamed. The course varies from mild localized infection to severe bacteremia ending in death. The pulmonary form, though rare, is serious and often fatal.

Leprosy (Hansen's Disease)

Leprosy is a common disease in tropical countries. In the United States, leprosy is seen in Southern California, Hawaii, and the southern states. It is caused by *Mycobacterium leprae,* an acid-fast bacillus that has not been cultured on artificial media.

The clinicopathologic features of leprosy are dependent on the immunologic reactivity of the host to the leprosy bacillus (see Chapter 5). There is a spectrum of disease pattern ranging from **tuberculoid** to **lepromatous,** with **borderline** being an intermediate pattern (Table 61–2).

A. Tuberculoid Leprosy: Tuberculoid leprosy occurs in patients who develop T cell hypersensitivity to the bacillus. The lepromin test, which measures the delayed (type IV) hypersensitivity response to injected leprosy antigen, is positive, and the organism is localized to the area of entry (macrophage migration inhibiting factor). The number of lesions is small, and bacteremic spread is rare. Clinically, the skin lesion is a hypopigmented macule. (A macule is a flat, well-defined area of discoloration of the skin.) Nerve involvement is characteristic and causes the macule to be hypesthetic. Involvement of large peripheral nerves (ulnar, common peroneal, greater auricular) produces palpable thickening and nerve palsies (wristdrop and footdrop are common presenting features). The skin lesion is characterized histologically by epithelioid cell granulomas, numerous lymphocytes, and small numbers of leprosy bacilli that may be difficult to demonstrate because of their paucity.

Tuberculoid leprosy is the least serious end of the clinical spectrum of leprosy. It has a slowly progressive course without treatment. It can often be successfully treated.

B. Lepromatous Leprosy: Lepromatous leprosy occurs in patients who have a low level of cellular immunity. The lepromin test is negative.

In the absence of an effective T cell response, the bacillus multiples unchecked in skin macrophages, forming large foamy "lepra cells" in which are found many acid-fast bacilli. Aggregation of macrophages causes thickening and nodularity of the skin. Lymphocytes are present but not numerous.

The bacillus also spreads via the bloodstream, causing widespread lesions in the skin, eye, upper respiratory tract, and testis. Leprosy bacilli grow preferentially at temperatures less than 37 °C, and internal viscera such as spleen and liver, which are at core body temperature, are rarely involved.

Lepromatous leprosy is a serious disease that causes extensive destruction of tissue. Involvement of the fingers, nose, and ears produces marked disfigurement. Treatment is unsatisfactory.

C. Borderline Leprosy: Borderline leprosy has features intermediate between lepromatous and tuberculous leprosy (Table 61–2).

D. Reactional Forms of Leprosy:

1. Erythema nodosum leprosum–This form is common in patients with lepromatous leprosy. Tender erythematous skin nodules develop in the extremities. Histologic examination shows a panniculitis (inflammation of the subcutaneous fat),

Table 61–2. Clinicopathologic types of leprosy.[1]

	Lepromatous	Borderline	Tuberculoid
Cell-mediated immunity	Deficient	Intermediate	Present
Lepromin test[2]	Negative	Positive or negative	Positive
Number of lesions	Numerous	Many	Few
Visceral lesions	Common	Uncommon	Absent
Skin lesion appearance	Nodular	Variable	Macular
Hypoesthesia of lesions	Rare	Rare	Common
Number of lymphocytes	Few	Intermediate	Numerous
Number of organisms	Numerous	Many	Few
Lepra cells	Numerous	Present	Absent
Distribution of macrophages	Diffuse	Aggregates	Granulomas
Erythema nodosum leprosum	Common	May occur	Rare

[1]Leprosy is characterized by a clinicopathologic spectrum whose extremes are called lepromatous and tuberculoid leprosy. Borderline leprosy is an intermediate form. Other intermediate forms, borderline-tuberculoid and borderline-lepromatous, are also recognized.

[2]The lepromin test consists of an intradermal injection of *Mycobacterium leprae* antigens. A positive response (induration) indicates the presence of type IV hypersensitivity against leprosy antigens.

with large numbers of macrophages (containing numerous leprosy bacilli), neutrophils, and an acute vasculitis involving dermal and subcutaneous arterioles.

2. Lucio's phenomenon–Lucio's phenomenon is a flare-up vasculitis that occurs in some patients with lepromatous leprosy; it is thought to be due to immune complex deposition (type III hypersensitivity). Small to medium-sized arteries of extremities are mainly affected. It is characterized by the presence of numerous bacilli in the vessel wall, marked intimal fibrosis, and narrowing of the lumen. Ischemic changes may occur in the tissues supplied by the involved arteries.

Other Mycobacterial Infections

A. Tuberculosis: *Mycobacterium tuberculosis* rarely infects the skin to cause **lupus vulgaris,** in which reddish patches occur on the face. **Scrofuloderma** is skin involvement over a tuberculous lymph node, usually in the neck. Both lesions are characterized by caseating granulomas from which *M tuberculosis* can be cultured.

B. *Mycobacterium marinum*–This is an atypical *Mycobacterium* sometimes found in seawater, swimming pools, and aquariums. It causes a chronic granulomatous nodular or ulcerative skin lesion in exposed areas (**"swimming pool granuloma"**). Culture is required to distinguish *M marinum* from *M tuberculosis.*

C. *Mycobacterium ulcerans*–This organism causes **Buruli ulcer,** which is common in parts of Africa. It is characterized by extensive ulceration of skin. Large numbers of acid-fast bacilli are present in the lesions. Culture of *M ulcerans* is diagnostic.

Spirochetal Infections

Syphilis is a common sexually transmitted disease (see Chapter 54) caused by *Treponema pallidum* that causes skin lesions in both early and late stages. In the primary stage, a primary chancre is present, most commonly on the external genitalia. The primary chancre is characterized by an indurated painless ulcer that exudes a serous fluid containing large numbers of treponemes. In the secondary stage, there are a large variety of skin rashes that affect the entire body. Most of these rashes have a nonspecific clinical and histologic pattern. **Condyloma latum** represents a specific skin lesion of secondary syphilis occurring in the anogenital region as a large, moist papule, the serous exudate of which contains large numbers of treponemes. In late syphilis, the skin is one of the sites in which gummas occur. These are nodular masses of granulomatous inflammation characterized by large central areas of gummatous necrosis. Treponemes are not usually demonstrable in gummas.

Yaws is caused by *Treponema pertenue,* a spirochete closely related to *T pallidum.* Yaws is an uncommon disease that is endemic in humid tropical countries around the world. It is transmitted by direct contact and is most prevalent among children. The early stage of the disease is characterized by the development of multiple raspberrylike papillomas of the skin that tend to heal after a varying period, resulting in atrophic epidermis and dermal scarring. The late stage of yaws, which occurs many years after onset of the disease, is characterized by ulcerative nodular masses resembling syphilitic gummas. Treponemes can be demonstrated in biopsies of early lesions.

Pinta is a disease endemic in Central America that is caused by *Treponema carateum.* It is transmitted by direct contact. In the early (primary and secondary) stages, there are multiple red-purple scaly papules. As the disease progresses, severe disfigurement may occur. Treponemes can be detected in biopsies of early lesions.

VIRAL INFECTIONS

1. EPIDERMOTROPIC VIRUSES

Viral infection of the epidermal cells leads to cellular degeneration and necrosis, resulting in formation of an intraepidermal vesicle (Fig 61–3). Diagnosis is by (1) clinical examination, including contact and travel history, incubation period, and distribution of lesions; (2) biopsy, looking for specific histologic changes such as inclusions and giant cells and demonstration of antigens by immunohistochemical techniques; (3) demonstration of virus by electron microscopy; (4) culture; and (5) serologic testing to detect the specific antibody response.

Smallpox (Variola)

The eradication of smallpox is a triumph of preventive medicine. Once the scourge of the world, smallpox has been eradicated by systematic vaccination. Smallpox has historical interest as the disease for which Jenner developed active immunization, showing that infection of humans with the relatively harmless cowpox virus (vaccinia) protected against smallpox. The term vaccination is derived from Jenner's experiment (L *vacca* "cow").

The smallpox virus enters via the respiratory tract and after an incubation period of 12 days disseminates via the bloodstream. Viremia coincides with the onset of fever. The skin rash begins as macules on the third day and progresses to vesicle formation. Confluent hemorrhagic lesions are typical. Severe viremia is common, and the mortality rate is high.

Histologic examination shows an intraepidermal vesicle (Fig 61–3). Infected cells contain eo-

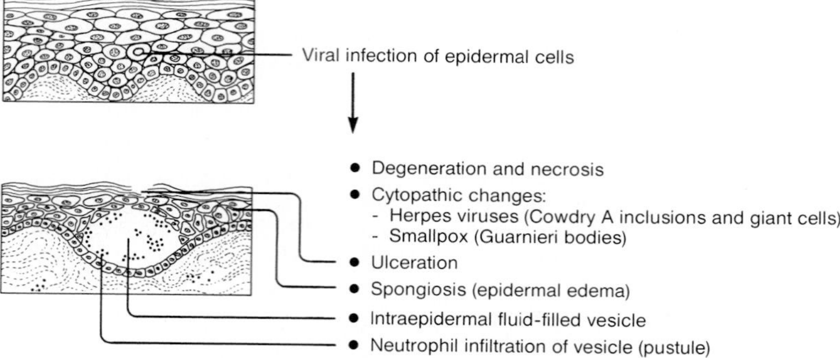

Figure 61-3. Epidermal viral infection leading to formation of an intraepidermal vesicle (as occurs in herpes simplex, chickenpox, zoster, and smallpox infections).

sinophilic cytoplasmic inclusions known as Guarnieri bodies.

Chickenpox (Varicella)

Chickenpox is a common childhood infection caused by varicella virus (also called varicella-zoster virus). The virus enters via the respiratory tract and after an incubation period of 13–17 days disseminates via the bloodstream, localizing mainly in the skin. The rash begins as a macule on the first day of fever and rapidly progresses to form intraepidermal vesicles. The rash is centripetal, the trunk being more affected than the extremities; and regionally heterogeneous, the lesions in a given area being at varying stages of evolution—both features in contrast with smallpox.

Histologic examination shows an intraepidermal vesicle in which cytopathic changes of herpesvirus may be seen, ie, giant cells and Cowdry A intranuclear inclusions (see Chapter 13).

Chickenpox is a mild and self-limited disease as a rule. Complications include corneal lesions, causing visual impairment; pneumonia; encephalitis; and disseminated disease, which occurs mainly in immunodeficient patients.

Herpes Zoster (Shingles)

Herpes zoster is also caused by the varicella-zoster (VZ) virus, the same herpesvirus that causes chickenpox. The virus reaches sensory ganglia during an attack of chickenpox and then remains dormant for long periods. Herpes zoster occurs mainly in patients over 50 years of age and represents activation of the dormant virus. Zoster is frequently precipitated by a debilitating disease such as cancer.

Reactivation leads to ganglionitis, associated with severe pain in the dermatome; and spread of virus down the sensory nerves to the skin, where it infects epidermal cells and produces vesicles. The distribution of vesicles corresponds to the dermatome supplied by the ganglion (Fig 61-4). Involvement of the ophthalmic branch of the trigeminal nerve causes corneal lesions and may lead to blindness.

The diagnosis is made clinically. The histologic features are identical to those of a chickenpox vesicle (Fig 61-3).

Since zoster is caused by reactivation of a dormant virus already present, the disease cannot be transmitted by a patient with chickenpox. However, the reverse may occur—a child may contract chickenpox from a patient with zoster.

Herpes Simplex

Two virus types, herpes simplex 1 and 2, are recognized as causing human disease. In general, herpes simplex type 1 (herpes febrilis) causes oral lesions and type 2 (herpes genitalis) causes genital lesions. There is, however, significant overlap.

Primary herpes simplex infection by type 1 vi-

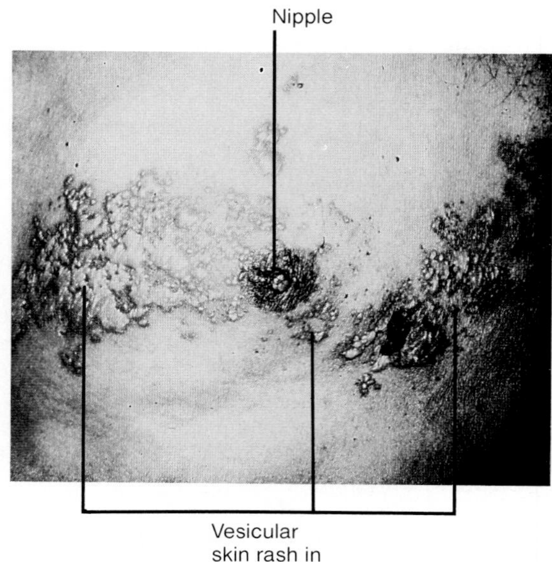

Figure 61-4. Herpes zoster of the chest wall, showing a vesicular skin eruption in a dermatomal distribution.

rus in children causes a severe ulcerative oral lesion with systemic symptoms known as acute gingivostomatitis. More rarely, keratoconjunctivitis occurs. The primary infection is self-limited. The virus is characterized by dormancy in a nearby ganglion with repeated recurrences.

Recurrent herpes simplex type 1 produces the familiar "cold blisters" or "cold sores" that occur in 20–30% of the population. These are typical intraepidermal vesicles (Fig 61–3) on the lips and buccal mucosa. They ulcerate easily to produce painful flat ulcers that heal without scarring or treatment.

Herpes simplex type 2 infection is currently an epidemic sexually transmitted disease in the United States. Herpes genitalis is highly infectious, causing recurrent blisters that may be almost symptomless on the cervix. The main danger is infection of the fetus during childbirth, leading to neonatal encephalitis.

Both types of herpes simplex produce identical histologic lesions, with intraepidermal vesicles, giant cells, and Cowdry A inclusions. The distinction from VZ virus lesions is possible on the basis of immunohistochemical demonstration of antigens specific for the virus types, demonstration of viral nucleic acid by in situ hybridization, clinical features, serologic tests, and culture.

Disseminated herpes simplex infections and encephalitis have a high mortality rate and occur in neonates and immunocompromised hosts. Herpes simplex is one of the viruses suspected of being associated with carcinoma of the uterine cervix.

2. DERMOTROPIC VIRUSES

Measles and rubella ("German measles") produce lesions in the skin, but in the dermis rather than the epidermis. As they do not infect epidermal cells, they do not produce vesicles. Involvement and inflammation around dermal small blood vessels produces an erythematous maculopapular rash.

FUNGAL INFECTIONS

Dermatophyte Infections (Tinea, "Ringworm")

Dermatophytes are a group of mycelial fungi that infect keratin of the stratum corneum, hair, and nails. They do not penetrate deeper parts of the skin. The 3 main species involved are *Trichophyton, Epidermophyton,* and *Microsporum.*

Clinically, the dermatophytes cause circular, elevated, red, scaly lesions that may exude fluid. The terms tinea and ringworm are used interchangeably, the latter because the lesion spreads outward in rings with healing in the center. Severe itching is the rule. Sites affected are the scalp (tinea capitis), the glabrous skin of the body (tinea corporis), the groin (tinea cruris), the feet (tinea pedis, or "athlete's foot"), the nails (tinea unguium), and the beard (tinea barbae).

The diagnosis is made clinically and confirmed by taking a scraping of the infected area. This material is mounted under a coverslip, and potassium hydroxide (KOH) is added to dissolve the keratin. The mycelial fungi can then be seen. Culture is necessary for species diagnosis.

Tinea Versicolor

This common infection is caused by *Pityrosporum orbicularis* (previously called *Malassezia*), which also infects only the stratum corneum; hair and nails are spared. It presents as an asymptomatic macule (area of discoloration, hyperpigmented in white-skinned races and hypopigmented in dark-skinned races). Multiple lesions are common and may cause facial disfigurement.

The diagnosis is made by examination of a KOH preparation of a scraping that shows mycelia and round spores ("spaghetti and meatballs").

Deep Fungal Infections

Deep fungal infections of the skin come about in 3 ways: **(1) Local inoculation** (puncture wounds, etc) is a common route of infection in chromoblastomycosis and sporotrichosis and, rarely, other fungal infections. **(2) Burnt or ulcerated skin** may harbor infection with a large number of opportunistic fungi such as *Candida* and *Aspergillus,* which may cause simple surface infections or may penetrate deeply, invade blood vessels, and result in fungemia. **(3)** Skin involvement secondary to **bloodstream spread** is usually from a primary focus in the lung. Such disseminated fungal disease may be manifested only in the skin or may be widespread, with numerous skin lesions plus organ involvement and severe systemic symptoms. Coccidioidomycosis, histoplasmosis, blastomycosis, and cryptococcosis all belong to this group.

Clinically, the skin lesions may be papular, pustular, or verrucous (wartlike). Multiple satellite pustules are often present and may coalesce to form larger lesions. Lymphangitic spread is characteristic.

Histologic sections show a mixed granulomatous and suppurative inflammation. In most cases, the fungus can be identified in tissue sections (sporotrichosis is the exception). Culture is diagnostic.

Mycetoma

This is a specific form of chronic suppurative inflammation that affects skin (Fig 61–5), causing extensive local tissue destruction without a tendency to disseminate in the body. It is caused by a variety of microorganisms other than fungi, including *Actinomyces* and *Nocardia* species (fila-

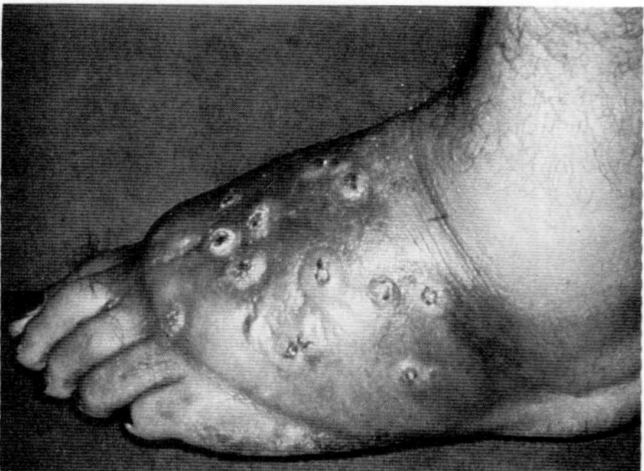

Figure 61–5. Madura foot, showing marked swelling, induration, and multiple sinuses draining purulent material and colonies of organisms. Gram stain and culture are necessary for specific microbiologic diagnosis.

mentous gram-positive bacteria) as well as several mycelial fungi, most commonly *Allescheria boydii.*

Clinically, mycetoma presents as an indurated abscess with multiple draining sinuses in the overlying skin. Colonies of the causative organism are frequently recognizable in pus from the draining sinuses as yellow ("sulfur") granules.

Histologically, there is extensive fibrosis, necrosis, and neutrophil infiltration. Special stains (Gram, acid-fast, silver) can help identify the organism. Diagnosis is made by culture of the granules.

PARASITIC INFECTIONS

Leishmaniasis

Leishmania trophozoites multiply in macrophages and result in diffuse accumulation of macrophages without granuloma formation. Massive enlargement of affected organs may occur. The diagnosis is made by finding the organisms (after Giemsa staining) in macrophages in a biopsy specimen or smear.

Three forms of leishmaniasis are caused by 3 different species of *Leishmania.*

Cutaneous leishmaniasis, caused by *Leishmania tropica,* is localized to the skin, producing a papule that progresses to a chronic ulcer. Oriental sore is an alternative name for the disease. This lesion heals spontaneously after about 1 year. Distribution is throughout the tropics, and this is the only form of the disease that is seen, albeit rarely, in the United States.

Mucocutaneous leishmaniasis, caused by *Leishmania braziliensis,* affects the face, nose, and oral cavity, producing marked nodular thickening with ulceration. Severe disfigurement occurs. It is endemic in Central and South America.

Visceral leishmaniasis (kala-azar) is caused by *Leishmania donovani* and is characterized by involvement of the reticuloendothelial system (liver and spleen). Skin involvement is rare. Kala-azar is endemic in the Mediterranean region and in South and East Asia.

Filariasis

Onchocerciasis (due to *Onchocerca volvulus* infection) is a common cause of skin and eye disease in Africa and a frequent cause of blindness. The disease is transmitted by the bite of the simulian fly. Onchocerciasis is characterized by subcutaneous nodules (onchocercomas) composed of a tangled mass of worms surrounded by fibrosis and inflammatory cells with large numbers of eosinophils. Microfilariae (larval forms) are present in the skin around the nodule but do not enter the bloodstream. The diagnosis is made by finding adult worms or microfilariae in a skin specimen.

Lymphatic filariasis (due to infection with *Wuchereria bancrofti* and *Brugia malayi*) is a common disease in South and Southeast Asia. Death of the lymphatic-dwelling filarial worms leads to an inflammatory reaction and lymphatic obstruction. The disease is transmitted by several species of mosquito. Changes in the skin are those of lymphatic obstruction, causing chronic lymphedema **(elephantiasis).**

Larva Migrans

Larva migrans is a rare disorder caused by larval forms of animal nematode parasites that accidentally gain entry to the human body; the common species are hookworms and roundworms of dogs and cats. Migration of the larvae in the skin **(cutaneous larva migrans)** or viscera **(visceral larva migrans)** evokes an inflammatory reaction—usually granulomatous with numerous eosinophils.

Scabies

Scabies is a common infection caused by the itch mite, *Sarcoptes scabiei.* The mite burrows into the stratum corneum, producing characteristic serpiginous burrows from which the mite can be extracted. As it moves, the mite lays eggs, which cause pruritus and lead to scratching, excoriation of the skin, and secondary bacterial infection.

Norwegian scabies is a variant seen in individuals with low resistance, such as children with leukemia, malnutrition, or Down's syndrome. It is characterized by widespread erythema, crusting, and scaling with no obvious burrows.

IMMUNOLOGIC DISEASES OF THE SKIN

Allergic Dermatitis (Eczema & "Contact" Dermatitis)

A large number of allergens produce dermatitis, acting either directly on the skin or via the bloodstream (after ingestion). In many cases, multiple allergens are involved, and in others the allergen is obscure. Type I and type III hypersensitivity mechanisms are involved, and acute dermatitis is the result (Fig 61–6). In type I reactions, patients have a high incidence of associated atopic disorders such as asthma and hay fever. Type IV hypersensitivity is responsible for chronic "contact" dermatitis, in which the area of dermatitis often corresponds exactly to contact with the allergen (eg, a bracelet, suspender, watch strap, etc).

Pemphigus Vulgaris

Pemphigus vulgaris is a chronic, severe, potentially fatal disease of middle age (40–60 years) characterized by formation of bullae (large blisters) in the skin and oral mucosa (Table 61–3). It is associated with IgG autoantibodies in the serum, which react against intercellular attachment sites of keratinocytes (Fig 61–7A), leading to separation of keratinocytes (acantholysis) and intraepidermal (suprabasal) vesicles that contain rounded-up acantholytic cells.

Clinically, the bullae of pemphigus vulgaris are large and flaccid and appear to arise on otherwise normal skin. They easily rupture, leaving tender, raw areas that progressively enlarge. **Nikolsky's sign** is positive (when the tip of the observer's finger is pressed on the skin of a patient with pemphigus, the horny layer can be felt to slide on the underlying basal layers because of the acantholysis).

Systemic symptoms such as fever and loss of weight are prominent. Without treatment, most patients die within 1 year. Treatment with steroids is effective in most cases.

Bullous Pemphigoid

Bullous pemphigoid is seen mainly in the elderly (aged 60–80 years). It resembles pemphigus clinically except that mucosal lesions are rare. It is associated with an IgG antibody that is deposited in linear fashion along the basement membrane of the skin, causing the basal cells to separate from the dermis to produce a subepidermal vesicle (Fig 61–7B). The vesicle contains a predominance of eosinophils.

Clinically, the vesicles are large and widespread. When they break, they produce denuded areas that show a tendency to heal. Nikolsky's sign is negative. The condition is relatively benign.

Dermatitis Herpetiformis

Dermatitis herpetiformis is a chronic disease characterized by erythematous vesicles and severe itching. It occurs in adults aged 20–40 years and is associated with granular deposits of IgA (contrast pemphigus and pemphigoid) at the dermoepidermal junction, especially at the tips of dermal papillae (Fig 61–7C). Dermatitis herpetiformis is associated with gluten-induced enteropathy ("celiac disease"), but the dermatitis does not improve with a gluten-free diet.

Histologically, there are subepidermal vesicles, with microabscesses at the tips of dermal papillae, and "nuclear dust" (disintegrating neutrophil nuclear material) in the upper dermis.

Clinically, dermatitis herpetiformis has a chronic course with spontaneous remissions and relapses. The patient's general health status is usually not affected.

Lupus Erythematosus

Lupus erythematosus is an autoimmune disorder that affects multiple systems and commonly shows skin involvement. It is associated with various immunologic abnormalities (see Chapter 68).

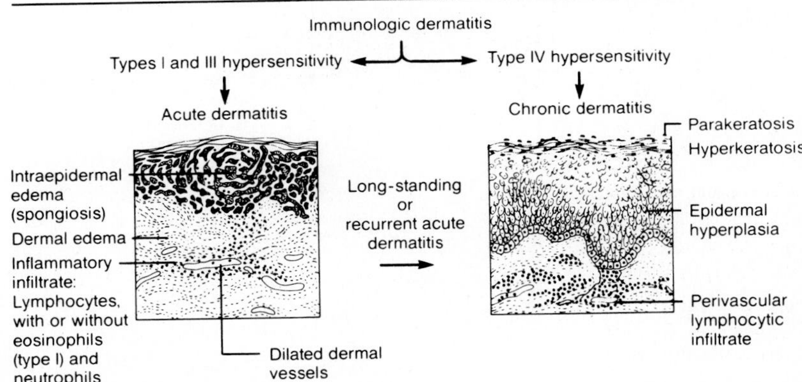

Figure 61–6. Immunologically mediated (allergic) dermatitis. In acute dermatitis, spongiosis, frequently accompanied by the formation of intraepidermal vesicles (not shown in this diagram), is the dominant feature. In chronic dermatitis, epidermal hyperplasia predominates. These histologic appearances are not specific.

Table 61-3. Common causes of blisters (bullae) in the skin.[1]

Site of Blister	Disease	Pathogenesis
Upper epidermal (subcorneal)	Impetigo (pustules) Burns, friction blisters	Infection Physical injury
Intraepidermal	Viral infection Acute dermatitis	Infection Immunologic mechanism
Suprabasal	Pemphigus vulgaris Benign familial pemphigus Darier's disease	Immunologic mechanism Inherited Inherited
Subepidermal	Bullous pemphigoid Dermatitis herpetiformis Epidermolysis bullosa Erythema multiforme Lichen planus	Immunologic mechanism Immunologic mechanism Inherited ?Immunologic mechanism Uncertain

[1]Differential diagnosis of bullae is important because of differences in etiology, prognosis, and treatment.

Skin lesions may occur either as isolated manifestations (discoid lupus erythematosus) or as part of systemic disease (systemic lupus erythematosus).

Systemic and discoid lupus erythematosus are identical histologically, characterized by epidermal atrophy, hyperkeratosis, follicular keratin plugs, liquefactive degeneration of the basal layers of the epidermis, and lymphocytic vasculitis in the dermis. However, systemic and discoid lupus erythematosus differ in that the former shows IgG and complement deposition in the basement membrane of both involved and uninvolved skin, whereas discoid lupus shows only deposition in clinically abnormal skin.

INHERITED DISEASES OF THE SKIN

Epidermolysis Bullosa

Epidermolysis bullosa includes several inherited variants characterized by onset in infancy and the formation of vesicles as a result of minor trauma.

Epidermolysis bullosa simplex is dominantly inherited. It is usually a mild disease, healing without scarring, and buccal mucosa is not involved. However, in the recessive-dystrophic form of

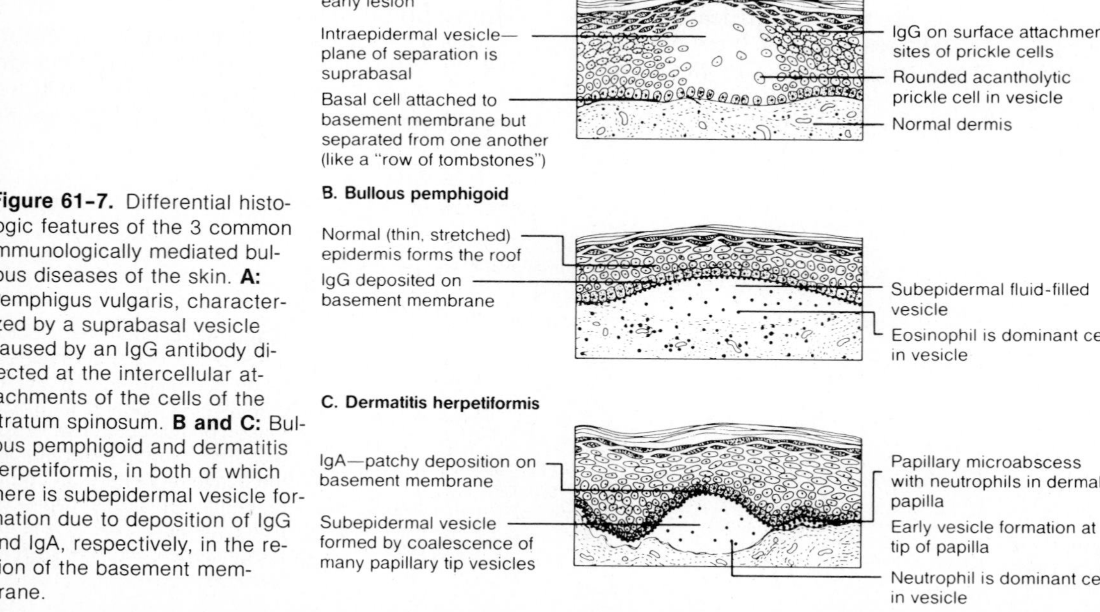

Figure 61-7. Differential histologic features of the 3 common immunologically mediated bullous diseases of the skin. **A:** Pemphigus vulgaris, characterized by a suprabasal vesicle caused by an IgG antibody directed at the intercellular attachments of the cells of the stratum spinosum. **B and C:** Bullous pemphigoid and dermatitis herpetiformis, in both of which there is subepidermal vesicle formation due to deposition of IgG and IgA, respectively, in the region of the basement membrane.

epidermolysis bullosa, there is extensive ulceration and scarring, and the oral mucosa is involved.

Histologically, vesicle formation occurs at various levels in the epidermis, probably as a result of defective intercellular attachments or defective anchoring of the basal cells.

Darier's Disease (Keratosis Follicularis)

Darier's disease is inherited as an autosomal dominant trait; cases without a family history represent mutations. The disease presents as a slowly progressive skin eruption consisting of hyperkeratotic crusted papules. Vesicles are rare.

Histologic features are characteristic and consist of acanthosis (thickening of epidermis), hyperkeratosis (increased keratin layer), dyskeratosis (abnormal keratinization), and suprabasal acantholysis, leading to the formation of clefts in the epidermis.

Benign Familial Pemphigus (Hailey-Hailey Disease)

Benign familial pemphigus is inherited as an autosomal dominant trait and characterized by localized eruption of vesicles, commonly in the skin of the axillas and groins. Histologically, there is acantholysis and vesicle formation but no immunoglobulin deposition.

Pseudoxanthoma Elasticum

This rare, recessively inherited disorder of elastic fibers produces soft yellowish plaques in the skin. The sides of the neck, the axillas, and the groins are most commonly affected. Histologically, there is accumulation of abnormal elastic fibers in the dermis.

Other sites where elastic tissue is found may also show involvement, ie, the ocular fundi and the arteries, leading to ischemia (coronary circulation), hemorrhage (commonly gastrointestinal), and abnormal peripheral pulses.

Ichthyosis

Ichthyosis exists in several forms with different inheritance patterns (dominant, recessive, X-linked) and varying degrees of severity. All are associated with hyperkeratosis, which may produce fishlike scales. Severe congenital forms may lead to early death.

IDIOPATHIC SKIN DISEASES

Many skin diseases have no known cause or pathogenetic mechanism. They are discussed here as a group under the heading idiopathic skin diseases. They are not related in any way other than in being of unknown origin.

Psoriasis Vulgaris

Psoriasis is common, affecting 1% of the population. It is a chronic disease characterized by remissions and exacerbations. The lesions of psoriasis are sharply defined papules and red plaques covered by silvery scales. Removal of the scales leads to multiple punctate hemorrhages. The nails are affected in 50% of cases.

The basic defect in the epidermis is an increase in the rate of maturation (Fig 61–8). It takes only

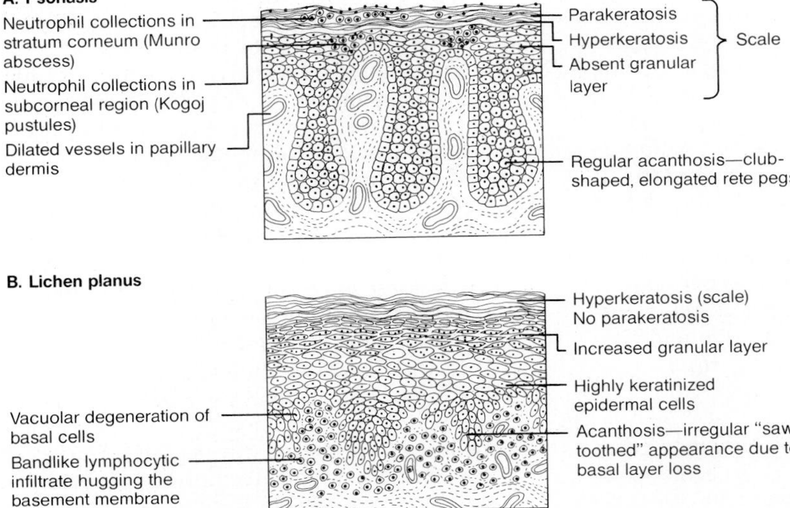

Figure 61–8. Contrasting features of psoriasis **(A)** and lichen planus **(B),** both of which are characterized clinically by the formation of papular skin lesions with silvery hyperkeratotic scales. Psoriasis is the result of an increased rate of epidermal cell turnover; lichen planus is the result of decreased epidermal cell turnover.

3 or 4 days for a psoriatic basal cell to become a parakeratotic cell in the horny layer, compared with the normal 2–4 weeks. The cause of this increased rate of cell turnover is unknown. Microscopic examination shows regular acanthosis with clubbing and fusion of rete pegs, hyperkeratosis with parakeratosis and an absent granular layer, and the presence of neutrophils in the epidermis with abscesses in the stratum corneum (Munro microabscesses) and subcorneal layer (Kojog spongiform pustules).

Psoriasis is rarely associated with a destructive joint disease resembling rheumatoid arthritis.

Lichen Planus

Lichen planus is a chronic disorder characterized by the appearance of violaceous, itching papules and plaques on the skin, oral mucosa, and external genitalia. Women are affected more frequently than men, and the maximal age incidence is 30–60 years.

The basic defect is a decrease in the rate of cellular proliferation (Fig 61–8), causing prolonged retention of cells in the epidermis with increased amounts of keratinization. Degeneration of the basal germinative layer is probably responsible for decreased cell turnover. The cause of basal layer degeneration is unknown. The presence of a dense lymphocytic infiltrate immediately below the basal layer suggests the possibility of a cell-mediated immunologic mechanism. Microscopic examination shows irregular acanthosis, hyperkeratosis, a prominent granular cell layer, vacuolar degeneration of basal cells, and a bandlike lymphocytic infiltrate in the upper dermis.

Erythema Multiforme

Erythema multiforme is a common skin disorder that may affect patients of any age. The cause and pathogenesis are unknown, though an immunologic mechanism is suspected. It is associated with a large variety of diseases, including many infections, drugs, cancers, and autoimmune diseases. It is characterized clinically by diverse lesions, including macules, papules, vesicles, and target lesions (red papules with a pale central area). Microscopically, erythema multiforme is characterized (1) by epidermal changes, including spongiosis, dyskeratosis, and epidermal necrosis; and (2) by dermal changes including vasculitis and edema.

Minor forms are self-limited. The major form of the disease **(Stevens-Johnson syndrome)** is characterized by high fever, extensive bulla formation and necrosis, ulceration of skin and orogenital mucosa, and a high mortality rate.

Erythema Nodosum

Erythema nodosum is the most common form of panniculitis (inflammation of subcutaneous fat). It may be associated with many diseases, including infections (β-hemolytic streptococcal infections, primary tuberculosis, fungal infections, leprosy), drugs (sulfonamides, iodides), sarcoidosis, acute rheumatic fever, inflammatory bowel disease, and cancer. However, most cases of erythema nodosum have no associated disease.

Clinically, there are multiple tender red nodules, commonly in the anterior tibial region. The disease remits spontaneously in 3 or 4 weeks without scarring.

Histologically, there is panniculitis characterized by cellular infiltration (mainly lymphocytes, histiocytes with a few granulocytes) of the connective tissue septa between lobules of subcutaneous fat, together with vasculitis.

Pityriasis Rosea

Pityriasis rosea is a common self-limited condition occurring in adults 20–30 years of age. It is suspected of having a viral origin, though no agent has yet been isolated.

The onset is typically with a "herald patch"—a sharply defined scaling plaque—followed by a generalized skin eruption consisting of oval salmon-pink papules covered by thin scales. Lesions tend to follow flexure lines.

Histologically, the features are those of nonspecific subacute dermatitis.

Acanthosis Nigricans

Acanthosis nigricans is characterized by velvety dark patches that involve especially the skin of the groin area in middle-aged patients, 50% of whom have associated visceral carcinoma. The mechanism for this association is unknown. Histologically, there is hyperkeratosis and papillomatosis, with some increase in melanin production by the melanocytes.

Melanocyte Disorders

Vitiligo is a relatively common disorder manifested by loss of pigmentation of the skin. Lesions are irregular in size and shape but sharply defined. They are more conspicuous in members of dark-skinned races. Histologically, there is total absence of melanocytes in the discolored areas, thought to be due to immune-mediated destruction (antimelanocyte antibodies are present in many cases). Vitiligo is distinct from **albinism,** in which pigmentation is absent throughout the body (skin, hair, eyes) owing to failure of melanin production by melanocytes.

Lentigo consists of small pigmented lesions in the young (lentigo simplex) or elderly (lentigo senilis, or "liver spots"). There is hyperplasia of the rete pegs, with increased numbers of melanocytes. These are not true neoplasms, and they are not premalignant.

Ephelides (freckles) are distinct from lentigo in that the increase in pigmentation is due to increased melanin production by normal numbers of melanocytes. Freckles are common in the young and have no sinister significance. They appear as small, flat, irregular brown lesions. They tend to increase with exposure to sunlight and begin to fade at puberty. A similar condition in pregnancy is called melasma or chloasma.

CYSTS OF THE SKIN

Epidermal Cyst & Pilar Cyst

Epidermal cysts are lined by keratinizing squamous epithelium and filled with laminated keratin. **Pilar cysts** (also called trichilemmal cysts) are similar but lack a granular layer and contain amorphous rather than laminated keratin. Pilar cysts are believed to develop from hair follicles.

Clinically, these common cysts are filled with thick yellow material and are often incorrectly called "sebaceous cysts."

Dermoid Cyst

Dermoid cysts are congenital cysts that occur at lines of embryonic skin closure and fusion, most commonly around the eyes (external angular dermoid). They are lined by an epithelium that shows various epidermal appendages, including hair follicles and sebaceous glands.

NEOPLASMS OF THE SKIN (Table 61-4)

NEOPLASMS OF KERATINOCYTES

1. BENIGN NEOPLASMS OF KERATINOCYTES

Verruca Vulgaris (Common Wart)

The common wart is caused by a papillomavirus and is transmitted from one site to another—and one person to another—by direct contact. It may occur anywhere in the skin, with the fingers the most common single site.

Histologically, the wart is a squamous papilloma with variable keratinization and conspicuous keratohyaline granules. Large vacuolated cells in the proliferating squamous epithelium stain positively for papilloma virus by the immunoperoxidase technique.

Condyloma Acuminatum

Condylomata acuminata are similar to large warts and are caused by a different serotype of papillomavirus. They occur in genital skin and mucosa and are sexually transmitted.

Molluscum Contagiosum

Molluscum contagiosum is caused by a virus of the poxvirus group. Lesions consist of small and discrete dome-shaped papules having an umbilicated center. They ultimately heal spontaneously.

Histologically, the epidermis bulges downward

Table 61-4. Neoplasms of the skin.

Cell of Origin	Benign	Malignant
Keratinocyte	Verruca vulgaris Condyloma acuminatum Molluscum contagiosum Keratoacanthoma	Carcinoma in situ (Bowen's disease) Squamous carcinoma Basal cell carcinoma
Skin adnexal cells	See Table 61-5	
Melanocyte	Nevocellular nevus Blue nevus	Lentigo maligna Superficial spreading malignant melanoma Nodular malignant melanoma
Merkel cell	...	Merkel cell carcinoma
Dermal mesenchymal cells	Dermatofibroma Fibroxanthoma Hemangioma Neurofibroma	Dermatofibrosarcoma protuberans Angiosarcoma Malignant schwannoma
Lymphocyte	...	Mycosis fungoides Sézary's syndrome
Mast cell	Urticaria pigmentosa Solitary mastocytoma	Systemic mastocytosis

into the dermis and the epidermal cells contain intracytoplasmic inclusion bodies known as molluscum bodies.

Seborrheic Keratosis

This lesion is very common, occurring on the trunk, extremities, and face, usually in elderly persons. The lesions are flat, raised, soft, sharply demarcated, and brown. Seborrheic keratosis is benign and probably not a true neoplasm.

Histologically, seborrheic keratosis is a flat, often pigmented squamous epithelial proliferation with many keratin-filled cysts (horn cysts).

Keratoacanthoma

Keratoacanthoma usually occurs in middle age, most commonly on the face or upper extremities. It is characterized by a rapid early growth phase, reaching maximum size in a few weeks, followed by a static phase (up to 1 year) after which the lesion spontaneously involutes with scarring. It is important to note that the benign keratoacanthoma has an early growth phase that is much more rapid than its malignant counterpart, squamous carcinoma.

Histologically, keratoacanthoma appears as a cup-shaped lesion with an irregular keratin-filled crater in the center. Though resembling invasion, the base of the lesion is smooth and does not penetrate deeper than the level of the hair follicles. The cells frequently show mild atypia, mitotic activity, and dyskeratosis, making histologic distinction from squamous carcinoma difficult.

2. PREMALIGNANT LESIONS OF THE SKIN

Actinic Keratosis

Actinic keratosis represents the effect of ultraviolet radiation of sunlight on skin. It occurs predominantly in fair-skinned individuals with a history of sunlight exposure (common in Australia, Southern and Southwestern United States, South Africa). Actinic keratoses appear as rough erythematous or brownish papules, usually small.

Histologically, there is dysplasia of the epidermis and degeneration of dermal collagen (so-called solar elastosis). Actinic keratosis is a premalignant lesion; the risk of carcinoma is directly proportionate to the degree of epithelial dysplasia.

3. MALIGNANT NEOPLASMS

Bowen's Disease (Carcinoma in Situ)

Bowen's disease may occur either on sun-exposed skin or on the vulva, oral mucosa, and glans penis. It is associated with visceral malignant disease. Rarely it is caused by chronic arsenic exposure.

Bowen's disease presents clinically as a slowly enlarging erythematous patch that on histologic examination shows extreme dysplastic change sufficient to warrant the term carcinoma in situ. By definition, there is no invasion of the basement membrane.

Basal Cell Carcinoma (Basal Cell Epithelioma)

Basal cell carcinoma is a common skin neoplasm, occurring usually in sun-exposed areas of light-skinned individuals over the age of 40 years. The face is the most common site. Rarely, multiple basal cell carcinomas arise in early life as part of an autosomal dominant inherited disorder in which abnormalities of bone, the nervous system, and the eyes coexist with the skin lesions (nevoid basal cell epithelioma syndrome).

Clinically, early basal cell carcinoma appears as a waxy papule with small telangiectatic vessels on its surface. Central necrosis produces a punched-out ulcer with pearly rolled edges (so-called rodent ulcer) (Fig 61–9). Melanin pigmentation is commonly present. A sclerosing variant presents as an indurated plaque without surface ulceration.

Histologically, basal cell carcinoma arises from the basal layer of the epidermis and invades the dermis as nests and cords of cells. The neoplastic

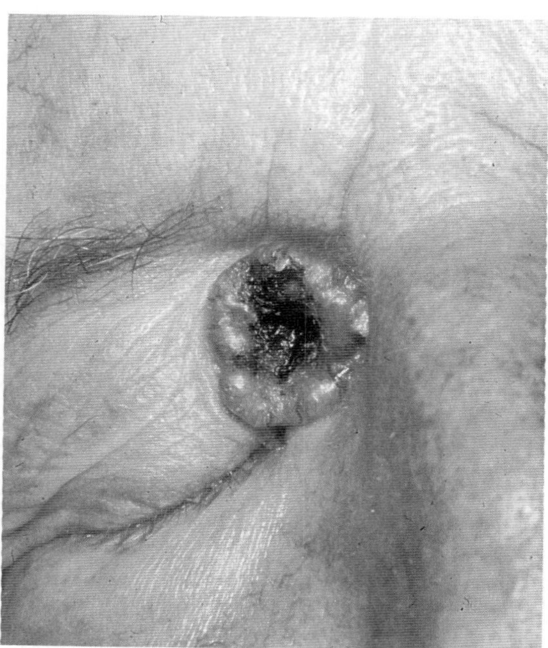

Figure 61–9. Basal cell carcinoma of the eyelid. This is the typical appearance, with a central punched-out ulcer surrounded by a raised edge that has a pearly appearance.

cells resemble basal cells, forming a palisade (basal layer) at the periphery of the tumor nests (Fig 61–10). In the sclerosing (morphealike) variety, proliferating connective tissue cells surround the neoplastic basal cells.

Basal cell carcinoma is locally aggressive; it may invade deeply to involve bone and muscle but almost never metastasizes. Wide surgical excision is curative, but the determination that the margins of resection are free of tumor requires multiple frozen section examinations at the time of surgery.

Squamous Carcinoma

Squamous carcinoma of the skin is also very common, especially in sun-exposed skin of elderly, fair-skinned individuals. It is a locally aggressive neoplasm that rarely metastasizes (1% of cases). Squamous carcinoma may also occur in relation to chronic ulcers, burn scars, and infected sinuses, in which case there is a much higher incidence of metastases (20–30%).

Clinically, squamous carcinoma presents as a shallow ulcer with a raised, everted, firm border.

Histologically, the tumor is composed of large polygonal cells with abundant pink cytoplasm (ie, they resemble cells of the prickle layer). Atypia, pleomorphism, and mitotic activity vary from minimal, in well-differentiated (grade 1) tumors, to marked in poorly differentiated ones (grade 3). Keratin-containing epithelial pearls are prominent in well-differentiated tumors. Invasion is present.

Wide surgical excision of squamous carcinomas arising in sun-exposed skin is usually curative. Radical lymph node dissection and other forms of adjuvant therapy may be necessary in management of other squamous carcinomas with a higher metastatic potential.

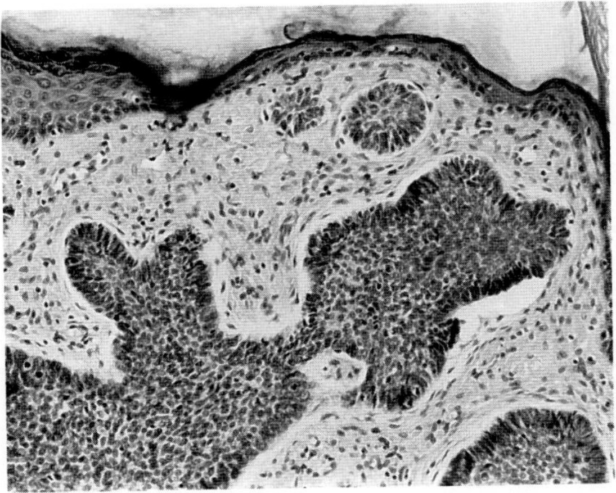

Figure 61–10. Basal cell carcinoma, showing irregular infiltrating nests of carcinoma cells in the dermis. The nests are composed of small cells that show peripheral palisading.

NEOPLASMS OF SKIN APPENDAGES

Neoplasms arising in skin appendages are usually benign and are identified by their distinctive histologic features and classified according to their differentiation as outlined in Table 61–5. All present clinically as painless skin nodules and are cured by simple surgical removal. Very rarely, adnexal skin tumors are malignant, with both locally infiltrative and metastasizing capability.

MELANOCYTIC NEOPLASMS (Fig 61–11)

There are 2 broad categories of melanocytic neoplasms.

(1) Nevi develop from clusters of melanocyte precursor cells (nevus cells) that are arrested during the terminal phase of their migration from the neural crest to the epidermis, where they form the melanocytes. Nevi develop in childhood but persist into adult life and are benign (see below).

(2) Malignant melanomas, by contrast, develop by neoplastic transformation of melanocytes in the epidermis and invade the dermis secondarily. They are relatively common in adults and rare in children.

Nevocellular Nevus (Melanocytic Nevus)

The term nevus (L *naevus* "mole") is used in a general sense for many cutaneous lesions present at birth. Melanocytic nevi are usually not present at birth but appear in childhood and stop growing soon after puberty. They are extremely common and are better regarded as hamartomatous growths rather than true neoplasms. They are benign and present clinically as flat, papular, papillomatous or pedunculated pigmented (black or brown) lesions (Fig 61–12). If a nevus changes its form in any way, malignancy should be suspected.

Histologically, moles are composed of nests of nevus (melanocytic) cells, which may be found in the dermis **(intradermal nevus),** at the junction between epidermis and dermis **(junctional nevus),** or in both locations **(compound nevus).** Junctional activity (melanocytic proliferation in the junctional zone) usually decreases after puberty; if it is prominent in an older patient or associated with cytologic atypia, malignant melanoma should be considered. In young patients, compound nevi may show marked cytologic atypia, pleomorphism, and junctional proliferation **(Spitz nevus)** with no implication of malignant behavior. When a Spitz nevus occurs in an older person, histologic differentiation from malignant melanoma is difficult.

Table 61-5. Classification of skin adnexal neoplasms.[1]

Neoplasm	Differentiation	Common Sites
Trichofolliculoma	Hair	Face, solitary
Trichoepithelioma	Hair	Face; may be multiple
Pilomatrixoma	Hair	All over body, mainly in children
Syringoma	Eccrine (sweat gland)	Lower eyelids, frequently multiple
Syringocystadenoma papilliferum	Eccrine	Face, scalp
Clear-cell hidradenoma	Eccrine	All over body
Eccrine poroma	Eccrine	Feet, hands; mainly in elderly
Eccrine spiradenoma	Eccrine	All over body
Hidradenoma papilliferum	Apocrine	Vulva in females
Cylindroma	Apocrine	Scalp; may be multiple
Nevus sebaceus	Sebaceous	Scalp, face; from birth
Sebaceous adenoma	Sebaceous	Rare

[1]These are all benign neoplasms. Their malignant counterparts occur very rarely, with sebaceous carcinoma being the most common.

Congenital Melanocytic Nevus

This uncommon lesion is present at birth but is not inherited. It presents as a pigmented, often hairy lesion occurring anywhere on the body (trunk, scalp and face, extremities). It may be very large and may be associated with many scattered smaller nevi (Fig 61–12).

Histologically, congenital melanocytic nevus is a compound nevus with a tendency to neural differentiation. It may predispose to the occurrence of malignant melanoma, which may be present at birth or may occur in infancy or later. The malignant potential of this lesion is thought to be very low.

Blue Nevus

Blue nevi are common skin lesions presenting as small, well-circumscribed, bluish-black nodules.

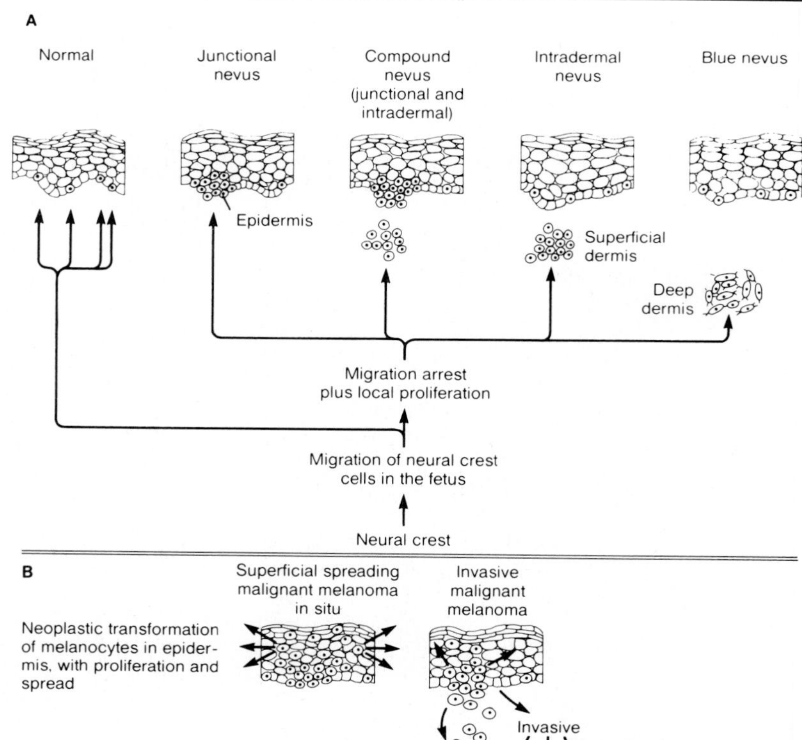

Figure 61–11. Melanocytic lesions. **A:** Melanocytic nevi that result from the arrest of melanocytic cells during embryonic migration from the neural crest, followed by proliferation, usually during childhood. These are hamartomatous rather than neoplastic lesions. **B:** Malignant melanoma, which arises from the neoplastic transformation of normally located melanocytes in the epidermis, followed by proliferation. Intraepidermal (in situ) and invasive phases of proliferation are recognized. Malignant melanomas commonly arise in older patients.

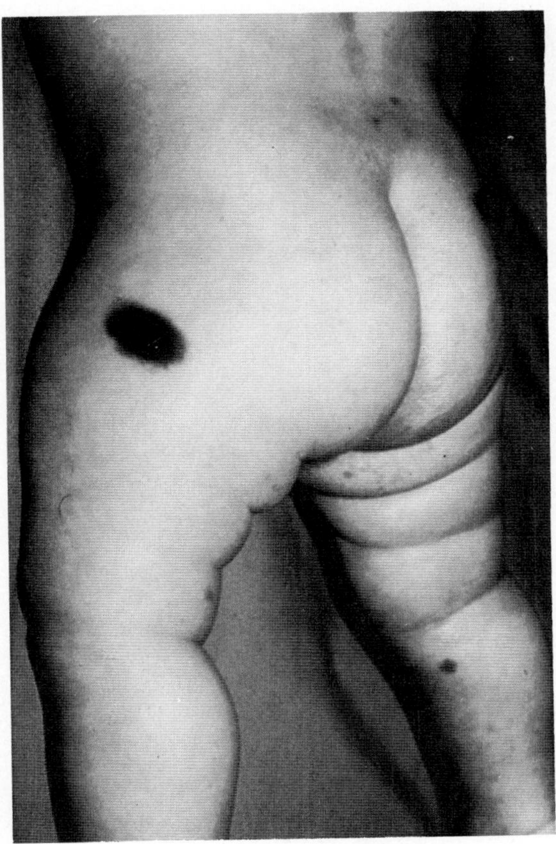

Figure 61–12. Congential melanocytic nevi of the skin. Note multiple lesions on the left thigh, right back, and right calf.

Histologically, the usual blue nevus is composed of a poorly circumscribed collection of heavily pigmented dendritic melanocytes deep in the dermis. The **cellular blue nevus** is a variant composed of large islands of spindle-shaped nevus cells with abundant cytoplasm and little or no melanin. Pleomorphism and mild cytologic atypia may be present, leading to confusion with malignant melanoma. Except in very rare instances, blue nevi are benign.

Malignant Melanoma in Situ (Noninvasive Malignant Melanoma)

A. Lentigo Maligna (Hutchinson's Freckle): Lentigo maligna occurs mainly in sun-exposed areas of skin in elderly persons. It presents clinically as an unevenly pigmented macule that becomes progressively larger.

Histologically, lentigo maligna is characterized by a marked increase in the number of melanocytes in the basal layer. The melanocytes are frequently spindle-shaped and show nuclear pleomorphism. Lentigo maligna tends to remain in situ for long periods (sometimes 10–15 years) before dermal invasion occurs. Dermal invasion is associated clinically with enlargement, induration, and nodularity of the macule.

B. Superficial Spreading Melanoma: This small pigmented and slightly elevated lesion occurs regardless of exposure to sunlight. The in-situ phase is much shorter than in lentigo maligna, and invasion frequently occurs within months after onset. Invasion is characterized clinically by the development of ulceration and bleeding.

Histologically, superficial spreading melanoma is characterized by the presence of nests of large, atypical, hyperchromatic neoplastic melanocytes in the lower epidermis. These cells often show extensive lateral intraepidermal spread (radial growth phase) prior to dermal invasion (vertical growth phase) (Fig 61–13).

Invasive Malignant Melanoma

Invasive malignant melanoma may arise de novo, in a previous lentigo maligna, in a superficial spreading melanoma in situ, in a congenital giant pigmented nevus, or in a nevocellular nevus.

Malignant melanoma occurs most often in skin, though extracutaneous melanomas do occur in a variety of sites: (1) the choroid layer of the eyes (common); (2) the oral cavity, nasal mucosa, and pharynx (rare); (3) the esophagus and bronchus (very rare); and (4) the vaginal and anorectal mucosa (very rare).

Malignant melanoma appears clinically as an elevated pigmented nodule (Fig 61–14) that grows rapidly and tends to bleed and ulcerate. Metastasis via the lymphatics and bloodstream tends to occur early. Rarely, malignant melanomas regress spontaneously.

Histologically, malignant melanoma is characterized by melanocytic proliferation originating in the basal epidermis. The cells show marked cytologic atypia, pleomorphism, nuclear hyperchromatism, and increased mitotic activity. Nuclei are large, with prominent nucleoli. The cytoplasm is abundant and usually contains melanin pigment. When no melanin is present, the term amelanotic or achromatic melanoma is used. In cases of amelanotic melanoma, the diagnosis may be established (1) by electron microscopy, which shows premelanosomes and melanosomes; and (2) by immunohistochemical demonstration of S100 protein or melanoma-related antigens (eg, HMB 45) in the melanocytes.

The tumor cells infiltrate into the dermis and extend upward into the upper part of the epidermis, frequently causing ulceration. The dermis shows a variable lymphocytic infiltrate around the invading melanocytes. Lymphatic involvement by the tumor may result in the formation of **satellite lesions** along the lymphatics.

The prognosis depends on several factors:

(1) The type of melanoma. Malignant mela-

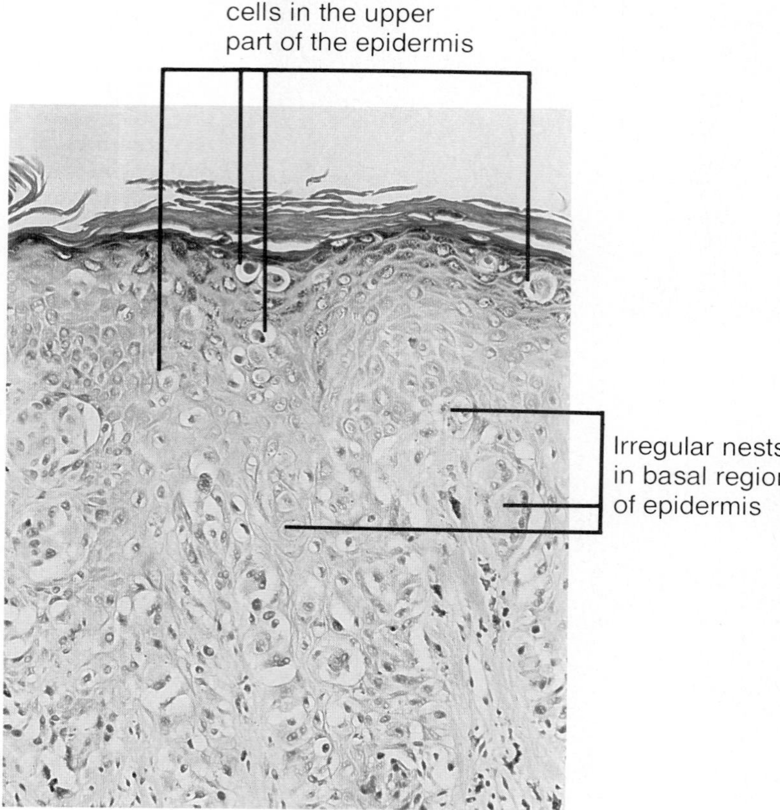

Figure 61-13. Malignant melanoma, superficial spreading type, characterized by nests of cells in the basal region and irregular single cells infiltrating into the upper part of the epidermis.

noma arising in lentigo maligna has a better prognosis than invasive superficial spreading melanoma. When no in-situ component is identified at the margin of the invasive tumor (nodular melanoma), the prognosis is even worse.

(2) The depth of invasion, determined by measurement of vertical extent of tumor below the stratum granulosum. Superficially invasive (< 0.75 mm) melanomas have a better prognosis than deeper invading neoplasms (Fig 61-15).

(3) The level of invasion (Clark) (Fig 61-15).

(4) The number of inflammatory cells. The greater the number of lymphocytes in the tumor, the better the prognosis.

(5) Clinical stage. The presence of lymph node metastases worsens the prognosis. When distant hematogenous metastases are present, the 5-year survival rate is less than 10%.

MERKEL CELL (NEUROENDOCRINE) CARCINOMA

Merkel cell carcinoma arises from Merkel cells, which are neuroendocrine cells situated in the basal epidermis. It presents as a nodular skin lesion and usually occurs in patients over 40 years of age. Histologically, it is composed of small cells with scanty cytoplasm and hyperchromatic nuclei arranged in nests and trabeculae, resembling small-cell undifferentiated carcinoma of the lung. The diagnosis of Merkel cell carcinoma can be confirmed by the finding of neurosecretory granules on electron microscopy and positive staining by immunoperoxidase techniques for neuroendocrine markers such as neuron-specific enolase and chromogranin. A few tumors have been reported to secrete serotonin and calcitonin. Lymph node and distant metastases occur early in the course in about 25% of cases. In the remainder, wide local excision results in cure.

NEOPLASMS OF DERMAL MESENCHYMAL CELLS

Dermatofibroma (Cutaneous Fibrous Histiocytoma)

This common neoplasm presents as a firm, slowly growing, nodular dermal lesion composed of fibroblasts, histiocytes, and collagen in varying amounts. It is benign.

A

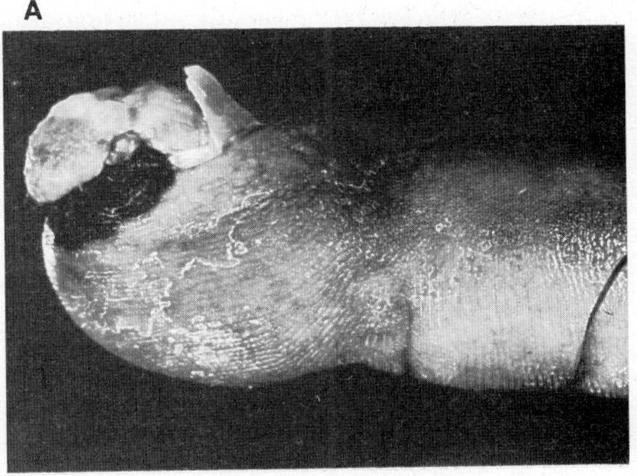

B

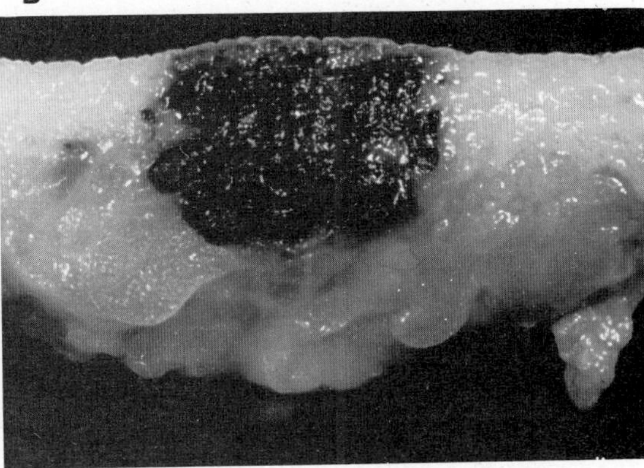

Figure 61–14. Malignant melanoma. **A:** Occurring in the subungual region. The partially pigmented mass has lifted the nail. **B:** A cross section of a lesion in the skin of another patient, showing deep dermal invasion.

Atypical Fibroxanthoma

Atypical fibroxanthoma is a nodular lesion that commonly occurs in a sun-exposed area, usually the head or neck, of an elderly patient. It is usually solitary and small.

Histologically, it is characterized by proliferation of fibroblasts and histiocytes, with marked atypia, pleomorphism, bizarre multinucleated giant cells, and numerous mitoses. The lesion is poorly circumscribed, with extension into subcutaneous fat and frequent ulceration of overlying epidermis. Despite its malignant appearance, the lesion does not metastasize; it may recur locally if inadequately excised.

Dermatofibrosarcoma Protuberans

This slowly growing nodular lesion may reach large size and result in ulceration of the overlying epidermis (Fig 61–16). It is locally invasive despite apparent gross circumscription. Surgical removal should include a wide margin of normal-appearing skin to avoid local recurrence. Metastases are rare but may occur after many years, especially in lesions that have recurred several times.

Histologically, dermatofibrosarcoma protuberans is characterized by proliferation of fibroblasts, showing cytologic atypia and increased mitotic activity. Irregular invasion of subcutaneous fat, fascia, and muscle may be present.

MALIGNANT LYMPHOMAS

Cutaneous malignant lymphoma may occur primarily in the skin or in the course of disseminated lymphoma (5–10% of patients with Hodgkin's lymphoma; 15–20% of patients with non-Hodg-

Table 61–6. Skin manifestations of systemic diseases.

Change	Associated Diseases
Hyperpigmentation	Addison's disease, hemochromatosis, heavy metal (arsenic, silver) poisoning, chronic renal failure, chronic liver disease
Hypopigmentation	Albinism, Chédiak-Higashi syndrome, tuberous sclerosis, hypopituitarism
Pigmented spots	Peutz-Jeghers syndrome, neurofibromatosis, Albright's syndrome
Yellow-orange discoloration	Jaundice, carotenemia
Pruritus	Chronic renal failure, obstructive jaundice, Hodgkin's disease
Petechial hemorrhages	Infective endocarditis, vasculitis, scurvy, thrombocytopenia, bacteremia
Bruising of skin	Coagulation disorders, leukemia, bacteremia, amyloidosis, Cushing's syndrome, scurvy
Telangiectases	Chronic liver disease, hereditary hemorrhagic telangiectasia
Hirsutism	Porphyria, Cushing's syndrome, androgen excess (many causes)
Hair loss	Hypothyroidism, systemic lupus erythematosus
Hyperkeratosis	Vitamin A toxicity, scurvy
Dermatitis	Phenylketonuria, pellagra, hypogammaglobulinemia, Parkinson's disease, vitamin A toxicity
Dermatitis herpetiformis	Celiac disease
Acanthosis nigricans	Associated with visceral carcinoma in 50% of cases
Dermatomyositis	Associated with visceral carcinoma in 30% of cases
Pyoderma gangrenosum	Ulcerative colitis, rheumatoid arthritis, myeloid leukemia
Erythema nodosum	Tuberculosis, streptococcal infections, rheumatic fever, leprosy

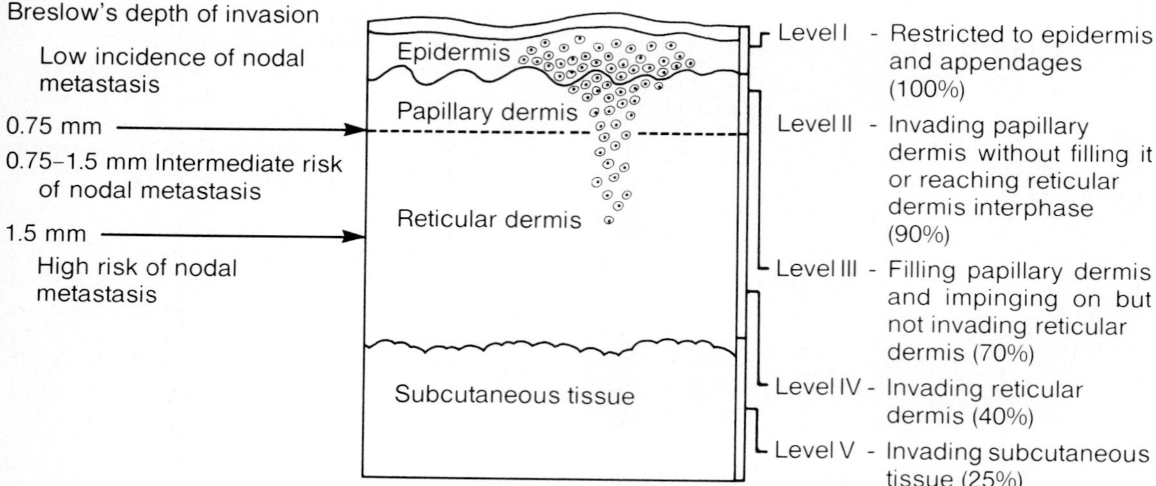

Figure 61–15. Two common methods of estimating the prognosis of malignant melanoma based on the degree of vertical invasion. On the left is Breslow's thickness, which is an actual measurement of the deepest invasion from the granular layer. On the right is Clark's level, which relates to involvement of different anatomic regions of the skin. The figures in parentheses given after individual Clark levels indicate disease-free 5-year survival rates. Note that metastasis, either lymph node or hematogenous, decreases survival drastically.

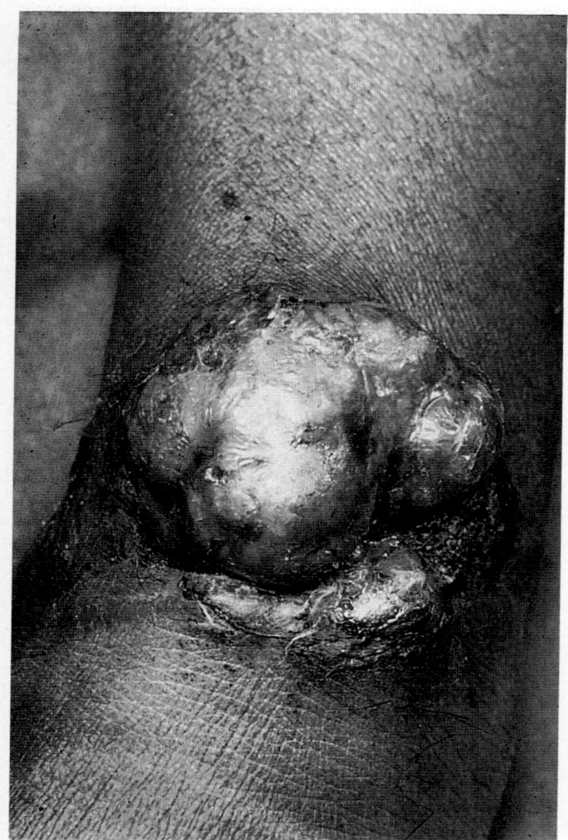

Figure 61–16. Dermatofibrosarcoma protuberans of the leg, showing the typical large exophytic mass.

kin's lymphoma). T cell lymphomas have a predilection for skin involvement.

Mycosis Fungoides (Cutaneous T Cell Lymphoma)

Mycosis fungoides is a T cell lymphoma that affects the skin primarily, with dissemination to lymph nodes and viscera occurring later in the course of the disease. It is characterized by large malignant T lymphocytes (called mycosis cells) that have hyperchromatic, irregularly lobulated, cerebriform ("brainlike") nuclei and a helper T cell phenotype.

Clinically, the disease can be divided into 3 stages:

A. Erythematous Stage: (Fig 61–17.) (Characterized by erythematous, scaling patches that itch severely.) Histologically, there is a perivascular lymphocytic infiltrate with upward extension into the epidermis (exocytosis) that is not diagnostic unless numerous mycosis cells are present. Patients may remain at this stage of the disease for several years.

B. Plaque Stage: (Characterized by well-demarcated, indurated erythematous plaques.) Histologic features are diagnostic and consist of a bandlike upper dermal polymorphous lymphocytic infiltrate in which numerous mycosis cells are present. Epidermal involvement, which appears as groups of mycosis cells (Pautrier's microabscesses), is pathognomonic.

C. Tumor Stage: (Characterized by reddish-brown nodules that ulcerate.) At this stage, mycosis fungoides resembles other lymphomas affect-

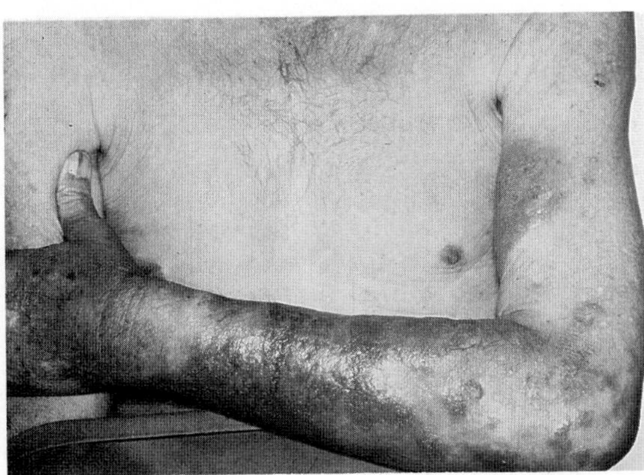

Figure 61-17. Mycosis fungoides (cutaneous T cell lymphoma), showing diffuse thickening and erythema of the skin of the upper extremity.

ing the skin both clinically and histologically. The tumor mass is composed of a polymorphous proliferation of mycosis cells. Lymph node and visceral involvement occurs in up to 70% of cases and signifies a poor prognosis. The overall 5-year survival rate is less than 10%.

Sézary's Syndrome

Sézary's syndrome may be regarded as a leukemic variant of mycosis fungoides. It is characterized clinically by generalized erythroderma with intense itching. Except for the fact that the erythroderma is generalized, the clinical and histologic features are identical to those of the erythematous stage of mycosis fungoides. Sézary cells (indistinguishable from mycosis cells) are present in the peripheral blood.

MAST CELL NEOPLASMS

Mast cells contain basophilic cytoplasmic granules that are best seen with metachromatic stains such as Giemsa's stain and toluidine blue. Release of histamine, serotonin, and other vasoactive substances from proliferating mast cells in the skin causes urticaria and flushing; such release may be induced by firm rubbing (Darier's sign; dermatographism). Rarely, vesicle formation occurs after minor trauma, particularly in infants.

Urticaria Pigmentosa

This type of cutaneous mastocytosis is seen in infants (infantile form) or adults. Clinically, there are multiple red-brown macules and papules all over the body. Increased numbers of mast cells are present around blood vessels in the upper dermis.

The prognosis is good; few patients develop systemic disease.

Solitary Mastocytoma

Mastocytoma is an uncommon benign lesion usually occurring at or soon after birth and presenting as a solitary nodular lesion; rarely, 2–4 lesions may be present.

Systemic Mastocytosis

Systemic mastocytosis is an uncommon disease that may occur at any age. Skin involvement may resemble urticaria pigmentosa or may produce lymphomalike masses composed of large numbers of mast cells. Visceral involvement occurs, characterized by mast cell infiltrates in bone marrow, liver, spleen, and lymph nodes. Systemic mastocytosis is a progressive malignant disease.

SKIN MANIFESTATIONS OF SYSTEMIC DISEASES

Many systemic diseases are manifested by skin lesions. Some of the more important ones are listed in Table 61–6.

Section XV.
The Nervous System

Cerebrovascular accidents (strokes, Chapter 64) are a common cause of death and disability in the USA. They commonly complicate atherosclerotic and hypertensive arterial disease (see Chapter 20). Cranial trauma (Chapter 64) is a major problem in road traffic accidents and is responsible for a significant proportion of deaths in the 10- to 30-year age group.

Bacterial meningitis, cerebral abscess and viral meningoencephalitis (Chapter 63) are the common infections of the nervous system. Infections related to AIDS are increasing in prevalence. Neoplasms of the nervous system constitute a significant proportion of cancers in children (see Chapter 17). In adults, metastatic neoplasms, glial neoplasms (Chapter 65), and peripheral nerve neoplasms (Chapter 66) occur but are less common.

62 The Central Nervous System: I. Structure & Function; Hydrocephalus; Congenital Diseases

STRUCTURE & FUNCTION

The Central Nervous System

The central nervous system is composed of the cerebral hemispheres, brain stem, cerebellum, and spinal cord. Microscopically, the principal cell types are neurons and neuroglial cells (Table 62–1). **Neurons** represent the basic functional unit of the nervous system and are found in the gray matter and ganglia. Each neuron is composed of a cell body plus cytoplasmic processes, including dendrites, which synapse with processes from other neurons; and axons, which carry impulses away from the cell body. The neuron has a large nucleus with a prominent nucleolus and an abundant pale eosinophilic cytoplasm in which the ribosomes form clumped masses (Nissl substance). Neurons are postmitotic (permanent) cells that have no mitotic capability.

Neuroglial cells form the supporting connective tissue of the brain. Neuroglial cells include astrocytes, oligodendroglial cells, and microglial cells. Neuroglial cells are capable of mitotic division and proliferate in a variety of conditions. Ependymal cells are specialized glial cells that line the ventricles and the central canal of the spinal cord. The normal brain has very little interstitial fluid.

The Peripheral Nervous System

The peripheral nervous system is composed of cranial and spinal nerves that originate in the brain stem or spinal cord and end in the periphery. The autonomic nervous system, with sympathetic and parasympathetic components, may be regarded as a specialized part of the peripheral nervous system with regulatory functions. Peripheral nerves are usually mixed motor and sensory nerves and are composed of bundles of nerve fibers that have their cell bodies in the motor nuclei (the anterior horn of the spinal cord or cranial nerve nuclei), the sensory nerve root ganglia, or the autonomic ganglia.

ANATOMIC & FUNCTIONAL DIVISIONS OF THE NERVOUS SYSTEM

The Cerebral Cortex

The cerebral cortex is represented by the outer neuronal layers (gray matter) on the surface of the cerebral hemispheres. The cortex is responsible for "higher" cerebral functions. Different areas subserve different functions (Fig 62–1).

The cortex of both hemispheres houses the major motor and sensory areas serving the opposite side of the body. The dominant hemisphere (the

Table 62-1. Principal cell types in the central nervous system and the common pathologic changes they undergo.

Cell Type	Basic Pathologic Change	Causes	Effects
Neuron (many subtypes)	Necrosis, usually liquefactive	Anoxia, commonly ischemic Hypoglycemia Toxins, including drugs Metabolites Infectious agents Neoplasm Trauma	Permanent loss of function subserved by neuron. Neurons have no regenerative capacity.
	Chromatolysis: swelling with loss of Nissl substance Neurofibrillary tangles Cytoplasmic inclusions Lipid Mucopolysaccharide Pick's bodies Lewy bodies Negri bodies Intranuclear inclusions Viral inclusions	Axonal injury Alzheimer's disease Lipid storage diseases Mucopolysaccharidoses Pick's disease Parkinson's disease Rabies (viral inclusion) Cytomegalovirus Herpes simplex virus Papovavirus	Associated with neuronal dysfunction.
Astrocyte	Degeneration, loss	Toxic states, eg, hepatic failure Infarction	No major known effect.
	Proliferation (nonneoplastic)	Variety of injuries	Associated with gliosis (analogue of fibrosis in the brain).
	Neoplasia	Astrocytomas	Most common primary central nervous system (CNS) neoplasm.
Oligodendroglia	Degeneration, loss	Demyelinating diseases	Oligodendroglial cells are responsible for myelination in CNS.
	Neoplasia	Oligodendroglioma	
Microglia	Proliferation and activation	Any cause of neuronal necrosis	Analogue of macrophages in CNS. Appear in activated state as swollen cells with foamy cytoplasm.
Ependymal cells	Neoplasia	Ependymoma	

left in righthanders) houses the motor and receptive speech area and areas relating to logic and mathematical activities. Much of the cortex of the nondominant hemisphere is believed to be responsible for creativity, including musical and artistic ability.

Only about 10% of the surface area of the cortex has known functions, and damage to these areas produces a recognizable functional deficit. The other 90% constitutes the so-called "silent areas" that can be removed without an easily detectable functional deficit. Neurosurgeons utilize these silent areas to gain access to the interior of the brain.

The various parts of the cerebral cortex are interconnected with each other and with the brain stem via cell processes (axons and dendrites) that originate in the neurons and pass across the deep white matter of the brain.

Effects of cerebrocortical destruction. Diffuse cortical neuronal loss produces dementia (organic brain syndrome), characterized by loss of memory—mainly for recent events—loss of intelligence, disorientation, and inappropriate social behavior. Damage to specific areas of the cerebral cortex may lead to abnormalities in speech (aphasia and dysphasia), cortical visual loss, motor paralysis, cortical sensory loss, etc. Lesser degrees of damage with focal scarring may lead to abnormal electrical activity and epilepsy.

The Cerebellum

The cerebellum is located in the posterior fossa and connected to the brain stem by the superior, middle, and inferior cerebellar peduncles. It is composed of the cerebellar cortex, the white matter, and the deep nuclei. The cerebellum receives afferent connections from the proprioceptor system and the pontine nuclei. Its main functions are maintenance of muscle tone and fine coordination of movements. The cerebellar efferents pass via the superior peduncle to the red nucleus, which plays an important role in the extrapyramidal system.

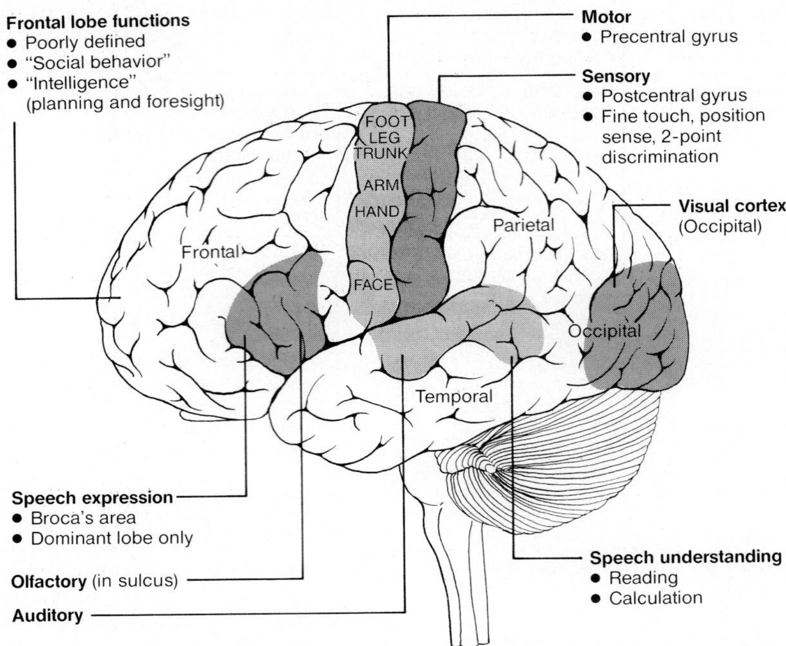

Figure 62–1. Major functional areas of the cerebral cortex.

Cerebellar dysfunction is manifested as failure of coordination of movements, decreased muscle tone, and intention tremors.

The Reticular Formation of the Brain Stem

The reticular formation is a poorly defined network of cells situated in the central part of the brain stem. It is responsible for maintenance of consciousness and is also associated with the pontomedullary centers that regulate cardiac and respiratory function. Dysfunction of the reticular formation (Table 62–2) produces alteration in the level of consciousness that may be transient and reversible, as in syncopal attacks ("fainting"), epilepsy, and concussion, or more severe, causing coma and death.

The Hypothalamus

The hypothalamus is situated in the floor of the third ventricle. It controls growth, sexual development and activity, sleep, hunger and thirst, body temperature, and endocrine functions of the pituitary gland. Hypothalamic lesions result in abnormalities relating to these functions.

The Motor System

Voluntary contraction of skeletal muscle is under the control of the motor system, which is composed of the upper and lower motor neurons (Fig 62–2) and regulated by the cerebellum and extrapyramidal nuclei (see below). The lower motor neuron, which represents the only source of stimulation of the skeletal muscle, is acted on by the

Table 62–2. Common causes of loss of consciousness.[1]

Circulatory failure (70%)
Vasovagal syncope (simple faint): pain, emotional stress
Decreased blood volume: blood loss, dehydration, shock
Venous pooling: prolonged standing, Valsalva maneuver
Orthostatic hypotension: elderly, antihypertensive drugs
Pulmonary embolism
Cardiac disease—decreased cardiac output (10%)
Arrhythmias: heart block, ventricular tachyarrhythmias
Myocardial infarction
Cardiac tamponade
Severe valvular disease, most commonly aortic stenosis
Aortic dissection
Metabolic causes (10%)
Hypoglycemia
Hypoxia
Hypercapnia (carbon dioxide narcosis)
Exogenous toxins, including drugs, alcohol
Endogenous toxins: diabetic coma, hepatic or renal failure
Primary disorders of the brain (10%)
Cerebrovascular accidents, especially cerebral hemorrhage
Epilepsy
Trauma: concussion
Hypertensive encephalopathy
Tumors ("space-occupying lesions")
Cerebral edema
Cerebral infections, especially viral encephalitis
Increased intracranial pressure

[1]Syncope when transient; coma when prolonged.

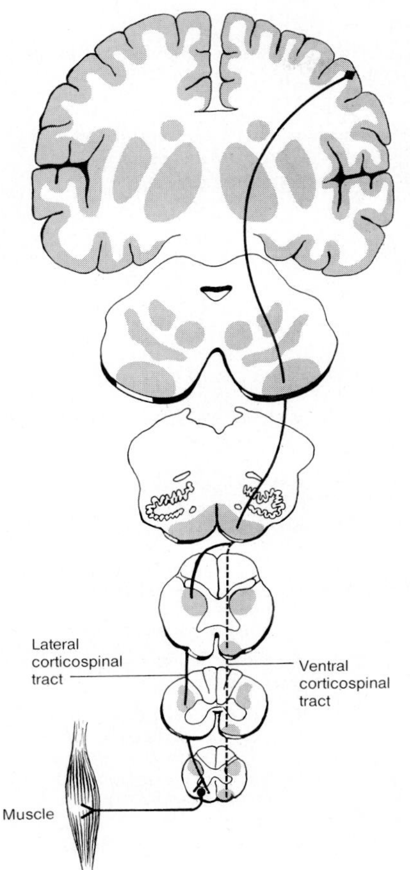

Figure 62–2. The motor (corticospinal or pyramidal) system. Note that the major motor innervation of the body decussates at the level of the medulla.

upper motor neuron, the spinal reflex arc, and the extrapyramidal system.

Lesions involving the motor system cause 2 types of muscle paralysis. **Upper motor neuron lesions** cause paralysis with increased tone (spastic paralysis) due to unopposed activity of the extrapyramidal system on the lower motor neuron; deep tendon reflexes are exaggerated, and the plantar reflex becomes extensor (Babinski response). **Lower motor neuron lesions** cause paralysis with absent tone (flaccid paralysis) and absent deep tendon reflexes. The plantar reflex is either abolished or flexor.

The Extrapyramidal System

The extrapyramidal system includes the basal ganglia, substantia nigra, red nucleus, and olivary nuclei. The efferent axons pass down the spinal cord and synapse with alpha and gamma motor neurons in the motor nuclei. The extrapyramidal system is responsible for maintenance of muscle tone and posture. It also plays a role in coordinating voluntary movements.

Lesions of the extrapyramidal system are characterized by increased muscle tone (rigidity), slowing of all motor activities (bradykinesia) and involuntary movements.

The Sensory System

The general sensory system (Fig 62–3) begins in specialized sensory nerve endings in the periphery from which sensory nerves pass to the cell body situated in the sensory dorsal nerve root ganglia of the spinal and cranial nuclei. Processes from these neurons then travel together as tracts to the thalamus and the sensory cortex of the opposite side. Pain fibers cross to the opposite lateral spinothalamic tract soon after they enter the spinal cord. Fibers subserving fine touch, vibration, and position sense pass in the ipsilateral posterior column of the spinal cord to the medulla, where they cross the midline in the decussating medial lemniscus. Proprioceptive fibers also pass to the cerebellum in the spinocerebellar pathways.

Visual fibers originate in the retina and pass via the optic nerves, chiasm, and radiation to the occipital cortex.

Fibers from olfactory nerve endings in the nasal

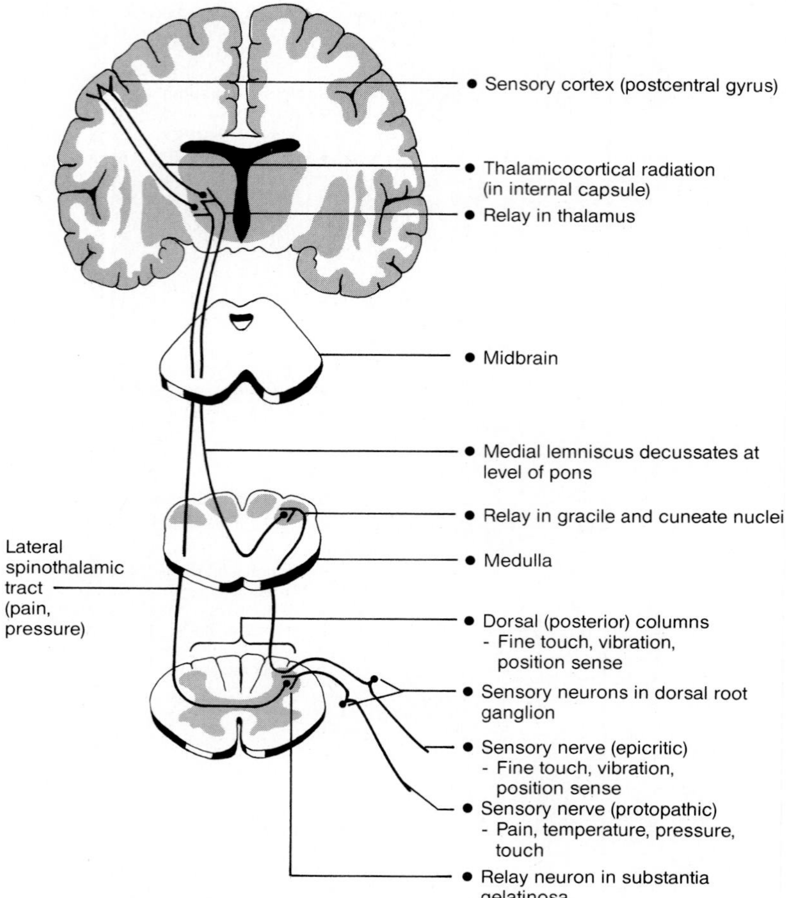

Figure 62-3. Principal sensory pathways. Note that the posterior (dorsal) columns are uncrossed up to the brain stem, whereas the nerves of the spinothalamic tracts cross near their points of entry into the spinal cord.

mucosa pass through the cribriform plate in the base of the anterior cranial fossa to the ophthalmic bulb and thence to the temporal lobe.

Auditory nerve endings are situated in the cochlea of the inner ear, from which nerves pass in the eighth cranial nerve to the medulla and thence to the temporal lobe.

Lesions involving the sensory system produce abnormalities in sensory perception that depend on the modality affected and the level of involvement. For example, a lesion affecting one side of the cord will impair vibration, joint position sense, and fine touch on the same side of the body due to involvement of the uncrossed posterior columns and impair pain sensation on the opposite side below the level of the lesion due to involvement of the crossed lateral spinothalamic tract.

METHODS OF ASSESSING NERVOUS SYSTEM STRUCTURE & FUNCTION

Clinical Examination

A detailed neurologic examination is the first step in assessing a patient with neurologic disease. Determination of the type and distribution of neurologic deficit, coupled with intimate knowledge of neuroanatomic pathways, often permits precise localization of disease.

Examination of Cerebrospinal Fluid

Lumbar puncture is generally a safe technique that permits collection of cerebrospinal fluid for chemical, microscopic, and microbiologic examination (Table 62-3). Lumbar puncture also permits measurement of the cerebrospinal fluid pressure, but it should not be done if raised pressure is suspected (eg, if papilledema is present).

Table 62-3. Cerebrospinal fluid abnormalities.[1]

	Normal	Abnormalities
Color	Clear, colorless	Yellow (xanthochromic): indicates old hemorrhage, high protein, complete subarachnoid obstruction. Red: subarachnoid hemorrhage (if traumatic puncture is excluded). Turbid (purulent): bacterial meningitis. Clear with clot on standing: high protein, common in tuberculous meningitis.
Protein	20–50 mg/dL	Marked increase: infection, hemorrhage, tumor causing subarachnoid block. Moderate increase: many causes.
Oligoclonal protein bands[2]	. . .	Multiple sclerosis, syphilis.
Serology	. . .	VDRL positive in neurosyphilis.
Glucose	50–80 mg/dL (~75% of blood glucose)	Marked decrease in bacterial meningitis; increased in hyperglycemic states.
Cells	0–5 (mostly lymphocytes); no neutrophils are present	↑ Neutrophils: bacterial infection. ↑ Lymphocytes: viral, fungal, tuberculous meningitis, syphilis, cysticercosis, degenerative diseases. Malignant cells: cancer (various types).
Gram stain of sediment	Negative	Useful test in meningitis; positive finding may provide immediate diagnosis.
Culture	Negative	Positive bacterial, mycobacterial, fungal, and viral cultures.

[1]Always check for evidence of raised intracranial pressure prior to lumbar puncture. If pressure is normal in a recumbent patient, remove 3-mL samples in 3 separate sterile containers (1) for chemistry/serology, (2) for culture, (3) for cell count and cytology.
[2]Oligoclonal protein bands: 2–4 immunoglobulin bands seen on electrophoresis of cerebrospinal fluid.

Radiologic Examination

Computerized tomography (CT) and magnetic resonance imaging (MRI) permit evaluation of ventricular size, shifts of neural structures, and mass lesions.

Carotid arteriography (injecting a contrast dye into the carotid artery) and ventriculography (injecting a dye into the ventricular system) are less frequently used. Myelography (injecting a dye into the lumbar subarachnoid space) remains a useful technique to evaluate spinal lesions.

Brain Biopsy

In the last decade, stereotactic brain biopsy has become increasingly popular as a means of diagnosis of mass lesions in the brain. This technique utilizes radiographic computer guidance to introduce a small biopsy needle into the mass. The procedure is performed under local anesthesia and is accurate in providing a precise histologic diagnosis of brain neoplasms.

Electroencephalography

The electroencephalogram (EEG) is generated from electrodes placed on the outer surface of the skull. Changes in the "brain waves" provide evidence of local masses or focal electrical excitability (epilepsy). Demonstration of a "flat" EEG is often used as a criterion for diagnosis of "brain death."

THE CEREBROSPINAL FLUID

The cerebrospinal fluid (CSF) fills the ventricular system of the brain, the central canal of the spinal cord, and the subarachnoid space.

CSF is secreted by the choroid plexuses situated in the lateral ventricles. From the lateral ventricles it passes through the foramen of Monro into the third ventricle and then through the cerebral aqueduct (aqueduct of Sylvius) in the midbrain into the fourth ventricle (Fig 62–4). The fourth ventricle houses the foramens of Luschka and Magendie, which permit the passage of CSF into the subarachnoid space. CSF then passes over the convexity of the brain to the region of the superior sagittal sinus, where it is absorbed into the venous system by the arachnoid villi.

HYDROCEPHALUS

Hydrocephalus is defined as abnormal dilatation of the ventricles (Fig 62–5). It is readily diagnosed by computerized tomography. Hydrocephalus may result from (1) increased secretion of CSF, as occurs very rarely with neoplasms of the

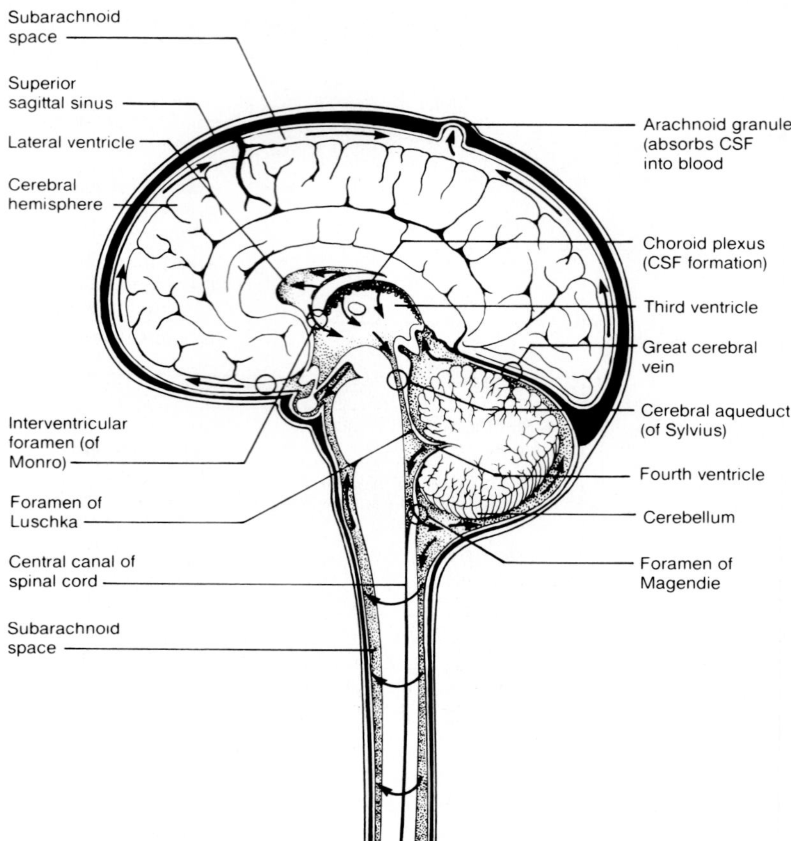

Figure 62–4. Production, circulation, and absorption of cerebrospinal fluid.

choroid plexus; (2) obstruction to the flow of CSF, either in the ventricular system or in the subarachnoid space; or (3) failure of absorption of CSF (Table 62–4).

Classification

A. Anatomic Classification:

1. Noncommunicating (obstructive) hydrocephalus occurs when there is an obstruction in the ventricular system that prevents CSF from passing into the subarachnoid space.

2. Communicating hydrocephalus occurs when CSF passes normally out of the ventricular system but flow is obstructed in the subarachnoid space or reabsorption is reduced.

B. Functional Classification:

1. High-pressure hydrocephalus is due to obstruction to CSF flow. If obstruction occurs after fusion of skull sutures, it causes an increase in intracranial pressure (see below). When it occurs in the fetus or infant before fusion of the sutures, it causes the skull to expand.

2. Low-pressure (or normal pressure) hydrocephalus is uncommon. There is slow dilatation of the ventricles associated with free flow of CSF, cerebral atrophy, and dementia. The cause is un-

Table 62–4. Causes of hydrocephalus.

Causes of hydrocephalus
Noncommunicating hydrocephalus
Congenital
Aqueductal stenosis and atresia
Dandy-Walker syndrome
Acquired
Neoplasms and cysts obstructing cerebral aqueduct and third ventricle
Gliosis and chronic inflammation involving aqueduct
Obstruction of fourth ventricle openings
Organized subarachnoid hemorrhage, obstructing flow at base of brain
Organized meningitis involving base of brain
Communicating hydrocephalus
Choroid plexus papilloma (increased secretion)
Arnold-Chiari malformation
Deficient absorption of cerebrospinal fluid
Dural sinus thrombosis
Organized subarachnoid hemorrhage
Organized meningitis
?Deficiency of arachnoid villi

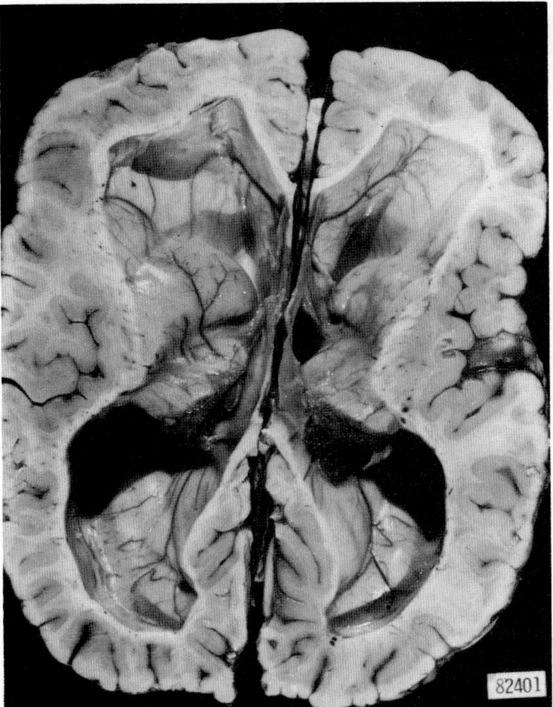

Figure 62–5. Congenital hydrocephalus. Section of whole brain, showing a markedly dilated ventricular system.

known in most cases. Recognition is important because symptoms may be reversed and progression halted if treatment by ventricular shunting is provided early.

INCREASED INTRACRANIAL PRESSURE

Increased intracranial pressure is defined as elevation of the mean CSF pressure above 200 mm water (15 mm Hg) when measured with the patient in the lateral decubitus position. Raised intracranial pressure is a common and important pathologic state; it is a frequent cause of neurologic symptoms and when severe can cause death.

Etiology (Table 62–5)

A. Due to Obstructive Hydrocephalus: See above.

B. Due to a Space-Occupying Mass Lesion in the Cranial Cavity: In general, the degree of elevation of intracranial pressure is proportionate to the size of the mass and the rate of expansion. For example, a slowly expanding subdural hematoma is associated with a lesser increase in intracranial pressure than a rapidly expanding extradural hematoma.

Table 62–5. Causes of increased intracranial pressure.

Hydrocephalus	(See Table 62–4)
Space-occupying lesions Hemorrhage or hematoma	Extradural, subdural, subarachnoid, or intracerebral
Infarction	With local edema or hemorrhage
Neoplasm	Primary or secondary (mass effect and local edema)
Infection	Abscess (mass effect and local edema)
Cerebral edema Cytotoxic	Anoxia of any cause; hypoglycemia
Vasogenic	Hypertensive encephalopathy; associated with altered capillaries of tumors, abscesses; toxins (eg, lead poisoning); uremia
Infection	Meningitis, encephalitis
Trauma	
Hypercapnia in chronic obstructive lung disease	

C. Cerebral Edema: Cerebral edema is accumulation of water in the brain.

1. Intracellular cytotoxic cerebral edema is an early manifestation of cell injury resulting from failure of normal energy production. It is most commonly seen in ischemic states.

2. Extracellular vasogenic edema is responsible for most cases of cerebral edema, occurring in infections, trauma, neoplasms, and metabolic disorders. Edema is caused by capillary damage, disruption of the normal blood-brain barrier, and leakage of fluid into the interstitium. New blood vessel formation in neoplasms or in the walls of abscesses causes edema because the new vessels are poorly developed and show increased permeability with lesser degrees of injury than normal vessels.

Pathology

Raised pressure occurring within the fixed volume of the bony cranial cavity causes displacement of the brain (Fig 62–6).

A. Supratentorial Lesions:

1. Caudal displacement of the entire brain stem may stretch the sixth cranial nerve (causing paralysis of the lateral rectus muscle) and may rupture vessels passing from the basilar artery to the brain stem. The resulting brain stem hemorrhages (Duret's hemorrhages; see Fig 62–7) inter-

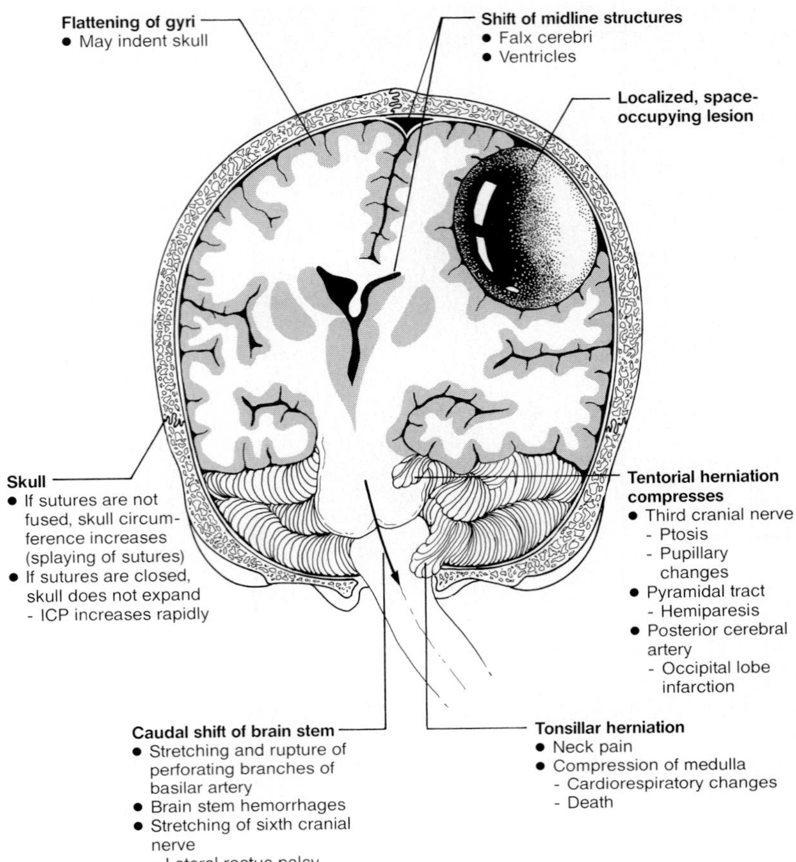

Figure 62–6. Possible consequences of raised intracranial pressure (ICP) resulting from a mass lesion in the right supratentorial compartment.

fere with vital centers and are a common cause of death.

2. Herniation of the uncinate gyrus of the temporal lobe through the tentorial opening (tentorial herniation) stretches the third nerve, causing eye muscle paralysis, ptosis, and pupillary changes. Compression of the pyramidal tract in the crus cerebri may also occur, causing motor paralysis in the contralateral side of the body.

B. Posterior Fossa Lesions: Posterior fossa lesions cause herniation of the cerebellar tonsils through the foramen magnum; late supratentorial lesions have a similar effect. Resulting compression of the medulla affects the cardiorespiratory centers, leading to death. Tonsillar herniation is particularly likely to occur if lumbar puncture is performed in patients with markedly raised intracranial pressure.

Clinical Features

Raised intracranial pressure presents with headache, vomiting, and papilledema. The headache is typically described as bursting, is present on waking in the morning, and is increased by coughing and straining, maneuvers that further increase the intracranial pressure. Vomiting is typically effortless, unaccompanied by nausea, and often projectile. Papilledema is edema of the optic disk, as shown by ophthalmoscopic (funduscopic) examination of the retina. The optic nerve is surrounded by a sheath of subarachnoid space into which the raised intracranial pressure is transmitted, thereby interfering with venous drainage of the optic disk and axoplasmic flow in the nerves, leading to edema followed by hemorrhage. Prolonged papilledema leads to atrophy of the optic disk (secondary optic atrophy) and blindness.

Raised intracranial pressure also produces "false localizing signs," caused by displacement of the brain. As noted above, sixth and third nerve palsies, pyramidal tract compression, and brain stem dysfunction are the commonest of these. Hemorrhage into the brain stem may cause unconsciousness and death.

The diagnosis of raised intracranial pressure is made by clinical examination. If raised intracranial pressure is suspected, lumbar puncture should not be performed because of the danger of precipitating tonsillar herniation.

Treatment

Raised intracranial pressure due to a mass le-

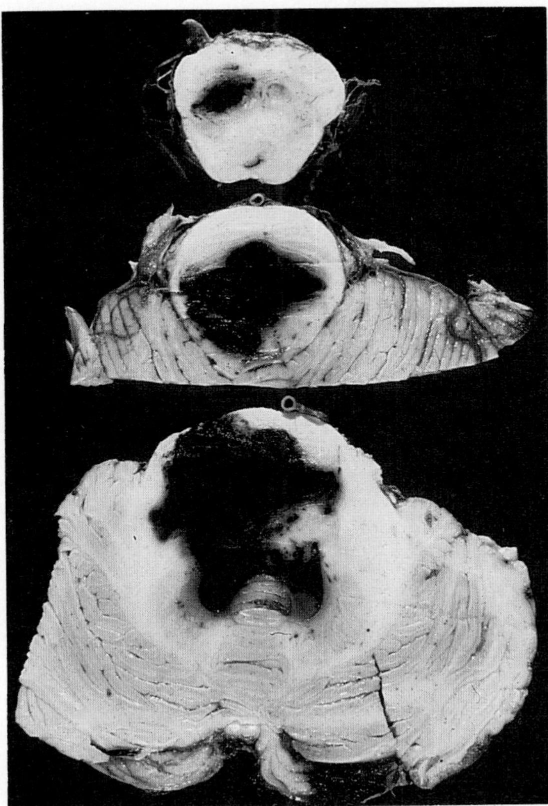

Figure 62-7. Duret's hemorrhages of the brain stem resulting from markedly increased intracranial pressure in a patient with a malignant neoplasm of the cerebral hemisphere. The brain stem hemorrhage was the immediate cause of death.

sion should be treated by removal of the mass. In cases of hydrocephalus caused by a lesion that cannot be removed, decompression of the dilated ventricles may be achieved by a ventricular shunt, which directs the CSF to an extracranial location such as the peritoneal cavity through a valved tube.

Raised intracranial pressure caused by cerebral edema may be treated with diuretics such as mannitol and with high doses of corticosteroids administered intravenously. Steroids appear to stabilize the blood-brain barrier and decrease cerebral edema.

CONGENITAL DISEASES OF THE NERVOUS SYSTEM

DEFECTIVE CLOSURE OF THE NEURAL TUBE

Embryology

The central nervous system develops from a specialized part of the dorsal ectoderm known as the neural plate, which in early fetal life folds along its length to form the neural tube. The surrounding mesoderm is destined to form the skull and vertebral column and is covered over by skin.

Defective closure of the neural tube may occur throughout its extent but is most common at either end.

A. **Defective Closure of the Caudal End (Spina Bifida):** Spina bifida is a general term for a group of disorders in which the vertebral arches of the lowest lumbar vertebrae are not fused posteriorly. All forms may be associated with Arnold-Chiari malformation and congenital hydrocephalus (see below). There are several degrees of severity (Fig 62–8).

1. **Spina bifida occulta** is the mildest form; it is characterized by failure of vertebral fusion only (the vertebral spine is bifid). The overlying skin often shows a dimple, a tuft of hair, or a fatty mass. In a few cases, a congenital dermal sinus passes from the epidermis through the vertebral defect into the spinal canal.

2. **Meningocele-**More severe degrees of spina bifida are associated with protrusion of a meningeal sac filled with CSF through the vertebral defect (Fig 62–9).

3. **Myelomeningocele** is a still more serious defect characterized by the presence of parts of the spinal cord in the sac and often associated with severe neurologic defects in the lower extremities, bladder, and rectum.

4. **Spina bifida aperta,** the most severe—and very rare—form of spina bifida, results from complete failure of fusion of the caudal end of the neural plate. The neural plate lies open on the skin surface. Severe neurologic defects in the legs, bladder, and rectum are invariably present.

B. **Defective Closure of the Cranial End:** Neural tube abnormalities at the cranial end are less common. Complete failure of development of the cranial end of the neural tube results in anencephaly, which is incompatible with life.

Occipital meningocele is protrusion of a CSF-filled sac of meninges through the skull in the occipital region. An encephalocele is similar but contains brain matter in the meningeal sac.

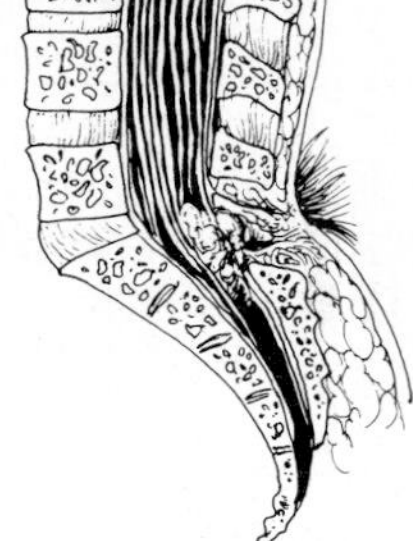

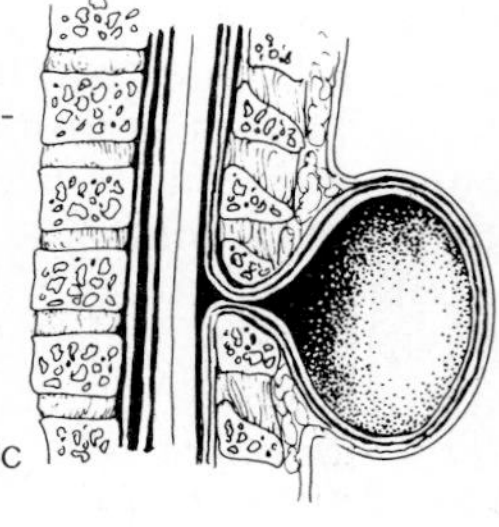

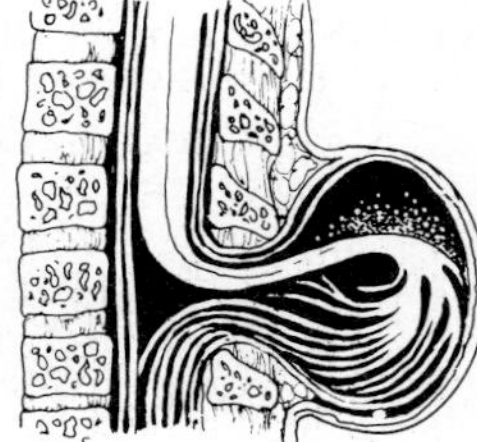

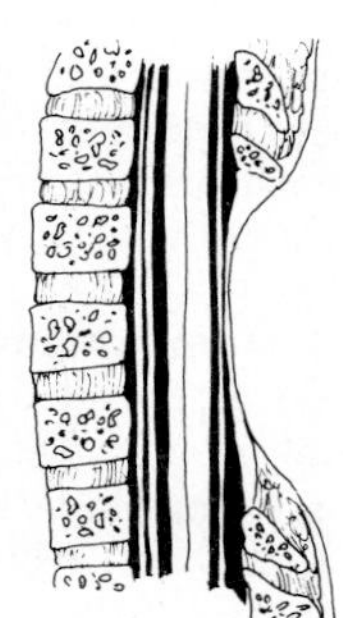

Figure 62-8. Spina bifida, showing different levels of involvement of skin, vertebral column, and neuraxis.

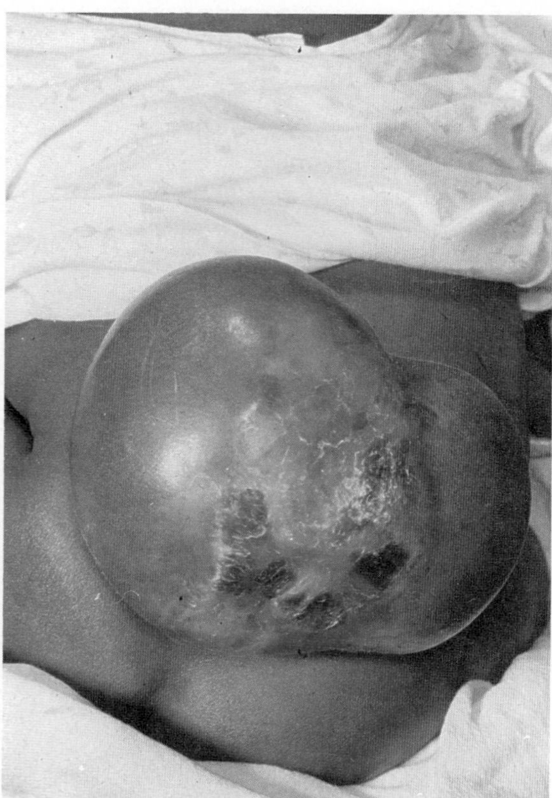

Figure 62-9. Meningocele of the lumbar region.

Clinical Features

Spina bifida occulta is a common abnormality that is usually asymptomatic and discovered when a radiograph of the lumbosacral spine is obtained. Rarely, these patients have an associated fistulous communication between the skin and the spinal canal that predisposes to recurrent meningitis in childhood. Also rarely, there may be a keratin-filled epidermal cyst in the spinal canal that may leak and cause chemical meningitis.

Meningocele, meningomyelocele, and spina bifida aperta present at birth with a detectable lesion in the lumbosacral region. Meningocele is cystic and translucent and is not associated with severe neurologic deficit. Meningomyelocele shows neural structures on transillumination of the cyst and is associated with lower limb weakness and with bladder and rectal dysfunction. Spina bifida aperta appears as a flat lesion in which the open spinal cord is visible and produces a profound neurologic deficit. All of these patients have an increased risk of meningitis and hydrocephalus from the frequently associated Arnold-Chiari malformation.

Anencephaly is incompatible with live birth. Occipital meningocele and encephalocele are similar to their spinal counterparts. The most common location of the cystic mass is the nape of the neck. When very large, an occipital meningocele may obstruct normal delivery of the baby.

Antenatal Diagnosis

Raised levels of alpha-fetoprotein (AFP) in the amniotic fluid are of value in the antenatal diagnosis of neural tube defects. Over 95% of fetuses with open defects will show elevation due to leakage of AFP through the skin defect into the amniotic fluid. AFP levels are routinely measured in the amniotic fluid whenever amniocentesis is performed.

Ultrasound examination of the fetus is also an effective method of demonstrating the anatomic abnormality before birth. All the clinically significant defects can be reliably detected.

Treatment

Meningocele, the commonest serious lesion, should be closed soon after birth before infection and ulceration occur. In many patients, surgical drainage of the associated hydrocephalus is required. Neurologic deficit in the legs in meningomyelocele presents a serious additional problem. The neural elements in the cyst are irreversibly damaged, with corresponding neurologic defects. Many of these children require numerous operations to correct deformities resulting from abnormal muscle action. Bladder and rectal incontinence may also be a major problem. Spina bifida aperta has a high mortality rate.

CEREBRAL PALSY

Cerebral palsy is a common disorder characterized by a disturbance of motor function, usually nonprogressive, that is manifest at birth or comes on in early infancy. The term cerebral palsy does not denote a specific disease but a variety of nonheritable motor disorders acquired in utero, during the birth process, or soon after delivery. Many patients with cerebral palsy reach adulthood, but life expectancy is shortened. The following fairly characteristic syndromes are recognized.

Spastic Diplegia (Little's Disease)

Spastic diplegia is characterized by spastic weakness of all 4 extremities. Two groups are recognized. Spastic diplegia associated with **prematurity** is characterized by predominant involvement of the legs, associated with minimal mental retardation. This type can be prevented by expert management of premature infants in neonatal intensive care units. Spastic diplegia associated with **full-term delivery and difficult labor** is believed to result from intrapartum asphyxia. The infant develops quadriplegia associated with severe mental retardation. The brain shows bilateral ischemic changes in the cortex and white matter.

Infantile Hemiplegia

Infantile hemiplegia usually results from unilateral infection or thrombosis of cerebral vessels that has occurred in utero or soon after birth. Mild mental retardation and convulsions are commonly associated. Pathologic changes consist of ischemic necrosis involving one cerebral hemisphere.

TRISOMY 13 (Patau's Syndrome)

Trisomy 13 is characterized by failure of normal development of the forebrain, leading to formation of a brain with a single frontal lobe and a single ventricle (holoprosencephaly), absence of the olfactory bulbs (arhinencephaly), a single median eye (cyclopia, from the Cyclops of Greek mythology), and failure of formation of nasal structures.

Patau's syndrome is usually fatal soon after birth.

CONGENITAL HYDROCEPHALUS

Hydrocephalus is a common abnormality, affecting about 0.1–0.5% of births. It is caused by several different congenital anomalies (Table 62–4).

1. AQUEDUCTAL STENOSIS & ATRESIA

Narrowing of the cerebral aqueduct is the commonest cause of congenital noncommunicating hydrocephalus. There is controversy about whether the narrowing represents a primary developmental abnormality or whether it is the result of an inflammatory process causing gliotic occlusion.

2. ARNOLD-CHIARI MALFORMATION

Arnold-Chiari malformation is the commonest cause of congenital communicating hydrocephalus. It is characterized by elongation of the medulla oblongata, so that the fourth ventricular foramens open below the level of the foramen magnum. Cerebrospinal fluid passing from these foramens cannot pass up to the arachnoid granulation for reabsorption, since the subarachnoid space is blocked at the level of the foramen magnum by an associated protrusion of the cerebellum into the foramen.

Arnold-Chiari malformation is commonly associated with flattening of the base of the skull (platybasia), abnormalities in the cervical vertebrae, spina bifida, meningomyelocele, and syringomyelia.

3. DANDY-WALKER SYNDROME

Dandy-Walker syndrome is a rare cause of congenital noncommunicating hydrocephalus characterized by failure of development of the cerebellar vermis and obstruction of the fourth ventricular foramens of Luschka and Magendie (Fig 62–4).

SYRINGOMYELIA

Syringomyelia is an uncommon disease of adults believed to result from abnormal development of the cervical spine and upper spinal cord. It is characterized by development of fluid-filled spaces in the spinal cord, mainly the cervical cord. Its exact pathogenesis is unknown, but many cases are associated with Arnold-Chiari malformation.

Pathologically, the cystic spaces occupy the central part of the cervical cord and may or may not communicate with the central canal. The spaces are lined by fibrillary astrocytes (gliosis). Clinical effects are quite characteristic, depending on the nerve fibers or tracts destroyed (Fig 62–10).

HEREDITARY HAMARTOMATOUS MALFORMATIONS

Multiple hamartomatous malformations involving the nervous system, skin, and blood vessels are not uncommon, and many are transmitted by autosomal dominant genes.

1. GENERALIZED NEUROFIBROMATOSIS (von Recklinghausen's Disease)

Neurofibromatosis is the commonest hereditary hamartomatous malformation, with an estimated prevalence of 1:3000 in the USA. It is inherited as an autosomal dominant trait with varying degrees of penetrance. The gene responsible is carried in chromosome number 17. The manifestations vary between asymptomatic disease characterized by a few skin lesions to severe disease that is fatal in early infancy.

Neurofibromatosis is characterized by café-au-lait ("coffee with milk") skin patches—well-demarcated flat areas of brown pigmentation. The presence of multiple (more than 5) or large (more than 5 cm) café-au-lait patches is diagnostic of generalized neurofibromatosis; they may be the only evidence of the abnormal gene in some patients. Multiple neurofibromas—benign hamartomatous proliferations of peripheral nerves—occur in the skin (Fig 62–11), intestine, autonomic nerve plexuses, and in relation to large peripheral nerve trunks. Extensive involvement of tissues by diffuse proliferation of nerve elements (plexiform neurofibromatosis) may cause massive enlargement of tissues, sometimes called elephantiasis neurofibromatosa ("Elephant Man disease"). One of the major complications is malignant transformation of neurofibromas to form neurofibrosarcomas in 5–10% of patients.

Neoplasms of the nervous system, including meningiomas, astrocytomas, and optic nerve gliomas, occur frequently in patients with neurofibromatosis.

2. TUBEROUS SCLEROSIS (Bourneville's Disease)

Tuberous sclerosis is a rare autosomal dominant disease usually presenting in young adults. It is characterized by multiple hamartomas in the brain, each composed of giant astrocytes. They form hard nodules that resemble raw potato tubers (hence the name). Intraventricular tumor masses composed of these giant astrocytes (subependymal giant cell astrocytoma) may act as space-occupying lesions causing CSF obstruction, hydrocephalus, and raised intracranial pressure. These are benign hamartomas and must be distinguished from malignant astrocytic neoplasms. Mental retardation and epilepsy are usual.

Small skin nodules composed of fibroblastic and vascular proliferation (adenoma sebaceum) involve mainly the face. Larger confluent papular

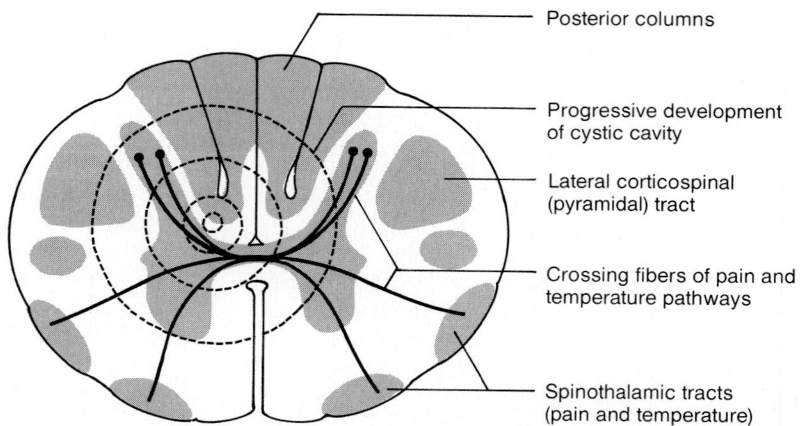

Figure 62–10. Syringomyelia. Transverse section of the cervical cord to illustrate the development of signs and symptoms. Dotted lines indicate the region where the cystic spaces develop, starting centrally and radiating outward. The initial symptoms are caused by involvement of the pain fibers crossing at the level of involvement from the dorsal nerve root to the spinothalamic tracts (shown). As the disease progresses, the more peripheral long tracts and the anterior horn are involved.

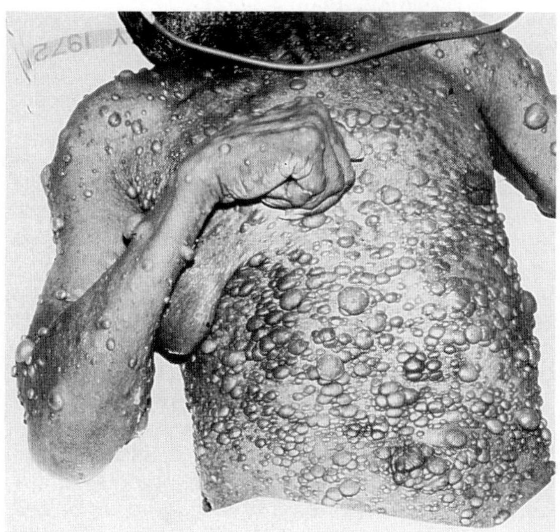

Figure 62–11. Generalized neurofibromatosis, showing large numbers of neurofibromas of the skin.

skin lesions called shagreen patches occur over the buttocks. Visceral lesions include rhabdomyoma of the heart, pancreatic cysts, and, most commonly, angiomyolipomas of the kidney (Chapter 49).

3. VON HIPPEL-LINDAU DISEASE

Von Hippel-Lindau disease, transmitted as an autosomal dominant trait, is characterized by multiple hemangiomas in the retina and brain, a benign neoplasm of the cerebellum called hemangioblastoma, and cysts in the kidneys and pancreas. There is an increased incidence of renal adenocarcinoma and pheochromocytoma. Cerebellar hemangioblastoma is associated with erythropoietin secretion, and many such patients develop polycythemia.

4. STURGE-WEBER SYNDROME

Sturge-Weber syndrome is very rare. It is characterized by a large unilateral cutaneous angioma ("port wine stain") of the face associated with a venous malformation involving the ipsilateral cerebral hemisphere and meninges. The cerebral angioma leads to cortical atrophy and epilepsy. The

Table 62–6. Types and causes of epilepsy.

Principal types of epilepsy	
Partial	
Motor (includes jacksonian)	Aura, motor movements, progressive spread
Sensory (visual or somatic)	Flashing lights or tingling, numbness
Temporal lobe	Emotional or autonomic responses, déja vu, smells, psychic phenomena
Generalized	
Grand mal	Aura, loss of consciousness, tonic-clonic movements
Petit mal (minor)	"Absence" attacks, brief lapses in activity or awareness
Myoclonic	Focal or generalized brief spasms, muscle twitching

Principal causes of epilepsy or seizures
A specific cause is identifiable more often with partial seizures than with generalized seizures.

	Neonate or Infant	Child	Young Adult	Elderly
Birth trauma or anoxia	+++	+	–	–
Congenital central nervous system malformation	++	+	–	–
Infection: encephalitis, meningitis, abscess	+++	++	+	+
Metabolic disease: hypoglycemia, hypocalcemia, uremia, aminoacidosis, lipidosis	++	+	+	+
Brain tumor, primary or secondary	–	+	++	++
Head injury with or without hematoma	–	+	++	+++
Cerebrovascular accident	–	–	+	+++
Drugs, alcohol, barbiturates	–	–	++	++
Degenerative disorders	+	–	–	++
Febrile seizures	+	+++	–	–
Idiopathic (cause unknown)	+	++	++	+

angioma is visible radiologically owing to its characteristic linear (''rail-track'') calcification.

CONGENITAL METABOLIC DISEASES

Many congenital metabolic disorders involve the central nervous system, either primarily or as part of a more generalized disorder. They are discussed in Chapter 64.

THE EPILEPSIES

The epilepsies are a group of disorders characterized by abnormal electrical discharges in the brain. Epilepsy is common: an estimated 1 million people in the USA are being maintained on lifetime anticonvulsant therapy.

Epilepsies may be classified according to type into partial and generalized epilepsy (Table 62–6). In **simple partial epilepsy,** the abnormal electrical discharge originates in the cerebral cortex, resulting in stimulation of that area without impairment of consciousness—eg, jacksonian epilepsy is characterized by focal motor seizure activity, and temporal lobe epilepsy is characterized by an abnormal smell or memory phenomenon. In **complex partial epilepsy,** the seizure begins as a simple partial seizure with evidence of cortical stimulation but is rapidly followed by impairment of consciousness as the abnormal electrical discharge spreads to involve the reticular formation. In **generalized epilepsy,** the abnormal electrical discharge begins in the reticular formation, leading to sudden loss of consciousness without evidence of a local cortical onset.

Two major forms of generalized epilepsy are recognized: **grand mal,** characterized by loss of consciousness followed by generalized clonic seizure; and **petit mal,** characterized by brief lapses of consciousness without clonic motor activity. In complex partial epilepsy, the cortical discharge spreads rapidly to the reticular formation and elsewhere, leading to seizures that closely resemble grand mal. In these cases, the initial cortical stimulation represents the aura of the epileptic attack.

Epilepsy may also be classified according to etiology (Table 62–6). Most cases of generalized epilepsy begin in childhood and have no detectable cause **(idiopathic epilepsy).** There is a familial tendency for the occurrence of idiopathic epilepsy without any well-defined inheritance pattern. Partial epilepsy is frequently caused by a cortical lesion **(symptomatic epilepsy).** In many cases, the cortical lesion is subtle and cannot be treated; eg, many cases of temporal lobe epilepsy are believed to result from cortical scarring as a result of birth injury. However, a significant number of cases of focal epilepsy—particularly those occurring for the first time after age 30 years—have a treatable cause, eg, infection, vascular malformation, contusion, brain neoplasm, or granuloma.

Electroencephalography (EEG) provides a means of detecting abnormal electrical activity in the brain. The type of activity differs in patients with idiopathic and symptomatic epilepsy. Computerized tomography is necessary to detect mass lesions.

The Central Nervous System: II. Infections

63

Infections of the nervous system are classified according to the tissue infected into (1) meningeal infections (meningitis), which may involve the dura primarily (pachymeningitis) or the pia-arachnoid (leptomeningitis); and (2) infections of the cerebral and spinal parenchyma (encephalitis or myelitis). In many cases, both the meninges and the brain parenchyma are affected to varying degrees (meningoencephalitis) (Fig 63–1).

MENINGEAL INFECTIONS

ACUTE LEPTOMENINGITIS

Acute leptomeningitis is an acute inflammation of the pia mater and arachnoid. Most cases are caused by infectious agents; rarely, release of keratinaceous contents from an intradural epidermoid cyst or teratoma causes a chemical meningitis. When the term meningitis is used without qualification, it means leptomeningitis.

Classification

Acute meningitis may be classified according to the type of inflammatory response.

A. Acute Pyogenic Meningitis: Pyogenic inflammation is caused by organisms that multiply extracellularly, mainly bacteria. The type of organism involved varies with the age of the patient (Fig 63–2).

Neonatal meningitis is acquired during passage of the fetus through the birth canal. Organisms found in the maternal birth canal, commonly *Escherichia coli* and *Streptococcus agalactiae* (a group B streptococcus) are responsible (Fig 63–2). Infection with *Listeria monocytogenes* is also common in the neonatal period.

In children up to 5 years of age, the most common pathogen causing meningitis is *Haemophilus influenzae*. In adolescents—in whom meningitis occurs most frequently—*Neisseria meningitidis* (meningococcus) is the commonest cause. *Streptococcus pneumoniae* (pneumococcus) causes meningitis in all age groups but most commonly at the extremes of life.

The fungi *Cryptococcus neoformans, Histoplasma, Blastomyces,* and *Candida albicans* may cause meningitis in immunocompromised patients. Free-living amebas belonging to the genera *Naegleria* and *Acanthamoeba* are rare causes of pyogenic meningitis.

B. Acute Lymphocytis (Nonpyogenic; Aseptic) Meningitis: A cellular response consisting predominantly of lymphocytes occurs in meningitis due to obligate intracellular organisms, most commonly enteroviruses, mumps virus, and lymphocytic choriomeningitis (LCM) virus. In about 30% of cases of acute lymphocytic meningitis, no virus can be isolated.

C. Tuberculous Meningitis: Tuberculous meningitis is typically chronic; however, in the early stages there may be an exudative phase that resembles acute meningitis.

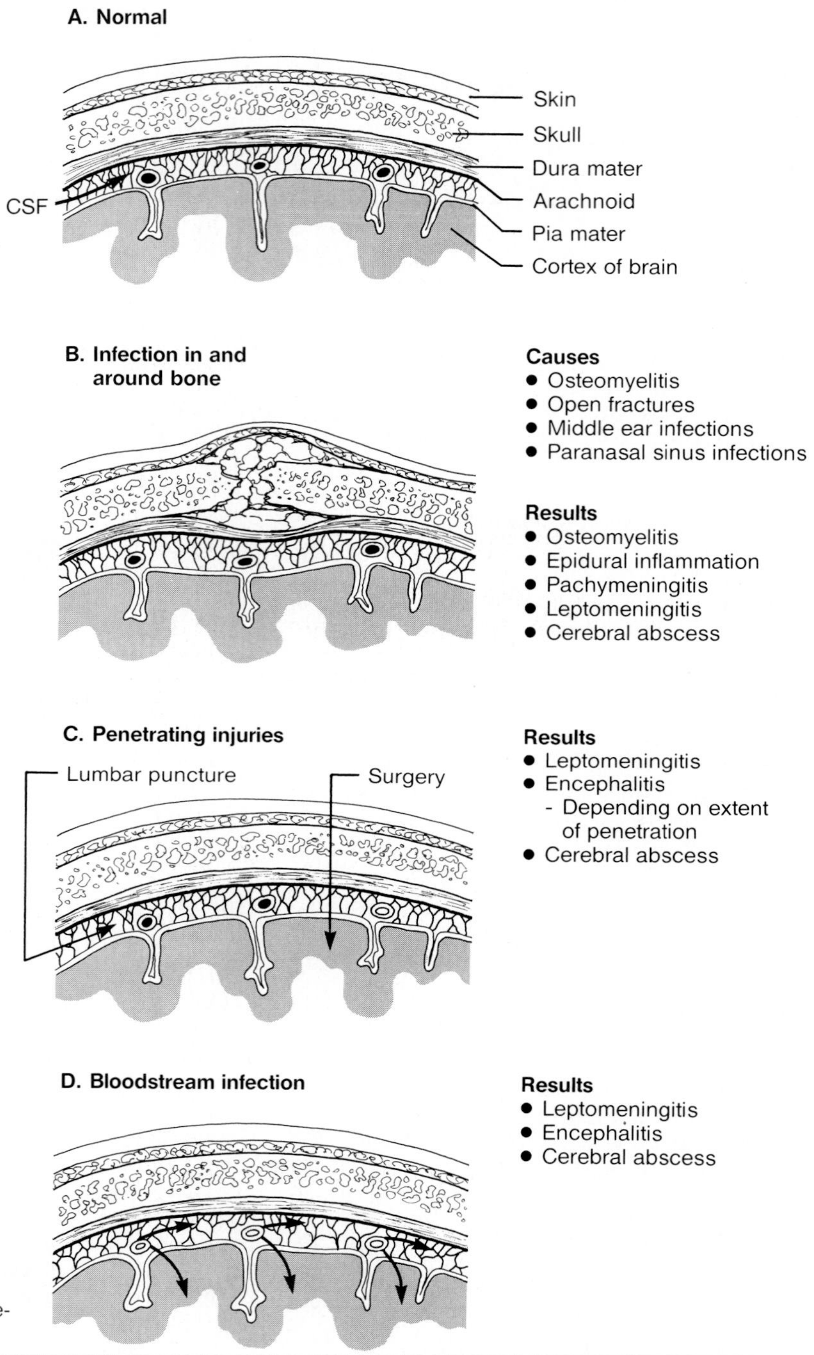

Figure 63-1. Pathogenesis of infection of the central nervous system and their common consequences.

Routes of Infection of the Meninges (Fig 63-1)

Bloodstream spread accounts for the majority of cases; the primary entry site of the organism may be the respiratory tract (*N meningitidis, H influenzae, S pneumoniae, C neoformans,* many viruses), skin (bacteria causing neonatal meningitis), or intestine (enteroviruses).

Meningitis may also result from direct spread of organisms from an infected middle ear or paranasal sinus, especially in childhood. Meningitis may be associated with skull fractures, especially those at the base of the skull that cause free communication between the subarachnoid space and the upper respiratory tract; brain surgery; or lumbar puncture. Organisms may also gain entry

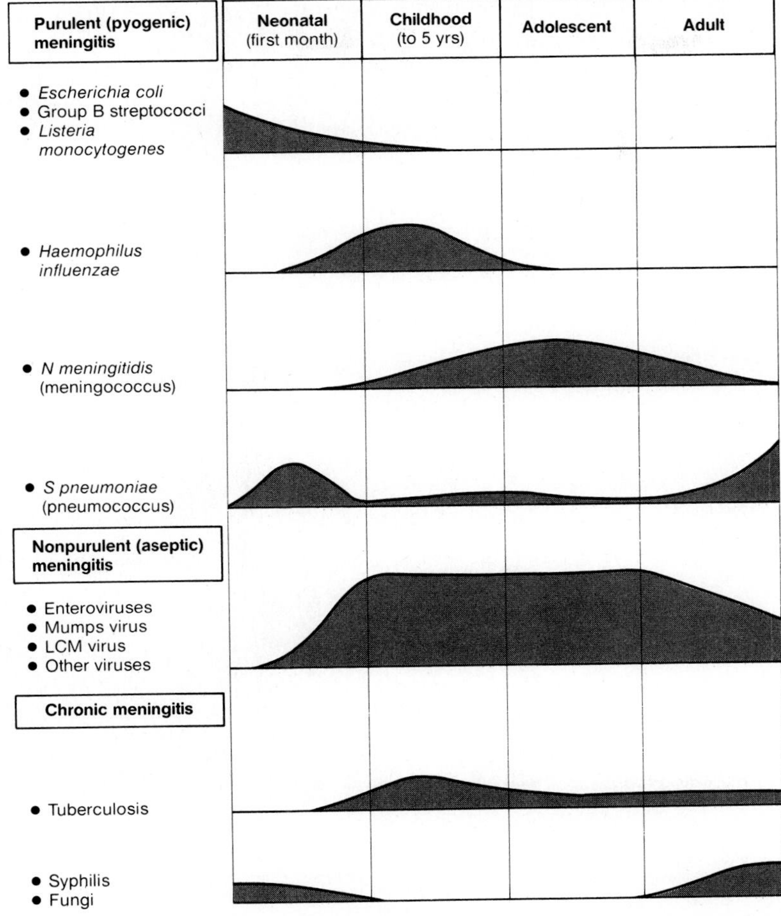

Figure 63-2. Leptomeningitis—principal types and pathogens.

through the intact nasal cribriform plate (eg, free-living soil amebas in stagnant swimming pools).

Tuberculous meningitis may occur during severe tuberculous bacteremia (miliary tuberculosis) or as a result of reactivation of a meningeal focus, in which case the patient may have no evidence of tuberculosis elsewhere.

Pathology

Grossly, the leptomeninges are congested and opaque and contain an exudate. Microscopically, acute meningitis is characterized by hyperemia, fibrin formation, and inflammatory cells. In pyogenic meningitis, neutrophils dominate (Figs 63–3A and 63–4); in acute lymphocytic meningitis, neutrophils are rare and lymphocytes dominate (Fig 63–3B). In acute tuberculous meningitis, there is an inflammatory exudate that contains increased numbers of both neutrophils and lymphocytes.

Clinical Features

Acute meningitis presents with fever and symptoms of meningeal irritation, which include headache, neck pain, and vomiting. Physical examination reveals neck stiffness and a positive Kernig sign (inability to straighten the raised leg because of pain), both of which are due to reflex spasm of spinal muscles, a consequence of irritation of nerves passing across the inflamed meninges.

In general, pyogenic meningitis is a serious disease with considerable risk of death while lymphocytic meningitis is usually a mild self-limited infection. Tuberculous meningitis has an insidious onset and a slow rate of progression but is fre-

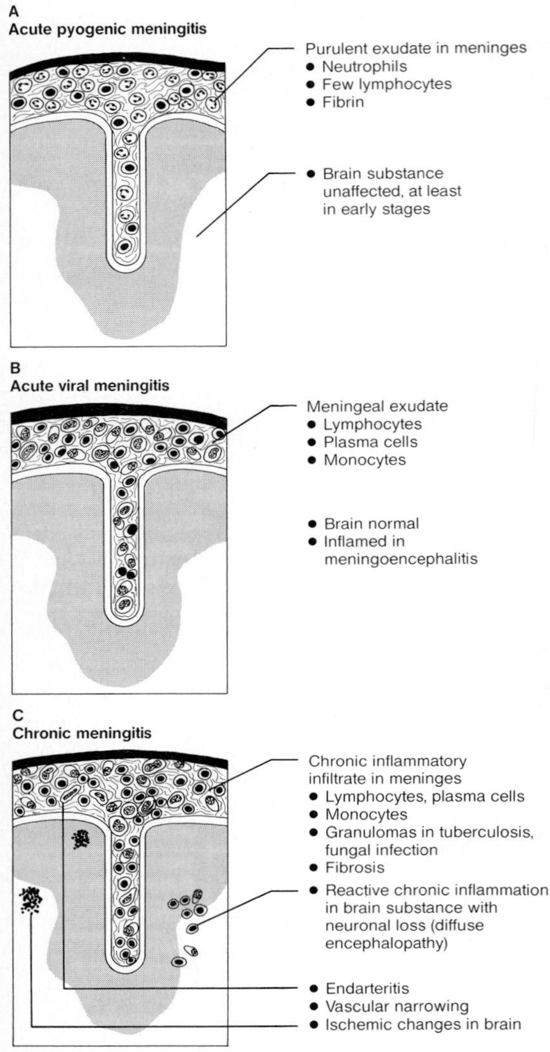

Figure 63-3. Contrasting histologic features in different types of meningitis.

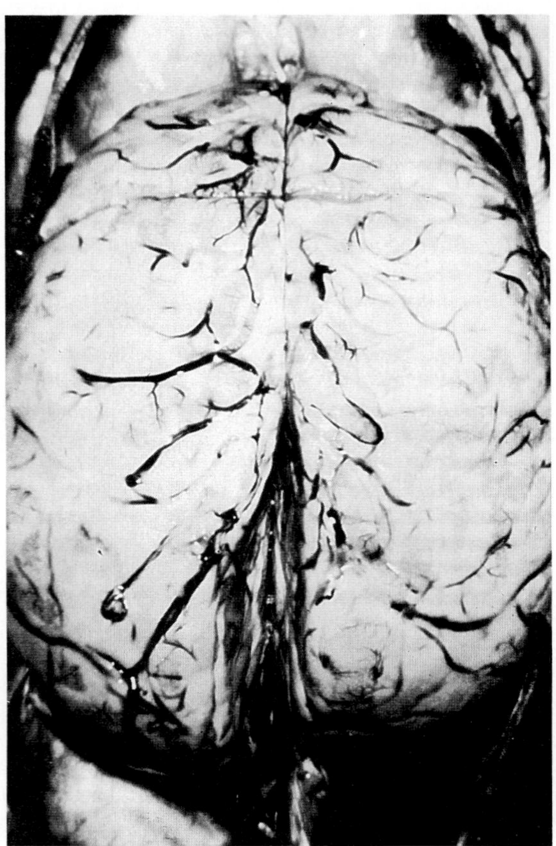

Figure 63-4. Pyogenic meningitis, showing obliteration of the gyri of the brain surface by the purulent exudate.

quently a severe illness with a fatal outcome if not treated.

Diagnosis

The diagnosis is made by examination of the CSF, a sample of which is obtained by lumbar puncture. The leptomeningeal exudate becomes admixed with the CSF, which reflects the type of inflammatory response and contains the infectious agent (see Table 63-1).

Treatment

Antibiotic treatment is urgent in pyogenic and tuberculous meningitis. The initial choice of antibiotic should be based on a presumptive etiologic diagnosis as suggested by the clinical features and CSF findings: chemical examination, type of inflammatory cells present, and Gram or acid-fast stain (Table 63-1). Drug treatment must be started immediately after lumbar puncture with a combination of antibiotics that are effective against all possible causative agents and the choice of drugs reconsidered if necessary when results of culture and sensitivity assays become available.

Viral meningitis usually requires only supportive treatment.

CHRONIC MENINGITIS

Chronic meningitis is caused by facultative intracellular organisms such as *Mycobacterium tuberculosis,* fungi, and *Treponema pallidum.* It is now relatively uncommon in the United States but more prevalent in parts of Africa, India, South America, and Southeast Asia.

Pathology & Clinical Features

Chronic tuberculous or fungal meningitis is characterized by caseous granulomatous inflam-

Table 63-1. Cerebrospinal fluid changes in infections of the central nervous system.

	Encephalitis	Bacterial Meningitis[1]	Viral Meningitis	Tuberculous (Chronic) Meningitis	Brain Abscess
Pressure	Raised	Raised	Raised	Raised	May be very high
Gross appearance	Clear	Turbid	Clear	Clear; may clot	Clear
Protein	Slightly elevated	High	Slightly elevated	Very high	Elevated
Glucose	Normal	Very low	Normal	Low	Normal
Chloride	Normal	Low	Normal	Very low	Normal or low
Cells	Lymphocytes or normal	Neutrophils	Lymphocytes	Pleocytosis[2]	Pleocytosis
Gram stain	Negative	Positive in 90%	Negative	Negative	Occasionally positive
Acid-fast stain	Negative	Negative	Negative	Rarely positive	Negative
Bacterial culture	Negative	Positive in 90%	Negative	Negative	Occasionally positive
Mycobacterial culture	Negative	Negative	Negative	Positive	Negative
Viral culture	Positive in 30% or less	Negative	Positive in 70%	Negative	Negative

[1]Amebic and cryptococcal meningitis are diagnosed by the finding of these organisms in the smear.
[2]Pleocytosis is the presence of both neutrophils and lymphocytes in cerebrospinal fluid.

mation with fibrosis (Fig 63-3). Marked fibrous thickening of the meninges is the dominant pathologic feature. The entire brain surface is involved, with the basal meninges more severely affected in cases of tuberculosis. The causative agent may be identified in tissue sections specially stained for acid-fast bacilli and fungi.

The meningovascular phase of syphilis also causes a basal chronic inflammation with marked fibrosis and obliterative vasculitis, with large numbers of plasma cells infiltrating the meninges; granulomas are not present.

Complications of chronic meningitis include (1) obliterative vasculitis (endarteritis obliterans), which may produce focal ischemia with microinfarcts in the brain and brain stem; (2) entrapment of cranial nerves in the fibrosis as they traverse the meninges, resulting in cranial nerve palsies; and (3) fibrosis around the fourth ventricular foramens, causing obstructive hydrocephalus.

Clinically, chronic meningitis is characterized by an insidious onset with symptoms of diffuse neurologic involvement, including apathy, somnolence, personality change, and poor concentration. These symptoms are thought to stem from a concomitant diffuse encephalopathy (Fig 63-3). Headache and vomiting are less severe than in acute meningitis, and fever is often low-grade. Focal neurologic signs and epileptic seizures result from ischemia, cranial nerve palsies, or hydrocephalus.

Diagnosis & Treatment

The diagnosis is established by lumbar puncture (Table 63-1). Serologic tests for syphilis performed on both serum and CSF are positive in meningeal syphilis. Culture is commonly positive in cases caused by tuberculosis and fungal infection unless the patient has received antibiotics prior to lumbar puncture. Skin tests for tuberculosis and fungal infection are positive unless the patient is anergic.

Antibiotic therapy is indicated once the organism is identified. Treatment begun after extensive fibrosis has occurred does not produce complete recovery.

INFECTIONS OF THE BRAIN PARENCHYMA

CEREBRAL ABSCESS

Cerebral abscess is a localized area of suppurative inflammation in the brain substance. The cavity contains thick pus formed from necrotic, liquefied brain tissue and large numbers of neutrophils and is surrounded by a fibrogliotic wall.

Etiology

Cerebral abscesses are caused by a large variety of bacteria; several organisms may occur in a single abscess, and anaerobic bacteria are common.

Cerebral abscesses occur as complications of other diseases (Fig 63-5).

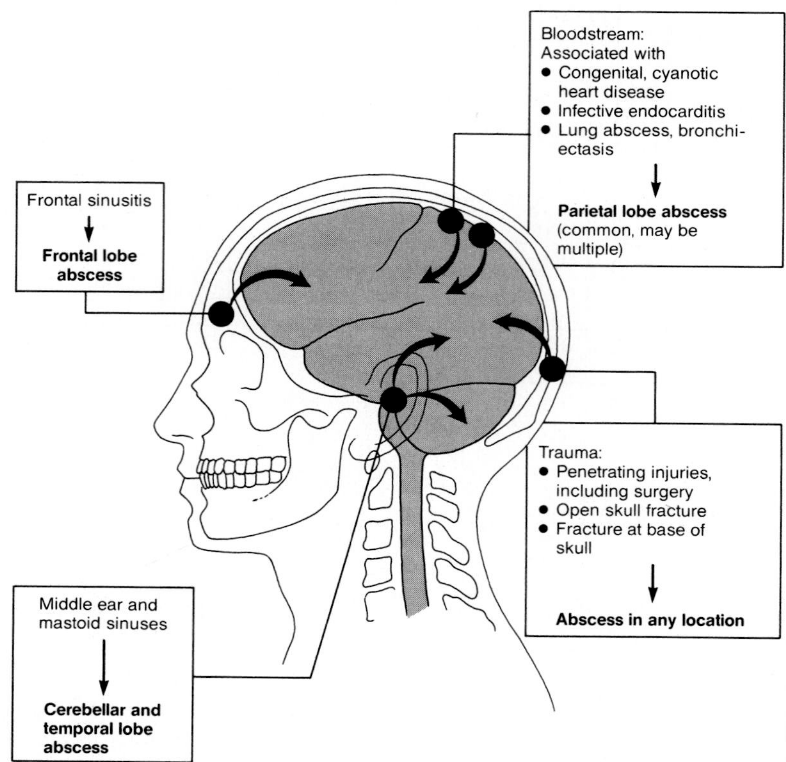

Figure 63-5. Cerebral abscess—common sites and routes of infection.

(1) Chronic suppurative infections of the **middle ear and mastoid** air spaces and of the **paranasal sinuses.** The middle ear is separated from the middle and posterior cranial fossa by thin bony plates that may be eroded by infection. The temporal lobe and the cerebellum are usually involved. Infections of the paranasal sinuses are occasionally associated with frontal lobe abscesses.

(2) Infective endocarditis with embolization to brain. These patients commonly develop parietal lobe abscesses, often small and multiple.

(3) Right-to-left shunts (eg, in patients with congenital cyanotic heart disease) may divert infected systemic emboli to the brain.

(4) Suppurative **lung diseases** such as chronic lung abscess and bronchiectasis are rarely complicated by embolization of infected material to the brain, leading to parietal lobe abscesses.

Pathology

Grossly, a cerebral abscess appears as a mass lesion in the brain. It has a liquefied center filled with pus and a fibrogliotic wall whose thickness depends on the duration of the abscess (Fig 63–6). The surrounding brain frequently shows vasogenic edema.

Clinical Features & Diagnosis

Cerebral abscess presents with (1) features of a space-occupying lesion, including evidence of raised intracranial pressure (headache, vomiting, papilledema) and focal neurologic signs, depending on the location of the abscess; (2) features relating to the source of infection, such as chronic otitis media, suppurative lung disease, and endocarditis; and (3) general evidence of infection,

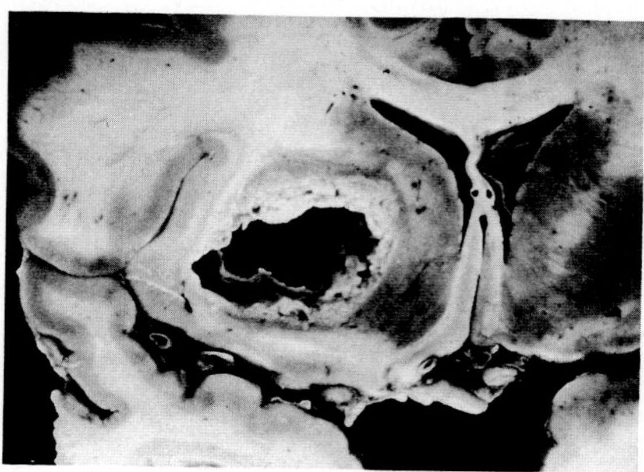

Figure 63-6. Cerebral abscess, showing a cavity in the region of the basal ganglia lined by inflammatory exudate. The cavity was filled with pus that drained when the brain was cut.

such as fever, rapid erythrocyte sedimentation rate, and weight loss in chronic cases.

In untreated cases, the abscess progressively enlarges and may cause death from increased intracranial pressure or rupture into the ventricular system.

The diagnosis of cerebral abscess is made clinically and confirmed by CT scan or MRI. Lumbar puncture is dangerous because of the risk of precipitating tonsillar herniation. The CSF may be normal or may show mild increases in protein, neutrophils, and lymphocytes (Table 63-1). CSF cultures may or may not be positive.

Treatment

Surgical evacuation of the abscess followed by antibiotic therapy is effective treatment and has reduced the previously high mortality rate of cerebral abscess to about 5–10%.

VIRAL ENCEPHALITIS

The frequency of viral encephalitis is difficult to estimate. In the United States, about 1500 cases are reported every year. Most of these are presumptive diagnoses—the etiologic virus is identified in only about 30% of cases. Worldwide, many cases of acute cerebral dysfunction in which no attempt is made to identify a virus probably go unreported.

Epidemics of encephalitis are most commonly the result of arthropod-borne viruses (arboviruses) (Table 63-2). Arboviruses have animal hosts, are transmitted to humans by arthropod bites, and have a distinctive geographic distribution. Sporadic cases of encephalitis may be caused by a large number of other viruses, most commonly herpes simplex virus.

Table 63-2. Causes of viral encephalitis.

Diffuse encephalitis
Epidemic (arbovirus) encephalitis
Eastern equine encephalitis
Western equine encephalitis
Venezuelan equine encephalitis
St. Louis encephalitis
California encephalitis
Japanese B encephalitis
Sporadic encephalitis
Herpes simplex
Enterovirus encephalitis
Measles
Varicella (chickenpox)
Encephalitis in the immunocompromised host
Herpes simplex
Progressive multifocal leukoencephalopathy
Cytomegalovirus
HIV (AIDS encephalitis)
Specific types of encephalitis
Poliomyelitis
Rabies
Subacute sclerosing panencephalitis
Slow virus infections

Pathology

The virus usually reaches the brain via the bloodstream. It infects brain cells, causing neuronal necrosis and marked cerebral edema, which in turn leads to acute cerebral dysfunction and increased intracranial pressure. Perivascular lymphocytic infiltration ("perivascular cuffing") is characteristic (Fig 63-7). In severe cases, hemorrhages occur.

Clinical Features

Viral encephalitis has an acute onset with fever, headache, and signs of brain dysfunction, the nature of which depend on the areas of brain involved. Convulsions may occur. There may be papilledema if cerebral edema is severe. In many cases of viral encephalitis, there is concomitant meningeal inflammation causing neck stiffness and CSF abnormalities typical of viral meningitis. The diagnosis is based on the clinical picture. Lumbar puncture with examination and culture of CSF may provide an etiologic diagnosis.

Treatment

Therapy is supportive. Control of cerebral edema with high doses of corticosteroids is important in preventing death from raised intracranial

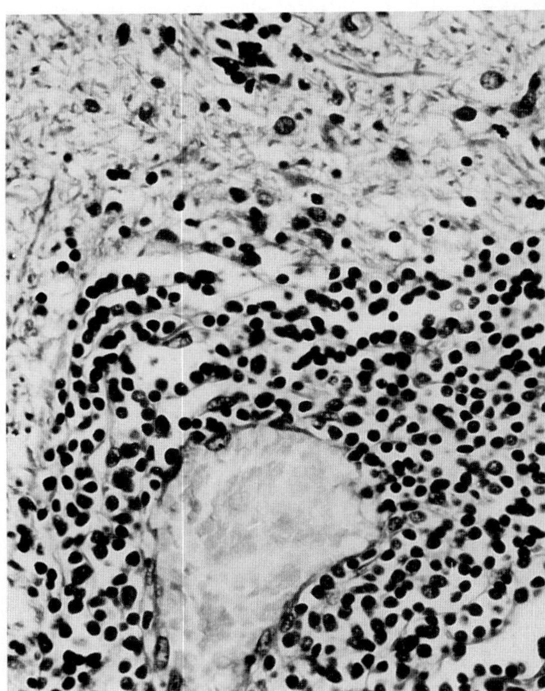

Figure 63-7. Viral encephalitis, showing perivascular lymphocytic cuffing.

pressure in the acute phase. The mortality rate from severe viral encephalitis is high, and patients who recover are frequently left with permanent neurologic deficits due to irreversible neuronal necrosis.

1. HERPES SIMPLEX ENCEPHALITIS

Incidence & Etiology

Herpes simplex encephalitis occurs in 3 classes of patients:

Neonates are infected during delivery in a woman with active genital herpes. The presence of herpes genitalis in the mother is an absolute indication for cesarian section. Herpes simplex type 2 is responsible for most cases.

Adults are infected through the bloodstream from a minor focus of viral replication, usually in the mouth. Herpes simplex type 1 is commonly involved.

Immunocompromised hosts, particularly patients undergoing chemotherapy for the treatment of cancer, have an increased susceptibility not only to become infected by herpes simplex virus but also to develop viremia and encephalitis.

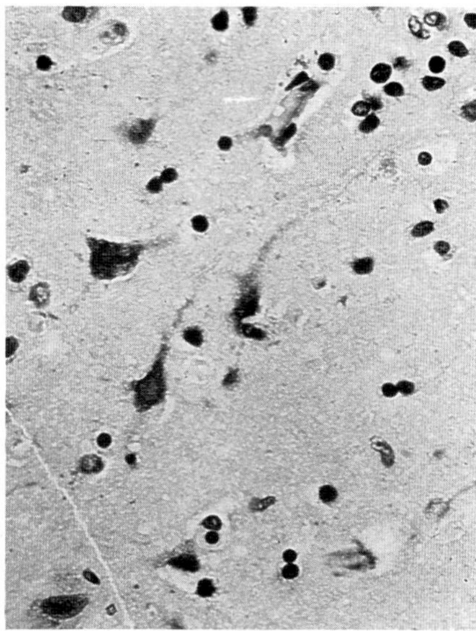

Figure 63-8. Herpes simplex encephalitis. This section has been stained for herpes simplex viral antigens by the immunoperoxidase technique. The darkly staining (positive) cells are infected with the virus.

Pathology

Herpes simplex encephalitis affects the temporal and inferior frontal lobes selectively, producing a necrotizing, hemorrhagic acute encephalitis that may rapidly cause death. Patients who survive frequently suffer permanent neurologic defects, the nature of which depends on the neuronal loss.

Diagnosis

The diagnosis may be made by brain biopsy, which shows cerebral edema, necrosis, lymphocytic infiltration, and the presence of intranuclear Cowdry A inclusions in infected cells. Electron microscopy or, preferably, immunohistochemical or in situ hybridization tests demonstrate the virus in the majority of cases (Fig 63-8).

Treatment

Treatment of herpes simplex encephalitis with antiviral agents such as vidarabine has improved survival in some series.

2. POLIOMYELITIS

Poliomyelitis is caused by the poliovirus, an enterovirus transmitted by the fecal-oral route. The virus enters the body through the intestine (Fig 63-9) and infects the brain and spinal cord via the bloodstream. Poliomyelitis was once common but has become rare in developed countries because of routine immunization during childhood. Poliomyelitis now occurs only in areas where childhood immunization is inadequate.

The poliovirus selectively infects (1) the meninges, producing acute lymphocytic meningitis; and (2) the lower motor neurons in the anterior horn of the spinal cord and medulla oblongata. Loss of motor neurons causes acute paralysis of affected muscles. The paralysis is typically asymmetric and flaccid, with muscle atrophy and loss of deep tendon reflexes. With time, the atrophic muscles may undergo fibrous contracture.

Poliomyelitis is a very serious disease associated with a significant mortality rate in the acute phase, when paralysis of respiratory muscle results in failure of ventilation. Patients who survive are commonly left with permanent muscle paralysis.

3. RABIES

Rabies is rare in humans but occurs in a variety of wild animals and domestic pets, including dogs and cats, in whom it causes a fatal illness called hydrophobia characterized by abnormal behavior, difficulty in swallowing, and convulsions. Humans are infected when bitten by an infected animal. The rabies virus enters the cutaneous nerve radicles at the site of inoculation and passes proximally to the central nerve system. The incubation period is 1–3 months, being shortest in facial bites.

Rabies virus causes a severe necrotizing enceph-

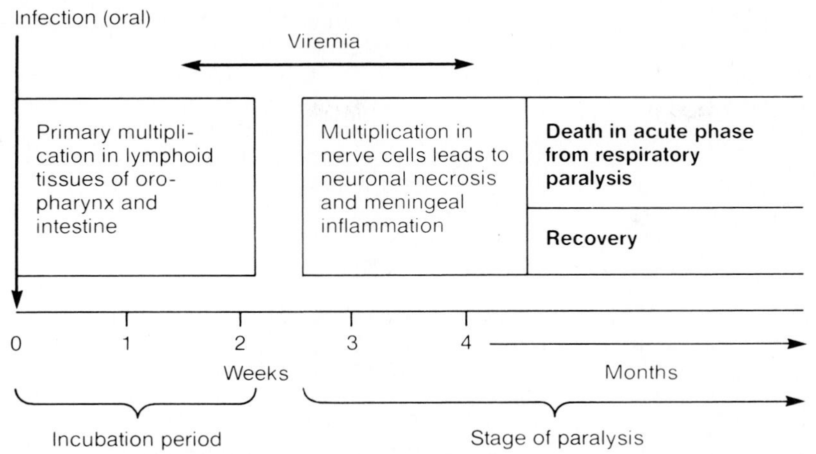

Figure 63-9. Poliomyelitis, showing the phases of infection. Patients who recover show a permanent neurolgic deficit that corresponds to the neuronal necrosis in the acute phase.

alitis that maximally affects the basal ganglia, hippocampus, and brain stem. Infected neurons show diagnostic eosinophilic intracytoplasmic inclusion bodies (Negri bodies). The virus can also be identified in the infected cells by electron microscopy and immunoperoxidase techniques.

Clinically, rabies presents with fever and generalized convulsions that are precipitated by the slightest of sensory stimulation such as a gust of wind, a faint noise, or the sight of water. Death is inevitable.

Since there is no treatment, prevention is essential and consists of controlling the disease in animals, rabies immunization of domestic pets, and administration of antirabies vaccine to humans immediately after exposure.

4. CYTOMEGALOVIRUS ENCEPHALITIS

Cytomegalovirus infection of the brain occurs in the fetus during the last trimester of pregnancy as a result of transplacental infection. Periventricular necrosis and calcification lead to microcephaly and mental retardation; chorioretinitis is common. Cytomegalovirus encephalitis occurs also in immunocompromised hosts, particularly patients with AIDS.

5. PROGRESSIVE MULTIFOCAL LEUKOENCEPHALOPATHY (PML)

PML is caused by papovarvirus SV40 and occurs usually in immunocompromised hosts, particularly patients with AIDS and those undergoing chemotherapy for cancer.

PML is characterized pathologically by widespread focal demyelination of cerebral white matter, with maximal involvement of the occipital lobe. Giant atypical astrocytes and intranuclear inclusions in oligodendroglial cells are typically present, along with a lymphocytic infiltrate. The papovavirus can be identified by immunohistochemical techniques.

Clinically, PML presents as an acute, rapidly progressive illness associated with multifocal cerebral dysfunction. The mortality rate is high.

6. SUBACUTE SCLEROSING PANENCEPHALITIS (SSPE)

SSPE is an uncommon disease that affects children several years after a known attack of measles. The measles virus, which has been demonstrated in the cerebral lesions of SSPE, is the causal agent. SSPE is therefore regarded as a chronic measles virus infection. The exact mechanism by which the virus causes encephalitis in this manner is unknown. Immunologic factors may play a role, or there may be some alteration of the measles virus itself.

Pathologically, SSPE is characterized by degeneration of neurons in the cerebral gray matter and basal ganglia. Intranuclear inclusions are present in infected cells. The white matter shows demyelination, reactive astrocytic proliferation, and perivascular lymphocytic infiltration.

Clinically, patients present with personality changes and involuntary myoclonic-type movements. The disease is relentlessly progressive, causing extensive brain damage leading to death, usually within 1–2 years after onset.

7. "SLOW VIRUS" INFECTIONS

"Slow virus" infections of the brain are characterized by a long latent period after infection followed by a slowly progressive disease ending in death. **Creutzfeldt-Jakob disease** and **kuru** are included in this category. **Scrapie,** an encephalopathy in sheep and goats, serves as the animal model for this group of diseases. Although the agents responsible have not been identified with certainty, there is growing evidence that a form of subviral transmissible agent known as a **prion** may be involved. Prions consist of protein only (no nucleic acid). The mode of transmission and whether or not cofactors are required are unknown. About 10% of cases of Creutzfeldt-Jakob disease appear to be dominantly inherited; a gene responsible for production of prion proteins has been located in chromosome 20.

Creutzfeldt-Jakob disease is important for pathologists because the agent is resistant to inactivation by formalin, imposing a great risk of infection from handling infected tissues. Kuru occurs mainly in cannibalistic tribes of Papua New Guinea, where the disease is believed to be transmitted by eating brain tissue of infected humans. Women in these tribes developed the disease because they were given the brain to eat, the muscle being reserved for the male tribal warriors.

Creutzfeldt-Jakob disease and kuru are both characterized by slowly progressive degeneration of the brain, with progressive neuronal loss, demyelination, and spongiform change in the cerebral white matter. There is no inflammatory cell infiltration. Kuru tends to affect the cerebellum and is characterized microscopically by the presence of "kuru plaques," which are amyloid bodies with radially arranged spicules. These appear to consist of filaments of prion protein.

Clinically, patients present with dementia, followed by ataxia that progresses slowly but relentlessly to a fatal outcome. There is no treatment.

NEUROSYPHILIS

Congenital syphilis and adult syphilis in its late tertiary phase may involve the nervous system in many ways (Table 63–3); it has, however, become relatively rare following the use of penicillin in the treatment of early syphilis.

The parenchymatous and meningovascular lesions of late syphilis may occur together in a given patient or separately.

Clinically, general paresis affects the cerebral hemispheres and is manifested by progressive dementia, overt psychosis, loss of memory, inappropriate social behavior, delusions (particularly delusions of grandeur), and hallucinations. Spirochetes are detectable in the brain. While penicillin may prevent further progression, it will not reverse deficits that have already occurred.

Tabes dorsalis causes chiefly degeneration of the dorsal nerve roots, dorsal ganglia, and posterior columns (see Chapter 64). No spirochetes can be demonstrated in these lesions.

Table 63–3. Neurosyphilis: Pathologic and clinical features.

Type of Disease	Time Elapsed After Primary Infection	Principal Pathologic Features	CSF	Clinical Features
Asymptomatic	2–3 years	Mild lymphocytic meningeal infiltrate	Positive VDRL[1]	Very common; discovered by routine lumbar puncture in patients with secondary syphilis; penicillin is curative
Meningovascular syphilis				
Diffuse	3+ years	Chronic inflammation of meninges with fibrosis and endarteritis	Increased protein; mild lymphocytosis; positive VDRL	Meningeal symptoms; cranial nerve palsies; penicillin may be effective in early stage
Focal	3+ years	Gumma formation	Positive VDRL; increased protein, lymphocytosis	Very rare; acts as a space-occupying lesion
Parenchymatous syphilis				
General paresis	10+ years	Diffuse cerebral cortical neuronal loss; chronic encephalitis; spirochetes present	Positive VDRL; mild lymphocytosis	Progressive dementia and psychosis; cerebral atrophy with ventricle dilatation; penicillin not effective
Tabes dorsalis	10+ years	Demyelination of spinal cord (posterior columns) and sensory nerve root; spirochetes absent	Positive VDRL; mild lymphocytosis	Lightning pains, sensory loss, hypotonia, areflexia; penicillin not effective

[1]VDRL = Veneral Disease Research Laboratory serologic test for syphilis. This is positive in about 50% of all cases of neurosyphilis. The more sensitive FTA-ABS (fluorescent treponemal antibody test) is positive in 90%.

Clinically, tabes dorsalis presents with (1) "lightning pains" in the extremities, due to abnormal stimulation of the degenerating dorsal nerve root fibers; (2) unsteady gait, due to loss of position sense (posterior columns); (3) loss of pain and temperature sensation, which leads to the development of trophic lesions in the skin and joints (Charcot's joints); (4) loss of deep tendon reflexes; (5) the typical Argyll Robertson pupils—small and irregular pupils showing brisk reaction to accommodation and no reaction to light; and (6) urinary and fecal incontinence and impotence.

Treatment with penicillin may prevent progression in the early stages but will not affect existing deficits.

GRANULOMAS OF THE BRAIN

Typical infectious granulomas due to *Mycobacterium tuberculosis* or fungi occur rarely in the brain. Granulomas present as mass lesions with increased intracranial pressure and focal neurologic signs depending on the location of the mass. Clinically and on radiologic examination, they resemble neoplasms. The diagnosis is made by biopsy, which shows typical histologic changes. The organisms can be identified with special stains and by culture.

PROTOZOAL INFECTIONS

TOXOPLASMOSIS

Toxoplasma gondii is a protozoan parasite that has its definitive cycle in the intestine of cats. Humans become infected through contact with cat feces containing infective forms of the parasite. Cerebral toxoplasmosis occurs in 2 distinct forms, congenital and acquired.

Congenital Toxoplasmosis

Fetal infection with *T gondii* occurs transplacentally in the third trimester of pregnancy. The organism infects the fetal brain and the retina, leading to extensive necrosis, calcification, and gliosis. Many infants die soon after birth, and those that survive have a variety of defects such as microcephaly, hydrocephalus, mental retardation, and visual disturbances. *Toxoplasma* pseudocysts can be identified in the brain and retinal lesions.

Acquired Toxoplasmosis

Acquired toxoplasmosis rarely causes cerebral lesions in normal individuals. It may, however, occur as an opportunistic infection in AIDS, and as such it is one of the criteria used for defining AIDS.

Cerebral toxoplasmosis in AIDS is characterized by the presence of multiple necrotic lesions ranging in size from 0.5 to 3 cm. *Toxoplasma* pseudocysts and tachyzoites may be seen in biopsies of lesions. Diagnosis in tissues is aided by staining for *Toxoplasma* antigens by immunoperoxidase techniques.

Clinically, patients present with fever and symptoms of acute cerebral dysfunction. Computerized tomography shows ring-enhancing mass lesions that are often multiple. Treatment with anti-*Toxoplasma* agents is effective.

CEREBRAL MALARIA

Cerebral malaria is caused by infection with *Plasmodium falciparum* and occurs only in regions where this species occurs. Clogging of cerebral capillaries by *P falciparum*-infected erythrocytes causes diffuse cerebral ischemia with edema, petechial hemorrhages, and necrosis. There is no direct infection of brain cells. Clinically, patients have fever and acute cerebral dysfunction with convulsions and progress rapidly to coma and death.

The diagnosis is made by finding *P falciparum* in erythrocytes in a peripheral blood smear. Treatment with antimalarial drugs is effective.

AFRICAN TRYPANOSOMIASIS ("Sleeping Sickness")

African trypanosomiasis is rarely seen outside Africa. It is caused by *Trypanosoma rhodesiense* (East Africa) and *Trypanosoma gambiense* (West Africa) and is transmitted by the bite of the tsetse fly.

Central nervous system involvement follows systemic dissemination after cutaneous inoculation. It is characterized by diffuse neuronal degeneration and perivascular lymphoplasmacytic infiltration. Clinically, patients have headache, severe drowsiness (hence, sleeping sickness), personality changes, convulsions, and coma. The disease has a high mortality rate.

OTHER PARASITIC DISEASES

Other parasitic diseases affecting the brain include cysticercosis, trichinosis, hydatid disease, and schistosomiasis. Very rarely, *Entamoeba histolytica* leads to brain abscesses.

64 The Central Nervous System: III. Traumatic, Vascular, Degenerative, & Metabolic Diseases

TRAUMATIC NERVOUS SYSTEM LESIONS

CEREBRAL INJURIES

1. PENETRATING (OPEN) INJURIES

Penetrating injuries are caused by gunshots and severe blunt trauma. They are associated with severe brain damage and a high incidence of infection. The symptoms and sequelae depend on the extent and area of damage.

2. NONPENETRATING (CLOSED) INJURIES

Nonpenetrating injuries, usually caused by blunt trauma, may produce several degrees of damage.

Cerebral Concussion ("Commotio Cerebri")

Cerebral concussion is transient loss of cerebral function—in most definitions including loss of consciousness—that immediately follows head injury. It is probably the result of relative motion between the brain stem and the cerebral hemispheres, causing temporary neuronal dysfunction in the reticular formation. The brain shows no gross or histologic abnormality. In severe concussion, coma may be prolonged, and in rare cases death may be the outcome.

Concussion is frequently associated with loss of memory for events occurring shortly before the traumatic episode (retrograde amnesia) or immediately afterward (posttraumatic amnesia). Recovery from concussion may be followed by recurrent headache, impaired ability to concentrate, and other minor neurologic symptoms (postconcussion syndrome). These symptoms are usually transient but in some cases may persist for years.

Cerebral Contusion

Rupture of small blood vessels in the brain near its surface and extravasation of blood into the brain substance is most commonly caused by movement of the brain relative to the skull (acceleration-deceleration injuries), causing it to strike bony prominences within the skull, such as those in the floor of the anterior cranial fossa or the internal occipital protuberance (Fig 64–1). Contusions also occur in the brain subjacent to the point of impact, particularly if there is a depressed skull fracture. Contusions may also occur on the side opposite the point of impact (contrecoup injuries).

Cerebral contusions appear initially as an area of subpial hemorrhage. Like an ordinary contusion (bruise) anywhere on the body, the lesion undergoes color change from red to brown as iron is deposited in the tissues. Cerebral contusions may serve as the focus for epileptic activity.

Cerebral Laceration

The most severe type of brain injury is tearing of cerebral tissue, resulting in acute hemorrhage in the subarachnoid or subdural space. Cerebral laceration is often associated with profound neurologic dysfunction and is associated with a high mortality rate.

SPINAL CORD INJURIES

Spinal cord injuries result from forced movements (such as the "whiplash" injury of the cervical cord) or vertebral fractures and subluxations. Road traffic accidents, diving into shallow water, and sports injuries are common causes.

The basic injuries in the spinal cord are similar to those in the brain: concussion, contusion, and laceration. Their clinical effects, however, are often more severe because of the concentration of neural pathways in the spinal cord. With high cervical cord injury, quadriplegia (paralysis of all 4 limbs) occurs; death may result from respiratory muscle paralysis. Thoracic cord injuries may lead to paraplegia (paralysis of lower body and legs) and dysfunction of the bladder and rectum.

MENINGEAL TEARS

Meningeal tears occur with fractures of the base of the skull and are manifested clinically as a leak of cerebrospinal fluid through the nose (CSF rhinorrhea) or ears (CSF otorrhea). The diagnosis of fluid draining from the nose or ear as cerebrospinal fluid may be made by chemical examination (low protein content and presence of glucose—un-

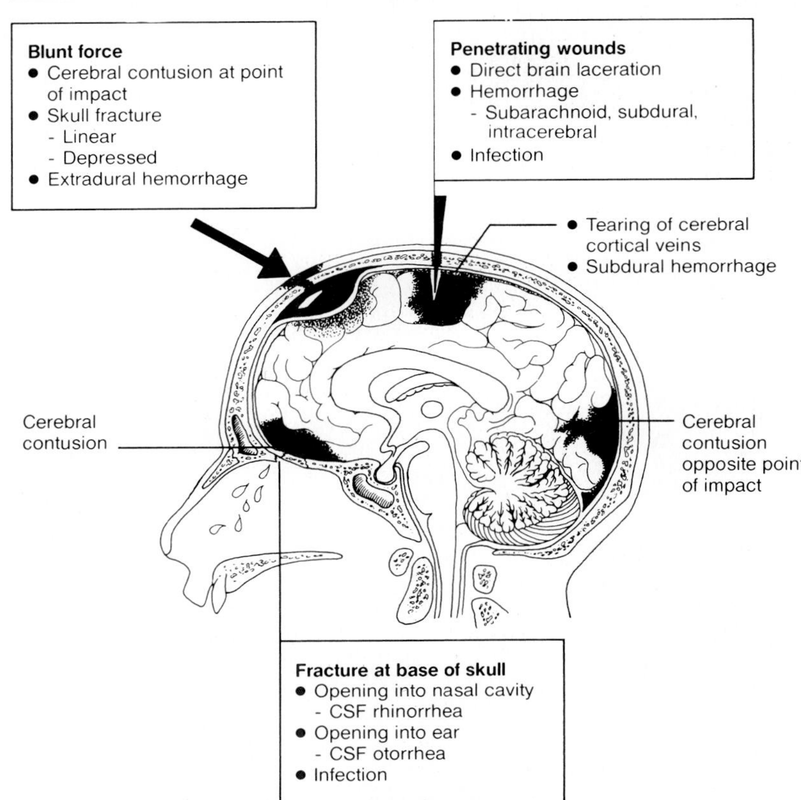

Figure 64–1. Direct effects of craniocerebral trauma.

like mucus, which is high in protein and contains no glucose). The main risk is that the tear will serve as a pathway for infection.

TRAUMATIC INTRACRANIAL HEMORRHAGE

1. ACUTE EXTRADURAL HEMATOMA

Extradural (epidural) hematoma is one of the commonest and most important complications of nonpenetrating head injuries. It is an accumulation of blood between the skull and the dura (Fig 64–2). In 90% of cases, bleeding is from a branch of the middle meningeal artery. In the remainder, the bleeding is of venous origin. Laceration of the middle meningeal artery is often associated with fracture of the temporal region of the skull.

With arterial bleeding, the hematoma expands rapidly, and symptoms appear within hours after injury; with venous bleeding, progression is less rapid.

The clinical history is characteristic. After a head injury—often associated with a variable pe-

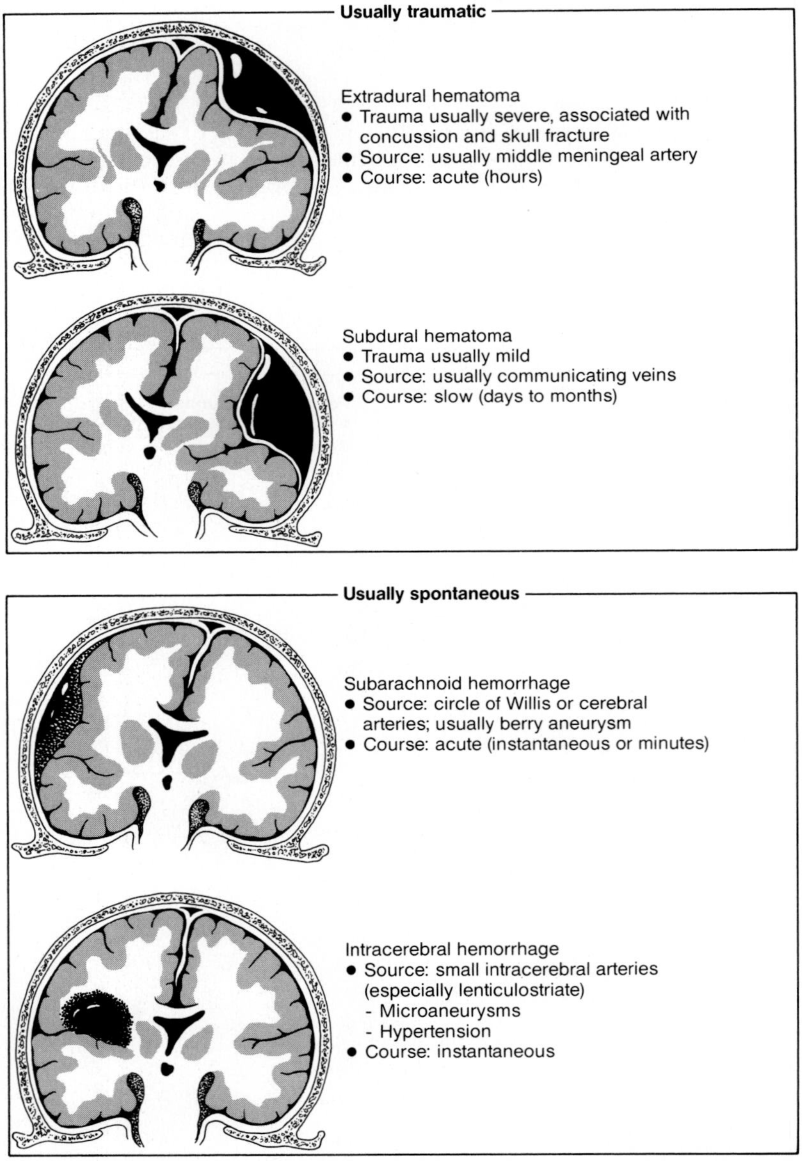

Figure 64–2. Common types of intracranial hemorrhage. Extradural and subdural hematomas are commonly caused by trauma, whereas subarachnoid and intracerebral hemorrhage are commonly the result of diseases involving the blood vessels.

riod of concussion— the patient appears normal for several hours. After this "lucid interval," the patient develops evidence of raised intracranial pressure with headache, vomiting, altered consciousness, and papilledema. Tentorial herniation rapidly follows, with oculomotor nerve palsy (pupillary inequality appears first, followed by failure of reaction to light) and pyramidal tract compression. Compression of the brain stem follows, resulting in changes in heart rate, blood pressure, and respiration. Coma and death rapidly ensue in untreated cases.

This condition requires urgent diagnosis, since treatment by surgical evacuation of the blood clot and hemostasis is successful if undertaken early.

2. CHRONIC SUBDURAL HEMATOMA

Chronic subdural hematoma is a common lesion characterized by accumulation of blood in the subdural space, separated from the brain by the arachnoid and subarachnoid space (Fig 64–2). It occurs mainly in elderly patients with some degree of cerebral atrophy. The amount of trauma required is minimal, and many patients give no history of head injury.

Bleeding is the result of rupture of veins passing from the cerebral cortex to the superior sagittal sinus. Rupture occurs when there is movement of the brain relative to the fixed superior sagittal sinus and is most likely when cerebral atrophy is present. Chronic subdural hematomas are frequently bilateral.

Bleeding is slow and often can be quickly controlled by normal hemostatic mechanisms. The blood clot in the subdural space then breaks down and exerts an osmotic effect that draws in fluid from the adjacent subarachnoid space. This imbibed fluid causes the lesion to expand slowly, compressing the brain.

Grossly, chronic subdural hematoma contains fluid of a brownish color and is lined by dura on one side and a new fibrous "membrane" on the leptomeningeal side. The thickness of this "false membrane" is proportionate to the duration of the hematoma.

Clinically, patients present with slowly increasing intracranial pressure, causing headache, vomiting, papilledema, and fluctuating levels of consciousness. Compression of the underlying brain may cause focal epileptic convulsions and neurologic symptoms, most commonly contralateral spastic paralysis. With prolonged but less severe compression, atrophy of the brain occurs and causes dementia.

Treatment by surgical evacuation of the fluid collection is curative. Return of brain function is variable, depending upon the duration and degree of cerebral atrophy that has occurred.

CEREBROVASCULAR ACCIDENTS (Strokes)

The term "stroke" denotes a wide variety of nontraumatic cerebrovascular accidents of abrupt onset. So defined, stroke has many causes (Table 64–1; Fig 64–3); cerebral thrombosis with infarction is responsible for about 90% of cases. Stroke is one of the leading causes of death and disease in developed countries, accounting for approximately 200,000 deaths per year in the USA and 80,000 in Great Britain.

ISCHEMIC STROKES (Cerebral Infarction)

Etiology

A. Atherosclerosis and Thrombosis: Cerebral thrombosis resulting from atherosclerotic arterial disease is responsible for most cases of cerebral infarction. Atherosclerosis tends to involve the large arteries (Fig 64–4). Sites of arterial branching (such as the carotid bifurcation) and curvature (the carotid siphon in the petrous temporal bone) tend to show severe atherosclerosis. Small arteries on the surface of the brain are rarely affected.

The circle of Willis at the base of the brain is a highly effective anastomotic system between the carotid and vertebrobasilar arteries. Occlusions proximal to the circle of Willis are usually compensated for by the collaterals in the circle. Arteries distal to the circle are functional end arteries,

Table 64–1. Classification and etiology of cerebrovascular accidents (CVA; "strokes").

Ischemic	Hemorrhagic
Cerebral infarction Nonocclusive Cerebral arterial thrombosis Cerebral embolism Transient ischemic attack Hypertensive encephalopathy with vasospasm Venous occlusion: in hypercoagulable states, infection Arteritis: polyarteritis nodosa, giant cell arteritis Dissecting aneurysm of the aorta Carotid injury	Intracerebral hemorrhage: hypertensive Subarachoid hemorrhage: berry aneurysms Associated with vascular malformations and neoplasms Associated with bleeding diathesis such as coagulation disorders, thrombocytopenia; anticoagulant therapy

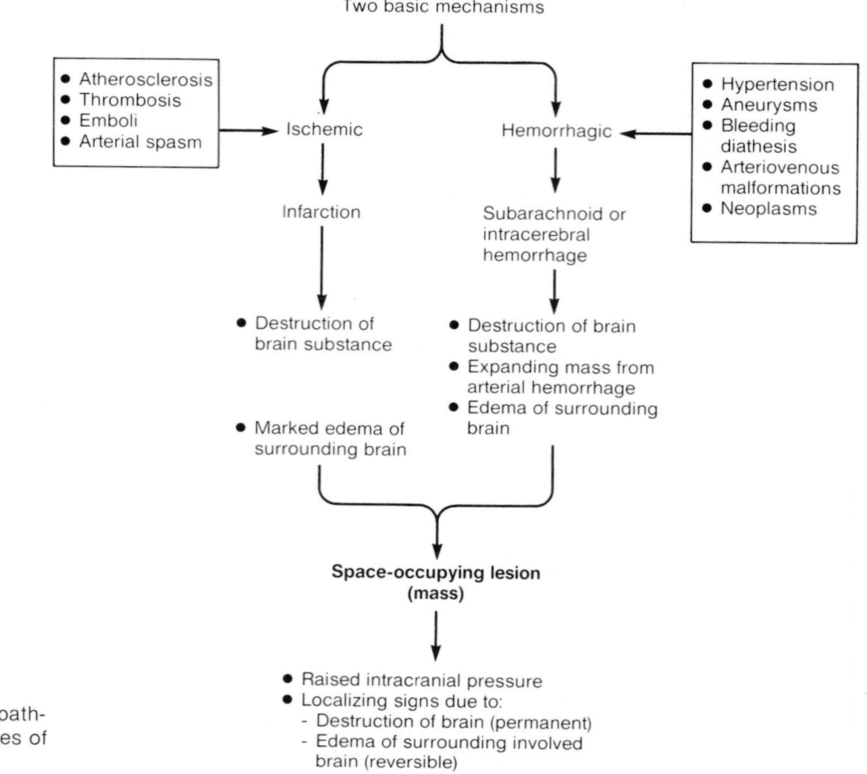

Figure 64–3. Etiology and pathogenesis of the 2 major types of cerebrovascular accident.

and their occlusion usually results in cerebral infarction.

Atherosclerosis may have several consequences: (1) narrowing in excess of 75% causes a significant decrease in blood flow; (2) thrombosis may occlude the artery—the most common site for thrombosis is at the carotid sinus and bifurcation; and (3) ulceration of an atherosclerotic plaque releases emboli into the distal circulation. These emboli are commonly composed of cholesterol or small platelet aggregates and may give rise to transient ischemic attacks (see below). Infarction follows any of the above if the blood supply falls below critical levels for a sufficiently long time.

B. Embolism: Small cerebral emboli are difficult to identify during life or at autopsy; they may be responsible for many cases of "nonocclusive" infarction. Recognizable emboli occur (1) after myocardial infarction due to detachment of mural thrombi; (2) with infective endocarditis due to detachment of valvular vegetations; (3) with prosthetic cardiac valves; (4) with mitral stenosis and atrial fibrillation; and (5) with atherosclerotic disease in the aortic arch, carotids, or circle of Willis.

C. Other Causes: Rarely, cerebral ischemia is the result of vasculitides such as polyarteritis nodosa and giant cell arteritis affecting cerebral arteries (Table 64–1). Cerebral venous occlusion is a rare cause of stroke but an important one since it occurs in hypercoagulable states or severe dehydration and is treatable if diagnosed early.

Pathology

The earliest gross change after infarction occurs at about 6 hours and is a softening of the brain with loss of the normal demarcation between gray and white matter (Fig 64–5). Microscopically, the neurons show nuclear pyknosis, cytoplasmic eosinophilia, and liquefaction. Glial cells disappear, and the myelin sheaths and axis cylinders in the white matter disintegrate.

At 48–72 hours the cerebral infarct is fully formed, appearing as a pale, soft area composed of liquefied necrotic cells. The surrounding brain shows edema. Ten to 20 percent of cerebral infarcts are hemorrhagic, due possibly to restoration of blood supply to the infarcted area, either by fibrinolysis or by fragmentation of the thrombus.

After a transient phase of neutrophil infiltration, macrophages appear in large numbers (Chapter 1). They phagocytose the dead tissue, becoming converted to large cells with abundant pale foamy cytoplasm called gitter cells or compound granular corpuscles.

After about 3 weeks, the debris has been cleared, producing a cystic fluid-filled cavity (Fig 64–6) surrounded by a zone of reactive gliosis.

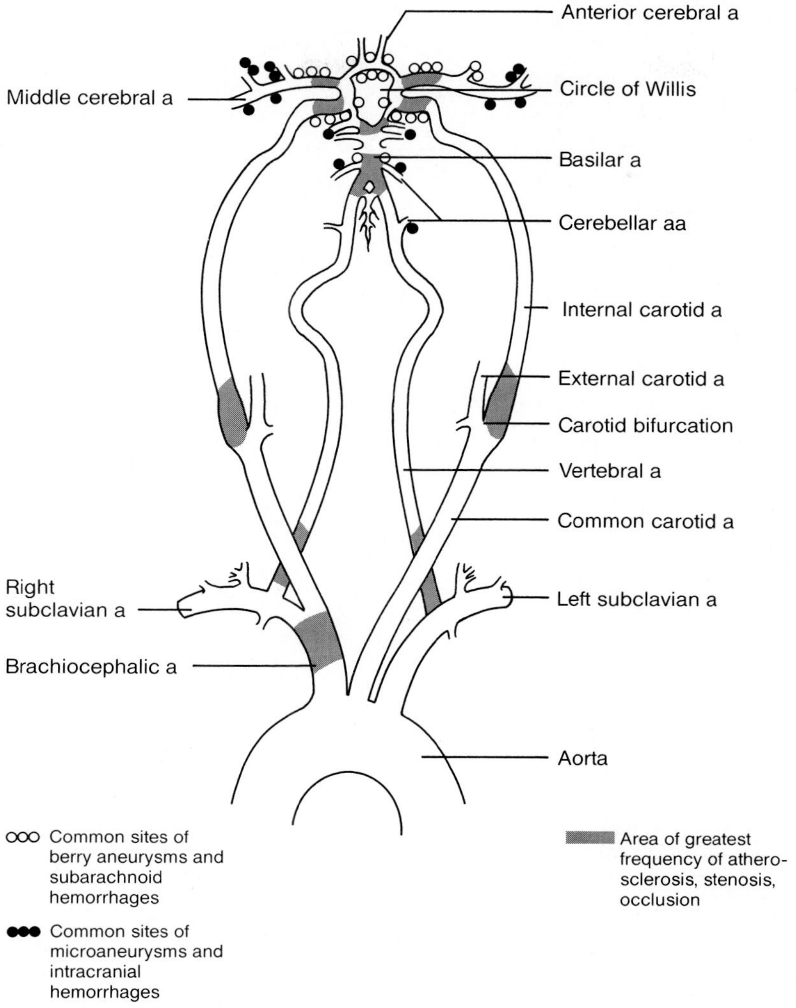

Anterior cerebral a
Middle cerebral a
Circle of Willis
Basilar a
Cerebellar aa
Internal carotid a
External carotid a
Carotid bifurcation
Vertebral a
Common carotid a
Right subclavian a
Left subclavian a
Brachiocephalic a
Aorta

ooo Common sites of berry aneurysms and subarachnoid hemorrhages

●●● Common sites of microaneurysms and intracranial hemorrhages

▬ Area of greatest frequency of atherosclerosis, stenosis, occlusion

Figure 64–4. Distribution of atherosclerosis, berry aneurysms, and microaneurysms in cerebral vessels.

Clinical Features

Cerebral infarction is characterized by a sudden loss of neurologic function corresponding to the area involved (Table 64–2). The onset may be acute but is usually not as explosive as in cerebral hemorrhage. In many cases the neurologic deficit progresses over several hours to days. Infarction secondary to thrombosis has a slower onset than that caused by embolism.

Most patients with infarction also show evidence of raised intracranial pressure due to the presence of edema around the infarct. The edema may cause additional neurologic deficits that are reversible—unlike the deficit produced by the infarct itself.

Treatment & Prognosis

Treatment is supportive. In the acute phase, corticosteroids and diuretics such as furosemide and mannitol are used to decrease cerebral edema and intracranial pressure.

The overall prognosis for recovery of neurologic function after cerebral infarction is reasonably good. Even in patients in whom the initial deficit is severe, considerable improvement may occur, with reversal of cerebral edema and recovery of function by ischemic but not necrotic neurons. Physical therapy is important to strengthen muscles that will then take over the function of paralyzed muscles. (The functions of neurons that have undergone necrosis are permanently lost, as these cells have no regenerative capability.)

TRANSIENT ISCHEMIC ATTACKS

Transient ischemic attacks are caused in many cases by platelet or cholesterol emboli originating

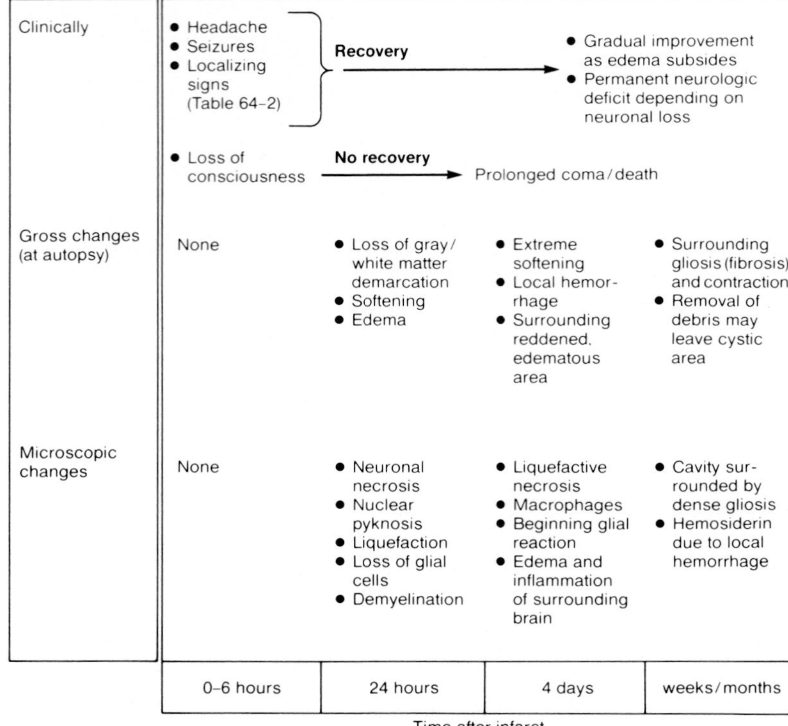

Figure 64–5. Cerebral infarction, showing clinical and pathologic changes observed at different stages.

from ulcerative atherosclerotic plaques in the carotid arteries or even the aorta. The neurologic dysfunction depends on the area of brain affected. Attacks last a few seconds to a few minutes; by definition, recovery (within 24 hours) is the rule. The frequency of attacks varies from several times a day to once in several months. In some patients, the diagnosis may be established by observing the embolic fragments in the vessels of the optic fundus. Cholesterol emboli have a bronze appearance, whereas platelet emboli are white. The brain shows no pathologic changes.

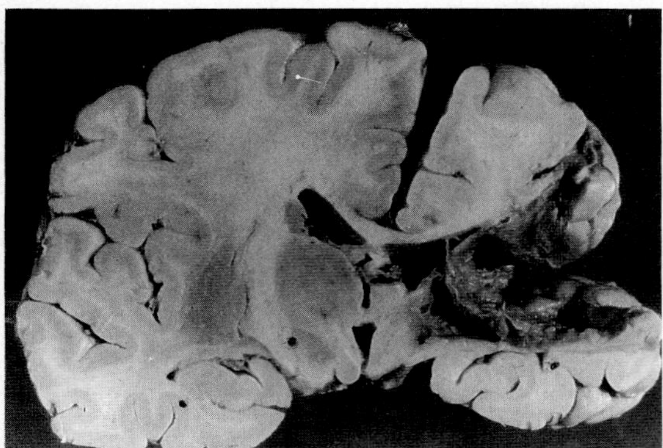

Figure 64–6. Cerebral infarct, showing a cystic space (which collapsed when the brain was cut) associated with loss of cerebral substance in the distribution of the middle cerebral artery. This is the typical appearance of an old infarct.

The occurrence of transient ischemic attacks indicates the presence of severe atherosclerosis in the cerebral arteries. Thirty percent of such patients will suffer cerebral infarction within 5 years; conversely, 30% of patients with cerebral infarction give a history of transient ischemic attacks. Patients with transient ischemic attacks should therefore be evaluated for surgically correctable vascular disease or for anticoagulant therapy. Aspirin has been used with some success in the treatment of transient ischemic attacks.

HYPERTENSIVE ENCEPHALOPATHY

Hypertensive encephalopathy results from cerebral ischemia due to arterial spasm precipitated by extremely high blood pressure. Spasm is temporary and results in cerebral edema, usually without necrosis.

Patients develop acute transient neurologic dysfunction, convulsions, and raised intracranial pressure. The condition requires immediate treatment to reduce blood pressure and decrease cerebral edema; recovery is then the rule.

Table 64–2. Localizing signs associated with occlusion of major cerebral arteries.

Artery Occluded	Area Infarcted	Clinical Effect
Anterior cerebral artery	Frontal lobe	Confusion, disorientation
	Motor and sensory cortex (leg area)	Contralateral weakness maximal in leg; cortical-type sensory loss, maximal in leg
Middle cerebral artery	Lateral surface of hemisphere	Contralateral hemiparesis, face > leg; contralateral cortical-type sensory loss
	Speech area (if dominant hemisphere)	Expressive aphasia
	Optic radiation	Hemianopia
Posterior cerebral artery	Occipital lobe	Cortical-type visual loss
Vertebrobasilar arteries	Cerebellum	Intention tremor, incoordination, hypotonia
	Brain stem	Contralateral hemiparesis and sensory loss; ipsilateral cranial nerve palsies

HEMORRHAGIC STROKES

Several factors may contribute to cerebral hemorrhage (Table 64–1). The site of the bleeding distinguishes intracerebral hemorrhages (small arteries deep in the brain substance, eg, lenticulostriate arteries) from subarachnoid hemorrhage (larger arteries traversing the subarachnoid space). In practice, the bleeding site may not be identifiable in large hemorrhages that involve both subarachnoid space and brain substance, and the distinction is then somewhat arbitrary.

1. SPONTANEOUS INTRACEREBRAL HEMORRHAGE

Cerebral hemorrhage is responsible for about 10% of strokes. Over 80% of intracerebral hemorrhages are secondary to hypertension. Most occur after age 40 years, and the most common site is around the basal ganglia and internal capsule from rupture of the lenticulostriate arteries (Fig 64–4).

Less commonly, intracerebral hemorrhage may result from rupture of arteriovenous malformations, particularly important as a cause in patients under 40 years of age. Bleeding diatheses such as thrombocytopenia and coagulation disorders are rare causes of intracerebral hemorrhage (Table 64–1).

Pathology

The site of rupture is frequently a microaneurysm (Charcot-Bouchard aneurysm) in the lenticulostriate arteries. Multiple microaneurysms occur at this location in a significant number (70%) of hypertensive patients (Fig 64–4). Rupture is commonly precipitated by a sudden increase in blood pressure. The rapidly expanding blood clot dissects and destroys brain tissue and may rupture into the ventricular system or subarachnoid space. Blood in the cerebrospinal fluid causes meningeal irritation.

The expanding hematoma (Fig 64–7) acts like a space-occupying lesion, causing rapid and marked increase in intracranial pressure and displacing the brain. Tentorial herniation is common and may cause death by compressing the brain stem.

Recovery from intracerebral hemorrhage is followed by breakdown of the blood and necrotic brain tissue, leading to an area of gliosis and cystic change that appears brown because of the numerous hemosiderin-laden macrophages.

Clinical Features

Intracerebral hemorrhage results in abrupt onset of headache, dense neurologic deficit, papilledema, and loss of consciousness ("cerebral apoplexy"). Since bleeding is commonly in the region of the basal ganglia, hemiplegia from pyramidal tract involvement in the internal capsule is

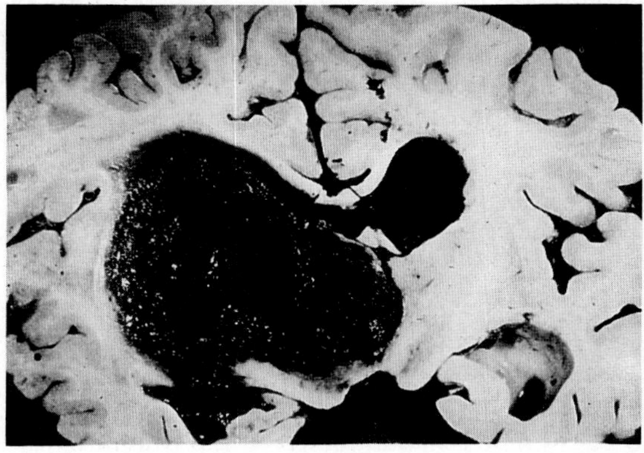

Figure 64–7. Intracerebral hematoma involving the region of the basal ganglia. This is the typical location of a hypertensive intracerebral hemorrhage caused by rupture of microaneurysms involving the lenticulostriate arteries.

the commonest neurologic deficit. Cerebral hemorrhage is associated with a high mortality rate.

2. SPONTANEOUS SUBARACHNOID HEMORRHAGE

Spontaneous subarachnoid hemorrhage is less common than spontaneous intracerebral hemorrhage and usually (95% of cases) results from rupture of a berry aneurysm (saccular aneurysm) of the cerebral arteries.

Berry aneurysms are also called congenital aneurysms, though they are not present at birth. There is, however, a congenital defect of the media of the artery, which becomes the site of the aneurysm in later life. Berry aneurysms are commonly located in the circle of Willis. The common sites are the anterior communicating artery (30%), the junction of the posterior communicating and internal carotid arteries (30%), the middle cerebral artery (10%), and the basilar artery (10%). In 10–20% of cases, multiple berry aneurysms are present (Fig 64–4).

Pathology

Rupture of a berry aneurysm may occur at any time but is rare in childhood. The frequency of rupture increases with age. Hypertension and atherosclerosis result in further weakening of the aneurysm and predispose to rupture. Actual rupture of an aneurysm may be precipitated by exercise (one of the recognized complications of jogging) and sexual intercourse. Many aneurysms never rupture and are found incidentally at autopsy.

When aneurysms rupture, they usually cause rapid bleeding into the subarachnoid space (Fig 64–8). Many aneurysms leak a little blood before they burst, leading to adhesions between the wall of the aneurysm and adjacent structures. If such adhesions tether the aneurysm to the brain surface, final rupture of the aneurysm may occur into the substance of the brain, presenting as an intracerebral hemorrhage rather than a subarachnoid hemorrhage.

Intact berry aneurysms may become large enough to cause focal symptoms, eg, third nerve paralysis due to compression by a large posterior communicating artery aneurysm.

Clinical Features

Subarachnoid hemorrhage presents with sudden onset of severe "bursting" headache associated with vomiting, pain in the neck, and rapid loss of consciousness. Marked neck stiffness is present as a result of the meningeal irritation caused by the blood. Raised intracranial pressure with papilledema is common. Blood courses along the subarachnoid sheath around the optic nerve and may be visible ophthalmoscopically as an area of hemorrhage in the retina below the optic disk.

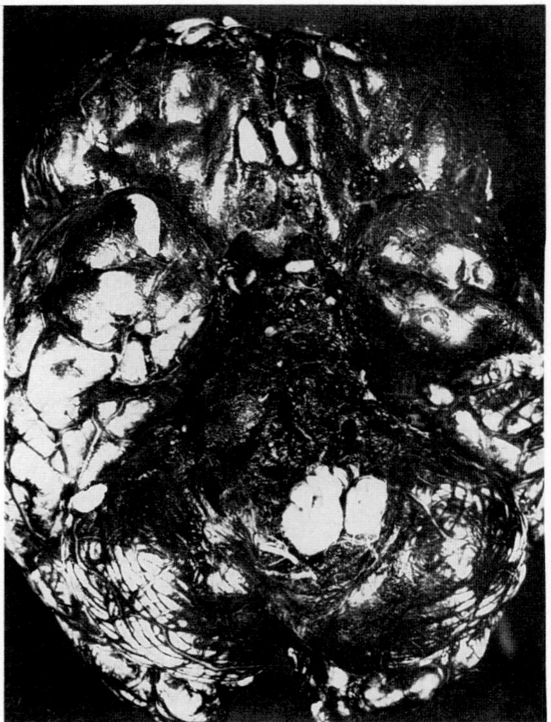

Figure 64–8. Subarachnoid hemorrhage, showing extensive bleeding into the subarachnoid space in a patient with a ruptured berry aneurysm.

The diagnosis is made clinically. Computerized tomography and magnetic resonance imaging are useful in demonstrating the blood as well as the aneurysm in many cases. Lumbar puncture, which may be performed after the presence of a mass lesion in the brain has been excluded, shows the presence of blood in cerebrospinal fluid.

Death may occur rapidly. In patients who recover, there is a high risk of recurrence, and surgical correction is urgent.

3. VENOUS OCCLUSION

Occlusion of cerebral veins and venous sinuses is an uncommon cause of cerebrovascular accident. In general, venous drainage of the brain has many collaterals, and occlusion of a large vein is necessary before clinical effects are produced.

Superior sagittal sinus thrombosis may occur in severely malnourished or chronically sick individuals. It is characterized by edema, hemorrhage, and infarction of both cerebral hemispheres.

Thrombophlebitis of the cortical cerebral veins rarely occurs in women after childbirth or abortion. When extensive, it causes fever, convulsions, and infarction of the cerebral hemisphere.

Thrombosis of the vein of Galen (internal cerebral vein) leads to hemorrhagic infarction of the thalamic region and deep white matter.

Cavernous sinus thrombophlebitis may result from spread of infection from the face and orbit and is associated with high fever, leukocytosis, orbital edema, congestion, and hemorrhage. This disorder presents with marked proptosis with pain and can result in blindness.

Lateral sinus thrombophlebitis may occur as a complication of suppurative otitis media. It is accompanied by severe bacteremia and associated with high fever and pain in the back of the head.

DEMYELINATING DISEASES

Demyelination is a common degenerative change in the nervous system (Table 64–3). It is most often secondary to neuronal or axonal injury, but in the group of diseases known as the demyelinating diseases, demyelination is the primary pathologic process.

MULTIPLE SCLEROSIS

Multiple sclerosis is the most common demyelinating disease. Its incidence varies greatly in different parts of the world, being most common in the Scandinavian countries, with a prevalence of 80:100,000 in Norway. The incidence progressively declines as one moves south (10:100,000 in southern Europe). A similar distribution is seen in the United States, Massachusetts having a higher incidence than Florida. Multiple sclerosis is rare in the tropics (1:100,000) and in Asia, even in the northern latitudes of Japan.

Individuals who migrate in early childhood from a low-risk to a high-risk area have the same risk of developing multiple sclerosis as those in the country they move to. If the same move is made after adolescence, the risk remains low. This suggests that environmental factors operating during childhood are responsible for causing multiple sclerosis; it has been postulated that infection by an as yet unidentified slow virus in childhood may be followed by a 10- to 20-year latent period prior to disease manifestation.

The onset of multiple sclerosis is usually in the years from 20 to 40. Both sexes are affected, and there is no racial predominance within geographic areas, but there is an increased family incidence plus an increased frequency of HLA-A3, -B7, and -DR2.

Etiology

Two closely related paramyxoviruses—measles virus and canine distemper virus—have been implicated in the etiology of multiple sclerosis. Patients suffering from multiple sclerosis have high measles antibody titers in the serum and cerebrospinal fluid. This antibody shows cross-reactivity to distemper virus, which has been linked epidemiologically to an outbreak of multiple sclerosis in the Faroe Islands off northern Scotland. In a few cases, electron microscopy has demonstrated structures resembling virus particles in affected brain; however, virus has not been consistently recovered. The serum, cerebrospinal fluid, and lymphocytes from patients with multiple sclerosis

Table 64–3. Demyelinating diseases.

Disease	Comments
Multiple sclerosis (MS)	Possible viral or immune mediated
Neuromyelitis optica (Devic's disease)	Variant of MS with lesions focused in optic nerves, brain stem, and spinal cord
Experimental allergic encephalomyelitis (EAE)	Demyelination induced in animals by immunization against brain tissue
Acute disseminated encephalomyelitis	Apparent human analogue of EAE; occurs postinfection with or postimmunization for smallpox, rabies, or pertussis
Guillain-Barré syndrome	Resembles EAE but demyelination involves nerve roots and peripheral nerves; typically follows virus infection
Progressive multifocal leukoencephalopathy	Papilloma virus infection (see Chapter 63)
Subacute sclerosing panencephalitis	Delayed injury caused by measles virus (see Chapter 63)
Diffuse sclerosis (Schilder's disease)	Several variants, familial and sporadic; present early in life; may include several different entities
Dysmyelinative disorders	Disorders of myelin metabolism; metachromatic leukodystrophy, lipidoses, phenylketonuria
Demyelination secondary to systemic disease	Anoxia, toxic agents, nutritional disorders (eg, vitamin B_{12} deficiency)

cause demyelination and cytolysis of oligodendrogial cells in tissue culture.

There is also evidence for immunologic hypersensitivity as a cause of multiple sclerosis. The brain lesions contain immunoglobulins, and most patients with multiple sclerosis have elevated levels of immunoglobulin in the cerebrospinal fluid with characteristic oligoclonal bands (Fig 64–9).

Pathology

Multiple sclerosis is characterized by the presence in the white matter of plaques of demyelination. These plaques appear as irregular, well-demarcated, gray or translucent lesions with a diameter varying from 0.1 cm to several centimeters. Multiple plaques, widely disseminated throughout the central nervous system, are common (Fig 64–10).

Any area of the brain can be affected. Sites of predilection are the optic nerves, paraventricular regions, brain stem, cerebellum, spinal cord, and deep cerebral white matter.

Microscopically, the plaques show demyelination (best seen in sections stained for myelin) and tangled masses of preserved axons (best seen in silver stained sections). Lymphocytic infiltration is present in areas of active and recent demyelination. Macrophages are present and contain phagocytosed myelin. There is reactive astrocytic proliferation at the edges of the plaque. Oligodendroglial cells are typically absent in the plaque.

Clinical Features

Multiple sclerosis is a chronic disease with an extremely variable clinical course, characterized by episodic relapses and remissions over several years. A minority of patients have a rapid course to death within months, and some appear to have only one or a few episodes from which they recover and have no further relapses.

The clinical manifestations depend on the area of brain affected and are therefore extremely varied. Common manifestations are abnormalities in vision, cerebellar dysfunction, paresthesias, weakness, and spinal cord dysfunction. The randomly disseminated nature of the lesions gives a characteristic clinical picture when multiple plaques are present.

The cerebrospinal fluid shows a mild increase in the number of lymphocytes, slightly elevated protein, and the presence of oligoclonal immunoglobulin bands on immunoelectrophoresis (Fig 64–9). Oligoclonal bands of IgG are not specific for multiple sclerosis, being seen also in neurosyphilis, subacute sclerosing panencephalitis, and Guillain-Barré syndrome (see below).

Treatment is limited to the management of complications. The course of the disease is not altered by treatment.

DEMYELINATION IN IMMUNOLOGIC INJURIES

1. EXPERIMENTAL ALLERGIC ENCEPHALOMYELITIS

In the experimental setting, acute demyelination of nerve fibers in the central nervous system can be produced in many animals by injection of a brain emulsion in Freund's adjuvant. The active antigen is myelin protein, and the disease is thought to be caused by the action of sensitized T lymphocytes.

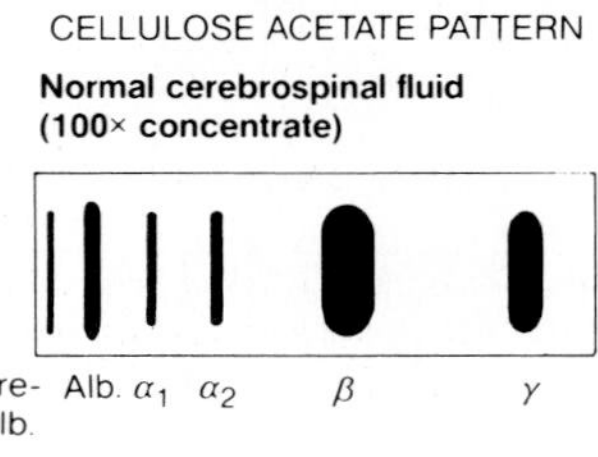

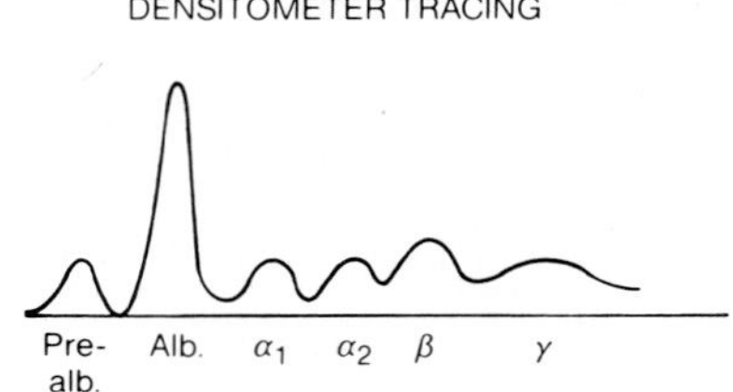

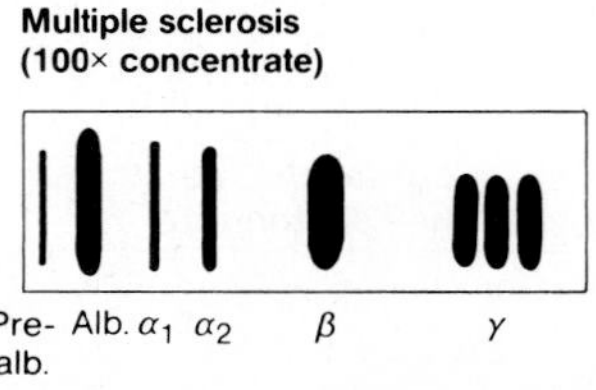

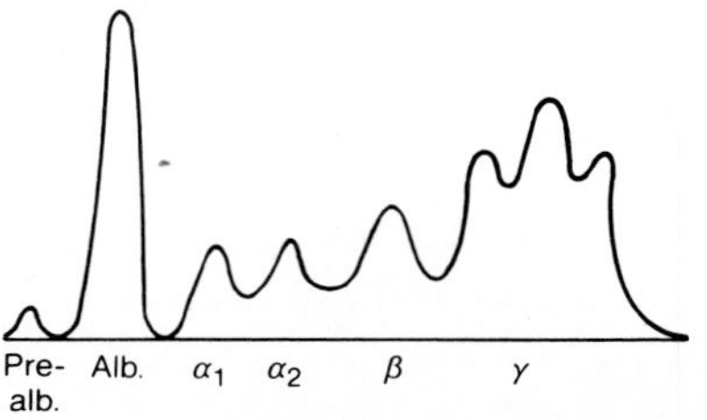

Figure 64–9. Protein electrophoresis of cerebrospinal fluid in normal patient (top) and a patient with multiple sclerosis (bottom), showing the presence of oligoclonal bands in multiple sclerosis. Note that this is not specific for multiple sclerosis and may occur in other diseases such as neurosyphilis.

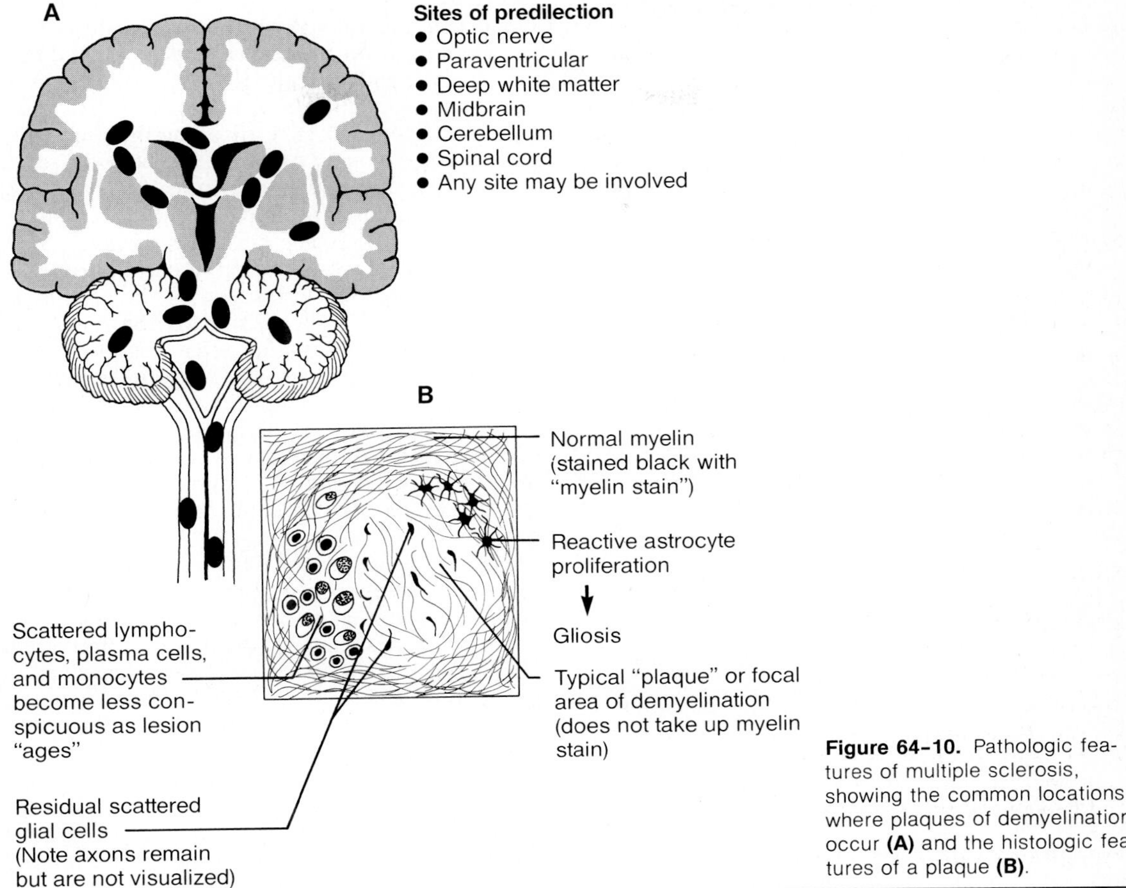

Figure 64–10. Pathologic features of multiple sclerosis, showing the common locations where plaques of demyelination occur **(A)** and the histologic features of a plaque **(B)**.

2. ACUTE DISSEMINATED ENCEPHALOMYELITIS

Acute disseminated encephalomyelitis is a group of diseases believed to have a pathogenesis similar to that of experimental allergic encephalomyelitis. Acute disseminated encephalomyelitis occurs after viral infections (postinfectious) and after immunization against smallpox, rabies, or pertussis (postvaccination). Lymphocytes from these patients exhibit cell-mediated immunologic reactivity against myelin protein in vitro.

Pathologically, there is extensive acute demyelination of the white matter of the brain and spinal cord. The manifestations and severity depend on the areas involved and the degree of involvement, but typically the mortality rate is high. Patients who survive improve slowly over several months, though many are left with neurologic deficits.

3. GUILLAIN-BARRÉ SYNDROME (Acute Idiopathic Polyneuritis)

Guillain-Barré syndrome is an uncommon disease believed to be the peripheral nervous system equivalent of experimental allergic encephalomyelitis. It follows viral infection in a majority of cases; less frequently, it is precipitated by injection of foreign proteins, immunization, or trauma. Well-documented cases were reported following the swine flu vaccination program of the 1970s. Experimentally, a similar disease—experimental allergic neuritis—can be induced in animals by injection of peripheral myelin protein P_2 with Freund's adjuvant; cytotoxic T lymphocytes develop that have the ability to produce demyelination in tissue culture.

Pathologically, Guillain-Barré syndrome is characterized by acute demyelination of multiple cranial and spinal nerve roots (polyradiculopathy), associated with lymphocytic infiltration of the involved nerves. The cerebrospinal fluid shows a typical change called cell-protein dissociation; the cell count is normal ($< 5/\mu L$), but the protein is markedly elevated.

Clinically, Guillain-Barré syndrome has a subacute onset with lower motor neuron type weakness, mainly in the lower extremities (flaccid paraparesis with urinary incontinence). Involvement of the upper extremities and respiratory muscles occurs in severe cases. Sensory impairment is much less than motor impairment, and many patients have no sensory loss. The paralysis progresses for 1–4 weeks and then slowly improves over several months because of the very slow rate of regeneration of axons within the restored myelin sheaths. Ninety percent of patients recover completely.

Treatment is supportive. There is evidence that plasma exchange (plasmapheresis) produces a beneficial effect, presumably by removing immunologically active elements from the patient's plasma. Plasmapheresis should be undertaken in severe cases or in the presence of respiratory compromise.

DEGENERATIVE DISEASES

CEREBROCORTICAL DEGENERATIONS

1. ALZHEIMER'S DISEASE

Alzheimer's disease is extremely common—responsible for more than 50% of all cases of dementia (Table 64–4). It is characterized by progressive loss of neurons in the entire cerebral cortex. The frontal lobe is involved preferentially. Neuronal loss leads to dementia, which is the characteristic clinical presentation.

The term Alzheimer's disease was initially applied to patients who developed dementia under 65 years of age (presenile dementia), and dementia occurring after age 65 was called senile dementia. It has now become clear that the changes seen in most patients with senile dementia are similar if not identical to those of Alzheimer's disease.

Table 64-4. Principal causes of dementia.

Alzheimer's disease: over 50% of cases
Chronic alcoholism
Tertiary syphilis (now rare)
Multiple cerebral infarcts
Creutzfeldt-Jakob disease
Huntington's chorea
Pick's disease
Chronic subdural hematoma
Aluminum toxicity, in chronic renal failure
Drugs
Deficiency of vitamins B_{12}, B_6, B_1
Hypothyroidism ("myxedema madness")
Chronic meningitis
Hydrocephalus, low pressure

Etiology

The cause is unknown. In some families, there is evidence of transmission as an autosomal dominant age-dependent trait. Recent cloning and sequencing of the complementary cDNA probe for the chromosome 21 gene encoding the β-amyloid protein of Alzheimer's disease (see below) has led to the claim that this gene is either defective or is duplicated in patients with Alzheimer's disease—ie, 3 copies of the gene are present instead of 2, owing to partial reduplication of chromosome 21. In such individuals, expression of the gene is increased, leading to deposition of the β-amyloid protein. The observation that patients with Down's syndrome (trisomy 21) who survive to adulthood also show an Alzheimerlike disease accords with the above observation, and the presence of a distinctive stable defect or microduplication of chromosome 21 could be invoked to explain the hereditary pattern displayed by some patients.

Many patients have deficiencies of the enzymes required to synthesize acetylcholine, and the levels of this neurotransmitter in the brains of many patients with Alzheimer's disease are decreased. High levels of aluminum have been described in the lesions, and some patients with Alzheimer's disease have increased serum aluminum levels. Furthermore, aluminum toxicity in chronic renal failure causes dementia. Despite this evidence, aluminum is not considered a likely etiologic agent in Alzheimer's disease. Finally, a viral origin has been proposed based on the occurrence of Alzheimer's disease and Creutzfeldt-Jakob disease (see Chapter 63) in the same families.

Pathology

Grossly, there is atrophy of the cerebral cortex with thinning of the gyri and widening of the sulci. The cortical gray matter is greatly thinned and poorly demarcated. The lateral ventricles show compensatory dilatation.

Microscopically, there is neuronal loss and disorganization of the cerebrocortical layers. Alzheimer's disease is characterized by the presence of **neurofibrillary tangles** in the cytoplasm of affected neurons (best seen in silver stains). These are complexly interwoven masses of paired helical filaments 10 nm in diameter consisting of various proteins. Also characteristic of Alzheimer's disease—and best seen on silver stains—are **argyrophilic plaques,** which are large (150 μm) extracellular collections of degenerated cellular processes disposed around a central mass of amyloid material (Fig 64–11). This β-amyloid protein appears identical to that present in Down's syndrome and in the elderly as senile amyloid.

Clinical Features

Alzheimer's disease usually occurs in patients over 50 years of age. The clinical symptoms are

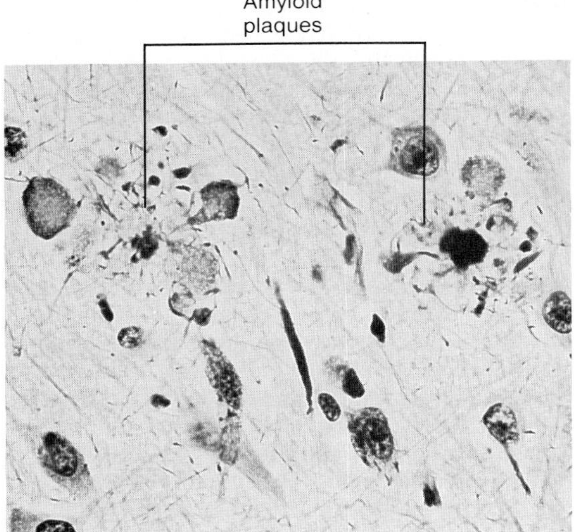

Figure 64–11. Amyloid plaques in cerebral cortex in Alzheimer's disease.

subtle at first, manifested as a loss of higher cortical functions. The loss of ability to solve problems, decreased agility of thought processes, and mild emotional lability are common early features. The dementia progresses inexorably over the next 5–10 years to an extent that the patient becomes unable to carry out daily activities. There is no effective treatment.

2. PICK'S DISEASE

Pick's disease is an extremely uncommon cause of presenile dementia, occurring in the age group from 40 to 65 years. The cause is unknown. The clinical course is indistinguishable from that of Alzheimer's disease. However, neurofibrillary tangles and argyrophilic plaques are not present; instead, affected neurons contain Pick bodies—round, lightly eosinophilic cytoplasmic inclusions that stain strongly positive with silver stains.

BASAL GANGLIA DEGENERATIONS

1. IDIOPATHIC PARKINSON'S DISEASE (Paralysis Agitans)

Idiopathic Parkinson's disease is a common disease, affecting 5% of persons over 70 years of age). The exact cause is unknown. There is degeneration of the pigmented nuclei of the brain stem, particularly the substantia nigra, producing dysfunction of the extrapyramidal system. Patients with Parkinson's disease have depletion of dopamine in the affected areas. Since dopamine is an important neurotransmitter in the extrapyramidal system, it has been postulated that failure of normal dopamine synthesis is responsible for the disease.

Pathology

Grossly, patients with Parkinson's disease have depigmentation of the substantia nigra. Microscopically, loss of pigmented neurons is accompanied by gliosis in the substantia nigra and other basal ganglia. Lewy bodies—rounded eosinophilic cytoplasmic inclusions—may be present in the remaining neurons; they are characteristic of Parkinson's disease.

Clinical Features

Onset is usually after the age of 50 years, and the disease is slowly progressive. It is characterized by extrapyramidal dysfunction, which causes increased rigidity of muscles, resting tremors, and slowness of movements (bradykinesia). Patients have a typical gait, walking stooped forward with short, quick shuffling steps (festinating gait). Up to 20% of patients with parkinsonism develop dementia. Slow, difficult speech is due to motor retardation.

Treatment with levodopa produces a good clinical response in most cases. However, the disease is progressive, and with time control becomes difficult. Transplantation of autologous adrenal medulla into the region of the basal ganglia has recently produced marked clinical improvement. Presumably, the implanted adrenal medulla serves as a source of dopamine. The overall prognosis is poor.

2. OTHER CAUSES OF PARKINSON'S DISEASE

Identical clinical features may be caused by several diseases that affect the extrapyramidal system.

(1) Postencephalitic parkinsonism, which occurred in association with the influenza epidemic of 1914–1918, tended to occur in younger individuals and is uncommon today.

(2) Ischemic damage to the basal ganglia is associated with atherosclerosis.

(3) Wilson's disease is due to deposition of copper in the basal ganglia (see Chapter 43).

(4) Damage to the basal ganglia may result from exposure to toxic agents such as carbon monoxide and manganese.

(5) Several drugs in therapeutic doses, notably the phenothiazines and reserpine, produce reversible Parkinson's syndrome.

(6) Shy-Drager syndrome is intractable hypotension with various autonomic defects and Parkinson's syndrome.

3. HUNTINGTON'S CHOREA

Huntington's chorea is a rare disease that is inherited as an autosomal dominant trait with complete penetrance but delayed appearance. Recently, DNA probes have become available for detection of the abnormal gene in childhood many years prior to the appearance of symptoms; since the disease is usually not manifested until after procreation, this test may be of value in assessing whether or not a member of an involved family should have children.

Huntington's chorea is characterized by atrophy and loss of neurons of the caudate nucleus and putamen, associated with variable cerebrocortical atrophy, particularly in the frontal lobe. Though inherited, the disease has its onset in adult life, usually between 20 and 50 years of age. It is characterized by depression and dementia, due to cerebral involvement, and choreiform involuntary movements, due to involvement of the basal ganglia. The disease is slowly but inexorably progressive, leading to death in 10–20 years.

SPINOCEREBELLAR DEGENERATIONS

These rare diseases are usually inherited as autosomal recessive traits. The most common is **Friedreich's ataxia,** in which there is degeneration of spinocerebellar tracts, posterior columns, the pyramidal tract, and the peripheral nerves (Fig 64–12). Clinical presentation is in late childhood, with incoordination and muscle weakness.

Olivopontocerebellar degeneration is another type of disease in which there is degeneration of

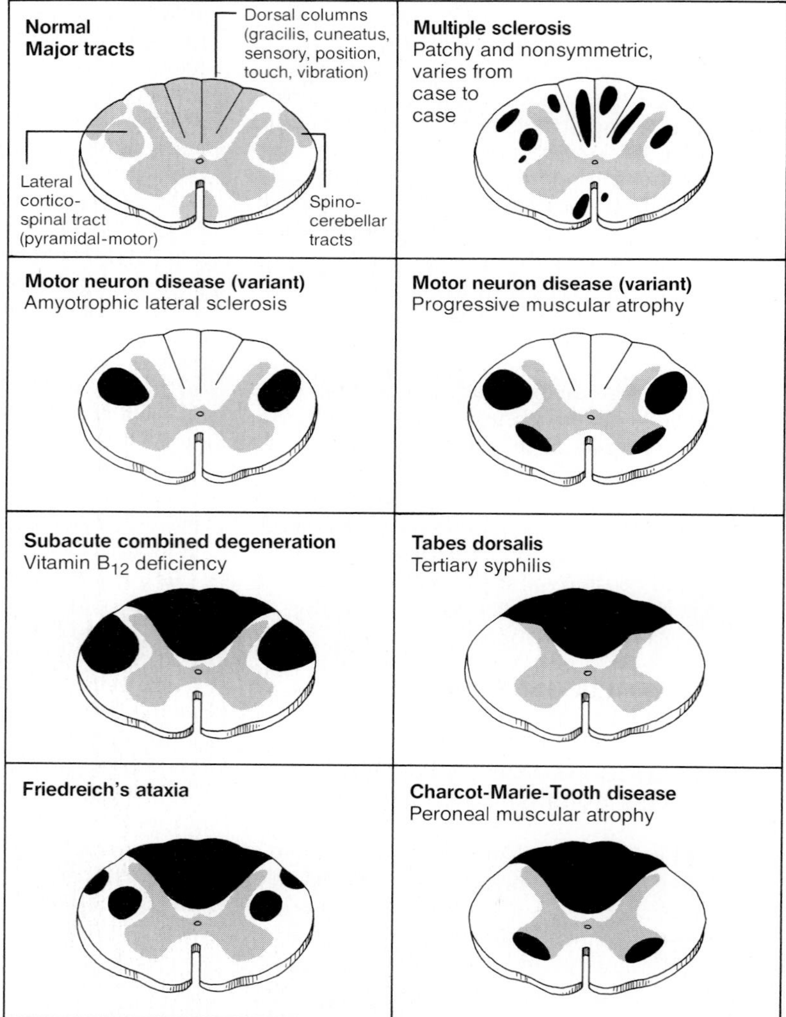

Figure 64–12. Sections of spinal cord, showing typical distribution of lesions in multiple sclerosis, motor neuron disease, Friedreich's ataxia, subacute combined degeneration, tabes dorsalis, and peroneal muscular atrophy.

neurons in the cerebellar cortex, cerebellar nuclei, olivary nuclei, and pons.

MOTOR NEURON DISEASE

Motor neuron disease is characterized by degeneration of both upper and lower motor neurons. The cause is unknown. Most cases occur in a sporadic manner. A high incidence of familial occurrence has been reported in Guam, the Marianas, and the Caroline Islands.

Typically, motor neuron disease affects individuals over the age of 50 years. The neurologic deficit is purely motor (Fig 64–12). Depending on the distribution of lesions, 4 clinical variants of the disease have been recognized.

(1) Amyotrophic lateral sclerosis is the commonest disease in this group. It is characterized by degeneration of the corticospinal tracts (lateral sclerosis) in the spinal cord, resulting in upper motor neuron paralysis in the extremities. The muscular paralysis is associated with absence of atrophy (amyotrophic), hypertonia, and exaggerated deep tendon reflexes.

(2) Progressive muscular atrophy shows preferential degeneration of anterior horn motor nuclei, causing lower motor neuron paralysis in the extremities. Neuronal degeneration is associated with irregular neuronal discharge, leading to muscle fasciculations, which is a feature of the disease. Fasciculation is followed by muscle atrophy. A similar disorder in infants is termed Werdnig-Hoffmann disease.

(3) Progressive bulbar palsy affects medullary motor nuclei, causing lower motor paralysis of the jaw, tongue, and pharyngeal muscles.

(4) Pseudobulbar palsy is a disorder in which bilateral upper motor neuron paralysis of the jaw, tongue, and pharyngeal muscles occurs.

Note that overlapping clinical features appear as the disease progresses toward the end stage, with severe deficits of both upper and lower motor neurons. Death usually occurs in 1–6 years from bronchopneumonia associated with respiratory muscle paralysis. The rate of progression is variable, and there is no specific treatment.

NUTRITIONAL DISEASES

SUBACUTE COMBINED DEGENERATION OF THE CORD

Deficiency of vitamin B_{12} (see Chapter 24) results in degeneration of several components of the nervous system. The commonest lesion is subacute combined degeneration of the cord (Figs 64–12 and 64–13), in which there is demyelination of (1) the posterior columns, leading to loss of position and vibration sense and interference with the reflex arc for the deep tendon reflexes; (2) the lateral columns, resulting in upper motor neuron paralysis; and (3) the peripheral nerves. Peripheral neuropathy or optic neuropathy may also occur as isolated lesions in patients with vitamin B_{12} deficiency. The diagnosis is important, since vitamin B_{12} therapy will prevent progression—though it does not repair the demyelinated fibers.

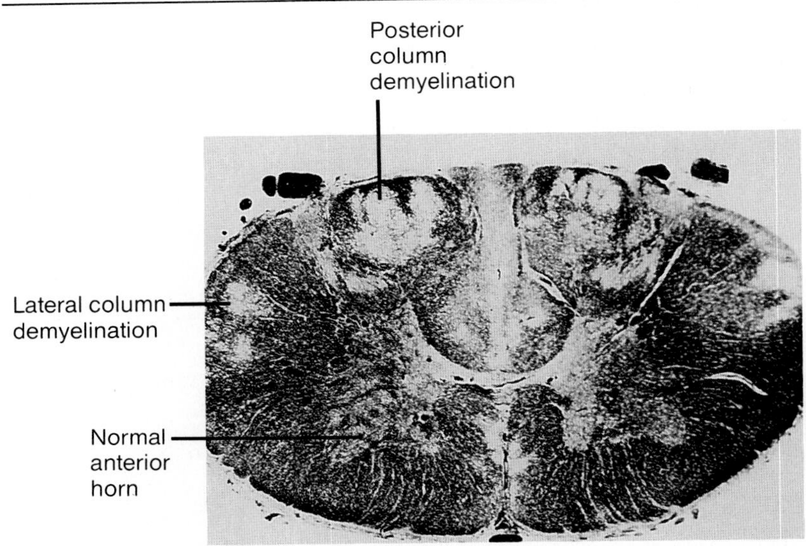

Figure 64–13. Subacute combined degeneration of the cord. Myelin-stained transverse section of the spinal cord, showing areas of demyelination involving the posterior and lateral columns.

WERNICKE'S ENCEPHALOPATHY

Thiamine deficiency (see Chapter 10) is commonly seen in malnourished individuals and chronic alcoholics. It causes involvement of the floor of the third ventricle and the periaqueductal region of the midbrain. The mammillary bodies are maximally involved.

The early lesion is characterized by petechial hemorrhages and capillary proliferation. This is followed by atrophy and degeneration of neurons. The atrophic areas in Wernicke's encephalopathy typically show a brownish discoloration because of hemosiderin pigment deposition.

Clinically, Wernicke's encephalopathy is manifested by confusion, ocular muscle paralysis, and nystagmus—an abnormal involuntary motion of the eyes. Wernicke's encephalopathy is frequently associated with a psychotic state (Korsakoff's psychosis), which is also related to thiamine deficiency.

PELLAGRA ENCEPHALOPATHY

Nicotinamide deficiency causes neuronal degeneration, affecting the cerebral cortex, pontine nuclei, cranial nerve nuclei, and anterior horn cells in the spinal cord. Dementia is the most common clinical manifestation.

METABOLIC DISEASES

KERNICTERUS

Kernicterus (see Chapter 1) is a rare disease of neonates resulting from deposition of bilirubin in the brain, particularly in the basal ganglia. The disease occurs in premature infants who develop unconjugated hyperbilirubinemia due to hemolysis of red cells. Rh incompatibility (hemolytic disease of the newborn) is the commonest cause. Bilirubin is toxic to neurons and causes cell death. Severe kernicterus has a high mortality rate. Patients who survive show evidence of basal ganglia damage characterized by extrapyramidal dysfunction. Bilirubin does not cross the blood-brain barrier after the neonatal period.

Table 64-5. Congenital metabolic diseases (inborn errors of metabolism) associated with mental retardation.

Defects of amino acid metabolism
Phenylketonuria (phenylalanine)
Maple syrup urine disease (valine, leucine, isoleucine)
Others (very rare)
Lipid storage diseases
Tay-Sachs disease
Mucopolysaccharidoses
Hunter-Hurler syndrome
Morquio's syndrome
Disorders of carbohydrate metabolism
Galactosemia
Glycogen storage diseases

WILSON'S DISEASE

Wilson's disease (see Chapter 43) is an inherited disorder characterized by deposition of copper in the liver (causing chronic liver disease) and the basal ganglia, especially the lenticular nuclei. Extrapyramidal symptoms due to lenticular neuronal degeneration occur in early life—commonly in the second decade—and include rigidity, involuntary movements, and slowing of movements (bradykinesia).

INBORN ERRORS OF METABOLISM (Table 64-5)

Numerous inherited enzyme deficiencies are associated with diffuse cortical neuronal loss and mental retardation (see also Chapter 15). They are rare.

The Central Nervous System: IV. Neoplasms

65

- Astrocytomas
  - Cerebral Hemisphere Astrocytoma
  - Juvenile Pilocytic Astrocytoma
  - Brain Stem and Spinal Cord Astrocytoma
- Oligodendroglioma
- Ependymal Neoplasms
  - Ependymoma
  - Choroid Plexus Papilloma
  - Colloid Cyst of the Third Ventricle
- Medulloblastoma
- Pineal Neoplasms
  - Pinealocyte Neoplasms
  - Germ Cell Neoplasms
- Meningioma
- Nerve Sheath Neoplasms
- Cerebellar Hemangioblastoma
- Malignant Lymphoma of the Brain
- Neoplasms Derived From Embryonal Remnants
  - Craniopharyngioma
  - Epidermoid Cyst
  - Chordoma
- Metastatic Neoplasms

Intracranial and spinal neoplasms may be primary or metastatic; in most autopsy series, metastatic tumors are more common. Primary intracranial neoplasms number about 13,000 new cases a year in the USA and represent about 2% of deaths from malignant neoplasms. They are the second most common group of neoplasms in children, after leukemia and lymphoma considered as one group. Taken overall, 65% of primary intracranial neoplasms are of glial origin (gliomas), 10% meningiomas, 10% acoustic schwannomas, 5% medulloblastomas, and 10% others. Primary malignant lymphomas of the central nervous system have recently increased in frequency because they are common in patients with AIDS. Tumors of neurons per se are extremely uncommon except in childhood (eg, medulloblastoma).

Classification

A. Histogenetic Classification: Classification on a histogenetic basis has great theoretic value and provides a means of logically remembering all the different kinds of intracranial neoplasms (Table 65–1).

B. Topographic Classification: When a patient presents with an intracranial neoplasm, its location can usually be ascertained by clinical examination and radiologic studies. According to their location, intracranial neoplasms may be classified as supratentorial or infratentorial. Further subdivisions in these main compartments are recognized (Table 65–2), leading to a topographic classification. When the location of the neoplasm is combined with the patient's age, a clinically useful differential diagnosis of the histologic type of the neoplasm can be arrived at. For example, if a child presents with a neoplasm in a cerebellar hemisphere, it is most likely a juvenile astrocytoma (Table 65–2).

C. Classification According to Biologic Potential: The criteria used to determine malignancy in neoplasms are somewhat different from those used elsewhere in the body:

1. Even highly malignant intracranial neoplasms generally do not metastasize outside the craniospinal axis (Fig 65–1). Metastasis within the craniospinal axis via the cerebrospinal fluid does occur, most commonly with medulloblastoma, pineoblastoma, malignant ependymoma, and glioblastoma multiforme.

2. Destructive infiltration of the brain is the major criterion of malignancy for intracranial neoplasms, and infiltration of brain substance usually prevents complete removal at surgery. All glial neoplasms invade brain, and all must be considered malignant. Neurologic deficits resulting from destructive invasion by malignant neoplasms are irreversible. Benign neoplasms, on the other hand, cause neurologic deficits due to compression; these often reverse when the neoplasm is removed.

3. The rate of growth of neoplasms also correlates well with malignant behavior. Rapidly growing neoplasms such as glioblastoma multiforme and medulloblastoma are highly malignant. Low-grade malignant neoplasms such as well-differentiated astrocytoma and oligodendroglioma grow slowly. Benign neoplasms usually grow very slowly, enlarging over several years.

4. Recurrence after treatment is almost invariable with malignant intracranial neoplasms. Recurrence also occurs with many benign neoplasms

Table 65-1. Classification of neoplasms of the nervous system on the basis of histogenesis.

Cell Type	Neoplasm
Cellular derivatives of the neural tube	
Glial cells	Glioma[1]
Astrocytes	Astrocytoma Glioblastoma multiforme
Oligodendroglia	Oligodendroglioma
Ependymal cells	Ependymoma Subependymoma Choroid plexus papilloma
Neurons	Medulloblastoma
Mixed glial and neuronal	Ganglioglioma
Pinealocyte	Pineocytoma Pineoblastoma
Cells derived from the neural crest	
Schwann cell	Schwannoma Neurofibroma
Arachnoid cell	Meningioma
Other cells	
Connective tissue cells	Sarcomas
Lymphoid cells	Malignant lymphoma
Vascular cells	Hemangioblastoma
Pituicytes	Pituitary adenoma
Embryonic remnants	
Ectodermal derivatives	Craniopharyngioma Epidermoid cysts Dermoid cysts
Notochordal remnants	Chordoma
Germ cells	Teratoma Germinoma
Melanocytes	Melanoma
Adipocytes	Lipoma
Metastatic neoplasms	
Tumors of bone (skull and vertebrae)	

[1]The term glioma has different applications. In its narrowest usage it is synonymous with astrocytomas; in its broadest usage it includes oligodendroglioma and ependymal neoplasms.

such as meningioma and craniopharyngioma, and recurrence of itself is not a criterion of malignancy.

5. The term "benign" for any intracranial neoplasm is probably inappropriate. Benign intracranial neoplasms frequently produce extremely serious clinical disease and may cause severe neurologic deficits and death unless treated. In fact, before craniotomy became a safe surgical procedure, almost all patients with "benign" intracranial neoplasms of any considerable size died from these tumors. The term benign is therefore used not in the sense that these neoplasms are harmless but rather to indicate that they are slow-growing and do not infiltrate the brain substance.

Pathology & Clinical Features (Fig 65-1)

The specific clinicopathologic features of intracranial neoplasms will be considered with the individual neoplasms. In general, intracranial neoplasms cause the following clinical and pathologic changes:

A. Compression: Compression of adjacent neural tissues occurs with all expanding neoplasms. When the rate of growth is slow, compression leads to atrophy, which may cause symptoms of dysfunction—eg, atrophy of the motor cortex adjacent to a meningioma causes upper motor neuron paralysis; compression of a cranial nerve may cause cranial nerve palsy. In general, relief of compression is followed by significant recovery of function. With long-standing compression, there may be a permanent deficit.

B. Destruction: Destruction of neural tissues by direct infiltration with a malignant neoplasm produces an irreversible deficit.

C. Cerebral Edema: Cerebral edema is commonly present around infiltrative neoplasms and may be severe. It is believed to result from neovascularization that accompanies malignant neoplasms. The new vessels have a poorly developed blood-brain barrier that permits exit of proteins and fluids more easily than normal vessels. Cerebral edema tends to be most marked in highly malignant neoplasms. Cerebral edema causes elevation of intracranial pressure that is additive to the mass effect of the tumor.

D. Irritative Effects: Irritation of neural tissues may occur with both compressing and infiltrating neoplasms. Abnormal stimulation is usually manifested as focal epilepsy. A neoplasm near the motor cortex may generate an abnormal electrical potential that causes motor stimulation of the entire contralateral half of the body (jacksonian epilepsy); activity may then spread to the brain stem reticular formation and cause loss of consciousness. Up to 5% of individuals with intracranial neoplasms experience one or more seizures. Note that although only a minority of cases of epilepsy are due to tumors, seizures should be fully investigated for tumor or other treatable disease, particularly when the onset is in adult life or when the seizure is focal rather than generalized (see Chapter 62).

E. Hydrocephalus: Neoplasms in the region of the third ventricle or in the posterior fossa may cause obstructive hydrocephalus. This causes marked elevation of intracranial pressure.

F. Raised Intracranial Pressure: Intracranial neoplasms cause increased intracranial pressure due to (1) the mass effect of the neoplasm itself, (2) cerebral edema, or (3) hydrocephalus. Many patients with intracranial neoplasms present with the effects of raised intracranial pressure—headache, vomiting, papilledema, and "false localizing signs" due to displacement of

Table 65-2. Common intracranial neoplasms classified according to location and age.

Location	Children	Adults
Supratentorial	**30%**[1]	**70%**[1]
Cerebral hemisphere	Rare	Glial neoplasms Meningiomas Metastases
Suprasellar	Craniopharyngioma Juvenile astrocytoma	Pituitary adenoma Craniopharyngioma Glial neoplasms
Pineal	Pineoblastoma Germ cell tumor (teratoma)	Pineocytoma Germ cell tumor (germinoma)
Infratentorial (posterior fossa)	**70%**[1]	**30%**[1]
Midline	Medulloblastoma Ependymoma	Brain stem glioma
Cerebellar hemisphere	Juvenile astrocytoma	Metastases Hemangioblastoma
Cerebellopontine angle	Epidermoid cyst	Schwannoma (acoustic neuroma) Meningioma
Spinal cord	**Rare**	**Common**
Epidural	Bone tumors	Metastases Bone tumors
Intradural but extramedullary	Rare	Neurofibroma Schwannoma Meningioma
Intramedullary	Ependymoma	Ependymoma Astrocytoma

[1]Percentages refer to frequency of intracranial neoplasms within each category; ie, in children, 70% of neoplasms are infratentorial and 30% are supratentorial, while in adults 70% of neoplasms are supratentorial and 30% are infratentorial.

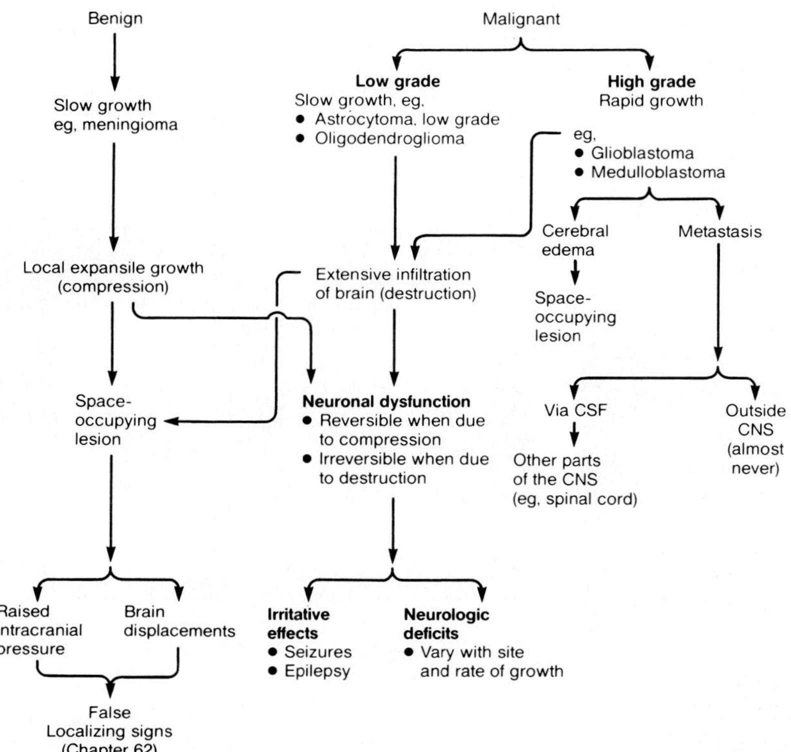

Figure 65-1. Clinical effects related to the biologic behavior of intracranial neoplasm.

stretching of cranial nerves (eg, sixth nerve palsy). Shift of structures can often be detected radiographically and provides a clue to the site of intracranial neoplasms.

ASTROCYTOMAS

CEREBRAL HEMISPHERE ASTROCYTOMA

Astrocytoma in the cerebral hemisphere is the commonest primary neoplasm of the brain and occurs chiefly in adults (Table 65–2). Astrocytomas originate from cerebral white matter astrocytes.

Well-Differentiated (Grade I) Astrocytomas

Well-differentiated (grade I) astrocytomas are infiltrative, slowly growing neoplasms that form firm, white ill-defined masses (Fig 65–2). Microscopically, they show slightly increased cellularity and astrocytes with cytologic features that deviate very slightly from normal. Neurofibrillary processes are present and, often, abundant (fibrillary astrocytoma). Well-differentiated astrocytomas, although low-grade malignant neoplasms, are practically impossible to excise surgically because of irregular extension beyond the apparent margin. They respond temporarily to radiation therapy and progress slowly to cause death after 5–10 years.

Anaplastic (Grade II & Grade III) Astrocytomas

Anaplastic astrocytoma is a more rapidly growing neoplasm that forms a white infiltrative mass in the cerebral hemisphere. Microscopically, it is composed of astrocytes that show greater cellularity, more pleomorphism, neovascularization with proliferation of endothelial cells, and an increased mitotic rate. They cause death after 1–5 years.

Glioblastoma Multiforme (Grade IV Astrocytoma)

Glioblastoma multiforme is the most common type of astrocytoma. It is also one of the most malignant and rapidly growing neoplasms of the brain. Grossly, glioblastomas appear as large infiltrative masses that typically extend across the midline as the so-called "butterfly" tumor. The cut surface commonly shows hemorrhage and necrosis (Fig 65–3). Microscopically, they are composed of highly pleomorphic astrocytic cells with frequent mitotic figures. Necrosis is an important indicator of aggressive behavior (Fig 65–4). Prominent neovascularization is common. Glioblastoma multiforme is highly malignant, with a median survival of 1 year after diagnosis.

JUVENILE PILOCYTIC ASTROCYTOMA

Juvenile pilocytic astrocytoma is a neoplasm of children and adolescents found most commonly in the cerebellar hemispheres. It accounts for 25% of intracranial neoplasms in children under age 10 years. Grossly, it is well circumscribed and often cystic. Microscopically, it shows slight hypercellularity and is composed of cytologically uniform fibrillary astrocytes. Microcystic change and the presence of enlarged astrocytic fibers (Rosenthal fibers) are characteristic features.

Juvenile cerebellar pilocytic astrocytoma is a very slowly growing tumor that is extremely well circumscribed. It is almost benign in its biologic

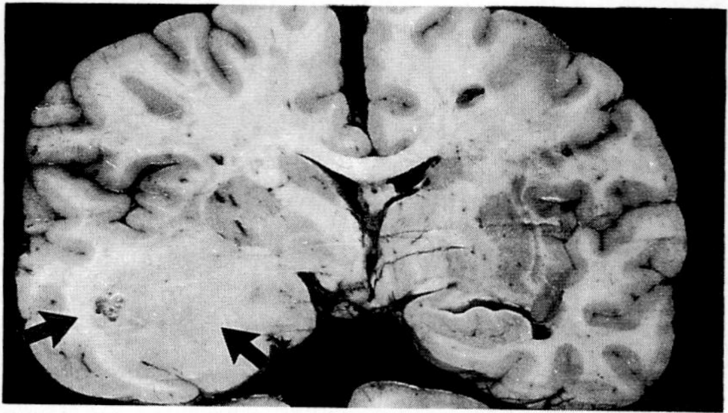

Figure 65–2. Well-differentiated (low-grade) astrocytoma of the left temporal lobe (arrow), characterized by poorly circumscribed homogeneous expansion of the white matter that has obliterated normal markings.

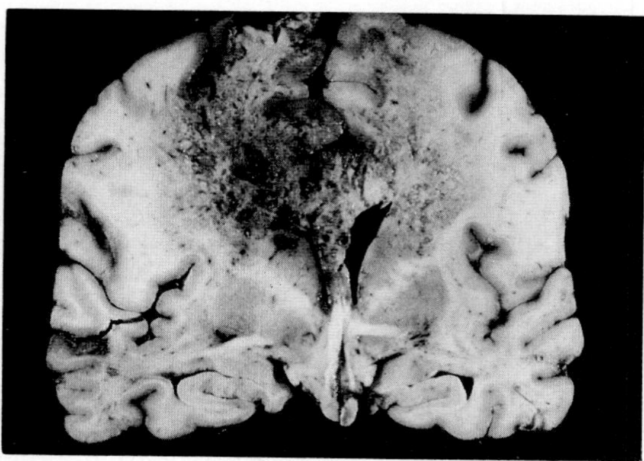

Figure 65–3. Glioblastoma multiforme of deep cerebral white matter, showing an extensively destructive and infiltrative mass extending across the midline to involve both hemispheres ("butterfly lesion"). Necrosis was present on microscopic examination.

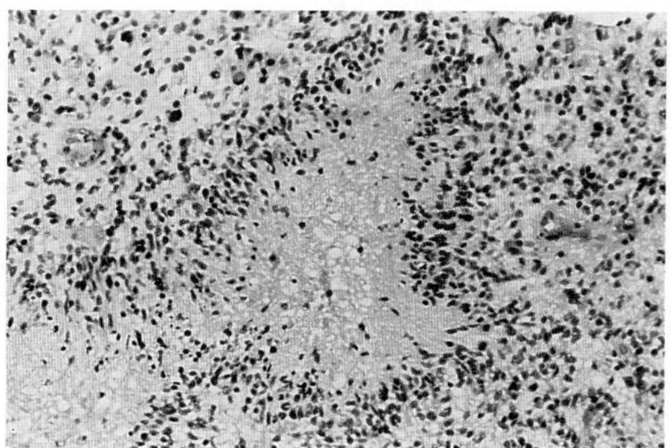

Figure 65-4. Glioblastoma multiforme, showing areas of necrosis surrounded by palisading neoplastic astrocytes.

behavior. Surgical removal results in permanent cure in most cases.

Juvenile pilocytic astrocytoma may also occur in the region of the hypothalamus. Though slowly growing and circumscribed, it is rarely possible to completely remove a hypothalamic pilocytic astrocytoma, and it frequently causes death.

BRAIN STEM & SPINAL CORD ASTROCYTOMA

Astrocytomas also occur in the brain stem and spinal cord and are analagous to the different types occurring in the cerebral hemispheres.

OLIGODENDROGLIOMA

Oligodendroglioma occurs in the cerebral hemisphere in adults 30–50 years of age. It is uncommon in pure form but more often is part of a mixed glial neoplasm with astrocytic and oligodenial components.

Grossly, oligodendrogliomas are well-circumscribed solid neoplasms. Seventy-five percent of oligodendrogliomas have speckled calcification that is visible on x-ray. Microscopically, the neoplasm is composed of numerous small uniform oligodendroglial cells. Mitotic activity is scarce.

Clinically, oligodendroglioma is a slowly growing neoplasm. The prognosis after surgical removal is good, though recurrence is common.

EPENDYMAL NEOPLASMS

EPENDYMOMA

Ependymoma is an uncommon neoplasm that occurs at all ages but is relatively more common in children. It accounts for 60% of intramedullary spinal cord neoplasms; in the brain, 60% occur in the fourth ventricle.

Grossly, ependymomas form well-circumscribed, reddish-brown nodular masses that occur in relation to the ventricular system. They grow slowly but have the ability to spread via the cerebrospinal fluid and should be considered as low-grade malignant neoplasms. Microscopically, ependymomas are highly cellular, with small polygonal cells that form ependymal tubules and perivascular pseudorosettes. Well-differentiated ependymomas tend to grow slowly and may be cured by complete surgical removal. Less well differentiated ependymomas infiltrate, grow rapidly, and have a bad prognosis.

A specific type of ependymoma called myxopapillary ependymoma occurs in the filum terminale and presents as a cauda equina tumor in young adults.

CHOROID PLEXUS PAPILLOMA

Choroid plexus papilloma is a rare neoplasm that tends to occur in the ventricles of young children. Grossly, it is characterized by a highly vascular papillary mass growing into the ventricle. Microscopically, the papillary processes have vascular cores and are lined by uniform columnar cells. Calcification may be present. Rarely, infiltration of brain, cytologic atypia, and increased mitotic activity justify a diagnosis of choroid plexus carcinoma.

Choroid plexus papillomas may sometimes secrete increased amounts of cerebrospinal fluid and give rise to communicating hydrocephalus.

COLLOID CYST OF THE THIRD VENTRICLE

Colloid cysts are believed to have an ependymal origin. They occur in the anterior third ventricle and are unilocular cysts lined by cuboidal epithelium and containing thick gelatinous fluid. As they enlarge, colloid cysts may block the foramen of Monro, producing acute obstructive hydrocephalus.

MEDULLOBLASTOMA

Medulloblastoma is derived from primitive neuroectodermal cells. It occurs mainly in children, accounting for 25% of all intracranial neoplasms in children under age 10 years. Its most common location is the midline cerebellar vermis in the posterior fossa.

Grossly, medulloblastoma appears as a grayish-white fleshy mass with infiltrative margins. Microscopically, the tumor is highly cellular and composed of sheets of small primitive cells with hyperchromatic nuclei and scant cytoplasm. Mitotic figures are frequently present.

Medulloblastoma is highly malignant and frequently seeds the cerebrospinal fluid to produce metastases around the spinal cord. The prognosis is poor.

PINEAL NEOPLASMS

The pineal gland is situated in the midline, dorsal to the midbrain and the posterior part of the third ventricle. It is composed of pinealocytes, which are modified neuroectodermal cells.

PINEALOCYTE NEOPLASMS

Pineocytoma is a benign or low-grade malignant neoplasm composed of well-differentiated pinealocytes. It occurs mainly in adults.

Pineoblastoma resembles medulloblastoma. It occurs in childhood and is highly malignant.

GERM CELL NEOPLASMS

Neoplasms arising from primitive germ cells in the nervous system occur most commonly in the pineal region. Germinoma, which resembles the testicular seminoma microscopically, is most common and typically forms a well-circumscribed mass that compresses the midbrain, causing abnormalities in ocular movement and hydrocephalus. Germinomas are malignant and tend to spread along CSF pathways. Germinomas are extremely radiosensitive neoplasms, and cures have been recorded following radiation therapy.

Other germ cell neoplasms occurring in the region of the pineal include teratoma, embryonal carcinoma, yolk sac carcinoma, and choriocarcinoma. All are very uncommon.

MENINGIOMA

Meningioma can occur at any age but is rare in childhood. Meningiomas occur most frequently in middle-aged women—the predominance in women is probably related to the presence of estrogen receptors on the tumor cells. The relationship of estrogens to growth of meningiomas is under study.

Pathology

Meningiomas usually arise outside of the brain substance and have an attachment to the dura. They present grossly as a firm encapsulated mass that compresses adjacent neural structures (Fig 65–5). Infiltration of the dura is usual and does not indicate malignancy. Meningiomas are frequently associated with hypertrophy of the overlying bone (hyperostosis); this may be so pronounced as to cause a palpable mass in the skull. Meningiomas may also infiltrate bone and extend into the scalp, a locally aggressive behavior pattern that still does not necessarily indicate malignancy. Rarely, meningiomas do not produce a distinct mass lesion but appear as a flat elevated plaque on the inner surface of the dura (meningioma en plaque). The term malignant meningioma is used when the neoplasm infiltrates the underlying brain.

Microscopically, meningioma is composed of sheets or whorls of meningothelial cells, which are plump spindle cells with oval nuclei and scant cytoplasm (syncytial or meningothelial meningioma). In some cases, the meningothelial cells are more elongated, resembling fibroblasts (fibroblastic meningioma). Psammoma bodies (round, laminated calcifications) occur in many meningiomas. Mitoses are rare. When there is necrosis, cellular pleomorphism, or a high mitotic rate, the term atypical meningioma may be used.

Angioblastic meningioma is a histologic subtype with a much more malignant biologic behavior. It is characterized histologically by a prominent vascular pattern resembling a hemangiopericytoma.

Biologic Behavior

Meningioma is a benign neoplasm. However, because of infiltration of dura and bone, complete surgical removal may be difficult in some cases, and there is a 10% recurrence rate. The recurrence rate increases in (1) atypical meningiomas (20–

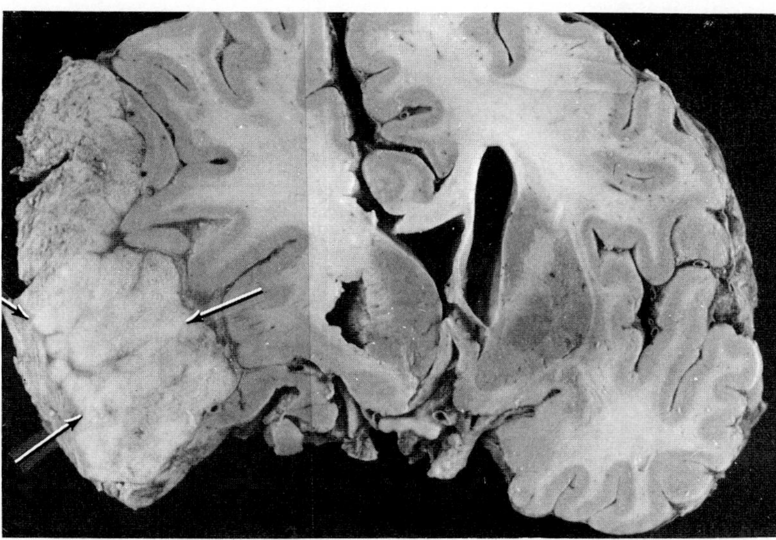

Figure 65-5. Meningioma of the convexity, causing marked compression of the underlying brain and shift of midline structures. Note the excellent demarcation between the cerebral cortex and the noninfiltrative neoplasm.

30% recurrence rate), (2) angioblastic meningiomas (75%), and (3) malignant meningiomas (90% without radiotherapy). Angioblastic meningiomas have also been reported to metastasize, particularly to bone.

Clinical Features

Meningiomas occur throughout the craniospinal axis, producing specific clinical features that depend on their location (Fig 65-6). Sites of predilection are (1) the parasagittal region and falx cerebri, giving rise to motor deficits; (2) the surface of the cerebral hemispheres, causing focal epilepsy and cortical dysfunction depending on exact location; (3) the olfactory bulb, compressing the optic nerve and causing blindness; (4) the sphenoidal ridge, compressing the cranial nerves passing into the orbit; (5) the posterior fossa, with features of a cerebellopontine angle tumor; and (6) the spinal cord, causing spinal compression.

NERVE SHEATH NEOPLASMS

Neoplasms arising in the nerve sheaths—schwannoma and neurofibroma—will be considered in the section on soft tissue neoplasms (Chapter 66). Nerve sheath neoplasms occur in relation to cranial and spinal nerve roots, particularly the sensory nerve roots.

The commonest intracranial example is the acoustic schwannoma (neuroma), which arises in the eighth cranial nerve and presents as a cerebellopontine angle mass. In this location, it compresses adjacent cranial nerves and cerebellum. Schwannoma less frequently arises from the fifth cranial nerve.

Neurofibromas are the commonest neoplasms occurring in the intradural but extramedullary compartment of the spinal column. They cause progressive spinal cord compression.

CEREBELLAR HEMANGIOBLASTOMA

Cerebellar hemangioblastoma is a benign neoplasm that occurs either sporadically or as part of von Hippel-Lindau disease (Chapter 62). It appears grossly as a well-circumscribed mass with cystic and solid components (Fig 65-7). Microscopically, numerous endothelium-lined vascular spaces are separated by trabeculae of cells with lipid-laden cytoplasm.

Clinically, presentation is with cerebellar dysfunction, hydrocephalus, or polycythemia (the tumor produces erythropoietin). Surgical removal is usually curative.

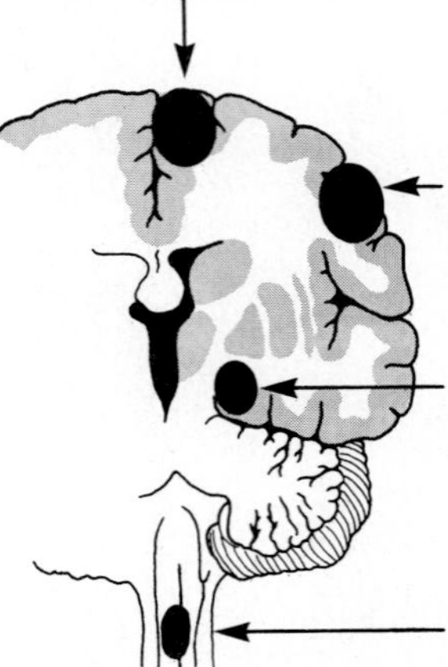

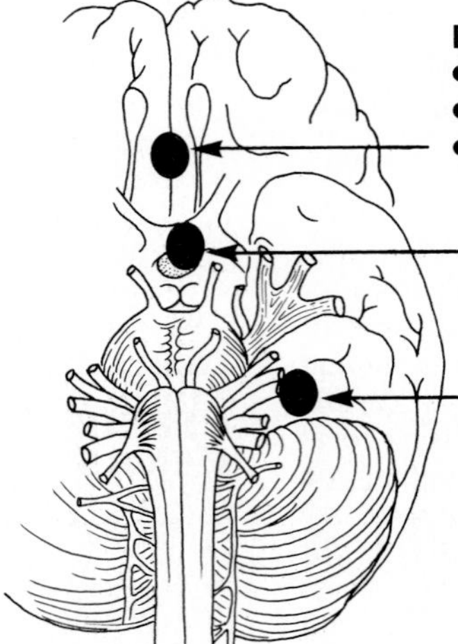

Figure 65-6. Intracranial meningiomas—common sites and symptomatology.

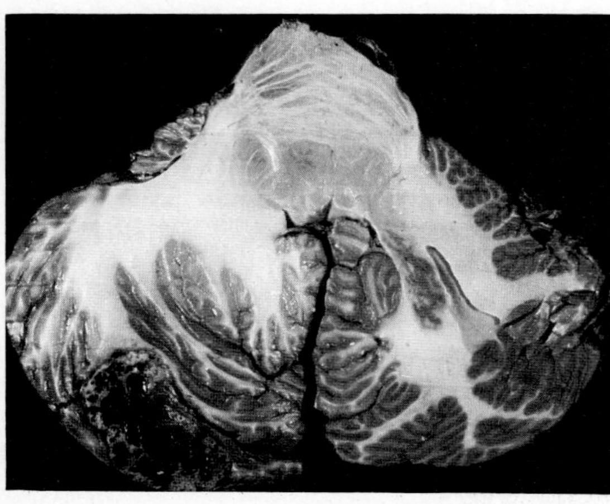

Figure 65-7. Cerebellar hemangioblastoma, showing a well-circumscribed hemorrhagic neoplasm in the cerebellar hemisphere.

MALIGNANT LYMPHOMA OF THE BRAIN

Primary malignant lymphoma of the brain is very uncommon in otherwise healthy individuals. Its incidence is greatly increased in immunocompromised patients, as in those with AIDS and after renal transplantation. In the past, brain lymphomas were called "reticulum cell sarcoma" or "microglioma"—until the lymphoid origin was proved by immunologic marker studies.

Intracranial lymphoma most commonly occurs in the deep cerebral hemispheres and is frequently multifocal. The commonest types are high-grade B cell lymphomas, most commonly B-immunoblastic lymphoma. Treatment with chemotherapy is of limited efficacy, and the prognosis is poor.

NEOPLASMS DERIVED FROM EMBRYONAL REMNANTS

CRANIOPHARYNGIOMA

Craniopharyngioma is believed to be derived from Rathke's pouch, the epithelial remnant of the foregut that contributes to the origin of the pituitary gland. It occurs mainly in childhood in the suprasellar region adjacent to the pituitary stalk.

Typically, craniopharyngioma is encapsulated and has cystic and solid components. In some cases, local infiltration makes complete surgical removal difficult. Microscopically, the cystic spaces are lined by stratified squamous epithelium and contain an oily fluid in which cholesterol crystals can be identified. The solid areas are composed of stroma and squamous epithelium that resembles tooth-forming ameloblastic epithelium. Calcification is usually present.

Craniopharyngiomas present with compression and destruction of (1) the pituitary, causing hypopituitarism—in children, growth retardation is a common finding; (2) the optic chiasm, causing visual field defects; and (3) the third ventricle, causing hydrocephalus. Treatment is surgical, often followed by radiation therapy in cases where complete surgical removal is not possible. The recurrence rate is high.

EPIDERMOID CYST

Epidermoid cysts are derived from rare embryonic epidermal remnants. The commonest locations are the cerebellopontine angle, the suprasellar region, and the lumbar region of the spinal cord in relation to spina bifida.

Epidermoid cysts are benign cystic structures lined by stratified squamous epithelium and filled with keratin. Surgical removal is curative.

CHORDOMA

Chordoma is a neoplasm derived from notochordal remnants found in the base of the skull and the dorsal aspect of the vertebral bodies. Chordoma occurs most commonly at either end

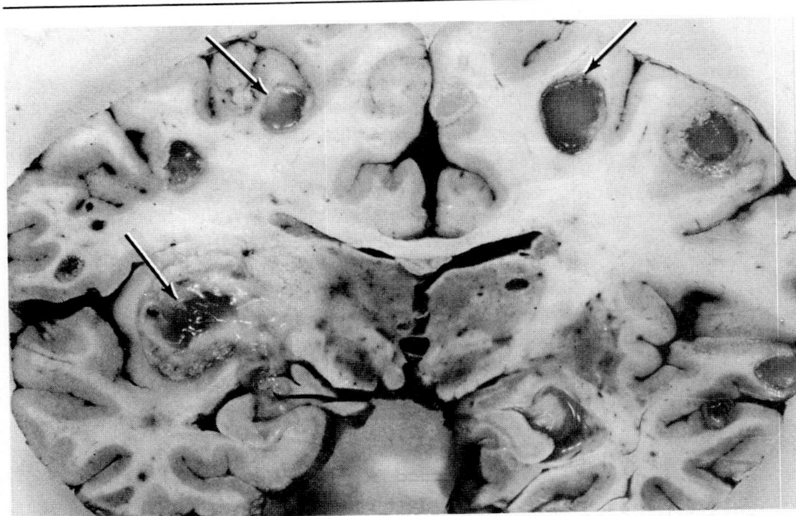

Figure 65-8. Multiple cerebral metastases from carcinoma of the lung.

of the notochord in the following locations: (1) in the sacrococcygeal region, where it causes compression of the cauda equina; (2) at the clivus, from which it extends into the posterior fossa, compressing the brain stem; and (3) in the suprasellar region, where it compresses the pituitary stalk and third ventricle.

Grossly, chordoma appears as a lobulated nodular mass that arises in bone and protrudes inward into the cranial cavity and spinal canal. It has a gelatinous appearance on cut section and histologically resembles the notochord, being composed of large cells with abundant bubbly cytoplasm (physaliphorous cells).

Chordomas are malignant neoplasms that grow slowly but inexorably. Complete surgical removal is rarely possible. Most patients die of their tumor, usually after several years.

METASTATIC NEOPLASMS

Neoplasms metastatic to the brain are common and may be derived from melanomas or from primary tumors in almost any primary location, most commonly the lung, breast, kidney, stomach, and colon. The brain metastasis may be the first manifestation of a previously occult malignant neoplasm, in which case differentiation from a primary intracranial neoplasm is difficult without biopsy. More frequently, metastasis to the brain occurs during the terminal phase in a patient with disseminated cancer (Fig 65–8).

Meningeal involvement by metastatic neoplasms occurs frequently in patients with acute leukemia. This presents a problem because the blood-brain barrier prevents chemotherapeutic agents from reaching the meningeal leukemic cells. The diagnosis of meningeal involvement can be made by identifying leukemic cells in cerebrospinal fluid. These patients can then be treated either with intrathecal chemotherapy or craniospinal irradiation.

The Peripheral Nerves & Skeletal Muscle

66

The peripheral nerves, neuromuscular junction, and skeletal muscle represent the final component of the lower motor neuron and are discussed together for that reason. Diseases involving these structure result in muscle weakness. The peripheral nerves also have sensory and autonomic fibers, and—unlike disease of muscle, which result in motor dysfunction alone—peripheral nerve diseases are manifested by a combination of motor and sensory loss.

DISORDERS OF PERIPHERAL NERVES

Peripheral nerves are composed of axons leading to and from sensory, motor, and autonomic neurons. Each individual axon is surrounded by a myelin sheath of varying thickness (Fig 66–1). The nerves contain Schwann cells, which form the myelin, and supporting connective tissue (endo-, epi-, and perineurium). The blood supply to peripheral nerves is by small arterioles called the vasa nervorum.

PERIPHERAL NEUROPATHY

Peripheral neuropathy is a clinical term that denotes nontraumatic disease of the nerves. Most peripheral neuropathies tend to affect the longest fibers first, producing a typical symmetric "glove and stocking" distribution of sensory loss and involvement of the muscles of the hands and feet. Sensory and mixed neuropathies are more common than pure motor neuropathy. Neuropathy affecting autonomic nerves results in autonomic dysfunction.

Two basic pathologic lesions occur in peripheral neuropathy: segmental demyelination and axonal degeneration. Both changes result in failure of nerve conduction. In the case of sensory nerves, the nerve damage results in degenerative changes in the neuron in the sensory nerve root ganglion. When neuronal loss occurs, the lesion is irreversible. There are many causes of peripheral neuropathy (Table 66–1).

Ischemic neuropathy tends to result in asymmetric involvement of a single nerve (mononeuritis) or scattered individual nerves (mononeuritis multiplex).

TRAUMATIC NERVE INJURIES

Peripheral nerve injuries resulting in transection of the nerve are common. Transection injury is characterized by loss of motor and sensory function in the distribution of the nerve, the severity of which depends on how many nerve fibers within the nerve are interrupted.

Recovery from a nerve injury depends on several factors, most importantly whether the continuity of the nerve sheath of the damaged axon is maintained. Where the nerve sheath is not disrupted, complete recovery is the rule. This takes a period of several weeks, because the axon and myelin sheath distal to the point of injury undergo wallerian degeneration and regenerate slowly (1–2 cm per week) from the proximal end. In such

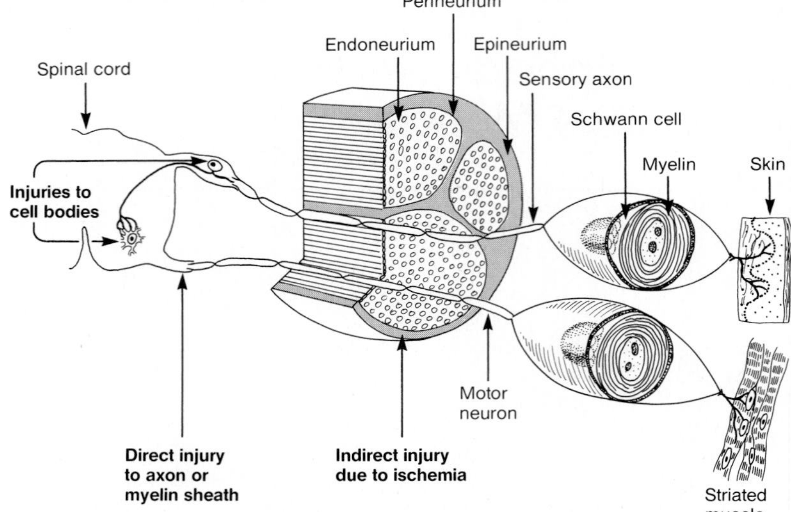

Figure 66–1. Diagram of peripheral nerve, showing the central and peripheral connections of nerves subserving a simple spinal reflex. The main types of injury that lead to peripheral nerve dysfunction are shown.

Table 66–1. Causes of peripheral neuropathy.

Hereditary neuropathies
Refsum's hypertrophic polyneuritis
Peroneal muscular atrophy (Charcot-Marie-Tooth disease): X-linked dominant inheritance; distal leg muscles involved
Neuropathies associated with heredofamilial amyloidosis
Ischemic neuropathies
Diabetic neuropathy[1]
Giant cell arteritis (high incidence of optic nerve involvement)
Systemic lupus erythematosus
Atherosclerosis
Toxic neuropathies
Drugs (isoniazid, nitrofurantoin)
Alcoholic polyneuropathy
Heavy metals: arsenic, lead, gold, mercury
Industrial substances: insecticides, solvents
Metabolic neuropathies
Deficiency of vitamins B_1, B_6, B_{12}
Diabetic neuropathy[1]
Porphyria
Amyloidosis
Infections and postinfection syndromes
Leprosy
Diphtheria toxin
Guillain-Barré syndrome
Carcinomatous neuropathy (noncompressive, nonmetastatic)

[1]Diabetic polyneuropathy may result from either axonal degeneration caused by the osmotic effect of sorbitol accumulating in the nerve or diabetic microangiopathy involving the vasa nervorum.

nerve injuries, return of effective function depends on the degree of secondary degeneration that occurs in the end organ (motor end plate, muscle, sensory receptor, etc), which depends on the time taken for reinnervation to occur.

More serious nerve injuries, which are much more common, are associated with transection of the nerve sheath as well as the axon (Fig 66–2). In most cases, the entire nerve trunk is severed. Wallerian degeneration occurs distally, with degeneration of axons and demyelination. The Schwann cells at the proximal end of the severed nerve fibers proliferate rapidly, and in some cases this process reestablishes continuity with the distal nerve sheath. Recovery of function is dependent on the number of nerve sheaths that reestablish continuity and permit axonal recovery. This depends mainly on the accuracy of apposition of the severed nerve ends. Effective functional recovery requires that the axon reestablish its original innervation. With complete transection of a mixed sensory and motor nerve, the chances of this occurring are slight.

The complications of nerve transection include (1) failure of return of function; (2) return of abnormal function, due to establishment of incorrect innervation, eg, proximal sensory fiber growing down a distal motor axon; and (3) development of a mass at the severed nerve end composed of proliferating Schwann cells—these resemble neurofibromas histologically and are called traumatic neuromas.

NEOPLASMS OF PERIPHERAL NERVES

Neoplasms of peripheral nerves are common. They may occur in any nerve and may be classi-

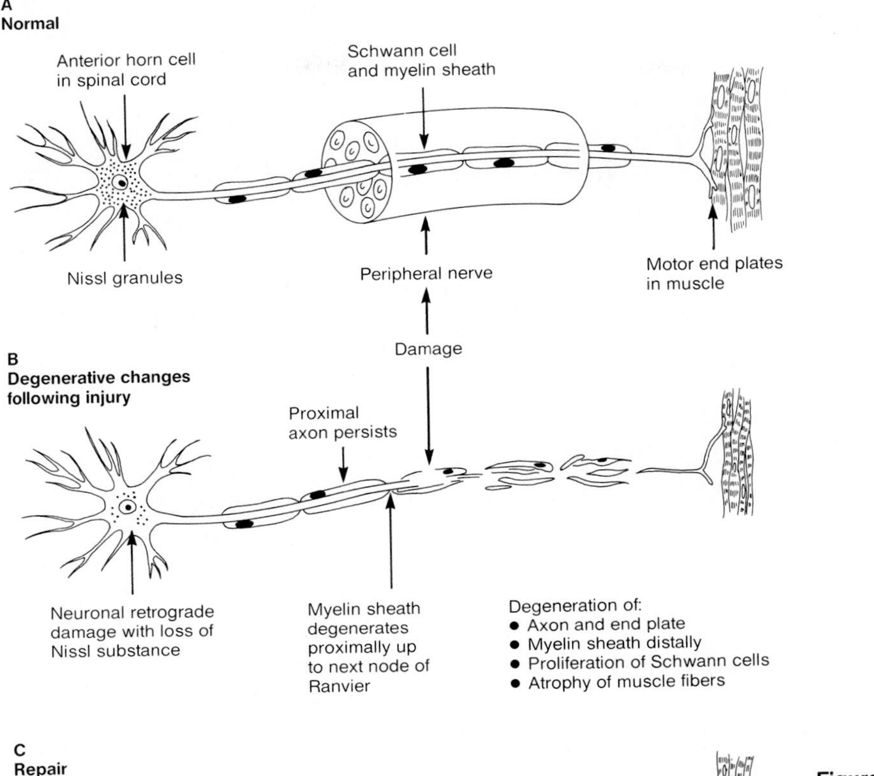

Figure 66–2. Wallerian degeneration and regeneration of a peripheral nerve after injury. The final functional result of nerve repair depends on the number of axons that reestablish their original innervation, which in turn depends on the type of apposition of the severed nerve ends and the distance of the nerve ending from the site of injury.

fied anatomically as (1) neoplasms within the skull or spinal canal; (2) neoplasms that involve both the spinal canal and the paraspinal soft tissue ("dumbbell" tumors, because of their shape—2 large masses connected by a narrow mass within the intervertebral foramen); (3) neoplasms arising in large nerve trunks in extraspinal or extracranial soft tissues; and (4) neoplasms in small peripheral nerve filaments that appear as soft tissue masses without obvious connections to nerves.

In all of these anatomic sites, neural tumors fall into 3 groups: (1) schwannoma, (2) neurofibroma, and (3) malignant peripheral nerve sheath tumor—a type of sarcoma also called malignant schwannoma and neurofibrosarcoma. Most neural neoplasms occur as sporadic lesions. In a small number of cases, multiple neural neoplasm occur as part of the familial generalized neurofibromatosis syndrome of von Recklinghausen (see Chapter 62).

1. SCHWANNOMA (Neurilemmoma) (Fig 66–3)

Schwannoma is a slowly growing benign neoplasm that commonly occurs in relation to large nerve trunks. Sensory cranial nerves (eighth and fifth nerve schwannoma) and the sensory root of spinal nerves are common locations. In the extra-axial soft tissues, they most commonly occur in the posterior mediastinum, the retroperitoneum, the head and neck, and the extremities. Schwannomas are usually solitary; multiple schwannomas

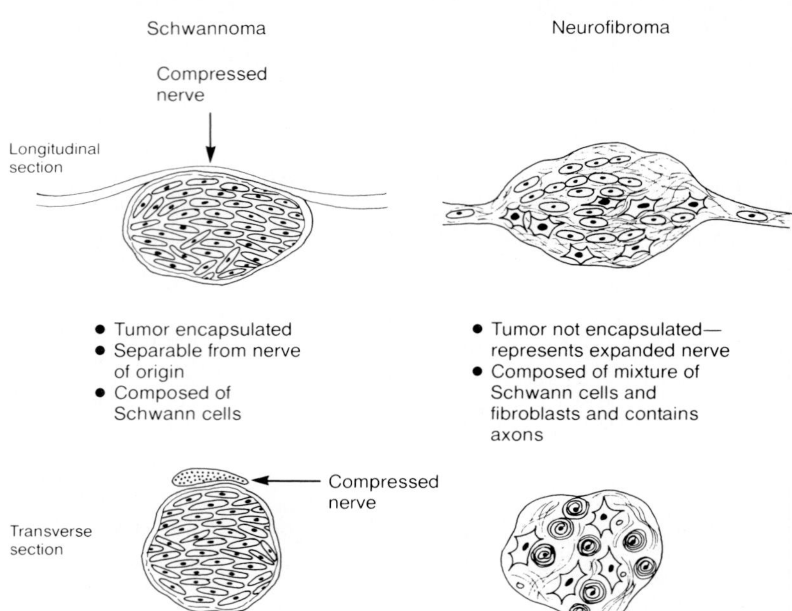

Figure 66-3. Differences between schwannoma (left) and neurofibroma (right). A schwannoma is a true encapsulated neoplasm, composed of Schwann cells, that compresses the nerve of origin. A neurofibroma is a hamartomatous proliferation of several cell types that expand the involved nerve.

may be associated with von Recklinghausen's neurofibromatosis.

Clinically, schwannomas present as a mass lesion, usually causing compression of surrounding structures. Compression of the nerve of origin causes irritative and paralytic symptoms—eg, acoustic schwannoma results in tinnitus followed by nerve deafness. Pain in the distribution of affected sensory nerves is a common finding.

On gross examination, schwannomas appear as encapsulated masses that compress the nerve of origin, which is frequently splayed out on one side of the mass. There is usually a plane of cleavage separating the nerve from the mass that may permit the tumor to be removed surgically without sacrificing the nerve. Areas of hemorrhage and cystic change are seen commonly in schwannomas; rarely, the neoplasm is composed predominantly of a cyst.

Histologic examination shows the tumor to be composed of Schwann cells arranged in 2 distinct patterns (Fig 66–4). The Antoni A pattern is characterized by highly cellular, compact, spindle-shaped cells arranged in short bundles or fascicles. Palisade arrangement of nuclei (nuclei of a fascicle of cells arranged one below the other) and Verocay bodies (structures formed by 2 rows of palisaded nuclei separated by an oval mass of pink cytoplasm) are characteristic histologic features. The Antoni B pattern is a loose, haphazard arrangement of Schwann cells in a richly myxomatous stroma. Large vascular spaces with hyalinized walls are a common feature. Nuclear pleomorphism and atypia, sometimes marked, may be present. Mitotic figures may also be present. Neither cytologic atypia nor mitotic activity indicates malignancy. Immunohistochemical studies show the presence of S-100 protein in the Schwann cells.

The malignant potential of schwannomas is very low.

2. NEUROFIBROMA (Fig 66-3)

Neurofibroma is a slowly growing benign neoplasm that occurs (1) in relation to large nerve trunks and (2) in peripheral tissues such as skin, where it arises from very small nerves. Neurofibroma most commonly occurs as a solitary neoplasm. In patients with von Recklinghausen's dis-

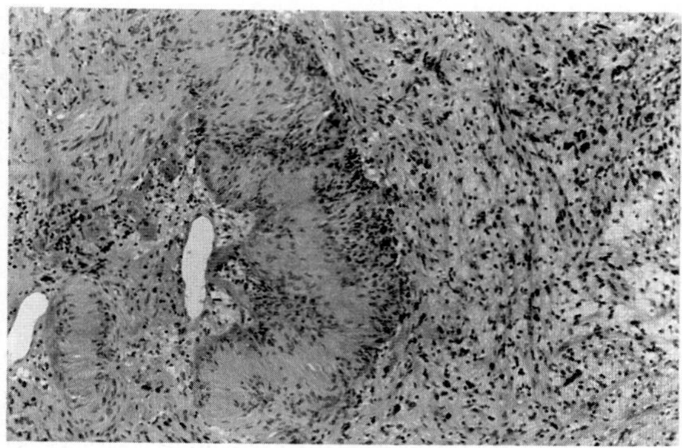

Figure 66-4. Schwannonma, showing compactly arranged Antoni A type of tissue with nuclear palisading (left half of photograph) and the loosely arranged Antoni B type of tissue (right half).

ease, there are multiple neurofibromas in the skin and viscera (Chapter 62).

Clinically, neurofibroma presents as a soft tissue mass. It is commonly associated with pain.

On gross examination, neurofibromas of large nerves appear as an expansion of the affected nerve (Fig 66-5). The mass is firm and rubbery, not demarcated from the nerve, and cannot be removed surgically without sacrificing the nerve. Cystic degeneration is common.

Histologic examination shows a varied spindle cell population composed of Schwann cells and fibroblasts. Cellularity is variable, and myxomatous change is commonly present in the stroma. Nuclear atypia and pleomorphism may occur. The presence of mitotic activity in a neurofibroma indicates a strong likelihood of malignant biologic potential. Immunohistochemical studies show the presence of S-100 protein; this is a reliable method of confirming the histologic diagnosis of both schwannoma and neurofibroma. Neurofibroma carries a low but significant risk of malignant transformation. Risk of malignancy is greatest in patients with von Recklinghausen's disease.

3. MALIGNANT PERIPHERAL NERVE SHEATH TUMOR

The term malignant peripheral nerve sheath tumor is applied to all malignant neural neoplasms and is synonymous with malignant schwannoma and neurofibrosarcoma. Most such tumors occur de novo; a few complicate preexisting neurofibroma, particularly in patients with von Recklinghausen's disease.

Malignant peripheral nerve sheath tumors appear clinically as soft tissue neoplasms. Any location may be affected, but most commonly the extremities and retroperitoneum. The rate of growth varies, being slow in low-grade neoplasms and rapid in high-grade ones. The tumors are diffusely infiltrative, frequently invading surrounding structures. Many patients have evidence of metastatic disease at the time of presentation. The common site of metastasis is the lung.

Grossly, malignant peripheral nerve sheath tumors are fleshy tumors, frequently large and showing extensive infiltration. Areas of necrosis and hemorrhage are common. Microscopically, they are highly cellular spindle cell sarcomas with marked cytologic atypia and pleomorphism and a high mitotic rate. The diagnosis of malignant peripheral nerve sheath tumor may be made (1) when a sarcoma has its origin from a large peripheral nerve, (2) when a sarcoma of appropriate histologic type occurs in a patient with von Recklinghausen's disease, (3) when S-100 protein is demonstrated in the tumor cells, or (4) when electron microscopy demonstrate features typical of Schwann cells. Less than 50% of malignant peripheral nerve sheath tumors are positive for S-100 protein.

DISORDERS OF SKELETAL MUSCLE

NORMAL SKELETAL MUSCLE (Fig 66-6)

Normal skeletal muscle is composed of fascicles of muscle fibers (myofibrils) that represent the cellular unit. A myofibril is a long, cylindric, multinucleate cell that is the contractile unit of the muscle. Myofibrils are invested by a delicate connective tissue (endomysium) that is continuous with the connective tissue present between the myofibrils (perimysium) and around the whole mus-

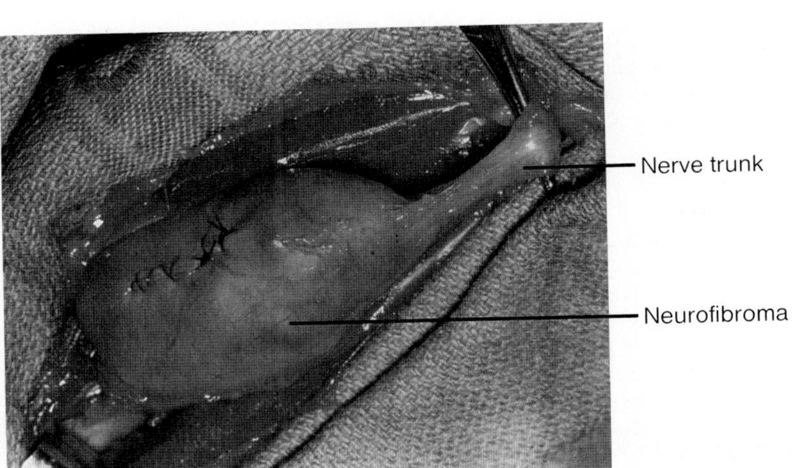

Figure 66-5. Neurofibroma arising in a large peripheral nerve.

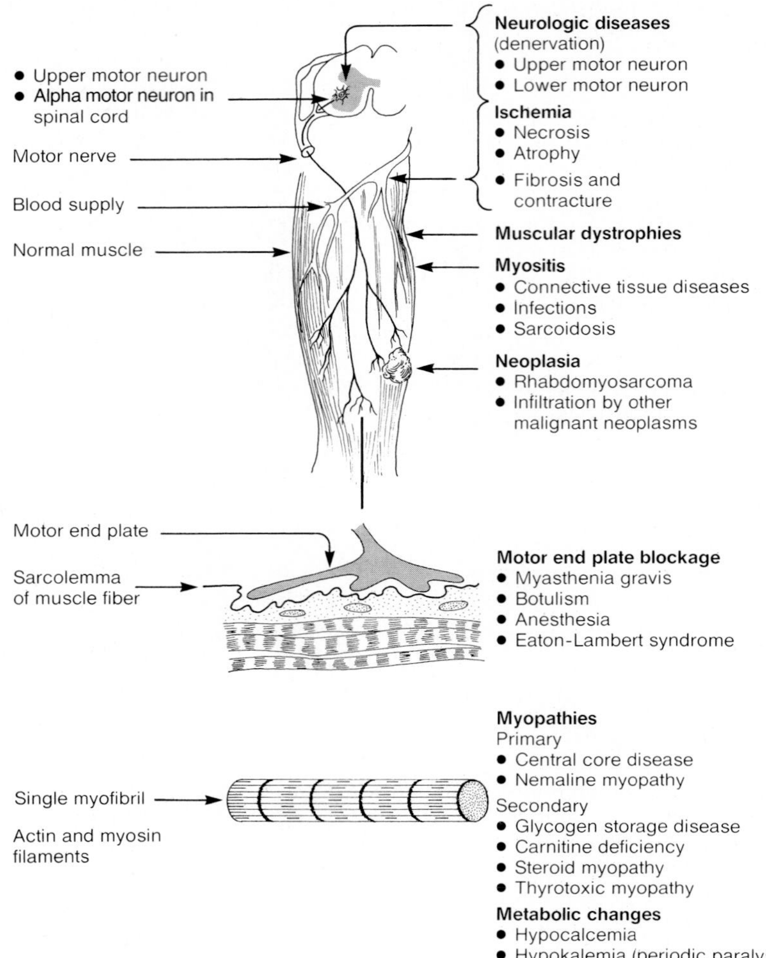

Figure 66-6. Structure and main diseases of skeletal muscle.

cle (epimysium). The connective tissue binds the myofibrils and is continuous at the ends of the muscle with the tendons with which muscles gain attachment to bone.

Each myofibril has a cell membrane (the sarcolemma) and shows cross-striations, because it is made up of regularly alternating bands of different refractility. Difference in refractility is related to the disposition of actin and myosin filaments in the myofibril.

Human muscle contains 3 different types of myofibril—red, intermediate, and white—based on color and biochemical features (Table 66-2). Red fibers are also called slow fibers because they have a slow conduction rate compared to white (fast) fibers. In humans, all 3 fiber types are present in different proportions in all muscles. The actual color of a given muscle depends on the proportion of the 3 fiber types present in the muscle. In birds, the pectoral muscle is predominantly

Table 66-2. Types of muscle fibers.[1]

Fiber Types	Cytochrome Oxidative Enzymes	ATPase	Glycogen	Myoglobin	Main Energy Source
Red: slow (type I)	+++	+	+	+++	Aerobic
Intermediate	++	++	++	++	. . .
White: fast (type II)	+	+++	+++	+	Anaerobic

[1]Type of fiber is determined by innervation: individual muscles contain a mixture of fiber types; individual nerve fiber innervates only one fiber type.

white ("white meat") and the muscles of the wings and legs are red ("dark meat").

CLINICAL FEATURES OF MUSCLE DISEASE

Muscle Weakness

Causes of muscle weakness include the following (Fig 66–6):

A. Neurologic diseases involving either the upper or lower motor neurons.

1. Lower motor neuron paralysis is characterized by muscle atrophy and loss of deep tendon reflexes; it may clinically resemble primary muscle diseases.

2. Upper motor neuron paralysis causes spasticity and brisk reflexes without significant muscle atrophy, at least initially.

B. Failure of neuromuscular transmission.

C. Disease involving skeletal muscle per se, including myositis, dystrophies, and myopathies.

Muscle Pain

Inflammatory lesions of muscle (myositis) are commonly associated with pain and tenderness in the involved muscles.

DIAGNOSIS OF MUSCLE DISEASES

Clinical Examination

The diagnosis of many muscle diseases is based on the distribution of involvement, family studies, and other clinical features.

Electromyography

Electromyography, which measures action potentials generated in muscles by means of an electrode inserted into the muscle belly, provides useful information regarding muscle function. The action potentials may be generated by voluntary contraction of the muscle or by stimulation of the nerve supply. The latter also permits evaluation of nerve conduction and neuromuscular transmission.

Serum Enzyme Levels

Serum levels of creatine kinase, aldolase, transaminases, and lactate dehydrogenase become elevated in many muscle diseases, especially the dystrophies and myositis (Table 66–3). Elevations of these enzymes, however, are not specific for muscle diseases, and clinical correlation is essential. Note that muscle atrophy secondary to neuronal lesions does not usually produce elevated enzyme levels. Mild elevation of serum enzyme levels may be present in normal individuals immediately after strenuous exercise.

Muscle Biopsy

Skeletal muscle biopsy is a highly specialized procedure. The preferred site for biopsy is the gastrocnemius. After removal the muscle should be placed in a special clamp before fixation to prevent contraction. In addition to routine light microscopy, muscle biopsies are examined by special histochemical methods—to assess their enzyme content—as well as by electron microscopy. Such techniques require special processing. Routine light microscopy shows features that permit differentiation of denervation atrophy, muscular dystrophy, and myositis (Fig 66–7).

PRIMARY MUSCLE DISEASES

1. MUSCULAR DYSTROPHIES

The muscular dystrophies are a group of rare inherited primary muscle diseases characterized by (1) onset in childhood, (2) distinctive distribution of involved muscles, and (3) nonspecific histologic changes (Fig 66–7) in muscle.

Types of Muscular Dystrophy (Table 66–4)

A. Duchenne Type Muscular Dystrophy: Duchenne muscular dystrophy (pseudohypertrophic muscular dystrophy) is the most common entity within this group. It is inherited as an X-linked recessive trait, with females carrying the abnormal gene and transmitting it to 50% of their male offspring, who manifest the disease.

Affected individuals are normal at birth and manifest the disease in early childhood. The disease progresses rapidly, with most children being disabled within a few years. Death commonly occurs by the end of the second decade.

Muscle weakness is symmetric and first affects the muscles of the pelvic girdle. This causes difficulty in getting up from a seated position, the child pushing up with the hands to compensate for pelvic girdle weakness. Walking become progressively more difficult, with a typical waddling gait, leading to a disability so severe as to confine the child to a wheelchair existence within a few years. A few patients with Duchenne muscular dystrophy have reduced intelligence and myocardial involvement. Death commonly results from involvement of respiratory muscles.

A typical feature of Duchenne muscular dystrophy is that the affected muscles appear larger than normal in the early stages. This is most easily seen in the calf muscles. Enlargement of muscle is caused by increased fat content (pseudohypertrophy); the myofibrils themselves show the randomly alternating muscle fiber atrophy and hypertrophy that characterizes all muscular dystrophies (Fig 66–7).

Table 66-3. Enzyme levels in diseases of muscle.[1]

	Myositis (Polymyositis)	Dystrophies	Myasthenia Gravis	Neurologic (Denervation) Disease	Myopathies	Comments
Creatine kinase (CK)	+++	++[2]	–	–	±	Three isoenzymes: BB, MB, MM. Muscle contains 90% MM, 10% MB. Thus elevated MM very good indication of muscle damage. MB is high in myocardial infarction.
Aldolase	++	+++[2]	–	–	±	Sensitive but not specific; high in liver disease and some psychoses. Present in red cells; hemolysis of specimen gives high value.
Transaminases (especially ALT [SGPT])	++	++	–	–	±	Elevated in many diseases, including cardiac and liver disease.
Lactate dehydrogenase (LDH)	++	++	–	–	±	LDH5 is especially muscle-related; high in liver, cardiac and other diseases. Present in red cells; hemolysis of specimen gives high value.
Other useful tests	Biopsy[3]	Electromyography (EMG), biopsy[4]	EMG, acetylcholine receptor antibody	EMG, biopsy	EMG, biopsy	

[1]Values given represent typical findings; some dystrophies give normal values at some stages of the disease, and neurogenic disorders may occasionally produce slightly increased values.
[2]More than half of female carriers of Duchenne muscular dystrophy show elevated levels.
[3]Will not reveal myositis if CK is normal.
[4]Requires special handling for analysis of enzymes.

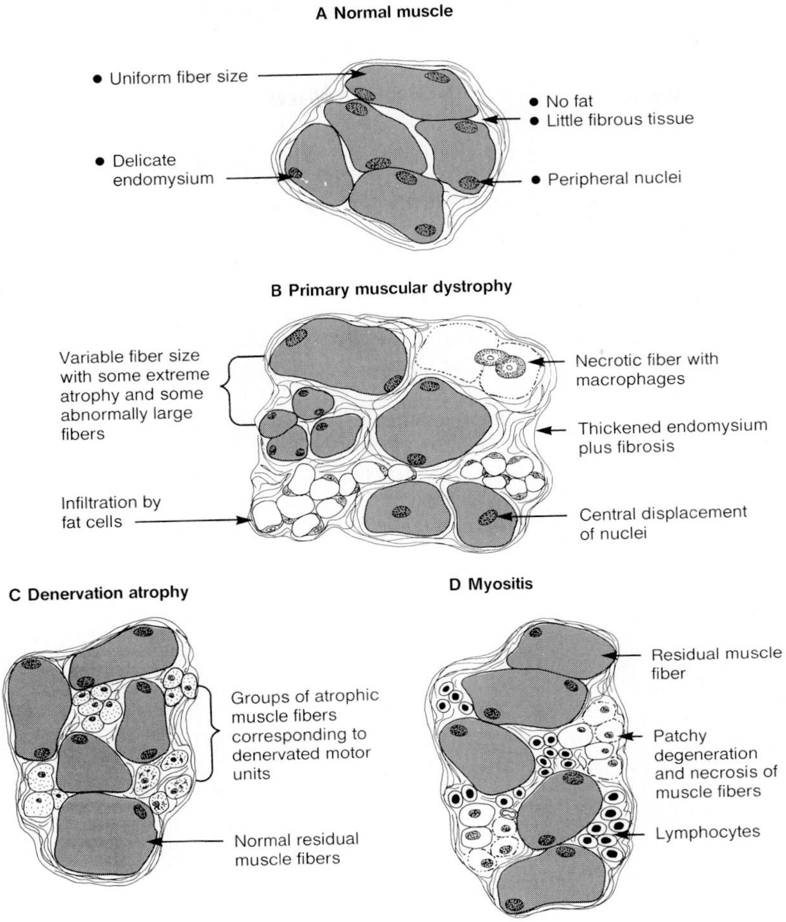

A Normal muscle

• Uniform fiber size

• Delicate endomysium

• No fat
• Little fibrous tissue

• Peripheral nuclei

B Primary muscular dystrophy

Variable fiber size with some extreme atrophy and some abnormally large fibers

Infiltration by fat cells

Necrotic fiber with macrophages

Thickened endomysium plus fibrosis

Central displacement of nuclei

C Denervation atrophy

Groups of atrophic muscle fibers corresponding to denervated motor units

Normal residual muscle fibers

D Myositis

Residual muscle fiber

Patchy degeneration and necrosis of muscle fibers

Lymphocytes

Figure 66–7. Histologic changes observed in the main groups of muscle diseases. **A:** Normal muscle. **B:** Variable sizes and patchy degeneration of individual fibers in primary muscular dystrophy. **C:** Motor unit atrophy in denervation. **D:** Inflammation associated with fiber loss in myositis.

B. Other Muscular Dystrophies: Many other types of muscular dystrophy are recognized and characterized according to the distribution of initial muscle weakness and inheritance patterns. Different entities have onset at different ages and different rates of progression of disease. Most are less severe than Duchenne muscular dystrophy. All are characterized by muscle weakness and atrophy, and histologic changes on muscle biopsy are identical.

One exception to these rules is **myotonic dystrophy,** which is characterized not by muscle weakness but by failure of relaxation of muscle after voluntary contraction. Onset is usually in adult life, and progression is very slow. Patients with myotonic dystrophy may have cataracts, gonadal

Table 66–4. Muscular dystrophies.

Type	Frequency	Inheritance[1]	Severity	Age at Onset	Distribution of First Involved Muscles
Duchenne (pseudohypertrophic)	Common	XR	Severe, fatal	0–12 years	Pelvis, legs
Becker	Rare	XR	Mild	10–70 years	Pelvis, legs
Facioscapulohumeral	Relatively common	AD	Mild	10–20 years	Face, shoulders
Limb girdle	Rare	AR	Moderate	Variable	Pelvis, shoulders
Distal	Very rare	AD	Variable	Adult	Hands, feet
Myotonic	Relatively common	AD	Variable, slow progression	Usually adult	Face, tongue, extremities

[1]X = X-linked; A = autosomal; R = recessive; D = dominant.

atrophy, mental retardation, abnormal insulin metabolism, and cardiac arrhythmias.

2. CONGENITAL MYOPATHIES

Congenital myopathies are a group of very rare primary muscle diseases characterized by (1) onset at birth or in early infancy, with muscle weakness and decreased muscle tone (''floppy infant syndrome''); (2) a very slowly progressive or nonprogressive course, with long survival being the rule; and (3) specific histologic changes on muscle biopsy that characterize individual entities within the group (Table 66–5). Most are inherited.

3. ACQUIRED MYOPATHIES

Many acquired diseases are associated with muscle weakness without causing histologic changes in the involved muscle. Common diseases causing acquired myopathies are thyrotoxicosis, hypercortisolism (Cushing's syndrome), acromegaly, and malignant neoplasia, in which myopathy occurs as a paraneoplastic syndrome. Hypocalcemia associated with osteomalacia and abnormal potassium metabolism associated with familial periodic paralysis also cause myopathy.

Table 66–5. Congenital and acquired myopathies (more common types only).

Disease	Histologic Characteristic
Central core disease	Amorphous central core in myofibrils with absence of myofilaments.
Nemaline myopathy	Elongated crystalline rods composed of tropomyosin present beneath sarcolemma; show periodicity on electron microscope.
Centronuclear myopathy	Nuclei occupy the central part of the myofibril, which lacks myofilaments.
Secondary congenital myopathies	Myopathy is a feature of some forms of glycogen storage disease and certain disorders of lipid metabolism (eg, carnitine deficiency).
Acquired myopathies	Endocrine diseases: thyrotoxicosis, corticosteroid excess (Cushing's syndrome, exogenous steroid administration), acromegaly; osteomalacia (hypocalcemia); familial periodic paralysis (potassium deficiency or excess); malignant neoplasms (paraneoplastic syndrome).

INFLAMMATION OF MUSCLE (Myositis)

A large number of infectious agents affect muscle, leading to myositis (Table 66–6). In **trichinosis,** muscle involvement characterized by severe muscle pain and swelling is the dominant clinical manifestation in the acute phase. **Bornholm's disease** is a coxsackievirus infection of chest wall muscles characterized by severe chest pain aggravated by breathing. Skeletal muscle involvement also occurs in exotoxic bacterial infections. In **diphtheria,** there is actual necrosis of muscle with inflammation. Muscle pain (myalgia) is a common clinical accompaniment of many viral infections, typhoid fever, and leptospirosis.

Inflammation of muscle is common in several autoimmune diseases. In polymyositis (often associated with skin involvement—dermatomyositis), inflammation of muscles is the dominant clinical manifestation (see Chapter 68). In other autoimmune diseases and in sarcoidosis, muscle involvement occurs as part of a general systemic illness. In myasthenia gravis, focal collections of lymphocytes (lymphorrhages) may be seen in muscle; they have little to do with the pathogenesis of the disease.

Myositis may also occur after high-dosage radiation (most commonly in treatment of cancer), is-

Table 66–6. Causes of myositis.[1]

Infectious diseases
- Bacterial
  - Local infection with pyogenic bacteria, usually secondary to trauma, intramuscular injection
  - Bacteremic myositis, eg, in infective endocarditis, typhoid fever, leptospirosis
  - Gas gangrene (clostridial infection)
- Viral
  - Coxsackievirus (Bornholm disease); affects mainly chest wall muscles
  - Influenza
  - Many other viruses
- Parasitic
  - *Trichinella spiralis* (trichinosis)
  - *Toxoplasma gondii*
  - Cysticercosis (*Taenia solium*)
  - *Trypanosoma cruzi* (Chagas' disease)
- Exotoxic
  - Diphtheria

Immune diseases
- Polymyositis-dermatomyositis
- Other autoimmune diseases: systemic lupus erythematosus, progressive systemic sclerosis
- Sarcoidosis
- Myasthenia gravis: associated with anti-striated muscle antibody in serum

Radiation

Ischemia

Myositis ossificans

[1]Myositis is characterized by the presence of inflammation on histologic examination.

chemia, and when muscle is infiltrated by malignant neoplasms. A specific form of myositis called **myositis ossificans** is characterized by bone formation in the involved muscle. This usually appears as a hard mass in the muscle that may be mistaken for a neoplasm.

DISORDERS OF NEUROMUSCULAR TRANSMISSION

1. MYASTHENIA GRAVIS

Myasthenia gravis is one of the commoner muscle diseases, affecting 1:40,000 persons in the USA. The commonest age at onset is 20–40 years. There is a female preponderance when the disease occurs under the age of 40 years.

Etiology

Myasthenia gravis is a clinical syndrome resulting from failure of neuromuscular transmission due to blockage of acetylcholine receptors by autoantibody (Fig 66–8). Myasthenia gravis is therefore an organ-specific autoimmune disease.

Acetylcholine receptor antibody is present in the serum of almost all patients. It is an IgG antibody and may cross the placenta in pregnancy, causing neonatal myasthenia in the newborn.

The reason for the production of anti-acetylcholine receptor autoantibody is unknown. Thymectomy often improves the condition, and it is believed that the thymus plays a role in the etiology of myasthenia gravis, either acting as a source of cross-reactive antigen or involved in the production of helper T cells or a cell-mediated immune response against muscle. The thymus is not the source of the antibody, which is produced by the peripheral lymphoid tissue.

Patients with myasthenia frequently have other autoantibodies in their blood. The commonest of these is anti-striated muscle antibody, which reacts with skeletal muscle fibers away from the motor end plate. This autoantibody also cross-reacts with myoid cells in the thymus.

Pathology

Specific morphologic abnormalities are not seen on gross examination or light microscopy. Focal collections of lymphocytes (lymphorrhages) may be seen in affected muscle. Immunohistochemistry demonstrates the presence of IgG and complement components on the motor end plate. Electron microscopy shows damage to the motor end plate with loss of the normally complex folds.

Thymic abnormalities are seen in many patients with myasthenia gravis. These include **thymic hyperplasia** (presence of reactive lymphoid follicles in an adult thymus) in 70% and thymomas in 15%.

Clinical Features & Diagnosis

Myasthenia gravis is characterized by muscle weakness that is typically aggravated by repeated contraction. Muscles with the smallest motor units are affected first, the most typical clinical presentation being weakness of ocular muscles (causing bilateral ptosis, or drooping of the eyelid, and diplopia or double vision). Twenty percent of patients with myasthenia have only ocular involvement (ocular myasthenia). In others, the disease progresses to include facial muscles, limb girdle muscles, and respiratory muscles (generalized myasthenia). Progression is variable but usually slow, with respiratory muscle involvement occurring 5–20 years after onset. Untreated, 40% of patients with myasthenia gravis will die of their disease within 10 years.

The clinical diagnosis of myasthenia gravis may

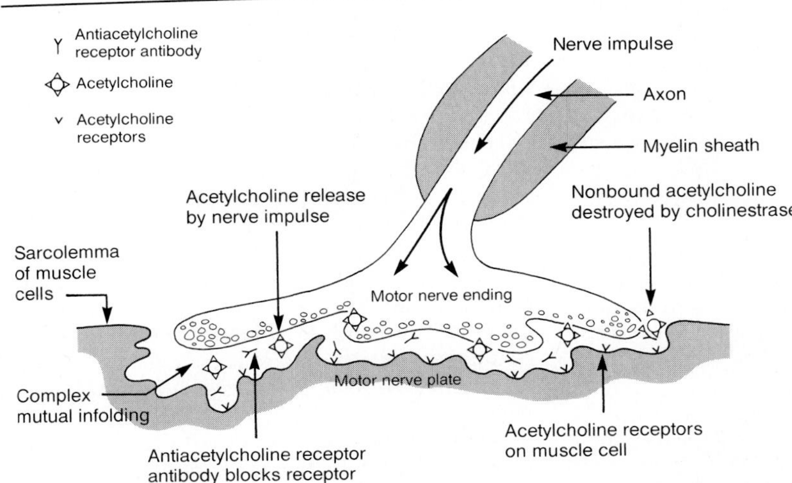

Figure 66–8. Pathogenesis of myasthenia gravis. Acetylcholine released at the nerve ending by the nerve impulse normally binds with acetylcholine receptors. This evokes the action potential in the muscle. In myasthenia gravis, antiacetylcholine receptor antibody binds to the acetylcholine receptor and inhibits the action of acetylcholine.

be confirmed by therapeutic testing, electromyography, and serologic testing: **(1) Edrophonium (Tensilon)** is a short-acting anticholinesterase drug that produces immediate improvement in muscle weakness when administered intravenously. **(2) Electromyography** shows a progressive decline in amplitude of muscle action potentials in patients with myasthenia gravis when the muscle is subjected to repeated voluntary contraction. **(3) Serum assay for acetylcholine receptor antibody** is a specific and sensitive test for the disease.

Treatment

Anticholinesterases, which increase the acetylcholine levels at the motor end plate and compensate for the receptor blockage, represent the mainstay of treatment. In crisis situations, the use of high-dosage corticosteroids and plasma exchange, which reduce antibody activity, have proved effective.

Thymectomy produces variable remission of the symptoms of myasthenia in many patients. The improvement is most pronounced in young women with recent onset of myasthenia and thymic hyperplasia. The improvement is least in patients with thymoma. The reason for remission of myasthenia after thymectomy is unknown.

2. OTHER CAUSES OF NEUROMUSCULAR TRANSMISSION FAILURE

Myasthenic Syndrome (Eaton-Lambert Syndrome)

Myasthenic syndrome is a paraneoplastic syndrome associated with cancer, particularly small-cell carcinoma of the lung. Very rarely, myasthenic syndrome occurs in patients without cancer.

Myasthenic syndrome is the result of an abnormality of acetylcholine release by nerve endings at the motor end plate. It is characterized clinically by weakness of muscles in a distribution similar to that of myasthenia gravis, with early involvement of ocular muscles. The muscle weakness is not aggravated by effort and on electromyography shows progressive increase of amplitude of action potentials upon repeated contraction (an effect opposite to that seen in myasthenia gravis).

Botulism

The exotoxin of *Clostridium botulinum* in minute doses blocks release of acetylcholine at the motor end plate. Generalized muscle weakness rapidly leads to respiratory paralysis and death.

Tick Paralysis

Ticks of the genus *Dermacentor—Dermacentor andersoni,* the Rocky Mountain wood tick; and *Dermacentor variabilis,* the American dog tick—secrete a toxin that inhibits acetylcholine release. Removal of the tick is curative.

Aminoglycoside Drugs

Aminoglycosides in high dosage, especially in the presence of renal dysfunction, inhibit acetylcholine release and cause muscle weakness. These antimicrobial drugs should be avoided in patients with myasthenia gravis.

NEOPLASMS OF SKELETAL MUSCLE

1. BENIGN NEOPLASMS (Rhabdomyoma)

Benign neoplasms of skeletal muscle (rhabdomyoma) are extremely uncommon. Cardiac rhabdomyoma occurs rarely in patients with tuberous sclerosis (see Chapter 62).

2. MALIGNANT NEOPLASMS (Rhabdomyosarcoma)

Rhabdomyosarcoma is an uncommon soft tissue sarcoma. Three histologic subtypes are recognized:

(1) Embryonal rhabdomyosarcoma is the most common type, especially in children under 10 years of age. It presents as a rapidly growing neoplasm involving the soft tissues of the extremities, retroperitoneum, orbit, nasal cavity, and a variety of organs. It is extremely infiltrative and tends to metastasize via the bloodstream at an early stage. A special variant of embryonal rhabdomyosarcoma occurring in the vagina in very young girls is known as **sarcoma botryoides**. This tumor appears as an enlarging mass that protrudes from the vagina, having the appearance of a bunch of grapes. Histologically, embryonal rhabdomyosarcoma is highly cellular, being composed of small round and oval cells with primitive hyperchromatic nuclei, scanty cytoplasm, and a high mitotic rate. Skeletal muscle differentiation can be demonstrated by (1) the presence of scattered cells with abundant pink cytoplasm (strap cells) that show cross-striations; (2) the presence of irregular Z bands on electron microscopy; and (3) the presence of muscle proteins such as myoglobin, myosin, actin, and desmin as shown by immunohistochemical studies. Sarcoma botryoides is composed of similar cells but shows areas of low cellularity with myxomatous change in the stroma and a characteristic layer of small primitive cells beneath the vaginal epithelium (cambium layer).

(2) Alveolar rhabdomyosarcoma is less common and occurs in the age group from 10 to 30 years, particularly around the shoulder and pelvis.

It is characterized by an alveolar arrangement of the small primitive neoplastic skeletal muscle cells. Like embryonal rhabdomyosarcoma, it is rapidly growing and highly malignant.

(3) Pleomorphic rhabdomyosarcoma is an uncommon neoplasm of soft tissue that mainly affects the extremities and retroperitoneum in elderly patients. It is highly malignant.

All 3 histologic types of rhabdomyosarcoma are high-grade malignant neoplasms showing rapid growth and early metastasis. New chemotherapeutic agents have improved the prognosis in embryonal and alveolar rhadomyosarcoma. Despite this, the overall prognosis for survival is still poor.

Section XVI. Bones, Joints, & Connective Tissue

A study of bone metabolism and its abnormalities (Chapter 67) should include a review of vitamin D metabolism (see Chapter 10) and the parathyroid glands (see Chapter 59). Bone fractures are a common consequence of trauma. Bacterial infections and neoplasms of bone are discussed in Chapter 67. Degenerative joint diseases, particularly osteoarthrosis (Chapter 68), is a common cause of disability in elderly persons. Many inflammatory diseases of joints and connective tissue have their basis in immunologic hypersensitivity (see Chapter 8). Neoplasms of connective tissue are considered in general here; many of the specific neoplasms have been discussed in other chapters, eg, vascular neoplasms in Chapter 20 and peripheral nerve neoplasms in Chapter 66.

67 Diseases of Bones

STRUCTURE & FUNCTION OF BONE

The skeleton is composed of flat bones and long tubular bones. Flat bones such as the skull, sternum, and pelvic bones develop from fibrous tissue **(intramembranous ossification),** whereas long tubular bones increase in length at a line of cartilage present near the growing ends of the bone known as the epiphyseal plate or growth plate. Anatomic regions of long bones relate to the growth plate and include the **epiphysis,** which is the region between the growth plate and the nearest joint; the **diaphysis,** which is the shaft region of the bone between the 2 growth plates; and the **metaphysis,** which is the region of bone adjacent to the growth plate on the diaphyseal side. The metaphysis is the area where new bone is laid down during growth, and in children it represents the most vascular and most metabolically active region of bone. For this reason, the metaphyseal region is the area most susceptible to infections and neoplasia in childhood (Fig 67–1).

All bones are composed of an outer (cortical) shell of compact bone and an inner meshwork of cancellous bone composed of bony trabeculae separated by vascular connective tissue, which contains fat and bone marrow. Both cortical and cancellous bone are composed of bone cells embedded in a matrix, which is mineralized. The main bone cells are osteoblasts, which secrete matrix protein, and osteoclasts, which resorb bone. The matrix of bone (called **osteoid**) is composed mainly of type I collagen. Other collagen types, other proteins such as osteocalcin and osteonectin (which may play a role in mineralization of the matrix), and glycoproteins complete the structure of bone matrix. The mineral phase of bone is composed predominantly of calcium hydroxyapatite with smaller amounts of calcium phosphate.

The main functions of bone are to act as a hard protective shell for vital structures (eg, skull, rib cage, pelvis), to provide support for the trunk and limbs, and to permit movement by the action of muscles attached to the bones. The long tubular bones of the limbs are ideal for their function because they are light and have high tensile strength. The bone mineral also acts as a massive storage for calcium and phosphorus.

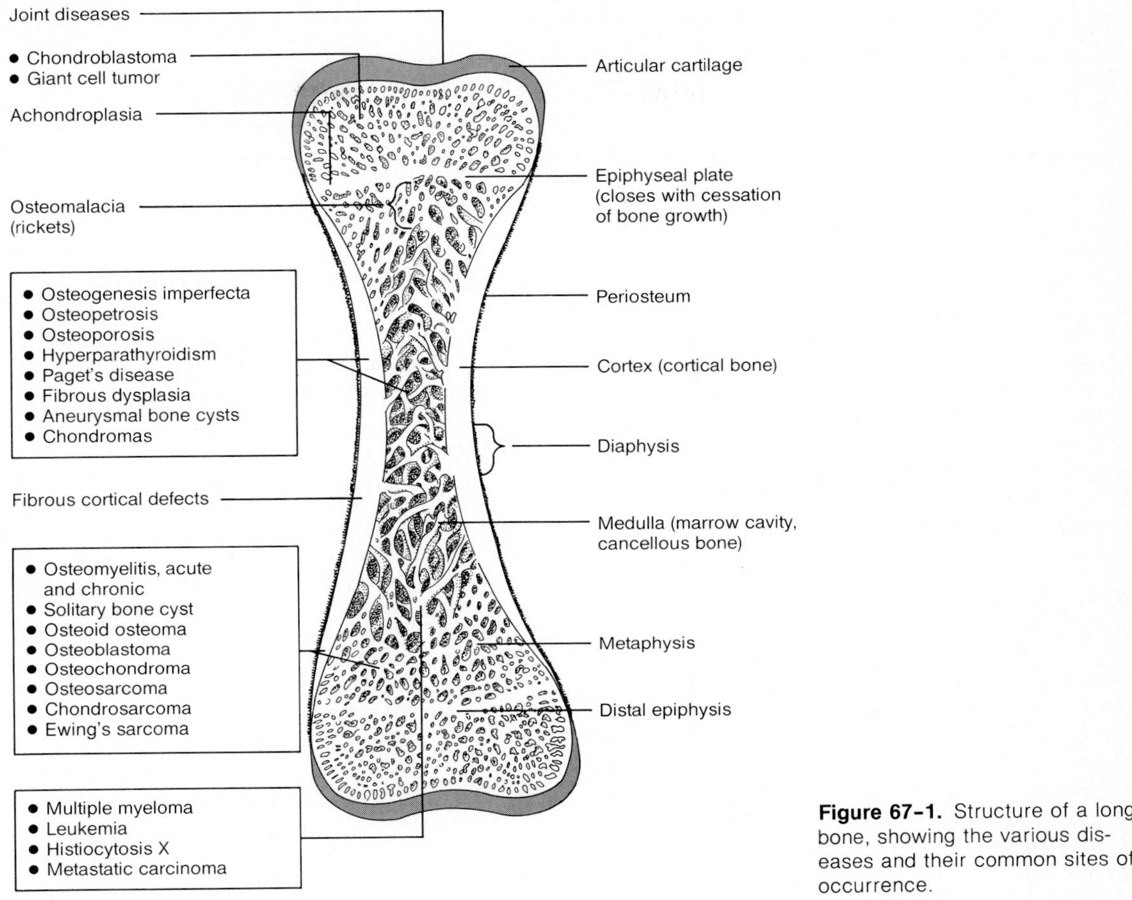

Figure 67–1. Structure of a long bone, showing the various diseases and their common sites of occurrence.

CLINICAL MANIFESTATIONS OF BONE DISEASE

Bone pain is usually localized to the site of the lesion. Acute inflammation, fractures, osteomalacia, and some bone neoplasms cause pain.

Bone deformity may result from (1) abnormal bone growth, as occurs in many congenital diseases; (2) fractures that heal improperly; and (3) softening of bone, as in rickets and osteomalacia.

Bone mass is the common mode of presentation of bone cysts and neoplasms.

Fracture of bone is commonly the result of trauma and usually occurs in normal bone when it is subjected to severe force. Fracture occurring in a previously abnormal bone—caused by relatively minor trauma or with no history of trauma—is called **pathologic fracture.**

Radiologic abnormalities, which may include masses, cysts, lytic areas, sclerotic areas, fractures, and deformities, may be detected incidentally or may confirm bone disease in a patient suspected of having a bone lesion. Pathologic evaluation of a **bone biopsy** must always be done with complete knowledge of the radiologic appearance of the lesion.

Laboratory evaluation of bone disease includes measurement of serum calcium and phosphorus, parathyroid hormone, vitamin D, and alkaline phosphatase. The serum alkaline phosphatase level increases in any bone disease in which there is increased osteoblast activity. In general, laboratory evaluation is of greatest value in metabolic bone diseases.

CONGENITAL DISEASES OF BONE

ACHONDROPLASIA

Achondroplasia is transmitted as an autosomal dominant trait. It is characterized by failure of cartilage cell proliferation at the epiphyseal plates of the long bones, resulting in failure of longitudinal bone growth and causing short limbs. Membranous ossification is not affected, so that the skull, facial bones, and axial skeleton develop normally. The result in adulthood is a normal-sized head and trunk but limbs that are much shorter than normal. Achondroplastic dwarfism is quite common. General health is not affected, and life expectancy is normal.

OSTEOGENESIS IMPERFECTA (Brittle Bone Disease)

Osteogenesis imperfecta (fragilitas ossium) usually has an autosomal dominant inheritance pattern with variable penetrance. It is characterized by defective synthesis of collagen by fibroblasts and osteoid by the osteoblasts. Abnormal collagen in joint capsules leads to loose-jointedness. Other manifestations include blue scleras, thin skin, development of hernias, and hearing loss in adults. Abnormal synthesis of osteoid leads to thin, poorly formed bones that tend to fracture easily.

Fractures usually begin to appear a few years after birth and often require internal fixation because they do not heal well. Survival into adult life is common. There is a rare autosomal recessive variant in which fractures begin at birth with death in the first year of life.

OSTEOPETROSIS (Marble Bone Disease; Albers-Schönberg Disease)

Osteopetrosis is very rare. There are 2 variants—a relatively mild autosomal dominant form and a lethal autosomal recessive form.

Osteopetrosis is characterized by bones that are greatly thickened due to overgrowth of cortical bone, with reduction or even obliteration of the marrow cavity. The vertebrae, pelvis, and ribs are more affected than extremities. Though thickened, affected bones are brittle and susceptible to fracture.

Patients present with recurrent fractures or anemia due to decreased hematopoiesis consequent upon the loss of bone marrow. The radiologic appearance of dense bones is characteristic.

INFECTIONS OF BONE

ACUTE PYOGENIC OSTEOMYELITIS

Pyogenic osteomyelitis is an acute inflammation of bone caused by bacterial infection. It occurs most frequently in children and young adults.

Etiology

Most cases of pyogenic osteomyelitis occur in previously healthy, active individuals and are caused by *Staphylococcus aureus,* which reaches the bone via the blood stream (Fig 67–2). The site of entry of the organism is usually not apparent, and the bacteremia is subclinical.

In a few cases, bone infection is a complication of compound fracture (ie, a fracture that breaks through the skin) or has spread to bone from a neighboring focus of infection, such as mandibular osteomyelitis occurring in dental infections.

Patients with sickle cell anemia have a special tendency to develop osteomyelitis caused by *Salmonella* species.

Pathology

The long bones of the extremities are most commonly involved. The infection tends to begin in the metaphyseal region, which is the most vascular area of the bone. It is believed that mild trauma associated with activity leads to small hematomas that become infected by blood-borne staphylococci.

Acute inflammation leads to marked increase in tissue tension within the confined bone space; suppuration and bone necrosis follow, with intrametaphyseal abscess formation. If not treated, the abscess extends to the surface (subperiosteal abscess), into an adjacent joint (pyogenic arthritis), or into the medullary cavity, leading to dissemination of the infection throughout the bone with extensive necrosis.

Clinical Features

The onset of acute osteomyelitis is rapid, with high fever and severe throbbing pain in the affected area. There is tenderness, swelling, and warmth over the inflamed bone. Very young children may not complain of pain but may manifest immobility.

There is almost invariably a neutrophil leukocytosis in the peripheral blood, and blood cultures are positive in 70% of patients. Radiographs may

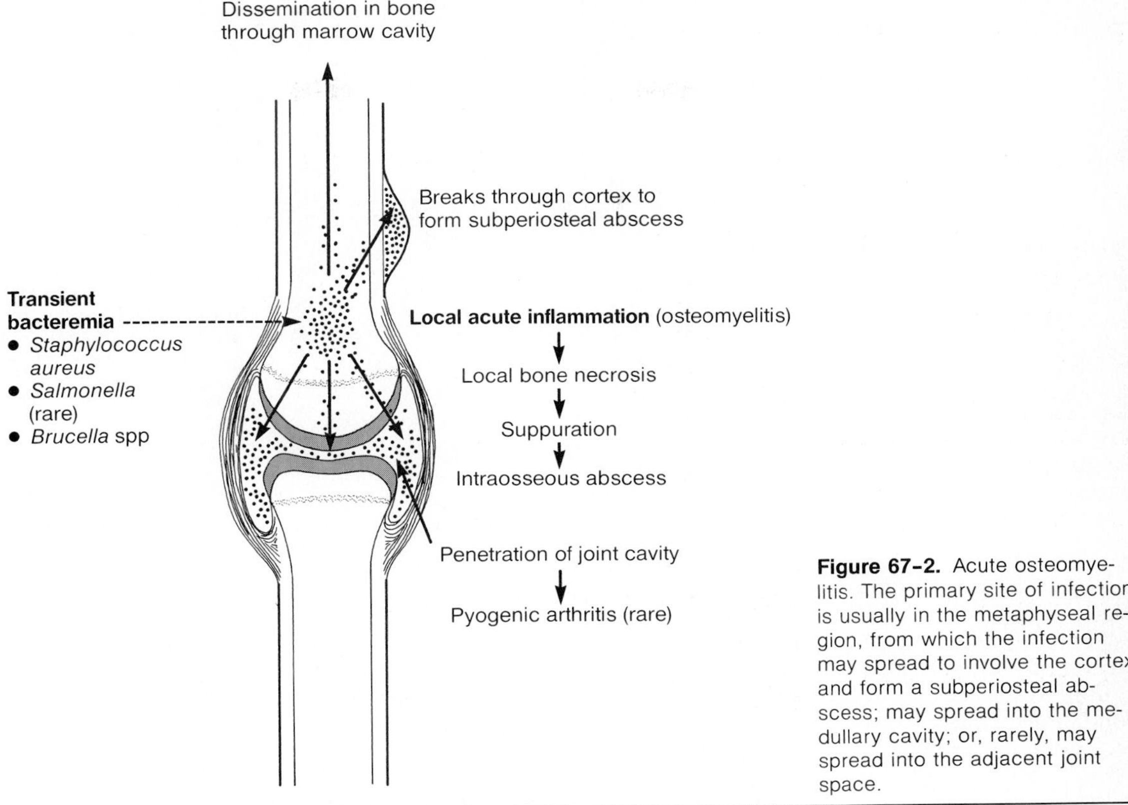

Figure 67-2. Acute osteomyelitis. The primary site of infection is usually in the metaphyseal region, from which the infection may spread to involve the cortex and form a subperiosteal abscess; may spread into the medullary cavity; or, rarely, may spread into the adjacent joint space.

be normal early; later, when bone necrosis occurs, areas of lucency appear.

Treatment & Prognosis

Early treatment by surgical drainage of pus plus antibiotics is essential. Culture of the pus provides guidance for antibiotic therapy. With effective treatment, less than 10% of cases are complicated by chronic osteomyelitis.

Complications

Untreated acute osteomyelitis frequently progresses to **chronic suppurative osteomyelitis,** in which necrotic bone forms a sequestrum of dead bone that perpetuates the infection. Reactive bone formation in the periosteum causes the sequestrum to be covered by irregular new bone (involucrum), with multiple draining sinuses through which pus escapes to the body surface (Fig 67-3). Complications of chronic osteomyelitis include secondary amyloidosis due to the persistent chronic suppuration and squamous epithelial hyperplasia and carcinoma of the overlying affected skin.

TUBERCULOSIS OF BONE

Tuberculous osteomyelitis has become rare in areas of the world where good control of pulmonary and intestinal tuberculosis has been achieved. It is still common in many developing countries. The vertebral column is the commonest site of disease (**Pott's disease** of the spine) (Fig 67-4).

Tuberculous osteomyelitis has an insidious onset, with low-grade fever and weight loss. Radiologic changes due to bone destruction can usually be demonstrated at presentation.

METABOLIC BONE DISEASE

Normal Bone Metabolism

Normal bone is composed of a protein matrix produced by osteoblasts. This matrix is called **osteoid** and is composed mainly of type I collagen. Osteoid becomes mineralized by deposition of calcium hydroxyapatite and calcium phosphate. The exact mechanism of mineralization is unknown

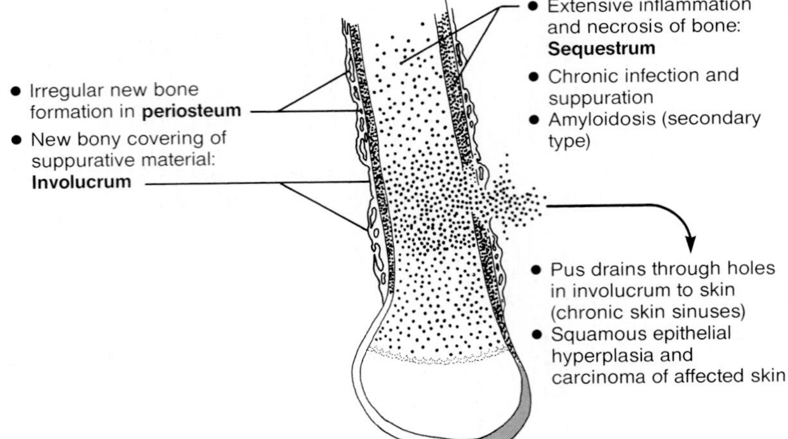

Figure 67–3. Chronic osteomyelitis, characterized by extensive suppurative necrosis of the bone, which forms a sequestrum. This is surrounded by an irregular mass of periosteal new bone (involucrum), which is perforated to permit drainage of the suppurative material into the skin via multiple sinuses.

but is dependent on the structure of osteoid, the presence of other proteins such as osteocalcin and osteonectin, and the calcium and phosphate concentrations in the blood.

Bone is an actively metabolizing tissue with a continuous turnover of osteoid and mineral. Bone resorption by osteoclasts is normally balanced exactly by bone deposition by osteoblasts. Abnormalities relating to bone metabolism cause the group of diseases known as metabolic bone diseases.

OSTEOPOROSIS

Osteoporosis is a decrease in the total mass of bone without other structural abnormalities; the term **osteopenia** is also sometimes used. Osteoporosis therefore represents a form of bone atrophy.

Etiology & Pathogenesis

Senile osteoporosis is present to some degree in most individuals over the age of 50 years. It is not

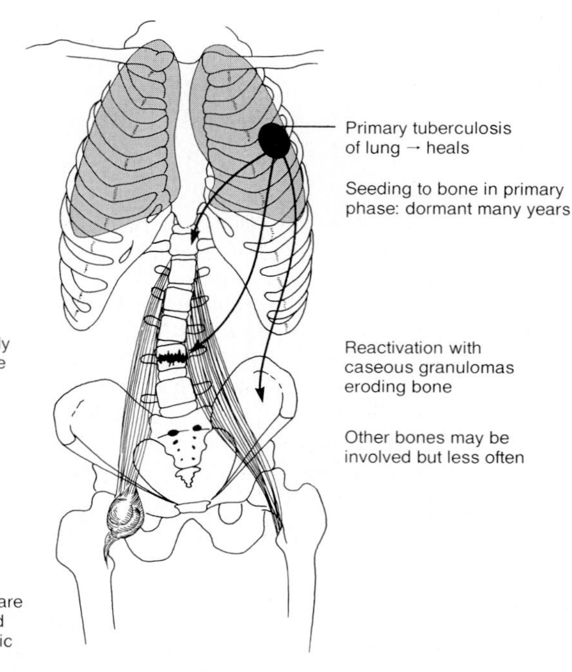

Figure 67–4. Pathogenesis and effects of tuberculosis of the spine (Pott's disease).

clear whether it is due to increased bone resorption or decreased bone formation (or both) or whether it is an integral part of the normal aging process. It is generally more severe in women after menopause (postmenopausal osteoporosis), probably a consequence of declining levels of estrogen. **Environmental factors** may play a role in osteoporosis in the elderly, eg, decreased physical activity and nutritional protein or vitamin deficiency.

Bone formation during remodeling is dependent on the presence of normal stress forces imposed during daily activities. Prolonged **immobilization** of any bone, by removing these normal stresses, causes disuse atrophy. A good example is the severe bone atrophy that occurs in hands of patients with severe rheumatoid arthritis whose inactivity contributes to the atrophy.

Osteoporosis also occurs in **endocrine diseases** such as Cushing's syndrome, hyperthyroidism, and acromegaly.

Many patients with osteoporosis are in **negative calcium balance,** due to decreased calcium absorption, increased urinary calcium loss, or both. While negative calcium balance is believed to play an important role, calcium supplements slow but do not reverse the process.

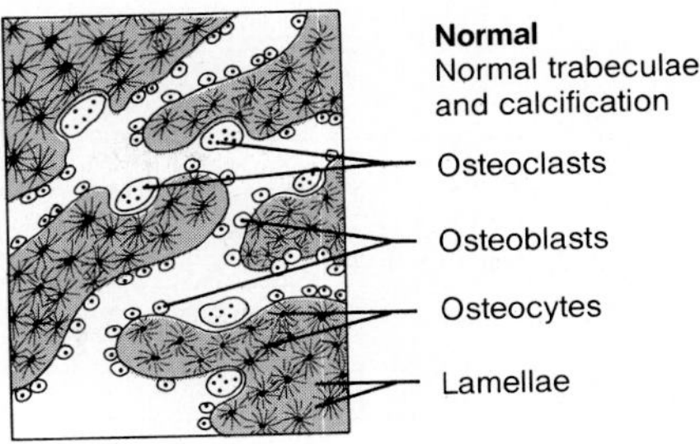

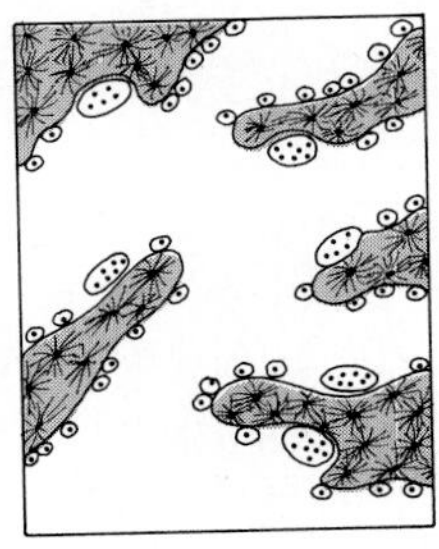

Osteomalacia
• Trabeculae normal in size but only partially calcified
• Surface shows "seams" of uncalcified osteoid
• Often increased osteoblasts
• Results:
- Soft bones
- Weakness
- Deformity
- Fracture

Hyperparathyroidism
• Increased osteoclasts erode bone
• Compensatory increase in osteoblasts insufficient to restore trabeculae
• Normal calcification of residual bone
• Fibrosis of marrow spaces with giant cells

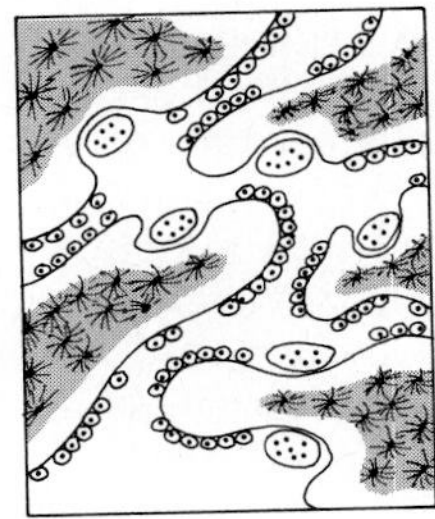

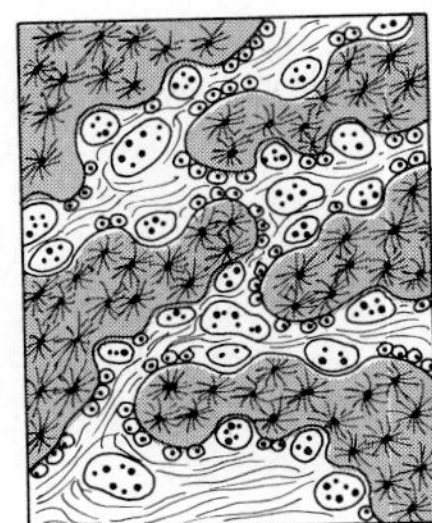

Figure 67–5. Pathologic changes in bone in metabolic bone diseases. In osteoporosis, the bone is qualitatively normal but decreased in amount; in osteomalacia and rickets, calcification does not occur normally in the osteoid produced by osteoblasts, resulting in wide uncalcified osteoid seams; in hyperparathyroidism, there is increased resorption of bone with proliferation of osteoclasts and fibrosis.

Pathology & Clinical Features

Osteoporosis affects all bones of the body but most commonly produces symptoms in the major weight-bearing and stress areas (vertebral bodies and femoral neck). The vertebral bodies show changes in shape, decreased height, and compression fractures. This results in a decrease in the overall height of the individual and abnormal vertebral curvature (kyphosis). Osteoporosis of the femoral neck predisposes to pathologic fractures (ie, fracture from minimal trauma), a common event in the elderly.

Affected bones have a decrease in their total mass and show thinning of the bony cortex and trabeculae (Fig 67–5). In mild cases, diagnosis is difficult because of the variation that exists in bone trabecular thickness in different "normal" individuals.

Diagnosis is possible both radiologically and histologically when severe osteoporosis is present. The structure of bone, as determined by chemical analysis of bone ash, shows no abnormality.

Patients with osteoporosis have normal serum levels of calcium, phosphate, and alkaline phosphatase (Table 67–1).

OSTEOMALACIA

Osteomalacia ("soft bone") is a structural abnormality of bone caused by defective mineralization of osteoid, which is produced in normal or increased amounts. Because it is not calcified normally, affected bones are soft.

Table 67-1. Laboratory findings in metabolic bone disease.

	Serum Calcium	Serum Phosphorus	Alkaline Phosphatase	Parathyroid Hormone (PTH)
Osteoporosis	N	N	N	N
Osteomalacia (rickets)	↓	↓(↑)[1]	↑	N(↑)
Primary hyperparathyroid bone disease	↑	↓	N↑	↑
Bone disease in renal failure—with secondary hyperparathyroidism	N↓	↑	↑	↑
Lytic bone neoplasms	N↑	N↑	N↑	N
Paget's disease of bone	N	N	↑	N

[1]Secondary increase in PTH production may elevate the serum phosphate level.

Etiology

Osteomalacia and its causes have been discussed in Chapter 10 with reference to vitamin D.

Pathology & Clinical Features

Microscopic examination of undecalcified bone shows the presence of **uncalcified osteoid,** usually in the form of wide seams on the outer aspect of bony trabeculae (Fig 67–5). This is diagnostic of osteomalacia. Note that the diagnosis is difficult if not impossible when the bone has been decalcified; special techniques to prepare sections of undecalcified bone are necessary.

Serum calcium levels are usually low in patients with vitamin D deficiency (Table 67–1). This may lead to increased secretion of parathyroid hormone and cause secondary elevation of serum phosphate.

Softening of bone leads to abnormal stresses in the bone, bone pain, and deformity. In the vertebral column, the vertebral bodies often become biconcave as a consequence of inward protrusion of the intervertebral disks. X-ray examination of bones shows deformities, decreased density of bones, and the presence of radiolucent bands (pseudofractures, or Looser's zones).

The changes of osteomalacia (except severe deformity) are reversible when **vitamin D** is replaced and calcium metabolism becomes normal.

HYPERPARATHYROIDISM (Osteitis Fibrosa Cystica)

Etiology

The etiology of hyperparathyroidism is discussed in Chapter 59. Bone changes are caused by elevated parathyroid hormone (PTH) levels and occur in both primary and secondary hyperparathyroidism.

Pathology

Increased PTH levels increase the rate of resorption of mineral from the bone, stimulating osteoclastic and fibroblastic activity in bone. The bone becomes thinned—best seen radiologically in the phalanges and in the mandible, where there is loss of the lamina dura (a radiopaque line normally present around the teeth).

Focal severe bone resorption may lead to cyst formation in the bone and to fibrosis (osteitis fibrosa cystica).

Microscopically, there is marked proliferation of osteoclastic giant cells and fibroblasts (Fig 67–5). When this is focal, nodular masses called brown tumors may occur in the bone. Brown tumors appear clinically as space-occupying masses and histologically resemble the neoplastic giant cell tumor of bone.

Clinical Features

Bone changes of hyperparathyroidism are usually asymptomatic and are usually observed as incidental radiologic findings in patients presenting with other features of hyperparathyroidism (Chapter 59). Rarely, bone pain, fractures, cysts, and mass lesions occur.

The bone changes regress when hyperparathyroidism is cured.

MISCELLANEOUS BONE DISEASES OF UNCERTAIN CAUSE

PAGET'S DISEASE OF BONE (Osteitis Deformans)

Paget's disease, which is characterized by thickening and disturbance of the architecture of bone, is very common: About 3% of the population over 50 years of age in the United States and Western Europe show radiologic evidence of Paget's disease. It is rare in blacks and in natives of Asia. Most cases are asymptomatic. The disease is rare in persons under 50 years of age. Men are affected somewhat more commonly than women.

Etiology & Pathology

The cause is unknown. The finding of viruslike particles in affected bones has led to the suggestion that Paget's disease may represent a slow virus infection of bone. Other studies have implicated measles virus.

Paget's disease may involve one bone (monostotic) or many (polyostotic). The bones most commonly involved are the pelvis, skull, spine, scapula, femur, tibia, humerus, and mandible.

The disease progresses through 3 stages: (1) In the first stage, there is irregular osteoclastic resorption of bone. (2) In the second stage, osteoblasts react by actively laying down new bone, which balances the osteolysis and maintains the total bone volume. The disease can be recognized at this stage by the irregular manner in which osteoblasts lay down trabeculae. The new bone is highly vascular, producing the physiologic effect of an arteriovenous fistula. (3) Finally, there is a sclerotic phase in which osteoblastic activity is greatly in excess of osteoclastic resorption, leading to marked thickening of bony trabeculae and cortex.

Histologically, affected bone shows thickened trabeculae with irregularly arranged cement lines (mosaic pattern). The irregularity of bone structure is best seen by polarized light. Abnormal mineralization of bone may produce focal collections of uncalcified osteoid.

Clinical Features

Early Paget's disease is asymptomatic. Pain in affected bone in the later stages is the most common symptom. Thickening of bone may cause deformities such as enlargement of the head—an increase in hat size is a common and perplexing symptom in patients who wear hats—abnormal vertebral curvatures, and bowing of the tibias and femurs. Fractures may occur, particularly in the spine.

Thickening of the bone may impinge on nerves that leave bony foramens, causing symptoms of nerve compression and radicular pain.

Serum calcium, phosphorus, and parathyroid hormone levels are normal. Serum alkaline phosphatase levels are greatly elevated, reflecting the marked osteoblastic activity (Table 67–1).

Complications

The arteriovenous fistula effect resulting from extreme hypervascularity in involved bones may be sufficient to cause high-output heart failure.

Paget's disease is associated with an increased risk (2–5%) of developing malignant neoplasms in the involved bones—most often osteosarcoma, with fibrosarcoma and chondrosarcoma occurring less commonly.

FIBROUS DYSPLASIA

Fibrous dysplasia is a focal slowly expanding lesion in which the bone is replaced by a mass of fibroblasts, collagen, and irregular bony trabeculae. Note that the term "dysplasia" here has a meaning different from its usual one, since fibrous dysplasia is not associated with cytologic abnormalities and there is no malignant potential.

Pathology & Clinical Features

Fibrous dysplasia occurs in 2 forms: monostotic and polyostotic.

A. Monostotic Fibrous Dysplasia: Fibrous dysplasia affecting a single bone is common and may occur at any age. Any bone may be involved, most often the lower extremities, skull, mandible, or ribs.

Pathologically, there is replacement of the affected area by proliferating fibroblasts in which are scattered trabeculae of irregular bone. The usual rim of osteoblasts around the bony trabeculae is absent. The lesion appears on x-ray as a well-defined circumscribed radiolucent area.

Clinically, fibrous dysplasia may produce pain, deformity, or pathologic fracture. Often it is detected radiologically as an incidental lytic lesion.

B. Polyostotic Fibrous Dysplasia: Rarely, fibrous dysplasia affects many bones, causing deformities and fractures. **Albright's syndrome** is a form of polyostotic fibrous dysplasia in which there are multiple unilateral bone lesions associated with endocrine abnormalities (precocious puberty is the commonest result) and unilateral pigmented skin lesions.

FIBROUS CORTICAL DEFECT

Fibrous cortical defect (sometimes called nonossifying fibroma or fibroxanthoma) is a common lesion that is believed to be of developmental origin. The term fibrous cortical defect is preferred over nonossifying fibroma and fibroxanthoma because the lesion is not a true neoplasm. It occurs in children, most commonly affecting the tibia, fibula, and femur.

Pathologically, a small area of the bony cortex is replaced by well-demarcated, soft, yellowish-gray tissue composed of fibroblasts, scattered foamy histiocytes, and giant cells. There is no new bone formation.

Patients present typically with nocturnal pain in the legs. Radiologic examination shows a circular, punched-out area of radiolucency surrounded by normal bone. The lesion is important to recognize because no treatment is necessary. Fibrous cortical defects disappear spontaneously after a variable interval.

BONE CYSTS

1. UNICAMERAL BONE CYST (Solitary Bone Cyst)

Unicameral bone cyst is an uncommon lesion affecting long bones in children and young adults. It is thought to result from a local developmental defect. The metaphysis is the favored site. The cyst contains clear or yellowish fluid and is lined by connective tissue, granulation tissue, collagen, and histiocytes, with hemosiderin deposition and cholesterol clefts.

Unicameral bone cyst commonly presents with pain, as a mass, or as a pathologic fracture.

2. ANEURYSMAL BONE CYST

Aneurysmal bone cyst is uncommon. It occurs most often in the age group from 10 to 20 years. It affects vertebrae and flat bones more commonly than long bones.

Pathologically, aneurysmal bone cyst usually appears as a large destructive lesion causing expansion of bone. It is usually multicystic and hemorrhagic, with a thin rim of bone at its outer surface. Microscopic examination shows large, endothelium-lined hemorrhagic spaces surrounded by proliferating cells bearing a close resemblance to giant cell tumor of bone. There are numerous osteoclastlike giant cells and smaller spindle cells.

The radiologic appearance is characterized by a well-circumscribed lytic lesion that greatly expands the involved bone.

NEOPLASMS OF BONE (Table 67-2)

By far the commonest neoplasm of bone, excluding leukemic involvement of bone marrow, is **metastatic carcinoma**. While any malignant neoplasm can metastasize to bone, the most frequent tumors that do so in adults are carcinomas of the lung, prostate, breast, thyroid, kidney, and colon. In children, neuroblastoma is the commonest skeletal metastasis. Eosinophilic granuloma and Hand-Schüller-Christian disease, part of the spectrum of histiocytosis X (see Chapter 29) also produce lytic lesions of bone, including the skull.

The more common **benign primary bone neoplasms** are osteochondroma, chondroma, and giant cell tumor. **Malignant primary bone neoplasms** tend to occur most often in children, with osteosarcoma and Ewing's sarcoma being the most common types. Chondrosarcoma is more common in adults.

The pathologic diagnosis of bone neoplasms should always be made with full clinical and radiologic correlation (When taking a specimen of a bone neoplasm to a pathologist, one should take the radiographs along.)

BENIGN NEOPLASMS OF BONE

1. OSTEOCHONDROMA

Osteochondroma (also called osteocartilaginous exostosis) is the commonest benign bone neoplasm. Most occur in children and young adults, and the common sites of involvement are the lower femur, upper tibia, humerus, and pelvis. The great majority are solitary. Rarely, multiple osteochondromas occur in familial distribution (called diaphyseal aclasis, multiple exostoses) with an autosomal dominant inheritance.

Osteochondromas vary in size, and the larger lesions may project outward from the cortex of the bone on a short stalk angled away from the growing end of the bone. Histologically, the stalk is composed of mature bone upon which there is a cap of hyaline cartilage.

Malignant transformation of solitary osteochondromas is very rare (the cartilage transforms into a chondrosarcoma). However, chondrosarcoma occurs more commonly (10% incidence) in patients with familial multiple osteochondromatosis.

2. CHONDROMA

Chondroma is a common benign neoplasm occurring most often in the diaphyseal medulla (enchondromas). The small bones of the hands and feet are the commonest sites, with ribs and long bones affected less frequently. About 30% of patients have more than one lesion. **Multiple enchondromas** may occur as a familial disease inherited as an autosomal dominant trait (Ollier's disease).

Enchondroma appears as a firm, well-circumscribed, glistening white mass that expands the bone from the center and causes thinning of the cortex. Microscopically, it is composed of lobules of hyaline cartilage of low cellularity.

Malignant transformation does not occur in solitary enchondromas. There is an increased risk of chondrosarcoma in patients with Ollier's disease.

Table 67-2. Bone neoplasms.

Neoplasm	Behavior	Age	Bones Commonly Involved	Location	Histologic Features
Neoplasms of osteoblasts					
Osteoma	Benign	40–50	Skull, facial bones	Flat bones	Dense, mature lamellar bone.
Osteoid osteoma	Benign	10–30	Femur, tibia, humerus, hands and feet, vertebrae	Cortex of metaphysis	Sharply demarcated with a nidus composed of highly vascular osteoblastic connective tissue and osteoid. Surrounded by sclerotic bone; smaller than 2 cm.
Osteoblastoma	Benign; rarely aggressive	10–30	Vertebrae, tibia, femur, humerus, pelvis, ribs	Medulla of metaphysis	Resembles the nidus of osteoid osteoma; larger than 2 cm.
Osteosarcoma	Malignant; 20% 5-year survival rate	10–25	Femur, tibia, humerus, pelvis, jaw	Medulla of metaphysis	Highly cellular, pleomorphic, abnormal osteoblasts with high mitotic rate; osteoid present; invasive.
Parosteal osteosarcoma	Malignant; 80% 5-year survival rate	30–60	Femur, tibia, humerus	Periosteal surface	Spindle cells alternating with bone-forming osteoblasts; well-differentiated.
Neoplasms of chondroblasts					
Chondroma	Benign	10–40	Hands and feet, ribs	Diaphysis	Well-differentiated hyaline cartilage.
Osteochondroma (exostosis)	Benign	10–30	Femur, tibia, humerus, pelvis	Cortex of metaphysis	Projecting mass composed of a bony stalk and cap of hyaline cartilage.
Chondroblastoma	Benign	10–25	Femur, humerus, tibia, pelvis, scapula, feet	Epiphysis	Uniform small round cells and giant cells; very cellular; chondroid areas.
Chondrosarcoma	Malignant; 30% (grade III) to 90% (grade I) 5-year survival rate	30–60	Pelvis, ribs, femur, vertebrae, humerus	Diaphysis and metaphysis	Malignant chondrocytes with variable anaplasia (grades I–III); chondroid stroma.
Unknown cell of origin					
Giant cell tumor	Benign; 50% recur locally	20–40	Femur, tibia, radius	Metaphysis and epiphysis	Very cellular; small spindle cells with numerous osteoclast-like giant cells.
Ewing's sarcoma	Malignant; 25% 5-year survival rate	5–20	Femur, pelvis, tibia, humerus, ribs, fibula	Diaphysis	Anaplastic small round cells with high mitotic rate.

3. CHONDROBLASTOMA

Chondroblastoma is an uncommon benign neoplasm of bone, occurring mainly in persons under the age of 20 years. There is a 2:1 male:female preponderance. Sites commonly affected are the distal femur, the proximal tibia, and the proximal humerus.

Chondroblastoma occurs in the epiphyseal region. Radiologically, it appears as a well-demarcated lucent lesion that may show calcification.

Microscopically, chondroblastoma is highly cellular. The dominant cell is an embryonic chondroblast that appears as a small uniform round cell with scant cytoplasm; these cells are quite uniform, with little mitotic activity. Multinucleated osteoclastlike giant cells are frequently present. Areas of cartilage formation are usually present. Calcification is common.

4. GIANT CELL TUMOR OF BONE (Osteoclastoma)

Giant cell tumor is a relatively common bone neoplasm that usually occurs in patients in the age group from 20 to 40 years. Sites commonly affected are the distal femur, proximal tibia, distal radius, and proximal humerus. The cell of origin is not known. The term giant cell tumor is preferred to osteoclastoma because the latter suggests an origin from osteoclasts.

Giant cell tumors are located in the epiphyseal region, with expansion of involved bone and thinning of the cortex. Extension into soft tissues occurs in about 20% of cases. Radiologically, giant cell tumors appear as a lytic mass traversed by thin sclerotic lines (''soap-bubble'' appearance).

Grossly, there is often hemorrhage and cystic degeneration (Fig 67–6). Microscopic examination (Fig 67–7) shows proliferation of small neoplastic spindle cells of unknown origin. Numerous osteoclastlike multinucleated giant cells are present but are probably not the critical neoplastic cells.

Most giant cell tumors are benign, but they have a high (50%) recurrence rate after surgical excision, leading some pathologists to regard them as locally aggressive neoplasms. Local recurrence cannot be predicted by the histologic features. Metastases occur in 10% of giant cell tumors, which must be regarded as being malignant. Malignancy correlates best with the presence of a high mitotic rate in the small stromal cells.

Giant cell tumor is difficult to differentiate histologically from aneurysmal bone cyst (see above) and brown tumor of hyperparathyroidism (Chapter 59). Careful clinical correlation, including the radiologic appearance and the serum calcium and parathyroid hormone levels, are often necessary to make the distinction.

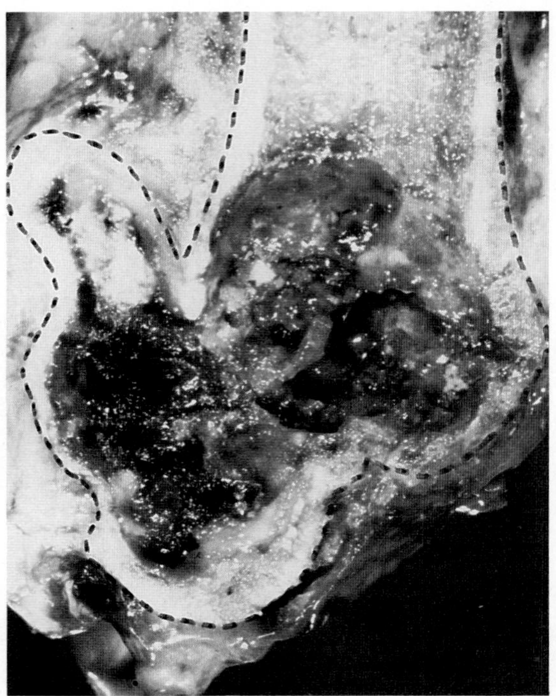

Figure 67–6. Giant cell tumor of the distal end of the femur, showing expansion of the bone end by a well-circumscribed mass composed of fleshy tumor that has replaced the bone. A thin rim of bone is present around the mass. The outline of the bone is indicated by the dotted lines.

5. OSTEOMA

Osteoma is an uncommon solitary benign neoplasm, almost totally confined to the skull and facial bones. Osteomas occur commonly in patients with Gardner's syndrome (familial colonic adenomatous polyposis with mesenchymal lesions). Osteoma is composed of a circumscribed mass of dense sclerotic bone.

6. OSTEOID OSTEOMA

Osteoid osteoma is an uncommon benign neoplasm of bone, occurring mainly in the 10- to 30-year age group. Males are more commonly affected than females. Favored sites include the cortices of the femur, tibia, and humerus. Patients typically present with severe pain. X-rays show a well-demarcated lucent area (up to 1.5 cm in diameter) in the cortex with a circumscribed rim of sclerotic reactive bone.

Microscopic examination shows the central nidus to be highly vascular, with numerous proliferating osteoblasts. Uncalcified osteoid is present in

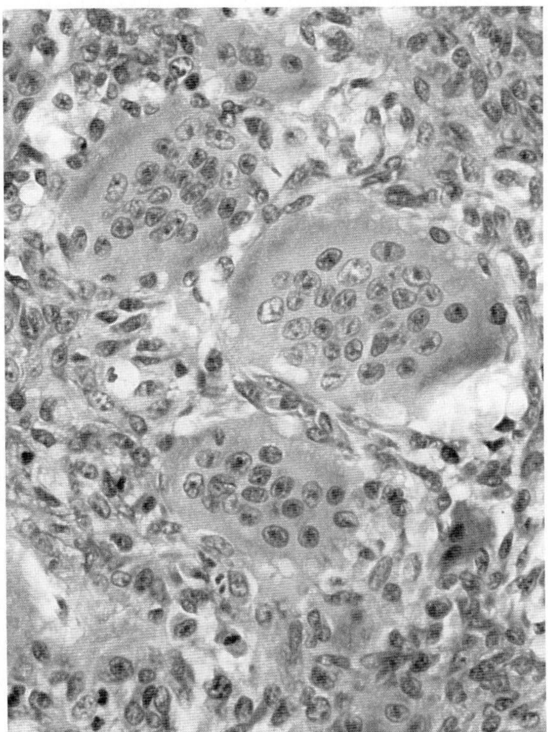

Figure 67–7. Giant cell tumor of bone, showing numerous osteoclastlike giant cells and intervening small spindle cells.

the central nidus. The nidus is surrounded by a rim of sclerotic bone.

Surgical removal is curative.

7. OSTEOBLASTOMA

Osteoblastoma is an uncommon bone neoplasm that occurs mainly in the age group from 10 to 30 years. Osteoblastomas occur all over the skeleton, the vertebrae being their commonest location. Patients usually present with pain and radiologically show an irregular lytic lesion.

Microscopically, osteoblastoma is indistinguishable from the central nidus of an osteoid osteoma—and for this reason, osteoblastoma is sometimes called giant osteoid osteoma. However, osteoblastoma differs from osteoid osteoma in that it is larger, usually exceeding 2 cm in diameter; it lacks the surrounding sclerotic reactive bone formation; and it arises in the medulla of the bone—in contrast to osteoid osteoma, which arises in the cortex.

Osteoblastomas are benign. Rarely, they behave in a locally aggressive manner, recurring after surgical removal. In some cases, the histologic distinction from well-differentiated osteosarcoma is difficult.

MALIGNANT NEOPLASMS OF BONE

1. OSTEOSARCOMA

Osteosarcoma is the commonest malignant neoplasm of bone. It affects mainly individuals in the age group from 10 to 25 years. There is a second peak in age incidence in the sixth decade, when osteosarcoma may complicate Paget's disease of bone.

Etiology

Several etiologic factors have been identified but account for only a minority of cases. An epidemic of osteosarcoma was reported in radium watch dial painters due to deposition of radioactive radium in bone (see Chapter 18). Thorotrast—a formerly used radiographic contrast medium that contained radioactive thorium dioxide—has been linked to the production of osteosarcoma as well as liver neoplasms.

Paget's disease of bone is complicated by mesenchymal neoplasms, most commonly osteosarcoma.

Pathology

Osteosarcoma arises most commonly in the medullary cavity of the metaphyseal region of long bones (Fig 67–8). The lower end of the femur, the upper tibia, and the upper humerus are the commonest locations. Rarely, osteosarcoma arises in the periosteum (periosteal osteosarcoma) or on its outer surface (parosteal osteosarcoma).

Grossly, osteosarcoma presents as a fleshy mass with areas of necrosis and hemorrhage (Fig 67–9). Bone and cartilage formation may be present. The involved bone is expanded by the tumor, which may infiltrate the medullary cavity and the soft tissues outside the bone. Radiologically, osteosarcomas present as irregular destructive lesions. The degree of calcification determines the radiopacity.

Osteosarcoma is an aggressive neoplasm that infiltrates widely. Hematogenous metastasis, most commonly to the lungs, occurs early. Lymphatic metastasis and tumor involvement of lymph nodes is rare.

Microscopically, osteosarcoma is composed of malignant osteoblasts with anaplasia and a high mitotic rate (Fig 67–10). Based on the degree of anaplasia, osteosarcomas are classified as grades I–III; patients with grade I tumors have longer survival.

Variable amounts of osteoid are produced by the tumor cells and may become calcified (tumor bone). The presence of osteoid in a malignant

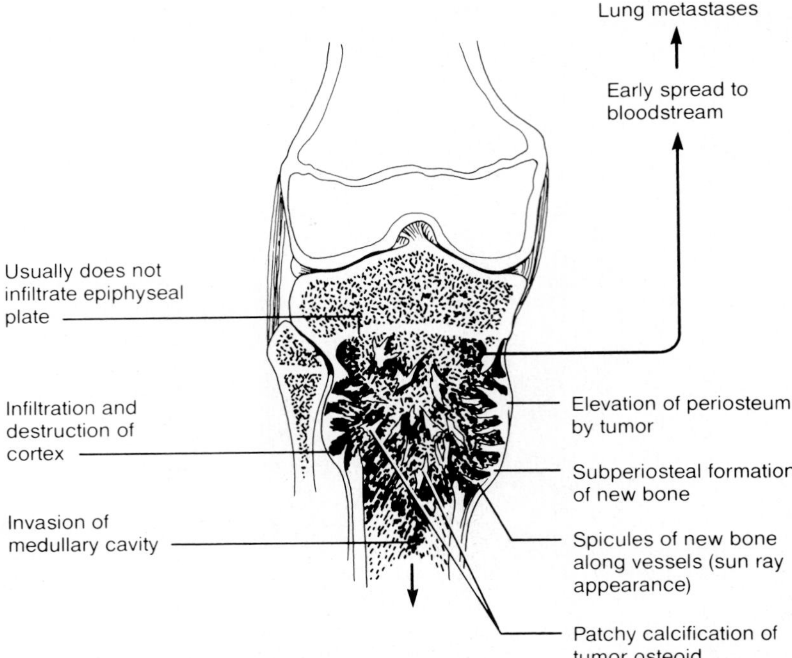

Figure 67-8. Osteosarcoma (diagrammatic), showing the typical metaphyseal location of the tumor, which destroys bone and induces reactive subperiosteal bone formation.

bone tumor establishes the diagnosis of osteosarcoma. Cartilage formation also is common and may be extensive (chondroblastic osteosarcoma). In some cases, numerous giant cells may be seen. In others, cavernous vascular spaces dominate the histologic picture (telangiectatic osteosarcoma).

Clinical Features

Osteosarcoma usually presents with a bony mass with or without pain. It is a rapidly growing tumor that tends to spread at an early stage via the bloodstream. It is not uncommon for patients to have evidence of metastases—most commonly pulmonary—at the time of presentation.

Osteosarcoma is sensitive to both radiation and modern chemotherapeutic agents but is not considered curable with these modalities. Surgery is the preferred treatment for early limb lesions. The 5-year survival rate is 25–30%.

2. CHONDROSARCOMA

Chondrosarcoma accounts for about 20% of primary malignant neoplasms of bone. It is most often seen in persons in the age group from 30 to 60 years, in whom it represents the commonest primary malignant bone neoplasm. Males are affected twice as frequently as females. Most cases occur as solitary neoplasms; a few cases occur in patients with familial multiple osteochondromatosis and familial enchondromatosis (Ollier's disease).

Pathology

The pelvic girdle, ribs, shoulder girdle, long bones, vertebrae, and sternum are affected—in decreasing order of frequency.

Grossly, chondrosarcoma appears as a large destructive mass with a characteristic translucent whitish appearance because of the chondroid stroma. Radiologically, chondrosarcomas are infiltrative masses that expand the bone. They commonly show flocculent calcification.

Microscopically, chondrosarcomas consist of malignant chondrocytes in a chondroid matrix. In the well-differentiated grade I chondrosarcomas, the number of cells is only slightly increased but the nuclei are enlarged, with many lacunae containing more than one cell. Differential diagnosis from enchondroma is difficult; the site of the lesion is helpful, because cartilaginous neoplasms in the hands and feet are almost always benign and those in the axial skeleton are usually malignant.

Grade II chondrosarcomas have increased cellularity and loss of differentiation. Grade III lesions are composed of malignant spindle cells with scant chondroid stroma.

Clinical Features

A bony mass or fracture may be the first indication of tumor. Metastasis occurs relatively late and usually through the bloodstream. Chondrosarcomas tend to be more radioresistant than osteosarcomas and do not respond to chemotherapy. Surgery is the principal means of treatment.

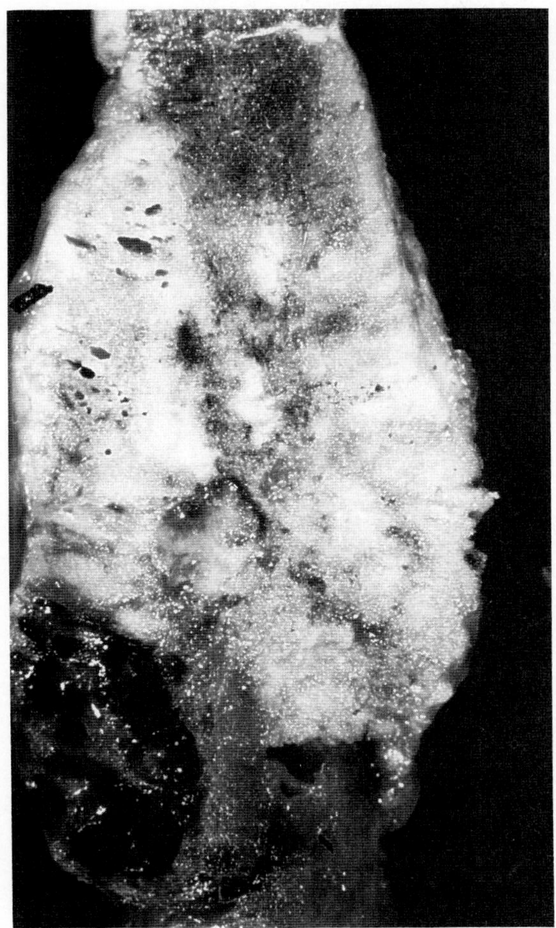

Figure 67-9. Osteosarcoma of the fibula, showing a solid destructive lesion involving the metaphyseal region.

The prognosis depends on the grade. Grade I chondrosarcoma has a 90% 5-year survival rate; grade III lesions have a 5-year survival rate of about 30–40%.

3. EWING'S SARCOMA

Ewing's sarcoma is uncommon. It occurs in children and young adults (5–30 years). Males are affected twice as frequently as females. Initially thought (by Ewing) to be of endothelial origin, this tumor is now believed to be derived from neuroectodermal cells—on the basis of neuron-specific enolase positivity, detectable cholinergic transmitter enzymes, and the consistent presence of a t(11–22) translocation, which has been reported in some other neuroepithelial tumors. The presence of the t(11–22) translocation is useful in distinguishing Ewing's sarcoma from neuroblastoma (which commonly shows partial monosomy 1). *C-MYC* expression is frequently detectable.

Ewing's sarcoma arises in the long bones, ribs, pelvic bones, and vertebrae and expands to destroy the medullary cavity, bony cortex, and surrounding soft tissues (Fig 67–11). Radiologically, it appears as a destructive radiolucent lesion in the diaphysis, infiltrating the cortex from within. Reactive periosteal bone formation may produce a laminated appearance.

Grossly, the neoplasm is soft and friable, with areas of necrosis and hemorrhage. Microscopically, it is characterized by sheets of proliferating small round to oval cells with a hyperchromatic nucleus and scant cytoplasm. Mitotic figures are numerous. The presence of glycogen in the cytoplasm (which gives a positive reaction with periodic acid-Schiff reagent) is a helpful diagnostic feature.

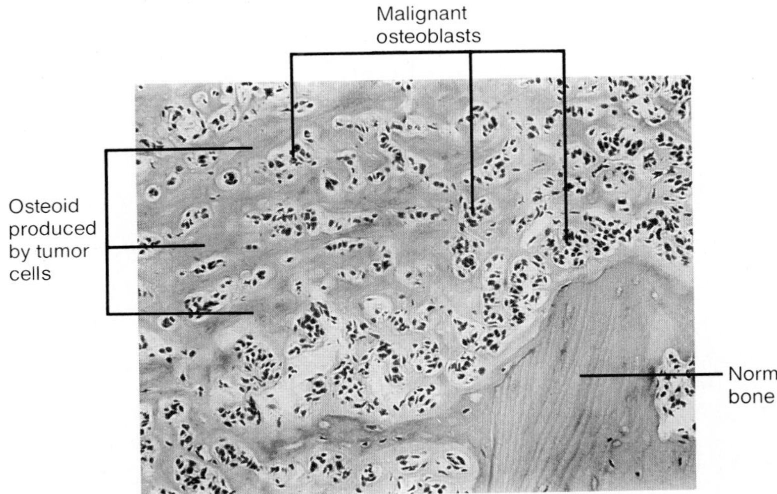

Figure 67–10. Osteosarcoma, showing small malignant osteoblastic cells surrounded by osteoid, which appears as a homogeneous material between the malignant cells. Contrast this with the residual normal bone spicule.

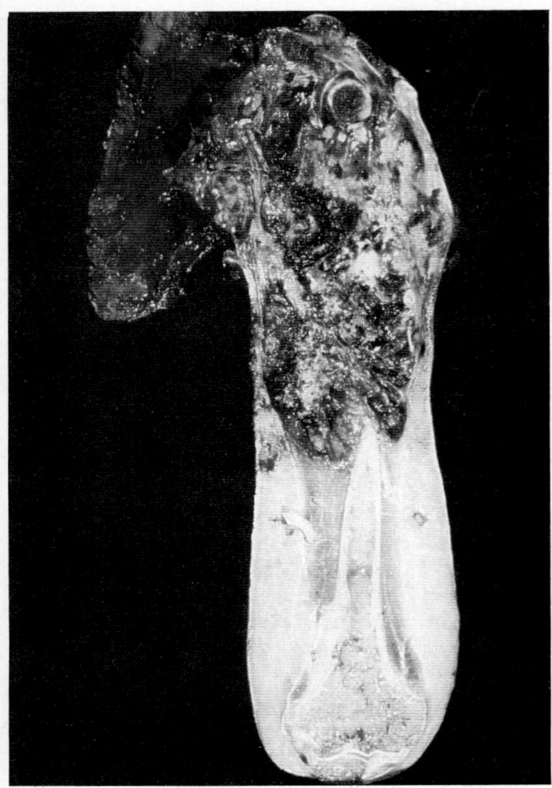

Figure 67-11. Ewing's sarcoma, showing complete destruction of the upper half of the humerus by a tumor that has extensively infiltrated the extraosseous soft tissues.

Ewing's sarcoma is a rapidly growing, highly malignant neoplasm that tends to spread via the bloodstream at an early stage. Response to both radiation and chemotherapy is poor; the 5-year survival rate is about 10%.

4. LYMPHOID NEOPLASMS

The leukemias, multiple myeloma, and neoplasms of bone marrow are described in Chapters 26, 29, and 30.

Diseases of Joints & Connective Tissue

68

I. DISORDERS OF JOINTS

STRUCTURE OF JOINTS

Joints are specialized areas of the skeletal system situated between 2 bones, permitting postural movements: flexion, extension, rotation, etc (Fig 68–1). The ends of the bone in the joint cavity are covered with smooth hyaline cartilage (articular cartilage). The joint is held together by a joint capsule composed of collagen, which is strengthened by ligaments. The inside of the joint capsule is lined by a layer of flat synovial cells that secrete synovial fluid. The synovial fluid in the joint cavity serves as a lubricant.

CLINICAL MANIFESTATIONS OF JOINT DISEASE

Joint Pain (Arthralgia)

Most joint diseases cause pain. The term arthralgia is used when there is joint pain without evidence of acute inflammation. When pain is accompanied by other features of inflammation such as swelling, redness, and increased temperature, the term arthritis is used.

Joint Swelling

Joint swelling is the result of an increase in synovial fluid volume. It may result from fluid exudation in inflammatory conditions or from bleeding. Swelling due to bleeding is called **hemarthrosis.** Fluid imparts a fluctuant feel and pro-

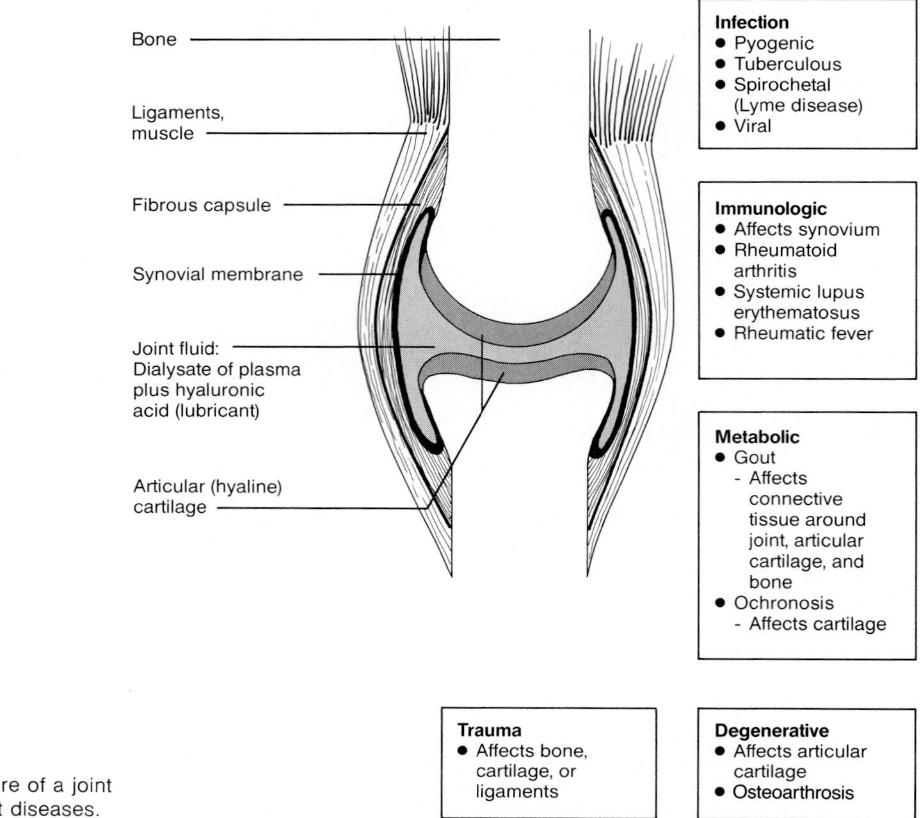

Figure 68-1. Structure of a joint and the principal joint diseases.

duces a wave when tapped that can be felt on the side opposite to tapping (fluid thrill).

Joint Mass Lesions

An increase in size of a joint may result from the presence of solid tissue within the cavity. This occurs in rare neoplastic lesions of joints. The distinction between a mass lesion and fluid can be made by x-ray examination, needle aspiration, and careful clinical examination: A mass lesion produces a "boggy" feel, compared to the fluctuant feel of fluid, and a fluid thrill is absent.

Joint Crepitus

The movement of one articular surface on another is normally smooth and silent. Crepitus is an abnormal sensation and sound of grating that accompanies joint movement. Since the articular cartilage represents the rubbing surface of a normal joint, crepitus occurs in diseases associated with loss of articular cartilage and exposure of subchondral bone.

Abnormal Joint Mobility

Most joint diseases result in restricted range of motion in the affected joints due to pain or stiffness. Rarely, the range of motion may be increased, as when structural components that hold the joint together are damaged. Tearing of cruciate ligaments in the knee and the general destruction associated with neuropathic joints are examples of disorders associated with an abnormal increase of joint mobility. Increased joint mobility may also be seen in congenital diseases characterized by abnormal collagen synthesis (eg, Ehlers-Danlos syndrome).

EVALUATION OF JOINT DISEASE

Physical Examination

Physical examination permits detection of acute inflammation which is characterized by swelling, redness, increased temperature, tenderness, and restriction of motion. The presence of joint swelling is best assessed by measurement of its circumference and comparing with the normal counterpart in the case of paired joints. With some joints (eg, atlantoaxial, intervertebral), the presence of inflammation may be difficult to establish. Joint swelling may be caused by fluid (fluctuant with a fluid thrill), blood, or solid mass.

Many joint diseases are characterized by abnormal mobility and crepitus.

X-Ray Abnormalities

The joint space as seen on an x-ray is occupied by articular cartilage, synovium, intra-articular ligaments, and synovial fluid, all of which are normally radiolucent. Radiologic abnormalities may include (1) an increase in the joint space when there is fluid, blood, a solid mass lesion, or proliferation of the synovium; (2) decreased joint space in diseases associated with degeneration of the articular cartilage; (3) abnormalities in articular cartilage, such as opacification, and subchondral bone, such as erosion and cyst formation; and (4) the presence of abnormal loose bodies in the joint space.

Laboratory Evaluation

Examination of aspirated synovial fluid is very useful in the diagnosis of inflammatory and metabolic diseases (Table 68–1). Fluid is cultured and examined chemically and microscopically for its protein content, specific gravity, the presence and type of inflammatory cells, and the presence of urate and calcium pyrophosphate crystals.

Many joint diseases cause serologic abnormalities. These are considered with the individual diseases.

Arthroscopic Examination

Insertion of a fiberoptic arthroscope into the joint space through a small incision in the joint capsule permits direct visualization of the joint. Biopsies may be taken of synovium and mass lesions. Arthroscopy also permits repair of intra-articular injuries.

Table 68–1. Changes in synovial fluid in disease of joints.

Disease	Findings
Pyogenic arthritis	Purulent fluid exudate; large numbers of neutrophils; culture positive for bacteria
Tuberculosus arthritis	Fluid exudate (high protein and specific gravity); neutrophils and mononuclear cells; culture positive for *Mycobacterium tuberculosis*
Rheumatoid arthritis	Clear fluid, high protein content; inflammatory cells: neutrophils and mononuclear cells; increased immunoglobulins and complement; rheumatoid factor present in many cases
Osteoarthrosis	Clear fluid, high protein content; no inflammatory cells
Gout	Urate crystals
Chondrocalcinosis	Calcium pyrophosphate crystals

CONGENITAL DISORDERS OF JOINTS

CONGENITAL DISLOCATION OF THE HIP

Deficient development of the acetabulum in an infant allows the femoral head to ride upward out of the joint socket (subluxation) when weight-bearing begins. This defect is much more common in females and shows a familial tendency. Unless it is corrected soon after birth, abnormal stresses cause malformation of the developing femoral neck, with a characteristic limp (if unilateral) or waddling gait (if bilateral).

Treatment requires early diagnosis with splinting of the hips in abduction during the first few months of life to allow development of the acetabulum.

TALIPES EQUINOVARUS & CALCANEOVALGUS (Clubfoot)

The 2 forms of clubfoot represent abnormal articulation of the small bones of the foot due to abnormal intrauterine forces, abnormal fetal muscle action, or defective ligament insertion. Treatment should be started at birth.

INFECTIOUS DISEASES OF JOINTS

PYOGENIC ARTHRITIS

Pyogenic arthritis is usually caused by *Staphylococcus aureus*. Less frequently, *Streptococcus pyogenes, Streptococcus pneumoniae, Neisseria gonorrhoeae,* and *Haemophilus influenzae* are responsible. The route of infection is hematogenous, and in most patients the primary access site of the pathogen is unknown. In a few patients, pyogenic arthritis complicates acute osteomyelitis (Chapter 67).

Pathology & Clinical Features

Pyogenic arthritis is an acute inflammation that commonly involves a single large joint such as the knee or hip, characterized by severe pain, tenderness, redness, swelling, and local warmth. There is marked restriction of movement. The joint space becomes filled with a purulent exudate. High fever, often with chills and a neutrophil leukocytosis, is present in most cases.

Diagnosis & Treatment

The diagnosis of pyogenic arthritis is made by clinical examination. Drainage of the joint forms part of the treatment and provides fluid for culture. Antibiotic therapy is usually effective. In untreated cases, infection spreads to the articular cartilage and adjacent bone, causing destruction and permanent disability. Life-threatening bacteremia may rarely develop.

TUBERCULOUS ARTHRITIS

Tuberculous arthritis has become rare in developed countries. It occurs in adults by reactivation of a dormant tuberculous focus in the joint and is often the only manifestation of tuberculosis in the body.

Tuberculous arthritis is characterized by involvement of a single large joint, most commonly the knee, hip, or wrist. The affected joint is swollen and painful, but other features of acute inflammation are not present. Diagnosis depends on culture of joint fluid or examination of a synovial biopsy specimen.

LYME DISEASE

Lyme disease is an infection caused by *Borrelia burgdorferi.* It was first described in Lyme, Connecticut. It is prevalent in northeastern USA, but cases have been reported elsewhere in the USA, in Europe, and in 20 countries on 6 continents. The disease is transmitted by ixodid ticks, which become infected by biting deer and mice, which are the common reservoirs of infection.

Lyme disease is characterized by development of a distinctive papular skin rash (erythema migrans) at the site of inoculation 1–4 weeks after the tick bite. The rash lasts several months and may be associated with spirochetemia and systemic disease. Migratory acute arthritis is one of the most common manifestations of systemic disease and may be followed by chronic arthritis. The synovial membrane shows thickening, with a lymphocytic and histiocytic infiltrate. Organisms are present in the walls of small blood vessels, blood, and synovial fluid. Myocarditis and neurologic abnormalities may also occur.

The diagnosis of Lyme disease is confirmed by serologic tests. Demonstration of the spirochete in blood or infected tissues is rarely successful. Treatment with penicillin or tetracycline is successful if started early in the acute phase and prevents chronic arthritis and other complications.

VIRAL ARTHRITIS

Viral infection of joints has been described in patients with rubella and viral hepatitis, but the incidence is low. Viral arthritis is usually transient and resolves completely.

IMMUNOLOGIC DISEASES OF JOINTS

RHEUMATOID ARTHRITIS

Rheumatoid arthritis is a chronic disease of unknown cause characterized by progressive and potentially deforming arthritis.

Incidence

Rheumatoid arthritis is common in the United States and Western Europe, affecting 1–3% of the population. Females are affected 2–3 times more frequently than males. The highest age incidence is between 30 and 50 years. Rheumatoid arthritis is uncommon in tropical countries.

Etiology

The exact cause of rheumatoid arthritis is unknown (Fig 68–2). Rheumatoid factor—an autoantibody (usually IgM) reactive against the patient's own IgG—is present in the plasma of about 90% of patients with rheumatoid arthritis, but its presence is not specific for rheumatoid arthritis (Fig 68–3). Immune complexes composed of rheumatoid factor and IgG have been found in the synovial fluid of some patients with rheumatoid arthritis. Complement levels are also frequently decreased in active disease, suggesting that complement activation by deposited immune complexes may play a role.

The synovial membrane in patients with rheumatoid arthritis is infiltrated by numerous lymphocytes and plasma cells.

Pathology

The synovial membrane of affected joints becomes swollen, congested, and thickened, with granulation tissue containing numerous lymphocytes and plasma cells (this fleshy tissue is termed **pannus**). Neutrophils are scarce in the synovial tissue but abundant in synovial fluid.

The pannus eventually erodes articular cartilage, subchondral bone, and periarticular ligaments and tendons. Progressive destruction of the

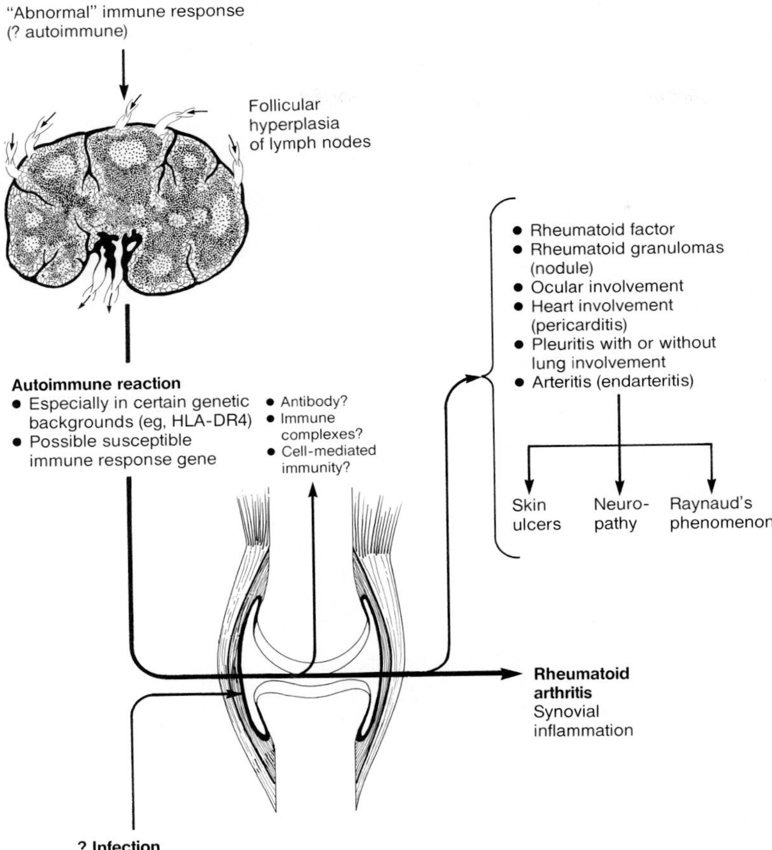

Figure 68–2. Proposed etiologic factors and pathologic effects of rheumatoid arthritis.

joint follows, with fibrosis, increasing deformity, and restriction of movement.

Clinical Features

Rheumatoid arthritis typically presents with symmetric involvement of the small joints of the hands and feet—classically, the proximal interphalangeal joints (Fig 68–4). Involvement of larger joints is the initial manifestation in a minority of patients.

Involved joints are swollen, painful, and stiff. Stiffness is maximal in the morning after the joint has been inactive during the night. The swollen joints are warm and tender, and movement is restricted. Swelling of the proximal interphalangeal joints of the fingers produces a typical spindled appearance of the fingers. Many patients have systemic symptoms such as low-grade fever, weakness, and malaise.

Joint deformity occurs early in severe cases. Restriction of movement may cause rapid disuse atrophy of muscles around the joint.

Extra-articular Manifestations

Rheumatoid arthritis is a systemic disorder. In a minority of patients, tissues other than joints show significant pathologic change (Table 68–2). Subcutaneous rheumatoid nodules are granulomas 1–2 cm in diameter seen commonly around the elbow, usually in patients with severe disease. They are characterized microscopically by an area of fibrinoid necrosis of collagen surrounded by palisading histiocytes (Fig 68–5).

Course & Prognosis

Rheumatoid arthritis is usually slowly progressive. In 10–20% of patients, the disease remits completely after the first attack. Most other patients go on to develop a chronic disease characterized by relapses and remissions, with slowly progressive disability from joint destruction. After 10 years of disease, about 10% of patients are severely disabled while about 50% are still fully employed.

Poor prognostic factors include a classic pattern of disease with high levels of rheumatoid factor in the serum, the presence of rheumatoid nodules, and onset of disease before age 30 years. In such patients, progress may be rapid.

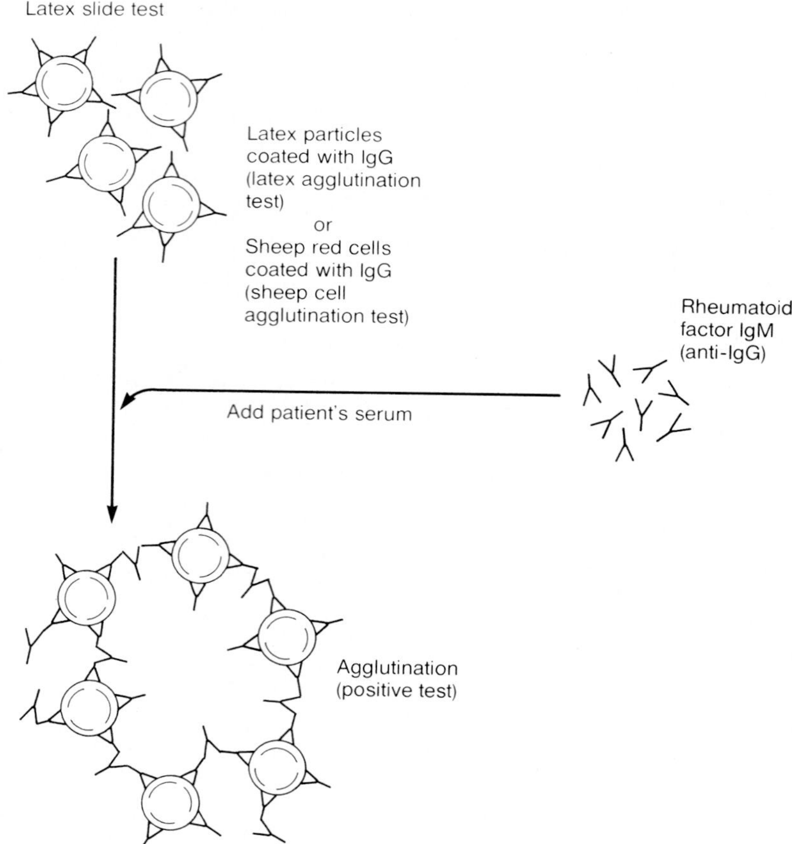

Figure 68-3. Principle of agglutination tests used to detect rheumatoid factor (which is an anti-IgG immunoglobulin) in the serum of patients.

VARIANTS OF RHEUMATOID ARTHRITIS

1. FELTY'S SYNDROME

Felty's syndrome occurs in older individuals with long-standing rheumatoid arthritis and high titers of rheumatoid factor. It is characterized by splenic enlargement and evidence of **hypersplenism** (destruction of blood cells in the enlarged spleen, resulting in granulocytopenia, anemia, and thrombocytopenia).

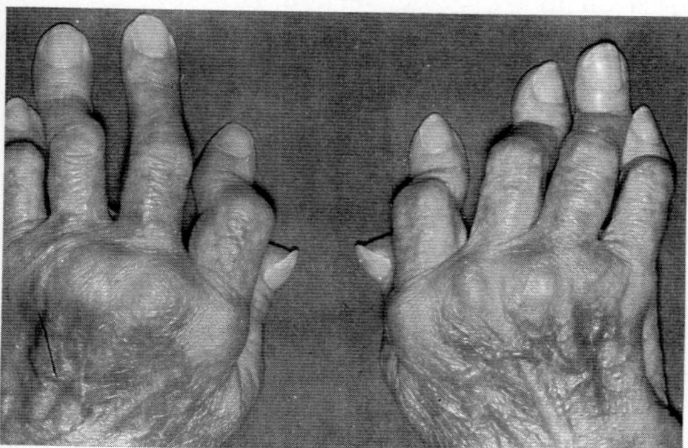

Figure 68-4. Rheumatoid arthritis (chronic phase, severe disease), showing symmetric involvement and severe deformity. Note dominant involvement of the proximal interphalangeal joint.

2. SJÖGREN'S SYNDROME

Sjögren's syndrome is commonly associated with rheumatoid arthritis. It is characterized by progressive destruction of salivary and lacrimal glands by an autoimmune lymphoid reaction, leading to dry mouth (xerostomia) and paucity of tears (keratoconjunctivitis sicca). The diagnosis may be made clinically by demonstrating the paucity of tears and confirmed histologically by lip biopsy, which shows infiltration of minor salivary glands in the lip with lymphocytes (see Chapter 31).

Sjögren's syndrome also occurs in isolation and may be associated with other collagen diseases, such as systemic lupus erythematosus and progressive systemic sclerosis. Rheumatoid factor and antinuclear antibodies are commonly present in the serum of patients with Sjögren's syndrome.

Table 68–2. Rheumatoid arthritis: Systemic manifestations and laboratory findings.

Systemic Manifestations	Description
Pyrexia, malaise	Mechanism unknown; ?lymphokines
Rheumatoid nodules	Subcutaneous granulomas with a central area of fibrinoid necrosis of connective tissue; tender 1- to 2-cm nodules at elbow and wrist particularly (see Fig 68–5)
Vasculitis	Particularly endarteritis; may lead to skin ulcers (ischemia), Raynaud's phenomenon, and peripheral neuropathy
Cardiac lesions	The myocardium is rarely involved (arrhythmias); pericarditis occurs in 10%
Lung lesions	Pleuritis, pleural effusions; large necrotizing rheumatoid nodules in lung; diffuse pulmonary fibrosis; nodular fibrosis of lung (in miners exposed to coal dust: Caplan's syndrome)
Neurologic lesions	Peripheral neuropathy (due to arteritis); mononeuropathy due to spinal nerve compression; carpal tunnel syndrome (median nerve compression); cervical cord compression (atlantoaxial joint involvement)
Ocular lesions	Keratitis, scleritis, granulomas, uveitis (iris inflamed)
Amyloidosis	Primary pattern of distribution (see Chapter 2)
Lymphadenopathy, splenomegaly	In up to 25% of cases, especially in juvenile form (Still's disease) and Felty's syndrome

Laboratory findings
- Positive rheumatoid factor (90% of classic adult cases but < 20% of childhood cases)
- Leukocytosis common (leukopenia in Felty's syndrome)
- Raised erythrocyte sedimentation rate
- Polyclonal hypergammaglobulinemia (in 50%)
- Positive ANA (antinuclear antibody), usually in low titer (10–40%)

3. JUVENILE RHEUMATOID ARTHRITIS (Still's Disease)

Still's disease is rheumatoid arthritis in a patient under 16 years of age. It is characterized by acute onset with high fever, leukocytosis, splenomegaly, arthritis, and skin rash. There may also be pericarditis and inflammation of the iris (uveitis). Rheumatoid factor is usually not present.

Patients with Still's disease commonly have monarticular involvement, frequently of a large joint. Growth abnormalities may occur if the disease strikes before the age of epiphyseal closure.

Fifty percent of patients with Still's disease undergo complete remission. Others progress to severe joint disease with extra-articular manifestations.

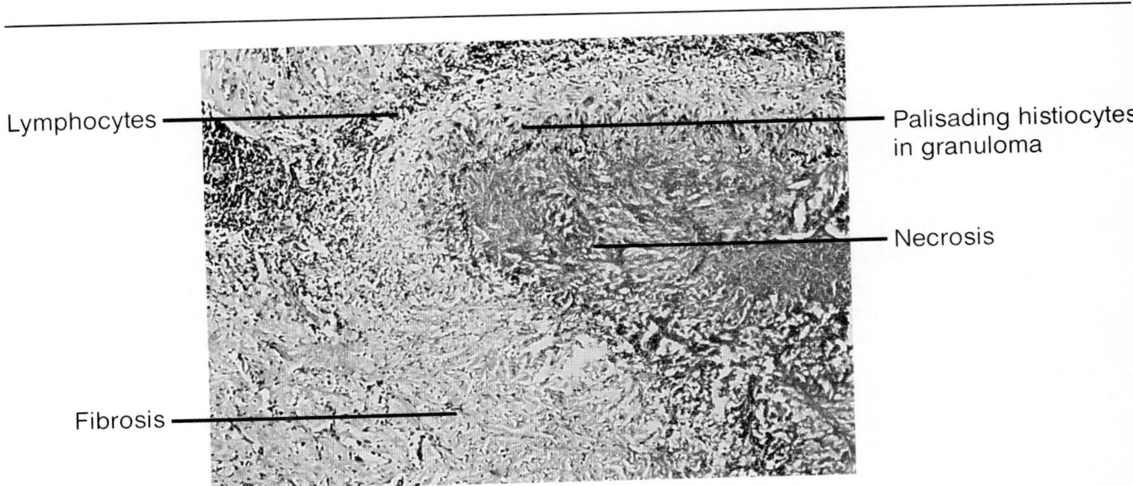

Figure 68–5. Subcutaneous rheumatoid nodule, showing a central area of necrosis of collagen surrounded by palisading histiocytes.

DEGENERATIVE JOINT DISEASES

ANKYLOSING SPONDYLITIS

Ankylosing spondylitis is a common disease (0.5% of the population in the USA) that predominantly affects young men (males:females 8:1), the maximum age incidence being between 15 and 30 years of age. The disease has a very strong association with HLA-B27, which is present in the cells of 95% of patients with ankylosing spondylitis, compared with 3–7% of the general population. The cause is unknown.

Pathology & Clinical Features

Ankylosing spondylitis maximally affects the sacroiliac joints. Chronic inflammation is associated with fibrosis and calcification, leading to bony fusion (ankylosis) of the joints.

Low back pain and stiffness are the common presenting symptoms. Calcification of the vertebral joints and paravertebral ligaments produces a characteristic radiologic appearance ("bamboo spine"; Fig 68–6) and marked immobility of the lower back.

Ankylosing spondylitis progresses slowly up the vertebral column. Involvement of the costovertebral joints and thoracic spine may result in restriction of chest expansion and rarely produces respiratory failure. Rheumatoid factor is typically absent.

A similar condition occurs in psoriasis, ulcerative colitis and Crohn's disease, and Reiter's syndrome, in which arthritis is associated with urethritis and conjunctivitis.

Extra-articular Manifestations

Patients with ankylosing spondylitis may show degeneration of the wall of the aorta, with dilatation and incompetence of the aortic valve. Aortic dissection and rupture may also occur. Twenty-five percent of patients have eye changes, most commonly iridocyclitis. Pulmonary fibrosis occurs in a few patients.

Course & Prognosis

Ankylosing spondylitis is a slowly progressive disease that causes increasing disability from pain and stiffness of the low back. Respiratory dysfunction and aortic disease represent life-threatening complications.

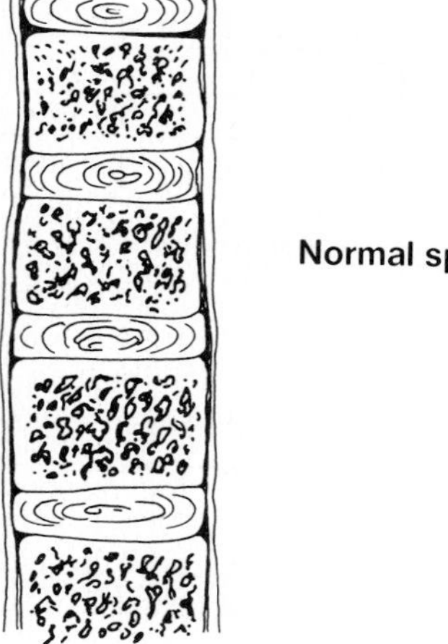

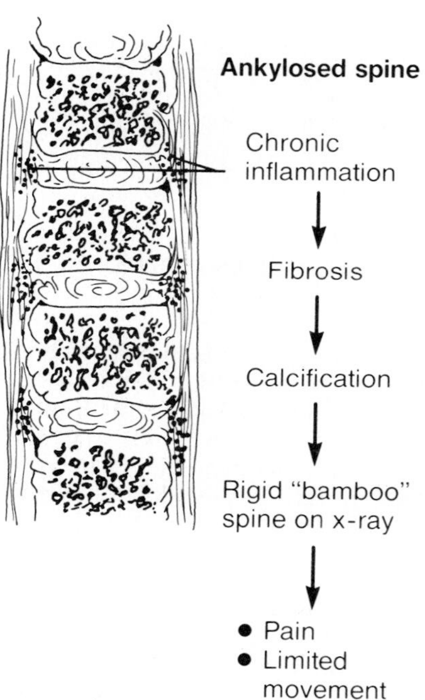

Figure 68–6. Pathologic features of ankylosing spondylitis.

OSTEOARTHROSIS (Osteoarthritis)

Osteoarthrosis is a common degenerative joint disease characterized by primary abnormalities in the articular cartilage. When assessed radiologically, changes of osteoarthrosis are present in over 90% of individuals over the age of 50 years of age. Though only a few of these patients are symptomatic, osteoarthrosis is the commonest cause of joint disability.

Osteoarthrosis is a disease of the elderly. When a younger individual develops osteoarthrosis, it is almost always secondary to a predisposing abnormality in the joint. Its clinical features are very different from those of rheumatoid arthritis (Table 68–3).

Table 68-3. Comparison of osteoarthrosis and rheumatoid arthritis.

	Osteoarthrosis	Rheumatoid Arthritis
Basic process	Degenerative	Immunologic, inflammatory
Site of initial lesion	Articular cartilage	Synovium
Age	50 plus	Any, but peaks at age 20–40 years
Sex	Male or female	Female > male
Joints involved	Especially knees, hips, spine; asymmetric involvement	Hands, later large joints; multiple symmetric involvement
Fingers	Herberden's nodes	Ulnar deviation, spindle swelling
Nodules	No	Rheumatoid nodules
Systemic features	None	Uveitis, pericarditis, etc.
Constitutional symptoms	None	Fever, malaise in some
Laboratory findings	None	Rheumatoid factor; ↑ erythrocyte sedimentation rate; anemia, leukocytosis, hyperglobulinemia
Joint fluid	Clear, normally viscous; no inflammatory cells	Clear; low viscosity, high protein; neutrophils, some lymphocytes; immunoglobulins, complement, rheumatoid factor

Osteoarthrosis is also frequently called osteoarthritis. The latter is an inaccurate term because it implies the presence of joint inflammation, which is not present.

Etiology

Osteoarthrosis is caused by degeneration of articular cartilage of joints (Fig 68–7). The exact cause of articular cartilage degeneration is not known. Abnormalities in the ground substance, collagen, increased lysosomal enzyme activity, and changes in water content have all been demonstrated in the articular cartilage in patients with osteoarthrosis, but their role in pathogenesis is unknown. The role of trauma and weight-bearing stresses is controversial. Osteoarthrosis occurs mainly in the weight-bearing joints, and it has been suggested that the disease may be the result of failure of repair of repeated minor trauma. A few cases of osteoarthrosis occur secondary to articular cartilage diseases (eg, alkaptonuria) and severe trauma (eg, in football players).

Pathology (Fig 68–7)

The large weight-bearing joints of the vertebral column, hips, and knees are most affected, along with the distal interphalangeal joints of the fingers. The primary abnormality is thinning and fragmentation of the articular cartilage. The normally smooth, white articular surface becomes irregular and yellow. Continued loss of articular cartilage leads to exposure of subchondral bone, which appears as shiny foci on the articular surface (eburnation). Fibrosis, increased bone formation, and cystic change frequently occur in the underlying bone. The loss of articular cartilage stimulates new bone formation, usually in the form of nodules (osteophytes) at the bone edges. Inflammation is absent.

Clinical Features

There is pain, stiffness, and swelling of affected joints, with no evidence of acute inflammation. Crepitus is a characteristic feature—a grating sound produced by friction between adjacent areas of exposed subchondral bone.

Osteophytes may be visible clinically—as bony masses such as those that occur over affected distal interphalangeal joints (Heberden's nodes)—or radiologically. They may cause compressive symptoms, most notably in spinal osteoarthrosis, in which nerve and spinal cord compression may occur.

Course & Prognosis

Osteoarthrosis is a slowly progressive, chronic joint disability. Eventually, elderly sufferers may become confined to wheelchairs; recent advancements in the technique of joint replacement with prostheses have improved the outlook of these patients considerably.

NEUROPATHIC JOINT (Charcot's Joint)

Neuropathic joint results from loss of sensory innervation to the joint, as occurs in peripheral neuropathy, tabes dorsalis, diabetic neuropathy, and syringomyelia. The lack of pain sensation deprives the joint of its normal protective muscle and postural responses when exposed to abnormal forces. Repeated trauma then leads to progressive destruction of the joint. Large joints such as the knees are usually involved. The affected joint is swollen, unstable, and frequently shows an abnormally increased range of motion resulting from destruction of intra-articular ligamentous restraints. The joint involvement is painless.

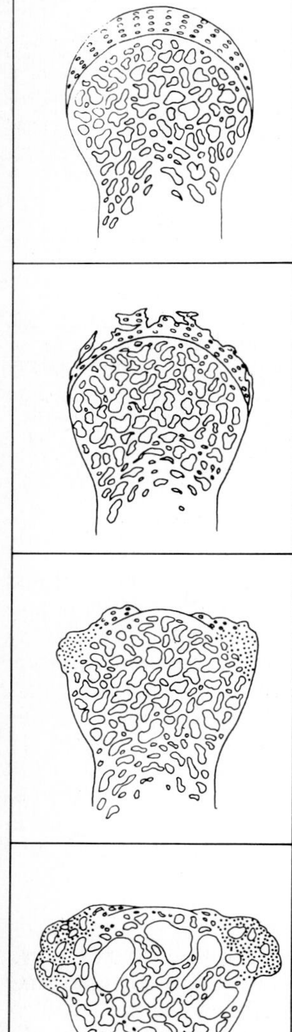

Figure 68–7. Pathologic features of osteoarthrosis. Degeneration of the articular cartilage may result in fragments of cartilage breaking free into the joint space as loose bodies ("joint mice").

METABOLIC DISEASES OF JOINTS

ALKAPTONURIA (Ochronosis)

Alkaptonuria is a rare autosomal recessive disease in which there is a deficiency of homogentisic acid oxidase. This defect blocks tyrosine metabolism and causes homogentisic acid to be deposited in collagen (dermis, ligaments, tendons, endocardium, the intimal surfaces of blood vessels) and cartilage (nose, ear, larynx, tracheobronchial tree, intervertebral disks, and joint spaces). All of these areas become black and radiopaque. Homogentisic acid is excreted in the urine; the urine is colorless when passed but darkens on exposure to air. In infants, this results in a blackish discoloration of diapers. Alkaptonuria is now routinely detected by neonatal screening tests.

The major clinical effect of alkaptonuria is degeneration of affected cartilages, resulting in juvenile osteoarthrosis.

GOUT (Gouty Arthritis)

Etiology

Gout is the result of deposition of urate crystals in connective tissues. Urate deposition commonly occurs in diseases in which abnormal uric acid metabolism causes elevated plasma uric acid levels **(hyperuricemia)**.

A. Primary Gout: Primary gout occurs mainly in elderly men and has a strong familial tendency. The basic abnormality in urate metabolism is not known. In one-third of patients, there is an increase in production of uric acid due to increased breakdown of purines, which are synthesized in excessive amounts in the liver. Lack of regulation of 5-phosphoribosyl-1-pyrophosphate (PRPP) aminotransferase, which catalyzes the first step in purine synthesis, is believed to be responsible for increased purine synthesis.

In another one-third of patients with primary gout, decreased renal clearance of uric acid is the major factor causing hyperuricemia.

In the remaining third of patients, hyperuricemia results from a combination of increased urate production and decreased urate excretion in the kidneys. Two rare X-linked diseases—deficiency of hypoxanthine guanine phosphoribosyl transferase and overactivity of PRPP synthesis—are associated with hyperuricemia and gout.

B. Secondary Gout: Secondary gout occurs in diseases in which excess breakdown of purines leads to increased uric acid synthesis. It is most commonly seen in patients with leukemia—particularly at the start of treatment, when there is marked cell necrosis, releasing nucleic acids that are catabolized to uric acid.

Effects of Urate Deposition

Two forms of sodium urate crystals may be deposited and produce 2 clinically distinct types of gout.

Acute gouty arthritis is caused by deposition of microcrystals of sodium urate in the synovial membranes of joints. For some unknown reason, the first metatarsophalangeal joint (big toe) is affected in 85% of cases. Urate microcrystals activate kinins, are chemotactic for neutrophils, and produce an intense acute inflammation. The urate microcrystals can be recognized in joint fluid as birefringent needle-shaped crystals under polarized light.

Chronic tophaceous gout is the result of deposition of sodium urate as large amorphous masses known as tophi. These evoke chronic—not acute—inflammation. Tophi occur commonly in the cartilage of the ear and around joints (Fig 68–8). Marked deformity may result. Gouty tophi appear microscopically as pale-pink amorphous masses surrounded by a foreign body type granulomatous reaction (Fig 68–9). Fixation in absolute alcohol followed by examination under polarized light permits identification of urate in tissue sections.

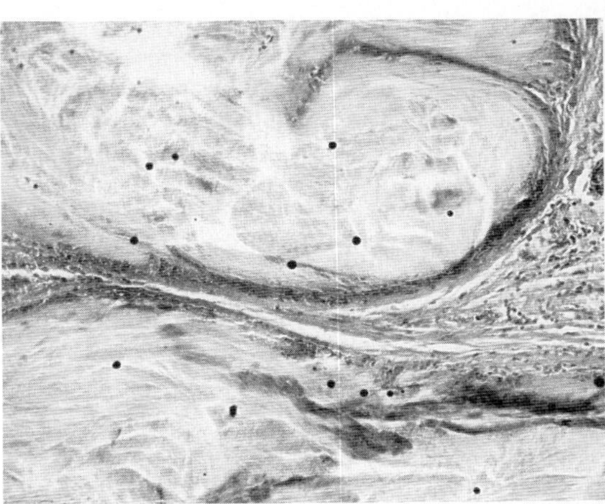

Figure 68–9. Gouty tophus, showing amorphous deposition of urate in connective tissue surrounded by inflammation.

CALCIUM PYROPHOSPHATE DEPOSITION DISEASE (Chondrocalcinosis; Pseudogout)

Calcium pyrophosphate deposition diseases is a degenerative joint disease characterized by deposition of calcium pyrophosphate in the joints. The cause is not known. Most cases involve the knee joints after trauma or surgery. Clinically, calcium pyrophosphate deposition is characterized by an acute arthritis involving one or many joints, most commonly the large joints of the lower extremity. The metatarsophalangeal joint is usually not affected. The arthritis is self-limited, lasting 1–4 weeks. The synovial fluid contains numerous leukocytes and calcium pyrophosphate crystals, which are short and rhomboid and can be distinguished from the longer, needle-shaped urate crystals by their polarization characteristics.

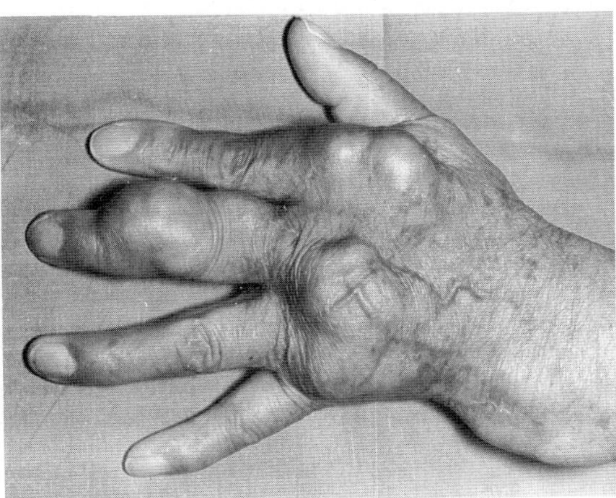

Figure 68–8. Chronic tophaceous gouty arthritis, showing deformity of the hand associated with multiple nodular tophi.

NEOPLASMS & NONNEOPLASTIC TUMORS OF JOINTS

PIGMENTED VILLONODULAR SYNOVITIS

Pigmented villonodular synovitis is an uncommon disease characterized by proliferation of the synovial membrane of joints. It occurs in adults and most commonly involves the knee joint. Clinically, there is pain, swelling, and progressively increasing joint disability.

The cause is unknown. It is believed that the lesion is inflammatory, though its histologic resemblance to giant cell tumor of tendon sheath has led to the suggestion that it is a benign neoplastic process.

Grossly, the synovial membrane is thickened and shows villous outgrowths that have a typical orange-brown color due to the presence of hemosiderin. Microscopically, the villi consist of proliferating synovial epithelial cells, lymphocytes, plasma cells, and histiocytes, many of which appear foamy and contain lipid and hemosiderin. Multinucleated giant cells are frequently present.

Surgical or arthroscopic removal of the abnormal synovium is effective treatment. Local recurrence may occur, probably due to incomplete surgical removal.

SYNOVIAL CHONDROMATOSIS

Synovial chondromatosis is an uncommon condition of unknown cause characterized by the occurrence of multiple foci of cartilaginous metaplasia in the synovial membrane. The cartilage appears as nodules that may undergo ossification and may become detached into the joint cavity as "loose bodies." The knee is commonly affected, with symptoms of pain, swelling, limitation of movement, and intermittent locking. Osteoarthrosis may result.

GANGLION

Ganglion is a common cystic lesion arising in the connective tissue of the joint capsule or in a tendon sheath. It most commonly occurs around the wrist. Microscopically, a ganglion is a cystic structure filled with myxomatous tissue and lined by collagen. It has no epithelial lining and is distinct from a synovial cyst.

Except for producing a lump, ganglions are of no significance clinically.

GIANT CELL TUMOR OF TENDON SHEATH

Giant cell tumor of tendon sheath is the only common benign neoplasm that involves the synovium. It occurs either inside the joint—usually the knee—or in relation to the tendon sheaths in the hands and feet. There is some controversy about whether giant cell tumor is a true neoplasm or whether it is inflammatory (nodular synovitis). The lesion presents as a mass that may become large and cause erosion of adjacent bone. Histologically, there is an admixture of foamy macrophages, multinucleated giant cells, and fibroblasts (benign fibrous histiocytoma is an alternative name).

Treatment is surgical removal, which is curative.

SYNOVIAL SARCOMA

Synovial sarcoma is a rare malignant neoplasm arising from synovial epithelial cells. Synovial sarcomas occur much more commonly in relation to bursae and tendon sheaths than within joints. They therefore tend to present as extra-articular soft tissue masses, most commonly near a joint in the extremities. Microscopically, they are highly cellular neoplasms with a biphasic pattern, being composed of spindle cells and epithelium-lined slit-like spaces resembling synovium. The cells contain keratin intermediate filaments in addition to vimentin, a point of distinction from other soft tissue sarcomas. Synovial sarcomas are high-grade malignant neoplasms with a high rate of local recurrence as well as metastasis. They have a 5-year survival rate of about 50% after optimal treatment.

II. DISEASES OF EXTRASKELETAL CONNECTIVE TISSUE

AUTOIMMUNE CONNECTIVE TISSUE DISEASES (Collagen Diseases)

Connective tissue diseases (also called collagen diseases) are a group of diseases characterized by (1) involvement of multiple tissues; (2) evidence for an autoimmune cause; (3) the presence of antinuclear antibodies in the serum (Table 68–4); and (4) inflammation of small blood vessels (vasculitis), frequently with fibrinoid necrosis of the wall.

Connective tissue diseases include lupus erythematosus, progressive systemic sclerosis, mixed connective tissue disease, and polymyositis-dermatomyositis. Polyarteritis nodosa (see Chapter 20), rheumatoid arthritis, and rheumatic fever (Chapter 22) also have some features of connective tissue diseases and are sometimes included within this category.

LUPUS ERYTHEMATOSUS

Lupus erythematosus is a connective tissue disease that exists in 2 clinical forms: (1) systemic lupus erythematosus (SLE), which is a progressive and often severe condition involving multiple systems; and (2) discoid lupus erythematosus, in which skin involvement dominates the clinical picture, usually without systemic disease (see Chapter 61).

Incidence

SLE is common in the United States, more so in nonwhites (particularly blacks) than whites. The disease is also common in Western Europe but less so in Asia.

Women are affected 10 times more frequently than men. The usual age at onset of disease is 20–40 years.

Table 68-4. Antinuclear antibodies in systemic lupus erythematosus (SLE) and other autoimmune connective tissue diseases.

	Pattern of Nuclear Immunostaining	Detects Antibodies Versus:	Diseases: Test Positive in:
Fluorescent antinuclear antibody (FANA) test **Screening test**	Variable	Many different nuclear antigens; one or several of these antibodies may be present together	99% SLE 85% Sjögren's syndrome 90% Systemic sclerosis 50% Rheumatoid arthritis plus many other connective tissue disorders; 20% or more of elderly "healthy" people and 20% of relatives of SLE patients
Additional information may be obtained from staining pattern			
FANA	Rim (shaggy)	Native double-stranded DNA (nDNA); nucleoprotein (soluble); histones	SLE (high-titer), less common and lower titers in other disorders
	Homogeneous	Nucleoproteins; histones	SLE, rheumatoid arthritis, systemic sclerosis, Sjögren's syndrome
	Speckled	Nuclear RNA-protein;[1] Sm antigen Scl-70[1] SS-8[1] Histone (H3)	SLE, mixed connective disease, others SLE (specific) Systemic sclerosis (specific) Sjögren's syndrome (specific) Undifferentiated connective tissue disease
	Nucleolar	Ribonuclear protein 6S-RNA	SLE, mixed connective tissue disease Systemic sclerosis (specific)
FANA (crithidial)	Kinetoplast of crithidial organism	nDNA only	Specific for SLE
Assays using other immunologic techniques	No staining by fluorescence	Single-stranded DNA (ssDNA) SS-A	All connective tissue diseases: Sjögren's syndrome, SLE, others

[1]Different antigens can only be distinguished by serial testing for separate nuclear components; this is a complex procedure not usually performed. Sm antigen = Smith RNA protein.

Etiology

The cause of lupus erythematosus is unknown (Fig 68–10). There is little doubt that it is mediated by an abnormal immune response associated with the presence of antinuclear antibodies and immune complexes in the plasma. The cause of this response is widely believed to be autoimmune, though there is evidence for viral and genetic influences.

A. Autoimmune Origin: There is considerable evidence that SLE is a type III autohypersensitivity (autoimmune) disease. The formation of **antinuclear antibodies (ANA)** is important in pathogenesis. A variety of antinuclear antibodies are present in the serum of all patients with systemic lupus erythematosus and are tested for and characterized by immunologic techniques (Table 68–4). The presence of antibody against double-stranded DNA is highly specific for lupus erythematosus, while antibodies against single-stranded DNA, RNA, and nucleoproteins are also found in other connective tissue diseases. A test utilizing *Crithidia* (a protozoon) as the DNA antigen is a simple method of detecting antibodies to double-stranded DNA; the kinetoplast of *Crithidia* is almost pure double-stranded DNA; whereas nuclei contain DNA, RNA, and many protein antigens.

Immune complexes formed between antinuclear antibodies and nuclear antigens are detectable in the serum and at sites of disease activity in the walls of small blood vessels, the skin, and glomerular basement membrane. Deposition of immune complexes in the tissue (Fig 68–10) activates complement and leads to inflammation by a type III hypersensitivity reaction. Serum complement levels are frequently reduced in the active phase of SLE.

Numerous **autoantibodies other than antinuclear antibodies** are also found in SLE. These include (1) rheumatoid factor (20–30%); (2) antibodies that give a false-positive reaction in serologic tests for syphilis; (3) antibodies against plasma coagulation proteins, most commonly factor VIII, producing bleeding diathesis; and (4) antibodies against antigens on erythrocytes, leuko-

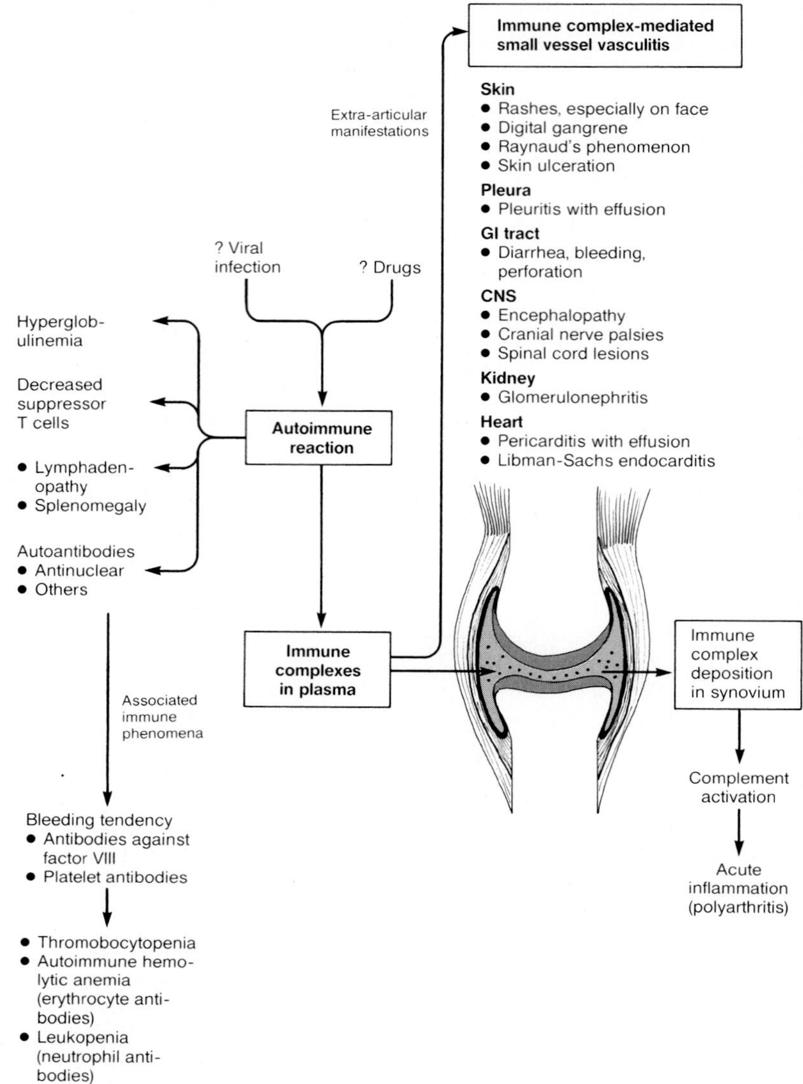

Figure 68–10. Etiologic factors and pathogenesis of systemic lupus erythematosus.

cytes, and platelets, which may lead to immune destruction of these cells in the peripheral circulation.

B. Drug-Induced Lupus: SLE is known to be precipitated by drugs such as hydralazine (an antihypertensive) and procainamide (used to control cardiac arrhythmias). Drug-induced disease may be similar to idiopathic SLE, including the presence of antinuclear antibodies, but renal disease is rare. Withdrawal of the drug often causes reversal of the disease and gradual disappearance of the antinuclear antibodies.

C. Viral Origin: Infectious agents—mainly viruses—have been suggested as causing lupus erythematosus, but no infectious agent has been isolated consistently from patients' tissues.

D. Genetic Factors: Genetic predisposition to SLE has been suggested because of the high concordance of clinical SLE in monozygotic twins and the increased frequency of the disease in first-degree relatives. HLA-DR2 is more common in SLE, leading to the suggestion that the presence of the corresponding immune response gene may predispose to the development of autoreactivity against nuclear antigens. The occurrence of SLE in patients with inherited deficiency of early complement factors (C1, C2, and C4) is also of interest, since the genes for C2 and C4 are known to be closely linked to the HLA-DR region.

Pathology & Clinical Features

Lupus erythematosus is a complement-mediated immune complex disorder. Sites of immune complex deposition show evidence of tissue necrosis and acute inflammation. The pattern of disease in an individual patient depends on where immune complex injury takes place. The presenting features are thus quite diverse (Table 68-5).

A. Small Vessel Vasculitis: Immune complex injury of arterioles is typical, with fibrinoid necrosis of the media and infiltration of the wall and perivascular tissue by neutrophils, lymphocytes, and plasma cells. Thrombosis is common and may lead to ischemia and tissue necrosis. In the skin, there may be digital gangrene and ulceration; and in the gastrointestinal tract, diarrhea, bleeding, intestinal obstruction, and perforation. These changes progress to intimal fibrosis, with a characteristic laminated ("onion skin") appearance.

B. Hyperplasia of the Lymphoid System: Enlargement of lymph nodes or spleen occurs in 50% of patients with SLE. This is due to nonspecific follicular and paracortical lymphocytic proliferation.

C. Skin: Immune complex deposition occurs in the basement membrane of the skin, where it can be perceived as lumpy deposits by electron microscopic and immunologic techniques. The resulting complement activation and inflammation lead to a skin rash, typically over the malar regions of the face ("butterfly rash"). Skin rash occurs some time in the course of the disease in 70% of cases.

In patients with discoid lupus erythematosus, the skin lesion is the sole abnormality. In discoid lupus, immune complex deposition is restricted to the area of the rash; in systemic lupus, immune complex deposition is widespread even in clinically normal skin.

Table 68-5. Clinical features of systemic lupus erythematosus (SLE).

	Presenting Feature[1] (%)	Prevalence (%)
Arthritis	50	90
Skin rashes	25	70
Fever[2]	20	80
Pleurisy or pericarditis	10	25
Renal disease[3]	5	65
Neurologic symptoms	5	25
Raynaud's phenomenon	2	10
Others: lymphadenopathy, malaise, weakness, weight loss		

[1]Note that in many patients, more than one of these features are present, eg, skin rash and arthritis.
[2]Fever is the only feature at presentation in 20% of patients. It is present in a larger number of cases in association with other features.
[3]Although not the most common presenting feature, renal disease occurs later and is the most common direct cause of death in SLE.

D. Joints: Joint inflammation (arthritis) or pain (arthralgia) occurs in 90% of patients with SLE. Both large and small joints may be involved, and initial involvement may resemble rheumatoid arthritis. Joint involvement in SLE is usually mild.

E. Heart: Cardiac lesions in patients with systemic lupus erythematosus include pericarditis with effusion, myocarditis, and Libman-Sachs endocarditis (see Chapter 22). These complications are usually not serious.

F. Nervous System: Clinical manifestations due to central nervous system vasculitis and ischemia occur in 25% of patients. Convulsions, mental disorders (emotional lability, dementia, psychosis), cranial nerve palsies, and spinal cord dysfunction may result. The cerebrospinal fluid in such patients often shows moderately increased protein levels and a mild increase in lymphocytes.

G. Kidneys: Renal involvement occurs in approximately two-thirds of patients and represents the most common mode of death in SLE. Renal lesions are due to immune complex deposition (see Chapter 48), producing proliferative and membranous types of glomerulonephritis.

Diagnosis

The diagnosis of lupus erythematosus is based on its clinical features and confirmed by demonstration of serum antinuclear antibodies (ANA), particularly anti-double-stranded DNA. The absence of ANA virtually rules out a diagnosis of SLE, because less than 5% of patients with SLE are ANA-negative (Table 68-4). Histologic examination of tissues such as the skin and kidney does not provide specific evidence of the disease but combined with the clinical features often leads to the diagnosis.

The LE cell test (an in vitro test to detect ingested nuclear debris in blood neutrophils) is now rarely used, being less sensitive than ANA tests. It is of historical significance because its discovery gave impetus to the concept of autoimmune diseases.

Course & Prognosis

The course of SLE is variable. Rarely, patients have a severe acute illness that is refractory to treatment. Most patients pursue a chronic course, with repeated exacerbations and remissions. Corticosteroid therapy is usually effective in controlling exacerbations, and with such therapy the survival rate is approximately 90% at 10 years.

Most deaths are due to renal failure followed by central nervous system disease. The complications of immunosuppressive drug therapy also account for significant morbidity and many deaths.

Patients with discoid lupus erythematosus have a chronic skin disorder. There is little danger of death unless systemic symptoms supervene (about 10% of patients develop SLE).

PROGRESSIVE SYSTEMIC SCLEROSIS

Progressive systemic sclerosis (previously called scleroderma) is an uncommon connective tissue disease characterized by vasculitis affecting small vessels and widespread deposition of collagen.

Progressive systemic sclerosis occurs more commonly in females and has its onset most frequently in the ages from 20 to 50 years.

Etiology

Progressive systemic sclerosis is probably an autoimmune disorder and is closely related to SLE. Antinuclear antibodies are usually present in the serum. The most characteristic antinuclear antibody for progressive systemic sclerosis has specificity against nucleolar RNA. Deposition of immune complexes in tissues has been demonstrated in renal and vascular lesions.

The mechanism underlying the excessive fibrosis is unknown.

Pathology

The pathologic changes in affected tissue include vasculitis, which is identical histologically with that seen in systemic lupus erythematosus; it tends to be more chronic. Marked fibrosis dominates the histologic appearance.

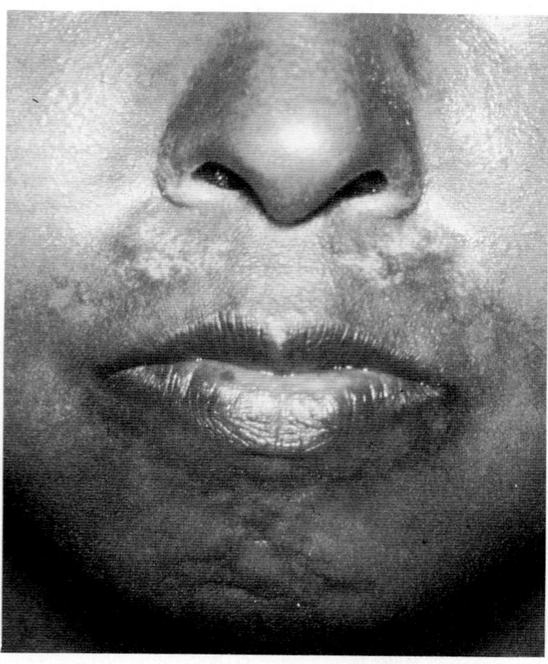

Figure 68–11. Progressive systemic sclerosis, showing scarring and stretching of the skin of the upper lip. Numerous small telangiectatic vessels were also present.

Clinical Features

Progressive systemic sclerosis usually has an insidious onset. Systemic symptoms are uncommon. In many patients, the disease is restricted to the skin for many years before visceral involvement occurs.

A. Skin: (Affected in 90% of cases.) The skin of the fingers and face is the most common first site of disease. Initially, the skin is edematous, with vasculitis and often petechial hemorrhages. Progressive fibrosis follows, involving the entire dermis and extending to the subcutaneous tissue. The epidermis becomes thin, and all adnexal structures (hair, sweat glands, etc) undergo atrophy. Enlarged vessels are frequently present and visible as telangiectases. Trophic ulceration of the skin is common, and dystrophic calcification may occur.

Severe skin changes lead to clawlike contracted hands and restriction of facial movements (Fig 68–11).

B. Gastrointestinal Tract: (60% of cases.) The entire gastrointestinal tract may be affected, with the esophagus and small intestine showing maximal disease. Dysphagia, deficient peristalsis, and malabsorption follow. **CREST syndrome** is a variant of progressive systemic sclerosis consisting of calcinosis, Raynaud's phenomenon, esophageal disease, sclerodactyly (involvement of the fingers), and telangiectasia. An autoantibody to centromeres is commonly present.

C. Kidneys: (60% of cases.) Glomerular changes result from immune complex deposition and include basement membrane thickening and mesangial hypercellularity. Small arterioles in the kidney frequently show intimal fibrosis, leading to glomerular ischemia, decreased glomerular filtration rate, and renal failure (Chapter 48).

D. Lungs: (20% of cases.) Pulmonary involvement in progressive systemic sclerosis takes the form of a diffuse interstitial pneumonitis and fibrosis identical to that seen in usual interstitial pneumonitis (see Chapter 35). The end stage is a honeycomb lung with respiratory failure.

Course

The clinical course is usually chronic. The occurrence of symptomatic visceral disease (especially renal disease) is an ominous sign. Treatment with immunosuppressive drugs is of limited value.

POLYMYOSITIS-DERMATOMYOSITIS

Polymyositis-dermatomyositis is an uncommon connective tissue disease affecting women twice as frequently as men. Onset of disease is maximal between the ages of 40 and 60 years.

The cause is unknown. An immunologic basis is likely, though the exact mechanism is not clear. Antinuclear antibodies occur in the serum of most patients, and immune complex deposition with complement activation can be demonstrated in many cases of dermatomyositis. Cell-mediated autohypersensitivity has also been implicated.

Patients with polymyositis-dermatomyositis are at increased risk for malignant neoplasms. Carcinoma of the lung is the most common, but carcinoma of the breast, kidney, stomach, and uterus also occurs. The incidence of cancer in these patients was originally reported to be around 25% but is now believed to be lower. The basis of the relationship between polymyositis-dermatomyositis and malignant neoplasia is unknown.

Pathology & Clinical Features

Polymyositis-dermatomyositis is a chronic disease that affects skeletal muscle in all cases and skin in 50% of cases. Visceral involvement is uncommon.

A. Myositis: (All cases.) Skeletal muscle is involved in all cases. The proximal muscles of the limb girdles are commonly the first affected, with involvement of pharyngeal and respiratory muscles in severe cases.

In the acute phase, affected muscle show edema, lymphocytic infiltration, myofibrillary necrosis, and phagocytosis of dead muscle. This is followed by muscle atrophy and fibrosis. Clinically, there is muscle weakness associated with pain and tenderness, the latter feature being useful in distinguishing polymyositis from muscular dystrophies. During the acute phase, serum creatine kinase and aldolase levels are greatly elevated, and creatinuria may be present when there is severe muscle necrosis.

Muscle biopsy, demonstrating inflammatory changes, permits distinction from muscular dystrophy and other causes of myositis (see Chapter 66).

B. Skin Changes: (Half of cases.) Skin changes are caused by vasculitis and typically take the form of a violaceous edematous rash (heliotrope rash) involving the upper eyelids, sometimes extending to the malar region of the face and neck. Dermal atrophy and calcification occur in the later stages. In 30% of patients, skin changes are associated with Raynaud's phenomenon.

Course

Polymyositis-dermatomyositis has a chronic course characterized by increasing disability from muscle wasting. The main danger of the disease is from the associated malignant neoplasms.

MIXED CONNECTIVE TISSUE DISEASE

Mixed connective tissue disease (MCTD) is an uncommon disease with clinical features that overlap with one or more of the other connective tissue diseases: systemic lupus erythematosus, progressive systemic sclerosis, and polymyositis ("overlap syndrome").

Mixed connective tissue disease is characterized by the presence in the serum of a high titer of antibodies against ribonucleoprotein (Table 68–4).

Mixed connective tissue disease should be distinguished from SLE because it tends to run a more benign course, mainly due to a lesser frequency of renal involvement.

SOFT TISSUE NEOPLASMS

Soft tissue neoplasms arise from any of the cells present in extraskeletal connective tissue, including fibroblasts, adipocytes, neural derivatives, vascular endothelium, smooth muscle of vessel walls, skeletal muscle, and other mesenchymal cells (Table 68–6). Neoplasms of blood vessels (see Chapter 20), nerves (Chapter 66), and skeletal muscle (Chapter 66) have been considered elsewhere.

Benign soft tissue neoplasms are very common. Lipomas and hemangiomas are among the commonest neoplasms occurring in humans. Malignant soft tissue neoplasms are rare.

Pathology

Soft tissue neoplasms occur in almost any tissue of the body. They are most commonly found in the extremities and retroperitoneum. Based on their biologic behavior, soft tissue neoplasms may be classified into 3 broad pathologic subgroups. The criteria for placing a given neoplasm in one of these subgroups varies with the cell of origin of the neoplasm.

A. Benign Soft Tissue Neoplasms: Benign soft tissue neoplasms appear as well-circumscribed encapsulated nodular masses that closely resemble the tissue of origin. Lipoma, for example, appears as a mass of mature adipose tissue distinguishable as a neoplasm only because it forms a mass and is encapsulated. Local excision is curative.

Rarely, neurofibromas and lipomas occur in families, being inherited as an autosomal dominant trait. **Generalized neurofibromatosis (von Recklinghausen's disease),** which is characterized by the occurrence of multiple neurofibromas throughout the body, is discussed in Chapter 62. **Generalized lipomatosis (Dercum's disease)** is rare and characterized by multiple lipomas, mainly subcutaneous. In these conditions, the neoplasms are usually too numerous to be removed surgically and can present a significant cosmetic problem. The benign neoplasms may rarely undergo malignant transformation into sarcomas; in neurofibro-

Table 68-6. Neoplasms of connective tissue ("soft tissue" neoplasms).

Cell of Origin	Benign[1]	Low-Grade Malignant,[1] Locally Aggressive	Malignant[1]
Fibroblast	Fibroma	Fibromatosis, fibrosarcoma (low-grade)	Fibrosarcoma (high-grade)
Adipocyte	Lipoma, hibernoma	Liposarcoma (well-differentiated and myxoid)	Liposarcoma (pleomorphic and round cell)
Nerve sheath	Neurofibroma, schwannoma, granular cell tumor		Malignant peripheral nerve sheath tumor
Fibrohistiocyte	Fibroxanthoma, dermatofibroma	Atypical fibroxanthoma, dermatofibrosarcoma protuberans	Malignant fibrous histiocytoma
Smooth muscle	Leiomyoma	Leiomyosarcoma (low-grade)	Leiomyosarcoma (high-grade)
Skeletal muscle	Rhabdomyoma		Rhabdomyosarcoma
Vascular	Hemangioma	Hemangiopericytoma, hemangioendothelioma (low-grade)	Angiosarcoma, Kaposi's sarcoma
Synovial	Giant cell tumor of tendon sheath		Synovial sarcoma
Unknown			Ewing's sarcoma (extraskeletal), alveolar soft part sarcoma, clear cell sarcoma,[2] epithelioid sarcoma

[1]Benign neoplasms are cured by surgical removal. Low-grade malignant soft tissue neoplasms are locally infiltrative and tend to recur locally after surgical removal. Their metastatic potential is low. Malignant neoplasms have a high metastatic potential as well as local infiltrative properties.

[2]Cells comprising clear cell sarcoma have been shown to contain melanosomes, and this neoplasm is now also called malignant melanoma of soft tissue.

matosis, 5–10% of affected patients develop malignant neoplasms.

B. Locally Aggressive Soft Tissue Neoplasms: Locally aggressive soft tissue neoplasms are intermediate in behavior between benign and malignant. They are locally infiltrative and tend to recur after surgical excision but rarely metastasize.

The best examples of this group are the **fibromatoses (desmoid tumors),** occurring in skeletal muscle. The commonest site is the rectus abdominis muscle, especially in women after pregnancy. Fibromatoses are slowly growing neoplasms that form large masses with extensive local infiltration along fascial planes. Unless excised with an adequately wide margin, the tumor recurs locally, often after several years, and considerable local destruction may ensue. Fibromatoses, despite their locally aggressive behavior, do not metastasize and in this way differ from sarcomas.

C. Malignant Soft Tissue Neoplasms (Sarcomas): Sarcomas are malignant neoplasms derived from mesenchymal cells, subclassified according to the cell of origin. They are generally much less common than carcinomas. The most common types of sarcomas are malignant fibrous histiocytoma and liposarcoma. Rhabdomyosarcoma, leiomyosarcoma, fibrosarcoma, malignant neural neoplasms, and angiosarcoma are rare. Sarcomas usually present as a soft tissue mass, often of large size (Fig 68–12). The extremities and retroperitoneum are the most common sites.

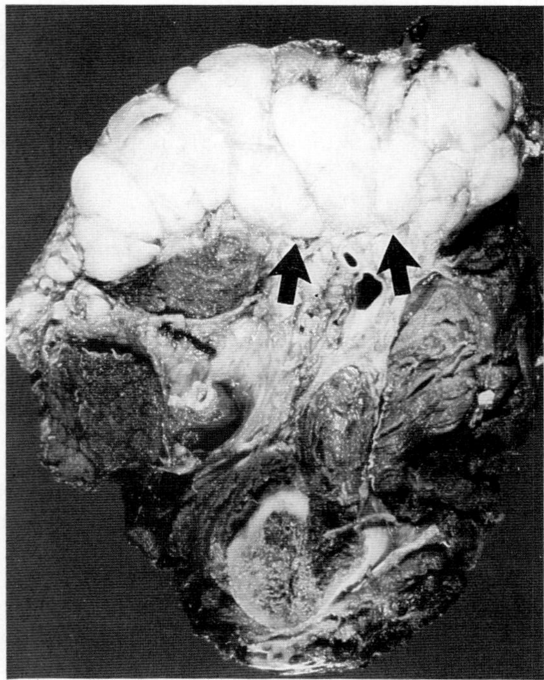

Figure 68–12. Transverse section of thigh, showing a large mass involving the subcutaneous and deep soft tissue (arrows). The mass is fleshy and poorly circumscribed. Histologic examination showed a high-grade malignant fibrous histiocytoma.

The biologic behavior of sarcomas is extremely variable.

1. **High-grade sarcomas** are highly cellular neoplasms, being composed of poorly differentiated mesenchymal cells. They show marked nuclear abnormalities and have a high mitotic rate. Because of their anaplasia, high-grade sarcomas are sometimes difficult to classify. The presence of lipoblasts (liposarcoma), cross-striations (rhabdomyosarcoma), or abnormal vascular channels (angiosarcoma) may be of help. Recognition of the cell of origin is sometimes possible by immunohistologic techniques, demonstrating factor VIII antigen (angiosarcoma) or myoglobin, desmin, and actin (myosarcomas) or keratin (synovial sarcoma). Electron microscopy is also of value in identifying the striated muscle, lipoblastic, or Schwann cell origin of an anaplastic sarcoma. High-grade sarcomas grow rapidly, show extensive local invasion, and tend to metastasize early through the bloodstream. Lymphatic spread is uncommon. High-grade sarcomas are usually fatal, and treatment is rarely successful.

2. **Low-grade sarcomas** are better-differentiated, less cellular, and tend to resemble the tissue of origin to some extent. Cytologic abnormalities are less prominent, and the mitotic rate is usually low. These tumors are characterized by a slower growth rate, a high risk of local recurrence after surgical removal, and a relatively low risk of metastasis. Patients typically survive a long time with repeated local recurrences after surgery. The behavior of low-grade sarcomas is similar to that of locally aggressive soft tissue neoplasms.

Treatment

Recognition that a given soft tissue mass may be malignant is extremely important. Simple excision of a sarcoma invariably leaves neoplastic cells behind and makes local recurrence certain. Sarcomas should be treated initially by incisional biopsy for pathologic diagnosis, followed by excision with a wide margin of normal tissue. Pathologic examination of the surgical margins at the time of surgery is advisable to ensure that the microscopic limit of the neoplasm has been reached in the excision.

Chemotherapy and radiotherapy are of limited value except for local control of recurrences. Recently, the use of preoperative intra-arterial chemotherapy, infusing the agent into the area via the artery of supply, has proved to be of some benefit.

Appendix I: Glossary

Abortion Termination of pregnancy before the 20th week of gestation.

Abrasion Injury to stratified squamous epithelium (skin or mucous membrane) involving scraping away of the superficial layers of the epithelium.

Abscess A walled-off collection of liquefied necrotic cellular debris, neutrophil leukocytes, and infectious agents.

Abruptio placentae Premature separation of the placenta from the uterine wall before the onset of labor.

Acanthocyte An erythrocyte characterized by irregular spikelike projections of the cell membrane.

Achalasia Failure of relaxation of a muscular sphincter.

Achlorhydria The absence of hydrochloric acid in gastric secretion even after maximal stimulation.

Acholuric jaundice Hyperbilirubinemia associated with absence of bilirubin in the urine.

Acidosis An increase in hydrogen ion concentration (= decrease in pH) of the blood, due either to accumulation of acid or loss of alkali.

Activated lymphocyte A lymphocyte that has reacted immunologically on exposure to an antigen.

Acute inflammation An immediate response to injury mediated by the microcirculation, characterized by vasodilatation, increased capillary permeability, exudation of fluid, and emigration of leukocytes. It is characterized clinically by redness, increased temperature, pain, swelling, and loss of function.

Addiction A state of strong dependence on a chemical substance to an extent that an abnormal clinical state results following abrupt abstention.

Adenocarcinoma A malignant neoplasm arising from glandular epithelial cells.

Adenoma A benign neoplasm arising from glandular epithelial cells.

Adenosis An abnormal, nonneoplastic proliferation of glands.

Agenesis Absence of an organ, resulting from failure of development of the anlage of that organ during embryogenesis.

Aging The gradual changes that occur in an organism with the passage of time that do not result from injury or disease.

Agranulocytosis Absence of mature granulocytes in the peripheral blood.

Albinism A congenital absence of melanin pigment in the skin, hair, and eyes, resulting from a failure of synthesis.

Alcoholism Abuse of alcoholic beverages to an extent that interferes with the drinker's health, social interactions, or work relationships or performance.

Alkalosis A decrease in hydrogen ion concentration (= increase in pH) of the blood, due either to accumulation of alkali or loss of acid.

Allele One of 2 or more alternative forms of a gene occupying corresponding loci on homologous chromosomes any 2 of which may be carried by an individual.

Allergy A state of abnormal immunologic hypersensitivity to a substance acquired by previous exposure to that substance.

Allergen An antigen that evokes a type I hypersensitivity response.

Allograft (= allogeneic graft) A transplant of tissue between individuals of the same species but of different genotypes.

Amenorrhea Absence of menstruation: **primary amenorrhea** if no menstrual periods have occurred by age 16 years; **secondary amenorrhea** if there is cessation of normally established menstruation.

Amniocentesis Withdrawal of fluid from the amniotic sac.

Amphophilic Having an affinity for both basic and acid dyes.

Amyloid Any of several types of amorphous eosinophilic extracellular protein, characterized by positive staining with Congo red (with apple-green birefringence in polarized light), a beta-pleated structure of x-ray diffraction studies, and a fibrillary appearance on electron microscopy.

Amyloidosis Deposition of amyloid in the interstitial space.

Anaerobe A microorganism that can multiply only in the absence of oxygen.

Anaphylaxis A systemic type I hypersensitivity reaction characterized by release of vasoactive substances into the bloodstream.

Anaplasia Failure of cells to differentiate and develop normal structure and function; commonly used for malignant neoplastic cells.

Anasarca Massive generalized edema associated with fluid accumulation in body cavities.

Anemia Decrease below normal of blood hemoglobin concentration.

Anergy A state of diminished immunologic reactivity to antigens.

Aneuploidy Any deviation from an exact multiple of the haploid number of chromosomes.

Aneurysm A localized abnormal dilatation of a blood vessel or of the heart.

Angina pectoris Ischemic myocardial pain, usually felt as a retrosternal tightening, that typically occurs on exertion and is relieved by rest.

Anisocytosis Variation in the size of cells, usually erythrocytes.

Ankylosis Restriction of movement of a joint owing to abnormal fibrous or bony union of the bone ends across the joint.

Anlage (= primordium) The earliest grouping of primitive embryonic cells from which an organ or tissue develops.

Anomaly A deviation from normal of the form, shape, or position of a structure, tissue, or organ.

Antibody An immunoglobulin molecule that contains specific amino acid sequences by virtue of which it reacts only with the antigen that induced its synthesis.

Antigen A molecule, usually protein or polysaccharide, capable of inducing a specific immune response and of reacting with the products of that response.

Antigenic determinant The structural component of an antigen molecule that is responsible for specific interaction with the antibody it induces.

Antitoxin An antibody that neutralizes microbial toxin.

Aplasia Complete failure of development of an organ or tissue from its anlage.

APUD An acronym—from amine precursor uptake and decarboxylation—for a system of neuroendocrine cells scattered throughout the body that secrete a variety of biogenic amines. (See also Neuroendocrine system.)

Arteriosclerosis Thickening, hardening, and loss of elasticity of an artery from any cause.

Arthus reaction A hypersensitivity reaction characterized by necrosis and acute inflammation at the site of antigen entry caused by the formation and deposition of immune complexes in the local microcirculation.

Ascites Excessive accumulation of free fluid in the peritoneal cavity.

Asthma A reversible condition caused by narrowing of the respiratory airways due to bronchial smooth muscle contraction.

Atelectasis Failure of the lungs to expand at birth or collapse of a previously inflated part of the lung.

Atheroma A lipid material deposited in the intima of arteries in atherosclerosis.

Atherosclerosis An arterial disease characterized by the formation of intimal plaques composed of lipid, smooth muscle, and collagen.

Atopy A localized type I hypersensitivity reaction resulting from release of vasoactive substances into the local tissues by mast cells.

Atrophy A decrease in the size of a cell, tissue, organ, or part, due either to a decrease in the size of individual cells or a reduction in numbers of cells.

Attenuation Reduction in the virulence of a microorganism.

Autoantibody An antibody that reacts with self antigens.

Autograft (= autogeneic graft = autologous graft) A transplant of tissue from one site to another in the body of an individual.

Autoimmune disease A disease resulting from a specific immune response directed against the body's own tissues.

Autoimmunity A state characterized by generation of a specific immune response against self antigens.

Autolysis Spontaneous liquefaction of cells or tissues by the action of their own enzymes.

Autopsy (= postmortem examination) The internal pathologic examination of a body after death.

Autosome Any chromosome that is not a sex chromosome.

Azoospermia Absence of spermatozoa in the semen.

Azotemia Elevation in blood levels of nonprotein nitrogenous compounds, mainly urea, uric acid, and creatinine.

B lymphocyte A lymphocyte that is primed in the bursa of Fabricius (in bird) or the bursa equivalent (fetal liver or bone marrow) in mammals. The B cell gives rise to plasma cells and is responsible for humoral immunity.

Bacteremia The presence of bacteria in the bloodstream.

Bacteriuria The presence of bacteria in the urine.

Band cell A neutrophil recently released from the bone marrow and characterized by an unsegmented nucleus that forms a continuous band.

Barr body A small, darkly staining mass of chromatin seen adjacent to the inner surface of the nuclear membrane in female cells during interphase.

Barrett's esophagus The presence of gastrointestinal columnar epithelium in the esophagus.

Basophilic Staining preferentially with basic dyes.

BCG (bacille Calmette-Guérin) An attenuated strain of *Mycobacterium bovis* that is used to actively immunize against tuberculosis and as a nonspecific immune stimulant.

Bence Jones protein Monoclonal immunoglobulin light chains detectable in the urine of some patients with B lymphocyte and plasma cell neoplasms.

Benign neoplasm One that does not infiltrate locally or metastasize.

Beta particle A particle emitted in radioactive decay consisting of either an electron or a positron.

Biopsy The surgical removal of cells, tissues, or fluids from the body for microscopic examination.

Blast cell A primitive precursor cell, usually applied to hematopoietic cells.

Blastema The primitive cells from which tissues are formed.

Blastocyst The ball of cells constituting the early embryo at the time of implantation in the uterus.

Blood coagulation The sequential process by which multiple plasma coagulation factors interact to finally cause the conversion of fibrinogen to fibrin.

Bronchiectasis Abnormal, permanent dilatation of bronchi.

Bruit (= murmur) An abnormal sound caused by turbulent blood flow in the cardiovascular system.

Bursa of Fabricius A small lymphoepithelial sac near the cloaca in birds that is critical to inducing B lymphocyte differentiation.

Cachexia A condition characterized by marked weight loss, wasting, anemia, weakness, and loss of appetite.

Calcification Deposition of crystalline calcium salts in tissues: **Dystrophic calcification** is deposition of calcium salts in abnormal tissues in persons whose plasma levels of calcium and phosphate are normal; **metastatic calcification** is deposition of calcium salts in tissues as a result of increased plasma levels of calcium or phosphate.

Calculus An abnormal concretion of crystalline material formed in the lumen of ducts and hollow organs.

Cancer Any malignant neoplasm.

Carcinogen An agent that causes malignant neoplasms.

Carcinogenesis The production of malignant neoplasms.

Carcinoma A malignant neoplasm derived from epithelial cells.

Carcinoma in situ A preinvasive stage of malignant epithelial neoplasms where the cytologic features of cancer are present but the neoplastic cells have not infiltrated through the basement membrane.

Carcinomatosis The presence in the body of widely disseminated cancer.

Cardiac tamponade A restriction of cardiac filling caused by accumulation of fluid in the pericardial sac.

Cardiomyopathy A primary myocardial disease of unknown cause characterized by ventricular enlargement in the absence of congenital, hypertensive, valvular, or ischemic heart disease.

CD (cluster designation) Terminology adopted for leukocyte surface antigens (eg, CD_4, CD_8).

Cell degeneration A reversible abnormality in cell structure.

Cellular (= cell-mediated) immunity The specific type of immune response that is mediated by T lymphocytes.

Cellular oncogene (C-*ONC*) Intrinsic cellular gene corresponding to a viral nucleic acid sequence (V-*ONC*) that is believed to play a role in cell growth regulation. Inappropriate expression may cause cancer.

Cellulitis A spreading acute inflammation of subcutaneous tissue.

Chalone A chemical substance released by a cell that inhibits cellular proliferation.

Chemotaxis Movement of a cell or an organism in response to a chemical concentration gradient.

Choristoma A developmental abnormality in which tissues not normally present in an organ grow in a disorganized fashion to produce a tumor. Not a true neoplasm. (Contrast with hamartoma.)

Chromatin A complex of nucleic acids and histones that constitute chromosomes.

Chronic inflammation The sum total of the response of the body to an injury that persists in the tissues. It is characterized by tissue manifestations of the immune response and by the phagocytic response and is associated with ongoing tissue damage and repair by fibrosis.

Chronic inflammatory cells Cells commonly present in the tissues in chronic inflammation, representing the effector cells of the immune response, phagocytosis, and repair (lymphocytes, plasma cells, macrophages, and fibroblasts).

Cirrhosis of the liver A diffuse chronic liver disease characterized by replacement of normal hepatic architecture by fibrosis and regenerative nodules.

Clonal deletion theory A theory advanced to explain natural tolerance to self antigens which states that clones of lymphoid cells which react against self antigens are permanently deleted on contact with the antigen during fetal life.

Clonal selection theory The hypothesis that a specific immune response is the result of selection, by reaction of the antigen with surface receptors on lymphocytes, of one or more clones of lymphocytes from a preexisting mass of many millions of lymphocyte clones.

Clone A number of identical cells (or nucleic acid sequences) derived from a single precursor.

Cloudy swelling Early reversible cell degeneration in states of injury, characterized by increased intracellular water; affected cells are swollen, and the cytoplasm appears cloudy.

Coagulative necrosis Cell death in which the cell becomes a homogeneous eosinophilic anuclear mass with retention of the basic cell outline.

Cold agglutinin An antibody that induces erythrocyte agglutination at temperatures below normal body temperature.

Collagen The fibrous protein formed in interstitial tissue from tropocollagen units secreted by fibroblasts.

Commensalism A natural state in which 2 organisms live together with benefit to one and no harm to the other, or with benefit to both (symbiosis).

Complement A series of plasma proteins that are activated in cascade fashion in certain immune reactions, leading to the release of vasoactive and chemotactic substances and resulting in the formation of a cytotoxic complex.

C-*ONC* See Cellular oncogene.

Concussion Transient loss of consciousness immediately following a head injury in the absence of detectable structural abnormality in the brain.

Congenital Present at birth.

Congestion (= hyperemia) The presence of an increased amount of blood in dilated blood vessels in tissues.

Consumption coagulopathy An acute reduction in blood coagulation factors resulting from their utilization in patients developing extensive intravascular coagulation.

Contact inhibition Cessation of cell proliferation that occurs when cells come into contact with one another.

Contraction Shortening or reduction in size

Contusion (= bruise) An injury characterized by extravasation of blood into the tissues without significant tissue disruption.

Coombs test (antiglobulin test) A method of detecting the presence of antibody fixed on the surface of erythrocytes.

Cowdry A inclusion body A large, round eosinophilic intranuclear inclusion body surrounded by a halo and occurring in cells infected by many viruses, most commonly herpesviruses.

Curling's ulcer Acute peptic ulceration of the stomach or duodenum following a severe burn on the surface of the body.

Cyanosis Bluish discoloration of the skin and mucous membranes owing to an increased concentration of reduced hemoglobin in the blood.

Cyst An epithelium-lined cavity containing fluid or semisolid material.

Cytopathic effect Morphologic changes that occur in cells during virus replication.

Cytotoxic Having a deleterious effect on cells.
Death The irreversible cessation of normal life processes. From a legal standpoint, death is usually defined as cessation of detectable electrical activity in the brain along with cardiac and respiratory arrest.
Debridement The surgical removal of devitalized tissue and foreign material from an area of injury until surrounding or underlying healthy tissue is exposed.
Definitive host In infectious disease, the host in which a parasite has its adult and sexual existence.
Degranulation The process in which cells lose their cytoplasmic granules.
Delayed hypersensitivity A type of immunologic hypersensitivity reaction that is manifested several hours (usually 24–72 hours) after exposure to the inciting antigen. The term is restricted in current usage to type IV hypersensitivity.
Deletion In genetics, a chromosomal abnormality characterized by loss of part of the chromosome.
Dementia An organic brain disorder characterized by progressive loss of cognitive functions and failure of memory.
Demyelination Loss of the myelin sheath of a nerve fiber without destruction of the axon.
Denudation Exposure of subepithelial tissues due to removal of the surface epithelium.
Desmoplasia Proliferation of fibroblasts with laying down of collagen; used particularly to denote production of a reactive fibrous stroma in neoplasms.
Diagnosis Determination of the nature of disease.
Diapedesis The passage outward of blood cells from a blood vessel to the interstitial space through an intact vessel wall.
Diarrhea An increase in the fluidity of bowel movements beyond what is usual for the individual.
Differentiation, cell The process by which immature cells mature morphologically to adult cells and become specialized to perform specific functions.
Differentiation, tumor The extent to which neoplastic cells are distinguished morphologically from their normal counterparts.
Diffuse Widely distributed.
Diploid Having 2 sets of homologous chromosomes.
Disease Any deviation of the normal structure or function of an organ that is manifested by a characteristic set of symptoms and signs.
Disseminated intravascular coagulation Formation of widespread thrombi in the microcirculation.
Diverticulum Protrusion of the lumen of a hollow viscus outside the normal plane of the adventitia. The luminal protrusion may be lined by mucosa alone **(false diverticulum)** or the entire wall **(true diverticulum).**
Dominant trait In genetics, a trait expressed when the abnormal allele is carried by only one of a pair of homologous chromosomes.
Doubling time (= generation time) The time required for all components of a cell culture to multiply by 2. In neoplasms, the time taken for the constituent number of cells to multiply by 2.
Drug Any chemical with therapeutic properties.
Drug abuse Excessive nontherapeutic use of a drug to the extent of developing dependence to the drug.
Drug dependence A state in which an established level of dosage or increasing doses of the drug are needed to prevent symptoms of withdrawal.
Dysentery Acute inflammation of the colon characterized by passage of liquid stools containing blood and mucus.
Dysfunctional uterine bleeding Excessive, disorderly menstrual bleeding resulting from hormonal imbalance.
Dysgenesis Defective development of an organ or tissue giving rise to an organ that is structurally abnormal.
Dyskeratosis The abnormal, often premature keratinization of squamous epithelial cells during maturation.
Dysmenorrhea Painful menstruation.
Dysphagia Difficulty in swallowing, usually manifested as a sensation of food becoming obstructed.
Dysplasia A cytologic abnormality in which affected cells have some of the criteria of malignancy but not enough to justify a diagnosis of carcinoma in situ (for epithelia) or malignant neoplasia.
Dyspnea Any alteration in breathing associated with awareness of respiratory effort.
Dystrophic calcification See Calcification.
Dysuria Pain or difficulty with urination.
Ecchymosis Hemorrhage into the skin that exceeds 3 cm in diameter.
Ectoderm The outer germ layer of the embryo that gives rise mainly to the skin and neural tissue.
Ectopic (= heterotopic) The occurrence of a structurally normal tissue or organ in an abnormal location.
Eczema An acute or chronic noncontagious inflammatory condition of the skin.
Edema Accumulation of excess amounts of fluid in the interstitial spaces.
Effector cells In immunology, lymphocytes that have been activated by antigen exposure which are the direct mediators of the immune response.
Effusion Escape of fluid into body cavities and joints.
Elephantiasis A clinical state caused by chronic lymphatic obstruction and characterized by lymphedema and hyperplasia of the skin.
Elliptocyte (= ovalocyte) An oval-shaped erythrocyte.
Embolism Occlusion of a blood vessel by an abnormal mass (called an **embolus,** which may be solid, liquid, or gaseous) that is transported by the bloodstream to that site from a different location in the body.
Emigration of leukocytes The active outward passage of leukocytes through the intact walls of the microcirculation.
Emperipolesis The penetration of and movement within a cell by another cell (usually a lymphocyte within a macrophage).
Emphysema Accumulation of air within a tissue.
Empyema A collection of purulent exudate in a body cavity or hollow viscus.
Endoderm See Entoderm.
Endometriosis The occurrence of endometrial glands and stroma in a location other than the endometrium.
Endotoxin A lipopolysaccharide component of the cell walls of gram-negative bacteria that has cytotoxic properties.
End-stage kidney A chronically damaged kidney in which the original underlying renal disease cannot be determined.

Enterotoxin An exotoxin produced by bacteria that has an adverse effect on the epithelial cells of the gastrointestinal tract.

Entoderm (= endoderm) The inner germ layer of the embryo that gives rise to the gastrointestinal tract, liver, pancreas, and respiratory tract.

Eosinophilic Having an affinity for the acidic dye eosin.

Epidemic Affecting a large number of persons in one geographic region at the same time.

Epidemiology The science concerned with the factors that determine the incidence and distribution of disease in a population.

Epilepsy A disorder characterized by recurrent seizures due to paroxysmal abnormal electrical discharges in the brain.

Epithelioid cell granuloma An aggregate of activated macrophages that superficially resemble epithelial cells, resulting from an immune response mediated by lymphokines produced by T lymphocytes.

Epitope An antigenic determinant, or that part of a molecule that reacts with the binding site of an antibody.

Erythrocyte rouleaux Aggregation of erythrocytes in the blood in a stacklike configuration resembling a pile of coins.

Essential hypertension Persistent elevation of the blood pressure without a discoverable underlying disease.

Essential nutrient A substance necessary for normal metabolism that must be supplied by food since it cannot be synthesized in the body.

Exotoxin A protein complex secreted by bacteria into the environment that has the potential for causing changes in cells at a location different from the site of infection.

Expressivity In genetics, the degree to which a heritable trait is manifested by an individual carrying the gene for the trait.

Exudation The outflow of increased amounts of fluid from the microcirculation into the interstitial spaces through vessels whose permeability is increased.

Facultative intracellular organisms Microorganisms that can multiply both extracellularly and intracellularly.

Fatty change The accumulation of lipid in the cytoplasm of cells.

Fc receptor A cell surface receptor present on some leukocytes that binds with the Fc (fragment, crystallizable) end of some immunoglobulin molecules.

Fibrillation The uncoordinated and ineffective contraction of single muscle fibers.

Fibrinoid A substance that accumulates in a variety of degenerative connective tissues characterized microscopically by a homogeneous, deeply eosinophilic staining reaction that resembles the staining properties of fibrin.

Fibrinolysis Dissolution of fibrin by enzymatic action resulting from activation of the enzyme plasmin in the bloodstream.

Fistula An abnormal passage that connects 2 epithelium-lined structures.

Focal Localized to a specific area.

Fomite (= fomes) An object harmless in itself that harbors infectious agents and may thus serve to transmit an infection.

Foreign body giant cell A multinucleated macrophage that has its nuclei dispersed haphazardly throughout the cytoplasm.

Foreign body granuloma A localized aggregate of macrophages around an inert, nonantigenic foreign body.

Fracture An injury characterized by a break in the tissue.

Free radical A highly unstable atom or molecule that has one or more unpaired electrons.

Friable Easily crumbled or broken into little pieces.

Frostbite Tissue injury resulting from exposure of the tissue to freezing temperatures.

Galactorrhea Flow of milk unrelated to lactation, usually caused by abnormally increased levels of prolactin.

Gamete A haploid germ cell—either an ovum or a spermatozoon.

Gamma ray A photon emitted by a radionuclide.

Gangrene Necrosis of tissue from any cause associated with bacterial infection.

Gene The fundamental unit of heredity that carries a single mendelian trait.

Genome The normal complement of chromosomes with the genes they contain.

Genotype The genetic makeup of an individual.

Germ layers The 3 fundamental embryonic divisions of cells—ectoderm, entoderm, and mesoderm—from which the organs and tissues are derived.

Giant cell A large multinucleated cell.

Goiter Any enlargement of the thyroid gland.

Goblet cell A mucin-secreting cell characterized by a large cytoplasmic vacuole filled with mucin.

Grade (in characterizing malignant neoplasms) A numerical representation of the degree of histologic differentiation of a malignant neoplasm.

Graft Any tissue that is transplanted from one site to another.

Graft-versus-host (GVH) disease A disease in which foreign immunocompetent cells introduced into a host react immunologically against host tissues.

Granulocytopenia (= neutropenia) A decrease in the number of neutrophil leukocytes in peripheral blood below 1500/μL.

Granulation tissue Pink, soft tissue that occurs in healing wounds composed of proliferating fibroblasts and new capillaries, frequently containing inflammatory cells.

Granuloma A nodular aggregate of macrophages involved in phagocytic and immune defense mechanisms.

Ground substance The acellular amorphous matrix of connective tissue, composed mainly of proteoglycans and water, in which cells are embedded.

Gumma A localized granulomatous mass that occurs in tertiary syphilis.

GVH disease See Graft-versus-host disease.

Gynecomastia Enlargement of the male breast.

Half-life The time taken for a substance to be reduced to half its original concentration by a process of natural decay or elimination.

Hamartoma A developmental abnormality in which the tissues normally present in an organ grow in a disorganized fashion to produce a tumor. Not a true neoplasm. (Contrast with choristoma.)

Haploid number The number of chromosomes in a gamete; in humans, the haploid number is 23.

Haplotype A group of genes that are so closely linked on the chromosome that they are inherited together as a group.

Haptens Small molecules that are not antigenic by themselves but can act as antigens when complexed with larger molecules.

Healing The process of restoration of integrity to injured tissue. **By first intention (= primary healing):** Healing of a skin wound where the wound edges are brought into apposition, and which is achieved with a minimum amount of scar formation. **By second intention (= secondary healing):** Healing of a large open skin wound achieved by granulation tissue ingrowth and extensive scarring.

Hematin The crystalline product of oxidation of heme from the ferrous to the ferric state.

Hematocrit (= packed cell volume) The volume of erythrocytes, expressed as a percentage of the volume of whole blood.

Hematoidin A golden-yellow crystalline material deposited in tissues as a result of breakdown of hemoglobin; it does not contain iron and has a structure similar that of bilirubin.

Hematoma A localized collection of blood in a tissue resulting from disruption of a blood vessel.

Hematopoiesis The production and development of blood cells.

Hemochromatosis A disorder characterized by iron overload and deposition of iron in parenchymal cells of various organs, resulting in cell necrosis.

Hemoconcentration An increase in the cell concentration of blood caused by a decrease in its fluid content.

Hemoglobinopathy A disorder caused by an alteration in molecular structure of hemoglobin.

Hemolysis The liberation of hemoglobin from erythrocytes.

Hemolytic anemia Anemia characterized by a shortened life span of erythrocytes.

Hemorrhage Escape of blood from the vascular system either into the tissues or the environment due to disruption of blood vessels.

Hemosiderosis The presence of increased amounts of stored iron in a tissue; differs from hemochromatosis in that there is no parenchymal cell necrosis.

Hemostasis The arrest of bleeding from a damaged blood vessel.

Hermaphroditism The presence of both testicular and ovarian tissue in one individual.

Hernia The protrusion of tissue through an opening in the surrounding tissue.

Heterograft (= heterologous graft = xenograft) A transplant of tissue between 2 animals of different species.

Heterozygous In genetics, having 2 different alleles of a particular gene.

Heterozygous carrier An individual who carries an abnormal gene for a recessive trait in one of the pair of homologous chromosomes; this individual does not manifest the disease but can transmit it the offspring.

Histocompatibility antigen A genetically determined antigen present on the cell surface of nucleated cells that induces an immune reaction when transplanted into a genetically different host.

Histology (= microscopic anatomy) The branch of anatomy concerned with the microscopic structure of cells and tissues.

HLA (human leukocyte antigen) complex A major group of histocompatibility antigens that is determined by genetic loci situated in the short arm of chromosome 6.

Homozygous In genetics, having 2 identical alleles of a particular gene.

Host (1) In infectious diseases, an animal or plant that harbors a parasitic microorganism. (2) In transplantation, the recipient of a graft.

Humoral immunity The component of the immune response that is mediated by B lymphocytes and immunoglobulin.

Hyalin An abnormal condensation of fibrillary proteins in the cytoplasm of liver cells, seen typically but not exclusively in acute alcoholic liver disease.

Hyaline Glassy and transparent.

Hydrocephalus A condition characterized by an increase in size of the ventricular system of the brain.

Hyperchromatism Excessive staining; usually used for nuclear hyperchromatism, which is a common microscopic feature of cancer.

Hyperemia (= congestion) The presence of an increased amount of blood in a tissue due to dilatation of blood vessels. **Active hyperemia** is the result of active arteriolar dilatation; **passive hyperemia** results from obstruction to venous outflow.

Hyperplasia An increase in the size of a tissue due to an increase in the number of constituent cells.

Hypersensitivity A state of altered reactivity in which the immune system reacts in an exaggerated way to an antigen, usually resulting in tissue damage. (See also Delayed hypersensitivity.)

Hypertension Elevation of blood pressure. (See also Essential hypertension, Malignant hypertension.)

Hyperthermia Abnormally high body temperature.

Hypertrophy Increase in size of a tissue due to an increase in the size of its constituent cells.

Hypervariable regions The 4 or more segments in the heavy and light chains of the immunoglobulin molecule that display marked variation in amino acid sequence and are responsible for conferring specificity to the antibody.

Hypoplasia Incomplete development of an organ from its anlage; the hypoplastic organ is smaller but structurally normal.

Hypovolemia An abnormal decrease in intravascular blood volume.

Hypoxemia A reduction in the amount of oxygen in arterial blood.

Hypoxia A reduction in the amount of oxygen available to tissues.

Iatrogenic illness An adverse condition resulting from actions of a physician.

Icterus (= jaundice) A yellow discoloration of tissues caused by an increase in the plasma bilirubin level.

Idiopathic Without known cause.

Idiotype An antigenic determinant present on and characteristic of a particular antibody molecule, located in the variable region (ie, the site of antigen binding).

Immediate hypersensitivity A type of hypersensitivity response that is manifested within minutes after exposure to the inciting antigen. The term is currently restricted in usage to type I hypersensitivity responses.

Immersion syndrome (= trench foot) Tissue injury caused by prolonged exposure of the tissue to nonfreezing cold water.

Immune complex The product of interaction between an antigen and an antibody; small, soluble immune complexes may be carried in the circulation to be deposited in tissues, leading to **immune complex diseases.**

Immune response The specific host response mediated by lymphocytes against a molecule that is recognized as foreign (the antigen).

Immune surveillance theory The theory that one major function of the immune system is to recognize and destroy neoplastic cells at their inception.

Immunity The ability of the host to defend against foreign antigens.

Immunization Production of a protective immune response by the deliberate introduction of foreign antigens into the host.

Immunoblast A large actively proliferating lymphoid cell that is formed as a result of antigen-induced transformation of a lymphocyte (both B and T lymphocytes); it is the immediate precursor of the effector cells.

Immunodeficient (= immunocompromised) Having an impaired immune response.

Immunoglobulin (= antibody) A protein synthesized by plasma cells that functions as a specific antibody reactive against the antigen that stimulated transformation of a B lymphocyte into that plasma cell.

Immunologic memory The capacity of the immune system to respond more rapidly and strongly to a subsequent challenge by an antigen to which the host has been previously exposed.

Immunologic tolerance An immunologic response characterized by the development of specific nonreactivity of the immune system to an antigen that is capable under other conditions of inducing an immune response.

Inborn error of metabolism A congenital biochemical abnormality resulting from the failure of synthesis of a protein (usually an enzyme) due to a specific genetic defect.

Incision An injury produced by a sharp instrument characterized by cutting of tissue.

Inclusion body A microscopically visible intracellular mass associated with intracellular viral or chlamydial replication.

Incubation period The time between exposure to an infectious agent and the first appearance of clinical symptoms due to that infection.

Induration The process of becoming hard.

Inert Not causing a reaction when introduced into the body.

Infarct A localized area of cell necrosis in a tissue caused by a reduction of arterial blood flow to the area.

Infection Multiplication of a microorganism in tissues.

Infectious disease A disease caused by infection.

Infectivity The ability to produce infection.

Inflammation See Acute inflammation, Chronic inflammation.

Initiation In carcinogenesis, the transformation of a cell into a neoplastic cell by a carcinogenic agent.

Inspissation The process of thickening of a fluid resulting from evaporation of water.

Interferon A group of proteins that inhibit viral replication and have a wide variety of effects on cells.

Interleukins Substances produced by leukocytes with activity on other leukocytes.

Intermediate host The host in which a parasite has its larval or nonsexual existence.

Intussusception The telescoping of a segment of intestine into a neighboring distal segment.

Invasion The extension by direct growth of a neoplasm into the adjacent normal tissues; a sign of a malignant neoplasm.

Involution A retrograde change in a tissue associated with decrease in size and number of parenchymal cells.

Ischemia Reduction of arterial blood supply to a part.

Jaundice (= icterus) Yellow discoloration of tissues caused by elevation of plasma bilirubin level.

K (killer) cell A lymphocyte that does not mark as either a T or a B cell and is the effector cell in antibody-dependent cell-mediated cytotoxicity.

Karyolysis Dissolution of the nucleus in a necrotic cell.

Karyorrhexis Disintegration of the nucleus into small, irregular, dark fragments in a necrotic cell.

Karyotype Systematic arrangement of the chromosomes of a cell achieved after arrest of mitosis of the cell in metaphase and separation of the chromosomes.

Keloid A nodular, enlarging scar resulting from excessive collagen deposition during healing of a skin wound.

Kernicterus A disorder characterized by deposition of bilirubin in the brain in neonates resulting in diffuse neuronal damage.

Kinins A group of chemical mediators derived from activation of precursor proteins in the plasma that act on blood vessels, smooth muscle, and pain-sensitive nerve endings (eg, bradykinin).

Kwashiorkor A form of protein-calorie malnutrition, usually in children, characterized by growth retardation, edema, and abnormal synthesis of plasma proteins and structural proteins of skin and hair.

Labile cell A cell that is continually dividing throughout life to replace cells that are being continuously lost from the body.

Laceration An injury characterized by tearing of tissue.

Langerhan's cell A specialized macrophage in skin.

Langhans' giant cells Multinucleated macrophages that have their nuclei arranged in a ring or horseshoe pattern at the periphery of the cell, typically seen in epithelioid cell granulomas.

Latent infection A phase of established infection during which the microorganism is dormant and there are no recognizable manifestations of disease.

Lesion Any structural or functional abnormality.

Leukemia A malignant neoplasm of hematopoietic cells.

Leukemoid reaction A severe reactive proliferation of neutrophil leukocytes that resembles leukemia.

Leukoplakia A clinical condition characterized by the development of thickened white patches on a mucosal surface.

Leukotrienes Vasoactive metabolites of arachidonic acid.
Lipofuscin A granular, brown, iron-negative pigment present in parenchymal cells of elderly and chronically ill individuals.
Liquefactive necrosis A type of necrosis characterized by enzymatic liquefaction of necrotic cells.
Locus The site of a gene on the chromosome.
Lymphadenopathy A general term used to denote enlargement of a lymph node due to any cause.
Lymphedema Progressive nonpitting edema of subcutaneous tissue caused by lymphatic obstruction.
Lymphokines A group of soluble proteins produced by T lymphocytes on exposure to antigen that play a role in cell-mediated immunity.
Lysis Liquefaction.
Macrocyte An erythrocyte with an increased corpuscular volume.
Macrophage A large cell derived from monocyte precursors in the bone marrow that functions in phagocytosis and the immune response.
Major histocompatibility complex The chromosomal region containing the genes that control the histocompatibility antigens (see HLA complex).
Malabsorption syndrome A group of diseases characterized by failure of absorption of dietary nutrients from the intestine.
Malformation A congenital structural abnormality of an organ.
Malignant Tending to become progressively worse and cause death; in neoplasia, the term signifies invasiveness and metastasis.
Malignant hypertension A condition characterized by severe hypertension and papilledema.
Malnutrition Any disorder of nutrition.
Marasmus A form of protein-calorie malnutrition, usually in children, characterized by growth retardation and wasting but usually with retention of appetite and mental alertness.
Margination Displacement of leukocytes from the central axial stream of blood flow to the periphery of the vessel, where they come into apposition with the endothelium.
Maturation The process whereby a primitive cell reaches its final structure and functional capacity.
Megaloblast A large abnormal erythrocyte precursor characterized by asynchrony of nuclear and cytoplasmic maturation.
Melena Darkening of stools due to the presence of blood.
Menarche The onset of cyclic menstruation in the adolescent female.
Menopause The period of life during which normal cyclic menstruation ceases.
Menorrhagia Excessive uterine bleeding coupled with normal cycle length.
Mesenchyme The embryonic tissue derived from the mesoderm that becomes the connective tissue of the body.
Mesoderm The middle germ layer of the embyro that gives rise mainly to the connective tissues.
Metachromatic A staining pattern in which tissue takes on a color different from that of the stain.
Metaplasia The replacement of one adult cell type by another.
Metastasis The process by which malignant neoplastic cells form secondary tumor deposits discontinuous with the primary tumor.
Metastatic calcification See Calcification.
Microangiopathy Any disorder affecting the microcirculation.
Microcyte An erythrocyte with a decreased corpuscular volume.
Microinvasion Limited invasion of the tissue subjacent to the basement membrane by the cells of a carcinoma.
Mitotic figure A cell undergoing mitotic division as identified by microscopic examination.
Monoclonal antibody Antibody of uniform specificity derived from a single clone.
Monoclonal cell population A group of cells derived from a single cell.
Monoclonal gammopathy A disease characterized by the presence of a large amount of one immunoglobulin type produced by a single clone of B lymphocytes.
Monosomy The absence of one of a pair of homologous chromosomes in an otherwise diploid cell.
M protein A term often used for the monoclonal immunoglobulin in plasma assocated with B lymphocyte and plasma cell neoplasms.
Mucin A viscous fluid composed of glycoproteins that is secreted by mucous glands.
Murmur (= bruit) An abnormal sound produced by turbulent blood flow in the cardiovascular system.
Mutation In genetics, a stable, heritable alteration in the genetic material of a cell, usually involving a single gene.
Mycosis A disease caused by fungi.
Mycosis fungoides A malignant T cell lymphoma of the skin; **not a fungal infection (therefore a misnomer).**
Mycotic aneurysm An aneurysm resulting from infection of the arterial wall. (***Note:*** The term *mycotic* covers all infections in this context and is not restricted to fungal infections; it is therefore a misnomer.)
Myeloid Pertaining to the granulocyte series of cells.
Myeloproliferative disorder A neoplastic proliferation of one or more cell lines of the bone marrow, including granulocytic, erythrocytic, and megakaryocytic precursors.
Myopathy A general term used to denote a muscle disorder.
Myxedema A condition associated with swelling of a tissue caused by accumulation of hydrated mucopolysaccharides.
Myxoid degeneration An abnormality in connective tissue characterized by an increase in the proteoglycan content of ground substance.
Natural killer (NK) cells Lymphocytes that do not mark as either B or T lymphocytes which are cytotoxic without being specifically sensitized against the target cell.
Necrosis Death of a cell or group of cells contained in living tissue.
Neoplasm An abnormal mass of cells whose growth is excessive and uncoordinated with that of surrounding cells and continues in the same excessive manner after withdrawal of the stimulus that initiated the growth.
Nephritic syndrome A condition characterized by oli-

guria, hematuria, proteinuria, hypertension, edema, and azotemia.

Nephrotic syndrome A condition in which increased glomerular permeability leads to heavy proteinuria, hypoproteinemia, and massive edema.

Neuroendocrine system (formerly APUD system) A system of cells scattered throughout the body that secrete biologically active peptide hormones and amines.

Neutropenia A decrease in the absolute neutrophil count of peripheral blood below 1500/μL.

Nondisjunction The failure of homologous chromosomes or sister chromatids to separate during meiotic or mitotic cell division.

Normoblast Nucleated precursor cells of the erythroid series.

Nosocomial Originating in a hospital.

Nuclear:cytoplasmic ratio The ratio of the diameter of the nucleus of the cell to the diameter of the cytoplasm.

Null cell A lymphocyte that does not have surface immunoglobulin and does not produce E rosettes when incubated with sheep red erythrocytes.

Obligate intracellular organism An organism that can grow and multiply only inside living cells.

Oligoclonal bands In cerebrospinal fluid protein electrophoresis, the presence of 2–5 distinct immunoglobulin bands.

Oliguria A decrease in urine output—in an adult, to less than 400 mL/24 h.

Oncofetal antigen A gene product that is expressed by fetal and neoplastic cells but suppressed in normal adult cells.

Oncogene The heritable genetic material carrying the potential for cancer. (See also Cellular oncogene, Viral oncogene.)

Oncogenesis The process by which neoplasms are produced.

Oncotic pressure The osmotic pressure exerted by colloids in a solution.

Opportunistic infection An infection caused by microorganisms of low virulence or by microorganisms considered nonpathogenic in the normal host, occurring in individuals with impaired immune defense mechanisms.

Opsonin A substance—usually an antibody or complement factor—that increases the susceptibility of bacteria and other cells to phagocytosis.

Organization Replacement of an area of injury by granulation tissue and collagen.

Organotropism The affinity of a pathogenic microorganism for particular organs or tissues of the body.

Osmotic pressure The force needed to counterbalance the force of osmotic flow across a semipermeable membrane.

Osteomalacia A condition in adults resulting from failure of mineralization of bone, leading to bone softening and excessive accumulation of uncalcified osteoid.

Osteoporosis A condition characterized by a reduction in total bone mass, usually manifested as thinning of trabecular bone.

Pandemic An epidemic disease that has an unusually wide distribution, usually involving more than one continent.

Pannus An abnormal mass of inflamed granulation tissue. The term is usually used in relation to the cornea and synovial membrane.

Papilledema Swelling of the optic disk.

Papilloma A benign epithelial neoplasm characterized grossly or microscopically by the presence of fingerlike projections from the epithelial surface.

Pap smear A cytologic preparation made from a scraping of the uterine cervix and stained with Papanicolaou stain.

Paraneoplastic syndrome Any complex of symptoms in a patient with cancer that cannot be directly attributed to the physical presence of either the primary tumor or its metastases.

Paraproteinemia Presence of increased amounts of a monoclonal immunoglobulin in the plasma, associated with a neoplasm of B lymphocytes or plasma cells.

Parasite An organism that lives upon or within another living organism and derives some advantage from the association.

Pathogen A disease-producing microorganism.

Pathogenesis The abnormal biochemical and pathophysiologic mechanisms that lead to disease.

Pathogenicity The capacity to produce disease.

Pathognomonic (= diagnostic) A clinical or pathologic abnormality specifically characteristic of one disease and no other.

Pavementing Adhesion of marginated leukocytes to the vascular endothelium as a prelude to their emigration out of the vessel.

Pellagra The disease resulting from niacin deficiency, characterized by dermatitis, dementia, and diarrhea.

Penetrance The frequency with which a heritable trait is manifested in individuals carrying the gene for the trait.

Perinatal Occurring at, shortly before, or immediately after birth.

Petechial hemorrhage A hemorrhage into the skin that is less than 3 cm in diameter.

Permanent cell A cell that has no capacity for mitotic division in postnatal life.

Phagocytosis The engulfment of microorganisms, other cells, and foreign particles by neutrophils and macrophages.

Phenotype The morphologic characteristics of an individual that result from interaction of genetic and environmental factors.

Phlebothrombosis Formation of a thrombus in a vein when inflammation is not the primary factor that induces the thrombosis.

Pinocytosis A method of active transport across the cell membrane characterized by formation of invaginations of membrane around extracellular fluid and contents which then close and pinch off to form pinocytic vesicles (pinosomes).

Plasma cell The effector cell resulting from antigen-induced transformation of B lymphocytes that produces specific antibody against the antigen that induced its formation.

Plasmid In bacteria, an extrachromosomal genetic element that contains autonomously replicating DNA distinct from the bacterial chromosome.

Pleomorphism In cytology, the presence of many different abnormal cell shapes, sizes, and nuclear appearances in a cell population.

Pluripotent Capable of differentiating into more than one cell type of one or 2 germ cell layers.

Pneumoconiosis A group of chronic diseases caused by inhalation of any of a large number of inorganic dusts.

Pneumonia Acute inflammation of the lung parenchyma.

Poikilocytosis The presence in the peripheral blood of erythrocytes with an abnormal degree of variation in shape.

Polyclonal cell population A cell population that is derived from many different cells.

Polycythemia A condition in which there is an increase in the erythrocyte count, hemoglobin concentration, and hematocrit of peripheral blood. In **Relative polycythemia,** the change is caused by a reduction in plasma volume; in **absolute polycythemia,** it is the result of an increase in erythrocyte numbers.

Polyp A circumscribed tumor that projects above the normally flat surface of an epithelium or mucous membrane.

Polyploidy An increase in the number of chromosomes by exact multiples of the number of chromosomes present in diploid cells.

Polyposis The presence of multiple polyps.

Portal of entry The site at which an infectious agent enters the body.

Precancerous (= premalignant) A pathologic process other than cancer that has an increased tendency compared with normal tissue to become a malignant neoplasm.

Premature baby A baby that weighs less than 2500 g at birth.

Preterm delivery The birth of a fetus before 34 weeks of gestation.

Primary amenorrhea See Amenorrhea.

Primordium See Anlage.

Prognosis The expected outcome of a disease process.

Promoter In neoplasia, a chemical substance that has no carcinogenic activity but is capable of increasing the incidence and rate of development of a neoplasm in a tissue previously exposed to a carcinogen.

Protein-calorie malnutrition Disease resulting from insufficient supply of protein and calories to the body.

Psammoma body A discrete, round, concentrically laminated, mineralized body seen in certain neoplasms.

Pseudocyst An abnormal fluid-filled cavity that is not lined by epithelium.

Pseudohermaphroditism The presence of gonads of one sex but internal and external reproductive organs that are either ambiguous or of the sex different from gonadal sex.

Pseudomembrane A flat plaque resembling a membrane on a mucosal surface that is composed of acute inflammatory exudate and necrotic epithelial cells.

Pseudopolyp In the intestine, a polypoid structure composed of inflammatory tissue and not neoplasm.

Purpura A disorder characterized by the occurrence of multiple small hemorrhages in the skin, mucous membranes, and serosal surfaces.

Purulent Consisting of, containing, or forming pus.

Pus A yellow liquid or semisolid substance composed of liquefied necrotic cells and neutrophil leukocytes.

Pyknosis A nuclear change associated with cell necrosis which is characterized by shrinkage and condensation of its chromatin.

Pyogenic Producing pus.

Pyrogen A chemical substance that acts on the temperature-regulating mechanism of the body and results in fever.

Radiation Emission of waves or particles from a source. **Ionizing radiation** has enough energy to displace electrons from atoms and lead to formation of unstable ions on interaction with tissues; **nonionizing radiation** does not have an adequate energy to cause ionization in tissues.

Radioactivity A phenomenon exhibited by unstable isotopes of chemical elements that undergo spontaneous decay, emitting various high-energy particles.

Radioresistant In tissues and neoplasms, indicating a relative resistance to the harmful effects of radiation in therapeutic dosage ranges.

Radiosensitive In tissues and neoplasms, indicating a relative sensitivity to the harmful effects of radiation in therapeutic dosage ranges.

Radiotherapy The use of ionizing radiation in the treatment of disease, usually cancer.

Raynaud's phenomenon The occurrence of transient and reversible ischemic changes in a tissue, usually an extremity, caused by spasm of small arteries.

Recanalization One end result of healing of a thrombus, characterized by organization and the formation of new vascular channels that serve to reestablish the circulation.

Recessive trait In genetics, a trait expressed when the abnormal allele is carried by both members of a pair of homologous chromosomes.

Reflux Backward flow of the contents of one hollow viscus to another.

Regeneration The replacement of parenchymal cells lost during injury by like cells.

Rejection An immune response against an antigenically incompatible transplanted tissue that leads to failure of function in the grafted tissue.

Relapse The return of symptoms or pathologic changes in a tissue with a chronic disease that has been kept in control.

Remission Abatement of the symptoms of a disease.

Repair The replacement of dead or damaged tissue by collagen (scar tissue).

Reservoir of infection An alternative host or passive carrier of a pathogenic microorganism.

Resolution The process by which a tissue returns to normal after an acute inflammatory response.

Reticulocyte An erythrocyte soon after its release from the bone marrow; it differs from other erythrocytes in being slightly larger and containing cytoplasmic RNA.

Reverse transcriptase An RNA-dependent DNA polymerase possessed by retroviruses that permits synthesis of a DNA copy of viral RNA.

Rickets A condition in children resulting from the failure of mineralization of bone, causing growth retardation and abnormal ossification.

Rouleaux See Erythrocyte rouleaux.

Sarcoma A malignant neoplasm of cells of mesodermal origin.

Scar A mass of collagen that is the end result of repair of an injury.

Schistocyte (= schizocyte) A deformed erythrocyte resulting from apposition of adjacent parts of the cell membrane.

Scirrhous Hard, indurated; usually used to describe the gross appearance of cancers that have a desmoplastic stromal response.

Sclerosis (= fibrosis) Deposition of collagen.

Scurvy The disease resulting from vitamin C (ascorbic acid) deficiency, characterized by abnormal collagen synthesis and vascular fragility.

Secondary amenorrhea See Amenorrhea.

Sensitivity In diagnostic pathology, The proportion of time a diagnostic test is positive in patients who have the disease or condition. A sensitive test has a low false-negative rate.

Sensitization The first exposure of an individual to an antigen leading to a primary immune response in cases where subsequent exposure to the antigen causes a hypersensitivity reaction.

Septicemia The systemic disease associated with the presence and multiplication of microorganisms or their toxins in the bloodstream.

Serology In infectious diseases, the detection of serum antibodies as evidence of a specific infection.

Serous Thin and watery, like serum.

Serum sickness A systemic immune complex-mediated disorder caused by the injection of foreign serum.

Sessile A descriptive term used for polyps denoting a broad base of attachment to the mucosa.

Sexually transmitted infection An infectious disease acquired through sexual contact.

Shock An acute generalized decrease of tissue perfusion caused by acute circulatory failure.

Sideroblast An erythroid precursor in the bone marrow that contains stainable iron in the form of ferritin in the cytoplasm.

Sign (= physical sign) Objective evidence of disease as observed or elicited by the physician.

Sinus An abnormal tract lined with granulation tissue that drains an inflammatory mass onto an epithelial surface.

Specificity In diagnostic pathology, the proportion of the time a diagnostic test is negative in patients who do not have the disease or condition. A specific test has a low false-positive rate.

Spherocyte An erythrocyte of decreased diameter recognizable on smears by the absence of the usual central area of pallor.

Sprue A disorder of the small intestine characterized by abnormal structure of villi and malabsorption.

Stable cell A cell that has a long life span and does not undergo mitotic division unless stimulated to regenerate.

Staging (= tumor staging) The classification of a malignant neoplasm based on its degree of spread, both local invasion and metastatic.

Stellate granuloma A specific morphologic type of epithelioid granuloma which has a central stellate zone of neutrophils.

Steatorrhea Excretion of a stool containing increased amounts of fat, in excess in 5 g/d. Steatorrhea is a typical clinical manifestation of maldigestion or malabsorption of fat.

Strangulation (intestinal) Occlusion of the blood flow to a loop of intestine leading to venous infarction.

Stricture Narrowing of the lumen of a hollow viscus by fibrous thickening of the wall or surrounding tissue, leading to obstruction of flow of luminal contents.

Suppuration Formation or discharge of pus.

Symptom A subjective manifestation of disease reported by the patient.

Syndrome A defined constellation of symptoms and signs comprising a clinical entity.

Tamponade See Cardiac tamponade.

Telangiectasia Dilatation of superficial small blood vessels in the skin and mucous membranes, resulting in small red lesions.

Tensile strength The ability to withstand stretching force.

Teratogen An agent acting on the fetus in utero during organogenesis that causes congenital structural anomalies.

Teratoma A neoplasm composed of a disorganized mass of different kinds of tissues representing all 3 germ layers (ectoderm, entoderm, and mesoderm).

Thalassemia A group of disorders characterized by quantitatively decreased or absent synthesis of one of the globin chains of the hemoglobin molecule.

Thrombocytopenia Decreased number of platelets in peripheral blood.

Thrombocytosis Increased number of platelets in peripheral blood.

Thromboembolism The transport of detached fragments of a thrombus in the circulation from its point of formation to another blood vessel, usually causing obstruction of the vessel at the point of impaction.

Thrombophlebitis Inflammation of a vein associated with thrombosis.

Thrombus A solid or semisolid mass formed from the constituents of the blood, primarily platelets and fibrin, in the vascular system during life.

T lymphocyte A lymphocyte that is primed by the thymus during its development in fetal life.

Tolerance The decreasing effect on the body of the same dose of a drug in response to continued use of the drug.

Tophus A tumorlike mass formed by the deposition of urate crystals in connective tissues.

Torsion Abnormality resulting when an object is twisted either upon itself or on a pedicle.

Totipotent Capable of differentiating into all the different types of tissues in the organism.

Toxemia The presence of bacterial toxins in the blood.

Toxoid A bacterial exotoxin that has been altered in such a way as to lose its toxicity while retaining its antigenicity.

Transformation In carcinogenesis, the change a cell undergoes that gives it neoplastic properties.

Transfusion Introduction of blood or blood components directly into the bloodstream.

Transfusion reaction Any adverse clinical effect that results from transfusion of blood or blood components.

Translocation A chromosomal abnormality resulting

from transfer of a segment of a chromosome to a nonhomologous chromosome.

Transplantation The grafting of tissues from one site to another or from one individual to another.

Transudation The outflow of an increased amount of fluid from the microcirculation into the interstitial space through vessels whose permeability is normal.

Trisomy The presence of an additional (third) chromosome of one type in an otherwise diploid cell.

Tropocollagen The molecular unit of collagen as it is secreted by the fibroblast.

Tumor Any swelling or abnormal mass of tissue.

Tumor markers Secretory products of neoplasms that are released into the blood or other body fluids, detection of which aids diagnosis of the tumor.

Ulcer A defect of the surface of an organ or tissue caused by sloughing of necrotic material.

Vaccination Administration of an antigenic preparation for the purpose of establishing immunity to an infectious disease in the recipient.

Varicose vein An enlarged, dilated, tortuous vein.

Vasoconstriction narrowing of a blood vessel resulting from contraction of medial smooth muscle.

Vasodilatation Increase in luminal diameter of a blood vessel resulting from relaxation of medial smooth muscle.

Vector An animal, usually an arthropod, that carries and transfers an infective agent from one host to another.

Vegetation A polypoid mass of thrombus formed on the endocardial surface of the heart, usually on a cardiac valve.

Venereal (= sexually transmitted) Resulting from sexual contact.

Viral oncogene (V-*ONC*) A nucleotide sequence carried by a virus that corresponds to a similar sequence in the DNA of mammalian cells.

Virilization The abnormal development of secondary male sexual characteristics in a female.

Virulence The degree to which a microorganism is capable of causing pathologic changes in tissues after infection.

Viscid Having a high viscosity, rendering the substance thick and sticky.

Viscus An organ situated in a body cavity.

Vitamins A group of organic essential nutrients that are necessary in trace amounts for normal metabolism.

Volvulus Rotation of a length of intestine about an axis that passes through the mesentery.

V-*ONC* See Viral oncogene.

Warthin-Finkeldey cell A multinucleated giant cell seen in tissues infected with the measles virus.

Withdrawal syndrome The clinical state caused by abstention from a drug an individual is addicted to.

Xanthoma A yellow skin lesion caused by deposition of lipids in dermal macrophages.

Xenograft Tissue transplanted between animals of different species.

Xerophthalmia A disorder characterized by dryness of the cornea, frequently associated with denudation and thickening.

Xerostomia Dryness of the mouth resulting from decreased secretion of saliva.

Zoonosis An infectious disease of animals that is transmissible to humans under natural conditions.

Zygote The diploid totipotent cell that results from union of the haploid male and female gametes.

Appendix II: References

The references provided in this bibliography are those that will be most useful to medical students who wish to indulge in additional reading. We have paid particular attention to listing atlases and texts that we have found are very helpful to the student. The bibliography is divided into two parts: general reference books and references that pertain to individual sections in the text. The general reference books are further divided into clinical texts and pathology texts. The books listed are widely used by senior medical students and physicians. The clinical texts provide excellent information relating to the clinical features, diagnosis, and treatment of all the diseases discussed in this book and should ideally be read as a means of complementing the basic clinical information provided. The pathology texts are specialized to a varying degree but will provide the interested student a means of complementing the basic information provided in this book of the pathologic features of disease. The references that pertain to the various sections are also predominantly general references that take the student to textbooks and review type journal articles that we think are most useful at this stage of study. We have resisted the temptation to provide papers relating to specific details of diseases and more controversial issues in medicine.

GENERAL REFERENCE BOOKS

Clinical

Behrman RE, Vaughan VC III (editors): *Nelson's Textbook of Pediatrics,* 13th ed. Saunders, 1987.

Braunwald E et al (editors): *Harrison's Principles of Internal Medicine,* 11th ed. (2 vols.) McGraw-Hill, 1987.

De Vita VT, Hellman S, Rosenberg SA (editors): *Cancer: Principles and Practice of Oncology,* 3rd ed. (2 vol.) Lippincott, 1989.

Hardy JD (editor): *Hardy's Textbook of Surgery,* 2nd ed. Lippincott, 1988.

Sabiston DC (editor): *Textbook of Surgery. The Biological Basis of Modern Surgical Practice,* 13th ed. Saunders, 1986.

Schroeder SA et al (editors): *Current Medical Diagnosis & Treatment 1990.* Appleton & Lange, 1990.

Way LW (editor): *Current Surgical Diagnosis & Treatment,* 8th ed. Appleton & Lange, 1988.

Wyngaarden JB, Smith LH (editors): *Cecil's Textbook of Medicine,* 18th ed. (2 vols.) Saunders, 1988.

Pathology

Anderson JR (editor): *Muir's Textbook of Pathology,* 12th ed. Arnold, 1985.

Ashley DJ: *Evans' Histological Appearances of Tumours,* 3rd ed. (2 vols.) Churchill Livingstone, 1978.

Chandrasoma P, Taylor CR: *Key Facts in Pathology.* Churchill Livingstone, 1986.

Cotran RS, Kumar V, Robbins SL: *Robbins Pathologic Basis of Disease,* 4th ed. Saunders, 1989.

Curran RC: *Color Atlas of Histopathology,* 3rd ed. Oxford Univ Press, 1985.

Fawcett DW: *Bloom and Fawcett: A Textbook of Histology,* 11th ed. Saunders, 1986.

Florey HW (editor): *General Pathology,* 4th ed. Saunders, 1970.

Giarelli L, Melato M, Antonutto G: *Color Atlas of Pathology.* Mosby, 1984.

Henry JB: *Clinical Diagnosis and Management by Laboratory Methods,* 17th ed. Saunders, 1984.

Kissane JM: *Anderson's Pathology,* 9th ed. Mosby, 1989.

Ludwig J: *Current Methods of Autopsy Practice,* 2nd ed. Saunders, 1979.

Roitt IM: *Essential Immunology,* 5th ed. Blackwell, 1984.

Rosai J: *Ackerman's Surgical Pathology,* 7th ed. (2 vols.) Mosby, 1989.

Rubin E, Farber JL (editors): *Pathology.* Lippincott, 1988.

Sandritter W, Thomas C: *Color Atlas and Textbook of Histopathology,* 6th ed. Year Book, 1979.

Sheldon H: *Boyd's Introduction to the Study of Disease,* 10th ed. Lea & Febiger, 1988.

Silverberg SG: *Principles and Practice of Surgical Pathology.* Wiley, 1983.

Smith LH, Thier SO: *Pathophysiology. The Biological Principles of Disease,* 2nd ed. Saunders, 1985.

Sodeman WA Jr, Sodeman TM (editors): *Pathologic*

Physiology: Mechanisms of Disease, 7th ed. Saunders, 1985.

Stites DP, Stobo JD, Wells, JV (editors): *Basic & Clinical Immunology,* 6th ed. Appleton & Lange, 1987.

Walter JB, Israel MS: *General Pathology,* 6th ed. Churchill Livingstone, 1987.

Wheather PR et al: *Basic Histopathology: A Colour Atlas and Text.* Churchill Livingstone, 1985.

REFERENCES BY SECTION

SECTION I: EFFECT OF INJURY ON TISSUES

Batlle DC, Kurtzman NA (editors): Symposium on acid-base disorders. Med Clin North Am 1983;67:751 [Entire issue].

Comporti M: Biology of disease: Lipid peroxidation and cellular damage in toxic liver injury. Lab Invest 1985;53:599.

Cormack DH: Part Two. Pages 27—134, in: *Ham's Histology,* 9th ed. Lippincott, 1987.

Farber JL: Biology of disease: Membrane injury and calcium homeostasis in the pathogenesis of coagulative necrosis. Lab Invest 1982;47:114.

Freeman BA, Crapo JD: Biology of disease: Free radicals and tissue injury. Lab Invest 1982;47:412.

Glenner GG: Amyloid deposits and amyloidosis: The beta-fibrilloses. (2 parts.) N Engl J Med 1980;302:1283, 1333.

Kim KM: Pathological calcification. In: *Pathobiology of Cell Membranes.* Trump BF, Arstila AU (editors). Vol 3. Academic Press, 1983.

McCord JM: Oxygen-derived free radicals in post-ischemic tissue injury. N Engl J Med 1985;312:159.

Narins RG et al: Diagnostic strategies in disorders of fluid, electrolyte and acid-base homeostasis. Am J Med 1982;72:496.

Schrier RW: Pathogenesis of sodium and water retention in high-output and low-output cardiac failure, nephrotic syndrome, cirrhosis, and pregnancy. (2 parts.) N Engl J Med 1988;319:1065, 1127.

Smith LH, Their SO: Section I: Cell biology. Pages 1–51 In: *Pathophysiology: The Biological Basis of Disease,* 2nd ed. Saunders, 1985.

Staub NC, Taylor AE (editors): *Edema.* Raven Press, 1984.

Trump BF, McDowell EM, Arstila AU: Cellular reaction to injury. Pages 20–111 in: *Principles of Pathobiology,* 3rd ed. Hill RB, LaVia MF (editors). Oxford Univ Press, 1980.

SECTION II: THE HOST RESPONSE TO INJURY

Adams DO: The biology of the granuloma. Pages 1–20 in: *Pathology of Granulomas.* Ioachim HL (editor). Raven Press. 1983.

Alper CA, Rosen FS: Inherited deficiencies of complement proteins in man. Springer Semin Immunopathol 1984;7:251.

Babior BM: Oxygen-dependent microbial killing by phagocytes. (2 parts.) N Engl J Med 1978;298:659, 721.

Barbul A et al (editors): *Growth Factors and Other Aspects of Wound Healing: Biological and Clinical Implications.* Liss, 1988.

Bomalaski JS, Williamson PK, Zurier RB: Prostaglandins and the inflammatory response. Clin Lab Med 1983;3:695.

Buckley RH: Immunodeficiency. J Allergy Clin Immunol 1983;72:627.

Dannenberg AM Jr: Macrophages in inflammation and infection. N Engl J Med 1975;293:489.

D'Ardenne AJ, McGee JO: Fibronectin in disease. J Pathol 1984;142:235.

Daughaday WH (editor): Tissue growth factors. (Symposium.) Clin Endocrinol Metab 1984;13:3. (Entire issue.)

DeVita VT Jr, Hellman S, Rosenberg SA (editors): *AIDS: Etiology, Diagnosis, Treatment and Prevention,* 2nd ed. Lippincott, 1988.

Frank MM: Complement in the pathophysiology of human disease. N Engl J Med 1987;316:1525.

Friedman-Kien AE: *Color Atlas of AIDS.* Saunders, 1989.

Gallin JI, Goldstein IM, Snyderman R (editors): *Inflammation: Basic Principles and Clinical Correlates.* Raven Press, 1988.

Herberman RB, Reynolds CW, Ortaldo JR. Mechanism of cytotoxicity by natural killer (NK) cells. Annu Rev Immunol 1986;4:651.

Leder P: The genetics of antibody diversity. Sci Am (May) 1982;246:102.

Levi R, Krell RD (editors): *Biology of the Leukotrienes.* New York Academy of Sciences, 1988.

Marsh J, Boggs D. Neutrophils. Pages 592–607 in: *Pathologic Physiology: Mechanisms of Disease,* 7th ed. Sodeman WA Jr, Sodeman TM (editors). Saunders, 1985.

Miller EJ: Chemistry of collagens and their distribution. Pages 1–39 in: *Extracellular Matrix Biochemistry.* Piez KA, Reddi AH (editors). Elsevier, 1984.

North RJ: The concept of the activated macrophage. J Immunol 1978;121:806.

O'Flaherty JT: Lipid mediators of inflammation and allergy. Lab Invest 1982;47:314.

Paul WE (editor): *Fundamental Immunology.* Raven Press, 1986.

Peacock EE Jr: *Wound Repair,* 3rd ed. Saunders, 1984.

Pick E (editor): *Lymphokines: A Forum for Immunoregulatory Cell Products.* Vol 3 of: *Lymphokine Reports: A Forum for Nonantibody Lymphocyte Products.* Academic Press, 1981.

Reinherz EL, Schlossman SF: The differentiation and function of human T lymphocytes. Cell 1980;19:821.

Reinherz EL et al: *Human B Lymphocytes.* Springer-Verlag, 1986.

Roitt IM: *Essential Immunology,* 5th ed. Blackwell, 1984.

Rosen FS: The acquired immunodeficiency syndrome (AIDS). J Clin Invest 1985;75:1.

Ryan GB, Majno G: Acute inflammation: A review. Am J Pathol 1977;86:183.

Samuelsson B, Paoletti R (editors): *Leucotrienes and Other Lipoxygenase Products.* Raven Press, 1982.

Schwartz RS: From molecular biology to the bedside: The example of immunoglobulin genes. (Editorial.) N Engl J Med 1984;310:521.

Selik RM, Dondero TJ, Curran JW: *Proposed Revision of the AIDS Case Definition: Proceedings of the Third International Conference on AIDS.* Washington DC, June 1–5, 1987.

Stites DP, Stobo JD, Wells JV (editors): *Basic & Clinical Immunology,* 6th ed. Appleton & Lange, 1987.

Szentivanyi A, Szentivanyi J: Pathophysiology of immunologic and related diseases. Pages 151–161 in: *Pathologic Physiology: Mechanisms of Disease,* 7th ed. Sodeman WA Jr, Sodeman TM (editors). Saunders, 1985.

Tauber AI: Current view of neutrophil dysfunction: An integrated clinical perspective. Am J Med 1981; 70:1237.

Wade BH, Mandell GL: Polymorphonuclear leukocytes: Dedicated professional phagocytes. Am J Med 1983;74:686.

SECTION III: AGENTS CAUSING TISSUE INJURY

Anderson RJ, Reed G, Knochel J: Heatstroke. Adv Intern Med 1983;28:115.

Aoki M, Hisamichi S, Tominaga S (editors): *Smoking and Health,* 1987. Elsevier, 1988.

Beaver PC, Jung RC, Cupp EW: *Clinical Parasitology.* 9th ed. Lea & Febiger, 1984.

Becker CE: Medical complications of drug abuse. Adv Intern Med 1979;24:183.

Bell WR, Simon TL: Current status of pulmonary thromboembolic disease: Pathophysiology, diagnosis, prevention, and treatment. Am Heart J 1982; 103:239.

Bellinger D et al: Longitudinal analyses of prenatal and postnatal lead exposure and early cognitive development. N Engl J Med 1987;316:1037.

Bennett J, Brachman PS (editors): *Hospital Infections,* 2nd ed. Little, Brown, 1985.

Bergquist LM: *Changing Patterns of Infectious Diseases.* Lea & Febiger, 1984.

Binford CH, Connor DH (editors): *Pathology of Tropical and Extraordinary Diseases.* (2 vols.) Armed Forces Institute of Pathology, 1976.

Chandler FW, Kaplan W, Ajello L: *Color Atlas and Textbook of the Histopathology of Mycotic Diseases.* Year Book, 1980.

Clowes GH: *Trauma, Sepsis, and Shock: The Physiological Basis of Therapy.* Dekker, 1988.

Cowley RA, Trump BF (editors): *Pathophysiology of Shock, Anoxia, and Ischemia.* Williams & Wilkins, 1981.

Doull J, Klaasen CD, Amdur MO: *Toxicology: The Basic Science of Poisons,* 3rd ed. Macmillan, 1986.

Feinstein DI: Diagnosis and management of disseminated intravascular coagulation: The role of heparin therapy. Blood 1982;60:284.

Fields BN et al (editor): *Fundamental Virology.* Raven Press, 1986.

Gawin FH, Ellinwood EH Jr: Cocaine and other stimulants: Actions, abuse, and treatment. N Engl J Med 1988;318:1173.

Grinspoon L, Bakalar JB: Adverse effects of cocaine: Selected issues. Ann NY Acad Sci 1981;362:125.

Hayry P: Immunobiology of transplant rejection. Ann Clin Res 1981;13:172.

Hunt JL et al: The pathophysiology of acute electric injuries. J Trauma 1976;16:335.

Klein J, Figueroa F, Nagy ZA: Genetics of the major histocompatibility complex: The final act. Annu Rev Immunol 1983;1:119.

Mandell GL, Douglas RG Jr, Bennett JH (editors): *Principles and Practice of Infectious Diseases,* 3rd ed. Wiley, 1990.

Manson-Bahr PE, Bell DR (editors): *Manson's Tropical Diseases,* 19th ed. Bailliére-Tindall, 1987.

Marcial-Rojas RA (editor): *Pathology of Protozoal and Helminthic Diseases, With Clinical Correlation.* Williams & Wilkins, 1971.

Myerowitz RL: *Pathology of Opportunistic Infections, With Pathogenetic, Diagnostic and Clinical Correlations.* Raven Press, 1983.

National Institutes of Health Consensus Development Conference Statement: Health implications of obesity. Ann Intern Med 1985;103:147.

Nelson TE, Flewellen EH: The malignant hyperthermia syndrome. N Engl J Med 1983;309:416.

Neu HC: What should the clinician expect from the microbiology laboratory? Ann Intern Med 1981;89:781.

Rose NR, Mackay IR (editors): *The Autoimmune Diseases.* Academic Press, 1985.

Rubin E (editor): Alcohol and the cell. Ann NY Acad Sci 1987;289:492.

Rubin RH, Young LS (editors): *Clinical Approach to Infection in the Compromised Host,* 2nd ed. Plenum Press, 1988.

Schwabe AD et al: Anorexia nervosa. Ann Intern Med 1981;94:371.

Shoenfeld Y, Schwartz RS: Immunologic and genetic factors in autoimmune diseases. N Engl J Med 1984;311:1019.

Smith TF: Clinical uses of the diagnostic virology laboratory. Med Clin North Am 1983;67:935.

Stites DP, Stobo JD, Wells JV (editors): *Basic & Clinical Immunology,* 6th ed. Appleton & Lange, 1987.

Strauss RH: Diving medicine. Am Rev Respir Dis 1979;119:1001.

Theofilopoulos AN, Dixon FJ: Immune complexes in human diseases: A review. Am J Pathol 1980; 100:529.

Theofilopoulos AN, Dixon FJ: Autoimmune diseases: Immunopathology and etiopathogenesis. Am J Pathol 1982;108:319.

Tuckerman MM, Turco SJ: *Human Nutrition.* Lea & Febiger, 1983.

United Nations Environment Programme: *Radiation: Doses, Effects, Risks.* United Nations Publications, 1986.

U.S. Department of Health, Education and Welfare. Smoking and Health. A Report of the Surgeon General. Publication No. (PHS) 79-50066, 1979.

Viteri FE, Torun B: Protein calorie malnutrition. In: *Modern Nutrition in Health and Disease,* 6th ed. Goodhart RS, Shils ME (editors). Lea & Febiger, 1980.

Wenzel RP: *Prevention and Control of Nosocomial Infections.* Williams & Wilkins, 1987.

West LJ et al: Alcoholism. Ann Intern Med 1984; 100:405.

SECTION IV: DISORDERS OF DEVELOPMENT & GROWTH

Arthur DC: Genetics and cytogenetics of pediatric cancers. Cancer 1986;58:534.

Beahrs OH et al (editors): *Manual for Staging of Cancer,* 3rd ed. Lippincott, 1988.

Behnke JA et al (editors): *The Biology of Aging.* Plenum Press, 1978

Brodeur GM et al: Clinical implications of oncogene activation in human neuroblastomas. Cancer 1986;58 (2 Suppl):541.

Burck KB, Liu ET, Larrick JW: *Oncogenes: An Introduction to the Concept of Cancer Genes.* Springer-Verlag, 1988.

Celis JE, Bravo R (editors): *Gene Expression in Normal and Transformed Cells.* Plenum Press, 1983.

Chu TM (editor): *Biochemical Markers for Cancer.* Dekker, 1982.

Cline MJ, Slamon DJ, Lipsick JS: Oncogenes: Implications for the diagnosis and treatment of cancer. Ann Intern Med 1984;101:223.

Crumpton MJ et al: The cell surface and its metabolism. J Pathol 1983;141:235.

Daar AS (editor): *Tumour Markers in Clinical Practice. Concepts and Applications.* Blackwell, 1987.

DeGrouchy J, Turleau C: *Clinical Atlas of Human Chromosomes.* 2nd ed. Wiley, 1984.

del Regato JA, Spjut HJ, Cox JD (editors): *Ackerman's Cancer. Diagnosis, Treatment and Prognosis.* 6th ed. Mosby, 1984.

De Vita VT, Hellman S, Rosenberg SA (editors): *Cancer. Principles and Practice of Oncology,* 3rd ed. (2 vols.) Lippincott, 1989.

Eisenstein BI: The polymerase chain reaction: A new method of using molecular genetics for medical diagnosis. N Engl J Med 1990;322:128.

Emery AE, Rimoin DL: *Principles and Practice of Medical Genetics.* Churchill Livingstone, 1983.

Franks LM, Teich NM: Introduction to the Cellular and Molecular Biology of Cancer. Oxford Univ Press, 1986.

Fries JF: Aging, natural death, and the compression of morbidity. N Engl J Med 1980;303:130.

Gowing NF: *Color Atlas of Tumor Histopathology.* Year Book, 1980.

Haskell CM: *Cancer Treatment,* 2nd ed. Saunders, 1985.

Holleb AI et al (editors): *The American Cancer Society's Complete Book of Cancer.* Doubleday, 1986.

Kelling W (editor): *Fetal and Neonatal Pathology.* Springer-Verlag, 1987.

Kemshead JT (editor): *Pediatric Tumors: Immunological and Molecular Markers.* CRC Press, 1989.

Kurzrock R, Gutterman JU, Talpaz M: The molecular genetics of Philadelphia chromosome-positive leukemias. N Engl J Med 1988;319:990.

Levitan M: *Textbook of Human Genetics,* 3rd ed. Oxford Univ Press, 1988.

Lewin B: *Genes,* 2nd ed. Wiley, 1985.

Liotta LA, Hurt IR (editors): *Tumour Invasion and Metastasis.* Martinus Nijhoff, 1982.

Lippman ME (editor): *Growth Regulation of Cancer.* Liss, 1988.

Maltoni C, Selikoff IJ (editors): *Living in a Chemical World: Occupational and Environmental Significance of Industrial Carcinogens.* New York Academy of Sciences, 1988.

Miller AB: *Screening for Cancer.* Academic Press, 1985.

Mitelman F: *Catalogue of Chromosome Aberrations in Cancer,* 3rd ed. Liss, 1988.

National Research Council: *Diet, Nutrition and Cancer.* National Academy Press, 1982.

Nicolson GL, Fidler IJ (editors): *Tumor Progression and Metastasis.* Liss, 1988.

Pitot HC: *Fundamentals of Oncology,* 3rd ed. Dekker, 1985.

Pitot HC: Oncogenes and human neoplasia. Clin Lab Med 1986;6:167.

Reed GB, et al (editors): *Diseases of the Fetus and Newborn: Pathology, Radiology and Genetics.* Mosby, 1989.

Ron E et al: Tumors of the brain and nervous system after radiotherapy in childhood. N Engl J Med 1988;319:1033.

Rubin P: *Clinical Oncology for Medical Students and Physicians. A Multidisciplinary Approach,* 6th ed. American Cancer Society, 1983.

Ruddon RW: *Cancer Biology,* 2nd ed. Oxford Univ Press, 1987.

Schweisguth O: *Solid Tumors in Children.* Wiley, 1982.

Scriver CR, et al (editors): *The Metabolic Basis of Inherited Disease,* 6th ed. McGraw-Hill, 1989.

Sell S, Reisfeld R (editors): *Monoclonal Antibodies in Cancer.* Humana, 1985.

Simpson JL (editor): *Disorders of Sexual Differentiation.* Academic Press, 1976.

Slamon DJ et al: Expression of cellular oncogenes in human malignancies. Science 1984;224:256.

Stanbury JB et al: *The Metabolic Basis of Inherited Disease,* 5th ed. McGraw-Hill, 1983.

Taylor CR: *Immunomicroscopy: A Diagnostic Tool for the Surgical Pathologist.* Saunders, 1986.

Vogel F, Motulsky AG: *Human Genetics: Problems and Approaches,* 2nd ed. Springer-Verlag, 1986.

Weiss L: *Principles of Metastasis.* Academic Press, 1985.

Wepsic HT: Overview of oncofetal antigens in cancer. Ann Clin Lab Sci 1983;13:261.

Willis RA: *Pathology of Tumors.* Butterworths, 1948.

SECTION V: THE CARDIOVASCULAR SYSTEM

Aretz HT et al: Myocarditis. Am J Cardiovasc Pathol 1987;1:3.

Ayoub EM: The search for host determinants of susceptibility to rheumatic fever: The missing link. Circulation 1984;69:197.

Becker AE, Anderson RH: *Cardiac Pathology.* Raven Press, 1983.

Braunwald E: *Heart Disease: A Textbook of Cardiovascular Medicine,* 3rd ed. Saunders, 1988.

Bulkley BH: The cardiomyopathies. Hosp Pract (June) 1984;19:59.

Cupps TR, Fauci AS: The vasculitic syndromes. Adv Intern Med 1982;27:315.

Davies MJ: *Color Atlas of Cardiovascular Pathology.* Oxford Univ Press, 1986.

Dec GW Jr et al: Active myocarditis in the spectrum of acute dilated cardiomyopathies: Clinical features, histologic correlates, and clinical outcome. N Engl J Med 1985;312:885.

Dillon MC et al: Diagnostic problems in acute myocardial infarction: CK-MB in the absence of abnormally elevated total creatine kinase levels. Arch Intern Med 1982;142:33.

Doroghazi RM, Slater EE (editors): *Aortic Dissection.* McGraw-Hill, 1983.

Fenoglio JJ Jr et al: Diagnosis and classification of myocarditis by endomyocardial biopsy. N Engl J Med 1983;308:12.

Fowler NO: Constrictive pericarditis: New aspects. Am J Cardiol 1982;50:1014.

Grundy SM et al: Coronary risk factor statement for the American public: A statement of the nutrition committee. Circulation 1985;72:1135A.

Hurst JW et al (editor): *The Heart,* 6th ed. McGraw-Hill, 1985.

Ishikawa K: Survival and morbidity after diagnosis of occlusive thromboaortopathy (Takayasu's disease). Am J Cardiol 1981;47:1026.

Julian DG, et al (editors): *Diseases of the Heart.* Saunders, 1989.

Kaplan NM: *Clinical Hypertension,* 4th ed. Williams & Wilkins, 1986.

Laragh JH: Atrial natriuretic hormone, the renin-aldosterone axis, and blood pressure-electrolyte homeostasis. N Engl J Med 1985:313:1330.

Little RC: *Physiology of the Heart and Circulation,* 3rd ed. Year Book, 1985.

Maseri A, Chierchia S: Coronary artery spasm: Demonstration, definition, diagnosis, and consequences. Prog Cardiovasc Dis 1982;25:169.

Pepine CJ (editor): *Acute Myocardial Infarction.* Dekker, 1989.

Perloff JK: *Physical Examination of the Heart and Circulation.* Saunders, 1982.

Peyeritz RE, McKusick VA: The Marfan's syndrome: Diagnosis and management. N Engl J Med 1979; 300:772.

Rahimtoola SH: Valvular heart disease: A perspective. J Am Coll Cardiol 1983;1:199.

Ross R, Glomset JA: The pathogenesis of atherosclerosis. (2 parts.) N Engl J Med 1976;295:369, 420.

Ross R: The pathogenesis of atherosclerosis: An update. N Engl J Med 1986;314:488.

Sande MA, Kaye D, Root RK (editors): *Endocarditis.* Vol 2: *Contemporary Issues in Infectious Diseases.* Churchill Livingstone, 1984.

Shulman ST et al: Prevention of bacterial endocarditis: A statement for health professionals by the Committee on Rheumatic Fever and Infective Endocarditis of the Council on Cardiovascular Diseases in the Young. Circulation 1984;70:1123.

Tarazi RC: The heart in hypertension (Editorial.) N Engl J Med 1985;312:308.

Thomas WA, Kim DN: Atherosclerosis as a hyperplastic and/or neoplastic process. Lab Invest 1983;48:245.

Veasy LG et al: Resurgence of acute rheumatic fever in the intermountain area of the United States. N Engl J Med 1987;316:421.

SECTION VI: THE BLOOD & LYMPHOID SYSTEM

Babior BM, Stossel TP: *Hematology: A Pathophysiological Approach,* 2nd ed. Churchill-Livingstone, 1990.

Bain BJ: *Blood Cells: A Practical Guide.* Lippincott, 1989.

Ballard MC: *Atlas of Blood Cells in Health and Disease.* U.S. Department of Health and Human Services, 1987.

Bennett JM et al: The French-American-British (FAB) cooperative group proposals for the classification of the myelodysplastic syndromes. Br J Haematol 1982;51:189.

Bloom AL, Thomas DP: *Haemostasis and Thrombosis,* 2nd ed. Churchill Livingstone, 1987.

Burke JS: Surgical pathology of the spleen: An approach to the differential diagnosis of splenic lymphomas and leukemias. (2 parts.) Am J Surg Pathol 1981;5:551, 681.

Gunz FW, Henderson ES (editors): *Leukemia,* 4th ed. Grune & Stratton, 1982.

Habeshaw JA, Lauder I (editors): *Malignant Lymphomas.* Churchill Livingstone, 1988.

Hardisty RM, Weatherall DJ (editors): *Blood and Its Disorders,* 2nd ed. Mosby, 1982.

Hoffbrand AV, Pettit JE: *Clinical Hematology Illustrated: An Integrated Text and Color Atlas.* Saunders, 1987.

Jaffe ES: *Surgical Pathology of Lymph Nodes and Related Organs.* Saunders, 1985.

Kaplan HS: *Hodgkin's Disease,* 2nd ed. Harvard Univ Press, 1980.

Koepke JA (editor): *Laboratory Hematology.* Churchill Livingstone, 1984.

Kyle RA, Bayrd EA: *The Monoclonal Gammopathies: Multiple Myeloma and Related Plasma-Cell Disorders.* Thomas, 1976.

Levine GD, Rosai J: Thymic hyperplasia and neoplasia. A review of current concepts. Hum Pathol 1978; 9:495.

Lichtman MA (editor): *Hematology and Oncology.* Grune & Stratton, 1980.

Lukes RJ et al: Immunologic approach to non-Hodgkin lymphomas and related leukemias: Analysis of the results of multiparameter studies of 425 cases. Semin Hematol 1978;15:322.

Robb-Smith AH, Taylor CR: *Lymph Node Biopsy.* Oxford Univ Press, 1981.

Rosenberg SA: National Cancer Institute-sponsored study of classifications of non-Hodgkin's lymphomas: Summary and description of a working formulation for clinical usage. Cancer 1982;49:2112.

Tavassoli M: Megakaryocyte-platelet axis and the process of platelet formation and release. Blood 1980; 55:537.

Travis WD, Pierre RV: Preleukemia dysmyelopoietic syndrome. Lab Med 1985:16:157.

van Assendelft OW: Reference values for the total and differential leukocyte count. Blood Cells 1985;11:77.
van der Twell JG, Taylor CR, Bosman FT: *Malignant Lymphoproliferative Diseases.* Leiden Univ Press, 1980.
Williams WJ et al (editors): *Hematology,* 3rd ed. McGraw-Hill, 1983.
Wintrobe MM et al: *Clinical Hematology,* 8th ed. Lea & Febiger, 1981.
Zucker-Franklin D et al (editors): *Atlas of Blood Cells: Function and Pathology,* 2nd ed. (2 vols.) Lea & Febiger, 1988.

SECTION VII: DISEASES OF THE HEAD & NECK

Barnes L (editor): *Surgical Pathology of the Head and Neck* (2 vols.) Dekker, 1985.
Batsakis JG: *Tumors of the Head and Neck: Clinical and Pathological Considerations,* 2nd ed. Williams & Wilkins, 1979.
Friedmann I (editor): *Nose, Throat and Ears.* Vol 1 of: *Systemic Pathology,* 3rd ed. Churchill Livingstone, 1986.
Gnepp DR (editor): *Pathology of the Head and Neck.* Churchill-Livingstone, 1988.
Joseph CE, Farnoush A: Current concepts of periodontitis. J Calif Dental Assoc 1984;12:43.
Meyer-Breiting E, Burkhardt A: *Tumours of the Larynx: Histopathology and Clinical Inferences.* Springer-Verlag, 1988.
Michaels L: *Ear, Nose and Throat Histopathology.* Springer-Verlag, 1987.
Newbrun E: Sugar and dental caries: A review of human studies. Science 1982;217:418.
Rootman J: *Diseases of the Orbit: A Multidisciplinary Approach.* Lippincott, 1988.
Silverman S Jr, Greenspan D: Early detection and diagnosis of oral cancer. J Calif Dental Assoc 1985;13:29.
Tabbara KF, Hyndiuk RA: *Infections of the Eye.* Little, Brown 1986
Yanoff M, Fine BS: *Ocular Pathology. A Text and Atlas,* 2nd ed. Harper & Row, 1982.

SECTION VIII: THE RESPIRATORY SYSTEM

Bone RC (editor): Symposium on respiratory failure. Med Clin North Am 1983;67:549 [Entire issue].
Crystal RG et al: Interstitial lung disease: Current concepts of pathogenesis, staging, and therapy. Am J Med 1981;70:542.
Dail DH, Hammar SP (editors): *Pulmonary Pathology.* Springer-Verlag, 1987.
Dunnill MS: *Pulmonary Pathology,* 2nd ed. Churchill Livingstone, 1987.
Ginsberg RJ, Feld R (editors): Proceedings of the IV world conference on lung cancer, Toronto, 25–30 August 1985. Chest 1986;89:199S [Entire issue].
Goldhaber SZ (editor): *Pulmonary Embolism and Deep Venous Thrombosis.* Saunders, 1985.
James DG, Williams WJ: *Sarcoidosis and Other Granulomatous Disorders.* Saunders, 1985.
Murray JF: *The Normal Lung: The Basis for Diagnosis and Treatment of Pulmonary Disease,* 2nd ed. Saunders, 1986.
Murray JF, Nadel JA (editors): *Textbook of Respiratory Medicine.* (2 vols.) Saunders, 1988.
Snider GL (editor): Symposium on emphysema. Clin Chest Med 1983;4:327 [Entire issue].
Spencer H: *Pathology of the Lung,* 4th ed. (2 vols.) Pergamon Press, 1985.
Thurlbeck WM (editor): *Pathology of the Lung.* Thieme, 1987.
Wilson AF (editor): *Pulmonary Function Testing: Indications and Intepretations.* Grune & Stratton, 1985.

SECTION IX: THE GASTROINTESTINAL TRACT

Appelman HD: *Pathology of the Esophagus, Stomach, and Duodenum.* Churchill Livingstone, 1984.
Berk JE (editor): *Bockus' Gastroenterology,* 4th ed. Saunders, 1985.
Correa P: Clinical implications of recent developments in gastric cancer pathology and epidemiology. Semin Oncol 1985;12:2.
Day DW: *Biopsy Pathology of the Oesophagus, Stomach and Duodenum.* Wiley, 1986.
Dworken HJ: *Gastroenterology: Pathophysiology and Clinical Applications.* Butterworths, 1982.
Gitnick G et al (editors): *Principles and Practice of Gastroenterology and Hepatology.* Elsevier, 1988.
Grossman ML (editor): *Peptic Ulcer: A Guide for the Practicing Physician.* Year Book, 1981.
Heyworth MF, Jones AL: *Immunology of the Gastrointestinal Tract and Liver.* Raven Press, 1988.
Johnson LR (editor): *Physiology of the Gastrointestinal Tract,* 2nd ed. Raven Press, 1987.
Kirsner JB, Shorter RG (editors): *Diseases of the Colon, Rectum, and Anal Canal.* Williams & Wilkins, 1988.
Kirsner JB, Shorter RG (editors): *Inflammatory Bowel Disease,* 3rd ed. Lea & Febiger, 1988.
Manuel PD, Walker-Smith JA, Tomkins A: *Infections of the Gastrointestinal Tract.* Churchill Livingstone, 1986.
Mitros FA: *Atlas of Gastrointestinal Pathology.* Lippincott, 1988.
Morson BC (editor): *Alimentary Tract.* Vol 3 of: *Systemic Pathology,* 3rd ed. Symmers WS (editor). Churchill Livingstone, 1987.
Morson BC: *Color Atlas of Gastrointestinal Pathology.* Saunders, 1988.
Morson BC, Dawson IM: *Gastrointestinal Pathology,* 2nd ed. Blackwell, 1979.
O'Brien MJ et al: Early gastric cancer: Clinicopathologic study. Am J Med 1985;78:195.
Santangelo WC, Krejs GJ: Gastrointestinal manifestations of the acquired immunodeficiency syndrome. Am J Med Sci 1986;292:328.
Sleisenger MH, Fordtran JS: *Gastrointestinal Disease,* 4th ed. Saunders, 1988.
Spechler SJ, Goyal RK: Barrett's esophagus. N Engl J Med 1986;315:362.

Steele G Jr et al (editors): *Basic and Clinical Perspectives of Colorectal Polyps and Cancer.* Liss, 1988.

Westergaard H: The sprue syndromes. Am J Med Sci 1985;290:249.

SECTION X: THE LIVER, BILIARY TRACT, & PANCREAS

Arias IM et al (editors): *The Liver: Biology and Pathobiology,* 2nd ed. Raven Press, 1988.

Kloppel G, Heitz PU (editors): *Pancreatic Pathology.* Churchill Livingstone, 1984.

Patrick RS, McGee JO: *Biopsy Pathology of the Liver.* Chapman & Hall, 1988.

Peters RL, Craig JR (editors): *Liver Pathology.* Churchill-Livingstone, 1986.

Schiff L, Schiff ER (editors): *Diseases of the Liver,* 6th ed. Lippincott, 1987.

Sherlock S: *Diseases of the Liver and Biliary System,* 8th ed. Mosby, 1989.

Zuckerman AJ (editor): *Viral Hepatitis and Liver Disease.* Liss, 1988.

SECTION XI: THE URINARY TRACT & MALE REPRODUCTIVE SYSTEM

Antonovych TT, Mostofi FK: *Atlas of Kidney Biopsies.* Armed Forces Institute of Pathology, 1980.

Brenner BM, Rector FC Jr (editors): *The Kidney,* 3rd ed. (2 vols.) Saunders, 1986.

Cameron JS, Glossock RJ (editors): *The Nephrotic Syndrome.* Vol 8: *Kidney Disease.* Dekker, 1988.

Gillenwater JY et al: *Adult and Pediatric Urology.* (2 vols.) Year Book, 1987.

Heptinstall RH (editor): *Pathology of the Kidney,* 3rd ed. (3 vols.) Little, Brown, 1983.

Hill GS (editor): *Uropathology.* Churchill-Livingstone, 1989.

Jacobi GH, Hohenfellner RF (editors): *Prostate Cancer.* Williams & Wilkins, 1982.

Johnson DE, Boileau MA (editors): *Genitourinary Tumors. Fundamental Principles and Surgical Techniques.* Grune & Stratton, 1982.

Klahr S, Schreiner G, Ichikawa I: The progression of renal disease. N Engl J Med 1988;318:1657.

Murphy WM: *Atlas of Bladder Carcinoma.* American Society of Clinical Pathologists, 1986.

Peterson RO, Stein B: *Urologic Pathology.* Lippincott, 1986.

Risdon RA, Turner DR: *An Atlas of Renal Pathology.* Lippincott, 1980.

Schrier RW, Gottschalk CW (editors): *Diseases of the Kidney,* 4th ed. (3 vols.) Little, Brown, 1988.

Talerman A, Roth LM (editors): *Pathology of the Testis and Its Adnexa.* Churchill Livingstone, 1986.

Tanagho EA, McAninch JW (editors): *Smith's General Urology,* 12th ed. Appleton & Lange, 1988.

Walsh PC et al: *Campbell's Urology,* 5th ed. (3 vols.) Saunders, 1986.

SECTION XII: THE FEMALE REPRODUCTIVE SYSTEM & BREAST

Coleman DV, Evans DM: *Biopsy Pathology and Cytology of the Cervix.* Chapman & Hall, 1988.

Danforth DN, Scott JR (editors): *Obstetrics & Gynecology,* 5th ed. Lippincott, 1986.

Donegan WL, Spratt JS: *Cancer of the Breast,* 3rd ed. Saunders, 1988.

Gusberg SB, Shingleton HM, Deppe G (editors): *Female Genital Cancer.* Churchill Livingstone, 1988.

Hendrickson MR, Kempson RL: *Surgical Pathology of the Uterine Corpus.* Saunders, 1980.

Hernandez E, Rosenshein NB: *Manual of Gynecologic Oncology.* Churchill-Livingstone, 1989.

Jones HW, Wentz AC, Burnett LS: *Novak's Textbook of Gynecology,* 11th ed. Williams & Wilkins, 1988.

Kurman RJ (editor): *Blaustein's Pathology of the Female Genital Tract,* 3rd ed. Springer-Verlag, 1987.

Page DL, Anderson TJ: *Diagnostic Histopathology of the Breast.* Churchill Livingstone, 1987.

Woodruff JD, Parmley TH: *Atlas of Gynecologic Pathology.* Lippincott, 1988.

Wynn RM: *Obstetrics and Gynecology: The Clinical Core,* 4th ed. Lea & Febiger, 1988.

SECTION XIII: THE ENDOCRINE GLANDS

Bloodworth JM Jr (editor): *Endocrine Pathology,* 2nd ed. Williams & Wilkins, 1982.

Davidson JK: *Clinical Diabetes Mellitus: A Problem-Oriented Approach.* Thieme, 1986

DeGroot LJ et al (editors): *Endocrinology,* 2nd ed. (3 vols.) Saunders, 1989.

Ghandur-Mnaymneh L et al: The parathyroid gland in health and disease. Am J Pathol 1986;125:292.

Ingbar SH, Braverman LE (editors): *Werner's The Thyroid. A Fundamental and Clinical Text,* 5th ed. Lippincott, 1986.

Kannan CR: *The Pituitary Gland.* Plenum Press, 1987.

Kini SR: *Guides to Clinical Aspiration Biopsy: Thyroid.* Igaku Shoin, 1987.

Mendelsohn G (editor): *Diagnosis and Pathology of Endocrine Diseases.* Lippincott, 1988.

Mulrow PJ (editor): *The Adrenal Gland.* Elsevier, 1986.

Slaunwhite WR Jr: *Fundamentals of Endocrinology.* Dekker, 1988.

Tindall GT, Barrow DL: *Disorders of the Pituitary.* Mosby, 1986.

Wilson JB, Foster DW: *Williams' Textbook of Endocrinology,* 7th ed. Saunders, 1985.

SECTION XIV: THE SKIN

Ackerman AB: *Histologic Diagnosis of Inflammatory Skin Diseases. A Method by Pattern Analysis.* Lea & Febiger, 1978.

Callen JP: *Cutaneous Aspects of Internal Disease.* Year Book, 1980.

Lever WF, Schaumburg-Lever G: *Histopathology of the Skin,* 7th ed. Lippincott, 1990.
Lookingbill DP, Marks JG: *Principles of Dermatology.* Saunders, 1986.
Mehregan AH: *Pinkus' Guide to Dermatohistopathology,* 4th ed. Appleton-Century-Crofts, 1986.
Schaumburg-Lever G, Lever WF: *Color Atlas of Histopathology of the Skin.* Lippincott, 1988.

SECTION XV: THE NERVOUS SYSTEM

Adams JH, Corsellis JA, Duchen LW (editors): *Greenfield's Neuropathology,* 4th ed. Wiley, 1985.
Adams RD, Victor M: *Principles of Neurology,* 3rd ed. McGraw-Hill, 1985.
Bannister R: *Brain's Clinical Neurology,* 6th ed. Oxford Univ Press, 1985.
Chandrasoma PT, Apuzzo ML: *Stereotactic Brain Biopsy.* Igaku Shoin, 1989.
Davis RL, Robertson DM: *Textbook of Neuropathology.* Williams & Wilkins, 1985.
Franks AJ: *Diagnostic Manual of Tumours of the Central Nervous System.* Churchill Livingstone, 1988.
McDonald WI, Silberberg DH (editors): *Multiple Sclerosis.* Butterworths, 1986.
Millikan CH, McDowell F, Easton JD: *Stroke.* Lea & Febiger, 1987.
Okazaki H, Scheithauer BW: *Atlas of Neuropathology.* Lippincott, 1988.
Schochet SS Jr, McCormick WE: *Neuropathology Case Studies,* 3rd ed. Medical Examinations Publishing Co, 1984.
Treip CS: *Color Atlas of Neuropathology.* Year Book, 1978.
Walton JA (editor): *Disorders of Voluntary Muscle,* 5th ed. Churchill Livingstone, 1988.
Walton JN: *Brain's Diseases of the Nervous System,* 9th ed. Oxford Univ Press, 1985.
Weller RO: *Color Atlas of Neuropathology.* Oxford Univ Press, 1984.

SECTION XVI: BONES, JOINTS, & CONNECTIVE TISSUE

Balow JE et al: Lupus nephritis. Ann Intern Med 1987;106:79.
Clough JD et al: Weighted criteria for the diagnosis of systemic lupus erythematosus. Arch Intern Med 1984;144:281.
Cohen AS (editor): *Laboratory Diagnostic Procedures in the Rheumatic Diseases,* 3rd ed. Grune & Stratton, 1985.
Cupps TR, Fauci AS: *The Vasculitides.* Saunders, 1981.
Enzinger FM, Weiss SW: *Soft Tissue Tumors,* 2nd ed. Mosby, 1988.
Fries JF: Disease criteria for systemic lupus erythematosus. (Editorial.) Arch Intern Med 1984;144:252.
Kelley WN et al: *Textbook of Rheumatology,* 2nd ed. (2 vols.) Saunders, 1985.
Krane SM, Simon LS: Rheumatoid arthritis: Clinical features and pathogenetic mechanisms. Med Clin North Am 1986;70:263.
Kuhlencordt F et al (editors): *Generalized Bone Diseases: Osteoporosis, Osteomalacia, Ostitis Fibrosa.* Springer-Verlag, 1988.
Mirra JM (editor): *Bone Tumors: Clinical, Radiologic, and Pathologic Correlations.* Lea & Febiger, 1989.
Moskowitz RW et al (editors): *Osteoarthritis: Diagnosis and Management.* Saunders, 1984.
Raisz LG: Local and systemic factors in the pathogenesis of osteoporosis. N Engl J Med 1988;318:818.
Rocco VK, Hurd ER: Scleroderma and scleroderma-like disorders. Semin Arthritis Rheum 1986;16:22.
Rodman GP, Schumacher HR (editors): *Primer on the Rheumatic Diseases,* 8th ed. Arthritis Foundation, 1983.
Scott JT (editor): *Copeman's Textbook of Rheumatic Diseases,* 6th ed. (2 vols.) Churchill Livingstone, 1986.
Unni KK (editor): *Bone Tumors.* Churchill Livingstone, 1988.
Zvaifler NJ: Pathogenesis of the joint disease of rheumatoid arthritis. Am J Med 1983;75:3.

Index

NOTE: Page numbers in bold face type indicate a major discussion. A *t* following a page number indicates tabular material and an *i* following a page number indicates an illustration. Drugs are listed under their generic names. When a drug trade name is listed, the reader is referred to the generic name.